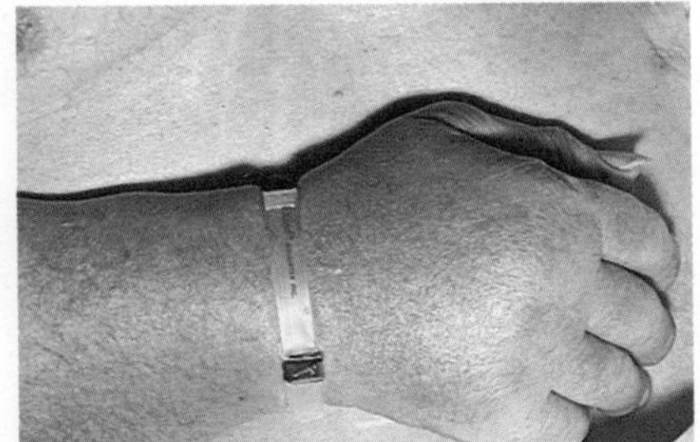

Plate 8. Dermatitis 2° penicillin.

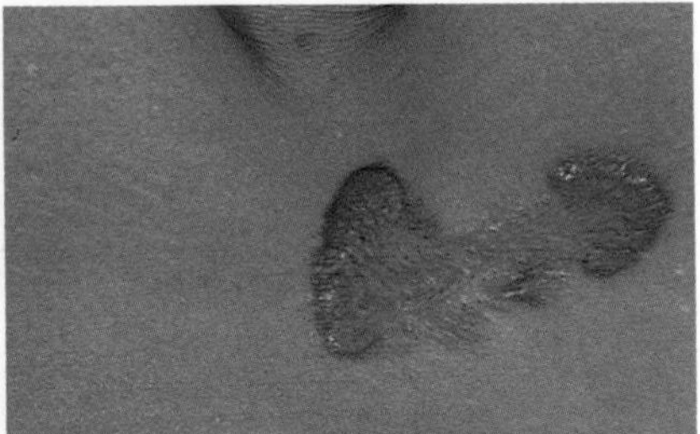

Plate 9. Keloid.

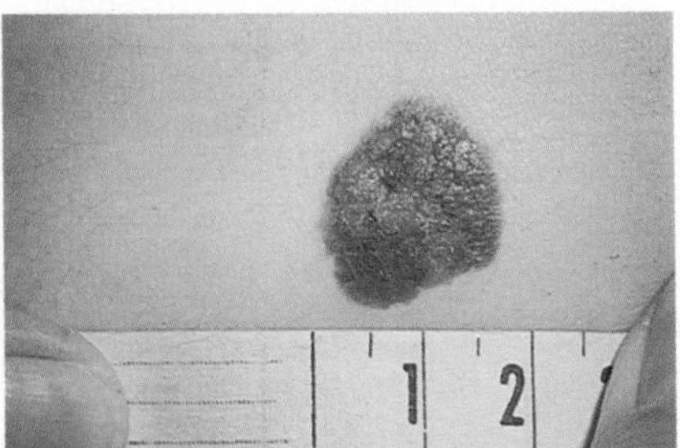

Plate 10. Melanoma.

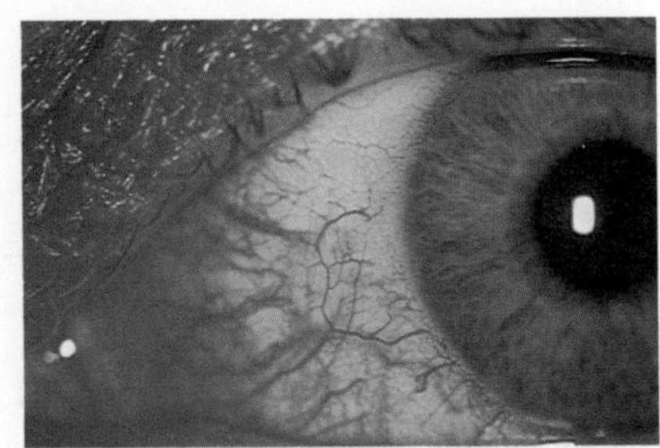

Plate 11. Conjunctivitis.

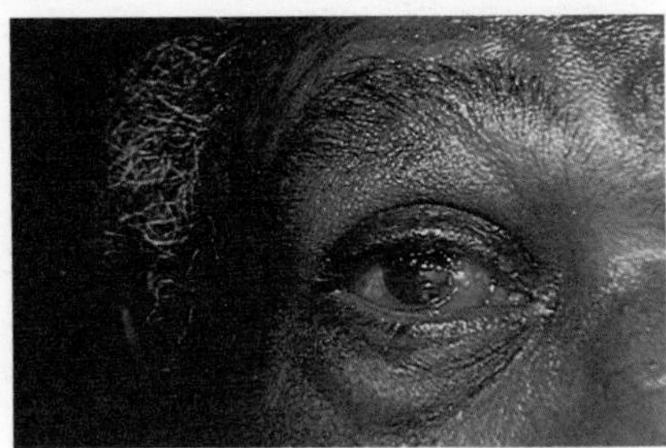

Plate 12. Eye hemorrhage.

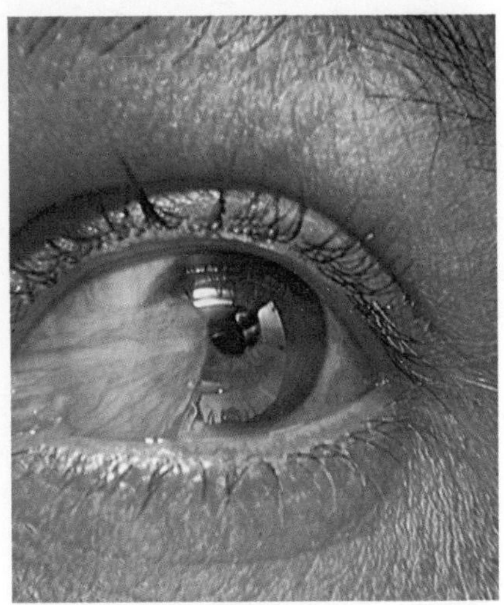

Plate 13. Pterygium.

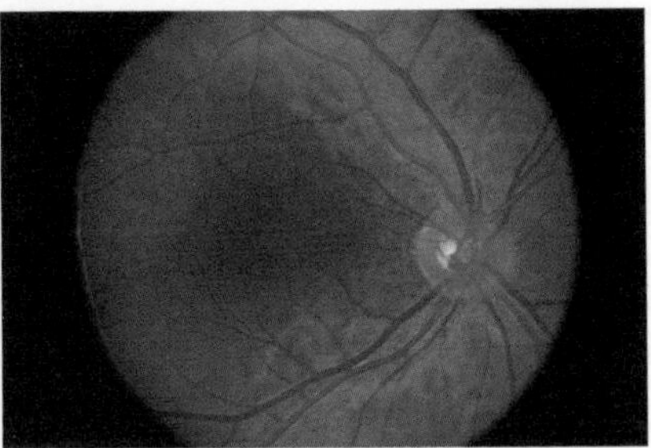

Plate 14. Normal Caucasian fundus.

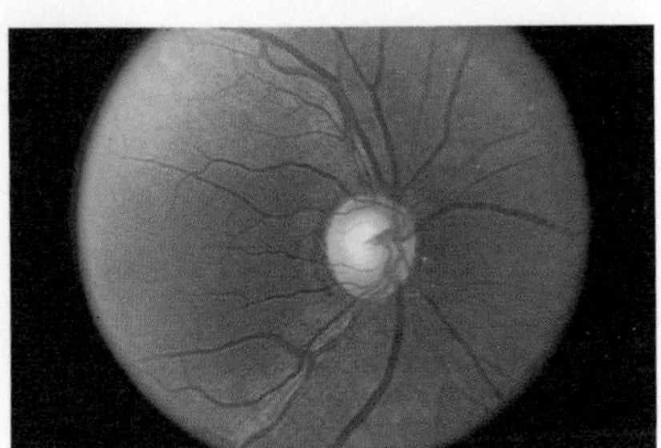

Plate 15. Normal Black fundus.

Health Assessment

IN NURSING PRACTICE

THIRD EDITION

Jorge Grimes, R.N., Ed.D.
State University of New York
Health Science Center
Syracuse, New York

Elizabeth Burns, R.N., Ed.D.
Niagara University
Niagara Falls, New York

Jones and Bartlett Publishers
Boston London

The selection and dosage of drugs presented in this book are in accord with standards accepted at the time of publication. The authors and publisher have made every effort to provide accurate information. However, research, clinical practice, and governmental regulations often change the accepted standard in this field. Before administering any drug, the reader is advised to check the manufacturer's product information sheet for the most up-to-date recommendations on dosage, precautions, and contraindications. This is especially important in the case of drugs that are new or seldom used.

Editorial, Sales, and Customer Service Offices
Jones and Bartlett Publishers
20 Park Plaza
Boston, MA 02116

Jones and Bartlett Publishers International
PO Box 1498
London W6 7RS
England

Library of Congress Cataloging-in-Publication Data

Grimes, Jorge.
Health assessment in nursing practice / Jorge Grimes, Elizabeth Burns.—3rd ed.
p. cm.
Includes bibliographical references and index.
ISBN 0-86720-312-9
1. Nursing assessment. I. Burns, Elizabeth, 1938– II. Title.
[DNLM: 1. Nursing Assessment. WY 100 G862h]
RT48.G74 1992
616.07′5—dc20
DNLM/DLC
for Library of Congress 91-20905
CIP

Printed in the United States of America
96 95 94 93 92 10 9 8 7 6 5 4 3 2 1

Contents

Acknowledgments

The authors would like to extend a special thank you to the following who have provided photographs and given permission for tables and illustrations.

6: Adapted from Don Fink, "Holistic Health: Implications for Health Planning," *American Journal of Health Planning,* July 1976.

7 (Fig. 1-4): From Barbara Blattner, *Holistic Nursing* (E. Norwalk, Conn.: Appleton-Century-Crofts), 1981.

10 (Fig. 1-5): From John A. Frederich, "Tension Control Techniques," in *Guide to Fitness After Fifty,* Roger Harris and Lawrence W. Frankel, eds. (New York: Plenum Press), 1977.

13 (Fig. 1-6): From C. Spielberger, R. Gorsuch, and R. Luschene, "Strait-Trait Anxiety Inventory" (Palo Alto, Calif.: Consulting Psychologists Press, Inc.), 1968.

13 (Fig. 1-7): Adapted with permission from D. Walters, Biofeedback Center, The Meninger Foundation, in Nola J. Pender, *Health Promotion in Nursing Practice* (E. Norwalk, Conn.: Appleton-Century-Crofts), 1982.

137 (Fig. 7-2): Reprinted with permission of Macmillan Publishing Company from *Physical Fitness: A Way of Life,* 3rd ed., by Bud Getchell (New York: Macmillan Publishing Co.), 1983.

147 (Fig. 7-3): Adapted from Bud Getchell and Wayne Anderson, *Being Fit: A Personal Guide* (New York: Wiley), © 1982.

160, 161, 173, 177, 180 (Fig. 9-8), 186 (Fig. 9-26), 188 (Fig. 9-29), 189 (Fig. 9-30), 195, 197 (Fig. 10-7), 203, 205 (Fig. 10-17 B and C), 212 (Fig. 11-4), 214 (Fig. 11-7), 216 (Fig. 11-12), 217, 248, 260, 261, 338 (Fig. 16-15), 353 (Fig. 17-11), 409 (Fig. 19-3), 411 (Fig. 19-7), 553: Used with permission from R. H. Kampmeier and T. M. Blake, *Physical Examination in Health and Disease,* 4th ed. (Philadelphia: F. A. Davis Company), 1970.

162–163, 172, 178, 180 (Figs. 9-9 and 9-11), 182 (Fig. 9-16), 186 (Fig. 9-23), 187, 188 (Fig. 9-28), 197 (Fig. 10-8), 205 (Fig. 10-17 A), 213 (Fig. 11-5), 215, 225–228, 245 (Fig. 12-19), 246 (Fig. 12-21), 311, 332 (Fig. 16-9), 347, 351–352, 353 (Figs. 17-10 and 17-12), 414, 418 (Fig. 19-17), 421 (Fig. 19-24), color endsheets: Courtesy Erie County Medical Center, Buffalo, New York.

181 (Fig. 9-15): From Abbott Laboratories, *Common Skin Diseases—An Atlas,* 1954.

182 (Fig. 9-17): From Braunwald et al., *Harrison's Principles of Internal Medicine,* 8th ed., © 1977 New York: McGraw-Hill. Reprinted by permission.

186 (Figs. 9-24 and 9-25), 235 (Fig. 12-5): From Abbott Laboratories, *Some Pathological Conditions of the Eye, Ear and Throat,* © 1946.

196 (Figs. 10-4 and 10-5), 212 (Fig. 11-3), 218, 245 (Figs. 12-17 and 12-18), 246 (Fig. 12-20), 247 (Figs. 12-23 and 12-24): From Mahlon H. Delp and Robert Manning, *Majors Physical Diagnosis* (Philadelphia: Saunders), 1981, by permission of the publisher.

247 (Fig. 12-22): From John A. Prior and Jack S. Silberstein, *Physical Diagnosis,* 6th ed. (St. Louis: C. V. Mosby), 1981, by permission of the publisher.

198, 233, 280 (Fig. 14-1), 354 (Fig. 17-13): Reprinted from the Revised Clinical Slide Collection on the Rheumatic Diseases, copyright 1981. Used by permission of the American Rheumatism Association.

348: From John A. Prior and Jack S. Silberstein, *Physical Diagnosis,* 5th ed. (St. Louis: C. V. Mosby), 1977, used by permission of the publisher.

432: From F. C. Battaglia and L. O. Lubchenco, "A Practical Classification of Newborn Infants by Weight and Gestational Age," *The Journal of Pediatrics,* August 1967, p. 161.

433: From C. H. Kempe, H. K. Silver, and D. O'Brien, *Current Pediatric Diagnosis and Treatment* (Los Altos, Calif.: Lange Medical Publications), 1980.

438–467: Photos courtesy of Mead Johnson Laboratories.

478–480: Courtesy William K. Frankenburg, M.D., University of Colorado, Denver.

500–501 (Figs. 21-5 through 21-8): Courtesy Ross Laboratories.

502, 505, 514 (Figs. 21-22 and 21-23): Daniel Bellack.

508: Courtesy National Society to Prevent Blindness, New York.

521: Joan Netherwood.

523: Courtesy NIH Gerontology Research Center.

552: Adapted from *Nutrition During Pregnancy and Lactation,* Maternal and Child Health Unit, California Department of Health, 1975, pp. 62–63.

Preface

Professional nurses are in a unique position to meet health care needs comprehensively because they respond to the total needs of the client, emphasizing health, the client's strengths, and the client's involvement in self-care. Professional nurses are committed to client and community education and to the promotion and maintenance of health, as well as to the restoration of health and the detection of illness. Today's nurse provides individuals and families with a humane and continuing point of contact with the health care delivery system.

We believe that maximizing the nurse's ability to provide care requires in-depth knowledge and skill in health assessment. The focus of this book is on providing a systematic approach to the health assessment of individuals of all ages.

The organizing framework integrates four major components of health assessment: social interaction, culture, mental health, and physical health.

Chapter 1 addresses social considerations in health and illness, holistic health, and the interrelationship of nursing and holistic health. It examines the roles of stress, environment, and social class and their relation to an individual's ability to maintain equilibrium. Chapter 2 focuses on cultural considerations in health assessment. The role that culture plays in an individual's health-promoting activities and response to illness is well recognized. Nurses need to understand culturally relevant approaches in care planning and delivery. Chapter 3 describes aspects of communication essential to comprehensive health assessment. This chapter also emphasizes self-awareness, trust, empathy, and respect, which are factors in the development of a therapeutic milieu.

Obtaining the health history is an important first step in assessing a client's health status. Chapter 4 is designed to provide the nurse with complete information on the client interview and on components of the health history. The assessment of health would be incomplete without attention to the individual's mental health. Chapter 5 provides guidelines for mental health assessment and the assessment of stressors such as anxiety and anger. Chapter 6 reviews the nursing process and provides information on how to analyze assessment data and develop a nursing diagnosis. Chapter 7, "Assessment of Wellness," outlines ways to help clients make choices leading to a more satisfying and healthful life.

Chapters 8 through 19 present steps in the physical assessment of all body systems. Of special assistance to the nurse are the learning objectives, discussion questions, and boxed overviews of the techniques of examination provided with every chapter. Following the systems chapters are three chapters that address assessment of clients at various age levels: Chapter 20, "Assessment of the Newborn"; Chapter 21, "Assessment of the Child and Adolescent"; and Chapter 22, "Assessment of the Older Adult". The remaining chapters focus on aggregates: Chapter 23, "The Assessment of Women's Health"; Chapter 24, "The Assessment of Men's Health"; and Chapter 25, "Family Health Assessment."

We wish to acknowledge the help of Judy Davis Grimes, Ph.D., licensed psychologist. Her contributions to the chapters on Communication in Health Assessment, The Health History, and Mental Health Assessment were extensive and helped make these chapters valuable guides for the nurse.

Jorge Grimes
Elizabeth Burns

CHAPTER 1

Sociologic Considerations in Health Assessment

LEARNING OBJECTIVES

1. Define the concepts of health and illness.
2. Discuss the psychosocial and physiological stages of illness.
3. Explain why loss of social role is traumatic.
4. Describe what is meant by the term Holistic Health.
5. Describe the role of nursing in Holistic Health and wellness.
6. Explain why and how stress affects health.
7. Identify tools the nurse can use to assess sociologic aspects of client's health.
8. Identify ways in which the environment affects health and illness.
9. Describe the relationship between social class and illness.

Several common sociologic factors that affect health such as stress, environment, and social class will be discussed in this chapter. Additionally, some concepts of health and illness with particular attention to Holistic Health care will be examined. It is important for you to keep in mind that the same standards of health cannot be applied to all. For example, a client with a chronic condition, such as diabetes mellitus, is viewed differently than a client without a chronic condition. Similarly, you need to relate to a client differently when he is relatively well as compared to when the client is experiencing the onset of illness or is recovering from illness. In Chapter 2 you will learn about cultural and ethnic factors that affect health.

Concepts of Health and Illness

According to Dunn (1959), health and illness are not discrete states of being. They are really part of a continuum, with optimum health or a high level of wellness at one end and illness and death at the other. Figure 1-1 shows this health continuum. Notice that there may be situations where the body operates with a dysfunction like diabetes mellitus, yet the overall level of wellness can be maintained through treatment. Therefore, a

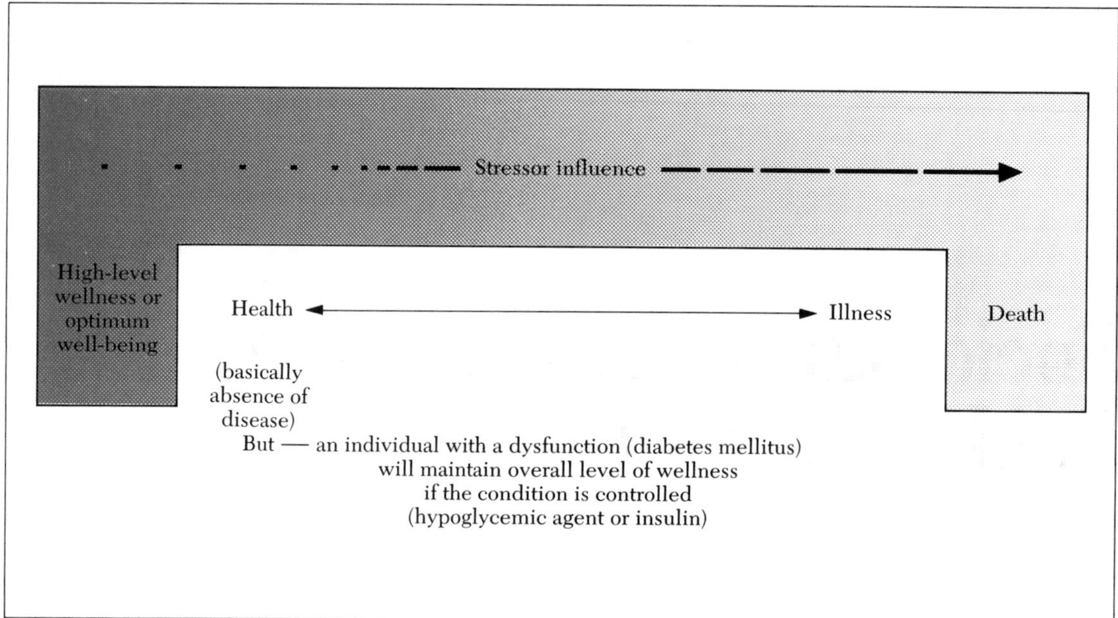

Figure 1-1 The health continuum.

client suffering from a chronic illness may, with the proper care, lead a healthy life.

Dunn's concept of health has since been criticized as being limited, because it's an either-or (wellness-illness) phenomenon. Nursing theorists have defined health in a variety of ways (Chinn & Jacobs 1987). Orem (1971) conceptualized health as a state of wholeness. Levine (1967) and Neuman (1974) talked of health as a holistic balance and a state of homeostasis, respectively. Some nursing theorists have thought of health as a process. Peplau (1952) defined health as a forward moving process. For Rogers (1970), health was a process of becoming. For King (1971) and Roy (1976), health was a process of adaptation. Whether conceptualized as a state or as a process, the common viewpoint of health seems to be that it is dynamic.

Because wellness and illness patterns are reflected in the gestalt of health, their characteristics, along with variables known to influence wellness and illness, are examined to assess health.

A person's level of wellness can be changed by stimuli that cause *stress*. These stressors can be physical, psychologic, or social. But no matter what the form of the stressor, the body responds holistically. Examples of physical stress are disease agents and conditions, such as particular bacteria, which might lead to tuberculosis or gastroenteritis, or damaged blood vessels, which might lead to kidney failure. Psychologic stress might ensue from the death of or separation from a loved one. Social stress might arise from a job or an environmental situation. Health would then be defined as the individual's ability to rally from and overcome these stresses and insults (Andy & Dunn 1974). As we will see later in this chapter, illness arises from the inability to cope with these threats to health.

An individual surrounds himself with protective devices that enable him to maintain health. These devices might be physical, such as clothing and housing; behavioral, such as diet, health habits, coping strategies, and hobbies; or psychosocial, such as family ties, love relationships, and a resilient attitude toward life. These protective devices may enable a person to easily overcome a stress and regain health. At other times, the stress will be too powerful and the individual will become ill and enter the stages of illness.

Figure 1-2 illustrates the physical and psychosocial stages of illness. There are two recognized physical stages of illness: the onset and the recovery. In addition, Martin and Prange (1962) have identified three psychosocial stages of illness that parallel the physical stages but lag behind them: (1) transition to illness, (2) acceptance of illness, and (3) convalescence. Additional time is needed (brown line) before a person can psychologically and socially assimilate the physical changes of illness (gray line).

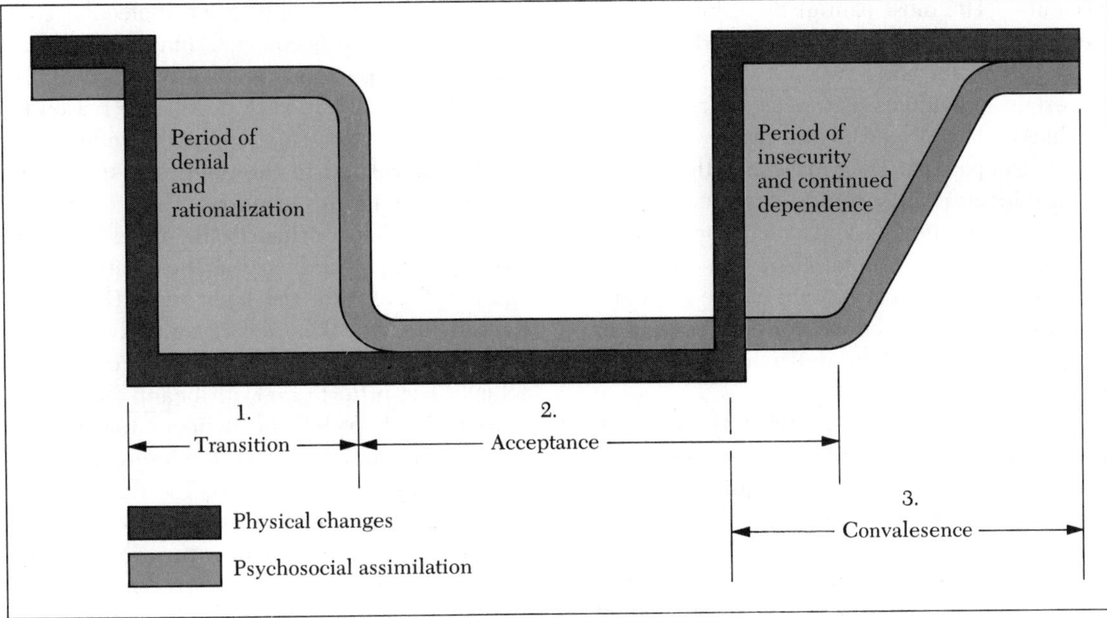

Figure 1-2 The physical stages of illness.

Two people can have the same illness and respond differently. Some rapidly identify the signs and symptoms of illness and then interrupt their activities. Others may continue to work in spite of pain and fever. These persons are using the major mental defense mechanism of the transition stage of illness: denial. Use of this mechanism may diminish the pain or alleviate it altogether. It is also quite common for the mechanism of rationalization to come into play at this time. The individual attempts to convince himself that he is *not* ill; he tells himself that he can't possibly be ill, or how could he have continued to unload a ton of cement blocks? Nor does a sick man play 18 holes of golf! The time lag between physical change and psychosocial assimilation is shown in Figure 1-2 by the shaded area, "period of denial and rationalization."

As the symptoms become more severe and more specific, the individual enters stage two (acceptance of illness). At this time he has acknowledged that he is ill and in most cases abandons the mechanisms of denial and rationalization. During this stage the individual begins to display regressive and passive behavior; he may lie down and request that someone take his temperature or get him a couple of aspirins or get the nurse or doctor, depending on the severity of the illness. This resting promotes the healing process. Generally, most people during this phase assume the position of cooperation fostered by the desire and the social obligation of getting well.

The third stage of illness (convalescence) is characterized by insecurity at the thought of relinquishing the protective world and all its accompanying attentions and kindnesses. At this stage the nurse must be careful not to reinforce the client's dependent behavior by continuing to feed and bathe him when he is capable of doing so himself. During this phase the nurse must encourage and support the client in steps to resume his independence. Figure 1-2 shows the time lag between the physical and psychosocial beginning of convalescence as the shaded area, "period of insecurity and continued dependence."

Not all individuals accept the role of cooperation during illness. Instead, a person may reject this role and become the "difficult" client. Why a person rejects the desired role requires study of the individual and his sociocultural system. There are numerous reasons why a person might choose to reject society's demand for cooperation.

The loss of social role is painful. It may be as traumatic as the illness itself. The sick mother will fret about not being able to meet her role obligations. The bank president may react angrily at feeling his need to be dependent and being told what to do by others. Disruption of role behavior may cause depression and mental torment—"The most painful thing for me is to see others running around and working. I've worked all my life and now . . ."

Certain individuals may react angrily or feel worthless when placed in the inactive, dependent role of patient. They may carry this feeling of worthlessness into their marriage relationship, believing they no longer have anything to offer their partner. Mental alienation, sickness, and injury place a heavy strain on life partners. The situation may produce constant friction or it may increase affection and tighten the interpersonal bond.

For some, illness may be used as an escape from social pressures and responsibilities. All the client has to do is relax and enjoy the dependent position. This type of client will resist returning to the "nonsick" role.

A variety of social, cultural, and biologic factors determine who will become ill and how ill persons will adjust to the sick role.

Holistic Health

Health professionals and laypeople are becoming increasingly aware that we must go beyond the goal of curing illness. Many illnesses appear to be caused, or at least encouraged, by the demands and conditions of our society and the lifestyles of individuals. Evidence indicates that the shift in emphasis should and can be toward the prevention of illness and the refinement of concepts of wellness and Holistic Health.

The movement in this direction has been slow for a number of reasons. The health care system has been and continues to a large extent today to be based on the Medical Model in which the focus of health care is on the treatment of illness. The reasons for this, of course, have been based historically on society's need to cure communicable disease. This goal has largely been accomplished, and at present the focus of the Medical Model is on the cure of life-threatening and chronic diseases such as hypertension, heart disease, stroke, diabetes, and cancer. Note the strides made by medicine in controlling disease through the use of sophisticated drugs and in the transplant of major organs. These advances are remarkable and will certainly save and prolong many lives.

The Medical Model bases its existence on the scientific method. This method reduces man to a physiologic and psychologic being, who can be further reduced to cellular and molecular components. Disease becomes a thing in itself, unrelated to the person's personality or way of life.

An additional and very persuasive reason for slowness in the movement toward a wellness orientation is related to the politics of the illness care system in this country. The health care industry, focused primarily on illness care, is the third largest industry in the United States and employs 6% of the labor force (Kalisch & Kalisch 1982, p. 93). According to Ivan Illich, a contemporary social critic, health care today actually has little to do with health (Kalisch & Kalisch, 1982, p. 93); he believes that it is an industry manipulated by vested interest groups, labor unions, and politicians. In addition most health care insurance is directed toward illness care. Little reimbursement is provided for providers and seekers of preventive health. The public is beginning, however, to demand care that will increase the level of wellness, reduce the cost of illness care, and enhance the quality of life.

Characteristics of Holistic Health

You need to understand the concept of holism before you can apply it to health and nursing. The philosophical concept of holism defines the whole as greater than the sum of its parts. A tremendous amount of literature related to holism has been generated over the years. Of particular import is the contribution of Jan Christian Smuts, in 1926, who in addressing the concepts of holism and evolution disagreed with the analytical method employed by the life sciences to study organisms. He knew there was more to learn about the human body than could be found by taking each cell part and studying it in isolation. He felt there is an organizing process that pulls everything together in harmony, causing the organism to maintain itself in a fluctuating environment. He referred to this process as "holism."

In the 1970s, D. C. Phillips incorporated the works of Smuts and others to develop a holistic framework that includes the following five points:

1. The analytic approach as typified by the physiochemical sciences proves inadequate when applied to certain cases—for example, a biological organism, society, or even reality as a whole.
2. The whole is more than the sum of its parts.

3. The whole determines the nature of its parts.
4. The parts cannot be understood if considered in isolation from the whole.
5. The parts are dynamically interrelated or interdependent. (Phillips 1976, p. 6)

Newtonian physics focuses on an assemblage of materials—particles, atoms. In this sense the "stuff of life" has the utilitarian value of control. The manipulation of "life" material has been "healing" in the Western world. Diagnosis and treatment are of the flesh—surgery, drugs, radiation. Western "healing" has been fixated on the incarnation of the flesh. The holistic perspective is not discontinuous of our heritage but unites Western science and traditional healing systems. In holism there exists a gestalt awareness. Wellness is conceptualized by a degree of awareness. Individuals consider themselves well when they have no illness complaints.

Philosophically, from the standpoint of holism in considering the whole to be greater than the sum of its parts, you need to pay attention to the interconnectiveness, the relationships, the awareness, the patterns of life and of self between the environment and within the universe. Primitive cultures were "in tune" with the earth and healing. The earth was sacred and a healer to the Indians. With the acceptance of the nature of life, illness, suffering, and death become an integral part of living.

Holistic Health is an approach to wellness that is person oriented rather than disease oriented. Holistic Health recognizes every aspect of the person interacting with the environment. Holistic Health practice emphasizes the prevention of illness and maintenance of health as well as the healing process. The average person does not maintain responsibility for health and has given over this responsibility to the health care system. As consumers we have come to believe that we can smoke, tolerate obesity, drink to excess, and drive carelessly; we expect that the effects of these excesses can be repaired by the health care system. The holistic perspective requires that the individual become an active participant in maintaining a healthy lifestyle. Another aspect of Holistic Health is the view that illness is a creative opportunity for the individual to learn more about himself, to evaluate goals and values, and to engage in a process of self-explanation.

Holistic Health Care concepts and practices include humanistic medicine, alternative health care, preprimary care, and altered provider-patient relationships (Fink, 1976, pp. 23–31).

Humanistic medicine deals with illness but focuses on the presence of health in the person who also happens to be ill. Humanistic medicine attempts to work within the health care system while encouraging it to move toward a more holistic approach. Using this approach, the professional is a technical specialist who supports clients in devising new approaches to health and in assuming responsibility for lifestyle choices.

Alternative health care permits and helps the client to choose among several possibilities. Examples of these alternatives are biofeedback, meditation, imaging, massage, rolfing, relaxation techniques, and therapeutic touch. Alternative care can also mean involvement in organized health systems that are not part of Western scientific medicine such as Chinese acupuncture, Black and Hispanic healing systems, and homeopathy.

Preprimary care is a health care system in which people manage their own health care problems. This includes the self-care and self-help movement.

There are five levels to be considered in the altered provider-patient relationship (see Figure 1-3). In the first level the patient is passive and the health practitioner relationship resembles the usual parent-child relationship. In level two the patient is ill but is aware and capable of following directions and making some choices. On the third level, mutual participation occurs such that the practitioner helps the individual to help himself. In this relationship the practitioner shares information with the individual. At the fourth level the practitioner is a consultant with the individual bearing responsibility for health or illness.

The highest level is that of self-care, which has captured the imagination and support of many in this country. Self-care is being encouraged by several health insurers as a means of containing health care costs.

Nursing and Holistic Health

Nursing historically has had a commitment to holistic health and wellness. From Florence Nightingale in the mid-1800s to the theorists of the last 30 years, nursing has focused on the promotion and maintenance of health. Concepts of wellness related to the individual, family, and community are addressed by nursing and include physical, psychosocial, cultural, spiritual,

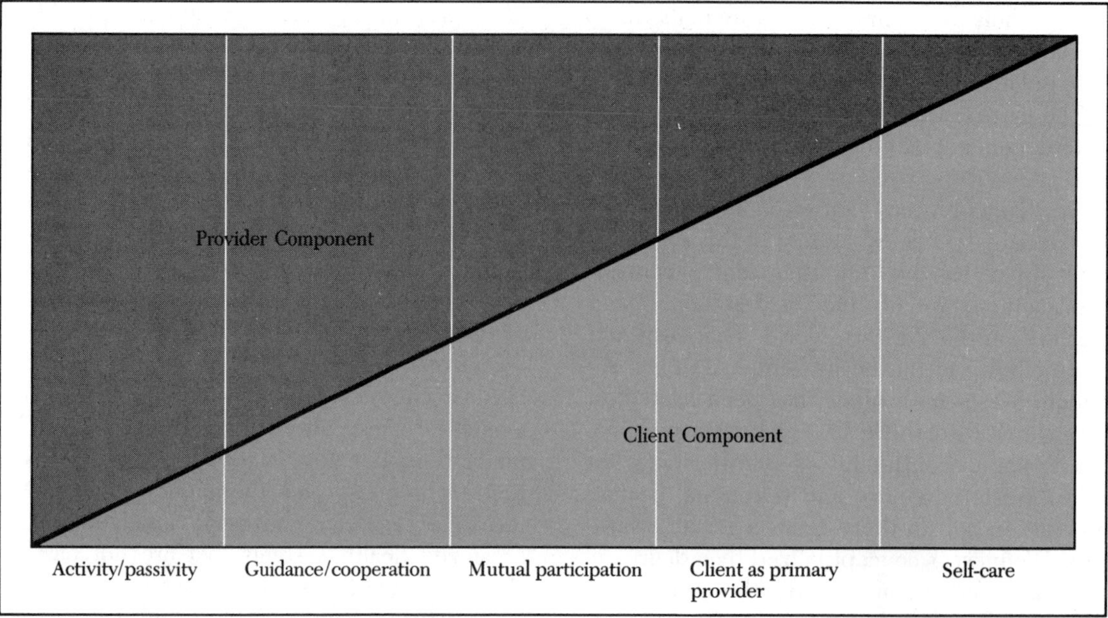

Figure 1-3 Altered provider-patient relationship model.

and environmental factors. The nursing process described by nursing leaders such as Orem, Roy, Peplau, King, and Neuman describe active client participation in goal setting. Smitherman (1981) in *Nursing Actions for Health Promotion* describes five processes: the communication process, the helping process, the problem-solving process, the teaching process, and the leadership process as means to assist the individual or family to attain optimal wellness.

Barbara Blattner (1981) has proposed a conceptual framework for holistic nursing (see Figure 1-4). She describes the goal of nursing as preventive, nutritive, and generative. High-level wellness is achieved by using nine life processes: self-responsibility, caring, stress, lifestyling, human development, problem solving, communication, teaching/learning, and leadership and change with self, client, and communities. These processes are focused in intrapersonal, interpersonal, and community systems. She describes the nurse who believes in and uses this conceptual framework as practicing holistic nursing.

Patricia Flynn has provided the nurse who wishes to integrate holistic practice suggestions related to the nurse and the client. The nurse as practitioner should exhibit "realness, empathetic understanding and unconditioned positive regard for the client" (Flynn 1980, p. 19).

She suggests that by gathering the following information, nurses will consciously integrate holistic principles in practice:

> We can attend to the part that our clients' lifestyle plays in their level of wellness. What is the way they live?
> How do their beliefs, values and needs fit their behavior?
> What are their relationships with others?
> How do they handle stress?
> Do they take care of their bodies?
> Do they recognize their philosophical and spiritual needs and are they comfortable with that aspect of their life? (Flynn 1980, p. 22)

Sociologic Factors Affecting Health

Health implies equilibrium, and reaching or maintaining this state is a goal for all people. However, many people find this task difficult and almost impossible because of numerous factors at work in their social environment. There are three main sociologic factors that can impede attaining a balanced life: stress, environment, and social class.

Stress

Our fast-paced competitive lifestyle is filled with stress. Our stressful environment, composed of both psychologic and socioecologic factors, cre-

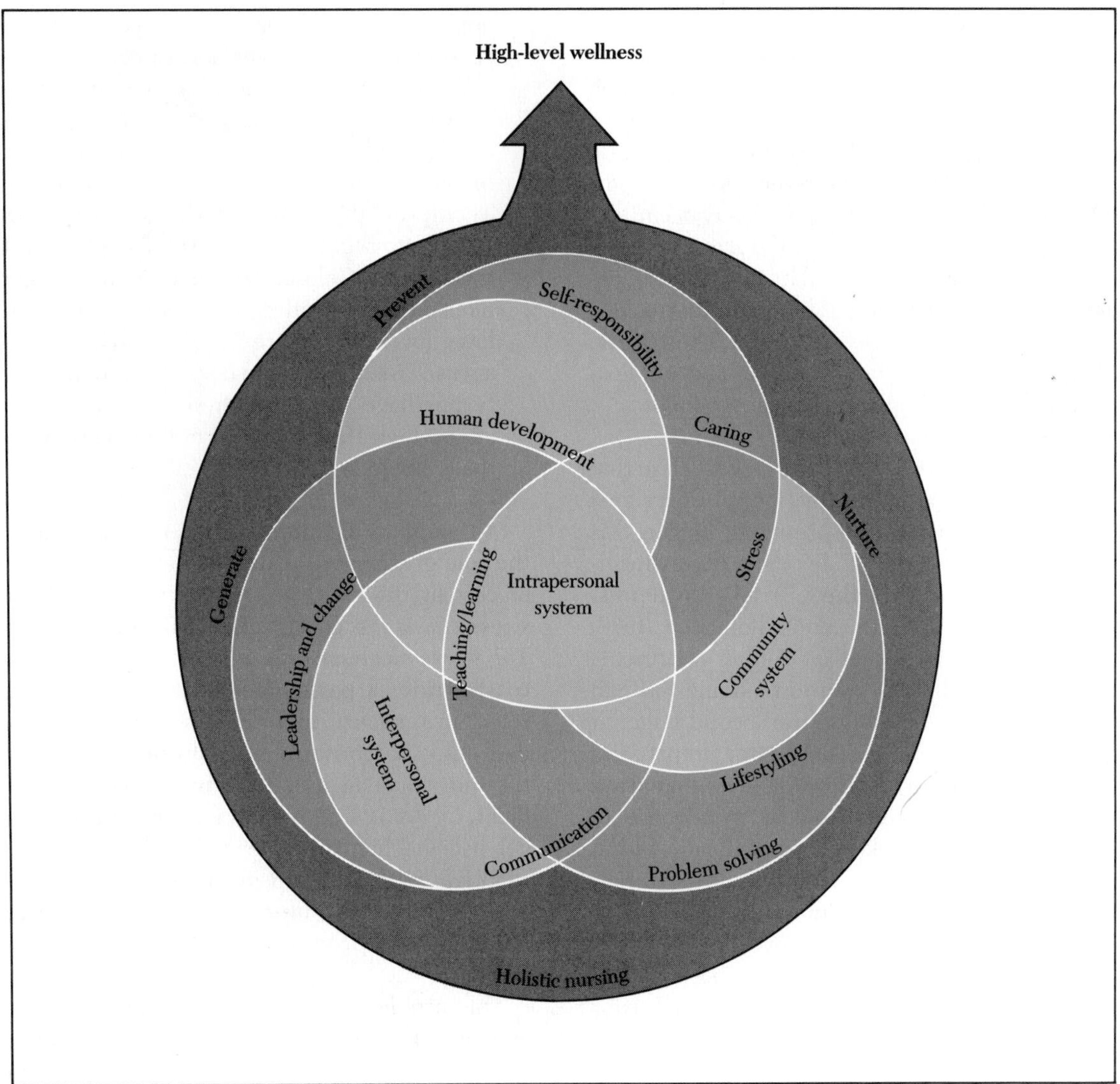

Figure 1-4 The holistic nursing model.

ates high levels of nervous tension and anxiety, which influence an individual's health. Excessive stress has been implicated in a long list of physical disorders, including hypertension, peptic ulcers, dermatitis, migraine headaches, asthma, rheumatoid arthritis, diabetes mellitus, obesity, and heart disease.

For example, research has found that populations living in rural or nonmodernized areas have lower blood pressure and an overall lower incidence of hypertension than populations living in urban or modernized environments (Ostfeld & Shekelle 1967). The implication is that the stress of urban areas can lead to high blood pressure. It should be pointed out, however, that other factors may be raising blood pressure, such as urban-rural differences in diet, rates of obesity, other chronic conditions, or genetic factors. It is true that short-term high levels of stress inflicted in experimental situations can raise blood pressure, but it has never been conclusively proven that chronic long-term stress can lead to permanently elevated blood pressure in anyone. Still, the findings of certain studies are suggestive that this may be the case (Harburg et al. 1973).

Stressors may be physical, psychologic, or social. No matter what the form, the person will be affected, as well as respond, holistically; both the body and mind will react. For instance, a physical illness produces behavioral changes that are quite obvious—anger, apathy, withdrawal. A social stressor, such as receiving a jail sentence, may exacerbate a dermatitis. The psychologic stress of taking a test can produce such physical symptoms as a migraine headache or stomach "upset." With extreme psychologic shock, such physical symptoms as hysterical blindness, deafness, or muteness may occur.

Regardless of the nature of the stressor, three physiologic stages, identified by Selye (1965), occur throughout the body. The only difference is in the degree of the stress response. These three stages, which have significant nursing implications for peoples of all cultures, are as follows:

1. The alarm reaction. A short trigger phase that sets the mechanism into action; an alert signal for the organism to get prepared. During this stage the Na^+ and Cl^- levels in the extracellular fluids fall while the K^+ rises. Blood pressure also falls. Byrne and Thompson (1978) have pointed out that explaining treatments to clients will assist them in moving through the alarm stage and into the second stage, at which time the clients are better prepared to tolerate the procedure. The explanation should not be given too far in advance of treatment, as the alarm stage will fade within a short time if the stressor does not materialize. If informed too far in advance, the client may become so apprehensive of the procedure that when it actually does occur, he or she may be even *more* vulnerable. In order to plan the most appropriate time for explanations of this type, you must consider the client's "behavioral stability, his adaptive capacity, as well as the nature of the stressor" (Byrne & Thompson 1978).
2. The resistance stage. Can be characterized by the statement, "I'm ready; let's get it over with!" This stage occurs when the organism adjusts to the stressor(s) with the aid of increased ACTH and glucocorticoids. At this time the electrolyte blood levels essentially return to normal, and the body attempts to combat the stress factors and to resist further organic damage.
3. The stage of exhaustion. The point at which, with prolonged stress, the organism can no longer maintain its adaptive energy resources. The organism becomes exhausted. The cholesterol stores in the adrenals are depleted, and the ACTH and glucocorticoid secretions dwindle. Many of the physiologic manifestations that may have originally appeared during the first stage begin to reappear—general malaise, headache, fever, anorexia. Reversal may or may not be achieved with external supports such as massive chemotherapy, psychotherapy, blood transfusions, and surgery (Byrne & Thompson 1978). Selye indicates that death is likely to occur if the stressor(s) continues at this stage. Cellular damage is no longer blocked; increased cellular permeability allows for rapid, extreme electrolyte imbalances. Tissue breakdown occurs, and massive hemorrhage into the adrenal gland ensues, after which the hormones of the gland eventually fail to be secreted.

Although much emphasis has been placed on the role of stress as a cause in the development of certain diseases, we should point out that stress can serve constructive purposes as well. The stress mechanism is initiated during a roller coaster ride, a passionate kiss, a jump off the street in response to an automobile horn, or a dash into the house in a rainstorm. It prepares the individual in a crisis situation for fight or flight; by doing so it reveals itself as a life-saving defense mechanism in league with such other adaptive body mechanisms as the healing process, the clotting mechanism of blood, the inflammatory process, and the immunologic response.

One problem in studying stress has been the difficulty of measuring stress in research subjects or clients. Events may be more or less stressful for different individuals, subcultures, or social groups. For example, the pregnancy of an unmarried teenage daughter may be an extremely stressful event for upper-middle-class parents who may worry about their daughter's future and the social stigma of the pregnancy. However, many lower-class families would find the pregnancy to be a less stressful event, for there is wider acceptance in this group of a mother taking charge of her offspring's children.

However, in assessing stress factors in a client's situation and in identifying areas for counseling, a nurse should be aware of the theory and methods postulated by Holmes and Rahe (1967). They suggested that significant stress in a person's life, both pleasant and unpleasant, would lower an individual's resistance to disease. From their study of several populations and analysis of the research data, they constructed the Social Readjustment Rating Scale

Table 1-1. Life Events and Weighted Values

Life event	Value	Life event	Value
1. Death of spouse	100	21. Change of responsibility at work	29
2. Divorce	73	22. Son or daughter leaving home	29
3. Marital separation	65	23. Trouble with in-laws	29
4. Jail term	63	24. Outstanding personal achievement	28
5. Death of close family member	63	25. Wife beginning or stopping work	26
6. Personal injury or illness	53	26. Beginning or ending school	26
7. Marriage	50	27. Revision of habits	24
8. Fired at work	47	28. Trouble with boss	23
9. Marital reconciliation	45	29. Change in work hours	20
10. Retirement	45	30. Change in residence	20
11. Change in health of family	44	31. Change in schools	20
12. Pregnancy	40	32. Change in recreation	19
13. Sex difficulties	39	33. Change in social activity	18
14. Gain of new family member	39	34. Mortgage less than $10,000	17
15. Change in financial state	38	35. Change in sleeping habits	16
16. Death of close friend	37	36. Change in number of family get-togethers	15
17. Change of work	36	37. Change in eating habits	15
18. Change in number of arguments with spouse	35	38. Vacation	13
19. Mortgage over $10,000	31	39. Minor violations of law	11
20. Foreclosure of mortgage	30		

From T. H. Holmes and R. H. Rahe, "The Social Readjustment Rating Scale," *Journal of Psychosomatic Research*, 11 (1967), 213.

Scoring the Life-Change Index

Score range	Interpretation
0–150	No significant problems, low or tolerable life change
150–199	Mild life change (approximately 33% chance of illness)
200–299	Moderate life change (approximately 50% chance of illness)
300 or over	Major life change (approximately 80% chance of illness)

From T. H. Holmes and R. H. Rahe, "The Social Readjustment Rating Scale," *Journal of Psychosomatic Research*, 11 (1967), 213.

(SRRS). This scale lists life events with assigned weighted values (see Tables 1-1 and 1-2). Their study revealed a significant relationship between the magnitude of life events and the time of the onset of disease. They also found a positive correlation between the magnitude of the event and the seriousness of the illness. For example, 80% of the study population who had received an SRRS score of over 300 in one year experienced heart attacks or developed other serious illnesses.

You can also use several other, less well-known measures to assess stress factors. John Friedrich has developed a Stress Symptom Checklist self-evaluation tool for monitoring stress (see Figure 1-5). Use of this checklist may be helpful to you and the client as you discuss the means to reduce stress (Friedrich 1977).

You can suggest that it would be helpful for the client to record stressful events and the symptoms experienced related to the events. After this has been done for several days or weeks, the client may be able to identify specific areas that need to be worked on to reduce stress. The diary should record time of day, the stressful event, and the symptoms that accompanied the event.

The State-Trait Anxiety Inventory provides an efficient, reliable means to assess feelings of stress occurring with clients (see Figure 1-6). This 40-item inventory contains 20 items related to state anxiety (that which the client feels at the moment) and 20 items related to trait anxiety (the way the client feels generally). The test can be obtained from Consulting Psychologists Press, Inc., Palo Alto, California.

Life stress review is part of the Menninger Foundation Biofeedback Center's stress man-

There are many symptoms of tension which imply a need for relaxation. In order to be able to cope with tension, it is helpful to become aware of some of these symptoms. By completing the following check list, you can gain further insight into your status regarding relaxation.

	Frequently (1)	Quite Often (2)	Seldom (3)	Never (−1)
1. Do you feel insecure?	______	______	______	______
2. Do you often feel over-excited?	______	______	______	______
3. Do you feel anxious?	______	______	______	______
4. Do you worry when you go to bed at night?	______	______	______	______
5. Is it difficult for you to fall asleep at night?	______	______	______	______
6. Do you find it difficult to relax when you want to?	______	______	______	______
7. Do you wake up in the morning feeling tired and loggy?	______	______	______	______
8. Do you find it difficult to concentrate on a problem?	______	______	______	______
9. Do you often feel tired during the day?	______	______	______	______
10. When playing a sport, do you find it hard to concentrate on it?	______	______	______	______
11. Is it hard for you to stay awake at work or in class?	______	______	______	______
12. Do you feel upset and ill-at-ease?	______	______	______	______
13. Do you lack self confidence?	______	______	______	______
14. Do you often worry during the day over possible misfortunes?	______	______	______	______
15. Do you frequently feel bored?	______	______	______	______
16. Do you often feel discouraged?	______	______	______	______
17. Do you have nervous feelings?	______	______	______	______
18. Do you feel depressed?	______	______	______	______
19. Do you have any type of twitch?	______	______	______	______
20. Do you have frequent headaches?	______	______	______	______
21. Do you have frequent colds, earaches, or sore throats?	______	______	______	______
22. Do you have any persistent pains in joints or feet?	______	______	______	______
23. If you feel yourself becoming tense, do you find it difficult to relax?	______	______	______	______
24. Do you notice that you seldom find time to relax or stretch during the day?	______	______	______	______
25. Do you exercise regularly?	______	______	______	______
26. Do you often find that you exhibit tension by scowling, clenching fists, tightening jaws, hunching shoulders or pursing lips?	______	______	______	______
27. Do your shoes, belt or other items of clothing fit too tightly?	______	______	______	______
28. When you notice any of the tension symptoms, do you find it difficult to stop or minimize them?	______	______	______	______
29. Are you unable to "let go" easily when you feel tense?	______	______	______	______

The foregoing was merely designed to bring attention to areas which may reflect tension in your daily life. If you wish to rate yourself, the following scale will reflect, to a degree, your tension potential. Score: Frequently (1), Quite Often (2), Seldom (3), Never (−1).

Score	**Rating**
0–19	Above average tension control
20–39	Average tension control
40–55	Low tension control
56–84	Poor tension control

Figure 1-5 Stress symptom checklist.

agement center. The stress charting exercise depicted in Figure 1-7 requires the client to list stressors and then place the corresponding number in the circle to depict the area of life in which the stress occurs. The center of the circle represents the client; the more anxiety-producing the stressor, the closer to the center of the circle the number is placed. Table 1-3 lists common stressors experienced in illness and hospitalization. The designated stress values aid in prioritizing interventions aimed at initially decreasing maximum level stressors. Each of these tests or a combination of them can be helpful to the nurse assessing the stress level of the client and, subsequently, in planning care activities to reduce the client's stress.

Environment

In the mid-eighteenth century, the French philosopher Rousseau (1913) espoused the idea that one's style of living is a main source of illness:

Table 1-3. Hospital Stress Rating Scale

Assigned rank	Stress value	Event	
1	13.9	Having strangers sleep in the same room with you	____
2	15.4	Having to eat at different times than you usually do	____
3	15.9	Having to sleep in a strange bed	____
4	16.0	Having to wear a hospital gown	____
5	16.8	Having strange machines around	____
6	16.9	Being awakened in the night by the nurse	____
7	17.0	Having to be assisted with bathing	____
8	17.7	Not being able to get newspapers, radio, or TV when you want them	____
9	18.1	Having a roommate who has too many visitors	____
10	19.1	Having to stay in bed or the same room all day	____
11	19.4	Being aware of unusual smells around you	____
12	21.2	Having a roommate who is seriously ill or cannot talk with you	____
13	21.5	Having to be assisted with a bedpan	____
14	21.6	Having a roommate who is unfriendly	____
15	21.7	Not having friends visit you	____
16	21.7	Being in a room that is too cold or too hot	____
17	21.1	Thinking your appearance might be changed after your hospitalization	____
18	22.3	Being in the hospital during holidays or special family occasions	____
19	22.4	Thinking you might have pain because of surgery or test procedures	____
20	22.7	Worrying about your spouse being away from you	____
21	23.2	Having to eat cold or tasteless food	____
22	23.3	Not being able to call family or friends on the phone	____
23	23.4	Being cared for by an unfamiliar doctor	____
24	23.6	Being put in the hospital because of an accident	____
25	24.2	Not knowing when to expect things will be done for you	____
26	24.5	Having the staff be in too much of a hurry	____
27	25.9	Thinking about losing income because of your illness	____
28	26.0	Having medications cause you discomfort	____
29	26.4	Having nurses or doctors talk too fast or use words you can't understand	____
30	26.4	Feeling you are getting dependent on medications	____
31	26.5	Not having family visit you	____
32	26.9	Knowing you have to have an operation	____
33	27.1	Being hospitalized far away from home	____
34	27.2	Having a sudden hospitalization you weren't planning to have	____
35	27.3	Not having your call light answered	____
36	27.4	Not having enough insurance to pay for your hospitalization	____
37	27.6	Not having your questions answered by the staff	____
38	28.4	Missing your spouse	____
39	29.2	Being fed through tubes	____
40	31.2	Not getting relief from pain medications	____
41	31.9	Not knowing the results or reasons for your treatments	____
42	32.4	Not getting pain medication when you need it	____

Continued on page 12

From Volicer, B. J.; and Bohannon, M. W. "A Hospital Stress Rating Scale." *Nursing Research*, *24*:352–359 (September–October 1975). Reprinted by permission of American Journal of Nursing Company.

Table 1-3. *Continued*

Assigned rank	Stress value	Event	
43	34.0	Not knowing for sure what illness you have	_____
44	34.1	Not being told what your diagnosis is	_____
45	34.5	Thinking you might lose your hearing	_____
46	34.6	Knowing you have a serious illness	_____
47	35.6	Thinking you might lose a kidney or some other organ	_____
48	39.2	Thinking you might have cancer	_____
49	40.6	Thinking you might lose your sight	_____
TOTAL			_____

> The great inequality in manner of living, the extreme idleness of some, and the excessive labour of others, the easiness of exciting and gratifying our sensual appetites, the too exquisite foods of the wealthy . . . the unwholesome food of the poor . . . all these, together with sitting up late, and excesses of every kind, immoderate transports of every passion, fatigue, mental exhaustion, the innumerable pains and anxieties inseparable from every condition of life, by which the mind of man is incessantly tormented; these are too fatal proofs that the greater part of our ills are of our own making, and that we might have avoided them nearly all by adhering to that simple, uniform and solitary manner of life which nature prescribed . . . What we think of the good constitution of the savages, at least of those whom we have not ruined with our spirituous liquors, and reflect that they are troubled with hardly any disorders, save wounds and old age, we are tempted to believe that, in following the history of civil society, we shall be telling also that of human sickness.

Rousseau spoke of activity. Exercise is a necessity for good health, yet our society encourages us to hop in the car to go but a city block or two to obtain a quart of milk or purchase a pack of cigarettes. So, too, our social environment encourages the habit of smoking by advertising its chicness (in lieu of the surgeon general's warning that it *is* dangerous to your health), by designating smoking areas, and by making ashtrays and matches easily available.

Rousseau also spoke of food. Most people are aware that diet has a direct influence on serum cholesterol and on obesity. A high correlation has been demonstrated between individual diet and cardiovascular diseases, liver and kidney diseases, and diabetes mellitus and other metabolic disorders (Lebowitz 1975). When Rousseau commented on the "too exquisite" foods of the wealthy, he was unknowingly identifying the excessive purine content, which may cause deposition of urate crystals in and about the joints and tendons in a pathologic condition known as gout.

While Rousseau noted that diet is socioculturally determined, the media realize that it is individually determined as well. Thus, when peddling their wares, many advertisers direct their appeal at the idea of promoting individual well-being. For instance, a person with a cardiac condition may be induced to buy Sizzlean, the nonbacon product that smells like bacon, tastes like bacon, but contains no cholesterol. But what the advertiser fails to relay to the consumer is that Sizzlean has a high sodium content that could prove to be hazardous to the health of a person with cardiovascular disease. Finally, malnutrition, especially the deficiency diseases, exists in our plentiful nation because of poor diets or lack of equal food distribution to all members of society.

The environmental effect on health that we are most aware of is pollution. The urban environment is rife with pollutants (Levin 1979). In a large city, an urban dweller may begin by drinking a glass of water run from pipes that have absorbed lead and other harmful metal fragments overnight. Stepping outside, the urban dweller takes a breath of "fresh" air. Again, the lead levels in the air from car exhausts and industrial plants may be dangerously high. In addition, there is the problem of carbon monoxide. On most days in New York City, for example, the carbon monoxide levels are well above the federally set standard of 9 parts per million. In mid-

Directions: A number of statements which people have used to describe themselves are given below. Read each statement and then blacken in the appropriate circle to the right of the statement to indicate how you *feel* right now, that is, *at this moment.* There are no right or wrong answers. Do not spend too much time on any one statement but give the answer which seems to describe your present feelings best.

① = not at all; ② = somewhat;
③ = moderately so; ④ = very much so

I feel at ease	①	②	③	④
I feel upset	①	②	③	④
I feel nervous	①	②	③	④
I am relaxed	①	②	③	④
I am worried	①	②	③	④

Directions: A number of statements that people have used to describe themselves are given below. Read each statement and then blacken in the appropriate circle to the right of the statement to indicate how you generally feel. There are no right or wrong answers. Do not spend too much time on any one statement, but give the answer that seems to describe how you generally feel.

① = not at all; ② = somewhat;
③ = moderately so; ④ = very much so

I wish I could be as happy as others seem to be	①	②	③	④
I am "calm, cool, and collected"	①	②	③	④
I feel that difficulties are piling up so that I cannot overcome them	①	②	③	④
I am inclined to take things hard	①	②	③	④
I am content	①	②	③	④

Figure 1-6 Sample items from the State-Trait Anxiety Inventory.

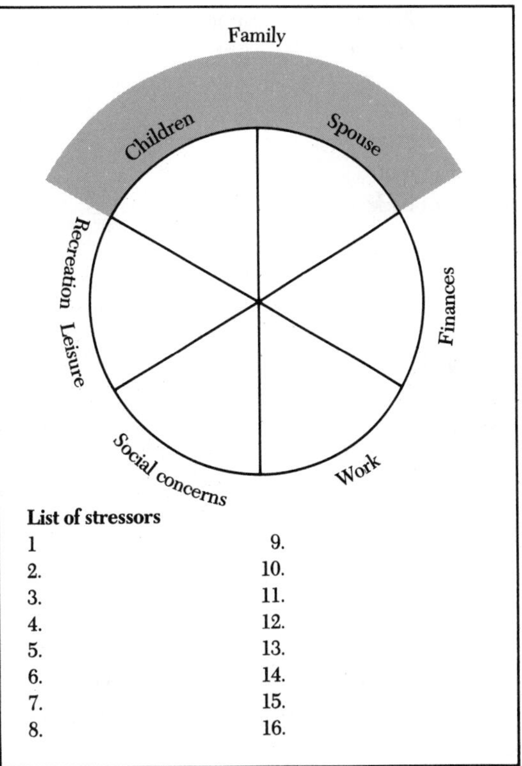

Figure 1-7 Stress charting.

town Manhattan levels of 30 to 40 ppm are not infrequent. An urban dweller's inhalation of this gas may produce high levels of carboxyhemoglobin, which can precipitate a heart attack.

Another pollutant in city air is asbestos. Large amounts of airborne asbestos can be found around construction sites. Asbestos is also a by-product of automobile use, as it can slough off from brake linings. Chronic exposure to asbestos has been linked to mesothelioma, a rapidly spreading cancer of the lungs and abdomen. Scientists used to believe that there was a safe threshold level of asbestos the body could take in and still be unharmed. Now they are not so sure. Still other air pollutants are the iron and steel dust and the ozone frequently found in subway air. This list could be added to indefinitely with the many petrochemicals that enter the air as by-products of industry.

Many urban dwellers have left the city to partake of the good life in the suburbs and the country. Recent studies have indicated that these areas may not be untainted. For example, reports have shown that the suburban development of Love Canal, in upper New York State, has offered a lethal environment to children. Some have died from liver and kidney damage that was possibly caused by PCB in the atmosphere. PCB (polychlorinated biphenyl) is a product of the petrochemical industry. How did the suburban children come in contact with the chemical? The development of Love Canal and the Love Canal Elementary School were built over a large chemical dump.

Other reports of rural pollution have recently come from small towns in Oregon where residents have come in contact with 2,4,5-T, a petrochemical used by the forestry industry to prepare areas for sapling planting. Exposure to 2,4,5-T has been linked to high rates of miscarriage in certain areas, short-term flulike ill-

Table 1-4. Percentage of Respondents in Each Social Class Recognizing Specified Symptoms as Needing Medical Attention

Symptom	Upper class (N = 51)	Middle class (N = 335)	Lower class (N = 128)
Loss of appetite	57	50	20
Persistent backache	33	44	19
Continued coughing	77	78	23
Persistent joint and muscle pain	80	47	19
Blood in stool	98	89	60
Blood in urine	100	93	69
Excessive vaginal bleeding	92	83	54
Swelling of ankles	77	76	23
Loss of weight	80	51	21
Bleeding gums	79	51	20
Chronic fatigue	80	53	19
Shortness of breath	77	55	21
Persistent headaches	80	56	22
Fainting spells	80	51	33
Pain in chest	80	51	31
Lump in breast	94	71	44
Lump in abdomen	92	65	34

From Earl L. Koos, *The Health of Regionville* (New York: Columbia University Press, 1954), p. 32. By permission of the publisher.

nesses, and possibly the rather high rates of cancer in these areas.

Many rural areas contain other possible health hazards as well: unsafe water supply, improper sewage disposal, unscreened windows, inadequate refrigeration or heating, lack of modern facilities in the kitchen and bathroom, and the scarcity of nursing and medical personnel and modern health facilities. Furthermore, the infant and maternal mortality rates are generally higher in rural areas. Rural health care is a national concern, and small-scale programs are being established in various regions to provide health personnel and mechanisms of communication and transportation to families living on isolated farms.

Social Class

Even though the United States lacks the sense of rigid social class that many European countries still have, class consciousness and the striving for upward mobility are clearly present. There are many indicators of social class: wealth, education, occupation, background, and neighborhood. Individuals or families may be stratified or ranked into different social classes on the basis of prestige, wealth, and power (Mausner & Bahn 1974). The United States government reports usually stratify on the basis of income. Income is not a bad way to gauge someone's health resources, as the amount of money earned determines how much an individual can afford to spend on doctor's visits, nutritious foods, and medical treatment. However, income is not always a strong predictor of educational background—a university professor and a skilled blue-collar worker can have the same income, yet they differ greatly in prestige and education. Therefore, certain socioeconomic rating scales take into account not only income but occupation and amount of education as well.

Different social classes are prone, because of their values, habits, and expectations, to different kinds of health problems. In general, persons of low socioeconomic status have more mental illness, higher morbidity rates, and lower life expectancies. There are, however, a few disease conditions in which high social class individuals have greater morbidity and mortality, including heart disease and leukemia (Mausner & Bahn 1974).

A major problem in the health care industry is that nurses and other health professionals tend to feel more comfortable with and to seek out clients from their own class and socioeconomic group. They are uncomfortable and have difficulty dealing with members of other groups. In the United States the majority of health professionals come from the middle and upper classes. Therefore, health care tends to be aimed at the client who has the same frame of reference as the health professional and the same expectations of health care. Thus, many health professionals misunderstand the expectations and concerns of lower-class clients, and they often come to view these clients as irresponsible.

It is the job of nurses and other health workers to try to understand the circumstances that make some of their clients seem irresponsible. For example, because health care costs are rising much faster than personal income, many lower-class people simply do not have money to pay for health care.

Many lower-class mothers lack prenatal and obstetric care. Their children rarely see a pediatrician or a dentist. The lower-class adult commonly resorts to a home remedy or drugstore tonic and rarely seeks medical attention outside of a major medical emergency. Koos (1954) found that the lower-class person identified specific symptoms as needing medical attention to a much lesser extent than members of the middle and upper classes (see Table 1-4).

Another problem facing the lower socioeconomic strata is substandard housing, with poor heating and ventilation systems. The children are tormented and bitten by rats as they lie in their beds. Communicable diseases spread like wildfire through the small crowded flats. Food is both scarce and of poor quality. The lower class has a higher occurrence of suicide, accidental deaths, homicides, delinquent behavior (Lebowitz 1975), infant mortality (Bernard & Thompson 1970), and adult mortality (Lebowitz 1975). With such a social environment, is it any wonder that people in the lower socioeconomic classes are ill more often, more seriously, and for a longer duration than those of the middle and upper classes?

An inverse relationship has been demonstrated to exist between educational level, family income, and the following pathologic conditions: chronic lung disease, heart disease, arthritis, kidney trouble, diabetes, and arteriosclerosis (Lebowitz 1975). Furthermore, a classic study of mental illness and social class conducted by Hollingshead and Redlich (1958) in New Haven showed that the rate of psychoses increased with the decline in social class. Fried's (1969) research concurred with this finding.

Summary

In this chapter we have considered the health-illness continuum and the various factors that control and influence the dynamic state of health. We described differences in clients' responses to the physiological and psychological stages of illness and the role the nurse should play in supporting the client.

Discussion Questions/Activities

1. Describe the differing responses of two different clients entering the health care system with the same problem, using Martin and Prange's framework of the stages of illness.
2. Use the Holmes and Rahe "Social Readjustment Rating Scale" to identify your own level of stress.
3. Choose a process described by a nursing leader and discuss how it can be used by the nurse to assist the client attain optimal wellness.
4. Explore one or several of alternative health care modes, e.g. biofeedback, meditation, imaging, massage, relaxation techniques, rolfing, therapeutic touch.
5. Describe the differences between the Medical Model and the Holistic Nursing Model.

CHAPTER 2

Cultural Considerations in Health Assessment

LEARNING OBJECTIVES

1. Define ethnocentrism.
2. Identify cultural areas of health assessment.
3. Discuss how values are formed.
4. List the steps in defining one's own values.
5. Explain what is meant by "The family is an expression of the culture in which it is found."
6. State examples of religious influence on health status.
7. Cite specific examples of ethnic-related practices that have an influence on health beliefs, practices, and health status.
8. Recognize that different cultural groups perceive their personal space differently.
9. Recognize that differences in customs exist between social classes.
10. Name examples of increased probability of disease in a particular population arising from the shared biological and/or cultural traits.
11. Implement health teaching that appeals to the values held by the client within the context of his culture.

The concept of culture is essential to nursing practice because the response of an individual to health and illness must be viewed in the context of culture. Health professionals are often dismayed to find that their well-intentioned health teaching, guidance, and planning appear to fall on deaf ears. Generally, this "failure to learn" is ascribed to lack of education, ignorance, or just plain not caring. If the situation were to be given further study, however, it might be found that what we consider high-level wellness has no meaning in certain cultures.

Knowledge of cultural differences must come from more than intellectual curiosity. Health assessment and nursing care, to be truly comprehensive, require active cultivation and use of this knowledge. Ethnocentrism, the tendency to use our own group and our own customs as the standard for all judgments, is counterproductive in intercultural communications. To avoid this narrow perspective, we need to view cultural factors as more than just addendums or last-minute considerations; they must become part of our thinking. This process should not be difficult if we become more aware that health and illness can be determined and influenced by an individual's cultural background. We are also operating within a cultural context and must understand how it affects our relations with others.

One way for us to do so is to examine our own cultural beliefs—how they affect our life, and how we may have thought and felt in the past when interacting with someone with beliefs different from our own.

How do we define culture and how does it relate to and affect health and illness? *Culture* includes those beliefs, values, attitudes, and customs that shape and color everything in our lives: education, occupation, marriage, family, and the way we experience health and illness. The United States contains many subcultures, including Blacks, Orientals, Hispanics, and Native Americans. As a nurse you will see many clients from various subcultures in performing health assessments. A general guide for cultural assessment is presented in Table 2-1.

Family

The nurse must not only be concerned with clients but must also take into account their frames of reference. Clients are social beings who function in a social environment composed of other people and who enter into certain relationships with these people. Clients' social environment continuously exerts influences upon them and shapes their human characteristics in health as well as illness. Therefore, it is important to view all clients as members of families and also as members of communities.

There are few nurses who do not subscribe to the notion that the family must be included in the planning for the care of the sick individual. How often, however, does the nurse fully investigate the kinship and family roles in specific cultural groups? Who makes the decisions in the family? In certain cultures it is the father; in others it is the mother or a designated elder or grandparent. To determine who makes the decisions in a particular subculture, a nurse may need to consult the literature, observe family interactions, or ask the family or group how decisions are made. More often than not, nurses view the family in the Western way or from an Anglo-Saxon viewpoint. Most American nurses tolerate involving the family in the health care scheme and invite them to be present only after it is determined that specific health teaching will assist the sick individual in the home situation. The major exception occurs when a child is ill. In this case the mother and father are encouraged to be present during the hospital stay.

The nurse must know the importance of family in particular subcultural groups and assist them in participating actively and knowingly in the health care process. Many cultural groups, notably Spanish Americans, Mexican Americans, and Native Americans, feel alienated when they are not surrounded by their entire family during illness. This attitude is also evident in Gypsy culture, where the entire clan comes to the hospital or clinic with the sick member. Such groups often avoid seeking medical attention because they fear separation. The Chinese design their hospitals so that families can remain with the sick person and help care for them.

As a nurse, you must be concerned with the client's perception—and his family's perception—of health and illness—Table 2-2 presents health views of four cultural groups. Superficially, health seems to be a personal and uniquely intimate experience rather than a "shared" sociologic one. But it is a sociologic phenomenon in that it involves not only the individual but the family, neighborhood, community, and society to which he belongs. Therefore, the client must be viewed in this framework, not in isolation. The nurse must learn to view wellness and illness not as isolated physiologic or psychologic phenomena but as parts of the context of family relationships and religious practice.

The family remains the basic social unit. The essence of family is living together as a unit—the grouping need not be permanent, conjugal (marriage-bound), or sanguineous (blood-related). However, the family is an expression of the culture in which it is found. In the United States there are a great number of subcultures that vary on the basis of race, ethnic origin, social class, religion, and occupation. Therefore, there are a great number of family types, and in our complex society one must first identify the subculture before attempting to describe a family. The family and lifestyle of a migrant fruit picker differ vastly from those of a state senator or of a factory laborer.

The traditional American family has been described as patriarchal, but this form is rapidly diminishing as more women are establishing careers and new life goals. Research has demonstrated a relationship between economic role and family role. In general, husbands exercise

Table 2-1. Cultural Assessment

Data categories	Guideline questions/instructions
Ethnic origin	Does the family identify with a particular ethnic group (e.g., Puerto Rican, African)?
Race	What is the family's racial background (e.g., black, Filipino, American Indian)?
Relocations	Where has the family lived (country, city)? How long? Has the family moved recently?
Habits, customs, values, and beliefs	Describe habits, customs, values, and beliefs the family holds or practices that affect its attitudes toward birth, life, death, health, illness, time orientation, the health care system, and health care providers. Does the family have special customs pertaining to the birth and naming of children? Is time in utero incorporated as part of the child's age (for example, is the child considered one year old at birth)? What is the family's degree of belief and adherence to its overall cultural system? Does an older child or adolescent adhere to these customs and beliefs?
Behaviors valued by culture	How does the family value privacy, courtesy, respect for elders, behaviors related to family roles, sex roles, and work ethics?
Cultural sanctions and restrictions	Sanctions—What is accepted behavior by the family's cultural group regarding expression of emotions and feelings, religious expressions, and response to illness and death?
	Restrictions—Does the family have any restrictions related to sexual matters, exposure of body parts, certain types of surgery, discussion of dead relatives, and discussion of fears related to the unknown?
Healing beliefs	Cultural healing system—What cultural healing system does the family predominately adhere to (e.g., Asian healing system, Raza/Latino curanderismo)? What religious healing system does the family predominately adhere to (for example, Seventh-Day Adventist, West African voodoo, Christian Scientist, Fundamentalist sect, Pentacostalist)?
	Cultural health beliefs—Is illness explained by the germ theory or cause-effect relationship, presence of evil spirits, imbalance between "hot" and "cold" or yin and yang, or disequilibrium between nature and human? Is good health related to success, ability to work or fulfill roles, reward from God, or balance with nature?
	Cultural health practices—What types of cultural healing practices does the family use?
	Cultural healers—Does the family rely on cultural healers?
Childrearing	How does the family discipline children? What behaviors are acceptable? What behaviors are unacceptable? How does the child show courtesy and respect for adults?
Childcare	What customs or beliefs influence care of the umbilical cord? What is the family's belief about when newborns should be taken outside the home? What customs or beliefs influence feedings, skin care, hair care, and other areas of personal hygiene?

Source: Adapted from Bloch's assessment guide for ethnic/cultural variations, by B. Bloch. In M. Orque, B. Bloch, and L. Monrroy (Eds.), *Ethnic nursing care: a multicultural approach*, pp. 49–75. Copyright © 1983 by The C. V. Mosby Co. Reprinted by permission.

less dominance over working wives than over nonworking wives, and unemployed husbands are far less dominant over working wives than are employed husbands. The degree of dominance over the wife increases with additional years of education and success of the husband (Blood & Wolfe 1960; Wolfe 1959).

There is increasing evidence that wives and mothers who have careers may experience health consequences—both good and bad. On

Table 2-2. Examples of Possible Beliefs and Practices of Some Members of Cultural Groups

	American Indian	Latino/Chicano	Asian	American Black
Views of health	Holistic view: God is seen as the giver of life and health	Holistic view: as a state of equilibrium; children may wear amulets for protection	Seen as a balance of energy, called Yin-Yang	Health means being able to work productively, being in a state of harmony with others in the universe
View of illness	Tied into religion	Has spiritual, social ramifications; good or "natural" diseases due to imbalance; "supernatural" diseases due to satanic forces	Seen as an imbalance of energy	Seen as a state of incapacitation, sense of disharmony, lack of communion
Resource person for treatment	Healing specialists, herbalists, diagnosticians	*Curanderos*, other types of healers	Healers, herbalists	Older woman with experience; the caregiver must develop a healing relationship with the ill person
Treatments	Herbs; sweat baths; a family conference if necessary to decide if a family member enters a hospital (Navajo)	Folk medicine; prayers; herbs; hot-cold foods and fluids to offset specific illnesses classified as derived from "hot" or "cold" causes	Herbs; nutrition; meditation; spiritual healing; massage; acupressure; acupuncture; hot-cold foods and fluids to counteract illnesses; moxibustion	Religious healing; folk remedies; herb teas; poultices
Views of children's health risks	Fear of strangers coming close to infants; fear of "witching" infant (Navajo)	If a stranger lavishes attention on but fails to touch a child, the child may develop "evil eye"; i.e., diarrhea, vomiting		A stout child is admired

From Servonsky/Opas: *Nursing Management of Children*, © 1987 Boston: Jones and Bartlett Publishers.

the one hand, executive women appear to suffer from an increased incidence of diseases that have long been known to plague male executives, including ulcers, heart disease, and respiratory problems resulting from excessive smoking (Mausner & Bahn 1974). On the other hand, the challenge and self-esteem arising from a career may lead to a decreased incidence of neurotic syndromes such as depression and anxiety (Chesler 1972). The children of career women may also experience health liabilities and benefits. It is possible that attending nursery school or day care at a young age may result in earlier infections of childhood diseases such as chicken pox and measles. However, earlier contact with other children in a play group situation may lead to greater social adjustment, increased independence, and an enhanced self-concept.

In Black families, decision-making power is often found to reside with the wife, who is usually dominant (Kephart 1961). This may mean that the wife will make the health decisions for the family, such as which health services to use and under which circumstances. Another difference in the Black family structure is the greater role of the grandmother, who may raise her daughter's or son's children and have the responsibility and control of seeing to their health and welfare (Williams 1975).

Another subculture and type of family that you may encounter is Spanish American or Mexican American. Margaret Clark (1970), in her studies of health practices among Spanish-speaking people in northern California, found that fathers are the dominant figures in the family. Childbearing is both the privilege and the obligation of the married women. Households are often large and may include not only a large number of offspring but grandparents as well.

Family size is another variable that may affect the health of individuals. In a study of 25,000 illnesses in a group of Cleveland families followed for 10 years, family size was found to be positively associated with the number of illnesses per person (Dingle, Badger & Jordan 1964). This is because there are more individuals present to introduce illness. For example, the rate for gastrointestinal diseases was 0.97 in three-person households and 1.89 in seven-person households. It must be noted that these families were upper middle class and were checked once a week. The situation in a lower-class family would be less healthy, for fewer illnesses would end in doctors' visits, which would mean that diseases would linger longer, exposing family members more frequently.

Religion

Religious beliefs, attitudes, and practices can also be strong cultural forces that affect health status and needs. For example, Jewish males are circumcised within a short time after birth. This widespread custom has been linked to the low incidence of cancer of the penis among Jewish males and cancer of the cervix among Jewish females (Damon 1977). Other religious groups that do not believe in early circumcision, such as Moslems, or that do not believe in circumcision at all, such as Hindus, have higher rates of these types of cancer. Low rates of cancer of the upper digestive tract and respiratory system among Jewish males are thought to be related to the moderate use of alcohol and tobacco advocated by the Jewish faith (Damon 1977). Total abstinence from tobacco smoking and alcohol drinking are thought to be associated with the low rates of certain types of cancer among the Mormons. One group of vegetarian Seventh Day Adventists, whose religion forbids them to use tobacco, alcohol, pork, caffeine-containing beverages, hot condiments and spices, and highly refined foods, was found to have significantly lower systolic and diastolic blood pressures than individuals from the general population (Armstrong, Van Merwyk & Coates 1977).

During crises such as severe illness or death, people tend to become more dependent on their religious faith. It is important for the nurse to be aware of the different religious sects in the community in order to facilitate the client's continuing practice of his religion and to recognize when religious beliefs conflict with scientific therapies.

Clients must be able to observe their religious practices during treatment. Such practices might involve talking with religious leaders or following dietary practices or other religious rules. It is essential for the nurse to recognize when beliefs and practices run counter to medical treatment or affect a client's perception of a health situation. For example, the Roman Catholic Church has recently reaffirmed its stand against Catholics using birth control measures. Although many Catholics in the United States do not heed the church's position, some do, and nurses must be aware of the fact. Other religious beliefs regarding medicine include the Jehovah's Witnesses' stand against blood transfusion and the Christian Scientists' opposition to surgical intervention. In fact, Christian Scientists rely heavily on faith healing and shun various kinds of medical help. It is not the nurse's role to resolve these conflicts but to assist the client and his family to reach appropriate decisions.

Ethnic Groups and Ethnomedical Systems

The ethnic group that one belongs to is a sociological variable over which the individual has no control. Within an American community there are often ethnic subcommunities—an Italian community, a Jewish community, a Black community, a Polish community, a Greek community, a Mexican American community, and so on. These ethnic groups have their own class structure, style of living, and entertainment (music and dance), and many may even still maintain their own language, food habits, and different conceptions of familial and personal roles. This maintenance of ethnic and cultural traditions is especially true in first- and second-generation immigrants, but remnants may also be found in beliefs and practices in many succeeding generations.

Studies have found that ethnic groups differ in reporting symptoms and in seeking medical aid (Mechanic 1968). They also vary in their willingness to accept psychologic interpretations of their complaints (Fink, Shapiro & Soldensohn

1969) and in their reactions to pain (Zborowski 1952). Zborowski found, for example, that of the four ethnic groups studied, Irish and Americans (those who had been in the U.S. for more than two generations) tended to be stoic in their response to pain, while Italians and Jews displayed more overt emotional behavior.

Most cultures have their own health norms and practices. Many groups continue to ascribe their illness to an "evil eye," sin, or failure to observe religious practice, while others perceive their condition as the "will of God" and therefore feel they cannot be treated. For example, the Italian grandmother who believes, even if half-heartedly, that her grandchild's headaches are caused by the "evil eye" (a curse) will perform the *malocchio*, a ceremony using oil and water, which will validate her suspicion of the presence of the "evil eye." The fact that the ceremony is performed provides the cure. Thus, the *malocchio* is a diagnosis as well as a cure.

Leininger (1970) discussed the Spanish American belief in the "evil eye," particularly in relation to children. Spanish Americans believe that disease occurs because someone has admired the child to an excessive degree. The treatment must then consist of having the person who has cast the *mal-ojo* (evil eye) touch or caress the child. This belief has implications for nursing in that the child should always be touched or caressed when being admired. Many Spanish Americans believe that illness is the will of God and that preventive measures are therefore of little value. Since the children are in God's hands, why should they have to be immunized? They see pregnancy as quite normal and as something health personnel should not disrupt. Thus, traditional nursing approaches would certainly be ineffective in relating with these people.

The Black folk medicine system has been described as including elements of African beliefs, folk and formal medicine, and modern scientific medicine, interwoven with factors from Christianity, voodoo, and sympathetic magic (Snow 1974). These medical beliefs are strictly adhered to by many Blacks. Illnesses are often treated within the community by individuals who try in their own fashion to restore equilibrium. Minsters, adult women, and in rural areas "root workers" (said to have supernatural powers granted by God) are active in providing health care (Dougherty 1976).

The Navajo Indian places strong credence in the power of spirits. Anthropologist Jeremiah Lyons has related an incident that occurred in a tuberculosis hospital in a western state. During a storm one evening a tree in the hospital courtyard was destroyed by lightning. By morning every Indian had left the hospital and would not return until a special ceremony was performed by the medicine man to appease the spirit they believed had destroyed the tree.

We cannot scoff at or disregard beliefs such as these. We must learn to provide health care that incorporates such beliefs, as they are strongly internalized values. Interestingly, medicine men, shamans, and *curanderos* provide a necessary and vital function within the cultural group. Often they are able to "cure" by providing emotional support, as they generally consider the whole person. Further, in many societies these people have been taught the basic skills of modern medicine, since they are frequently contacted first by the ill person or family. As a nurse, you must encourage people to seek out medical attention, but you must also be aware of the important role these people have in the cultural lives of certain groups. You must learn to provide meaningful health care and still respect, and more importantly understand, the value system operating within the culture. It may be helpful and necessary to include the client's folk medicine practitioner when providing care.

You also need to consider the fact that many folk remedies are therapeutic. It is important to recognize that herb and plant remedies can be helpful and to interfere only to avoid overdoses or in cases where incompatibility with prescribed drugs may occur. Such practices as wearing garlic to ward off spirits or wearing copper bracelets to alleviate the symptoms of arthritis should not be ridiculed. Furthermore, a nurse should not ignore clients' fears of spells and hexes.

Communication and Personal Space

Verbal and nonverbal communication are extremely important in health assessment. The ability to communicate effectively is essential. Fluency in the other's native language is particularly important. Many Americans express annoyance when other cultural groups do not know how to speak English. Such an attitude creates anxiety in the nurse-client relationship. The usual expectation is that the client should speak English, not that the nurse should speak the language of the client. This attitude implies that the client should meet the expectations of the nurse, and it often results in poor cooperation and resentment between the two. Certainly nurses cannot expect to be fluent in all languages, but if they are actively involved with a specific cultural group, they should be able to communicate in that group's language.

Another problem with language communication may arise from the client's lack of understanding of medical terminology. The nurse should be quite sure that the client understands directions for medical procedures and prescriptions. In the hospital setting, the patient may be confused or awed and agree quickly to instructions while not having any real understanding of the information being relayed. In order to be sure that the client has a good understanding of what is happening, the nurse may have to spend more time in what seems a repetitive conversation, but the result may be a better health outcome for the client.

Communicating effectively also means listening to what the client brings to the encounter and may necessitate taking on another vocabulary. Loudell Snow (1976) has pointed to this need in dealing with Black or White low-income patients. In such cases, the practitioner should be aware of such terms as a "risin" (boil), "tizik" (tuberculosis), or "the smothers" (inability to breathe easily). Southern patients may also refer to a class of problems having to do with the state of their blood; "bad blood," "high blood," and "low blood" are all terms that have specific meaning for the client, who may be confused when the nurse talks about other medically perceived syndromes such as low or high blood pressure. Table 2-3 contains some folk illnesses in Hispanic and Black cultures.

Knowing the language, although important, does not guarantee effective communication; the nurse must also take into account concepts of nonverbal communication and personal space. For example, nurses should not assume that eye contact and touching are good means of positive reinforcement with clients. Some cultural groups view these behaviors as intrusions on their privacy. Prolonged eye contact is considered very disrespectful among Eastern and Oriental cultures: "The Indian believes that to touch someone violates his body boundary and takes something away from him as a person" (Fire & Baker 1976). Spanish Americans, however, feel more comfortable if eye contact is maintained. The Japanese use nonverbal communication very effectively, as they place great store in silence. Laughing or smiling in their culture often does not mean happiness, as it might to Westerners. For the Japanese it may be an indication of anger or grief. Emotions are rarely expressed facially, and direct eye contact often makes the Japanese uncomfortable. The Black American has developed a highly effective means of communicating nonverbally through body movements, expressions, and gestures. Many Black children are taught not to look an adult directly in the eye, as this communicates disrespect.

The use of personal space is an aspect of culture that frequently serves as a means of nonverbal communication (Hall 1960). Different cultural groups perceive their personal space differently. For example, the Germans are quite particular about preserving their private sphere; they need to have their own space. The German culture puts heavy emphasis on orderliness; they even consider open doors to be sloppy and disorderly. The Polish people, on the other hand, appear to like a little disorder, and the "private sphere" is not nearly so rigid. The English are conditioned to sharing space but have learned to erect behavioral barriers that allow for privacy.

Hospitals, clinics, and nurses rarely take these spatial differences into account. Nurses who have a compulsion to keep things neat and orderly may in fact be creating a nontherapeutic environment—orderly, uncrowded rooms are thought by the Navajo to indicate impending death. The neat and orderly look may in fact discourage effective communication. In Western culture individuals are more comfortable when they maintain a considerable distance between each other during social contact. They avoid touching except in special situations. Latin Americans and Arabs, on the other hand, relate to each other in very close proximity, and the Japanese appear to be quite comfortable in crowded situations. "Spatial changes give a tone to a communication, accent it, and at times even override the spoken word" (Hall 1973, p. 180).

Accurate and effective health assessment cannot be made without effective communication. If this important aspect of nursing practice is

Table 2-3. Folk Illnesses in Hispanic and Black Cultures

Culture	Folk illness	Etiology	Behaviors	Practitioner	Treatment
Hispanic	*Susto* (fright)	An individual experiences a stressful event at some time prior to the onset of symptoms. The stressor may vary from death of a significant person to a child's nightmare to inability to adequately fulfill social-role responsibility. Children are more susceptible to *susto*. It is believed that the soul or spirit leaves the body.	Restlessness during sleep Anorexia Depression Listlessness Disinterest in personal appearance	*Curandero* or *Espiritualista* (*Espiritista*)	A ceremony is performed using branches from a sweet pepper tree and a candle. Motions by the ill person and the curer are performed that form a cross. Three Ave Marias or credos (Apostles' Creed) are said.
	Empacho	Bolus of undigested food adheres to the stomach or wall of intestine. The cause may be the food itself, or it may be due to eating when one is not hungry or when one is stressed.	Stomach pain Diarrhea Vomiting Anorexia	Family member *Sabador* *Curandero*	Massage of the stomach or back until a popping sound is heard. A laxative may be given.
	Caida de la Mollera (fallen fontanel)	Trauma—a fall or blow to the head or the rapid dislodging of a nipple from an infant's mouth causes the fontanel to be sucked into the palate.	Inability to suckle Irritability Vomiting Diarrhea Sunken fontanel	Family member *Curandero*	One or more of these practitioners insert a finger into the child's mouth and push the palate back into place. Hold the child by the ankles with the top of the head just touching a pan of tepid water for a minute or two. Apply a poultice of soap shavings to the fontanel. Administer herb tea.
	Mal de ojo (evil eye)	A disease of magical origin cast by a person who is jealous or envious of another person or something the person owns. The evil eye is cast by the envious person's vision upon the subject thereby heating the blood and producing symptoms. Usually a beautiful child is envied or admired but is not touched by the admirer and the evil eye can be inflicted. The admirer may not be aware of the damage done. If the child is admired and then touched by that person the evil eye is not inflicted.	Fever Diarrhea Vomiting Crying without apparent cause	*Curandero* *Brujo*	Passing an unbroken egg over the body or rubbing the body with an egg to draw the heat (fever) from the body. Prayers such as the Our Father or Hail Mary may be said simultaneously with the passing of the egg. The egg is then broken in a bowl, placed under the head of the bed and left there all night. By morning if the egg is almost cooked from the heat of the body this is a sign that the sick person had *mal deojo*.
	Mal Puesto (evil)	Illness caused by a hex put on by a *brujo*, witch, or *curandero*, or other person knowledgeable about witchcraft.	Vary considerably Strange behavioral changes Labile emotions Convulsions	*Curandero* *Brujo*	Varies, depending on the hex.

Source: From Folk health and illness beliefs, by M. A. Hautman, *Nurse Practitioner: The American Journal of Primary Health Care* 4(4):27 (1979). Reprinted by permission.

Table 2-3. *Continued*

Culture	Folk illness	Etiology	Behaviors	Practitioner	Treatment
Black	High blood (too much blood)	Diet very high in red meat and rich food. Belief that high blood causes stroke.	Weakness, paralysis, vertigo, or other behaviors related to stroke	Family member or friend of Spiritualist or self (the latter does this after referring to a Zodiac almanac)	Take internally lemon juice, vinegar, epsom salts, or other astringent food to sweat out the excess blood. Treatment varies depending on what is appropriate for each person according to the Zodiac almanac.
	Low blood (not enough blood—anemia is conceptualized)	Too many astringent foods, too harsh a treatment for high blood. Remaining on high blood-pressure medication for too long.	Fatigue Weakness	Same as for high blood	Eat rich red meat, raw beets. Stop taking treatment for high blood. Consult the Zodiac almanac.
	Thin blood (predisposition to illness)	Occurs in women, children, or old people. Blood is very thin until puberty and remains so until old age except for women.	Greater susceptibility to illness	Individual	Individual should exercise caution in cold weather by wearing warm clothing or by staying indoors.
	Rash appearing on a child after birth (no specific disease name—the concept is that of body defilement)	Impurities within the body coming out. The body is being defiled and will therefore produce skin rashes.	Rash anywhere on the body; may be accompanied by fever	Family member	Catnip tea as a laxative or other commercial laxative. The quantity and kind depend on the age of the individual.
	Diseases of witchcraft, hex or conjuring	Envy and sexual conflict are the most frequent causes of having someone hex another person.	Unusual behavior not normal for the person Sudden death Symptoms related to poisoning (i.e., foul taste, fall off [weight loss], nausea, vomiting) A crawling sensation on the skin or in the stomach Psychotic behavior	Voodoo Priest(ess) Spiritualist	"*Conja*" is the help given to the conjured person. Treatment varies depending on the spell cast.

neglected, valuable knowledge—as well as rapport between the client and nurse—will be lost.

Socioeconomic Factors

Yamamoto and Goin (1966) report that clients from the lower socioeconomic groups more frequently fail to keep appointments, a behavior that greatly irritates and frustrates most professionals, who tend to view the client's behavior superficially and out of context. Try, for a moment, to imagine what a clinic visit would be like. You have just completed a number of application papers; no one has bothered to ask you how you feel today. They just want to get your address, phone number, and so forth—the same information that you supplied during your previous visit. You wait for hours in a crowded, noisy hall sitting on a hard wooden chair that has uneven legs. Maybe, you think, they've lost your chart or perhaps the nurse didn't get your name.

You try to tell her your name as she runs by . . . "Yes, yes. Just go sit down and wait your turn." You go back and continue to rock on the uneven legs of the miserable chair. Finally, you hear your last name called out, and you get your 3 to 5 minutes with a blasé and impersonal nurse or physician. Your stomach is upset, and you're uncomfortable. It's late afternoon, and you remember how much better you felt when you arrived here at the clinic at 8 A.M., shortly after your breakfast. Within your precious 3 to 5 minutes you are reprimanded for not adhering to your prescribed weight reduction diet. You explain that the dietetic foods you were instructed to buy were too expensive and that you didn't have the money. "We can't help you if you don't want to follow instructions." Then you are dismissed nonchalantly as a hopeless case and waste of time. The nurse shouts, "Doctor, do you want to see this client next week?" An uninterested reply, "Yeah . . . I guess. . . same day."

Teresa Bello (1976) has wisely pointed out that "attitudes about the poor also interfere with cultural sensitivity. Many health professionals think poor people are hopeless in that they are poorly educated (academically and health-wise)." We must continually ask ourselves whether the behaviors we see are representative of the customs of a particular social class or are perhaps occasioned by the circumstances a lower-class client must endure to receive health care. The only way to answer this question is to provide time, interest, and understanding for each client.

A study of 865 Caucasian working-class and middle-class high school seniors conducted by Kilwein (1975) indicated that social-class differences in family attitudes have diminished among young people. The participants in the study were reported to be representative of what the literature describes as more "middle class." What was particularly alarming to the researcher was that "so many males, particularly blue-collar males, considered it wrong for husbands to express the emotions of fear and tenderness." Kilwein urges us to emphasize the normalcy of basic emotional expression by males and to provide a nonthreatening atmosphere in which emotions such as these can be "wholesomely" expressed. Although this study showed convergence of class values, generally there are wide differences in the customs between the various class levels.

The members of each class level have their own set of values, system of behavior, and terminology and way of communicating. Members "culturize" their children, colleagues, students, or neighbors to their held beliefs and accepted modes of behavior. Examine, for example, your own socialization into the occupational culture of nursing—have your value system, behavior, communication style, and jargon changed at all?

Bernard and Thompson (1970) described a number of differences in customs between social classes. They noted that Kinsey reported sexual behavior to be associated with social classes stratified according to education and occupation. Certain sexual behaviors condoned by one class were viewed indifferently or with censure by another, and vice versa. They further pointed out that child-rearing patterns, attitudes toward cleanliness, and attitudes toward education are quite dissimilar between classes. They noted that some social classes encourage the development of aggressiveness, whereas others discourage it. For example, an elementary school nurse found that her office was constantly filled with students, particularly Black children, who were referred to her as behavioral problems on the basis of loud, disruptive or aggressive behavior. When the White middle-class teachers were told that aggressiveness is encouraged and valued as a personal attribute in many Black families, they were then able to view the behavior in a different light from the generally far removed perspective of the White middle class.

Nurses, physicians, and other allied health workers also tend to share a middle-class ethnocentrism. Health providers engaged in private practice or employed in private institutions are most likely to deal with clients from the middle and upper socioeconomic levels—clients who share their emphasis on preventative health measures and medical care. Clients identify better with health workers who share the same social class and common life experiences. Rosenthal and Frank (1958) reported that psychiatrists tended to refer those clients for psychotherapy who were most like themselves. Thus, they referred significantly more White than Black clients, the better educated, and those in the upper rather than the lower income range. Generally, health professionals tend to view the health practices and concerns of lower-class clients as haphazard and irresponsible. When they find themselves interacting, sometimes not too successfully, with clients having a cultural orientation quite different from their own, they often seem to ignore the sociologic variables that influence the value system of these clients. Although some believe that such health workers simply do not care or try to understand, we feel that perhaps the basic problem stems from the fact that most health workers, including nurses, are not knowledgeable about the social factors and dynamics at work in the different social classes.

Although statistics indicate that overall family income and earnings are steadily increasing, this does not apply to all families, nor do increases keep pace with the rise in the cost of living in all cases. Many families that were once economically stable are now treading a fine line between adequate and inadequate income. It is this marginal position that "tends to increase family vulnerability to crisis events. When family expenditures equal or exceed their income, unexpected costs of illness can jeopardize the family's precarious financial balance" (Hill 1968). Furthermore, families have less money to spend on health care.

Health Teaching

In providing health teaching to persons of varying cultural backgrounds, you should keep in mind that not all are eager to participate in health care planning and illness prevention. Because some groups may not be future oriented, your health teaching must appeal to immediate concerns rather than long-range goals. For example, it may be more important to stress the active treatment of obesity than to focus on the long-range effects of being obese. The teaching must appeal to the values held by the individual within the context of his culture. Otherwise, the client may not comply with treatments, and lengthy and expensive health care measures may consequently be ineffective.

The Puerto Rican has a fatalistic attitude toward life, which results in the belief that there is little control over life. Predominant reasons for illness are "God's will" or that someone has done something wrong and must suffer. The illness is outside of one's sphere of influence. Several studies have been carried out related to powerlessness. Seeman (1963) found that patients who scored above the mean on his Powerless Scale (indicating a high level of powerlessness) scored significantly lower on a test of knowledge of tuberculosis than did a matched sample of patients who scored below the mean. Another study looked at the relationship between powerlessness and knowledge of self-care, and found that those patients with a higher degree of powerlessness had less knowledge about caring for themselves. Since this feeling of powerlessness is part of the Puerto Rican way of life, it has implications for planning educational programs to assist this ethnic group in controlling disease and promoting wellness. The powerlessness has resulted in individuals not seeking help until a disease has progressed to a severe stage.

Brosnan (1976) suggested techniques that would enhance the health-teaching efforts of the nurse. As part of the plan God's will and fate should be emphasized. To the Puerto Rican, suffering is part of life and chronic illness is considered a fate that one must resign oneself to. An attempt should be made to establish yourself as a friend of the household and not attempt to advocate any public health measures unless asked. Visits to the home should be scheduled at night so that the husband who is the head of household will be there. You need to also be aware of the belief that injections are considered the best medicine while pills are the least effective. Worst of all is no medicine. Whenever an individual is sick, a purgative is in order to throw the disease out of the body.

Louie (1976), writing about Chinese Americans, described the processes of explanatory thinking and how they relate to concepts of health and illness in the Chinese American illness situation. These processes, picking up and linking, are believed to "normalize" symptoms. Picking up is defined as that process in which the individual selectively receives notes and retains information from the specific environment. Linking is the process of making connections, or integrating or creating relationships within oneself. This mechanism assists the Chinese American in making the transition between Chinese and American health belief systems, and you should be familiar with these cultural concepts when attempting to develop a teaching plan.

There are numerous studies in the nursing and anthropological literature that you can re-

BIOLOGICAL AND CULTURAL VARIATIONS

An Introduction

Specific population groups have higher incidence rates of certain diseases, genetic conditions, and psychobehavioral disorders. Some well-known examples of genetic disorders associated with certain population groups are Tay-Sachs disease among Ashkenazic Jews and sickle-cell anemia among Black Americans of West African origin. This is not to say that these diseases occur in everyone in the specific population group or that they are restricted to that population group. For example, although the incidence of Tay-Sachs disease is 100 times higher among Ashkenazic Jews than among non-Jews, it still occurs in 1 out of 500,000 non-Jewish births.

Knowledge that there is a higher probability of a certain disease appearing in a particular population group can be useful to diagnosticians and health planners. For example, a diagnostician presented with a case of abdominal pain, fever, and increased white blood cell count would do well to note the population group to which the patient belongs (Damon 1977). In a patient of Mediterranean background, the symptoms might be due to a crisis of familial Mediterranean fever or glucose-6-phosphate dehydrogenase deficiency, both of which are largely found among Syrians, Armenians, Greeks, Italians, and Sephardic Jews. In a Black American or Black African, the same symptoms might be due to a crisis of sickle-cell anemia. In a Native American or person of Western European origin, these may be symptoms of a gallbladder inflammation. Knowledge of disease patterns in different populations aids the clinician in making the diagnoses and, in this case, might prevent unnecessary surgery. Knowing the population a disease is likely to occur in is also useful to health planners, for it helps them to allocate services and money for health screening and health care. Information on population variation in disease incidence will be found in some of the following chapters under the heading "Biological and Cultural Variations."

We prefer to use the term "population group" rather than "racial group" or "ethnic group." "Racial group" has been used to define a breeding population with distinguishing biological characteristics and certain genes in common. "Ethnic group" is used to denote a breeding population sharing cultural characteristics, such as attitudes, religion, and dietary habits. Obviously, there is no such thing as a completely distinct racial or ethnic group, because individuals tend to marry individuals from other groups. Also, although biological characteristics may be present to a different degree in different racial groups, all biological traits generally occur to some degree in each group, as we saw

search so that your teaching is meaningful to the specific cultural group. If this is not done, little learning will occur.

Culture and Values

Values represent a system of ideas, attitudes, and beliefs about the worth of an entity or concept. They consciously and unconsciously bind together individuals and families in a common culture (Parad & Caplan 1965, p. 58). Values function as general guides to behavior. They help the individual or group to understand the nature and meaning of the world and how they fit into that world.

Development of Values

Socialization is the process by which values are instilled in individuals. Values, emerging over time, result from personal experience, interpersonal relationships, and the circumstances of the times in which one lives. Individual value systems reflect culture, society, personal needs, and significant reference groups (Rokeach 1973, p. 5). The fully functioning self develops and in the case of genes for Tay-Sachs disease. Finally, there is variation in the extent to which cultural characteristics are shared by the members of an ethnic group. Thus, we have chosen to use the term "population group" to encompass the meaning of both "racial group" and "ethnic group." A *population group* is an aggregation of individuals who have an increased likelihood of mating with each other and tend to have biological and/or cultural characteristics in common. Increased probability of disease in a particular population group thus arises from the shared biological and/or cultural traits.

In some cases a disease has a strictly biological transmission and arises from genes found in the population group, such as the gene for producing the deficient enzyme glucose-6-phosphate dehydrogenase in Mediterranean peoples. And sickle-cell anemia is due to a variation in the hemoglobin gene that originally occurred in West African populations and is carried by Black Americans of West African ancestry.

Other diseases result from the interaction of biological and cultural factors in the population group. Black Americans have higher rates of morbidity and mortality from hypertension. There seems to be an underlying genetic predisposition to develop high blood pressure in this group, but it is probably exacerbated by the lower socioeconomic status, varying dietary patterns, and potentially higher levels of stress among Black Americans. Among other conditions that are probably due to the interaction of biological and cultural characteristics are lactase deficiency among Orientals and Blacks and atherosclerosis among White Americans.

In addition, cultural or socioeconomic factors may lead to higher or lower incidences of disease within a population group. For example, the greater incidence of infectious diseases such as pneumonia, tuberculosis, and syphilis among non-White Americans is related to the greater proportion of low-socioeconomic-status individuals in this group. In some cases a disease that was formerly thought to be due to biological factors is now seen to result from cultural or socioeconomic conditions. For example, because Native Americans have high rates of alcoholism, many investigators have researched the possibility that biological differences in alcohol metabolism might be the cause. However, it now seems that differences in cultural attitudes about alcohol use and drinking behavior may explain the higher Native American alcoholism rates.

These and other examples of biological and cultural variations in disease patterns will be considered in the following chapters.

holds human values. Everyone holds some values. Values come about through the life an individual lives, which determines what that person cares about (Kelley 1977, p. 300).

Values are hierarchical. Some values are more central, molding or influencing aspects of an individual's life. Other values, which are more peripheral, have less influence. Therefore certain values have a greater priority at a given time in the individual's life. According to Rokeach:

> To say that a person has a value is to say that he has an enduring prescriptive or proscriptive belief that a specific mode of behavior . . . is preferred to an opposite mode of behavior. . . . This belief transcends attitudes toward objects and toward situations; it is a standard that guides and determines action, attitudes . . . and comparisons of self with others. Values serve adjustive, ego-defensive, knowledge and self-actualizing functions. (Rokeach 1973, p. 51)

A nursing assessment without analysis of the client's values is incomplete. What does the client believe about illness, health, and wellness? Does the client believe that he has the ability to shape events and that certain behaviors can provide a fuller, happier health? Does the client believe that what is happening is an act of God? Has an evil eye been cast on the individual and the family? An individual's or family's values are a reflection of the community in which the individual lives and the subculture(s) with which they identify. Most persons belong to a number of subcultures based on social class, ethnic background, occupational groups, peer groups, and religious affiliations (Friedman 1981, p. 172). These subgroups are very influential in the development of the values held by the individual.

Many observers today are concerned that the values held by health professionals are not congruent with the values held by a large number of their clients. As a result the relationship with the client resembles a tug of war in which the health professional usually wins. Thus, once the client leaves the health care facility he is unlikely to follow the prescribed treatment regimen because it is useless to his lifestyle and goals.

If you are aware of the client's cultural values, this awareness becomes an excellent predictive basis for determining behavior and planning the most effective nursing interventions. You must also be aware of subcultural values as well as the values of the dominant culture (Leininger 1978, p. 92). Most nurses subscribe to Anglo-American middle-class values, which stress individuality, material wealth, physical beauty, democracy, cleanliness, work, education, science, and the legal system. You should be aware of personal value orientations as you are assessing the health behavior of clients. Some basic values of cultures with selected cultural examples are shown in Table 2-4.

Assessing Values

Leininger identified several ways by which the nurse can assess values:

1. as a theme or patterns of recurrent behavior of an individual or of groups
2. as patterns of interrelated behavior among many elements of a culture
3. as a single isolated bit of individualized behavior that needs further validation under similar circumstances
4. as a combination of the three methods, in which behavior should be validated by checking with the people on each aspect of the data collected. (Leininger 1978, p. 92)

It is extremely important that you understand the cultural background of the client. Since this information may not be at your fingertips, you must review literature pertinent to the particular client. Much can also be learned about the manifest values of the individual's cultural group by observing the verbal and nonverbal communication occurring during the assessment. You can thereby inquire how the client perceives health, illness, wellness, religion, family, friends, and other areas that often are value laden.

Of increasing usefulness, too, is values clarification. Values clarification is a process that helps the individual to understand what is meaningful. Throughout this process a professional assists the individual in examining which values are important to the individual's life and which are not. Values clarification can facilitate decision making and problem solving in the area of health by promoting behavior consistent with health-related values. You can use several tools to determine the value hierarchies of individuals (Kavanagh 1980). Shostrum (1963) reviewed six value instruments for examining personal values in the counseling setting:

- The Allport-Vernon-Lindzey Study of Values (SV)
- The Survey of Personal Values (SPV)
- The Survey of Interpersonal Values (SIV)
- The Differential Value Profile (DVP)
- The Personal Orientation Inventory (POI)
- Ways to Live

The Mental Measurements Yearbook provides information about the scope of the instruments, reliability, validity, qualifications for administration, and publishing source.

As nurses we can try to determine, but we cannot always be certain, what values or style of life is most suitable for any client. As health care givers we value health, and hopefully we can influence other individuals and groups to value health. We can assist the client in the process of valuing health and health-related practices in the following ways:

1. Encourage them to make more choices and to make them freely.

2. Help them to discover alternatives when faced with choices.
3. Help them to weigh alternatives thoughtfully, reflecting on the consequences of each.
4. Encourage them to consider what they prize and cherish.
5. Provide opportunities to affirm choices.
6. Encourage them to act and live in accordance with their choices.
7. Help them to be aware of repeated behaviors or patterns in their life (Raths, Harmin & Simon 1978).

Table 2-4. Basic Values of Cultures with Selected Cultural Examples

Value	Range of beliefs	Example of cultural/subcultural group adhering to value
Human nature (What is innate nature of man?)	A. The person is basically *evil but capable of achieving goodness* with self-control and effort.	Puritan ancestors. Protestants of Pentecostal or Fundamentalist background. Appalachian subculture.
	B. The person is a *combination of good and evil*, with self-control necessary but lapses in behavior understood.	Most people in the United States.
	C. The person is basically *good.*	
Man-nature (What is relation of man to nature or supernature?)	A. The person is *subjugated to nature* and cannot change whatever is destined to happen.	Spanish-American culture. Appalachian subculture.
	B. The person lives in *harmony with nature*; man-nature-supernature exist as a whole entity.	Oriental cultures. Navajo Indian culture.
	C. The person is to *gain mastery over nature*; all natural forces can be overcome.	Most people in the United States.
Time (What is temporal focus on human life?)	A. *Past time* is given preference; most important events to guide life have happened in the past.	Historic China.
	B. *Present time* is the main focus; people pay little attention to the past and regard the future as vague.	Spanish-American cultures. Appalachian subcultures.
	C. *Future* is the main emphasis, seen as bigger and better; people are not content with the present.	Most people in the United States.
Activity (What is the main purpose in life?)	A. *Being orientation.* The person is important just because he is and may spontaneously express impulses and desires.	Appalachian subculture. While no culture allows complete expression of impulses and all cultures must have some work done, the Mexican fiesta and Mardi Gras in New Orleans are manifestations of this value.
	B. *Becoming-in-being orientation.* The person is important for what he is, but he must continue to develop.	Most religious cultures. Native American subcultures.
	C. *Doing orientation.* The person is important when he is active or accomplishing something.	Most people in the United States.

Continued on page 32

From Murray Beckmann, Ruth Zentner, and Judith Proctor, *Nursing Concepts for Health Promotion*, 3rd ed. (Englewood Cliffs, N.J.: Prentice-Hall, 1985), pp. 437–438.

Table 2-4. *Continued*

Value	Range of beliefs	Example of cultural/subcultural group adhering to value
Relational (What is man's relation to other men?)	A. *Individualistic relations* emphasize autonomy of the person; he does not have to fully submit to authority. Individual goals have primacy over group goal.	Most Gemeinschaft societies, such as folk or rural cultures. Yankee and Appalachian subcultures. Middle class America, with emphasis on nuclear family.
	B. *Collateral relations* emphasize that the person is part of a social and family order and does not live just for himself. Group or family goals have primacy.	Most European-American ethnic groups, especially Italian-American. Spanish American culture. Native American tribal subcultures. Most cultures adhere to somewhat through sibling relations in family.
	C. *Lineal relations* emphasize the extended family and biological and cultural relationships through time. Group goals have primacy.	Cultures that emphasize hereditary lines. Upper class America. Oriental cultures. Middle-East cultures.

By recognizing the client's values and cultural orientation, you are able to carry out an in-depth and meaningful assessment, which can enhance the helping and caring process.

Summary

We have briefly examined the essential components of culture that you must consider in assessing the health of a client. For instance, a person's ethnic group affects attitudes toward health and illness. The best scientific methods and intentions may have a negative effect, if they contradict a client's expectations and beliefs. Family groups from various cultures respond in certain culturally specific ways to the illness of a family member. Contributing to these responses are religious beliefs, values, and folk medicine practices. You must also take into consideration such factors as health teaching, personal space, and socioeconomic differences when providing care for different cultural groups.

Discussion Questions/Activities

1. In what ways do your ideas, beliefs, practices, and so on differ from those of your parents? From those of your grandparents? How can you account for the differences?
2. Identify some groups with which you have been associated. How have they influenced you and your lifestyle?
3. Discuss the implications for nursing of the following statements: (a) Cultural behavior is not present at birth but is acquired through learning over a period of years. (b) Cultures are not static but are subject to change.
4. How has your education reflected, influenced, and/or modified your culture?
5. Share examples of folk medicine practices you are aware of within your own culture and in various other cultures. Identify at least five examples.
6. Identify and discuss at least eight examples of nursing care planning that would incorporate the cultural beliefs and religious practices of various clients.
7. Consider the following nursing situation: Ora Morningstar has been admitted for chest surgery in the morning. She is 62 years old and has lived on the Indian reservation all of her life. This is the first time she has been admitted to a hospital. It is customary to consult a medicine man prior to surgery to insure a successful operation. A ritual is performed that takes a couple of hours. There are many preoperative measures to be completed this evening prior to the surgery. What would your approach be to Ms. Morningstar? It is now 10 P.M. and visiting hours are over ac-

cording to hospital policy. As you see the medicine man leave the corridor you enter Ms. Morningstar's room to find that there are still nine relatives in the room. The client tells you that they will be staying with her tonight. You realize that it is customary for members of an Indian family to remain with an ill member. How would you handle this situation?

8. Describe your own health values.

Checklist for Cultural Assessment

Age
Sex
Race
Developmental stage and tasks of the individual
Ethnic group
Social class
Occupation and education
Financial status
Religious orientation and practices
Communication
- Verbal/language
- Nonverbal behavior
- Time and space

Roles/responsibilities
Family
- Family developmental stage
- Child-rearing beliefs and practices
- Kinship
- Decision-making power

Community structure/neighborhood
Occurrence of stressful life events
Health care practices/Healing practices
Restrictions in health care
Explanation of cause (belief) of illness

CHAPTER 3

Communication in Health Assessment

LEARNING OBJECTIVES

1. Describe communication from the standpoint of the concept of life field and the context of perceptual psychology.
2. List factors that distort communication.
3. State three general principles of communication.
4. Identify unresolved feelings and needs that may interfere with your interactions with clients.
5. Incorporate trust, empathy, and respect into fostering a therapeutic milieu for clients.
6. Recognize examples of unproductive and productive patterns of communication.
7. Discuss the use of silence as an interview technique.
8. Recognize body language as a form of nonverbal communication.

This chapter introduces you to some aspects of communication that are essential to a successful health assessment. We will begin by discussing in general what communication is and then move to three aspects of communication that are important to keep in mind in working with clients. The central part of the chapter is devoted to factors that foster a therapeutic milieu and to a detailed examination of unproductive and productive patterns of communication that can occur in performing a health assessment. All of us have unconscious ways of relating to people, some of which are more effective than others. It is important to become aware of the patterns you use and how they affect the person you are encountering. The final part of the chapter discusses kinesics, the study of body language.

What Is Communication?

We all think that we know what communication is and that we are fairly good at it. We commonly think that if we have "command of the language" we "have it made." Yet if you think back over the past days, chances are that you will be able to recall situations where you or someone else misunderstood what the other meant to communicate. How did this situation affect you? How must the other person have felt—anxious? frustrated? Have you ever had the experience of completing a time-consuming assignment only to discover that you did not understand the communiqué and did the wrong assignment? How many times in the past week did you hear the words, "Oh I thought you meant . . ."?

Communication is commonly defined as the process of transmitting a message or idea. This definition may seem quite simple and clear to you, but it is not as simple as you may think. There are many definitions and theories of communication. For our purposes, it seems most logical to begin with the derivation of the word *communication* and view it within the context of perceptual psychology.

The word *communication* comes from the Latin word *communis,* meaning to make common to many, to share. Therefore, it could be said that successful verbal or nonverbal communication has taken place when an experience of mutual "meaning" of thoughts, feelings, and ideas has been shared with another. The words or behavior are nothing in themselves; they only "become" when a commonness has been established. Thus, communication is the process of transmitting *meaning.* It is this meaning that you must search for during health assessment.

As we discussed in Chapter 2, our personal cultural group provides us with many of our ways of communicating. Therefore, we need to keep in mind that the "meanings" being communicated will vary from person to person, depending on such influencing factors as culture, environment, and life experiences. No two individual experiences are ever alike. Most people would agree that our differing experiences are the cause of misunderstandings in communication. However, the true meanings of communication can be more closely reached if we try to see things from the other person's perspective—if we practice empathy along with other communication skills.

Two basic concepts in perceptual psychology as set forth by Combs fit well with our definition of communication as the transmission of meaning. First, the focus of the perceptual psychologist is on the meaning of the events to the individual. Combs wrote that "the individual's behavior is seen as a direct consequence, not of the fact or stimulus with which he is confronted, but the meaning of events in his perceptual field" (Combs, Avila, & Purkey 1971, p. 118). Therefore, the aim is to understand the behavior from the person's own viewpoint. Second, the individual's meaning is formed as a result of "how he sees the situation he is in and how he sees himself" (p. 119). It seems, then, that self-concept, as well as events, has great impact on behavior and indirectly on communication.

The schema of communication in Figure 3-1 has been constructed from a particular definition of communication—the concept of *life field*—and from concepts of perceptual psychology. The life field is the molder of meaning of the events an individual experiences. Figure 3-1 shows the primary constructs of the life field: culture (feelings, beliefs, attitudes, values), the environment, life experiences, and self-concept. These forces not only direct the content of our thought but create a way of thinking. The results of the process are expressed by the sender in verbalizations or nonverbal behavior. The sender's expression may be further influenced by certain distortion factors before being received cognitively by the receiver. Although several distortion factors (noise, lighting, and so on) are identified in the figure, they do not by any means constitute a complete list. The judgment or interpretation aspect of the meaning is in turn influenced by the life field of the receiver. Whether or not "successful" communication has occurred cannot be established unless the receiver sends feedback to the sender for validation. If the sender responds appropriately to the feedback, it is assumed that a close degree of meaning has been mutually shared. Obviously *absolute* communication can never be achieved.

Principles of Communication

In order to assist you in improving your communication with others we have selected three basic principles for detailed discussion.

1. *People communicate in a variety of ways.* They communicate via spoken or written symbols. They use body language, such as smiling, covering one's face, shrugging one's shoulders, or winking an eye. People also communicate by touch, such as a handshake,

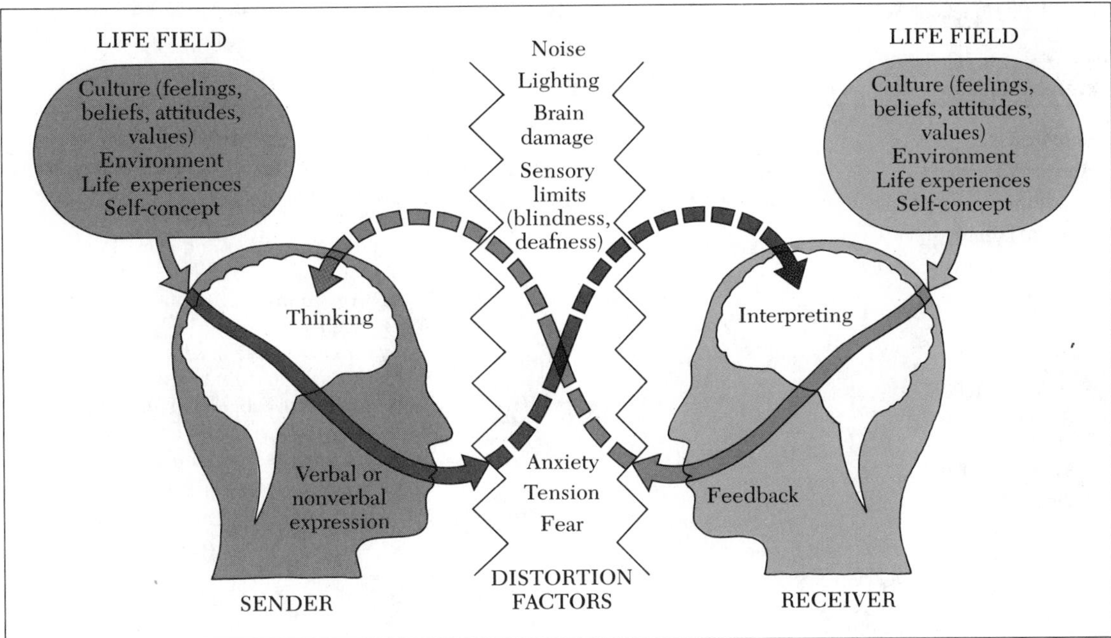

Figure 3-1 A model of communication.

a pat on the back, a soft caress, a slap in the face. Nonverbal communication is commonly drawn attention to in remarks such as "You could read his expression," "His face was an open book," or "If looks could kill, I'd be dead." All these ways of communication are expressed and experienced in the context of each individual's life field.

2. *If understanding is absent, communication has not occurred.* During health assessment, it is important for you to communicate clearly to obtain the needed information. By using words appropriate to the client's level of understanding and avoiding medical/nursing jargon, you will foster understanding. You should not hesitate to question the client as to whether he understands. Furthermore, using a question like "What do you mean when you say . . ." may help you to understand something the client is attempting to communicate to you. It is wise to remember that the meaning being sent is not always the meaning received. Because nonverbal communication is often a more reliable reflection of an individual's true meaning, your client's meaning may become more clear if you take note of such factors as tone of voice, voice inflections, the loudness and amount of speech, and accompanying gestures. In addition, the context (the specific setting, event, or person) may give relevance to the meaning. When a woman says "I've gotta run!" her exclamation is best interpreted in light of whether she is in a hurry or has a problem with her pantyhose.
3. *Listening is a principal route to awareness and understanding of communication.* "A good listener is not only popular everywhere, but after a while he knows something." This insightful comment was made by Wilson Mizner (1955). To be a good listener, you need to exercise your full concentration and listen not only for facts but for the overall meaning being expressed by the client. Tune in to the main ideas and topics of the client's conversation, along with the choice of words and repetition of key words. Take note of any hesitations and any aggressive expression of words and ideas.

Careful attention is the highest form of compliment you can pay your client. Basically, you are conveying "I care and want to understand"; this attitude helps to promote a positive and supportive psychologic climate in which the client feels free to express himself. Listening and not talking is difficult for most of us. We often cut off communication by quickly jumping to conclu-

Table 3-1. Effects of Self-Image on Counseling Interaction

Potential problem area and unresolved feelings and needs	Attitude about self	Possible counseling behaviors
Competence Incompetence Inadequacy Fear of failure Fear of success	1. Pollyanna; overly positive—fearful of failing	Structures counseling to maintain Pollyanna attitude, avoiding conflicts by: 1. discounting negative feedback 2. giving "fake" feedback 3. avoiding or smoothing over "heavy stuff"
	2. Negative; overly self-critical—fearful of succeeding	Structures counseling to maintain negative self-image by: 1. avoiding positive interactions 2. discounting positive feedback 3. giving self overly negative feedback 4. making goals and expectations too high 5. making self-deprecating or apologetic comments
	3. Not masculine enough or not feminine enough	Structures counseling to make self feel more secure as a male or female by: 1. overidentifying with or rejecting very masculine or very feminine clients 2. seducing clients of opposite sex 3. overreacting to or misinterpreting both positive and negative reactions from male and female clients

From Cormier/Cormier/Weisser, *Interviewing and Helping Skills for Health Professionals*, © 1986 Boston: Jones and Bartlett Publishers.

sions and offering friendly advice or by giving judgmental comments of approval or disapproval. When you recognize this behavior in yourself, you can often overcome the tendency by consciously substituting a nod of the head, a gesture that usually communicates "I am listening" to the client. As Mark Twain once said, "A good memory and a tongue tied in the middle is a combination which gives immortality to conversation."

Fostering Therapeutic Milieu

The climate for communication must be viewed as an integral part of the therapeutic milieu. Every day communication takes place with little thought or genuine response. However, communication, which is at the crux of the interview process and interactions with clients, deserves thoughtfulness and analysis. Attention must be given, not only to what transpires between you and the client, but also to the creation of a climate for effective communication. You are both an integral part of this climate and a "molder" of the climate. Understanding yourself will place you in a better position to effect a therapeutic milieu.

Self-Awareness

Understanding yourself can greatly enhance your ability to interact effectively with clients. Cormier and Cormier (1979) have identified three potential problem areas regarding self-image and have explored how these problems could affect your interactions with clients. These potential problem areas are unresolved feelings and needs in respect to competence, power, and intimacy (see Table 3-1 and Figure 3-2).

If you don't feel competent in your professional role, this attitude and self-image may be communicated to your client. This is a common self-image perspective of beginning nursing students. Their interactions with clients often proceed in a manner that meets the needs of the novice rather than the client. Many first interactions with clients are focused on self more than the client. Problem feelings in the area of competence are incompetence, inadequacy, fear of failure, and fear of success. A fear of failure can provoke you into ignoring negative and heavy topics and keeping the conversation at a super-

Table 3-1. *Continued*

Potential problem area and unresolved feelings and needs	Attitude about self	Possible counseling behaviors
Power Impotence Control Passivity Dependence Independence Counterdependence	1. Omnipotent—fearful of losing control	Structures counseling to get and stay in control by: 1. persuading client to do whatever counselor wants 2. subtly informing client how good or right counselor is 3. dominating content and direction of interview 4. getting upset or irritated if client is resistant or reluctant
	2. Weak and unresourceful—fearful of control	Structures counseling to avoid taking control by: 1. being overly silent and nonparticipatory 2. giving client too much direction, as in constant client rambling 3. frequently asking client for permission to do or say something 4. not expressing opinion; always referring back to client 5. avoiding any other risks
	3. Lifestyle converter	Structures counseling to convert client to counselor's beliefs or lifestyle by: 1. promoting ideology 2. getting in a power struggle 3. rejecting clients who are too different or who don't respond 4. "preaching"
Intimacy Affection Rejection	1. Needing warmth and acceptance—fearful of being rejected	Structures counseling to make self liked by: 1. eliciting positive feelings from client 2. avoiding confronting or offending client 3. ignoring negative client cues 4. doing things for client—favors and so on
	2. Needing distance—fearful of closeness, affection	Structures counseling to maintain distance and avoid emotional intimacy by: 1. ignoring client's positive feelings 2. acting overly gruff or distant 3. maintaining professional role as "expert"

ficial or social conversation level. Fear of success is reflected by a depreciative self-image, accompanied by apologies of self-identified shortcomings, and the interaction is structured to maintain a negative self-image. Also, inadequacies in feelings of masculinity or femininity may possibly cause you to behave in ways that make you feel more secure as a woman or man—for example, seductive behaviors.

Unresolved feelings and needs regarding power are reflected in attitudes of omnipotence and being fearful of control. A power struggle between you and the client is likely to occur if you are fearful of losing control. On the other hand, if you are weak and avoid taking risks, you may find yourself giving the client "free reign" in order to avoid assuming responsibility.

Lastly, problem areas within the realm of intimacy involve feelings and needs for affection and rejection. If you have needs for being valued and liked by the client, you may find yourself subtly seeking positive strokes from the client; selective hearing will tune out any expressions of client dissatisfaction. Taped role play may aid you in identifying this problem area. Fear of intimacy could result in a "strictly business" attitude, wherein you may find yourself behaving aloof and somewhat impersonable. Being yourself and using humor when appropriate is therapeutic.

Instructions: The following learning activity may help you explore some of your feelings and attitudes about yourself and possible effects on your counseling interactions. The activity consists of a Self-Rating Checklist divided into the three areas of competence, power, and intimacy. We suggest you work through each section separately. As you read the items listed for each section, think about the extent to which the item accurately describes your behavior *most* of the time (there are always exceptions to our consistent behaviors). If an item asks about you in relation to a client and you haven't had much counseling experience, try to project yourself into the counselor's role. Check the items that are most descriptive of you. Try to be as honest with yourself as possible.

Self-Rating Checklist

Check the items that are most descriptive of you.

I. *Competence Assessment*

___ 1. Constructive negative feedback about myself doesn't make me feel incompetent or uncertain of myself.
___ 2. I tend to put myself down frequently.
___ 3. I feel fairly confident about myself as a helper.
___ 4. I often am preoccupied with thinking that I'm not going to be a competent counselor.
___ 5. When I am involved in a conflict, I don't go out of my way to ignore or avoid it.
___ 6. When I get positive feedback about myself, I often don't believe it's true.
___ 7. I set realistic goals for myself as a helper that are within reach.
___ 8. I believe that a confronting, hostile client could make me feel uneasy or incompetent.
___ 9. I often find myself apologizing for myself or my behavior.
___ 10. I'm fairly confident I can or will be a successful counselor.
___ 11. I find myself worrying a lot about "not making it" as a counselor.
___ 12. I'm likely to be a little scared by clients who would idealize me.
___ 13. A lot of times I will set standards or goals for myself that are too tough to attain.
___ 14. I tend to avoid negative feedback when I can.
___ 15. Doing well or being successful does not make me feel uneasy.

II. *Power Assessment*

___ 1. If I'm really honest, I think my counseling methods are a little superior to other people's.
___ 2. A lot of times I try to get people to do what I want. I might get pretty defensive or upset if the client disagreed with what I wanted to do or did not follow my direction in the interview.
___ 3. I believe there is (or will be) a balance in the interviews between my participation and the client's.
___ 4. I could feel angry when working with a resistant or stubborn client.
___ 5. I can see that I might be tempted to get some of my own ideology across to the client.
___ 6. As a counselor, "preaching" is not likely to be a problem for me.
___ 7. Sometimes I feel impatient with clients who have a different way of looking at the world than I do.
___ 8. I know there are times when I would be reluctant to refer my client to someone else, especially if the other counselor's style differed from mine.
___ 9. Sometimes I feel rejecting or intolerant of clients whose values and life-styles are very different from mine.
___ 10. It is hard for me to avoid getting in a power struggle with some clients.

III. *Intimacy Assessment*

___ 1. There are times when I act more gruff than I really feel.
___ 2. It's hard for me to express positive feelings to a client.
___ 3. There are some clients I would really like to be my friends more than my clients.
___ 4. It would upset me if a client didn't like me.
___ 5. If I sense a client has some negative feelings toward me, I try to talk about it rather than avoid it.
___ 6. Many times I go out of my way to avoid offending clients.
___ 7. I feel more comfortable maintaining a professional distance between myself and the client.
___ 8. Being close to people is something that does not make me feel uncomfortable.
___ 9. I am more comfortable when I am a little aloof.
___ 10. I am very sensitive to how clients feel about me, especially if it's negative.
___ 11. I can accept positive feedback from clients fairly easily.
___ 12. It is difficult for me to confront a client.

Figure 3-2 Self-image learning activity.

Trust

In a trusting relationship information shared will be of a honest and often an intimate nature. However, a trusting relationship may not be easily had; the establishment of such a relationship is dependent on a variety of factors. Each client will react differently to the sharing of information depending on past experiences, beginning with parent bonding and the developmental stage of trust versus mistrust, and past experiences with health professionals. The media also influences attitudes and perceptions. If the client believes the television image of gossiping nurses on the soap operas, he is unlikely to divulge little private information. The client is also assessing you. He is asking himself, "How much can I tell this nurse? Can I trust her/him?" The client may spend considerable energy in testing you. He may be very observant of how you handle information given to you. Therefore it is extremely important that you specify with whom you will need to share information. Carelessness in handling information and messages must be avoided. Information given in confidence must be honored else trust will be broken. When legitimate sharing of information about a client is taking place with another health professional or in a learning setting, privacy must be attended. This type of interchange should not take place in public as in a hallway, nurses' station, restroom, lounge, public dining area, or even an office if the door is ajar. Furthermore, inadvertently talking to a client about staff or another client indiscriminantly will cause distrust. Many times it is helpful to give a client situation as an example, but the example need not be so explicit as to reveal the individual's identity. For interactions, communication, and history-taking to be as meaningful and accurate as possible, the client must feel free to be open and honest and to trust the nurse. Likewise, the nurse must be aware of and adhere to ethical guidelines established by the professional organization (American Nurses Association Code of Ethics) in regard to confidentiality.

Respect

An essential ingredient in promoting a therapeutic milieu is respect; the client must feel this respect from you. This can be conveyed in such ways as properly addressing the client by title and name—for example, Ms. Jackson, Dr. Harris, and Judge Davis. Respect also entails listening attentively when the client speaks, being nonjudgmental and accepting of the client as he is, placing your own bias and values on the "back shelf," and affording the client common courtesies.

We may not like everyone with whom we come in contact. In light of this, we must admit to our feelings and examine them in the context of what they mean to us and our client. If they block the relationship, it may be best for another professional to work closely with the client.

Empathy

Empathy is identification with another's feelings. It means recognizing the other person's perspective or frame of reference, as if these feelings were your own—without ever forgetting the "as if." An example of forgetting the "as if" is when you identify so closely with the feelings of a client that you cannot differentiate your own feelings from those of the client. In this case you may find it hard to maintain the professional role and provide the guidance and support your client needs. The more the client is like you (in age, sex, and background), and the more the situation is similar to one you have experienced, the more likely this may happen to you. Even though you wish to continue working with this client, you may not be able to be objective. In this case it would be best to refer the client to another professional. Be aware that this is no reflection on your professional capabilities; indeed it is a reflection of your skill in recognizing your own limitations. This in itself is a mark of a professional. On the other hand, you must be careful not to use this as a "cop-out" whenever you experience uncomfortableness with a client. You need to examine the uncomfortableness. Many times dealing with the identified cause will allow you to experience personal growth.

To foster understanding you should attempt to look at life and events from the client's perspective. Obviously your bias and values exist, but to empathize with a client does not mean that you agree with or hold the same values as the client. The process of empathizing is sharing your recognition of the feelings held by the client; it is an additional means of conveying respect. Often sharing your feelings and experiences with the client can lead to further disclosure. More disclosure can lead to a deeper relationship and understanding.

Patterns of Communication

Most of the time talking occurs without thinking. For instance, the person asking, "How are you?" does not *really* want to know, in most cases, and the individual responding, "Fine," may not be fine at all! Such automatic verbalizations are predominant in social conversation but have little value in the health assessment process. A comprehensive health assessment requires a certain degree of communication skill.

One step toward improving your communication skills is to become aware of your use of such automatic responses and of your personal verbal patterns. Another is to learn the principles of various therapeutic communication patterns. A third step is to plan and evaluate your interactions, and a fourth is to make a conscious effort toward replacing unproductive patterns with productive ones. This last step is perhaps the most difficult, as it takes more energy to "unlearn" than to learn. However, you will discover that the application and use of productive patterns will become easier with practice. In turn, your use of unproductive patterns will slowly diminish. The key is conscious attention and effort.

Unproductive Patterns

Many negative verbal patterns are already a part of most people's communication habits. Therefore, we will begin with the negative to help you identify whether you have any of these undesirable habits. These negative patterns are useless for obtaining information, and most actually inhibit communication because of their psychologic undertones. If any of these patterns characterize your interactions with others, try to "catch" them in the future—it is no crime to stop and think before you respond.

The Value Judgment Pattern

The indiscriminate or constant use of words such as "good," "fine," and "excellent" figuratively places your stamp of approval on the client's actions or ideas. If the client should change his mind and make another decision, he would be in opposition to your sanctioned action or thought. Clients frequently exhibit "nurse-pleaser" behavior. They find it difficult to contradict you because they depend on you in varying degrees and feel they must remain in your good graces should they need you at a future time. Have you ever ceased to create waves to remain on the "right" side of someone at one time or another?

Clients with little self-worth will only suffer more ego deflation if they reject their idea to cling to yours or if they are no longer capable of performing your sanctioned behavior. Even clients with a strong self-concept may avoid telling you they have changed their mind about something. Thus, you unknowingly lose out on "sharing," and some communication bonds between you are severed. It is better for you to help the client explore his own feelings about his actions and ideas. You can use such prompters as "I see you are able to comb your hair (feed yourself, shave) today . . . How do you *feel* about it?" or "Are you presently comfortable with . . . ?" This latter pattern allows the client the freedom to change his mind and feelings should he become uncomfortable with decisions he has made.

Conversely, disapproval, expressed in such statements and questions as "That's wrong!" "You shouldn't do that!" "I don't believe you want to say (do) that, do you?" or "You don't have syphilis, do you?" forward your values. If the client's values differ or if he has a disorder you disapprove of, he infers that he is "bad." Again, the client has been set up either to experience ego deterioration (I'm wrong . . . I'm bad) or to become defensive. Defensiveness will only tend to strengthen the client's ideas, and he will fight for them all the more. When you impose your values and judgments on the client, you are in essence inhibiting his growth.

You also inhibit the client's growth when you give him advice. This does not mean that it is wrong to offer suggestions, but giving advice is an entirely different thing. By giving advice, you imply that you know best, and you take away the client's opportunity to solve the problem, usurping a responsibility that belongs to him. You may direct the client's thoughts toward other alternatives by asking, "Have you considered these possibilities?" or "Have you weighed the advantages and disadvantages of . . ." Should the client ask you what he should think, do, or feel about a certain situation, rather than jump to conclusions and offer friendly advice, you should help the client to do his own decision making. This process can be initiated by reflecting the request back to the client: "What are *your* feelings about . . ." or "What do *you* think?" This technique not only stimulates the client to rethink the situation but also implies that *his* thinking has value. One of the therapeutic aims in health assessment and any nurse-client interaction is to free the client, help him grow, and assist him to come to his own conclusions and decisions.

The Insecure Pattern

Hearing of another's anxieties tends to make you uncomfortable. This is what is meant by the expression "anxiety is contagious." In order to ease your own discomfort, your first tendency may be to offer a quick shot of what you believe to be "courage-builder" or to give false reassurance to the anxious client: "Chin up!" "Keep on smiling!" "Don't worry," "Just listen to the doctors and nurses, and you'll do fine!" "You have a good doctor," "We have the latest and finest equipment," "Things always turn out all right in the end," or "You think you're bad off, just think about all the . . ." Such attempts at solace may ease *your* anxiety somewhat. You are let off the hook, as these comments have an air of dismissal and will usually cut off any further communication on the subject.

Rather than reject the client and his anxieties by use of these familiar clichés, you can offer your empathy and understanding through the use of touch, such as holding the client's hand or placing your arm around his shoulder. With this support, the client can begin to explore and further express his feelings. You can initiate and facilitate this process by questions or statements such as, "This seems very hard for you," "You must feel very bad," "What makes you say (do) this?" "Would you like to talk about it?" or "Perhaps if you talk about it we can discover what it is that makes you feel anxious."

The Defensive Pattern

It is very difficult to accept criticism of oneself. Even though you may have groomed the attitude of listening and taking into account what others say, at times you may find yourself knee-deep in rationalizing or defensive behavior. When you work closely with other health care workers and with a particular institution, you become identified with them and their cause. In essence, then, an attack on them is an attack on the extension of your "self." Because of the frustrations that you may have personally suffered in the bureaucratic system, you may jump to the conclusion that a client's criticism is unfair. Indeed, it may be unjust, but the client needs to express such hurt or angry feelings nonetheless. These feelings exist now for the client, whether or not they are truly justified. Some of the common responses you may have used or heard being said to a "complaining, ungrateful, hostile" client are "Ms. McKay would never leave you on the bedpan for two hours!" "Dr. Crane is very understanding and a well-known practitioner!" or "Beacon General has an excellent reputation!" If you understand the principles of anxiety and you are a fairly secure individual, you will be able to accept the client's feelings without becoming defensive and to help him express them more fully: "You sound angry (hurt)," "What happened to cause you to feel this way?" or "Will you try to trace the sequence of events leading up to the point when you began to feel this way?"

Productive Patterns

The following therapeutic patterns, when used appropriately, will greatly facilitate the health assessment process. It will be helpful to both you and your clients for you to become familiar with these patterns and to use them consciously in your interactions with others. You will find that with experience you will develop better timing and use of these patterns.

The Open-ended Pattern

Generally, when given the chance, a client will overtly or covertly talk about his concerns. But many clients don't know where and how to begin or progress; they may not be sure of what their role is in the interaction. An open-ended question or statement not only demonstrates your concern and interest but points out that it is the *client* who is the topic of conversation. Examples of open-ended patterns are: "What brought you to the clinic today?" "What do you hope to get from this therapy?" "Tell me about yourself," or "A penny for your thoughts."

At times a client may test your interest to see whether he truly is the focus of conversation. A "needy" nurse will fall prey to such testing and begin to talk about him/herself. If this happens to you, you are falling short of fulfilling your role as a professional nurse. For example, the client may say, "I see you are not wearing a wedding band." You should not ignore the client's comment but simply acknowledge that he has made a correct observation and redirect the focus back to him: "No, I'm not, but we're not here to talk about me, so I would like to continue with the major purpose of the interview, which is . . ." If the client persists, you can reiterate your interest in him as a client by saying something like, "I cannot see of what benefit my personal life would be to you, and I do see my role as trying to help you. I feel that in order to do so I must learn more about you."

The General Lead Pattern

The general lead pattern assures the client that

you are listening, interested, and following him. General leads also encourage the client to continue and elaborate. General leads include nodding the head, raising the eyebrows at appropriate times, and making such comments as, "Uh huh," "I see," "Continue," "Go on," "And then?" or "Really?"

Did you ever notice the comment made about an individual who uses general leads appropriately? It is said that he is "a great conversationalist"!

The Reflective Pattern

When you reflect a word, thought, feeling, or idea back to a client, you are doing one or more of the following four things.

1. You may be stimulating elaboration or more thought on a particular point, behavior, or feeling that the client has expressed: "It's faster?" "I see you're biting your nails," or "You seem to be uncomfortable (anxious, angry, sad, downtrodden, and so on)." By stimulating elaboration, you keep the conversation flowing and help the client to recognize, explore, and begin to deal with his emotions. Do not hesitate to use the word "feelings," as in "What are your *feelings* regarding . . ." "How do you *feel* about . . ." or "How does this make you *feel?*"
2. You may be clarifying your understanding of what the client has just said: "Are you saying that . . . ?" or "In other words . . ." If you are not sure what is being communicated or if you have "lost" the progression of thought, you should inform the client that you are not following what he is saying and ask him to repeat what he has just said. Perhaps the client has used a phrase that is unclear to you. For instance, if a client states, "I'm going in circles," what does he mean by this? What is he experiencing? You may begin clarification by reflecting his entire statement: "You're going in circles?" If this approach leads nowhere, perhaps you can help him pinpoint his experience by being more specific: "You're feeling confused (frustrated, dizzy)?"
3. You may be clarifying the use of dubious pronouns. Take the following dialogue:

   Client: They told me not to take this medicine.

   Nurse: They?

   Client: Mr. Pine, the head nurse.

   Careless use of pronouns happens with both clients and nurses alike. Many clients have difficulty with self-identity, and you may unknowingly compound this problem by careless use of pronouns and by not keeping your identity separate from that of the client. How many times have you heard a nurse say something like, "We are going to take our tub bath now." The client could rightly reply, "Who is going to get in first?" or "I doubt if the two of us will fit in that tub!" Clarification of the use of "we–us, they–them" by either the client or you is always necessary.
4. You may be summarizing an interaction or requesting a conclusion. You may reflect what has taken place with such openings as, "During the past 15 minutes you and I have been discussing . . ." or "What would you say was the main point or focus of what you and I have been talking about?" Use of the reflective pattern in this way allows you and the client to clearly view the experience and to part with the same idea in mind.

The Silence Pattern

The use of silence following the use of a therapeutic pattern of communication is quite effective; it gives the client time to think over what has just been expressed and to organize his thoughts for response. It is also a golden opportunity for you to assess the interaction and form alternative plans of response and further communication. In addition, silence coupled with attention can convey acceptance and interest in the client; this attitude will encourage the client to continue his communication.

Most people, particularly Americans, have a difficult time handling silence. Our culture is action oriented. Because silence is not an overt form of action, many people have the impression that nothing is happening, when basically a lot of mental "wheels" are turning furiously. It is important for you to be aware of this fact in order to appreciate the value of silence in communication and to feel more comfortable with using silence therapeutically.

An awareness of common nontherapeutic and therapeutic patterns of communication will in itself serve as a guide for use in the interviewing process of health assessment. The time and conscious effort you spend to limit the use of nonproductive patterns and replace them with more productive ones will be repaid time and time again.

Body Language

Kinesics, the systematic study of body motion and position as a means of communication, is intriguing. What whets the appetite even more is the thought that body language, kinesic behavior, may be a more accurate barometer of true feelings and may actually contradict verbal communications. A question of interest is, Does everyone speak the same language when communicating in or by body language? Ekman, Sorenson and Friesen (1969) conducted cross-cultural studies (U.S., Brazil, Japan, New Guinea, and Borneo) and found that facial expressions of emotions are similar regardless of culture. In their studies the subjects identified sameness of emotion when shown a standard set of facial photographs—for example, they could say that this man expresses happiness, sadness, surprise, and so on. However, body language entails more than facial expressions. One speaks with eye and mouth movements, motion in gestures, movement of total body, posture, distance and position in a room. The narrowed eye or quivering lip must be viewed within the context of the client's idiosyncracy. The narrow eye could be the squinting of happiness or a sinister glance; the quivering lip could be reflective of sadness or anxiety. The waving back and forth (left and right) of the hand with extended index finger tells the receiver, "no, no." Worry, anxiety, impatience—all could be expressed by rocking the total body back and forth in a chair. Slouched shoulders and bowed head could mean sadness, reverence, or, perhaps, exhaustion. Closer than 3 to 5 feet in American culture creates tension and discomfort—the client may feel encroached upon. Sitting in a corner or apart from a group may express shyness or desire to be left alone.

Interpretation of body language is not simple and clear cut. The complexity of this interpretation is increased by the fact that body language is a reflection of each individual's experiences; environment (the body language, as verbal expressions, differs in urban and rural communities); socioeconomic group (affluent versus poverty class body expressions); and cultural group, which includes not only ethnic groups but countercultures such as drug societies and religious cults. Thus, kinesic behaviors cannot be examined in isolation but must be analyzed in conjunction with what occurred prior, during, and after the presenting body behavior as well as in conjunction with accompanying verbal communication. To aid you in increasing your awareness and understanding of body language, Table 3-2 lists some selected behaviors and associated *possible* and *probable* meanings.

Table 3-2. Inventory of Nonverbal Communication

Nonverbal dimensions	Behaviors	Description of counselor-client interaction	Possible effects or meanings
Eyes	Direct eye contact	Client is Anglo-American. Client has just shared concern with counselor. Counselor responds; client maintains eye contact.	Readiness or willingness for interpersonal communication or exchange; attentiveness
	Lack of sustained eye contact	Client is Anglo-American. Each time counselor brings up the topic of client's family, client looks away.	Withdrawal or avoidance of interpersonal exchange; or respect or deference
		Client is a Mexican-American who demonstrates intermittent breaks in eye contact while conversing with counselor.	Respect or deference

Continued on page 46

From Cormier/Cormier/Weisser, *Interviewing and Helping Skills for Health Professionals*, © 1986 Boston: Jones and Bartlett Publishers.

Table 3-2. *Continued*

Nonverbal dimensions	Behaviors	Description of counselor-client interaction	Possible effects or meanings
		Client mentions sexual concerns, then abruptly looks away. When counselor initiates this topic, client looks away again.	Withdrawal from topic of conversation; discomfort or embarrassment; or preoccupation
	Lowering eyes—looking down or away	Client talks at some length about alternatives to present job situation. Pauses briefly and looks down. Then resumes speaking and eye contact with counselor.	Preoccupation
	Staring or fixation on person or object	Counselor has just asked client to consider consequences of a certain decision. Client is silent and gazes at a picture on the wall.	Preoccupation; possibly rigidness or uptightness
	Darting eyes or blinking rapidly—rapid eye movements; twitching brow	Client indicates desire to discuss a topic yet is hesitant. As counselor probes, client's eyes move around the room rapidly.	Excitation or anxiety; or wearing contact lenses
	Squinting or furrow on brow	Client has just asked counselor for advice. Counselor explains role and client squints, and furrows appear in client's brow.	Thought or perplexity; or avoidance of person or topic
		Counselor suggests possible things for client to explore in difficulties with parents. Client doesn't respond verbally; furrow in brow appears.	Avoidance of person or topic
	Moisture or tears	Client has just reported recent death of father; tears well up in client's eyes.	Sadness; frustration; sensitive areas of concern
		Client reports real progress during past week in marital communication; eyes get moist.	Happiness
	Eye shifts	Counselor has just asked client to remember significant events in week; client pauses and looks away; then responds and looks back.	Processing or recalling material; or keen interest; satisfaction
	Pupil dilation	Client discusses spouse's sudden disinterest and pupils dilate.	Alarm; or keen interest
		Client leans forward while counselor talks and pupils dilate.	Keen interest; satisfaction
Mouth	Smiles	Counselor has just asked client to report positive events of the week. Client smiles, then recounts some of these instances.	Positive thought, feeling, or action in content of conversation; or greeting
		Client responds with a smile to counselor's verbal greeting at beginning of interview.	Greeting

Table 3-2. *Continued*

Nonverbal dimensions	Behaviors	Description of counselor-client interaction	Possible effects or meanings
	Tight lips (pursed together)	Client has just described efforts at sticking to a difficult living arrangement. Pauses and purses lips together.	Stress or determination; anger or hostility
		Client just expressed irritation at counselor's lateness. Client sits with lips pursed together while counselor explains the reasons.	Anger or hostility
	Lower lip quivers or biting lip	Client starts to describe her recent experience of being raped. As client continues to talk, her lower lip quivers; occasionally she bites her lip.	Anxiety or sadness
		Client discusses loss of parental support after a recent divorce. Client bites her lip after discussing this.	Sadness
	Open mouth without speaking	Counselor has just expressed feelings about a block in the relationship. Client's mouth drops open; client says he or she was not aware of it.	Surprise; or suppression of yawn—fatigue
		It has been a long session. As counselor talks, client's mouth parts slightly.	Suppression of yawn—fatigue
Facial expressions	Eye contact with smiles	Client talks very easily and smoothly, occasionally smiling; maintains eye contact for most of session.	Happiness or comfortableness
	Eyes strained; furrow on brow; mouth tight	Client has just reported strained situation with a child. Then client sits with lips pursed together and a frown.	Anger; or concern; sadness
	Eyes rigid, mouth rigid (unanimated)	Client states she or he has nothing to say; there is no evident expression or alertness on client's face.	Preoccupation; anxiety; fear
Head	Nodding head up and down	Client just expressed concern over the status of his or her health; counselor reflects client's feelings. Client nods head and says "That's right."	Confirmation; agreement; or listening, attending
		Client nods head during counselor explanation.	Listening; attending
	Shaking head from left to right	Counselor has just suggested that client's continual lateness to sessions may be an issue that needs to be discussed. Client responds with "No" and shakes head from left to right.	Disagreement; or disapproval

Continued on page 48

Table 3-2. *Continued*

Nonverbal dimensions	Behaviors	Description of counselor-client interaction	Possible effects or meanings
	Hanging head down, jaw down toward chest	Counselor initiates topic of termination. Client lowers head toward chest, then says he or she is not ready to stop the counseling sessions.	Sadness; concern
Shoulders	Shrugging	Client reports that spouse just walked out with no explanation. Client shrugs shoulders while describing this.	Uncertainty; or ambivalence
	Leaning forward	Client has been sitting back in the chair. Counselor discloses something about herself or himself; client leans forward and asks counselor a question about the experience.	Eagerness; attentiveness, openness to communication
	Slouched, stooped, rounded or turned away from person	Client reports feeling inadequate and defeated because of poor grades; slouches in chair after saying this. Client reports difficulty in talking. As counselor pursues this, client slouches in chair and turns shoulders away from counselor.	Sadness or ambivalence; or lack of receptivity to interpersonal exchange Lack of receptivity to interpersonal exchange
Arms and hands	Arms folded across chest	Counselor has just initiated conversation. Client doesn't respond verbally; sits back in chair with arms crossed against chest.	Avoidance of interpersonal exchange or dislike
	Trembling and fidgety hands	Client expresses fear of suicide; hands tremble while talking about this.	Anxiety or anger
		In a loud voice, client expresses resentment; client's hands shake while talking.	Anger
	Fist clenching to objects or holding hands tightly	Client has just come in for initial interview. Says that he or she feels uncomfortable; hands are clasped together tightly.	Anxiety or anger
		Client expresses hostility toward boss; clenches fists while talking.	Anger
	Arms unfolded—arms and hands gesturing in conversation	Counselor has just asked a question; client replies and gestures during reply.	Accenting or emphasizing point in conversation; or openness to interpersonal exchange
		Counselor initiates new topic. Client readily responds; arms are unfolded at this time.	Openness to interpersonal exchange
	Rarely gesturing, hands and arms stiff	Client arrives for initial session. Responds to counselor's questions with short answers. Arms are kept down at side.	Tension or anger

Table 3-2. *Continued*

Nonverbal dimensions	Behaviors	Description of counselor-client interaction	Possible effects or meanings
		Client has been referred; sits with arms down at side while explaining reasons for referral and irritation at being here.	Anger
Legs and feet	Legs and feet appear comfortable and relaxed	Client's legs and feet are relaxed without excessive movement while client freely discusses personal concerns.	Openness to interpersonal exchange; relaxation
	Crossing and uncrossing legs repeatedly	Client is talking rapidly in spurts about problems; continually crosses and uncrosses legs while doing so.	Anxiety; depression
	Foot-tapping	Client is tapping feet during a lengthy counselor summary; client interrupts counselor to make a point.	Anxiety; impatience—wanting to make a point
	Legs and feet appear stiff and controlled	Client is open and relaxed while talking about job. When counselor introduces topic of marriage, client's legs become more rigid.	Uptightness or anxiety; closed to extensive interpersonal exchange
Total body	Facing other person squarely or leaning forward	Client shares a concern and faces counselor directly while talking; continues to face counselor while counselor responds.	Openness to interpersonal communication and exchange
	Turning of body orientation at an angle, not directly facing person, or slouching in seat	Client indicates some difficulty in "getting into" interview. Counselor probes for reasons; client turns body away.	Less openness to interpersonal exchange
	Rocking back and forth in chair or squirming in seat	Client indicates a lot of nervousness about an approaching conflict situation. Client rocks as this is discussed.	Concern; worry; anxiety
	Stiff—sitting erect and rigidly on edge of chair	Client indicates some uncertainty about direction of interview; sits very stiff and erect at this time.	Tension; anxiety; concern
Distance	Moves away	Counselor has just confronted client; client moves back before responding verbally.	Signal that space has been invaded; increased arousal, discomfort
	Moves closer	Midway through session, client moves chair toward helper.	Seeking closer interaction, more intimacy
Position in room	Sits behind or next to an object in the room, such as table or desk	A new client comes in and sits in a chair that is distant from counselor.	Seeking protection or more space
	Sits near counselor without any intervening objects	A client who has been in to see counselor before sits in chair closest to counselor.	Expression of adequate comfort level

Summary

This chapter has focused on some concepts of communication essential to effective health assessment. There are three important aspects of communication to keep in mind: (1) people communicate in a variety of ways; (2) if understanding is absent, communication has not occurred; and (3) listening is a principal route to awareness and understanding of communication. Trust, empathy, and respect were described as essential to the creation of therapeutic milieu. Patterns of communication were discussed and specific examples of unproductive and productive patterns were given. Body language, an important manner of communication, was identified as an index of assessment.

Discussion Questions/Activities

1. Describe communication from the standpoint of the concept of life field and the context of perceptual psychology.
2. List factors that distort communication.
3. What is meant by the following statement: "If understanding is absent, communication has not occurred."
4. Role-play an interview session with a colleague. Have another colleague note your communication patterns and interview technique. Role-play or actual interview could be audiotaped or videotaped.
5. Discuss the use of silence as an interview technique. Why is the technique of silence difficult for many people?
6. Describe body behaviors observed in a selected setting and give rationale for interpretation of the kinesics.

CHAPTER 4

The Health History

LEARNING OBJECTIVES

1. Recognize the importance of the health history as a component of the assessment of health status.
2. Describe the components of the health history.
3. Recognize nursing behaviors that assist in developing a trusting relationship with a client.
4. Describe the three phases of the interview structure.
5. Identify guidelines designed to elicit information about the client's current health status or history of present illness.
6. Describe the areas of the client's lifestyle that are investigated during health history-taking.
7. Differentiate lifestyle factors that enhance health status from those that are a risk to health status.
8. Identify the purpose of the review of systems used in health history-taking.

The health history is a chronologic and detailed health record of the client. Its purpose is to elicit information regarding all the variables that may affect the client's health status. These data are then used to develop nursing diagnoses and subsequent plans for individualized care. For the ill client, the health history serves as background material related to the development of present symptoms and associated difficulties. For the well client, such as a student who is having a routine physical assessment and health history update, it supplies data by which you can provide health preventive/maintenance/promotion counseling and establish need for immunizations and eye or dental care. In the latter situation, your time with the client is usually limited, and there is a great deal of information to gather to complete the record. Thus, you need to be skilled in the interview technique in order to best guide the client through the process in a logical order. Increasingly, many aspects of the health history are being tabulated through health history forms or checklists that the client fills out himself and that are then quickly validated at the beginning of the interview. Further, computer technology is enhancing the collection and recording of accumulated health history records.

Health is not static; therefore, there is a need for continuous review and reassessment of client health status. This review is necessary not only to detect changes and possible problems but to update the record on both interim illnesses and health promotion activities, such as incorporating jogging into the daily pattern of living. Baseline laboratory data are also part of the client's health history record and should be carefully reviewed or compared to recent laboratory tests performed.

Client Interview

The interview is the first step in assessing the health status of the client. The health history obtained during the interview is a crucial component in the client's total health assessment. It is also at this point that the nurse-client relationship is initiated. The interview serves as the arena in which rapport is established between nurse and client and from which a trusting relationship can develop. The interview is also a means of mental health assessment and offers insight into possible or existing problems.

The interview provides the principal basis for nursing diagnoses and guides the focus of the physical assessment process. For example, if a client complains of headaches, vertigo, and syncope, you would conduct a more highly scrutinizing physical assessment of the head and neck and of the cardiovascular and neurologic systems.

In order to obtain information, you must convey sensitivity toward the client's needs and feelings, creating a climate of warmth and support. Once this climate is established, you will be able to more fully explore the client's attitudes about health and illness. These attitudes and feelings will further provide data from which you can determine a client-centered plan of care. Through the interview process, you will be able to elicit information about the client's past and present health status that will be of great value in making subsequent nursing judgments.

To elicit important information you may want to use open-ended patterns of communication, such as, "How do you feel about your family life?" or "How do you feel about your illness?" Questions such as these are less limiting than ones such as, "Do you feel your health is poor?" where the client is not encouraged to express his feelings.

It may sometimes be necessary for you to ask direct questions about family relationships, financial status, personal habits, and daily life patterns. Allow the client sufficient time to answer these questions. Hurrying to the next question may make the client feel that you are only interested in completing the interview efficiently. Be sensitive to the fact that certain aspects of physical status may be uncomfortable and embarrassing to the client. In addition, some aspects of personal life, ethnic background, and religious beliefs may have cultural implications that make it more difficult for the client to be open about answering some questions.

If the client demonstrates marked anxiety over any topic, you should not press your inquiries merely to be "thorough" in completing an established assessment outline—especially if doing so would sacrifice the client's comfort in any way. Investigation into sensitive areas might better be left until a time when rapport has been better established, unless it is of extreme import to the client's immediate situation, in which case the client should be made aware of why this information is necessary for you to efficiently carry out the nursing process. Such sensitive areas may include sexual deviations, secret drinking, family quarrels, or parental attitudes.

During the interview you must be supportive of the client by being nonjudgmental and accepting of the client's feelings and attitudes. The client's nonverbal behavior frequently provides cues for interpreting his verbal messages. You need to listen to what the client says or *does not say.* Total involvement is necessary for attentive listening. It is also essential that you use words and sentences that the client can comprehend. Many people do not understand such terms as C.V.A., M.I., or ADL (activities of daily living). It is often necessary to rephrase a question or assist the client in returning to the topic. Straying from the question may be an indication that the client is anxious or is trying to avoid disturbing topics. Assure the client that you are not prying, but are attempting to gain information that will be useful in developing a plan of care. Avoid false reassurances and pep talks. Statements such as, "Don't worry about it," "Everything will be just fine," or "Pull yourself together" can create frustration for the client. The client's questions should be answered honestly and directly. Leaving concerns unanswered tends to create anger and anxiety and may destroy the process of interaction.

Confidentiality and privacy are essential and should be maintained for the client. Any transgression could break down or inhibit the establishment of trust in the nurse-client relationship. Trust is important in all interpersonal relationships, but it is especially important when interacting with children. You should be truthful in all things with children. Perhaps one of the most difficult things to tell a child is that something is going to hurt, but doing so maintains and strengthens the trust between nurse and child. By being honest you also show the child what he can expect of a nurse, and you aid in building the image of the nurse as a "helping" individual.

When you are gathering assessment data, relatives and friends should be asked to leave the room. They should be allowed to remain only at the request of the client. Once you and the client are alone, you can ask whether the client wishes to have anyone present. In this way no social or family pressures bear upon the client's decision.

Although the client is the best source of information, there are times when the family or a friend must provide the needed information, such as when the child is a young child or is unable to respond because of injury or illness. In such situations you must develop the same trusting relationship with the individuals being interviewed. When you wish to talk to friends and family members about a particular topic regarding an adult client, you should obtain his permission first.

For additional suggestions when interviewing the child and adolescent refer to Chapter 21.

Interview Structure

The interview is not social conversation; it is a goal-directed process of communication. In most cases, it is structured. Basically, the interview structure is composed of three phases: an *introduction*, a *focus*, and *termination*. How and when these phases are initiated depends on such variables as available time, environmental circumstances, and the age, education, and emotional/physical condition of the client.

Introduction

When you first meet someone in a social context, questions usually flow back and forth for the purpose of discovering whether the two of you have anything in common. The mutual interests, values, and experiences that you discover may form the basis for a friendship. Within this type of relationship, each individual generally tries in varying degrees to meet certain needs of the other. But in your professional role you are concerned with assisting the client in meeting *his* needs; you must use ways, means, and persons other than the client to meet *your* needs.

In the introduction phase the information you give the client and your demeanor reflect the expertise you are offering. It is important that you call the client by name and introduce yourself and your status: "Hello, Mr. Ralph Ray? (pause) I'm Mr. Burns, the head nurse (student nurse, registered nurse, nurse specialist)." It is also necessary to introduce by name and status any health worker who may be accompanying you and to ask the client's permission if others are to be present during the interview. You should state the purpose of the interview at the beginning to clarify the client's participation, and, if applicable, you should share your specific role and responsibilities with the client. This latter step informs the client more specifically about what you may be called upon to do or what areas you may be consulted on. Depending on the situation, additional contractual information and arrangements may be made, such as regarding time limitations on the interaction(s), fees (the particulars of cost, payment, the client's ability to pay, and available financial assistance), and subsequent interactions (time, place, and expectations of client participation).

In the initial introduction, you must approach the subject of confidentiality, which is vital in maintaining trust and rapport with the client. The client must understand that any information he gives will be shared with other health team members for the purpose of providing the best health care possible. If during the interview the client asks you to keep something to yourself, you need to inform him that you cannot honor such a request if the information negatively affects his well-being or that of another. In all interactions you need to evaluate what specific information to record. It may be unnecessary to chart certain information that can be kept confidential between you and the client, and you need only record your interpretation of the information.

You need to establish a comfortable climate for the interview, as setting can greatly influence the quality of the interaction. The setting should afford privacy and should be free of interruptions and distractions (such as radio, TV, bright colors, extensive decorations, glaring lights or inadequate lighting, offensive odors, uncomfortable room temperature, poor ventilation and humidity, and a "cluttered" environment). You should make every attempt to promote the client's comfort. If possible, the client should be seated in a comfortable chair so that he can relax. Sitting on a straight chair for prolonged periods can be as uncomfortable as sitting on a cactus.

Most people find communication more difficult if direct eye contact is not maintained; however, there are cultural groups who consider this practice to be disrespectful. It is best for you to be on the same level and face to face with the client during the interview. If it is necessary to interview the client in bed, you should be seated in a chair at the bedside so you will be at the client's eye level. In a standing position you would loom over the client and perhaps appear as an imposing, threatening figure. The standing posture may also imply the attitude of "one foot out the door" to the client. This "too busy" appearance can hamper the interview.

Focus

The focus of an interview is the health assessment of the client. You can learn much by observing the client's behavior—and he can learn much from observing yours. You need to be alert to your own behavior and what it may convey to the client. Gazing out a window may indicate lack of interest to the client; nervous gestures such as finger tapping and leg swinging may be interpreted as impatience.

It is best to encourage the client to initiate the discussion. Once the client begins to talk and places his concerns in the open, his anxiety level will gradually decline. Then you will be able to focus his energies toward any necessary problem solving. As the client relaxes, he will tend to talk more freely. You can assist the client to relax and begin the discussion by using open-ended communication patterns more frequently at the onset of the interview. The next step is to keep the ball rolling by interjecting timely general leads. The overall communication flow of the interview is optimally free.

Strict adherence to a question-answer format is very mechanical. Consistent use of this format is often symptomatic of a nurse who is uncomfortable in dealing with clients' anxieties, as it can serve as a means of easily circumventing these anxieties. Furthermore, it creates an atmosphere in which the client may find it difficult to seek advice and support for underlying personal problems. Both clients and inexperienced nurses may become preoccupied with the questions and answers of an established interview form as an unconscious escape from facing the real demanding and threatening problems. In other words, it is the process that becomes the main focus, and for the most part, the anxieties go unnoticed. There are times, however, when a modification of this question-answer format is necessary, usually when time is at a premium.

During the interview you must give guidance to the conversation; you should not allow the client to ramble aimlessly. If you are passive, you may miss pertinent issues, and your passivity may increase rather than reduce the client's anxiety level. Also, the client may interpret passivity as evidence of lack of concern or competence. Rambling is nonproductive and detrimental to the assessment process, particularly when time is limited and there are several pertinent areas to be investigated. A helpful technique for directing the client to specific areas is to use more closed-ended questions that require a yes-no response or short answer. When using this communication pattern, you need to avoid the common error of asking more than one question at a time.

If during the interview the client does not respond to a specific question, you may try a related question. Should the client state that he would rather not answer or discuss that particular topic, it is generally best to drop the line of inquiry. In this way you show acceptance of his right to privacy. By having asked the question, you have indicated your interest in the topic, should he care to share information with you at a later time. Marked probing tends to place the client on the defensive and may propel him away from charged areas.

The more sensitive areas of investigation are best pursued in the later part of the interview. By this time a greater degree of rapport has been established with the client, which will facilitate the sharing of more intimate information. Also by this time you will have collected most of the information relevant to assessing the client's health status, so little data will be lost should the client decrease his communication or become silent in response to the investigation of these demanding areas.

Part of the interview focus may be on health teaching. In this regard it is important to remember not to overload the client's circuits; rather, use short learning periods with rest (and practice) breaks. It is sometimes easy for a nurse to become overzealous with a wealth of information and go berserk with endless, intense explanations and descriptions in order to get the message across.

Termination

Sadly, termination is a neglected phase of many interviews and nurse-client interactions. Most of us do not enjoy the feeling of "hanging at loose ends." The termination phase allows you and the client to reflect on your experience and the work you have accomplished together. It is a time of recapitulation, in which there is some degree of completeness as you and the client evaluate whether your objectives have been fulfilled. It may be a time of establishing future goals, renegotiating contracts, referring the client to another health worker or agency, or ending the relationship.

Sudden termination without warning may cause difficulty for the client in developing trusting relationships in the future. If you know that there is a time limit to your relationship or that you will be going on vacation or having days off, you should share this with the client as soon as possible. The dependent client—which many "ill" clients are—may be severely distressed at the disappearance of "his" nurse.

In single interview sessions, you should remind the client when the meeting is coming to an end: "We are going to have to end our discussion in 10 minutes. Is there anything in particular you would like to talk about or are there any specific questions you have at this time?" If you and the client are meeting for a specific number of sessions, the client should be reminded a few sessions from the terminating session: "After today we have three more sessions left in this series." The chief purpose of the termination phase is to allow people time to adjust and plan for change in order to minimize the stress that is inherent in change.

Checklist for the Interview Structure

- Introduction
  - Give your name and status
  - Give name and status of accompanying health worker(s)
  - State purpose of the interview
  - Clarify your role to the client
  - Clarify the client's role and expectations
  - Discuss contractual arrangement
    - Times
    - Finances
  - Discuss the parameters of confidentiality
  - Setting
    - Privacy
    - Environmental controls
    - Comfort of client
  - Maintain eye contact (when culturally appropriate)
- Focus
  - Body language conducive to the interview process
  - Productive patterns of communication
    - Open-ended
    - General lead
    - Reflection
    - Silence
- Termination
  - Advise client of approaching termination
  - Recapitulate the interview
  - Remind client of the number and times of future sessions (if appropriate)

Components of the Health History

To assist you in gathering a health history, most forms follow a relatively standardized format. Although these history forms may vary slightly, they contain essentially the same basic information. In addition, there are specific sections for obtaining the health history of an infant or a child (containing questions related to growth and development patterns and to school and social history) and for obtaining an obstetric history from a female client.

As a general rule, the following sequence is followed in a health history interview or on a self-completed checklist:

1. Biographical data.
2. Reason for seeking health evaluation or chief complaint.

3. Current health status or history of present illness.
4. Personal history and patterns of living.
5. Previous experience with illness.
6. ROS (review of systems).
7. Client profile.

Biographical Data

The client's biographical data are helpful to you in anticipating the special needs of the client and in comparing his background with epidemiologic studies. The health record should contain the client's home address, sex, age, and birth date. It should also contain information about his marital status, current occupation, religion, race, and ethnic origin. The client's level of education and whether he is able to read and write are important for you to know—more than once a client has been given written instructions, only to reveal on subsequent contact that he did not understand or follow the instructions because he was unable to read them!

As we saw in Chapter 2, knowing a client's cultural traditions, ethnic background, and religion is important because these factors can influence the client's health and his attitudes toward health care. Also, the client interprets his current situation on the basis of values and norms that exist within a social and cultural structure. Knowing this background will assist you in understanding why the client responds as he does toward health, illness, hospitalization, and the individuals responsible for providing health care delivery.

Although the four leading causes of death in the United States are heart disease, cancer, cerebrovascular disorders (stroke), and accidents, in specific age groups the leading causes are quite different (Damon 1977). In children ages 1 to 14, the four leading causes of death, in order, are accidents, cancer, congenital malformations, and influenza and pneumonia. It is obvious that children have low rates of chronic circulatory diseases and tend to die from acute problems such as accidents or respiratory infections. Of course, overall mortality for children is much lower than that for middle-aged or old adults. If the community population is composed largely of teenagers, the nurse may expect to find an increased incidence of venereal disease, drug abuse, smoking, accidents, suicide, and juvenile crime. Statistical data also tell the nurse what specific areas should be assessed to determine adequacy of treatment, prevention, and educational measures. In a predominantly middle-aged population, for instance, the prevalent health problems may be peptic ulcers and coronary artery disease.

Disease incidence may vary by population group as well as by age. Although both Black and White American middle-aged males tend to die of problems involving the circulatory system and the heart, the cause of death tends to be different in these two population groups. Black middle-aged males tend to die of the secondary effects of hypertension, such as stroke, kidney failure, or myocardial infarctions (Mausner & Bahn 1974). White middle-aged males, however, tend to die of coronary failure associated with chronic heart disease and atherosclerosis. This difference in mortality patterns is probably due to a combination of factors, including population genetic differences, socioeconomic differences, and such subcultural differences as lifestyle and dietary habits.

Childhood morbidity and mortality also vary by subculture. For example, Native American children, whose families are poorer and tend to live in areas with poor sanitation and housing, are most likely to die from accidents, pneumonia, congenital malformations, gastroenteritis, and other infective and parasitic diseases (Wallace 1973), and their rate of death from all these causes (excluding congenital malformation) is at least twice as high as that for the population as a whole. It is obvious that poverty and differences in lifestyle result in high rates of infectious disease.

Because such age-specific health problems occur in various population groups, your awareness of these differences can assist you in conducting a more thorough health assessment.

Marital status can be viewed in light of epidemiology; for example, more single males attempt suicide than married males. It also has important bearing on possible economic problems, rehabilitation potential, and future health needs of the family. Current and past occupation has both epidemiologic and economic significance.

Should someone other than the client provide the health history information, his name and his relationship to the client must be identified on the record. In most cases this will be a parent, spouse, friend, or relative. In the case of accident, it may be a total stranger who may give an eyewitness account of what happened to the

Checklist for Biographical Data

- Name
- Address
- Sex
- Age/birth date
- Marital status/compatibility and adjustment
- Current occupation
- Religion/practice and attitude toward religion
- Race
- Ethnic origin
- Level of education/ability to read and write
- Health history informant and reliability

client. Whatever the case, you should make a statement about your perceived reliability of the informant, describing his mental status (such as alert, well oriented, confused, or anxious). Confusion or anxiety, for example, may alter the accuracy of the record.

Reason for Seeking Health Evaluation or Chief Complaint

It is necessary to identify the reason for which the client is seeking health care attention. It may, for example, indicate his attitude toward health and health practices, as when a client wants an annual physical checkup or employment health clearance. Those clients who seek help because of illness often experience symptoms for some time before they seek attention. Why they seek help on a particular day may be related to changes in these symptoms. Knowing this information may be important to you in evaluating the client's perception of the situation as well as in establishing guidelines for further investigation.

It is vital that the client be allowed to describe the reason or complaint in his own words. Particularly with illness, the nurse might have the tendency to make assumptions that are not related to the client's immediate reason for seeking help. It is thus best to use open-ended questions or statements at this point in the gathering process, allowing the client to talk freely without interruption. At the end of his explanation you will have obtained most of what the client views as important complaints or reasons for seeking health evaluation. Generally, by this time you will also have a basic feeling for his attitude toward health care services and personnel. In addition, you will most likely be able to evaluate his ability to organize his thoughts and ideas.

Checklist for the Reason for Seeking Health Evaluation or Chief Complaint

- Annual check-up
- Employment health clearance
- Follow-up care and evaluation
- Signs and symptoms that led client to seek health care
- Monitoring of existing health problem(s)

Record the chief complaint in the client's own words. Sometimes the client will say something like, "I have heart trouble," "I have cancer," or "I have multiple sclerosis." When the client uses such terms or diagnoses, have him elaborate. Ask him what symptoms led him to his conclusion or what he means by multiple sclerosis. Many times a client will self-diagnose if he manifests a sign or symptom similar to something his neighbor, relative, or friend has been medically diagnosed as having. Further investigation will usually produce a chief complaint such as "I've had chest pains for the past 2 hours," "I've lost 60 pounds in the past month," or "I've had muscle cramps and weakness in my legs for 4 months."

From these examples you can see that the chief complaint is a brief statement of only one or two signs or symptoms and their duration. (A "sign," such as weight loss or weakness, is objective—you can weigh the client or test muscle strength; a "symptom," such as pain or cramps, is subjective—you are unable to observe it.) Should the client use vague terms such as "bowel trouble" or "not feeling well," clarify what he means: "What is it that makes you say you have bowel trouble (are not feeling well)?" or "What is happening that causes you to say this?" These questions may produce such concrete responses as "vomiting and diarrhea for the past 4 days," or "headache and general weakness for the past 2 days."

In recording *do not* alter the client's chief complaint into medical terminology, such as "Occipital lobe headache—intermittent for 2 months' duration."

Current Health Status or History of Present Illness

Ask the client to describe his general health, using a general question such as, "How would you describe your health up until this time?"

The client who has described numerous past illnesses and then describes his state of health as "good" may be trying to minimize or deny certain problems. Whether the client describes his health as "terrible" or "good," you should ask for some clarification, as for example, "What do you mean by terrible?" How individuals perceive their general health has bearing on how well they are able to participate in their health care planning.

If the client should have a major complaint, you must elicit all factors that relate to this complaint. This is a painstaking process in which you must encourage the client to provide a factual account of the illness. You must remember not to jump to conclusions or to bias the account by adding professional judgments or opinions. Questions should be phrased so that the client will not give a simple "yes" or "no" answer. Many clients are very suggestible. If you use questions like, "You have more pain when you sit up?" or "Your illness began just a short time ago?" they might agree even if the answer is not exactly true. It is better to ask "What brings on the pain?" or "How long have you been ill?" so the client has the opportunity to qualify the information.

A thorough investigation of a particular sign or symptom is accomplished by using certain guidelines designed to elicit essential information. One effective guideline is the "Seven Variables of Investigation" suggested by Morgan and Engel (1969):

1. Bodily location.
2. Quality.
3. Quantity.
4. Chronology.
5. Setting.
6. Aggravating and alleviating factors.
7. Associated manifestations.

Bodily Location

Where is the symptom located? It can be a small, well-defined area or a larger, more diffuse one. Ask the client to indicate the location and outline it, if possible, with a finger or hand. It is not enough for the client to indicate pain in the abdomen, since the abdomen is a large area covering a great number of structures. Is the pain located in a right lower quadrant? around the umbilicus? below the sternum? Does the pain radiate to other areas? Ask the client to indicate the path of radiation. The client should also describe whether the pain is superficial or deep.

Quality

Ask the client to describe the quality of the symptom. For example, pain may be described as dull, sharp, achey, gnawing, churning, or throbbing. Is this the worst pain he has experienced? Often clients will compare the pain to another experience, such as like "having a baby," like the pain of an abscessed tooth, or like "when I broke my wrist 2 years ago." The client's posture and facial expression can often give you a clue to the type of pain. For example, the client may grimace or bend over during the interview.

This kind of measurement also applies to other types of symptoms, such as "I'm really nervous," or "I'm dizzy." For the client who complains of being nervous, you might reflect, "Nervous?" or ask, "What makes you say this?" If the client has difficulty describing the nervousness, you might ask, "Do your hands shake?" "Are you unable to sleep?" or "Is it difficult to sit still or concentrate?" If you can see possible manifestations of his statement in his behavior, you might reflect such observations: "I see you have been tapping your fingers since we began talking." With a complaint of dizziness, you should determine the degree. Does he feel faint? Does he seem to be spinning, or does the room seem to spin about him? Is his vision blurred or is there ringing in his ears? Does the dizziness cause him to lose his balance? Is it accompanied by nausea or vomiting?

Quantity

Terms such as frequency, volume, number, size, and extent can be used to quantify the severity or intensity of the symptom. How has the symptom affected patterns of living? Is there anything the client cannot do now that he was able to do prior to the onset of the symptom? Has it affected his everyday bodily functions, such as eating, walking, lifting? Has it altered his activities, such as job performance, family relationships, sexual activity, recreation?

Chronology

When did the symptom first appear? It is helpful if the client can pinpoint the date and can tell whether the onset was gradual or abrupt. The pain associated with arthritis may occur gradually over a period of months or years, whereas the pain associated with kidney stones is usually abrupt. How long has the symptom persisted (duration)? Is it constant or intermittent? Did it occur abruptly and last for several weeks, or does it occur periodically (exacerbations and remissions)? If the complaint is an exacerbation of an already established medical condition, the client's knowledge and understanding of his condition should be assessed. This line of questioning leads directly to the next variable.

Setting

Setting refers to the precipitating factors and circumstances under which the symptom occurs; it could be a particular place, activity, or person. Setting can be determined by asking the client such questions as, "Where were you when this occurred?" "Where were you prior to this?" "What were you doing (prior to) at the time?" "Who was with you?" "Were you with anyone else prior to this happening?" "Does the symptom occur when you are lying down, sitting, exercising?" "Is it related to tension at work or in the home?" "Does it follow the ingestion of a meal?" Certain gastrointestinal complaints might occur after a meal; a tension headache might follow an argument or upsetting home or business situation. It is thus important to investigate the circumstances that surrounded the client before and during the onset of a sign or symptom.

Aggravating and Alleviating Factors

At this point you are interested in determining what, if anything, causes the complaint to become better or worse. Aggravating factors might include physical exertion, position, ingestion of spicy foods or cold liquids, cold weather, or loud noises. Ask about alleviating factors, such as home remedies and medical treatment: "What have you tried to relieve the problem? Has it worked?" The client with a headache may obtain relief by taking aspirin every 3 to 4 hours or he may say that lying down quietly is some help.

Associated Manifestations

With the exception of generalized symptoms such as chills, fever, weakness, or fatigue, it is most unusual for a symptom to occur without other related manifestations. Most symptoms suggest disturbances in one or more body systems. As you are listening and guiding the client in describing his illness, you should cluster symptoms together and begin thinking of possible causes of the problem. You then can pursue certain areas of investigation. For example, swelling of the ankles and feet may suggest that you ask questions related to both cardiac and renal function. Shortness of breath following activity should prompt you to determine the amount of activity necessary to cause dyspnea, to inquire whether the client experiences orthopnea or paroxysmal nocturnal dyspnea, and to ask whether the client has a history of respiratory problems or symptoms.

When you have identified possible involvement of a certain body system, you can proceed to reviewing the entire system at this time instead of waiting until the review of symptoms (ROS) portion of the health history interview. For example, if the complaint is abdominal upset, you can ask specifically whether there have been accompanying episodes of pain, nausea, vomiting, diarrhea, changes in bowel habits, melena, clay-colored stools, and so on. Because many gastrointestinal dysfunctions have related skin manifestations (for example, cirrhosis is often accompanied by pruritus, spider angiomas, and palmar erythema), the ROS for the integumentary system may be completed at this time. The urinary system may also be reviewed here, as gastrointestinal signs and symptoms sometimes reflect renal problems; nausea, vomiting, and diarrhea commonly accompany such kidney conditions as nephritis and uremia. Here laboratory data become quite enlightening.

Knowing which systems to review in relation to the present illness requires not only a thorough knowledge of pathophysiology and pathopsychology but also a great deal of experience. However, any apprehensions you may have should be somewhat relieved by realizing that

Checklist for Current Health Status or History of Present Illness

- Location
- Quality
- Quantity
- Chronology
- Setting
- Aggravating and alleviating factors
- Associated manifestations
- Effect on ADLs and other life areas
- Review of relevant body system(s)

the routine ROS will identify disorders in systems other than those you consider significant and review during the investigation of the present illness. Thorough documentation of your findings will be vital to the further analysis of the client's data base by the nurse specialist or physician.

Personal History and Patterns of Living

The next component of the health history deals with the client's lifestyle; its aim is to determine the kind of environment the client is accustomed to. What are the client's personal habits, daily activities, and financial status? These facts are of great importance in determining a plan of care because the conditions and the way in which people live often contribute to illness. Information is obtained relating to occupational history, financial status, family history of illness, geographic exposure, and lifestyle.

Occupational History

What is the client's work history? Are days of work missed because of illness, inability to "get going" on Monday mornings, or a variety of reasons for not being able to get to work on time? Does the client have a history of accidents while on the job? A poor work history showing any of these symptoms could be an indication of beginning illnesses, or it could be an indication of problem drinking.

Is the client presently employed or unemployed? If unemployed, it may be beneficial to determine which type of unemployment situation the client is facing. For example, if the unemployment is due to seasonal fluctuation such as common in the construction industry, the client's mental health status and stress levels may be more adaptive to the situation than that of the client facing chronic or long-term unemployment. Some clients may be unemployed due to the economy or supply and demand of the job market. This client may be facing the issue of whether to remain in the present geographical location or relocate, and complicating the issue will be the age of the client. For the worker over age 50, the possibility of employment or career change may appear bleak. These factors, either in combination or singly, can alter the client's stress levels, thus lowering the client's resistance to illness, both physical and psychological.

Is the client retired or soon to be retired? The client's ability to work, despite an impending or existing state of retirement, has implications for an individual's feeling of well-being. It may also be helpful to determine if the client is or was retired voluntarily (worker chose to retire) or involuntarily due to health problems or age. The worker who voluntarily chooses to retire is usually more prepared for the retirement life than the worker who was involuntarily retired, and thus may have more coping skills. Another factor that may contribute to the worker's mental and physical well-being is the opportunity to participate in preretirement workshops.

What are the occupational hazards of the client's job? Knowing that a client who is complaining of pain in the chest and coughing has worked with industrial solvents for some years may help pinpoint a contributing factor to the illness. Where is the geographic location of the work site? If the employment area is out of doors, environmental pollutants such as soot, coal dust, and other airborne particles may aggravate an already existing condition. What kind of stress does the individual perceive in his work role? What is the level of the client's job satisfaction? As we saw in Chapter 1, such stressors can have major consequences for health.

What means does the client have for support? Will the amount of support be adequate? Will he be able to pay for treatment, medications, and medical care? There are a multitude of important avenues the nurse can explore in relation to the client's occupation.

Financial Status

Financial status is closely related to occupation. The ability to meet financial obligations relative to personal needs, family, food, and housing is often a major cause for concern. Is the client employed in a job paying minimum wage? Is the client holding down more than one job? Does the client's income fall just above the cutoff for social supports such as food stamps, access to well-baby clinics, or other low cost health care facilities? An example of this might be the young divorced mother with dependent children, who may postpone health care for herself because of the inability to pay for it.

Other victims of difficulties with financial status are people living on low fixed incomes; this may include both the young and the elderly. Food and shelter are basic necessities of life, but for these people, many times shelter takes priority over food. Because they are unable to eat

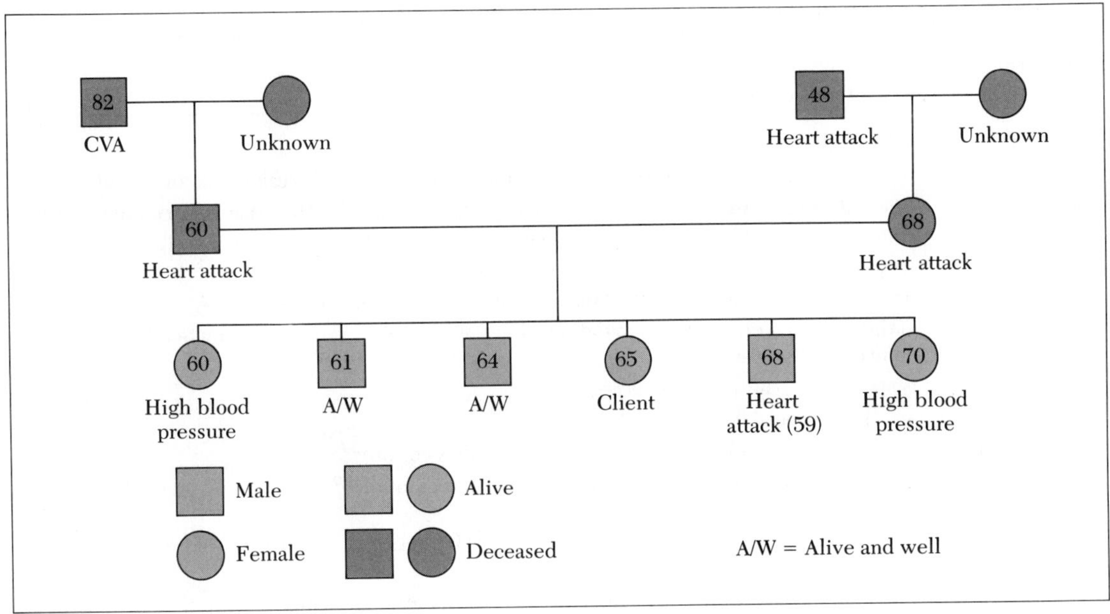

Figure 4-1 Family genogram

properly, they are often weak and anemic or obese and malnourished. For persons in the lower financial/income areas, clothing is many times a luxury, and the lack of proper or adequate clothing decreases protection and opens the individual to recurring illnesses. Another result of lower financial status may be the inability to afford proper or adequate sanitation, heat, or utilities such as electricity and gas. The best way to determine financial status is to use open-ended questions, such as "How would you describe your financial status?" Information regarding salary is often considered personal; asking the client outright what his salary is may create blocks to communication.

Family History of Illness

General background and familial tendencies are related to the development of many illnesses. Information about the family can provide important evidence about the client's complaints. As Figure 4-1 demonstrates, this information should include the ages of siblings, parents, and grandparents, their current state of health, and if they are deceased, the cause of death. Special attention should be paid to such disorders as heart disease, hypertension, cancer, diabetes, obesity, allergies, jaundice, bleeding, ulcers, migraine, alcoholism, arthritis, and tuberculosis. If absent, these items are recorded as pertinent negatives, that is, no history of heart disease, hypertension, cancer, diabetes, and so on.

Geographic Exposure

With the ease of world-wide travel, there is increased exposure to diseases that are indigenous to foreign lands. Therefore, you should ask the client about any travel to foreign lands. Inquiring about military service may reveal a tour of overseas duty. Sometimes the birthplace of an individual provides additional clues.

Lifestyle

The investigation of an individual's lifestyle will give you some idea of factors that can be used for health maintenance or restoration. The sample questions in Table 4-1 will aid in assessing some cultural values and practices related to health care.

Sexuality Assessment of sexuality is done about as frequently as rectal examinations. In fact, it is probably the most neglected area of health assessment; it is not even addressed in most instances, whereas the existence of the rectal examination as part of health assessment is at least acknowledged, if only by the words "referred" or "not done." Some nurses believe that sexual matters are personal and should not be explored. Others ignore assessment of sexuality because of their own discomfort. Furthermore young nurses may find it difficult to discuss sexuality with persons who are older than themselves. They may also find it difficult to think of men and women late in life as having sexual feel-

Table 4-1. Assessment of Cultural Values and Practices Related to Health Care

Cultural factor	Assessment questions
Language	What is the first language of the family?
	If English is not spoken, is there a family member or friend who can speak for the others?
	Is an interpreter necessary? Should language cards be used? (These cards are pictures with appropriate statements or questions in a specified foreign language.)
Diet	Does the family have cultural food preferences?
	Are any foods forbidden by the family's cultural or religious beliefs?
	Is there special etiquette surrounding eating practices (for example, a practice that eating is done only in privacy)?
	Is special preparation of foods required?
	Are there special foods for certain occasions?
	What are the customary mealtimes in the family's culture?
Health and illness beliefs	How are health and illness described in the family's culture? Do all family members hold these beliefs?
	What are the family's beliefs about the causes of illness (e.g., punishment for sin, an imbalance of the body system)?
	Whom does the family respect as a health practitioner (e.g., a physician, public health nurse, grandmother, *curandero*, spiritualist, herbalist, acupuncturist)?
	What are the usual remedies used by the family for illness (e.g., home remedies, over-the-counter medications, herbs, prayers, prescription drugs)?
	What are the family's customs and beliefs related to death?
Child-family relationships	Are there religious practices surrounding birth, illness, and death? What are they?
	How is the birth of a child received in the family?
	What are the family's goals for the child? What approach does the family take to help the child reach those goals?
	What health care practices for the child's welfare does the family value? Are there cultural objections to any practices (e.g., immunizations, dental care, teaching of hygiene and other self-care practices)?
	From what source does the family derive its greatest support (e.g., extended family, religion, friends)?
	What role does the extended family play?
	What are the major values of the family (e.g., education, wealth, spiritual life, sports)?

From Bellack/Bamford: *Nursing Assessment: A Multidimensional Approach*, © 1987 Boston: Jones and Bartlett Publishers.

ings, needs, and relationships. Well-being and sexual functioning are interrelated. If the client is sick or in poor shape, energy, enthusiasm, and interest for sexual activity are generally decreased. Including the assessment of sexual functioning near the end of history-taking allows you and the client to feel more comfortable in the roles of nurse and client—that is, in exploring sexuality in relation to health status and in divulging the information.

Sexuality is an identity fashioned greatly by morality, which in turn is developed by the direct influence of the guidance and values of parents and significant others (such as peers, other adults, and teachers) generally in concordance with accepted roles and formal laws of religion and society. Thus, there exists a wide variation cross-culturally in attitudes toward sexuality and in sexual behavior. See Table 4-2.

Ebersole and Hess (1981, p. 329) define sexuality as "love, warmth, sharing, touching between people, not just the physical act of coitus." Intercourse is only a part of sexuality. It is being a woman. It is being a man. It is being sensual. It is the total personality (Griggs 1978).

Using Maslow's hierarchy, a well-known model, allows the nurse to see that sexuality is a part of the person's total being, as shown in Figure 4-2. Maslow (1954) has postulated that human behavior is motivated by certain categories of basic needs that are arranged in a hierarchical fashion. In a gestalt mode all needs and levels of need exist simultaneously; however, in most circumstances, the primary or lower level needs

Table 4-2. Some Cultural Aspects Affecting Sexuality Assessment

Culture/ subculture	Religious/ family orientation	Privacy/ modesty needs	Other
Mexican-Americans	Family and religion important. Few decisions made without husband. May utilize only a Catholic obstetrician.	Very modest: Male unlikely to undress, provide urine specimens, or allow examination by female; Male likely to remain with female during obstetric or urologic exams. Body in general is considered private, even sacred, and is not to be exposed.	Believe males should have higher education and more privileges than females.
Puerto Ricans	Often matriarchal, large, with strong home orientation. Religion often important.		
American Indians	Religion and medicine are intertwined. Decisions often made by the family as a unit.	Privacy important for their medicine ceremonies. Very modest: May require permission to touch body; e.g., to bathe, brush hair; unlikely to undress with someone in room.	Avoid eye contact because believe one sees into the soul through the eyes and may take soul away. Heavy labor often part of female life; so must consider when providing instructions regarding limitations of activities.
Orientals	Often patriarchal; husband may speak for wife.	Very modest.	Schools are sex segregated from childhood on.
Blacks	Not necessarily matriarchal as often believed. Husband and wife work together. Children valued. Often a strong religious orientation.		
Appalachians	Strong family orientation; often bring whole family to hospital or clinic.		Upper and middle classes are similar to general U.S. upper and middle classes. Poor and working classes may differ: "neutrality" ethic prevails; nonassertive, nonaggressive, avoid eye contact, "mind own business" attitudes are valued.

Adapted from *Human Sexuality: A Nursing Perspective*, by R. Hogan (Ed.). Copyright © 1980 by Appleton-Century-Crofts. Reprinted by permission.

take priority over seeking satisfaction of the higher level needs. The primary physiologic needs include those such as oxygen, food, water, shelter, elimination, activity, rest, pain avoidance, and sexual activity. The emphases of sexuality at the primary level can be viewed as

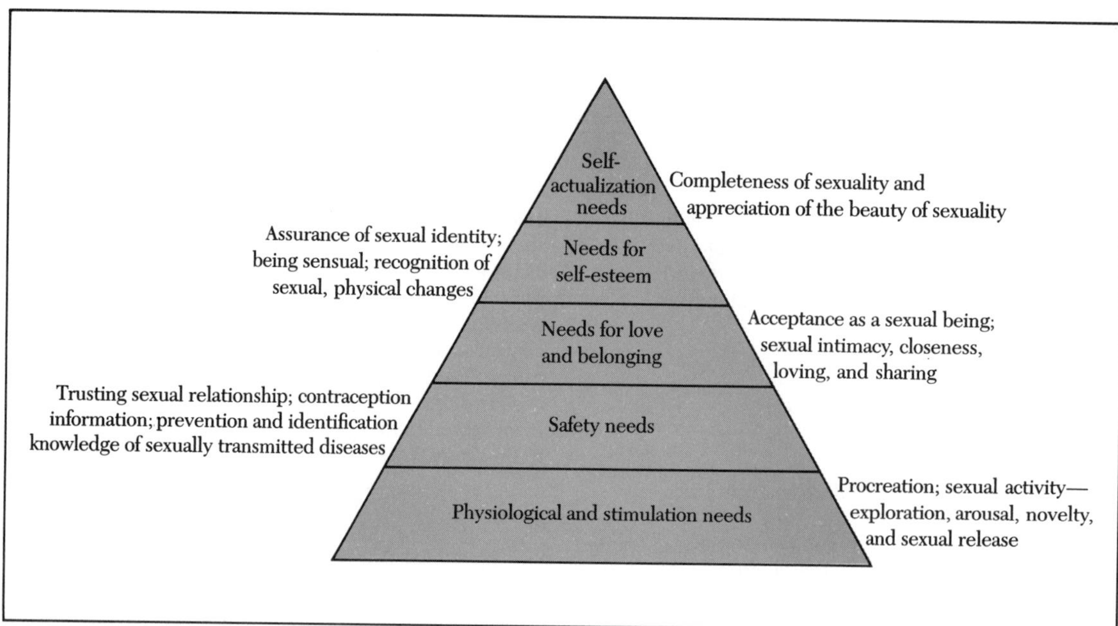

Figure 4-2 Schema of Maslow's hierarchy of needs with identification of sexuality emphases throughout.

procreation and sexual activity, including sexual exploration, arousal, novelty, and sexual release. Safety and security needs in light of sexuality are the desire for trusting sexual relationships and acquisition of knowledge regarding contraception and the means to prevent and recognize sexually transmitted diseases. Sexually, the needs for love and belonging are reflected in behaviors of sexual intimacy, wherein closeness, loving, and sharing abound, and the need to be accepted as a sexual being at no matter what age. The need to have a sexual identity and to feel that one is sensual satisfies the need for self-esteem in regard to sexuality; this includes the recognition of sexual, physical changes. The pinnacle of Maslow's hierarchy is self-actualization; this encompasses aesthetic needs, and in the sphere of sexuality is represented by the feelings of sexual completeness and an appreciation of the beauty of sexuality.

Alterations in sexual functioning may occur because of social barriers, myths, or effects of illness. Table 4-3 lists diseases and medical therapies that may interfere with sexual health. For example, diabetes can have a significant effect on sexual functioning. Men with diabetes may experience absence of emission or a "dry orgasm" caused by diabetic neuropathy wherein the semen is forced back into the bladder (retrograde ejaculation). Surgical penile implants are used for maintaining erection. For the diabetic female the most common problem affecting sexual functioning is fungal infections of the vagina. Treatment of the infection ends painful intercourse. Medications may also affect sexual functioning. See Table 4-4. The client should be educated about the possible side effects of decreased or increased libido. If this is distressing to the client, perhaps the possibility of alternative treatment could be discussed with the physician. Often the client is just relieved to know that sexual dysfunction is caused by the medication and that sexual powers have not been lost. The knowledge alone of increased or decreased libido due to a medication may be sufficient. For additional information on sexual dysfunctions in men see Chapter 24.

Keeping in mind the nursing goal of promoting and maintaining health status and having background knowledge of sexuality will enable you to pursue this pertinent area of health assessment with your clients. Assessment of the client's knowledge, assets, needs, and losses in the area of sexuality will help you provide measures for expression of sexuality—for example, use of cosmetics; attractive clothing; opportunities for closeness, touching, kissing, and holding. When sexual activity is not desired or available, suitable substitute activities are listening to music, dancing, relaxing in a rocking chair, and stroking a pet. Alternative choices or options available to sexual intercourse are masturbation,

Table 4-3. Physiologic Interferences with Sexual Health

Interferences	Hypothesized mechanism of action
Systemic diseases Pulmonary disease Renal disease Malignancies Infections Degenerative diseases Some cardiovascular diseases	Debility, pain, and depression probably interfere with libido as well as sexual expression
Metabolic disruptions Cirrhosis Mononucleosis Hepatitis	Hepatic problems in the male result in estrogen buildup related to inability of the liver to conjugate estrogens; similar processes occur in the female along with general debility
Hypothyroidism Addison's disease Hypogonadism Hypopituitarism Acromegaly Feminizing tumors Cushing's disease Diabetes mellitus	By depression of the CNS function, general debilitation, and depression, libido may be decreased, and impaired arousal in the female and impaired erectile abilities in the male may result. With diabetes there is a hypothesized relationship between neuropathic and vascular damage and retrograde ejaculation and impotence or secondary orgasmic dysfunction, dyspareunia, or adolescent amenorrhea
Genital interferences Priapism Peyronie's disease Balantitis Phimosis Genital herpes Trauma to the penis Vaginal infections Senile vaginitis Vulvitis Leukoplakia Bartholin cyst Allergic response to vaginal sprays, deodorants Vaginitis following radiation therapy Pelvic inflammatory disease Fibroadenomas Endometriosis Uterine prolapse Anal fissures, hemorrhoids Pelvic masses Ovarian cysts Reduced vaginal lubrication, postpartum or with aging	Each of these problems involves damage to the genital organs, which may result in painful intercourse
Prostatitis Urethritis	Local irritability, damage to genitals, and consequent interference with reflex mechanisms involved in erection and ejaculation
Medical or surgical castration Orchiectomy Radiation therapy Ovariectomy, adrenalectomy	Lowered androgen levels depress libido and lead to impotence, retarded ejaculation, and/or impaired sexual responsiveness

Adapted from Kaplan, H. S. *The New Sex Therapy*. New York: Brunner/Mazel, Inc. 1974; and Phipps, W.; Long, B.; Woods, N. F. and Cassmeyer, V. *Medical Surgical Nursing: Concepts and Clinical Practice*, 4th ed. St. Louis: C. V. Mosby, 1991, p. 1520.

Table 4-4. Potential Effects of Drugs on Sexual Function

Drug or drug category	Effect	Probable mechanism of action: Physiologic	Probable mechanism of action: Psychological
Recreational drugs			
Alcohol	Small amounts transiently positive		Reduced inhibitions
	Large amounts or prolonged use negative	CNS depressant Impotence Premature ejaculation Associated with fetal alcohol syndrome in pregnancy	
Amphetamines and cocaine	Transiently positive	CNS stimulant Rapid and long-lasting erection Intensification of orgasm Decreased fatigue	Mood enhancement Increased mental alertness
	Enduring–negative	Impotence Decreased vaginal secretions resulting in painful intercourse	Decreased libido
Amyl nitrite*	Questionable	Peripheral vasodilation may enhance orgasm but can also produce dizziness, headache, and syncope.	
Caffeine	Transiently positive	Central nervous system stimulant—may reduce fatigue	
	Large amounts or prolonged use–negative	May produce a "nervous reaction"	
Canthoris (Spanish fly)	Negative	Irritation and inflammation of GU tract, systemic poisoning	
Hallucinogens	Questionable		Alters perceptions with either heightened sexual sensations or inability to focus on sexual activity
Nicotine	Negative transient effects	Vasoconstriction with decreased oxygen level and decreased blood flow to sex organs	
	Negative enduring effects	Decreased spermatogenesis Decreased sperm motility Increased incidence of abortion, stillbirths and small-for-gestational age babies	

*Also considered a therapeutic drug.

Adapted from Wood, J.S. "Drug Effects on Human Sexual Behavior." *In:* Woods, N. F. (Ed.). *Human Sexuality in Health and Illness,* 2nd ed. St. Louis: C. V. Mosby, 1979, pp. 378–379; Ball, W.D. "Drugs That Affect Sexuality." *In:* Hogan, R., (Ed.). *Human Sexuality: A Nursing Perspective.* New York: Appleton-Century-Crofts, 1980, pp.712–726; and Partridge, R. V. "Sexuality and Drugs." *In:* Lion, E. M., (Ed.). *Human Sexuality in Nursing Process.* New York: John Wiley & Sons, 1982, pp. 331–339.

Table 4-4. *Continued*

Drug or drug category	Effect	Probable mechanism of action: Physiologic	Probable mechanism of action: Psychological
Opiates*	Transiently positive	Central nervous system depression	Reduced inhibitions
Codeine Heroin Methadone Morphine	Negative–enduring effects	Impotence Decreased ejaculate volume Decreased sperm motility	Decreased sexual enjoyment Decreased libido
Opium		Amenorrhea, dysmenorrhea, infertility, increased incidence of abortion	
Potassium nitrate (saltpeter)	Questionable	Diuresis	
Sedative-hypnotics* Compazine Librium Marijuana	Transiently positive	Central nervous system depressant Tranquilization Relaxation	Reduced inhibitions
Mellaril Thorazine Valium	Large doses negative	Lethargy Decreased coordination	Decreased libido
Therapeutic drugs			
Antidepressants	Negative and positive	Central nervous system depression Impotence Inhibited ejaculation Orgasmic difficulties	Increased libido if depression is reduced
Antihistamines	Transiently negative	Central nervous system depression Decreased vaginal secretion	Decreased libido
Antihypertensives	Negative	Peripheral blockage of innervation of sex organs Decrease or absence of ejaculate; retrograde ejaculation; impotence; orgasmic difficulties; breast tenderness; menstrual irregularities; gynecomastia	Decreased libido
Antipsychotics	Transiently negative	Dry ejaculation Erectile difficulties Gynecomastia Decreased vaginal lubrication Spontaneous flow of milk from breasts Amenorrhea	Decreased responsiveness
Antispasmodics	Negative	Vasoconstriction Ganglionic blockage of innervation of sex organs impotence Decreased vaginal lubrication	

(continued on page 70)

Table 4-4. *Continued*

Drug or drug category	Effect	Probable mechanism of action: Physiologic	Probable mechanism of action: Psychological
Therapeutic drugs *continued*			
Corticosteroids	Negative–enduring	Decreased spermatogenesis Can precipitate latent diabetes mellitus	
Cytotoxins	Negative, usually only transient	Decreased spermatogenesis Amenorrhea	Decreased libido and potency
Diuretics	Transiently negative	Impotence Gynecomastia Amenorrhea Breast tenderness	
Hormones			
Sex hormone preparations	Negative	Antiandrogenic effects	Decreased libido Decreased potency
Oral contraceptives	Usually positive	Anovulation Amenorrhea	Concern regarding conception separated from sexual activity
Clomid	Usually positive	Increased testosterone in male Stimulation of ovulation	Decreased libido Decreased potency
L-Dopa and P-chorophenylalanine	Questionable		Improvement of wellbeing
Selenium	Questionable	Supports fertility in laboratory animals	
Strychnine	Questionable	Stimulation of neuraxis Priapism	
Vitamin E	Questionable	Supports fertility in laboratory animals	
Yohimbine	Questionable	Stimulation of lower spinal nerve centers	

sexual fantasies, oral stimulation, and homosexual relationships. If sexual intercourse is fatiguing to the client due to a chronic illness or handicap, use of vibrators may be of benefit. Your suggestions will depend on the client's values, medical condition, psychological health, and social situation. An important role will be to assist the client to accept normal changes in sexuality and to appreciate alternative practices of maintaining sexuality and sexual functioning.

Personal Habits Information should be obtained regarding use of cigarettes, alcohol, over-the-counter drugs, and drugs prescribed in the past. Smoking must be described in "pack years," which is calculated by multiplying the number of packs the client has smoked each day by the number of years the client has smoked. For example, the client who smokes 1½ packs a day and has smoked for 20 years, is said to have smoked 30 pack years.

People vary greatly in the amount of alcohol they consume and in the body's ability to process this consumption. The rate of metabolism of alcohol is influenced by a variety of factors, including total body weight, sex, age, poly drug use, and physical condition. The tolerance level of the individual also needs to be considered when trying to determine the degree of a drinking problem. An individual with a low tolerance level for alcohol, meaning he may be able to handle only one drink every hour or two, is an indication of low alcohol consumption. On the other hand, the person who can handle three or four drinks per hour is indicative of an experienced drinker. As previously stated, tolerance levels relate to body weight, sex, and experience. However, as alcohol consumption accelerates, the tolerance level does not rise uniformly. First, as consumption increases, the tolerance level also rises, but only until it peaks. Then the tolerance level decreases as the consumption increases. This explains why the novice drinker and the alcoholic become drunk quicker than the more experienced drinker.

Social drinking is usually described as a few drinks now and then, but the distinction between the problem drinker and the alcoholic is less clearly defined. To pinpoint the extent of your client's social drinking or drinking problem, you must go beyond asking the number of cans of beer consumed per week or the number of cocktails consumed on a weekend. Questions regarding the time of day the drinking begins, a hidden supply of alcohol, a switch from a popular alcoholic drink or beverage to a less popular drink or beverage in order to protect the supply, family problems due to drinking, job loss or work time lost due to drinking, gulping drinks, blackouts (blackouts are loss of memory not loss of consciousness), sore gums, and malnourishment are all good indicators that the client may be experiencing drinking problems as opposed to social drinking.

Questions about alcohol are often omitted with the young client, yet teenage alcoholism is a very real problem today. Alcohol-related highways fatalities are the number-one killer of America's youth; to play ostrich when it comes to adolescent drinking is foolhardy, to say the least. In addition, the number of women experiencing drinking problems and alcoholism is on the rise, opening up another new area of concern—fetal alcohol syndrome. A full understanding of the effects of alcohol on the fetus is not yet known, but what is known is that as few as two drinks of alcohol per day (not an average of two drinks per day) can cause damage to the fetus. This damage is mainly in the form of abnormalities and mental retardation or learning disabilities. Many of your pregnant clients may be unaware of this potential problem.

It is essential to determine how many and what kinds of over-the-counter (OTC) drugs the client buys and uses regularly, as well as whether he uses street drugs. For characteristics of psychoactive chemical abuse see Table 4-5. Many clients who take OTC drugs do not think they are important enough to mention in a health interview. However, aspirin accounts for the largest part of drug overdoses. Women are particularly prone to taking nonprescriptive diet pills and OTC diuretics. Another abused drug is caffeine, which is a stimulant. Because using stimulants provides longer periods of intellectual functioning, many students drink excessive amounts of coffee or take caffeine-containing drugs. They may not consider such practices dangerous and therefore may not mention them unless questioned directly. As a drug, caffeine can become addictive and withdrawal symptoms such as tremors and headache may be experienced 18 to 24 hours after the last ingestion of the drug. Caffeine is a diuretic and can cause insomnia, restlessness, dizziness, irritability, chronic headache, agitation, anxiety, and psychophysiological disorders. It has been shown that there is a high correlation between drinking over five cups of coffee per day and heart disease. Moreover, caffeine has also been linked to other disorders such as peptic ulcer, hiatal hernia, bladder cancer, birth defects, noncancerous fibrocystic breast disorders, and menstrual cramps. Caffeine is present in a variety of products ranging from coffee and tea to colas and over-the-counter preparations for headache, allergy, and cold symptoms. It can even be obtained from a chocolate bar. Caffeine consumers come from all socioeconomic levels, but the greatest consumers are also high users of minor tranquilizers, sedative-hypnotics, alcohol, and tobacco (cigarettes).

Diet At first glance questions about diet may seem straightforward and directed mainly at determining whether the client's diet is well balanced. However, knowing a person's diet, eating habits, and eating patterns provides additional invaluable information. Food preferences reflect cultural background, age, financial status, self-image, body image, and a number of other significant factors. A client's eating patterns may be the clue to a problem of obesity or may be the signal that the malnourished or underweight client may be suffering from psychological problems leading to anorexia or bulimia. In either case, further investigation into the eating patterns of the client and the client's self-image or body image would be warranted. In addition to the client's eating patterns, the client's eating habits may also direct you to areas for further assessment; for example, the adolescent who ex-

Table 4-5. Characteristics of Psychoactive Chemical Abuse

Psychoactive substance[a]	Common terms[b]	Usual route of administration	Abuse: signs/symptoms	Overdose: signs/symptoms	General comments
Narcotics					
Opium derivatives					
heroin	H, Harry, Horse, brother, scag, smack, junk	Intravenous Intranasal	Pupil constriction, euphoria followed by CNS depression (impaired coordination, lethargy, cyanosis, coma)	Respiratory arrest, death	Relatively small proportion of youth abuse this Schedule I–controlled substance. Tolerance and a strong physical and psychological dependence usually develop rapidly. Potential for perinatal/neonatal addiction and/or effects exists.[c]
morphine	M, white stuff	Intravenous Oral Intranasal	Euphoria, pupil constriction, constipation, nausea, skin flushing, sweating, respiratory depression, cyanosis, coma	Coma, respiratory arrest, death	Schedule II–controlled substance with high physical and psychological dependence capability. Tolerance develops rapidly, and naloxone hydrochloride (morphine antagonist) will precipitate *withdrawal symptoms*: (muscle cramps, stomach cramps, diarrhea, rhinitis, restlessness, and convulsions). Potential for perinatal/neonatal addiction and/or effects exists.[c]
codeine	Schoolboy	Oral	Mild euphoria, constipation, nausea	Depressed blood pressure and respirations	Schedule II–controlled substance, less likely to produce physical dependence. Large doses produce paradoxical stimulation. Less frequently abused drug by youth except in combination with other substances—e.g., a *Load* is 3 Doriden and 3 codeine.
Synthetic opiates					
methadone (Dolophine)	Meth, dollies	Oral (preferred) Intravenous	Euphoria, nodding-dozing state, restlessness	Respiratory depression, convulsions, or death	Schedule II–controlled substance causing *severe withdrawal symptoms* including diarrhea, stomach pain, hot and cold flashes, insomnia, and sweating. Tolerance develops slowly, but all components of addiction occur. Potential for perinatal/neonatal addiction and/or effects exists.[c]

meperidine (Demerol)		Intravenous	Pupil constriction, sweating, respiratory depression, cyanosis	Cold, clammy skin; depressed respirations; decreased blood pressure; shock; coma; death	Schedule II–controlled substance available in hospitals; therefore, abuse potential for medical personnel. Tolerance and physical and psychological dependence develop. Potential for perinatal effects (depressed infant) and perinatal addiction exists.[c]
pentazocine (Talwin)	Ts	Oral Intravenous		Similar to opiate overdose, particularly respiratory depression May be lethal if combined with barbiturates or alcohol	Schedule IV–controlled substance for which tolerance and psychological dependence develop after prolonged use.
Depressants Alcohol (ethanol)	Booze, hootch, suds, juice	Oral	Progressive stages of intoxication: euphoria, loss of inhibition, emotional lability, impaired judgment, aggressiveness, hostility, incoordination, lethargy, and stupor	Coma, death (especially when combined with barbiturates and some tranquilizers—e.g., diazepam)	Alcohol-induced judgment impairment and incoordination are highly correlated with moving vehicle accidents during adolescence. Alcohol dependence is a progressive disease. Psychological dependence precedes physical dependence.

(*continued on page 74*)

[a]The list covers only the major chemicals or drugs abused.

[b]Common terms vary from area to area across the country.

[c]This is conclusive evidence of the effect on the neonate.

[d]A potential risk of neonatal effects exists. These may be subtle neurological effects, such as hyperactivity or learning problems, that are not detected until later childhood.

From Servonsky/Opas: *Nursing Management of Children*, ©1987 Boston: Jones and Bartlett Publishers.

Table 4-5. *Continued*

Psychoactive substance[a]	Common terms[b]	Usual route of administration	Abuse: signs/symptoms	Overdose: signs/ symptoms	General comments
Depressants Alcohol (ethanol) *continued*			Blackouts (drug-related memory failure without loss of consciousness, i.e., amnesia)		Tolerance develops at varying rates, and high tolerance is suggestive of alcoholism. Blackouts are indicative of alcoholism. Some adolescent ethanol deaths have been reported due to a single large intake episode. *Withdrawal*: Anxiety, tremors, hallucinations, hyperreflexia, convulsions, and death. Brain damage (subtle to pronounced), liver damage. Transmitted through placenta, fetal alcohol effects (FAE) may occur as well as Fetal Alcohol Syndrome (FAS).[c]
Barbiturate Sedative-hypnotics	Barbs, downers	Oral Intravenous	Slurred speech, ataxia, slowed reflexes, constricted pupils, short attention span, impaired judgment, combativeness, violence, paranoid delusions	Respiratory depression, coma, death	Schedule II–controlled substance. Tolerance and physical and psychological dependence develop. High potential for homicide or other violence with intravenous use. Combined with alcohol can cause extreme violence or coma or death. *Withdrawal*: hyperreflexia, irritability, convulsions, death. Transmitted through placenta: perinatal barbiturate effects include inattentiveness and permanent neurological sequelae with excessive amounts.[c]
secobarbital (Seconal)	Reds, red devils, red birds				
pentobarbital (Nembutal)	Nembies, yellow jackets				
amobarbital (Amytal)	Blues, blue heavens				

Nonbarbiturate Sedative-hypnotics methaqualone (Quaalude)	Quads, Sopers, ludes	Oral	Euphoria, irritability, sleeplessness, delirium tremors	Convulsions, cutaneous and pulmonary edema, shock, respiratory arrest	Schedule II–controlled substance with high abuse potential. Tolerance and physical and psychic dependence develop. *Withdrawal*: Similar to barbiturates; often fatal if detoxified without medical supervision. (If convulsions are not treated, status epilepticus usually develops.)
glutethimide (Doriden)		Oral	Dilated pupils	Prolonged coma, absence of reflexes, fever, and death	Schedule III–controlled substance. Tolerance and physical dependence develop fairly rapidly. Psychic dependence occurs. Potentiated effect with alcohol or other sedatives (e.g., Loads), can cause fatal respiratory and circulatory failure.
Minor tranquilizers chlordiazepoxide (Librium) diazepam (Valium) meprobamate (Equanil)	Tranks	Oral Intravenous	Occasional disinhibition, various nonspecific symptoms	Similar to barbiturate or alcohol intoxication Depressants, including alcohol, potentiate effects and may cause coma and death	Schedule IV–controlled substance. Prolonged use can result in tolerance and physical dependence. Moderate to high potential for psychological dependence. *Withdrawal*: Tremor, abdominal and/or muscle cramping, sweating, and convulsions may occur as late as 14 days following discontinuation of the drug. Sometimes used following stimulant abuse to counteract the effects; rarely used alone by youths. *Special pediatric concerns*: Accidental and nonaccidental tranquilizer poisonings of young children have been reported. Potential for perinatal/neonatal effects and/or addiction exists.[d]

(continued on page 76)

Table 4-5. *Continued*

Psychoactive substance[a]	Common terms[b]	Usual route of administration	Abuse: signs/symptoms	Overdose: signs/symptoms	General comments
Stimulants Amphetamines amphetamine sulfate (Benzedrine) dextroamphetamine (Dexedrine) methamphetamine (Methedrine)	Uppers, bennies, dexies, pep pills, speed, crystal	Oral Subcutaneous Intravenous	Hypertension, weight loss, dilated pupils, sweating (if injected), psychological and motor stimulation, insomnia, pronounced euphoric state	Cardiac failure, convulsions, coma, cerebral hemorrhage	Schedule II–controlled substance. Tolerance and psychic dependence develop. *Prolonged use*: impaired judgment, pronounced euphoric state, paranoid psychosis. *Withdrawal*: severe depression with suicidal tendency. Potential for perinatal/neonatal effects exists.[d]
Cocaine	Coke Snow Crack Rock	Intranasal Intravenous Intrapulmonary (Smoking)	Hypertension, tachycardia, hyperreflexia, hyperactivity, intense euphoria	Tachycardia, hallucinations, nausea, vomiting, muscle spasms Respiratory failure, convulsions, coma, and circulatory collapse	Schedule II–controlled substance. Powerful psychological dependence usually develops. Stimulation is more pronounced than with amphetamines, accompanied with illusion of great physical strength and mental capacity. Expense factor is decreasing as cocaine is being made into a smokable form. Probability of abuse increases with greater financial resources and availability. *Withdrawal*: severe depression. Potential for perinatal/neonatal effects exists.[d]
Hallucinogens cannabis (marijuana, hashish)	Joint, grass, pot, weed, reefer, Mary Janes, stick, hash	Intrapulmonary (smoking) Oral	Mild euphoria, intoxication, heightened sensory awareness, drowsiness, tachycardia, delayed response time, poor coordination, occasional depressed or anxiety reactions	Physical exhaustion, convulsions, anxiety, and paranoia (bad trip)	Schedule I–controlled substance. Classified as hallucinogen but closer to an intoxicant in effect. Physical dependence does not occur but psychological dependence may. Marijuana, as a substance of abuse for adolescents and children is on the increase. A major problem is that use

			Large doses produce hallucinatory effects		of this or other psychoactives may retard individual and group social development—i.e., the substance becomes the recreational focus. Moderate to heavy use is correlated with amotivational syndrome in adolescents and is hazardous to normal personality development. *Withdrawal*: irritability, sleep disturbances, sweating, anorexia, gastrointestinal upset, weight loss
Phencyclidine Lysergic acid N-N-dimethyltryp-tamine 2,5-dimethoxy-4-methyamphetamine	PCP Angel Dust LSD Acid DMT Cohoba STP, DOM	Intrapulmonary (smoking) Oral	Dilated pupils, reddened eyes, occasionally hypertension, hyperthermia, piloerection, euphoria, heightened sensory awareness, hallucinations, confusion, paranoia	Hypotensive crisis, intracerebral hemorrhage, convulsions, death	Schedule I–controlled substances. Physical dependence does not occur, but tolerance probably does. PCP, STP, DMT and LSD are major street drugs; LSD may be a deliberate contaminant as a substitute for other substances. *Psychiatric complications*: drugs intensify latent psychotic tendencies, panic, suicide potential, flashbacks (particularly with LSD). Potential for perinatal/neonatal effects exists.[d]
Inhalants and organic solvents hydrocarbons and fluorocarbons (glue, cleaning fluid, aerosol sprays, nail polish remover, gasoline)		Intranasal	Some degree of short-term intoxication, euphoria, impaired perception and coordination, loss of consciousness	Moderate overdosage: unconscious, in no immediate danger of death High overdosage: adrenergic crisis, status epilepticus, respiratory failure	Some degree of psychological dependence in the broad sense—i.e., abuser becomes dependent on the euphoric state. Most often seen with younger substance abusers. Users have an increased probability of alcohol or other substance abuse. Medical complications: asphyxia from plastic bags used to inhale fumes, ventricular fibrillation or other arrhythmias, secondary trauma. Lead poisoning. Possible irreversible damage to central nervous system, kidneys, liver, and bone marrow. Psychosis, similar to that evoked by hallucinogenic drugs may occur.

ists on fad foods may develop skin problems, obesity, or anemia, while the elderly person subsisting on tea and toast may be in fluid and electrolyte imbalance and malnourished. Some specifics to take into consideration include:

1. Is the client subject to food fads?
2. How much does the client eat?
3. Does the client think he is too fat?
4. Does the client binge eat and then vomit?
5. What is the typical diet on a normal day?
6. How many meals does the client have per day?
7. Does the client eat snacks? If so, how many a day and of what kind?
8. Does the client have free access to snacks?
9. Who prepares the client's meals?
10. Is the client on a special diet? If so, for how long? Does he understand and feel comfortable with the diet?
11. Does the client take vitamins or diet pills? If so, what is the variety of pills taken and the number of each variety?
12. Has the client had any disturbances in digestion, chewing, or swallowing?

Sleep and Rest Patterns The most common sleep disorder is insomnia. Clients with psychoses and neuroses suffer from insomnia. As psychological states (such as distress, obsessive behavior, depression, or anxiety) lessen, the client will sleep for longer periods of time. Initial insomnia occurs when the client has difficulty falling asleep. Emotional factors like excitement or anxiety may be the cause. At one time or another all of us have tossed and turned and been unable to fall asleep quickly before a trip or celebration day, such as the night before Christmas. Sudden and diverse stimuli, such as strange noises, may also interfere with falling asleep. Nutritional disorders and excessive alcohol or caffeine intake can also affect sleep. Initial insomnia tends to occur in clients when they are first admitted to the hospital.

Intermittent insomnia is when the client awakes frequently throughout the night; it may result from some of the same sources (clanging bedpans, loud voices, slamming doors) as well as from physical causes such as poor ventilation and illness symptoms. The more prevalent physical predisposers to insomnia are chronic pain, diabetes mellitus, hyperthyroidism, angina pectoris, gastric ulcer, and respiratory disorders. Terminal insomnia is when the client awakes in the early morning and cannot return to sleep. Excitement, anxiety, and change in sleeping habit may be causes of terminal insomnia. An example of the latter would be the client who is wideawake at 4 A.M. However, since being hospitalized, he has been going to sleep earlier in the evening or napping during the day and, therefore, has had a good night's sleep by that time. If the client does not display sleep deprivation symptoms or exhaustion, his need for sleep has most likely been met. Some physical characteristics that may indicate troubled sleeping patterns are dark circles under the eyes, puffy eyelids, bloodshot eyes, irritability, headache, fatigue, and decreased attention span.

Sleep and rest clearly affect the total well-being of the client. The following types of questions will aid you in assessing the sleep and rest patterns of your clients:

1. When do you usually retire and awake each day?
2. How many hours do you generally sleep?
3. Have you experienced any difficulty in sleeping?
4. If the client has experienced difficulty, what remedies have you tried?
5. Has anything happened recently to which you might attribute your sleeping difficulty?
6. What comfort measures do you usually employ that help you sleep well? Examples might include read before retiring, watch TV, set the radio on automatic "off," open the window, drink a warm beverage, have a glass of wine, take a sleeping medication, and so forth.
7. Do you have trouble falling asleep?
8. Do you wake up often during the night? If so, can you easily fall back to sleep?
9. Do you wake early in the morning feeling fatigued?
10. Do you nap during the day?
11. Do you experience nightmares? sleepwalking? bedwetting?

Sleep patterns specific to age are discussed in the appropriate age-related chapters of the text.

Activities of Daily Living When assessing daily activities, you are actually gathering the client's perception of any difficulties he may be experiencing in the basic activities of eating, grooming, dressing, elimination, and locomotion. At this time you may want to discuss the effects of handicaps on the client's abilities, or he may reveal any covert handicaps.

You should also determine whether the client is independent in performing daily activities or whether he needs supervision or assistance:

1. Is he unable to carry out certain activities?
2. How much assistance does he need?
3. Does he require adaptive devices or prostheses to perform certain activities?
4. Can the client feed himself? Does he need help cutting meat and opening containers? Does he need to be fed? Does he eat at the table? in a dining room? in bed?
5. Is the client independent in grooming himself? Can he bathe (bed, tub, shower)? Can he brush his teeth? Can he comb and wash his hair?
6. Can he care for his nails? Shave? Is he able to apply cologne, deodorant, or cosmetics?
7. Does dressing present any difficulties to the client?
8. Is the client able to go to the bathroom by himself?
9. Is he able to care for altered routes of elimination if they are necessary (colostomy, ureterostomy)?
10. Can he get out of bed (transfer)?
11. Can he get into and out of a chair?
12. Does he have any difficulty with standing? walking? stairs?
13. If wheelchair bound, is he able to propel the chair himself?

Home and Neighborhood The client's physical and emotional environment may create problems or it may provide an atmosphere conducive to well-being. It is therefore important to determine the conditions of the home and neighborhood and the services available. For example, do the drug stores accept Medicare and Medicaid? Do the grocery stores accept food stamps? Are there community services available to meet the needs of the disabled—food services, modified access routes, transportation?

Investigation of the client's housing conditions and facilities may reveal surprises. Many economically deprived elderly persons live in unheated flats or rooms with few comforts and little food. If there are children in the home, it is important to evaluate safety measures regarding such things as poisons, bare electrical wires, and other home accident factors.

Your investigation of the client's homelife may be opened by asking the client whether he lives alone. Next you can ask how he feels about this

Checklist for Personal History and Patterns of Living

Occupational history
Financial status
Family history of illness/past and present
Pertinent negatives of specific illness in family
Example: No history of hypertension, strokes, TB, ulcers, mental illness, alcoholism, epilepsy, gout, bleeding disorders
Significant for diabetes, heart disease, cancer, arthritis, ulcerative colitis
Geographic exposure
- Places
- Date and length of time

Lifestyle
- Sexuality
  - Values
  - Self-image
  - Sexual function
  - Sexual difficulties
- Personal habits
  - Smoking—type and pack years
  - Alcohol—type and amount
  - Drugs—type, amount, and pattern of use
- Diet
  - Mealtimes
  - Prepared by
  - Special diet/type and when started
  - Vitamins and/or diet pills
  - Specific difficulties
- Sleep and rest patterns
  - Hours of sleep and awakening
  - Naps
  - Difficulties/remedies tried
- Activities of daily living
- Home and neighborhood
  - Living arrangements/resources
  - Quality of interpersonal relationships
- Recreation/hobbies

arrangement. This line of questioning easily leads into an exploration of the support systems—family, friends—available to the client. The quality of these support relationships can then be assessed. Is a relationship characterized by trust, distrust, mutual support, competition, dominance, submission? Has it been harmonious, strained, or interrupted? A client who expresses concern about a family member might be encouraged to elaborate if you offer a general lead such as, "Tell me more about it." Investigating such aspects of the relationship as amount of time spent at home and away, sharing of values and goals, and planning of family activities will shed light on the client's health status. To get at specific relationships you might ask, "How would you describe your mother?" and "How would your mother describe you?"

Recreation/Hobbies Recreation is generally considered a part of an individual's lifestyle. Discussion might include such things as exercise activity and tolerance, hobbies and other interests, vacations, and even the amount of time spent with family and friends. In the case of a child, you would also be interested in whether his play is generally isolated, parallel, or interactive. The play style should then be assessed according to developmental criteria based on the child's age.

Because lifestyles are so varied in this country, you need to be open, imaginative, and tactful in your collection of data and to sort out the information necessary for a health history that is truly in the interest of the client's health status. Table 4-6 is a self-test for wellness life-style.

Previous Experience with Illness

Knowledge of previous illnesses can often be useful in interpreting the significance of the client's present status and his reactions to illness and therapy. Direct questioning may be necessary to obtain the information in the areas of childhood illnesses, immunizations, allergies, and medical history.

Childhood Illnesses and Immunizations

It is not sufficient to ask whether the client has had the "common" childhood illnesses because what is common to one age group is not to another. He should be specifically asked about measles, mumps, chickenpox, diphtheria, and smallpox. Dates of these diseases must be carefully documented. For more information on childhood infectious diseases see Appendix C. Many older people have difficulty remembering a specific disease but can recall having had a high fever with their skin peeling off or an uncomfortable rash that left scars.

The dates and types of all immunizations should be recorded. This information is difficult for many to recall; at least try to pinpoint at what age the client received the immunization(s). Record information about such immunizations as diphtheria, tetanus, pertussis (whooping cough), rubella (German measles), measles, mumps, and poliomyelitis. Table 4-7 is a schedule for first vaccinations based on the recommendations of the American Medical Association and the American Academy of Pediatrics (1989).

Individuals over 65 years of age and clients with chronic illness (heart disease, lung disease, diabetes) are generally advised to have an influenza vaccination in the fall for temporary protection. Because the medium used for the production of the flu vaccine is eggs, vaccination against influenza is not recommended for those individuals who are allergic to eggs. It is also recommended that adults get a combination tetanus-diphtheria booster every 10 years. Students, health workers, and military personnel are most likely to have had recent immunizations. People who have traveled abroad are likely to have received immunizations, the types depending on where they have traveled.

Allergies

Allergic responses to any substance, including drugs, food, pollen, clothing, and chemicals, should be explored. What does the client do for relief of these allergies? Allergic reactions should be documented as to time, place, treatment, and number of occurrences. Information about allergies can be important in diagnosis and treatment of other disorders. For example, the client who has severe "hay fever" may be more susceptible to upper respiratory infections. Allergies to drugs like penicillin or to preparations containing iodine or eggs are significant, as the client may be unable to be treated or tested with these substances.

Medical History, Surgical History, and Traumatic Injuries

All statements regarding past illnesses should be thoroughly investigated, including symptoms, course treatment, and hospitalization. Many dis-

Table 4-6. Self-Test for Parents' Wellness Life-Style

Behavior		Scoring:	Almost always	Sometimes	Almost never
Cigarette smoking	If you never smoke, enter a score of 10 for this section and go to the next section "Alcohol and Drugs."		2	1	0
	1. I avoid smoking cigarettes.		2	1	0
	2. I smoke only low-tar-and-nicotine cigarettes OR I smoke a pipe or cigars.		2	1	0
		Smoking Score:	___	___	___
Alcohol and Drugs	1. I avoid drinking alcoholic beverages OR I drink no more than 1 or 2 drinks a day.		4	1	0
	2. I avoid using alcohol or other drugs (especially illegal drugs) as a way of handling stressful situations or the problems in my life.		2	1	0
	3. I am careful not to drink alcohol when taking certain medicines (for example, medicine for sleeping, pain, colds, and allergies) or when pregnant.		2	1	0
	4. I read and follow the label directions when using prescribed and over-the-counter drugs.		2	1	0
		Alcohol and Drugs Scores:	___	___	___
Eating Habits	1. I eat a variety of foods each day, such as fruits and vegetables, whole-grain breads and cereals, lean meats, dairy products, dry peas and beans, and nuts and seeds.		4	1	0
	2. I limit the amount of fat, saturated fat, and cholesterol I eat (including eggs, butter, cream, shortenings, fat on meats, and organ meats such as liver).		2	1	0

(continued on page 82)

Table 4-6. *Continued*

Behavior		Scoring:	Almost always	Sometimes	Almost never
Eating Habits continued	3. I limit the amount of salt I eat by cooking with only small amounts, not adding salt at the table, and avoiding salty snacks.		2	1	0
	4. I avoid eating too much sugar (especially frequent snacks of sticky candy or soft drinks).		2	1	0
		Eating Habits Score:	____	____	____
Exercise and Fitness	1. I maintain a desired weight, avoiding overweight and underweight.		3	1	0
	2. I do vigorous exercises for 15 to 30 minutes at least 3 times a week (examples including running, swimming, brisk walking).		3	1	0
	3. I do exercises that enhance my muscle tone for 15 to 30 minutes at least 3 times a week (examples include yoga and calisthenics).		2	1	0
	4. I use part of my leisure time participating in individual, family, or team activities that increase my level of fitness (such as gardening, bowling, golf, and baseball).		2	1	0
		Exercise and Fitness Score:	____	____	____
Stress Control	1. I have a job or do other work that I enjoy.		2	1	0
	2. I find it easy to relax and express my feelings freely.		2	1	0
	3. I recognize early, and prepare for, events or situations likely to be stressful for me.		2	1	0
	4. I have close friends, relatives, or others whom I can talk to about personal matters and call on for help when needed.		2	1	0

Table 4-6. *Continued*

Behavior		Scoring:	Almost always	Sometimes	Almost never
	5. I participate in group activities (such as church and community organizations) or hobbies that I enjoy.		2	1	0
		Stress Control Score:	____	____	____
Safety	1. I wear a seat belt while riding in a car.		2	1	0
	2. I avoid driving while under the influence of alcohol and other drugs.		2	1	0
	3. I obey traffic rules and the speed limit when driving.		2	1	0
	4. I am careful when using potentially harmful products or substances (such as household cleaners, poisons, and electrical devices).		2	1	0
	5. I avoid smoking in bed.		2	1	0
		Safety Score:	____	____	____
		Total Scores:	Cigarette Smoking		____
			Alcohol and Drugs		____
			Eating Habits		____
			Exercise/Fitness		____
			Stress Control		____
			Safety		____
			Total:		______

Interpretation of scores for each category:

Scores of 9 and 10: Excellent! Your answers show that you are aware of the importance of this area to your health. More important, you are putting your knowledge to work for you by practicing good health habits. As long as you continue to do so, this area should not pose a serious health risk. It's likely that you are setting an example for your family and friends to follow. Since you get a very high test score on this part of the test, you may want to consider other areas where your scores indicate room for improvement.

Scores of 6 to 8: Your health practices in this area are good, but there is room for improvement. Look again at the items you answered with a "Sometimes" or "Almost Never." What changes can you make to improve your score? Even a small change can often help you achieve better health.

Scores of 3 to 5: Your health risks are showing! Would you like more information about the risks you are facing and why it is important for you to change these behaviors? Perhaps you need help in deciding how to successfully make the changes you desire. In either case, help is available.

Scores of 0 to 2: Obviously, you were concerned enough about your health to take the test, but your answers show that you may be taking serious and unnecessary risks with your health. Perhaps you are not aware of the risks and what to do about them. You can easily get the information and help you need to improve—if you wish. The next step is up to you.

Source: Test developed by United States Public Health Service. National Health Information Clearinghouse, Washington, D.C.

Table 4-7. Schedule for Childhood Immunizations

Disease	Number of doses	Age for first series	Booster
Diphtheria Tetanus Pertussis (whooping cough)	5 doses (DTP)	2 months 4 months 6 months 18 months 4–6 years	At 4–6 years, before entering school, as recommended by physician, 14–16 years, and every 10 years thereafter
Rubella (German measles)	1 vaccination (MMR)*	15 months*	None
Measles	1 vaccination (MMR)*	15 months*	None
Mumps	1 vaccination (MMR)*	15 months*	None
Polio (oral vaccine)	4 doses (OPV)	2 months 4 months 6 months** 18 months	At 4–6 years, before entering school, as recommended by physician
Haemophilus influenza	1 vaccination (Hib)	18 months	None
Tuberculosis		May be recommended at 1 year	
Tetanus and Diphtheria (adult type) toxoid	1 dose (Td)	14–16 years	Repeat every 10 years

*Rubella, measles, and mumps vaccines can be given in a combined form at about 15 months of age with a single injection (MMR).

**Trivalent oral polio vaccine may be given in areas of high poliomyelitis epidemicity.

eases have an acute phase earlier in life and then reappear at a later time. For example, an individual who had rheumatic fever as a child may now demonstrate such symptoms as shortness of breath, weakness, and swelling of ankles and feet.

The mental status of the client is next to be discussed. Often clients will not volunteer such information because mental illness is still considered by some to have a social stigma. Ask the client if he has ever had a nervous breakdown, frequent crying spells, depression, or emotional problems. If he has, you must examine the course of the illness, precipitating factors, and treatment.

Information related to all past surgical procedures is an important part of the history. The dates of all operations and the places where they were performed should be recorded. This information is often essential in evaluating the client's present situation. Many times clients who have had surgery know little about the exact nature of the operation or the findings. Transcripts of the client's chart should be sought if more information is needed. This same kind of inquiry should be made regarding all major injuries.

The surgical history of the client should include every operation he has ever undergone, including a tonsillectomy. All operations should be dated and the recovery period following surgery explored. The client should also be asked if he has ever had a blood transfusion and, if so, when, why, how many, and whether there were any adverse reactions. The client should then be asked whether he has ever had any traumatic injuries or has been involved in an accident. In-

Checklist for Previous Experience with Illness

Childhood illnesses
Immunizations
Allergies—type, response
Past illnesses
Surgery
Blood transfusions
Trauma

quiry as to whether he has ever been seen or treated in an emergency room may stimulate recall of such injuries. Remember, every bit of information that the client is able to offer may have a bearing on the diagnosis and subsequent planning for the current problem.

Review of Systems

The purpose of the review of systems is to be sure that no important clues have been overlooked by the client or nurse. If, in the history of present illness, you have already reviewed one or more systems, do not review them again. Some of the questions will seem repetitive and annoying to clients, so make sure you explain the purpose of the review. If the client identifies one or more symptoms that have not previously come to light, they should be explored in depth. The review should eventually be memorized, but the beginning nurse interviewer might use 3 × 5 cards for some assistance. The absence as well as the presence of symptoms should be recorded. In the example that follows, the review is stated in terms understandable to the general population. In the recording of these data, medical terminology is used, so we have included medical terms in parentheses.

1. *General health.* Ask whether the client has now or has lately experienced any: fever, weight loss, being easily fatigued, weakness, mood changes, night sweats, profuse perspiration (diaphoresis), intolerance to heat or cold, excessive thirst (polydipsia), being easily bruised, or bleeding tendencies.
2. *Skin, hair, and nails.* Has he had a history of skin diseases, changes in skin pigmentation, excessive dryness or moisture, jaundice, eczema, psoriasis, dandruff (seborrhea), hives, acne, rashes, bruising (ecchymosis), itching (pruritus), moles (nevi) that have changed in color or size, open sores that are slow to heal, itchy scalp, frequent loss of hair, hirsutism, nail biting?
3. *Head.* Unusually frequent or severe headaches, trauma?
4. *Eyes.* History of infections, visual changes, eye pain, double vision (diplopia), blurring, excessive tearing (lacrimation), sensitivity to light (photophobia), itching, spots in front of eyes or halo-rainbows around things? Does he wear glasses? For near or far vision? Bifocals? When was his last eye examination?
5. *Ears.* History of infections, loss of hearing, pain, discharge, ringing in the ears (tinnitus), hearing noises, dizziness?
6. *Nose, nasopharynx, and paranasal sinuses.* Discharge, frequent colds, nosebleeds (epistaxis), allergies, loss or poor sense of smell, obstruction, postnasal drip, pain, tenderness?
7. *Mouth and throat.* Bleeding gums; frequent sore throat; soreness or lesion of the mouth, lips, or tongue; persistent white spots in the mouth; difficulty swallowing (dysphagia); voice change; hoarseness; toothaches; cavities (dental caries)? Does he wear dentures? When was his last dental appointment? What are his dental hygiene practices?
8. *Neck.* Pain, swelling (edema), limitation of movement, swollen glands?
9. *Breasts.* Nipple discharge, scaling and cracks (fissures) around nipples, dimpling of skin, masses, pain (mastodynia), skin discoloration or lesions, practice of SBE (self-breast examination)?
10. *Cardiorespiratory system.* Swelling, persistent cough, frequent pneumonia, sputum, shortness of breath (differentiate between dyspnea, orthopnea, and paroxysmal nocturnal dyspnea), pain in the chest, palpitation, fainting (syncope), wheezing,

coughing up blood (hemoptysis), high blood pressure, anemia, heart attack, murmur, varicosities? Does he know anyone with TB? Has he ever had a chest x-ray? an EKG? When? Results?

11. *Gastrointestinal system.* Nausea, vomiting, loss of appetite (anorexia), indigestion (dyspepsia), heartburn (pyrosis), food intolerance, bright blood in stools, tarry-black stools (melena or iron supplements?), gas (flatulence), pain, diarrhea, constipation, piles (hemorrhoids), rectal pain? What are his bowel habits (every day, every third day, etc.), color of stool, consistency of stool (hard, soft, formed, liquid)?
12. *Genitourinary system.* Frequency, urgency, urination at night (nocturia), difficulty in starting stream, blood in urine (hematuria), dribbling, unable to control bladder (incontinent), pain or burning upon urination, excessive amounts of each urination (polyuria)? Has he had a venereal disease (may need to be said in lay terms, i.e., gonorrhea—"clap," "morning drip"; syphilis—"bad blood")?

    For male clients: Any penile discharge? Are you able to have erection, ejaculation? Are you sexually active? Does sex play an important role in your life? "Clients with your illness (excessive stress, diabetes, alcoholism, renal shutdown on dialysis, neurosis, schizophrenia, heavy drug use, priapism, neurologic damage) or on medications like yours (antispasmodics, antihypertensives, tranquilizers, narcotics, psychotropics) often have difficulty in sexual functioning. How has this influenced your life?"
13. *Gynecologic and obstetric.* Menarche (onset age of menstruation), last menstrual period (L.M.P.), regularity of cycle, duration of menstrual flow, volume (amount) of daily flow, painful menstruation (dysmenorrhea), bleeding between periods (metorrhagia), excessive bleeding (menorrhagia), bleeding following intercourse, pain during intercourse (dyspareunia), vaginal discharge (color, amount, consistency), vaginal pruritus, number of pregnancies (para), live births (gravida), any labor or delivery or after-delivery (puerperium) complications, abortions (spontaneous or induced; gestation), stillbirths, method of birth control, menopause (treatment)?
14. *Musculoskeletal system.* Muscular pain, swelling, lameness, weakness, soreness in joints, leg cramps, flat feet, arthritis, broken bones (fractures), dislocations, sprains, congenital defects? Corrections?
15. *Neurologic system.* Unconsciousness, difficulty walking, nervousness, anxiety, fits or spells (convulsion, seizure), dizziness (vertigo), pain in the arms or legs, paralysis, numbness, tingling, burning, "crawling" sensations (anywhere in body), decreased strength in arms or legs, weakness on one side of the body, unclear thinking, forgetfulness, nightmares, tremors, changes in emotional state, speech problems?

Checklist for Review of Systems (ROS)

General health
Integument
Head and neck
Breasts
Cardiorespiratory
Gastrointestinal
Genitourinary
Gynecologic/obstetric
Musculoskeletal
Neurologic

Client Profile

The client profile is a brief summary of your impression of the client based on the information obtained during the process of gathering the health history. It serves to personalize the data and to communicate a concise picture of the total person. Examples of client profiles are given in Figure 4-3.

Summary

In this chapter the health history was discussed in detail. Elements of the client interview and the components of the health history were pre-

Client profile: Ms. J. is a 29-year-old Caucasian woman who appeared anxious during the interview. This was noted in her inability to maintain eye contact and constant wringing of her hands. She expressed concern because she has no health insurance.

Client profile: Mr. G. is a 38-year-old Black male who appeared calm and comfortable during the interview. He has a good understanding of his current health status. His reason for seeking health assessment is for health maintenance.

Figure 4-3 Examples of client profiles.

sented, as well as the rationale and techniques for careful recording of biographical data and the chief complaint. Guidelines to enhance the investigation of signs and symptoms were discussed. Emphasis was placed on the sensitivity needed in exploring the personal history and the five specific areas within this portion of the history. The chapter concluded with investigating previous experiences with illness and a detailed description of the review of systems. The information gathered in each of the component areas of the health history is useful for interpreting the client's present status and for planning individualized nursing care. An example of a completed health history is provided.

Discussion Questions/Activities

1. What is the purpose of the health history?
2. Give examples to demonstrate the use and purpose of the specific information included in the biographical data section of the health history.
3. Describe how the chief complaint is recorded.
4. List and discuss Morgan and Engel's seven variables of investigating present illness.
5. What information would you obtain relating to the client's personal history and patterns of living?
6. What is the rationale for the review of systems?
7. Why is it important to identify pertinent negatives in the health history recording, particularly with the review of systems and the family health history?
8. Role play and videotape an initial interaction with a client; then critique it in regard to the principles inherent in the three phases of the interview structure.

Checklist for Health History

1. Biographical Data
   - Name
   - Address
   - Sex
   - Age/birth date
   - Marital status/compatibility and adjustment
   - Current occupation
   - Religion/practice and attitude toward religion
   - Race
   - Ethnic origin
   - Level of education/ability to read and write
   - Health history informant and reliability
2. Reason for Seeking Health Evaluation or Chief Complaint
   - Annual check-up
   - Employment health clearance
   - Follow-up care and evaluation
   - Signs and symptoms that led client to seek health care
   - Monitoring of existing health problem(s)
3. Current Health Status or History of Present Illness
   - Location
   - Quality
   - Quantity
   - Chronology
   - Setting
   - Aggravating and alleviating factors
   - Associated manifestations
   - Effect on ADLs and other life areas
   - Review of relevant body system(s)
4. Personal History and Patterns of Living
   - Occupational history
   - Financial status
   - Family history of illness/past and present
   - Pertinent negatives of specific illness in family
   - Example: No history of hypertension, strokes, TB, ulcers, mental illness, alcoholism, epilepsy, gout, bleeding disorders
   - Significant for diabetes, heart disease, cancer, arthritis, ulcerative colitis
   - Geographic exposure
     - Places
     - Date and length of time
   - Lifestyle
     - Sexuality
       - Values
       - Self-image
       - Sexual functioning
       - Sexual problems
     - Personal habits
       - Smoking—type and pack years
       - Alcohol—type and amount
       - Drugs—type, amount, and pattern of use
     - Diet
       - Mealtimes
       - Prepared by
       - Special diet/type and when started
       - Vitamins and/or diet pills
       - Specific difficulties
     - Sleep and rest patterns
       - Hours of sleep and awakening
       - Naps
       - Difficulties/remedies tried
     - Activities of daily living
     - Home and neighborhood
       - Living arrangements/resources
       - Quality of interpersonal relationships
     - Recreation/hobbies
5. Previous Experience with Illness
   - Childhood illnesses
   - Immunizations
   - Allergies—type, response
   - Past illnesses
   - Surgery
   - Blood transfusions
   - Trauma
6. Review of Systems (ROS)
   - General health
   - Integument
   - Head and neck
   - Breasts
   - Cardiorespiratory
   - Gastrointestinal
   - Genitourinary
   - Gynecologic/obstetric
   - Musculoskeletal
   - Neurologic
7. Client Profile

EXAMPLE OF A HEALTH HISTORY

Name: Mary Jones
Address: 234 Any Street, Anytown, Anystate
Sex: Female
Age: 35
Birthday: 7/17/57
Marital status: Married—states "happily married"
Occupation: Part-time clerk in variety store
Religion: Protestant (attends church on irregular basis)
Race: Caucasian
Ethnic origin: Polish
Education: High school graduate
Informant: Client; reliable historian
Chief concern: Lump in left breast of two days duration

History of present illness: Client first noticed lump in left breast two days ago while bathing. Denies pain or tenderness. No history of trauma to the area. Describes lump as being soft and about the size of peach pit. States there has been no change in the size of her breasts and no skin discoloration. Denies nipple drainage. Very anxious concerning the "lump" as mother died of breast cancer in 1968. Client feels she is in good health except for the "lump." Knowledgeable of SBE procedure but does it sporadically.

Personal history and patterns of living: Has worked part-time as a clerk in a variety store for 4 years (yard goods dept.). Prior to this time remained home caring for family since birth of first child in 1978. Husband employed at steel company (salary: $29,500). Her salary: $8,000. Describes financial status as adequate for personal and family needs. Two-car family with $36,000 house mortgage. No unusual debts. Blue Cross and Blue Shield Health Insurance.

Family health history: Denies family history of diabetes, arthritis, TB, alcoholism, bleeding disorders, mental illness, stomach problems, liver disorders, kidney diseases. Family history significant for cancer, heart disease, hypertension.

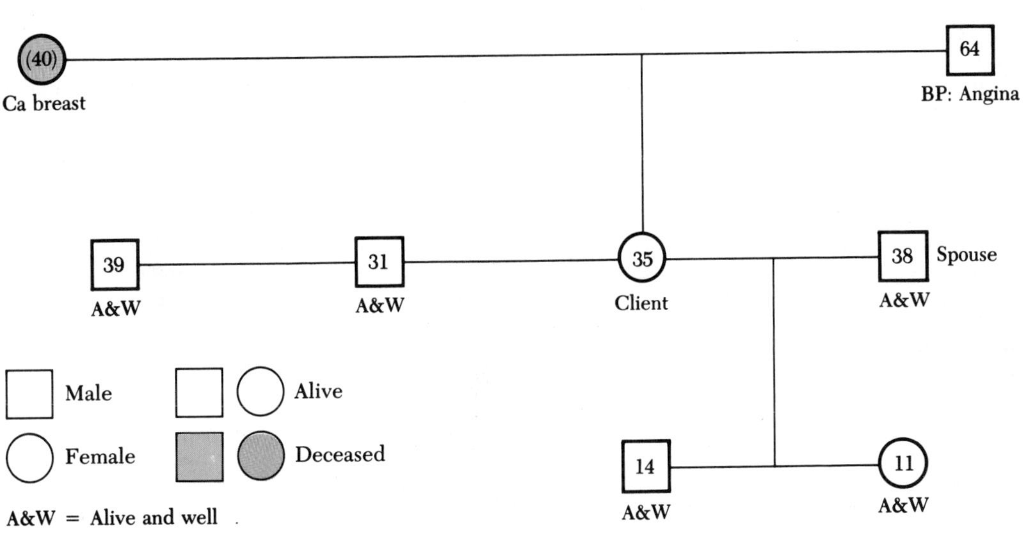

Geographic exposure: Has never traveled out of state.

Lifestyle:

1. Sexuality—traditional values of monogamy. Worried about image as woman as she states "I am worried how my husband will react if I must have a mastectomy." Satisfactory sexual activity—no expressed difficulties.
2. Personal habits—Smokes 1½ ppd (25½ pk yrs.). Beer or whiskey—no more than 3 drinks at the most. Takes over-the-counter cold pills (2 × /yr) when necessary. Coffee—4 cups/day. Coke—2 bottles/day.

(continued on page 90)

3. Diet—Client does most of cooking. Family eats three meals/day. Breakfast—fruit, coffee, toast. Lunch—(brown bag) sandwich, cookies, buys ice cream and coke in vending machine. Dinner—meat (5×/wk), potatoes or noodles, bread, vegetable (beans, peas), dessert almost every night (cookies, cake). Family usually snacks at bedtime (crackers, chips). Denies dieting or diet pills. Occasionally takes multi-vits during cold weather. No apparent difficulty with diet, i.e., no indigestion or swallowing difficulties.
4. Sleep and rest patterns—Denies any sleeping difficulties in general but since discovery of lump in breast has awakened several times in the past night and had difficulty falling back asleep. Usually sleeps 7½–8 hrs/day.
5. Activities of daily living—No difficulties caring for self and carrying out her responsibilities of living.
6. Home and neighborhood—Home in middle-class neighborhood. Living arrangements more than sufficient for family needs (2 bathrooms, each child has own bedroom).
7. Interpersonal relationships—Describes family relationships as close and very good. No family tensions. Keeps close to extended family members on both sides of the family. Annual family reunions.
8. Recreation—No regular active recreation. Watches TV most evenings. Picnics on Sunday afternoons during the summer months. Likes to knit.

Previous experience with illness:
Childhood illnesses: Measles, chickenpox, scarlet fever, rheumatic fever (not sure of exact age—10?).
Immunizations: Smallpox (age 6); oral polio vaccine (1969).
Allergies: Denies any known allergies.
Past illness, injuries, surgery: No significant illnesses or injuries until car accident (1978) in which she sustained concussion, broken nose, and multiple bruises to both legs. Was hospitalized 5 days. Appendectomy (1975).

Review of systems:
1. General health—Denies weight loss, fatigue, weakness, changes in mood, night sweats, diaphoresis, intolerance to cold, polydipsia, being easily bruised, and bleeding tendencies.
2. Integument—No history of skin diseases. Denies any changes in skin pigmentation, excessive dryness or moisture, jaundice, eczema, psoriasis or seborrhea, hives, acne, rashes, ecchymosis, pruritis, nevi that have changed in color or size, open sores that are slow to heal, itchy scalp, frequent loss of hair, and nail biting.
3. Head—Denies unusually frequent or severe headaches. Concussion (1978)—see past injuries (car accident).
4. Eyes—No history of infections or pain. Wears eyeglasses for close work. Last eye exam 1991. Denies diplopia, blurring, excessive lacrimation, photophobia, pruritis, and spots before eyes or halo-rainbows about lights. Has eye exam every 2 years.
5. Ears—No history of infections. Denies loss of hearing, pain, discharge, tinnitus, auditory hallucinations, and vertigo.
6. Nose, nasopharynx, and paranasal sinuses—No discharge, colds 1–2×/yr. Denies epistaxis, allergies, loss of smell, obstruction, postnasal drip, pain and tenderness.
7. Mouth and throat—Denies bleeding gums, frequent sore throat, soreness of the mouth, lips, or tongue, dysphagia, voice change, hoarseness, toothaches, dentures. Last dentist appointment—can't remember: "long ago." Visits dentist only when experiencing dental "problems." Brushes and flosses every A.M.
8. Neck—Denies pain, edema, limitation of movement, swollen glands.
9. Breasts—(see HPI).
10. Cardiorespiratory system—Nonproductive morning cough since 1977. Last chest x-ray in 1978 (neg.). No history of pneumonia. Denies sputum, dyspnea, orthopnea, and PND. No chest pain, palpitation, syncope, wheezing, hemoptysis, or contact with anyone having TB. No history of anemia, heart attack, and varicosities. Was told she had slight murmur when given physical examination in high school; no follow-up on this was ever done.
11. Gastrointestinal system—Denies nausea and vomiting, anorexia, dyspepsia, pyrosis, food intolerance, bright blood in stools, melena, flatulence, pain, hemorrhoids and rectal pain. Soft formed brown stool every AM after hot coffee.
12. Genitourinary system—Denies frequency, urgency, nocturia, difficulty in starting stream, hematuria, dribbling, incontinence, pain or burning upon urination, polyuria, and VD. Sexually active 2×/wk and is satisfied with sex life.
13. Gynecologic and obstetric—Menarche age 12. LMP 2/22/87. Reg. 28-day cycle. Flow duration of 5 days—1st day heavy flow (4 pads) (av. 3 tampons other days). Denies dysmenorrhea, metorrhagia, menorrhagia, dyspareunia, bleeding following intercourse, vaginal discharge, and mastodynia. Para 2, gravida 2. No labor or puerperal complications. No abortions. Birth control—uses diaphragm.

14. Musculoskeletal system—Denies muscular pain, edema, lameness, weakness, joint soreness or pain, leg cramps, flat feet, arthritis, fractures (other than nose in 1978 car accident), dislocation, sprains, and congenital defects.

15. Neurologic system—No history of unconsciousness. Denies difficulty walking, convulsions, vertigo, pain in arms or legs, numbness, paralysis, tingling or burning anywhere in body, decreased strength in arms or legs, weakness in one part of the body, nightmares, tremors, changes in emotional states, and speech problems. Has felt nervous and anxious past 2 days since discovered lump in breast. Some forgetfulness manifested during these past 2 days.

Client profile: Mrs. Mary Jones, 35-year-old female, appears apprehensive. Speech is rapid; logical thought processes. Tears in eyes. Very concerned about breast lump due to mother's cancer of breast and subsequent death at age 40. Otherwise appears in good health generally. Seems anxious for help.

CHAPTER 5

Mental Health Assessment

LEARNING OBJECTIVES

1. List the seven (7) mental functions by which to assess mental functioning.
2. Identify the various levels of consciousness.
3. Discuss the techniques used to assess mental functioning.
4. Describe examples of maturational and situational crises.
5. Describe Kübler-Ross's stages of dying.
6. Recognize signs and symptoms and areas of assessment for situations involving violence, addiction, and loss or impending death.
7. Describe behaviors significant of mild to extreme anxiety states.
8. State the principles important in interactions with depressed and/or suicidal clients.

Everyone has his "ups" and "downs" and his "good" and "bad" days. The key to health is a happy medium—a balance. As we saw in Chapter 1, stress has a tremendous impact on this equilibrium. Both body and mind attempt to cope with the impact of stress through their own protective means. The body musters up energy stores and the mind makes increased use of mental defense mechanisms. The mentally healthy person uses these protective devices to regain homeostasis and is able to function socially; he constructively deals with major tragedies by overcoming misfortunes and using them beneficially. It is when these protective devices fail to recapture homeostasis that illness or an "unhealthy" state exists. In mental illness these signs and symptoms of dysfunction are part of the client's life and interfere with his ability to function socially.

What is mental health? What constitutes a state of mental well-being? Are there criteria available to assess a client's presence of or lack of mental illness? To date no concrete definition exists for the term *mental health*. However, the general consensus is that a mentally healthy individual is one who is able to perform the tasks required by his culture, has the ability to maintain social relationships, and is able to establish and maintain intimate relationships. Mental health does not mean that there is freedom from stressors. The mentally healthy individual is the individual who actively practices coping strategies and is able to face life's problems.

While many attempts have been made at defining mental health, the surfacing factor in each of these definitions is that an assessment of mental health of an individual is made in the context of his or her culture or subculture. For instance, in the eyes of the assessor, folkways and home remedies, such as those of the rural Appalachians, may seem detrimental, and ways of coping with stress or crisis may appear as defeating the purpose or even maladaptive. However, when taken in the cultural context of the client, the behavior and coping mechanisms appear to be adaptive, and the client is fully functioning and mentally healthy.

Of course, the presence of signs and symptoms of dysfunction may not necessarily indicate mental illness but in fact may represent a means of coping with a temporary stress situation. The assessment of the client's mental health must encompass not only the signs and symptoms of dysfunction but also their preponderance, degree of severity, duration, and extent of interference with social functioning.

Additional data from the client's health history will shed light on the mental health assessment. The historical background provides a dynamic perspective for the survey of the nature of the client's current behavior. A review of the client's history in terms of previous personality and characteristic modes of behavior should reveal adaptations that the client has made to life stresses (medical and nonmedical) in the past. The history will indicate whether the client has a family history or past medical history of mental illness, whether he has demonstrated an ability to form close relationships, how he views himself, the nature of his interpersonal relationships, his degree of dependence-independence, his existing and available support systems, and his degree of successful living (jobs, family, friends/scope). These are aspects that are investigated with every client.

Mental status is evaluated whenever you have multiple interview sessions or subsequent interactions with a client. It is important to remember that because of stress, the client's emotional state may be markedly different from one contact to another. Thus, mental health assessment is an ongoing process—it is never "complete," except for the moment. Method and approach are important. You need to be aware that relentless searching for "psychopathology" can prove to be a barrier to further assessment and can only serve to anger and alienate the client.

Mental Functioning

The evaluation of mental functioning is part of the mental health assessment. Because mental functioning is an internal process, it is not directly available to observation; therefore, you need to assess it indirectly by analyzing the *ABC's* of observable data: *appearance, behavior,* and *conversation.* In most cases you will have gathered adequate observable data on the client's appearance, behavior, and conversation in the routine course of interviewing to serve as a base to assess his mental functioning. This assessment is accomplished by viewing the client's appearance, behavior, and conversation in relation to seven mental functions:

1. *Attitude.* What is the general overall presentation of the client's behavior? How cooperative is he? Does he engage in solitary activity? Parallel activity? Group activity? What is the extent of his participation in interpersonal relationships?
2. *Affect/mood.* Affect is the emotional state of the client—the way he *appears* to others. Mood is what the client *says* in regard to how he is "feeling"—happy, sad, and so on. Is the client's affect appropriate to the situation? For example, a client who walked about with a constant grin would be displaying inappropriate affect and would not be experiencing his total environment. Appearance may belie feelings. When this happens—as when the client feigns cheerfulness when he actually feels depressed—the affect and mood are in disharmony. Are mood swings present—does the client cry one minute and laugh the next?
3. *Speech characteristics.* Does the client's speech include circumstantiality, scattering, a loosening of thought associations, a degree of vagueness, a tendency to overgeneralize, the use of global pronouns lacking specific

referents (terms such as "they" and "them"), and an inability to describe participation in an experience? These are some of the characteristics of speech that help you to detect the presence or absence of difficulties with thought processes.

4. *Thought processes.* Does the client's conversation flow in a logical sequence? Does his conversation make sense? How does the client experience the world around him? Is he in contact with reality? Does he experience hallucinations (sensory impressions that lack external stimuli)? Does he experience delusions (false beliefs not based on fact)?
5. *Sensorium and reasoning.* Is the client aware of his immediate situation? Is he alert? Is he oriented to time, place, and person? Do his recent and remote memories appear to be intact? Is he able to perform simple calculations? Is he able to conceptualize and make appropriate judgments? Does he understand his condition and the situation in which he finds himself? Does he know things that would be considered common knowledge?
6. *Potential for danger.* Does the client display a positive self-concept? Has he ever thought about harming or has he actually harmed himself or others? Does he have a history of uncontrollable temper? Has he ever been in trouble with the law? Is he able to cope with situations that are not to his liking? What life stresses has he experienced? How has he handled or responded to these?
7. *Psychological assets.* The outcome of an illness depends as much on the client's assets as on the nature of the pathology. Does the client have a positive self-image? a repertoire of coping mechanisms? interested and supportive significant others? financial stability? satisfying interests and hobbies? the ability to get along with others?

If, after evaluating your ABC data in light of the seven mental functions, you suspect mental dysfunction, you will need to carefully pursue a more detailed investigation. Signs of disturbances in the client's sensorium, thought processes, or interpersonal relationships would prompt you to further investigate these specific aspects of mental functioning. This investigation requires more extensive techniques designed specifically for securing an in-depth evaluation. These special techniques are inherent in the following discussions of each of the ABC's of mental status and functioning.

Manifestations of Mental Dysfunction

We will now examine the ABC's of mental health assessment: appearance, behavior, and conversation. Each of these areas can provide insight into the client's mental functioning.

Appearance

An individual's general appearance can reveal a great deal about him. However, it must be kept in mind that the description of a client is highly subjective. To exaggerate, a nurse who is as "neat as a pin" may view the "open collar" client as carelessly dressed; a nurse who is a casual dresser may describe the "neat as a pin" client as being obsessed with neatness.

Note the client's body build. Is he or she short, tall, shapely, thin, obese, muscular? Body build may have significant influence on the client's self-esteem and behavior. Body communication is also important to notice. Is the client's posture relaxed, tense, erect, or slouched? A tense, erect posture accompanied by laughter, fidgeting, or tremors may indicate anxiety. You may want to consider the possibility of thyrotoxicosis when such anxiety symptoms exist.

Does the client appear unkempt, careless, and dirty, or is he clean, neat, and tidy? An unkempt appearance often occurs with chronic organic brain disorder and with certain neuroses and psychoses. A severe physical condition or physical handicap could also be responsible for what may appear to be neglect of physical appearance.

Is the client dressed appropriately for the occasion and for his age? Is the dress appropriately applied? For example, clients with chronic organic brain syndrome often have difficulty dressing themselves and may apply their outer garments first and their undergarments on top. The colors of the client's clothing, whether bright or subdued, often tell the nurse something about his personality. Eccentric combinations in dress and inappropriate use of cosmetics are commonly found in clients with schizophrenic or manic personalities.

Is the client's facial expression mobile, fixed,

Checklist for Mental Health Assessment: Appearance

This table presents a *range* of signs and symptoms that *may suggest* dysfunction. They are not in themselves necessarily reflective of mental illness, nor are they all necessarily confined to a specific area of appearance, but may overlap with behavior and conversation.

Mental functions	Appearance	Mental functions	Appearance
1. Attitude a. Cooperativeness b. Interpersonal relationships	Client is aloof, unclean, disheveled, indifferent	4. Thought processes a. Logical b. Coherent c. Perceptual	Client is inattentive, easily distracted, preoccupied
2. Affect/mood a. Appropriate b. Harmony c. Swings	Client has masklike face; is apathetic, flat, rigid, labile, euphoric, depressed, suspicious, hostile; displays inappropriate affect; shows physical signs of anxiety (flushing, sweating, tremors, respirations)	5. Sensorium and reasoning a. Levels of consciousness b. Orientation c. Memory (recent, remote) d. Calculation e. Abstract thinking f. Judgment/ insight g. Intelligence	Client displays decreased or absent physiologic reflexes, disinterest, peculiarity of dress, bewilderment
3. Speech characteristics a. Description b. Speed c. Quantity	Client is soft-spoken, loud, boisterous; has monotonous, slow, or rapid speech	6. Potential for danger a. Self-concept b. Harm to self/ others	Client is docile, sad, hostile, angry, apathetic
		7. Client's psychologic assets	Few or no physical assets

bland, furrowed, tense, worried, sad, angry, sneering, suspicious, in pain, frightened, dreamy, laughing, smiling? A flat, masklike face may be a sign of parkinsonism or of certain psychoses.

If possible, you should also make observations when the client is unaware of being observed. Under such circumstances, the client may manifest a different appearance. For instance, a client who is normally quite animated and abrasive may be overly docile and polite in an assessment interview, where he is under close scrutiny. It is important to recognize that clients often act and appear in a particular manner in order to please the nurse and significant others.

Behavior

One of the best indicators of the degree of mental functioning is the *level of consciousness.* There are four basic levels:

1. Conscious and alert.
2. Obtundent—has slowed mental processes, lethargy, sleepiness.
3. Semicomatose or stupor—is unconscious but can be aroused sufficiently to respond to verbal commands.
4. Comatose or unconscious—cannot be aroused; does not respond to painful stimuli; often has accompanying abnormal reflexes and respirations.

Structural (organic) brain damage that would alter the client's level of consciousness can result from vascular pathology, alcoholic psychoses, toxic psychoses (particularly drug induced), general paresis, meningitis, encephalitis, brain tumors, head injuries, and degenerative disorders (adult hydrocephalus, Pick's disease, Alzheimer's disease, Huntington's chorea).

Any situation that alters the normal electrolyte content and pH of the body (acidosis and alkalosis) affects the level of consciousness. Such situations include hypoglycemia, starvation, persistent vomiting, dehydration, cardiorespiratory disease, renal disease, cirrhosis, burns, pyrexia, and use of illicit drugs or improper use of prescribed medications. A cloudy sensorium and confusion are more frequently related to toxic or structural damage than to functional (psychodynamic) factors.

The client's state of orientation should be determined. Is he oriented in the three spheres—person, place, and time? Disorientation in place and person implies cerebral disorder. Such disorientation is commonly observed in elderly clients with circulatory impairments and cerebral degeneration due to the aging process. Coupled with these circulatory and degenerative changes is cerebral hypoxia, observed in elderly clients undergoing general anesthesia. Many an oriented elderly client is sent to surgery only to return postoperatively in a disoriented state of mind caused by hypoxia.

Radical change in environment (from home to hospital room to operating room to recovery room to intensive care unit, and so on) adds to a client's disorientation. Hospitalization and other forms of institutionalization, as well as the separation from one's home and loved ones, upsets the client's routine activities. Without the predictability of these daily activities, the client may become bewildered. He is faced with a new set of stimuli that are strange and sometimes frightening.

Disorientation can also result from sensory deprivation. Sensory deprivation can occur following ocular surgery, because of the bandages covering the client's eyes, or as a result of isolation, flotation therapy, or immobilization. Again, the elderly individual in our society is more prone to disorientation and other mental disorders because of developmentally related circumstances, such as the loss of spouse and friends by death, social isolation, job retirement, financial deprivation, decreased physical capacity, and decreased resistance, resulting in acute and chronic illnesses.

Dysfunctional behavior patterns are most likely to be detected or suspected during the routine history-taking process. Difficulties may become apparent when investigating such areas as employment, school, and family life. Problems with interpersonal relationships may emerge in exploring the client's ability to work with others, his attitude toward his employer or teachers, his attitude toward rules and regulations, his aspirations, and his attitudes toward his parents.

In assessing the client's family dynamics it may be helpful to ask the client to compare himself to his siblings in regard to role, responsibilities, aggressiveness, passivity, intelligence, success, failure, likes, dislikes, and so on. Such conditions among family members as alcoholism, drug dependency, antisocial personality, mental retardation, and psychopathology may be revealed at this time. At this point you may also want to discuss significant life crises and the client's response to them (adaptation/coping patterns).

If the client reveals sexual problems during the sexual history or if such problems emerge while you are investigating his relationships with others and his lifestyle, you should try to determine their etiology in order to best direct further exploration. Sexual problems can result from physical illness, surgery, neuroses, psychoses, and behavioral management problems. Behavioral management problems tend to produce sexual promiscuity, whereas the other etiologies tend to result in a decrease or cessation of sexual activity. For example, the schizophrenic client, who has unstable interpersonal relationships, is actually fearful of getting too close to anyone; even the thought of sexual contact with another may be terrifying to him.

Cadoret and King (1974) have categorized some specific psychiatric syndromes into three groups of behaviors. Following are the three groups and some examples (for further elaboration see their text, *Psychiatry in Primary Care*):

1. *Recent changes in personality or behavior:* (a) Forgetfulness, emotional lability, disorientation, inattentiveness, decreased alertness (organic brain syndrome). (b) Inattentiveness, temper outbursts, poor grades, school truancy (drug abuse or dependency).
2. *Lifelong, often chronic, difficulties in behavior:* Home and school discipline problems, sexual promiscuity, poor job history, trouble with the law, drug and alcohol abuse (antisocial personality).
3. *Medical symptoms:* (a) Somatic preoccupation, fatigue, headaches, anorexia, constipation, weight loss, insomnia, decreased libido (depressive syndrome). (b) Intermittent attacks of cardiac symptoms and fear; rarely beginning after age 40 and commonly seen in the emergency room setting (anxiety neurosis).

Jenkins (1971) suggests that there may be psy-

Checklist for Mental Health Assessment: Behavior

This table presents a *range* of signs and symptoms that *may suggest* dysfunction. They are not in themselves necessarily reflective of mental illness, nor are they all necessarily confined to a specific area of behavior but may overlap with appearance and conversation.

Mental functions	Behavior	Mental functions	Behavior
1. Attitude a. Cooperativeness b. Interpersonal relationships	Client is negativistic, uncooperative, hostile, belligerent, passive, drooping, withdrawn, impulsive; has slow gait	4. Thought processes a. Logical b. Coherent c. Perceptual	Client avoids anxiety, displays phobic behavior, compulsiveness, echopraxia
2. Affect/mood a. Appropriate b. Harmony c. Swings	Client is overactive, underactive; cries or laughs easily; wrings hands; paces floor; strikes head with hands; holds fixed posture for prolonged periods; has silly smile	5. Sensorium and reasoning a. Levels of consciousness b. Orientation c. Memory (recent, remote) d. Calculation e. Abstract thinking f. Judgment/insight g. Intelligence	Client displays stupor, lethargy, coma, confusion, agitation, delirium panic, twilight state, behavior problems, conduct disorder
3. Speech characteristics a. Description b. Speed c. Quantity	Client grimaces, stammers, stutters; displays uncoordinated or exaggerated movement, mutism, echolalia	6. Potential for danger a. Self-concept b. Harm to self/others	Client has made suicide attempts; is malingering, withdrawn, assaultive, combative, violent; lacks temper control; displays antisocial or criminal behavior (arrests), irritability, explosiveness, excitability, maladaptive coping
		7. Client's psychologic assets	Few or no behavioral assets

chological "risk factors" for coronary artery disease in addition to the established physical risk factors of age, sex, blood pressure, obesity, and cigarette smoking. Clients with coronary artery disease tend to be serious, shy, and conforming, but self-sufficient. In many cases they are experiencing rejection, marital difficulties, or general dissatisfaction with their job. Cassem and Hackett (1971) reported that nearly a third (32.7%) of clients admitted to a coronary care unit were referred for psychiatric consultation because of sexual acting-out, hostile behavior, and noncompliance with the treatment regimen, in addition to anxiety or depressive symptoms.

Conversation

Observing the content, manner, and process of the client's conversation is essential to the assessment of mental functioning. For example, the client with a depressive character disorder will have a pessimistic attitude and will avoid certain topics. Because guilt and self-hate are central to depression, the depressed client will tend to talk of guilt, sin, or unworthiness. You may notice disharmony between the client's affect and his thought content. For instance, the client may manifest silly behavior when his attitude should be one of concern.

Speech characteristics can be significant. A

client with manic psychosis will speak in a rapid, pressured manner, whereas a client who is depressed or has myxedema may speak in a slow monotone. The client with multiple sclerosis will have a staccato pattern of slurred speech.

While observing the client's conversation, the nurse should examine his stream of mental activity. Is his conversation appropriate? Is it consistent? Does he ramble, or is he able to proceed logically and to develop a point? Is his conversation spontaneous and coherent?

Exaggeration and confabulation (making up for memory gaps by substituting falsehoods) are characteristics of clients with Korsakoff's psychosis, amnesia, and other disorders in which clients attempt to hide their memory defects. A blocking or sudden stop in conversation for no apparent reason may result from preoccupation with or interference by delusional thoughts or hallucinations. Circumstantiality ("beating around the bush" before coming to the point) and tangentiality (going off on a tangent and never reaching the goal, despite refocusing by the interviewer) are manifestations of either neuroses or psychoses. Autistic speech (talking in one's own made-up language), incoherent speech, flight of ideas, and neologisms (self-coined words) are characteristic of schizophrenia.

Hallucinations can result not only from psychoses but from use of various drugs and can occur in delirium tremens, severe myxedema, uremia, and hepatic encephalopathy. A person who is very thirsty, very hungry, severely fatigued, or highly tense may also have hallucinations.

The client with a paranoid psychosis is quite concrete in his thinking and generally exhibits delusions of persecution. He will most likely be suspicious of you in the interview session. Delusions of influence or alien control (by other people or by strange voices) are more characteristic of the client with schizophrenia, as is the delusion that everyone knows what he is thinking.

Most of the client's sensorium and reasoning can be evaluated through analysis of conversation. The entire process of history-taking affords continuous opportunity for evaluating the client's memory. The reliability of the information received from the client can be checked by follow-up, cross-validation questioning, talking with friends and family, reading past records, and questioning other health personnel who have had contact with the client. These practices will aid in identifying confabulation and memory dysfunction. Loss of memory is an early sign of pathology of the cerebral cortex in general and of the temporal and occipital lobes in particular. Recent memories are those most affected, since remote memory is seldom disturbed and tends to survive disease. A specific test of recent memory is to give the client a name and address to remember. Have the client repeat the name and address until he has them memorized. Five minutes later, ask him to recall the information.

The loss of the ability to perform simple mental arithmetic calculations is a sensitive index of parietal lesions and diffuse cerebral disease. Depression, psychosis, and severe anxiety can also interfere with this intellectual function. You can indirectly test the client's ability to perform mental calculations by asking questions that require the client to calculate his age in a particular year or the number of years since a particular occasion. In this way you can avoid putting the client in a "testing" situation. Failure under a testing-type environment, which in itself usually promotes apprehension, might only serve to increase the anxiety level of the client.

If the client appears to have difficulty in calculation, you can tell him that you would like to test his ability to concentrate. Then ask the client to count forward by adding 3's (1 + 3 = 4, 4 + 3 = 7, 7 + 3 = 10, 10 + 3 = 13, . . .). In most cases, you need not go further than 22 or 25 in order to gauge his ability. Another commonly used test is to ask the client to start at 100 and subtract 7 from each successive answer (93, 86, 79, 72, 65, . . .). This test is known as "serial 7's."

The ability to think abstractly and to conceptualize can be reduced in advanced psychoses and in acute confusional states (inflammatory, metabolic, toxic, or traumatic cerebral disease). Such states also diminish a client's judgment and knowledge base (intelligence). Problems with abstract thinking can also be seen with amnesia, aphasia, schizophrenia, and brain lesions. Clients with such problems may have ideas but can't manipulate them, and their thinking tends to be quite literal. Abstract thinking is commonly fine-tested by asking the client, "What do these sayings mean to you?"

1. People in glass houses shouldn't throw stones.
2. Don't count your chickens before they're hatched.
3. A stitch in time saves nine.
4. No use crying over spilt milk.
5. A rolling stone gathers no moss.
6. You can lead a horse to water, but you can't make him drink.

Each set of two proverbs is at a higher level; numbers 5 and 6 require greater abstract thinking ability. A further test is to ask the client how the following terms are alike: coat/dress, axe/saw, table/chair.

If, in the context of conversation, the client seems to display poor judgment, you can further test this ability by saying that you would like to have him answer a few questions that you routinely ask all clients. Then ask such questions as: Why should people pay taxes? Why should a promise be kept? Why are laws necessary? Why do we have child labor laws? Why pay bills with checks?

During the history-taking session you can ease into assessing the client's general knowledge by asking the client whether he keeps up with the news. Most clients of average intelligence will be able to tell you the name of the president of the United States, the state governor, and the city mayor and will be able to answer such questions as "How many days in a week?" "Where does the sun set?" and "What animal does wool come from?"

Because impaired abstract thinking, judgment, and decision making tend to interfere

Checklist for Mental Health Assessment: Conversation

This table presents a *range* of signs and symptoms that *may suggest* dysfunction. They are not in themselves necessarily reflective of mental illness, nor are they all necessarily confined to a specific area of conversation but may overlap with appearance and behavior.

Mental functions	Conversation	Mental functions	Conversation
1. Attitude a. Cooperativeness b. Interpersonal relationships	Client avoids topics; is pessimistic	4. Thought processes a. Logical b. Coherent c. Perceptual	Client displays phobias, obsessions, paranoid ideas, illogical flow; has feelings of strangeness, depersonalization, hallucinations, delusions (somatic, grandeur, persecution, alien control)
2. Affect/mood a. Appropriate b. Harmony c. Swings	Client displays disharmony with thought processes; talks of guilt, sin, or unworthiness		
3. Speech characteristics a. Description b. Speed c. Quantity	Client displays exaggeration, confabulation, blocking of thought, circumstantiality, tangentiality, autistic speech, incoherence, flight of ideas; is overtalkative; uses neologisms	5. Sensorium and reasoning a. Levels of consciousness b. Orientation c. Memory (recent, remote) d. Calculation e. Abstract thinking f. Judgment/insight g. Intelligence	Client displays aphasia, memory defect, disorientation, poor judgment, lack of insight, inability of abstract thinking and calculations
		6. Potential for danger a. Self-concept b. Harm to self/others	Client has ideas of self-accusation and condemnation, self-depreciation, suicidal ideations
		7. Client's psychologic assets	Few or no conversational assets

greatly with the client's ability to function at his job and manage his household, examination of his work and home problems may further reveal such impairment.

Finally, you should try to determine whether the client's conversation reveals suicidal tendencies. You must be particularly alert for suicide when hyperactivity is coupled with low narcissism or when the client is severely depressed. With all clients you should inquire, tactfully and at an appropriate time, whether they have ever entertained the idea of suicide: "Are you sometimes so discouraged that you feel there is no use in going on?" "Are you ever troubled by thoughts of hurting yourself?" "Have you ever made plans to end it all?" It is also important to investigate avenues that may reveal antisocial behavior: "What kind of temper do you have?" "How do you get along with people?" "Do you feel you drink too much for your own good?"

In mental assessment it is quite helpful if you can observe the client interacting with family, with friends, and in other settings and to compare your interactions with the client to those of other health team members.

When you record the conclusions of the mental health assessment, including mental functioning, it is desirable to include verbatim wordings and body language samples. With mute clients, you need to keep in mind that they communicate by body language, so the main means you have of evaluating them is nonverbal behavior.

Crisis Assessment

Webster defines a crisis as "a turning point for better or worse in an acute disease or fever . . . or emotionally significant event or radical change of status in a person's life . . . the decisive moment . . . an unstable or crucial time or state of affairs."

A crisis can be the end of a decade, like turning 40, or a rite of passage, such as the onset of menstruation for the adolescent female. A crisis can be a marriage or a divorce. It can be a terminal illness diagnosis or an abused spouse or child. Crises range from happiness to violence.

Situational Crisis

Crises of this type arise when the environment in which the client lives is altered dramatically. The homeostasis of the individual is threatened, and bodily responses are usually generated. Three kinds of situational crises are violence, addiction, and loss.

Checklist for Assessing Crisis

1. Is the client's chief complaint indicative of internal discomfort?
2. Did the symptoms appear rapidly?
3. Will the situation take time to resolve?
4. Can you identify an event leading up to or contributing to the situation?
5. Does the client show any physical or behavioral signs of disturbance?

If the answers are yes, the client may be facing a crisis. Many times the client may only need support, someone to talk to who will listen and reflect both the content and feeling of the client's statements. In some cases, however, the crisis may become intense and referral for therapy may be warranted.

Violence

Victims of violent acts and of continuous physical and/or emotional abuse can be found in every community. They include the physically assaulted, rape victims, children who are verbally and physically punished or threatened into submission, spouses who stay in the home and allow beatings to continue out of fear for their safety or the safety of their children, and the elderly who are bullied, pushed, shoved, and sometimes beaten by other members of society, including their own children. Many times clients who experience physical violence show signs of repeated beatings or shovings. The telltale bruises, black eyes, multiple fractures, or missing teeth are clues that something is amiss. However, the verbal assaults and threats are more difficult to detect. Consider the child whose eyes fill with tears of fear or who cowers in the corner when his or her name is called. Also be suspect when the elderly grandparent begins to tremble or displays other symptoms of anxiety when you ask about his children, grandchildren, or neighbors. You may encounter, too, a middle-aged woman who insists on going home despite an extreme state of anxiety. These are only a few examples of violence crises and reactions. A screening tool for child abusers is seen in Figure 5-1.

Addictions

Addiction and crisis assessment usually consists of two components: the crisis of the addict and

Index of Suspicion: Screening for Child Abusers

Item	Index Score
1. *Attitude in dealing with staff*	
__ Irrationally hostile	3
__ Situationally hostile	1
__ Verbally paranoid (project all blame on others)	3
__ Combative	5
__ Abusive	5
2. *Family structure*	
__ Family together	0
__ Divorce	1
__ Separation exists	4
__ Child/parent role reversal	5
__ Foster home	3
__ One spouse deceased	1
__ Uncontrolled sibling rivalry	3
__ Rigid, compulsive structure	2
__ Loose, ill-defined structure	2
3. *Family problems (parental figures)*	
__ Alcoholism	5
__ Drug abuse	5
__ Frequent visitors to emergency ward	3
__ Evidence of sexual promiscuity	3
__ History of parental figures being abused as children	5
__ Chronic organizational problems in the home because of child	5
__ Psychiatric history	3
__ Unstable job pattern	5
__ Documented assault and/or battery	5
__ Hypertension	2
__ Ulcers	2
__ Past suicide attempt	5
4. *Religious affiliation*	
__ None	5
__ Strong	0
__ Lukewarm	2
5. *Labor and delivery*	
__ High-risk pregnancy	3
__ Low birth weight	5
__ Mental retardation in child, mother, or father figure	5
__ No prenatal care	5
__ Isolation from mother during newborn period	3
__ Born out of wedlock	5
6. *Cultural factors*	
__ Bicultural home	3
__ Interracial marriage	3

Item	Index Score
6. *Cultural factors (continued)*	
__ Patrilineal authority	5
__ Jewish	0
__ Caucasian	3
__ Black	3
__ Hawaiian	1
__ Polynesian	1
__ Chicano	2
__ Puerto Rican	2
__ First generation European immigrant	1
__ Arab	1
__ Matrilineal authority	3
__ Jewish	1
__ Caucasian	3
__ Black	1
__ Hawaiian	0
__ Polynesian	0
__ Chicano	0
__ Puerto Rican	1
__ First generation European immigrant	3
__ Arab	3
__ Metropolitan residency	4
__ Rural residency	2
7. *Child or siblings*	
__ Frequently admitted to hospital	5
__ Diagnosis:	
__ Long bone fractures	5
__ Head injuries	5
__ Hematomas	5
__ Failure to thrive	5
__ Malnourishment	3
__ Bruises (multiple) in various stages of healing	5
__ Multiple scratches	2
__ Burn sites, varying healing stage	5
__ Described by parent figures as discipline problems	5
__ One child or more under 3 years of age	3
__ Parents contradict themselves when describing illnesses and injuries of children	5
__ History of not visiting children when admitted to hospital	5

When the interview for the Index of Suspicion is completed, points assigned the parent for each item are added and the total is ranked: low risk—0 to 40 points, moderate risk—41 to 75 points; high risk—76 to 115; very high risk—116 to 149; and extreme risk—150 points or more.

Figure 5-1 Olson's index of Suspicion: Identification of parents who are potential child abusers. *Source:* Olson, R. S. Index of Suspicion: Screening for Child Abusers, *American Journal of Nursing*, January 1976, 108–110. Used with permission.

Checklist for Assessing Situational Crisis (Violence, Addiction, Loss, or Impending Death)

Assessment for Violence

1. Physical findings suggesting violence/abuse:
   - Bruises
   - Burns (cigarette, rope, hot water, fire)
   - Broken bones
   - Excessively bitten nails
   - Welts on the body
   - Missing hair (excessive hair-pulling)
   - Puffy face
   - Black eye(s)
   - Signs of malnutrition
   - Lumps on the head, trunk, or extremities
   - Concussion
   - Clothing inappropriate for environmental conditions
   - Body twitches when touched
   - Rigid body position, tense muscles
   - Reluctance to go home
   - Unwillingness to disrobe for physical examination
   - Crying uncontrollably

2. Historical findings suggesting violence/abuse:
   - Expression of fear
   - Heightened emotional arousal—e.g., sudden defensiveness or hostility to specific questions
   - Multiple expressions of self-hate
   - Expressions of low self-esteem and insecurity
   - Request that you not report your observations

Assessment for Addiction

1. Physical findings suggesting addiction:
   - Needle marks on arms, legs, trunk, or between fingers and toes
   - Malnourishment
   - Bad breath caused by inability to brush teeth due to extremely sore gums
   - Delerium tremors (DT's) (uncontrollable, heavy shaking)
   - Pupils dilated
   - Evidence of nausea and/or vomiting
   - Slurred speech
   - Unkempt appearance
   - Compulsive alcohol consumption
   - Hallucinatory behavior
   - Memory loss

2. Historical findings suggesting addiction:
   - Inability to maintain employment
   - Loss of family and friends
   - Inability to display socially acceptable behaviors
   - High value given to the addicting substance—e.g., will give up anything for the drug
   - Confused state of alertness
   - Appearance of intoxication but insistence on having "only a couple" drinks
   - Craving for the substance
   - Lies told about drinking patterns; attempts made to minimize the amount consumed; incongruency in answering similar questions
   - Alcohol consumption begun in the morning

Assessment for Denial of Loss or Impending Death

1. Physical findings suggesting loss or impending death:
   - Signs of grieving
   - Signs of advanced, acute, or terminal illness

2. Historical findings suggesting loss or impending death:
   - Refusal to seek medical diagnosis
   - Refusal to follow prescribed treatment plan
   - Avoidance of conversations related to the loss, illness, or individual who is deceased
   - Avoidance of interaction with family members and friends
   - Rejection of suggestions to join support groups
   - In the case of the death of a loved one, behavior continuing as if that significant other is still alive

the crisis of the addict's family. For the addict, the realization that he or she is truly addicted to a substance can be overwhelming. Because of the devastating probabilities, the addict may likely have lost his job, spouse, family, and community support as well as his self-respect, and possibly his identity. In addition to the physical needs of the addict, the psychological needs must be assessed and addressed. What does the addict see for himself in the future? What does he want? Is he willing to begin treatment? Is he willing to work toward recovery?

When assessing the needs of the addict, particularly the alcoholic, it is important to keep in mind that the client is sincere in his expressed desire for recovery and fully intends to honor the commitments he is about to make. Realistically a lot of backsliding generally occurs. Therefore an assessment of the addict's living environment is important. Will moral support and help be available, or will backsliding be met with criticisms and put-downs?

Loss

Diagnosis of a terminal illness, advanced aging, accidental death of a family member, or the fear of death itself can initiate a crisis situation in an individual. Kübler-Ross has outlined a model consisting of five (5) stages that can be used to assess adjustment to death, disability or loss of something or someone.

- *Stage 1: Denial* In this stage the client denies the existence of the loss. "It can't happen to me!" or some other form of disbelief is expressed. One of the dangers in this stage is that by denying the existence, for example, of an illness, the client may neglect treatment until it becomes too late and little can be done to alter the course of the disease. In addition to the client, a family member or close friend may also become involved in denial. This person refuses to accept the possibility of illness, or in the case of an accidental death, refuses to acknowledge it. He, too, may retreat into his own world and pretend that it never happened. Thus, he continues on as before, but with the unresolved or pending crisis looming over him.
- *Stage 2: Anger* In this stage the client expresses anger at life. He is angry because "it" has happened to him, not to others; he can turn the anger inward, cutting off communications necessary for maintaining support, and thus, alienating family and friends. However, in some cases, this can work to the client's advantage if you are able to redirect this anger. The client may begin to fight for himself. Hence, in the case of injury or disability, the restoration process can be enhanced.
- *Stage 3: Bargaining* In this stage the client or family member tries to strike a bargain with God or some other deity. The client will do anything, such as change his way of living or give more to charity or the church, if only this affliction will be taken away. The family member, too, makes concessions and promises to be carried out if only his loved one will be saved or if only the pain and agony of the loved one's situation be spared. When the attempts prove futile, the next stage, depression, is entered.
- *Stage 4: Depression* Here the client or family member becomes ambivalent and perhaps uncaring. Usually one of two types of depression is demonstrated: reaction or preparatory. In reaction depression the client or family member reacts to his environment or life change. In many cases this type of depression can be maladaptive—locking the individual in this stage and preventing him from resolving his crisis. In preparatory depression the client or family member can be observed working through the crisis situation—for example, putting his life in order and, primarily for the terminal client, preparing to die. In contrast to reaction depression, preparatory depression can be adaptive in that it allows the client or family member to work toward and possibly accomplish crisis resolution.
- *Stage 5: Acceptance* In this, the final stage, the client or family member has worked through the previous stages and accepted his fate. He has resolved the crisis and is ready to continue living. He now appears to become more sociable and content.

When assessing the client and his acceptance of loss or impending death of self or of a significant other, keep in mind that it is not necessary to progress through all the stages nor is it necessary to pass through them in any prescribed order. Also the client may vacillate back and forth many times between several of the stages.

Maturational Crisis

Maturational crises are keyed to the human growth and development process. In some cultures they are celebrated as the rite of passage from childhood to adulthood, adulthood to old age. For the early adolescent female, menarche (first menstrual cycle) signals the beginning of womanhood. For the male, first ejaculation announces the passage into manhood. Adolescence is the time of physical and emotional growing—of exploring, searching, questioning, and sorting out values to be weighed against those of the parent. Adolescence is the time of wondering who am I, where do I belong, and how do I fit in. It is the time for trying out roles to see which one fits. Likewise it is the time for decision making and planning one's life. It is a time for doing "my own thing," which may result in rejection by parents and, sometimes, society. It's a time for recognizing that double standards do exist, and the law will not turn its head when violated. The adolescent faces a multitude of crises as he precariously makes his way from the world of the child to that of the adult. However, reaching the world of the adult does not signal the end of everyday crises.

Some crises are more typical of one sex or one age group. Women, for example, face a crisis or turning point in their lives when their child or children leave home. In what has been labeled the "empty nest syndrome," these women suddenly find themselves with only their spouse to care for. After years of nurturing, parenting, and teaching their children the ways of their culture and society, they find a void in their lives. Some fill this void by returning to the world of work, seeking volunteer work, or returning to school. Others are engulfed within the void, becoming withdrawn, lonely, or depressed. It is at this point, too, that crises in husband-wife relationships arise. For women this usually happens after years of cooking, ironing, washing, and cleaning, and perhaps becoming dependent on their children to fulfill their needs at the expense of their spouse.

At about this same time the man, too, experiences his own crises. He may have reached the point in his life where he is "taking an assessment" of himself. What were his goals when he was young? Where does he stand now in relation to those goals? Can he progress upward? Many times males feel dissatisfied with their accomplishments in life. They become unhappy with their work and disenchanted. They feel an urge to take risks, to try new adventures before it's too late. In addition to evaluating themselves relative to their employment and occupational success, they also evaluate other accomplishments. Have they been "good" parents? "good" spouses? In their eyes has their life been rewarding? And generally they must face retirement just around the corner.

Retirement, often associated with aging, brings with it body image crises. While body image is important throughout the life span, the sudden realization that body changes have taken place can be a crisis for some. By the natural process of maturing, the body tends to slow down. Gray hairs appear; bald spots become evident; the youthful figure reflects padding. For some persons these natural changes are taken in stride. For others, these changes remind them that they are mortal, and the fear of senility and/or death grows out of proportion. The inability to understand and cope with the physical and emotional changes that occur as a result of maturation can present a crisis situation. When assessing the maturational crisis situation, remember that usually a combination of events, not just one, has precipitated the event.

Checklist for Assessing Maturational Crisis

1. Are anxiety-arousing or tension-producing events occurring in the client's environment (home, school, workplace)?
2. Have recent changes occurred in the client's lifestyle?
3. Has there been a recent loss of a loved one or significant other through divorce, moving, or death?
4. Does the client have good rapport with family and friends?
5. Is the client satisfied in his/her occupation? If not, how would he/she like it to be?
6. Is the client accepted by his peers?
7. Are there free-flowing lines of communication in the home between husband and wife, parents and child, and between siblings?

Assessment of Internal Stressors

Anxiety

While many psychological definitions of anxiety exist, and the construct of anxiety remains obtruse, the consensus is that anxiety results from a stimulation, either physical or emotional, in the environment, which produces a reaction (physical and/or emotional) within the organism. Anxiety ranges from mild to extreme, and various physical and psychological reactions correspond to the various degrees of anxiety.

The degrees of anxiety range on a continuum from adaptive or reactive to maladaptive anxiety. There are certain times when anxiety is beneficial and appropriate to the situation, and times when the level of anxiety reaches such proportions as to be detrimental to the person. A common example of this is in the performing arts. Adaptive (mild) anxiety serves as a stimulus to practice, or to perfect the art, but when the stimulus becomes so intense that the person panics or loses confidence in his ability to perform, the performance may turn into a failure. Thus, the anxiety becomes maladaptive in nature. Another example of reactive anxiety may be seen when persons are forced into situations for which they are unprepared. In these situations, the level or degree of anxiety may reach extreme proportions quickly; this depends on the individual's level of competence and coping skills. The client may demonstrate physical symptoms ranging from increased heart rate to incapacitation resulting from fear.

In cases of extreme anxiety the client may experience anxiety attacks. These attacks may be in the form of body tremors, respiratory difficulty, heart palpitations, and a choking sensation. Other degrees of anxiety can produce increased perspiration, clammy palms, gastric distress, diarrhea, loss of appetite, and inability to concentrate.

In the hospital setting, clients waiting to undergo tests or surgery generally exhibit symptoms of anxiety. Note whether the client's body tenses or flexes when you touch him. This could be indicative of increased response to stimuli due to fear of the unknown. Unfortunately,

Checklist for Assessing the Degree of Anxiety

Mild Anxiety

1. Client demonstrates an increased sense of alertness and attentiveness.
2. Client is focused more on others than himself.
3. Client displays an interest in the people and objects surrounding him.
4. Client desires to assume responsibility for his own hygiene.
5. Client may become interested in activities.
6. Client may exhibit symptoms such as restlessness, a desire to talk, repeated questions, joking, and procrastination.

Moderate Anxiety

1. Client may demonstrate either an increase in the use of his capacities or demonstrate an unawareness of activities in his immediate environment.
2. Client may indicate a desire to move away from others—to withdraw or isolate himself.
3. Client may display acting-out behavior in the form of complaining constantly, arguing, or excessive teasing.
4. Client may exhibit physical symptoms such as nausea, headache, or low back pain.

Severe Anxiety

1. Client demonstrates inability to make rational decisions; exhibits a state of confusion.
2. Client demonstrates a loss in the body's ability to restore itself.
3. Client appears extremely concerned regarding his condition. This is evidenced through constant questioning, focusing on details, and an impairment in his ability to perceive the situation clearly.
4. Client becomes extremely concerned with routine TPR checks.
5. Client displays automated behaviors such as aimlessly pacing or walking about, picking at clothing and bedding, or conversing without purpose.

Extreme Anxiety

1. Client exhibits a loss of control, and emotions surface.
2. Client can no longer perceive, remember, make decisions, control affect or motor activity, think, or test reality.
3. Client displays relative helplessness.
4. Client may seek escape from life or threats by using rash behaviors.
5. Client may demonstrate the need for comfort from a nonthreatening individual.
6. Client may demonstrate the need for a nonstimulating environment.

Symptoms of Anxiety

- Change in tone of voice
- Increase or decrease in rate of speech
- Change in posture
- Change in pattern of gestures or motions
- Intellectual or emotional preoccupation
- Nonreceptive to communications
- Increased perspiration
- Body tremors
- Lump in throat or choking sensation
- Sinking feeling in abdomen
- Diarrhea
- Vomiting
- Changes in heartbeat, pulse, respirations
- Change in appetite
- Dry mouth
- Sweaty palms
- Increased muscle tension
- Focus on detail
- Physical withdrawal
- Inability to function
- Inability to attend to immediate surroundings
- Immobility or paralysis

heightened anxiety can lead to complications or reactions to drugs. In the surgical area the client in such a heightened state of anxiety may require more anesthesia than usual to produce the desired effect. Once the desired effect is produced, the danger of overdose exists. Anxiety also has the ability to increase blood pressure and pulse and respiration rates; in some instances, high levels of anxiety can alter test results.

Anger

Anger is a very powerful emotion. It is the lashing out at or releasing of hostilities aimed at some other object. It is a forceful self-assertion, which tends to be destructive in nature. It is a way of venting frustration and confusion associated with a lack of effective coping skills. The behaviors are highly charged and emotionally filled. If these pent-up hostilities are released on others, physical and/or emotional abuses may result. But if these hostilities are held within the person, physical consequences may result. Blood pressure tends to rise as temper flares. Other physical effects include ulcers, gastric disturbances, sleep disturbances, tension headaches, and increased body tension.

In the clinical setting you may encounter the client who resists some or all forms of treatment. Instead of countering his hostility with yours, you may be able to defuse the situation and gain his cooperation if you listen to his reasons for his anger. Perhaps he is angry with himself for being ill. He may be feeling self-guilt or helplessness. Keep in mind that the client who feels threatened or out of control of the situation may well demonstrate hostility and aggression or anger. For this client, your empathy, caring, and understanding of his needs and concerns may make a difference.

Checklist for Assessing Anger

1. Is the client able to control his faculties?
2. Can the client think through the situation?
3. Is the client rational?
4. Is the client becoming physically destructive?

Type A/Type B Personality

The Type A personality is the emotionally charged, ready-to-go person. He is the first to go when the red light changes green, he is a half hour early for appointments, and he completes tasks well in advance. Everything must be done ahead of time. He is anxious, impatient, and must always feel in control. When threatened by a stressful situation, he struggles to regain the control he feels he lost. Type A personality with underlying feelings of anger is highly correlated with coronary disease, angina pectoris, and myocardial infarction. This person tends to work faster, strive harder, and become more aggressive than the Type B person.

The Type B personality, on the other hand, remains calm when threatened by stressors. He refrains from frantically trying to gain control and maintains energy under prolonged stress. He has been labeled the noncoronary-prone person, who tends to be more relaxed, more accepting of events, and less rushed. While the two types of personalities exist, each falls at the opposite end of a continuum, with the majority of persons falling somewhere in between.

Checklist for Assessing Type A Personality

1. Is the client competitive?
2. Does the client work in a stressful, demanding position?
3. Is the client impatient and always in a hurry?
4. Is the client impulsive?
5. Is the client aggressive?
6. Does the client appear to be a workaholic?

Assessment of Coping Methods

Everyone has his own method of coping with stress; some are more adaptive than others (see Table 5-1). Defense mechanisms or ego defenses are used to protect the ego from undue stress. The following are commonly used defense mechanisms:

1. *Denial.* Denial is a way of hiding, or burying deeply within oneself, thoughts and feelings. It is a way of pushing these thoughts and feelings into one's unconsciousness. It is a means that can protect one from painful memories; once repressed, these memories remain in the unconsciousness despite efforts to retrieve them. With denial certain aspects of reality are blotted out. An example of denial is the person who upon receiving bad or un-

Table 5-1. Coping Strategies

Affective-oriented coping strategies	Problem-oriented coping strategies
Hope that things will get better	Try to maintain some control over the situation
Eat; smoke; chew gum	Find out more about the situation
Pray; trust in God	Think through different ways to handle the situation
Get nervous	Look at the problem objectively
Worry	Try out different ways of solving the problem to see which works best
Seek comfort or help from friends or family	Draw on past experience to help you handle the situation
Want to be alone	Try to find meaning in the situation
Laugh it off, figuring that things could be worse	Break the problem down into "smaller pieces"
Try to put the problem out of your mind	Set specific goals to help solve the problem
Daydream, fantasize	Accept the situation as it is
Get prepared to expect the worst	Talk the problem over with someone who has been in the same type of situation
Get mad; curse; swear	Actively try to change the situation
Go to sleep, figuring things will look better in the morning	Settle for the next best thing
Don't worry about it, everything will probably work out fine	Do anything just to do something
Withdraw from the situation	Let someone else solve the problem
Work off tension with physical activity	
Take out your tensions on someone or something else	
Drink alcoholic beverages	
Resign yourself to the situation because things look hopeless	
Do nothing in the hope that the problem will take care of itself	
Resign yourself to the situation because it's your fate	
Blame someone else for your problems	
Meditation, yoga, biofeedback	
Take drugs	

From Jalowiec, A.; and Powers, M. J. "Stress and Coping in Hypertensive and Emergency Room Patients." *Nursing Research*, *30*:13 (January–February 1981). Reprinted with permission, American Journal of Nursing Company.

welcomed news of an event rejects it, pretending it never happened and continues living as if nothing had changed. For instance, the parents who are unable to accept the death of a child may keep the child's room intact for years to come, and they may talk about the child as if he were still alive.

2. *Projection.* Projection is attributing your feelings or thoughts to another person. Often a person unconsciously recognizes some characteristics about himself that make him feel guilty. He then projects, or attributes these characteristics to someone else, thus releasing himself of guilt and responsibility for these characteristics. An example might be an aggressive wife who tells you how hostile her husband is and that she feels she must retaliate in some way. Another example is the mother, married at a very early age, who refuses to allow her daughter to date before mid to late adolescence.
3. *Introjection.* Introjection, which is a way of coping with a threatening situation, involves taking ideas or thoughts incongruent with your own and making them your own. It's a sort of "If you can't beat them, join them" type of behavior. This coping mechanism can come into play in situations where a threatening issue is in conflict with your set of moral values; in order to resolve this issue, you make a compromise.
4. *Reaction Formation.* In reaction formation one expresses the opposite of one's true feelings. This is a means of protection from one's guilt. For instance, when one family member has a deep dislike for another family member, he may go out of his way to express love and caring for the disliked member.

5. *Isolation.* In isolation, the thought and act connected with the thought are separate, and only the thought is allowed to surface. For example, suppose you have an unpleasant task to do on a beautiful, sunny, summer day. While performing the task, your mind is filled with thoughts of pleasant things that you like to do on these kinds of days. In some cases the content of the thoughts is socially unacceptable. For instance, suppose someone toward whom you feel animosity is in danger. Suddenly you are filled with feelings of hostility, and this prevents you from taking swift, appropriate action to help.
6. *Intellectualization.* To intellectualize is to practice exaggerated thinking over feeling. A person using this defense mechanism discusses issues in a very cool, abstract way, without expressing feelings that most persons would express. An adolescent often uses this mechanism when discussing sensitive issues, such as sex. By using this mechanism, he is able to resolve many of the conflicts he must face while growing up.
7. *Undoing.* This is a way of behaviorally making amends for something you wish that you had not done. Shakespeare's Lady MacBeth continuously washed her hands after making arrangements for the death of the king, which was her way of undoing her evil act. It is a way of negating guilt.

There are coping strategies other than the ego defense mechanisms. One way most people cope with difficult situations is to talk to someone—a family member or spouse, friend, or religious leader. Some clients seek professional help, but usually after alternative sources have failed to provide help. By talking the problem over with someone, the client is able to see the issues from a different perspective, lay the issues out on the table, examine them from all sides, and generate some alternative solutions to the problems at hand.

Another coping strategy is involvement in hobbies or volunteer activities. Frequently people find clubs, church or civic groups, and volunteer agencies helpful and rewarding for providing companionship and filling gaps in their lives. For many, these type of activities provide a change in the daily routine and something to which they can look forward.

Other strategies that are used to release pent-up energies include physical exercise, long quiet walks, and meditation/relaxation techniques. These help the client relax his body and provide time for rethinking or reexamining his dilemma.

Many people turn to their religion as a source of support and a way to cope with daily stressors. They find strength and assurance through their faith in addition to fellowship and friendships formed with other members. Many times a sharing of experiences proves beneficial for all parties involved.

These are only several of the many coping mechanisms used to solve everyday or crisis situations. Remember that facing the problem situation rather than retreating from it or denying its existence is more important than the coping mechanism used to handle the situation.

Checklist for Assessing Coping

1. Does the client confront situations or withdraw?
2. Does the client deny or accept situations?
3. Does the client have a confidant—someone to talk to?
4. Does the client use defense mechanisms to "get over the rough spots," depend on them for an extended period of time, or use them every time rather than face issues?

Depression

Described as a feeling of sadness, depression ranges from mild to severe. It occurs irrespective of age; however, it tends to occur most often within the adolescent and aging populations. Some depressed clients may appear sad and withdrawn or preoccupied with a serious life event. They appear lethargic and lacking energy and interest. On the other hand, some depressed clients may appear very active, constantly talking and displaying extensive body activity. They may even appear inappropriately happy. When assessing the underlying causes of the depression and the range of depression, you should consider several areas: depression due to loss, lack of skills, low self-esteem, illness, and behaviors of depression.

Depression Due to Loss

Depression due to loss can result from many things: loss of a spouse or significant other through separation, divorce, or death; loss of a limb or limbs; total or partial body paralysis; and loss of a job, home, or prestige within a community. When assessing the client suffering from loss and depression, keep in mind that given a sufficient amount of time, most clients will be able to work through the grieving process described earlier in this chapter and resolve their crisis. Be a good listener and try not to offer platitudes to the client. Above all, do not tell the client that he should not feel depressed, that he has no good reason to feel depressed, or that things always work out for the best. In the eyes of the client, he has every reason to feel sad and depressed. For many clients, depression may result from a combination of issues.

Lack of Skills

Another contributor to depression is lack of skills, including such common skills as those of communication, problem solving, and social. Begin by investigating the client's support system. Does he have someone to talk to, and does he have the skill and vocabulary to express himself? The depressed client may withdraw from family and friends, because he may feel that if he opens up to a family member, he will be rejected.

For adolescents, the lines of communication between parent and child are often tense, if not severed. A special effort needs to be made to help the adolescent understand that you are listening without judging or moralizing and that you are trying to understand. Frequently, when the client is assisted in verbalizing the problem or area of concern, he is able to examine the situation and formulate some viable alternatives.

For the older adult, particularly men, support networks may have been established only with the spouse or the spouse and one or two significant others. When death of one of these support figures occurs, the network weakens or vanishes altogether; the survivor may not have the skills to establish a new network. In this case your listening, empathy, understanding, and encouragement may help to raise the client's level of self-confidence and enable him to take the risks needed in meeting new friends. If a lack of problem-solving skills exists, this may only add to the state of depression. The more the client ruminates over the problem, the more intense the depressed state may become, and, in his efforts to solve or resolve a conflict, the client may easily succumb. Helping the client identify the problem or face the issue and generate some realistic, concrete solutions may begin to lead him out of his depression.

Low Self-Esteem

The feelings of uselessness, helplessness, and worthlessness may be overwhelming to a client; he may have depended on a significant other for reinforcement and a feeling of self-worth. Now he may have to face life without a substitute reinforcer. He may easily fall into a trap of self-pity, or, because he has low self-esteem, he may feel incapable of making decisions or coping with the situation. He may feel helpless to change his environment, or he may feel that the situation is out of his control. This would be especially true in the case of an older adult who is suddenly told that he is incapable of making critical decisions in his life with regard to finances, living arrangements, lifestyle, and food.

Illness

Illness, especially one that may require modifying or changing one's lifestyle, may contribute to depression. Questions regarding the prognosis and long-term effects or duration of the illness, plus a lack of understanding of the disease, can contribute to excessive dwelling on the issue by the client. Unexpressed fear can also be a contributor. While assessing the client for depression, make an attempt to encourage the client to discuss the issue(s), express his concerns and fears, and ask any questions he may have.

Behaviors of Depression

In the traditional sense the depressed client is thought to be solemn and withdrawn, very quiet, and preoccupied with himself; he looks anxious and yet sad, fearful of the unknown, and lacking self-confidence. But keep in mind that other behaviors are indicative of depression. For example, a client experiencing depression may be dressed quite gaudily, act bubbly and talkative, and display a lot of body movement as she tells you about the situation in which her husband just ran off with another woman. She says that she is left with no job and no skills, and she tells you that she feels depressed. She is indeed a depressed client! The surface value seems to tell you not to believe the client; but, in truth,

Checklist for Assessing Depression

1. Does the client appear withdrawn?
2. Has the client been confronted with a crisis situation in the recent past?
3. Does the client appear excessively active and inappropriately attired (excessive body movements and gaudy attire)?
4. Does the client appear overly talkative and excessively happy for a given set of adverse circumstances?
5. Does the client demonstrate behavior appropriate to the situation?
6. Does the client appear to have difficulty reaching a decision regarding his situation?

the effervescence is only a charade—an act that allows the client to hide this difficulty of exposing her true feelings to the world.

Indecisiveness may also be a reflection of a depressed state. The client is aware of his situation or his reason for feeling depressed, but is not able to make a decision regarding what kind of action, if any, he wishes to take. Other behaviors observed with depression are over- or undereating, insomnia, prolonged sleeping pattern, headache, confusion, or preoccupation.

Suicide

When depression becomes severe, the client may not be able to think rationally. He wants the situation to end. He is tired, frustrated, and confused. Suicide seems to be the only choice. Suicide is an individual act and, like depression, is no respecter of age. The methods used in suicide attempts vary according to sex, and this accounts for the fact that while women attempt suicide more than men, men are more successful in their attempts. Men use more lethal methods such as guns, hanging, and jumping out of windows whereas women use drug overdose more often. However, with the women's liberation movement has come an increased use of more lethal methods of suicide by women. A suicide attempt is a cry for help, and the actual attempt is a last resort. Prior to the attempt the client usually has been giving out signals or hints. For assessment you need to be aware of these cues.

Culture and ethnic background are reflected in the suicide rates. The American Indian has a suicide rate above the national average; in some traditional Oriental cultures, if you have been disgraced, you are expected to take your own life. However, in American society today, suicide is viewed as a tragedy and, in some cases, a disgrace to the family.

Checklist for Assessing Suicide

1. Does the client talk of suicide? He might say things like, "I won't be here to bother you," or "You won't have to put up with me much longer," or "I wish I were dead," or "No one cares whether I live or die." He may ask how you would feel if he were dead.
2. Does the client appear extremely depressed; does he want to talk but is reluctant to do so?
3. Is he beginning to give away his most cherished possessions? This is a big clue.
4. Does he appear to have made a big decision and is now at peace with himself? Is his turmoil or crisis over? It is at this point that the danger of successful suicide exists. Up to this point family and friends have been keeping a close watch on the client, but they relax their vigil because they mistakenly think nothing will happen. But the decision to make the attempt has now been made, the method chosen, and the time and place picked out.
5. Has the client attempted suicide and failed? He will most likely try again . . . and succeed.

Severe depression may culminate in suicidal attempt. The client will most likely be found to have a history of long-standing problems, which had escalated and eventually had reached a point where they were unbearable; the latter point in time generally will occur two to three days prior to the suicidal attempt. The approach for assessment is to establish a nonjudgmental relationship in which you listen and reflect the client's feelings. Confrontation is an important part of the assessment. Ask the client if he is thinking about committing suicide. Assess the lethality of the situation. Ask the client if he has a plan, and what that plan might be. Promote catharsis; allow and encourage the client to explore and express his feelings. Try to get the client to reach a decision and express an interest and commitment to live. If you feel that the client may attempt suicide, be sure that someone is with him at all times, and refer him for treatment. Even make the appointment and take the client if necessary.

BIOLOGICAL AND CULTURAL VARIATIONS

Populations More Prone to Suicide

Urban dwellers more than rural
Protestants more than Catholics
Singles more than family group members
Divorced persons
Unemployed persons
Ill persons
Men, who are five times more successful at suicide than women
Psychotic clients, some of whom have voices telling them to kill themselves

Clients with a history of the following:
- Early loss of family member (especially father)
- Parent-child conflict
- Sibling conflict
- Substance abuse including alcoholism
- Socioeconomic concerns
- Death of another family member or significant other by suicide

Table 5-2 is a brief analysis of disease conditions delineating the characteristics of common psychopathologies. Table 5-3 gives an overview of the definition, dynamics, symptomatology, and bases of nursing care for psychoneurotic reactions. Some tools for assessing mental health are seen in Appendix D.

Summary

This chapter has presented several factors necessary in completing a mental health assessment. Mental functioning is an internal process and is not directly available to observation. Such aspects as attitude, affect/mood, speech, thought processes, sensorium and reasoning, potential for danger, and the psychologic assets of the client are reflectors of mental functioning. Manifestations of mental dysfunctions are revealed in the client's appearance, behavior, and conversation. Situational and maturational crises were presented. In particular, the situational crises of violence and addiction were examined. Sources of internal stress, such as anxiety, anger, and personality, were discussed along with the ego defense mechanisms and other coping strategies. The symptoms of depression and cues for suicide were highlighted. A brief descriptive analysis of disease states that may be reflected in mental dysfunctioning was presented in a table.

One last note: The pathologic conditions and medical diagnoses mentioned in this chapter were not presented for the purpose of providing you with knowledge in order to establish etiologies or medical diagnoses of mental dysfunctions; rather, they were used to emphasize the fact that ABC data need to be carefully evaluated in terms of need for nursing intervention and/or referral.

Discussion Questions/Activities

1. Discuss the importance of noting the client's appearance in relation to altered mental states.
2. Identify factors that can affect level of consciousness.
3. Name ten findings in mental health assessment that require the client to be referred to a specialist in the area. Compare and discuss these with your peers.
4. Discuss examples of situational and/or maturational crises that you have personally experienced or have been involved with—such as those of a relative, friend, or client. Do not reveal the person's identity.
5. Identify your personal ways of coping with stress.
6. Role-play a crisis situation and have an observer note your interpersonal and communication techniques. Critique the role-play.

Table 5-2. Descriptive Analysis of Disease Conditions

	Psychoneurosis	Psychophysiologic autonomic and visceral disorders (psychosomatic)	Personality disorders	Psychosis	Acute and chronic brain disorders
Definition	A psychological disability resulting from an individual's inability to cope with emotional conflicts or stressful environmental problems.	A maladaptive emotional reaction in which the symptoms are expressed in organs innervated by the autonomic nervous system producing physiologic change concurrent with psychological disequilibrium.	Entrenched, chronic, maladaptive characterologic patterns in which an individual experiences little or no anxiety or guilt.	Psychogenic reactions in which the individual experiences severe personality disorganization and disintegration along with marked distortions of reality.	A disorder in which the individual sustains psychological and physiological dysfunction as a consequence of damaged brain tissue.
Types	Anxiety neurosis Phobic neurosis Conversion neurosis Dissociative neurosis Depressive neurosis Obsessive-compulsive neurosis	Gastrointestinal reactions a. Peptic ulcer b. Ulcerative colitis Cardiovascular reactions a. Essential hypertension b. Migraine Respiratory reactions a. Bronchial asthma b. Hyperventilation syndrome Genitourinary reactions a. Impotence or frigidity b. Amenorrhea Musculoskeletal reactions a. Functional backache b. Rheumatoid arthritis Skin reactions a. Psoriasis b. Neurodermatitis	Personality disorders a. Schizoid b. Paranoid c. Inadequate d. Passive-aggressive e. Antisocial Sexual deviation Alcoholism Drug dependence Maladjustment reactions to living	Schizophrenia a. Simple b. Hebephrenic c. Catatonic d. Paranoid e. Schizoaffective f. Chronic undifferentiated g. Childhood schizophrenia Major affective disorders a. Manic-depressive: manic b. Manic-depressive: depressed Involutional melancholia Paranoid states	Delirium tremens Korsakoff's syndrome Cerebral arteriosclerosis Intercranial neoplasms Brain trauma Encephalitis Systemic intoxication or poisoning and others

(continued on page 114)

From H. Kreigh, and J. E. Perko, *Psychiatric and Mental Health Nursing: A Commitment to Care.* Reston, Va.: Reston Publishing Co., 1979.

Table 5-2. *Continued*

	Psychoneurosis	Psychophysiologic autonomic and visceral disorders (psychosomatic)	Personality disorders	Psychosis	Acute and chronic brain disorders
Types *continued*		Endocrine reactions a. Diabetes mellitus b. Hyperthyroidism			
Etiology	Disruption in the developmental pattern or in interpersonal experiences. Multiple, intrapsychic conflicts resulting from unresolved guilt, fear, prolonged stress or crisis. Conflict between what patient believes society expects and the bipersonal self. Underlying and sustained conflict arising from the dichotomy of bicultures and subcultures.	Internalization of feelings. Internalization of negative emotions. Internal discharge of negative emotions. Constitutional organ susceptibility.	Faulty or arrested emotional development which interferes with adequate social control or superego formation. Constitutional predisposition. Deprivation of basic needs in early childhood. Physical and/or emotional trauma in childhood or adolescence.	Multiple causality, most likely a combination of biochemical, social, and psychological factors.	Any condition or agent which produces central nervous system pathology and cerebral tissue impairment.
Characteristics	A strong sense of personal discomfort; heightened levels of anxiety. Major personality organization remains intact. Maintains contact with reality. Maintains usual roles, activities, or employment. Decreased productivity and creativity.	Organ pathology. Physical illness is the expression of prolonged or intense emotional stress. Physical rather than emotional symptoms dominate the clinical picture. Excellent ability to overtly mask stress and conflict. If unchecked and unresolved, physical symptoms may be fatal.	Lifelong, repetitive, maladaptive and often self-defeating behavior. Anxiety is not apparent. Seldom seeks help on own initiative. Tolerance to frustration and stress is low. Occasional intellectual insight. Pathology is directed outward toward and against others.	Major personality disorganization. Marked interference with ability to function, personally and interpersonally. Significant discrepancies between thoughts, feelings and behavior. Substitution of fantasy for reality. Presence of delusional and hallucinatory systems.	Reversible or irreversible. Deficits in intellectual functioning. Impaired orientation. Lability of affect. Primary and secondary personality changes. Alterations in the levels of consciousness. Memory and/or speech impairment.

	Fixed attitudes, affections and/or mannerisms. Excessive dependency or domination. Correlation between thought and feeling content.		Frequent confrontation with society's mores, norms and laws.	Disorientation in the three spheres. Regression.	
Dynamics	Unresolved emotional conflict is complicated with underlying feelings of guilt resulting in overwhelming anxiety. Unsatisfactory relationships with parents, siblings or peers in the developmental process. The resultant symptomatology offers the individual an external means of expressing repressed material thereby allowing both primary and secondary gains for the ego.	Psychological stress is converted into anxiety which is directed internally through the nervous system. The individual experiences pathophysiological functional or structural changes of the organs. Sustained or prolonged conflict causes internalization of fear, hostility and/or guilt.	The individual operates from an egocentric viewpoint and remains narcissistic. Interpersonal relationships are not important unless they can be used to achieve specific need gratification. A concealed "taking" relationship predominates as opposed to a mutual "give and take" relationship. Avoidance of expectations, discomfort and/or stress-producing situations. Disproportionate projection and accusations toward persons, places and objects in the environment.	Loss of ego boundaries. Denial of reality. Severe regression. Security and identity are threatened. Interpersonal relationships are superficial. Failure or inability to trust self or others.	Interference with or destruction of cerebral tissue. Libidinal energy is released as a result of organic changes. Loss of ability to control libidinal drives. Interruption of learning and coping potential.
Concepts and principles for nursing care	The presence of anxiety is a universal phenomenon. Knowledge and understanding of "normal anxiety" will provide the nurse with a	Any attitude, behavior or situation which produces a sense of insecurity arouses anxiety. The overt expression of feelings alleviates internal stress.	A firm, calm, consistent, quiet approach is most effective and will produce the least amount of manipulative or explosive response behavior.	The attitude of personnel makes or breaks the possibility of recovery for the psychotic patient. Care must be directed toward the maintenance of reality relationships.	Cerebral damage produces physiological and psychological malfunctioning. Organic conditions produce mental dysfunction, alteration in mood, physical

(continued on page 116)

Table 5-2. *Continued*

	Psychoneurosis	Psychophysiologic autonomic and visceral disorders (psychosomatic)	Personality disorders	Psychosis	Acute and chronic brain disorders
Concepts and principles for nursing care *continued*	base to assess the level of patient dysfunction. The symptom picture is usually indicative of the underlying conflict. Rituals are accompanied by profound dread and apprehension. All behavior is meaningful. Nursing care is directed toward the relief of physical and psychological symptoms. The patient's self-esteem is enhanced by the nurse's demonstration of acceptance, respect and concern for his well-being. Positive, satisfying experiences are introduced to correct developmental and maturational deficits.	Disturbed family relationships play an important role in the development and outcome of the patient's illness. In psychosomatic illness interpersonal factors and physical disease are woven together into a single process. Effective treatment depends on a dual emphasis, physical and psychological. A planned schedule of social and recreational activities provides release from tension. Diversion deflects mental preoccupation with self and disability. Know the source or cause of the stresses, tensions or problems creating the physical reactions. Give priority to the exploration of the primary causes of repressed feelings with the patient.	The nurse must protect other patients from being manipulated or exploited by an individual with a personality disorder. Give clear, concise explanations and directions to avoid verbal entanglements with the patient. Uniform scheduling and consistent application of firm limit setting offers positive guidance toward establishing self-control. Consistency in decision making enables the nurse to maintain an objective viewpoint.	Genuine interest, honesty, warmth and optimism are essential for establishing contact with psychotic persons. Physical and psychological needs merit equal attention. Familiar routines and persons contribute to security. As a social being, man's psychological equilibrium needs to be maintained through satisfying relationships with others, both individually and in groups.	manifestations and disrupted interpersonal relationships. Acute conditions require immediate interventive techniques to maintain life. Chronic conditions require supportive care coupled with an attitudinal approach of hopefulness. Patients with impaired judgment are unable to function independently and therefore require close observation and protective supervision. Familiarity with the environment promotes feelings of security while change produces frustration. Loss or impairment of physical functioning contributes to increasing the level of fear, anxiety, and confusion.

Table 5-3. An Overview of Psychoneurotic Reactions

Condition	Definition	Dynamics	Symptom picture	Concepts and principles for nursing care
Anxiety neurosis	A reaction in response to no apparent or insufficient environmental stimulus.	Persistent overuse of *repression* to control emotionally charged thoughts and feelings. The presence of socially unacceptable thoughts, feelings, wants or desires that if actualized would cause loss of approval, acceptance or love from others. Fear of censure, disapproval or rejection threatens the self-concept.	Free floating and recurrent acute anxiety. Dramatic increase in the level and diffusion of anxiety. Somatic symptoms are associated with the autonomic nervous system. Decreased ability to focus on the situation at hand. Interruption of judgment. Sudden onset of panic.	Intervention is imperative before anxiety mounts and becomes uncontrollable. Remaining with the patient and providing a warm, concerned human environment enhances the patient's security and reduces the level of anxiety. The nurse listens carefully to the expression of somatic concerns and does not challenge or cast doubt on their validity.
Phobic neurosis	A reaction of intense recurrent, unreasonable fear attached to a specific object or situation.	Incomplete repression with *displacement* of anxiety onto an external focus which the individual can then avoid. Particular phobias assume a *symbolic* significance with respect to underlying emotional conflicts or unacceptable desires.	Intense, prolonged irrational and disabling fear. Common phobias include fear of the dark; open and closed spaces; heights; animals and birds; and dirt or germs. Avoidance of socializing behavior and frequent reclusiveness results in eccentricities.	Phobias are *real* to the individual. The nurse demonstrates acceptance of the patient's avoidance patterns as being necessary for his survival. The nurse assumes initiative in seeking out the patient and provides opportunities for the verbal expression of feelings. Assisting the patient in exploring the "source" or primary painful life experience or trauma that eventuated in displacement.

(continued on page 118)

From H. Kreigh and J. E. Perko, *Psychiatric and Mental Health Nursing: A Commitment to Care.* Reston, Va.: Reston Publishing Co., 1979.

Table 5-3. *Continued*

Condition	Definition	Dynamics	Symptom picture	Concepts and principles for nursing care
Conversion neurosis	A reaction in which the individual unconsciously transforms his underlying conflict into specific kinds of motor or sensory dysfunction.	*Conversion* of anxiety into somatic symptoms, *symbolic* of the underlying conflict. Primary gain is relief from emotional tension. Secondary gain is the advantage the symptom provides in meeting the need for dependency. Outcome is the avoidance of responsible, independent functioning. Avoidance of an anticipated, emotionally and/or physically painful experience. *Denial* of an unpleasant and/or uncomfortable reality in one's life.	Physical manifestations in the form of blindness, deafness, aphonia, laryngitis and convulsions. Displays a lack of concern or indifference toward the existing symptom. Minimal observable anxiety.	The individual does not consciously invent or choose the condition. Conversion involves the voluntary and sensory systems. The physical symptoms serve to lessen any consciously felt anxiety. Nursing care is focused on the individual and his feelings, not on his symptoms.
Dissociative neurosis	A reaction in which certain aspects of the individual's personality are split off, separated or detached from his conscious awareness.	Employs mechanisms of *dissociation, conversion* and *symbolism.* Ego attempts to protect itself from critical and/or dangerous pain. *Denial* is used to escape from reality.	Alterations in the state of consciousness, in the person's identity or memory. Depersonalization. Overwhelming anxiety. Manifested through amnesia, fugues and twilight states.	The nurse must view the patient's emotional functioning as the outcome of his growth and developmental process. It is necessary for the nurse to understand the patient's feelings and behavior and not pass judgment on his actions. Understand the dynamics of this problem to maximize interventive techniques.

Table 5-3. *Continued*

Condition	Definition	Dynamics	Symptom picture	Concepts and principles for nursing care
Obsessive-compulsive neurosis	A reaction in which the individual experiences persistent, distressing thoughts or impulses resulting in irresistible acting-out behavior	Unsuccessful repression is reinforced through the use of such defensive responses as: *displacement*, *reaction formation*, *undoing* and *symbolism*.	Ambivalence. Doubt. Vacillation. Persistent, recurring ideation. Repetitive, stereotyped, motor activity.	The patient recognizes the unreasonableness of his obsessions and compulsions. Rituals release tension, and temporarily reduce the level of anxiety. Interruption of ritualistic behavior increases the patient's anxiety and guilt. Protect patient from ridicule. Assist the patient to develop new interests outside self.
Depressive neurosis	A reaction in which the individual experiences a state of sadness due to disappointment, an upsetting life event or a loss of a significant person, possession or position.	Damage to self-esteem with associated repressed anger. Disparity between the superego value system and the ego activity which results in guilt. Feelings of inadequacy and inferiority are more pronounced due to exaggerated ego ideal. Depressive features existent throughout the life experience.	Marked ambivalence. Diffused anger and hostility. Fluctuations in mood. Difficulty in concentration. Reduction in psychomotor activity. Reality oriented. Appetite and sleep disturbances. Somatic complaints. Pessimism. Vacillation between ability to function and immobility. Numerous suicidal threats. Accidental death.	Provide external structure and milieu that gradually allow the patient to assume responsibility for his life experiences. Verbal or behavioral expression of anger or hostility provides a release for internalized emotion. Persuasion is a useful tool for meeting the needs for acceptance and attention. Reassurance is conveyed through the setting of realistic limits. Feelings of adequacy can be promoted by opportunities for achieving small goals. Allow patient to experience success and accomplishment via a short-term project.

CHAPTER 6

Data Analysis and Nursing Diagnosis

LEARNING OBJECTIVES

1. Give examples of dependent, interdependent, and independent nursing practices.
2. Explain the concept of health assessment in nursing practice.
3. Describe the phases of the nursing process.
4. Explain the concept of data analysis.
5. Differentiate nursing assessment and diagnosis from medical assessment and diagnosis.
6. Define nursing diagnosis.

Information can be gathered about a client, but before it can be of use, it must be analyzed. Data compiled about one aspect of the client must be analyzed not only individually but in relationship to all other aspects, for the whole is greater than the sum of the parts. It must be remembered that health assessment data, although made up of content from cultural, mental, and physical areas, encompass the whole individual, family, or community at any given moment of time. It is via the analysis and synthesis of the data that nursing diagnoses are arrived at.

Where does health assessment fit in the context of roles in nursing practice? How is health assessment viewed within the framework of the nursing process? What is the concept of data analysis? How does nursing assessment and diagnosis differ from medical examination and diagnosis? What is the nature of nursing diagnoses? This chapter pursues these primary questions.

Nursing Practice Roles

Dependent, interdependent, and independent roles exist in nursing practice. The *dependent* role comprises nursing activities that are dependent on medical orders. To execute any activities within this category without medical orders is to practice outside legal bounds established by state nurse practice acts. Because nurse practice acts vary from state to state, the nurse needs to become familiar with the definitions of nursing practice within the state(s) where he or she is practicing. Examples of dependent nursing activities include administration of medically prescribed medications, intravenous fluids, and electrolytes, and application of medically prescribed treatments.

Interdependent nursing roles include activities such as consultation, referral, and the planning and coordination of client care with other health care workers as well as other members of the nursing team, such as counselors, social workers, psychologists, physicians, pharmacists, and allied health therapists (physical therapists, occupational therapists, radiology therapists, recreational therapists, inhalation therapists). Although the resources exist, nursing practice, unlike medical practice, has not yet evolved to the level of consultative practice between the experts of specific areas of nursing practice. However, consultation does seem to occur on an informal basis when "like a good neighbor" we ask our nursing friends and colleagues for input and suggestions. The consultation process is somewhat more formal if the institution employs nurse clinicians (experts in various aspects or knowledge areas of nursing), whose role is to serve as consultant for nursing care within the institutional setting. The accepted fee-for-consultation practice of medicine does not presently occur in nursing.

Independent nursing roles encompass those nursing activities that are prescribed and performed by the nurse. These are activities that are not dependent on medical prescription or supervision. Examples of independent nursing functions are those actions that are client supporting and that assist the client in decision making and coping with stresses, such as providing comfort measures, health teaching, counseling, networking for health enhancement resources, and modifying environmental factors detrimental to health.

Health assessment is an independent nursing activity. It provides the foundation for the nurse to make nursing diagnoses and to perform tasks and responsibilities within the framework of "casefinding, health teaching, health counseling, and provision of care supportive and restorative of life and well-being" (New York State Nurse Practice Act, Article 139 of the Education Law, Section 6902).

The Nursing Process

The *nursing process* is a means of problem solving within the context of nursing practice. It is a purposeful process with the ultimate goal of helping to improve the health status of a client or assisting the client in maintaining or returning to his or her optimum level of functioning and wellness. The phases of the nursing process are generally described as assessment, planning, intervention, and evaluation. These four phases are not linear but rather evolve as information is critically processed by the nurse. In other words, as the nurse assesses, validation and evaluation constantly come into play. Throughout each additional phase, ongoing assessment and evaluation take place.

Assessment has generally been referred to as the foundation of the nursing process. It is a complex concept, and, like the total nursing process, it is not a linear phenomeon. Knowledge and experience affect the quality of the assessment performed. The greater the knowledge and experience base of the nurse, the greater the potential for accuracy and comprehensiveness of the assessment. With a data base that is plagued with incorrect or sparse information, there is a greater chance of coming to erroneous conclusions. Knowledge aids the nurse in determining when a behavior or response needs to be pursued to collect additional pertinent information, and it also helps the nurse recognize interrelationships of findings and identifying patterns. When the time available for assessment is short, knowledge and experience dictate the priorities for investigation in light of the presenting behavioral responses. During the data collection phase as well as during the analysis and synthesis of data, knowledge sets the stage by organizing frames of reference. In health assessment some of the commonly used theories that provide such frames of reference are Maslow's hierarchy of needs, Selye's general adaptation syndrome, Erikson's psychosocial development theory, Havighurst's developmental tasks, Duvall's stages of family development, Piaget's cognitive developmental theory, and Lewin's field phenomenon. Such theories, plus knowledge of normal ranges and normal variations, provide guidelines for understanding clients and their environments and for decision making that occurs in collecting data about the client's health status and in analyzing and synthesizing the data base.

Assessment establishes the client as a person—as a unique individual—and therefore facilitates the individualization of care.

Assessment

Data collection is inherent in the assessment phase and is directed toward information relative to health status. To afford a systematic framework for the assessment of a client's health status, indicies or areas of importance to health status are identified. There is much similarity among nursing tools available to guide health status data collection and to document findings. Some tools offer a head-to-toe approach; others are organized around the physiologic systems. More recently a functional-pattern approach is being developed. Data collection requires interpersonal and communication skills, the ability to empathize, a knowledge of nursing and related sciences, and skillful use of the senses in observation (seeing and smelling), palpation (feeling/sense of touch), percussion (feeling and hearing), and auscultation (hearing).

Data collection is a process of ongoing analysis of interaction, historical aspects, physical findings, and client behaviors. Tentative nursing diagnoses are made. Indicies related to specific diagnoses are explored. Information, behaviors, feelings, and thoughts are clarified and validated and are revised as warranted. The assessment is both a phase of the nursing process and a process in itself. It is dynamic and ever-occurring throughout the nursing process.

Generally data are classified as being either objective or subjective. *Objective* data are measurable by the nurse, and they can be similarly observed and measured by another individual. Examples of objective data include vital signs, deformities, skin lesions, drainage, emesis, edema, feces, urine volume, asymmetry, distention, and laboratory test results (blood chemistry, urinalysis, sonogram, ECG, EEG, x-ray, and so on). A "sign" is objective data—you can see, smell, touch, hear, or obtain a standardized measurement of it. A "symptom," on the other hand, is considered subjective data. *Subjective* data are observable only by the client. Examples include pain, nausea, vertigo, palpitations, and mood. The nurse may observe facial expressions or characteristic body positioning or gestures that might be clues that the client is experiencing a particular symptom, but the nurse will never really know what the client is experiencing except by the client telling her or him during the process of validation. Subjective data are influenced by personal feelings and personal perspectives. They are any data reflecting what the client says or what others (family members, health professionals, even the nurse) say about the client.

Analysis and synthesis of data are paramount to assessment. The interpretation at times may stimulate further data collection. Accuracy takes precedence. The more thorough and comprehensive the data base, the greater the potential for insight regarding the client or situation. No matter how complete the data base, the data are virtually useless without skillful and knowledgeable analysis to arrive at nursing diagnoses. The nursing diagnoses in turn give direction to nursing prescriptions (Nsg Rx), the product of the second phase of the nursing process.

Planning

Following assessment, the analysis and synthesis of the data base, and the formulation of nursing diagnoses, nursing goals are established and priorities are determined. The first task is to decide what to do about the nursing diagnoses. The decision making must be within ethical boundaries and must take into consideration the health status assessment, the client's rights, and the nurse's legal responsibilities within a nonbiased context of respect and acceptance of the client. The American Hospital Association (AHA) published "A Patient's Bill of Rights" (see box) to communicate the rights of clients to all concerned. Professionals must protect and facilitate the client's exercise of ethical and legal rights. The American Nurses' Association (ANA) has published a Code for Nurses that establishes guidelines to ethical behaviors and responsibilities in nursing practice (see box). In the eyes of the law, the nurse is legally bound to render a certain standard of nursing care contingent on educational level. This expected level of care is judged by what nurses of similar education would do in the client situation. It is assumed that educational programs are similar enough for nurses with similar educational back-

A Patient's Bill of Rights

The American Hospital Association presents a Patient's Bill of Rights with the expectation that observance of these rights will contribute to more effective patient care and greater satisfaction for the patient, his physician, and the hospital organization. Further, the Association presents these rights in the expectation that they will be supported by the hospital on behalf of its patients, as an integral part of the healing process. It is recognized that a personal relationship between the physician and the patient is essential for the provision of proper medical care. The traditional physician-patient relationship takes on a new dimension when care is rendered within an organizational structure. Legal precedent has established that the institution itself also has a responsibility to the patient. It is in recognition of these factors that these rights are affirmed.

1. The patient has the right to considerate and respectful care.
2. The patient has the right to obtain from his physician complete current information concerning his diagnosis, treatment, and prognosis in terms the patient can be reasonably expected to understand. When it is not medically advisable to give such information to the patient, the information should be made available to an appropriate person in his behalf. He has the right to know, by name, the physician responsible for coordinating his care.
3. The patient has the right to receive from his physician information necessary to give informed consent prior to the start of any procedure and/or treatment. Except in emergencies, such information for informed consent should include but not necessarily be limited to the specific procedure and/or treatment, the medically significant risks involved, and the probable duration of incapacitation. Where medically significant alternatives for care or treatment exist, or when the patient requests information concerning medical alternatives, the patient has the right to such information. The patient also has the right to know the name of the person responsible for the procedures and/or treatment.
4. The patient has the right to refuse treatment to the extent permitted by law and to be informed of the medical consequences of his action.
5. The patient has the right to every consideration of his privacy concerning his own medical care program. Case discussion, consultation, examination, and treatment are confidential and should be conducted discreetly. Those not directly involved in his care must have the permission of the patient to be present.
6. The patient has the right to expect that all communications and records pertaining to his care should be treated as confidential.
7. The patient has the right to expect that within its capacity a hospital must make reasonable response to the request of a patient for services. The hospital must provide evaluation, service, and/or referral as indicated by the urgency of the case. When medically permissible a patient may be transferred to another facility only after he has received complete information and explanation concerning the needs for and alternatives to such a transfer. The institution to which the patient is to be transferred must first have accepted the patient for transfer.
8. The patient has the right to obtain information as to any relationship of his hospital to other health care and educational institutions insofar as his care is concerned. The patient has the right to obtain information as to the existence of any professional relationships among individuals, by name, who are treating him.
9. The patient has the right to be advised if the hospital proposes to engage in or perform human experimentation affecting his care or treatment. The patient has the right to refuse to participate in such research projects.
10. The patient has the right to expect reasonable continuity of care. He has the

right to know in advance what appointment times and physicians are available and when. The patient has the right that the hospital will provide a mechanism whereby he is informed by his physician or a delegate of the physician of the patient's continuing health care requirements following discharge.

11. The patient has the right to examine and receive an explanation of his bill regardless of source of payment.
12. The patient has a right to know what hospital rules and regulations apply to his conduct as a patient.

No catalogue of rights can guarantee for the patient the kind of treatment he has a right to expect. A hospital has many functions to perform, including the prevention and treatment of disease, the education of both health professionals and patients, and the conduct of clinical research. All these activities must be conducted with an overriding concern for the patient and, above all, the recognition of his dignity as a human being. Success in achieving this recognition assures success in the defense of the rights of the patient.

Courtesy American Hospital Association.

American Nurses' Association Code for Nurses

1. The nurse provides services with respect for human dignity and the uniqueness of the client unrestricted by considerations of social or economic status, personal attributes, or the nature of health problems.
2. The nurse safeguards the client's right to privacy by judiciously protecting information of a confidential nature.
3. The nurse acts to safeguard the client and the public when health care and safety are affected by incompetent, unethical, or illegal practice of any person.
4. The nurse assumes responsibility and accountability for individual nursing judgments and actions.
5. The nurse maintains competence in nursing.
6. The nurse exercises informed judgment and uses individual competence and qualifications as criteria in seeking consultation, accepting responsibilities, and delegating nursing activities to others.
7. The nurse participates in activities that contribute to the ongoing development of the profession's body of knowledge.
8. The nurse participates in the profession's efforts to implement and improve standards of nursing.
9. The nurse participates in the profession's efforts to establish and maintain conditions of employment conducive to high-quality nursing care.
10. The nurse participates in the profession's effort to protect the public from misinformation and misrepresentation and to maintain the integrity of nursing.
11. The nurse collaborates with members of the health professions and other citizens in promoting community and national efforts to meet the health needs of the public.

grounds to make nursing judgments that are reasonably the same.

Outcomes are desired changes in clients' health status developed in response to the nursing goals. For example, a nursing diagnosis of "fluid volume deficit related to persistent diarrhea" may have the outcome "moist lips, good skin turgor, and 3000 ml oral intake in 24 hours." The nursing prescriptions are the means, planned mutually by the client and the nurse, to help the client achieve the specific outcomes. An important aspect of outcomes is that they are able to be observed and measured.

Nursing prescriptions promote and strengthen the client's coping strategies and health resources; they are directed toward the prevention of health problems and of complications of illness or treatment measures. They are prescribed to eradicate, modify, and control the cause or etiology of a health problem and to prevent further debilitation. Creative thinking must be used when determining nursing prescriptions. Brainstorming (generating ideas with no holds barred) will aid in identifying multiple alternative prescriptions, which can then be evaluated theoretically for appropriateness and potential effectiveness, inherent advantages and disadvantages, and end results. This process leads to determination of the specific nursing prescriptions to be implemented.

Client participation in the identification of concerns, the setting of priorities, and the determination of the plans of action is extremely important. Clients' concerns or what they may see as priorities may go unattended if the client is not actively involved in planning. As a result, the clients' perspective persists and frequently interferes with medical and nursing diagnoses and priorities and related medical and nursing prescriptions. Client participation increases client compliance with nursing and medical treatment. The nurse needs to be aware of what the client's priorities are and to work from that point.

Sometimes the client is unaware of health enhancement priorities because of knowledge deficit. Health teaching provides the client with an opportunity for learning about his or her health status and alternative means of enhancing it. The additional knowledge gives the client a different perspective and more information on which to evaluate the situation. The added knowledge may affect how the client views his concerns and priorities. Furthermore, the client's perspective may come more in line with that of the nurse or the physician.

Sometimes prescriptions made in the absence of the client's participation may prove to be more harsh than necessary. For instance, if a client on bedrest develops bowel elimination concerns, he may be given a laxative ordered by the physician in anticipation of decreased peristalsis. The nurse in planning with the client may discover a less harsh solution. It may well be for this particular client that a class of prune juice or apple cider in the morning and evening will do the trick just as well as the laxative.

Intervention

Once the nursing prescriptions have been determined, they must be carried out. This implementation of nursing plans is the action phase of the nursing process. This intervention phase is based on scientific rationale underpinning each purposeful action performed by the nurse or the client. Concomitant assessment, analysis, and evaluation are done with the initiation of each step of the plan. The interventions may be reflective of one or all of the types of nursing functions (dependent, interdependent, and independent). The effectiveness of the intervention in assisting the client to achieve outcome objectives is evaluated.

Evaluation

The evaluation phase judges the degree to which the client's status has progressed toward the established outcomes. In order to evaluate, the nurse must again collect data regarding the client's health status. Whether this status has been maintained or improved or whether it has actually regressed will help in determining the effectiveness of the nursing interventions.

Care must be taken not to compare apples and oranges. For example, nursing actions directed toward alleviating stress or perhaps pain may be effective in spite of the client's overall physical deterioration resulting from a debilitating disease process. In such a case, the nursing interventions may be promoting wellness aspects of health status even though the physical illness aspect of health status may be progressive.

Should the desired outcomes relative to the specific nursing diagnosis and nursing prescriptions not be realized, analysis is necessary to determine whether the data or decisions were correct, whether enough time was allotted to realistically achieve the established outcomes, whether the client was motivated in the direction of the outcomes, and whether adequate resources were available for optimum implementation of the nursing prescriptions (see Figure 6-1). A host of variables, many unique to the individual situation, could be influencing regression and need to be evaluated.

Evaluation is the phase of the nursing process in which the nurse determines whether a specific nursing diagnosis has been resolved or continues to exist and, if still present, to what degree. Evaluation may lead to reformulation of nursing diagnoses and nursing prescriptions. It is by the evaluation process that improvement in the quality of nursing care is promoted.

The interrelatedness of the phases of the nursing process is illustrated in Figure 6-2.

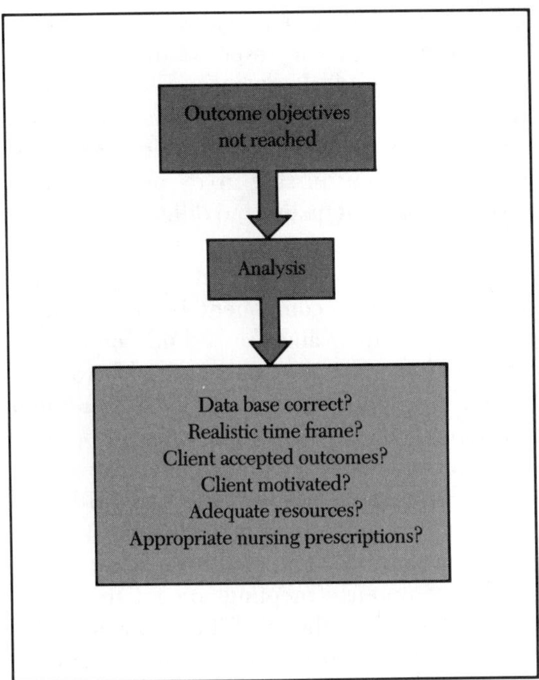

Figure 6-1 Some analytic questions to consider when the desired outcomes are not achieved.

Data Analysis

Data analysis occurs continuously throughout all phases of the nursing process. Behavioral responses are emitted constantly. As the nurse interviews the client, interacts with the client, plans care with the client, renders care for the client, evaluates participation of the client in his or her own care, and evaluates the effectiveness of the nursing interventions, the process of data analysis is ongoing.

Analysis of the client's health situation has a different flavor when performed by the nurse than when performed by the physician. The physician screens the client with the goal of ascertaining whether there are existing pathologies that require medical or surgical care. The nurse assesses the client's health status in regard to responses. A client response can be a reaction to or a result of a medical problem. The nurse's focus is on nursing care for the total human being in all phases and life functions.

The nurse also screens for signs and symptoms that deviate from norms and may indicate illness that requires medical referral; in this aspect nursing assessment overlaps with medical screening of health status. If pathology requiring medical or surgical intervention exists, the nurse is responsible for medical referral, but it is not within the legal practice of the nurse to make a medical diagnosis of the disease state and prescribe medical treatment. Nurse practice acts hold the nurse responsible for case finding and for having the client seek medical attention when needed. Recognizing deviations from the norm and seeking medical consultation or initiating medical referral is reflective of ethical practice and accountability in nursing practice. These legal obligations require the nurse to have knowledge of norms, of differences in norms as influenced by age, race, and gender, and of com-

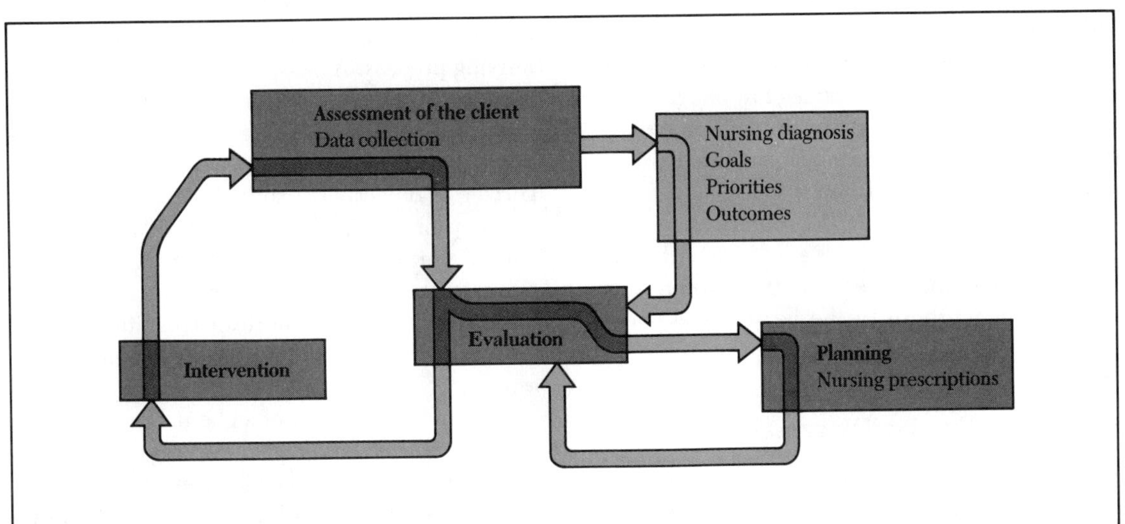

Figure 6-2 The phases of the nursing process are not linear but intertwine. Initial data collection generates nursing diagnoses; data collection following intervention leads to evaluation of nursing prescription effectiveness or to reformulation of the planning phase.

mon normal variations that may be observed, such as cherry angioma or Adie's syndrome.

Analysis of the data should also focus on identification of the client's assets. These strengths are what help the client maintain balance or restore equilibrium when imbalances in health status occur. Strengths might include such things as a healthy constitution (resistance or decreased vulnerability to illness, minimal medical history), decreased exposure to illness-causing variables, good nutrition and exercise habits, vital signs and weight within norm, temperance in all things, absence of detrimental habits such as smoking, drug abuse, or alcohol abuse, a solid support system, a love of life, a thriving spirituality, stable sexuality, leisure and hobby interests, ability to learn quickly and be flexible, financial security, insurance, employment, self-esteem, and self-care capabilities. When the situation is viewed by the client and the nurse in light of the client's assets, the outlook may not be as dismal as first thought. For instance, a client who has had a limb amputated as a result of an accident would have a lot to work with and a brighter outlook if his many assets were recognized than if the focus was merely on the limb loss and the limitations resulting from it.

In a larger context, data analysis can lead to the discovery and development of new knowledge and new theoretical frameworks. It can assist in identifying populations at risk. It can aid in the endeavor to develop and perfect assessment tools, to categorize knowledge, to improve nursing prescriptions and the implementation and evaluation of nursing care, and in this way, to make more efficient and effective use of the nursing process in the practice of nursing.

Analysis determines patterns of client behavior. A presenting pattern may designate existing risk factors, responses to an actual health problem, the potential of a health problem or complication occurring, or wellness enhancement practices. Nursing diagnoses are the products of analysis and synthesis of the health assessment data base.

Nursing Diagnoses

Most nurse practice acts state that it is the legal responsibility of the licensed registered nurse to make nursing diagnoses. Nursing diagnoses determine the scope and specificity of nursing prescriptions needed in an individual client's case as they are developed in response to the nursing goals and desired client outcomes. Carpenito (1983) stated that "nursing diagnosis can provide a solution to the quest of nursing because it serves to: define nursing in its present state, classify nursing's domain, and differentiate nursing from medicine."

A nursing diagnosis generally has two components. The first component is the actual or potential problem, and the second component consists of what the potential or actual factors are that may be contributing to the health problem (see Table 6-1). The first conference to be held for the purpose of developing a classification system for nursing diagnoses was held in 1973. The left column in Table 6-2 lists the diagnostic categories that have accumulated from several subsequent conference meetings on nursing diagnoses. The right column of Table 6-2 lists the chapters of the textbook that describe the assessment techniques and skills for primary data that might lead to a particular nursing diagnosis. This column should not be considered inclusive of all data that may be necessary for arriving at a specific nursing diagnosis. Obviously data from various assessment indices in multiple chapters may be necessary because of the interrelatedness of data.

Summary

Health assessment is an independent nursing function in contrast to dependent and interdependent nursing functions. It is the base of the nursing process. Assessment is the first phase of the nursing process and includes data collection, nursing diagnoses, nursing goals, setting priorities, and outcome objectives. Data can be categorized as objective or subjective.

Decision making by the nurse must take place within ethical and legal boundaries. Nurse practice acts, the American Nurses' Association Code for Nurses, and the American Hospital Association's "Patient's Bill of Rights" delineate these aspects.

Nursing assessment of a client's health status and nursing diagnoses are different from those of medicine. Analysis of data focuses on identifying actual or potential problems and client assets. Nursing diagnoses are the products of the analysis and synthesis of the data base.

Table 6-1. Examples of Nursing Diagnoses

Actual or potential problem		Contributing actual or potential factor
Ineffective breathing	related to	retained secretions
Alteration in urinary elimination	related to	incontinence
Alteration in sexual functioning	related to	side effects of sedatives
Knowledge deficit	related to	low-salt diet
Acute anxiety	related to	impending surgery
Self-care deficit: feeding	related to	right side paralysis
Decreased self-esteem	related to	unemployment
Inadequate bowel elimination	related to	immobility inadequate fluids lack of fiber in diet
Noncompliance with diabetic diet	related to	lack of knowledge inadequate finances
Potential for injury	related to	decreased visual acuity muscle weakness throw rugs absence of handrails
Social isolation	related to	depression due to death of spouse
Anticipatory grieving	related to	loss of right leg

Table 6-2. Nursing Diagnoses Accepted by the North American Nursing Diagnoses Association

Nursing diagnoses patterns			Primary data chapters
Human response pattern: choosing			
*Y00	Family Coping, Impaired		Family Health Assessment (25) Mental Health (5) Neurologic System (18)
	Y00.0	Compromised	
	Y00.1	Disabled	
Y01	[Health Seeking Behavior]		
	Y01.0–9	Health Seeking Behaviors, (Specify)	Health History (4)
*Y02	Individual Coping, Impaired		
	Y02.0	Adjustment, Impaired	Family Health Assessment (25) Mental Health (5)
	Y02.1	Conflict: Decisional	Sociologic Considerations (1)
	Y02.2	Coping: Defensive	Sociologic Considerations (1)
	*Y02.3	Denial, Impaired	Sociologic Considerations (1)
	Y02.4	Noncompliance	Cultural Considerations (2) Health History (4) Mental Health (5)
Human response pattern: communicating			
Y10	[Communication, Impaired]		
	Y10.0	Verbal	Cultural Considerations (2) Communication (3) Mental Health (5) Neurologic System (18) Family Health Assessment (25) Health History (4)
Human response pattern: exchanging			
Y20	[Bowel Elimination, Altered]		Abdomen (16)
	Y20.0	Bowel Incontinence	
	Y20.1	Constipation: Colonic	
	Y20.2	Constipation: Perceived	
	Y20.3	Diarrhea	
*Y21	Cardiac Output, Altered		
Y22	[Fluid Volume, Altered]		Health History (4) Integument (9) Genitals and Rectum (19)
	Y22.0	Deficit	
	Y22.1	Deficit: Risk	
	Y22.2	Excess	

(continued on page 130)

Table 6-2. *Continued*

Nursing diagnoses patterns			Primary data chapters
Human response pattern: exchanging *(continued)*			
*Y23	Injury: Risk		Health History (4)
	*Y23.0	Aspiration	
	*Y23.1	Disuse Syndrome	
	*Y23.2	Poisoning	
	*Y23.3	Suffocation	
	*Y23.4	Trauma	
Y24	[Nutrition, Altered]		Health History (4) Mental Health (5) Wellness (7) Abdomen (16) Neurologic System (18)
	Y24.0	Less than Body Requirement	
	Y24.1	More than Body Requirement	
	*Y24.2	More than Body Requirement: Risk	
Y25	[Physical Regulation, Altered]		Introduction to Physical Assessment (8) Neurologic System (18)
	Y25.0	Dysreflexia	
	Y25.1	Hyperthermia	
	Y25.2	Hypothermia	
	*Y25.3	Infection: Risk	
	*Y25.4	Thermoregulation, Impaired	
Y26	[Respiration, Altered]		Health History (4) Integument (9) Thorax and Lungs (13) Cardiovascular System (14) Neurologic System (18) Assessment of Men's Health (24)
	*Y26.0	Airway Clearance, Impaired	
	*Y26.1	Breathing Pattern, Impaired	
	Y26.2	Gas Exchange, Impaired	
Y27	Tissue Integrity, Altered		Health History (4) Integument (9) Ear, Nose, Mouth, and Pharynx (12)
	*Y27.0	Oral Mucous Membranes, Impaired	
	Y27.1	Skin Integrity, Impaired	
	Y27.2	Skin Integrity, Impaired: Risk	
Y28	Tissue Perfusion, Altered)		Health History (4) Integument (9) Thorax and Lungs (13) Cardiovascular System (14) Abdomen (16) Neurologic System (18) Genitals and Rectum (19) Assessment of Men's Health (24)
	Y28.0	Cardiopulmonary	
	Y28.1	Cerebral	
	Y28.2	Gastrointestinal	
	Y28.3	Peripheral	
	Y28.4	Renal	
Y29	Urinary Elimination, Altered		Health History (4) Genitals and Rectum (19) Assessment of Men's Health (24)
	Y29.0	Incontinence: Functional	
	Y29.1	Incontinence: Reflex	
	Y29.2	Incontinence: Stress	
	Y29.3	Incontinence: Urge	
	Y29.4	Incontinence: Total	
	*Y29.5	Retention	
Human response pattern: feeling			
Y30	Anxiety		Health History (4) Mental Health (5)
Y31	[Comfort, Altered]		Health History (4)
	Y31.0	Pain, [Acute]	
	Y31.1	Pain, Chronic	
Y32	Fear		Mental Health (5)
Y33	[Grieving]		Health History (4) Mental Health (5)
	Y33.0	Anticipatory	
	Y33.1	Dysfunctional	
Y34	Post-Trauma Response		Mental Health (5)
	Y34.0	Rape Trauma Syndrome	
	Y34.1	Rape Trauma Syndrome: Compound Reaction	
	Y34.2	Rape Trauma Syndrome: Silent Reaction	
*Y35	Violence: Risk		Health History (4) Mental Health (5) Neurologic System (18)
Human response pattern: knowing			
Y40	[Knowledge Deficit]		Cultural Considerations (2) Health History (4) Mental Health (5) Neurologic System (18)
	Y40.0–9	Knowledge Deficit (Specify)	
Y41	Thought Processes, Altered		Health History (4) Mental Health (5)
Human response pattern: moving			
Y50	[Activity, altered]		Health History (4) Mental Health (5) Thorax and Lungs (13) Cardiovascular System (14) Musculoskeletal System (17) Neurologic System (18)
	Y50.0	Activity Intolerance	
	Y50.1	Activity Intolerance: Risk	
	Y50.2	Diversional Activity Deficit	
	Y50.3	Fatigue	

Table 6-2. *Continued*

Nursing diagnoses patterns			Primary data chapters
	Y50.4	Physical Mobility, Impaired	Health History (4) Mental Health (5) Thorax and Lungs (13) Cardiovascular System (14) Musculoskeletal System (17) Neurologic System (18)
	Y50.5	Sleep Pattern Disturbance	Health History (4)
*Y51	Bathing/Hygiene Deficit		Health History (4) Musculoskeletal System (17)
*Y52	Dressing/Grooming Deficit		Neurologic System (18)
*Y53	Feeding Deficit		
	*Y53.0	Breastfeeding, Impaired	
	Y53.1	Swallowing, Impaired	
Y54	Growth and Development, altered		
Y55	Health Maintenance, Altered		Sociologic Considerations (1) Health History (4) Health History (4)
Y56	Home Maintenance Management, Impaired		Health History (4) Mental Health (5) Neurologic System (18)
*Y57	Toileting Deficit		
Human response pattern: perceiving			
Y60	[Meaningfulness, Altered]		Mental Health (5)
	Y60.0	Hopelessness	
	Y60.1	Powerlessness	
Y61	[Self Concept, Altered]		Sociologic Considerations (1) Cultural Considerations (2) Health History (4) Mental Health (5) Assessment of Men's Health (24)
	Y61.0	Body Image Disturbance	
	Y61.1	Personal Identity Disturbance	
	Y61.2	Self-Esteem Disturbance: Chronic Low	
	Y61.3	Self-Esteem Disturbance: Situational	
*Y62	[Sensory Perception, Altered]		Mental Health (5) Neurologic System (18)
	Y62.0	Auditory	
	Y62.1	Gustatory	
	Y62.2	Kinesthetic	
	Y62.3	Olfactory	
	Y62.4	Tactile	
	Y62.5	Visual	
	Y62.6	Unilateral Neglect	
Human response pattern: relating			
Y70	Family Processes, Altered		Family Health Assessment (25)
Y71	Role Performance, Altered		Sociologic Considerations (1) Health History (4) Mental Health (5) Child and Adolescent (21) Health History (4)
	Y71.0	Parental Role Conflict	
	Y71.1	Parenting, Altered	
	Y71.2	Parenting, Altered: Risk	
	Y71.3	Sexual Dysfunction	
Y72	Sexuality Patterns, Altered		Health History (4) Mental Health (5) Genitals and Rectum (19) Older Adult (22) Assessment of Men's Health (24)
Y73	[Socialization, Altered]		Family Health Assessment (25)
	Y73.0	Social Interaction, Impaired	
	Y73.1	Social Isolation	Mental Health (5) Older Adult (22)
Human response pattern: valuing			
Y80	[Spiritual State, Altered]		Sociologic Considerations (1) Cultural Considerations (2) Health History (4) Mental Health (5)
	Y80.0	Spiritual Distress	

Discussion Questions/Activities

1. Discuss the key words used in the nurse practice act in your state.
2. Generate nursing diagnoses and contributing factors from a nursing history and compare and discuss them in a group of peers who did the same using the identical nursing history.
3. Choose eight nursing diagnoses and list possible contributory factors and possible signs and symptoms that may occur as a result of each contributory factor.
4. Take the same eight nursing diagnoses and related contributory factors and develop client outcome objectives.

CHAPTER 7

Assessment of Wellness

LEARNING OBJECTIVES

1. Describe the techniques of anthropometric measurement.
2. Cite specific examples of undernutrition.
3. Explain what is meant by subclinical malnutrition.
4. Describe body density, lean body weight, and body fat.
5. Describe methods for determining body density and body fat.
6. Review tests used to measure cardiovascular function, strength, and flexibility.

Aesculapius, the Greek God of Healing, had two daughters, Panacea and Hygeia. Panacea believed the best way to help people was to treat all illness. Hygeia believed the best way was to teach people how to live so that they did not become ill. The approach of Hygeia is related to the focus on wellness in our society. Wellness can be viewed as a process through which individuals become aware of and make choices toward a more satisfying and healthful existence. Wellness assessment includes mental and physical assessment; in addition, it is a review of lifestyle and the identification of health-related beliefs. The culmination of the wellness assessment is reached by helping clients gain increased control over their health. They do this by improving their personal health habits, lifestyle, and environment. Mental assessment was discussed in Chapter 5. This chapter will focus on nutritional and physical fitness assessment.

Nutritional Assessment

Good nutrition is a major prerequisite to health. An adequate and carefully planned diet can alleviate and modify disease states and prevent disease. Many scientists believe that reducing calories, fat, cholesterol, sugar, and salt and eat-

Table 7-1. Ideal Body Weights Using the Height-Frame Rule

Frame size	Height data	Weight (lb) Men	Weight (lb) Women
Medium	First 5 feet	106	100
	Each inch above 5 feet	6	5
Large	Each inch above 5 feet	110/100 × weight calculated for medium-frame person	
Small	Each inch above 5 feet	90/100 × weight calculated for medium-frame person	

From H. Y. Hui. *Human Nutrition and Diet Therapy* (Boston: Jones and Bartlett, 1983), p. 294.

ing more whole grains, fruits, and vegetables will reduce heart disease, cancer, and strokes. There is evidence that the public is becoming more interested in human nutrition as demonstrated by the number of new books dealing with eating better and staying healthy and thin. Increasing media attention has been devoted to food safety, exercise and diet, world hunger, drug and diet interaction and the mental and physical effects of long-term nutritional excess or deprivation. Since it is believed that an improper diet and sedentary lifestyle are the major risk factors leading to disease and early death, it is only sensible that attention to these factors be an important part of wellness assessment and in the subsequent planning with the client for proper and healthful nutrition.

Four major areas must be included in nutritional assessment:

1. Anthropometric measurement
2. Clinical examination
3. Dietary evaluation
4. Biochemical data evaluation

Anthropometric Measurement

This assessment involves measurement of height, weight, mid-arm and chest circumference, skinfold thickness, and—in infants and young children—head circumference. Height and weight tables can be used to determine normal values for specific sex, age, and body frame (see Appendix B). Care should be taken in determining whether a client is overweight or underweight based on these tables alone since they do not take into consideration the quality of body weight. For example, an athlete with well-developed muscles might be overweight according to the tables, yet he may not have excessive adipose tissue. Another individual, on the other hand, may be considered only slightly underweight according to the tables, but he may actually have lost significant body protein, which could be life threatening (Lewis 1984, p. 125). A method of determining ideal body weight is shown in Table 7-1.

Skinfold measurement is a method for determining body density, body fat, and lean body weight (see Figure 7-1). Body density describes the compactness of the body. Body fat refers to fat that is subcutaneous and stored in adipose tissue. Lean body weight is the body weight minus the fat stored in the adipose tissue. There are two ways to take skinfold measurements. The first is referred to as the "scientific pinch." Since most body fat is subcutaneous, the thickness of a "pinch" of skin and fat can be a good indicator of total body fatness. Pinch the skin and fat on the back of the arm over the triceps muscle, at the lower tip of the shoulder blade, and at the abdomen. The thickness of these folds should average not more than ¾ inch. As the saying goes, if you can pinch an inch, you are too fat. A more accurate method is to measure the skinfolds with calipers and then use formulas to calculate body density and fat (Table 7-2).

Table 7-2. Triceps Skinfold Thickness Indicating Obesity (mm)

Age (yr)	Males	Females
5	≥12	≥15
10	≥13	≥17
15	≥15	≥20
20	≥16	≥28
25	≥20	≥29
30 and above	≥23	≥30

From C. C. Seltzer and J. A. Mayer. "Simple Criterion of Obesity." *Post Graduate Medicine,* August 1965.

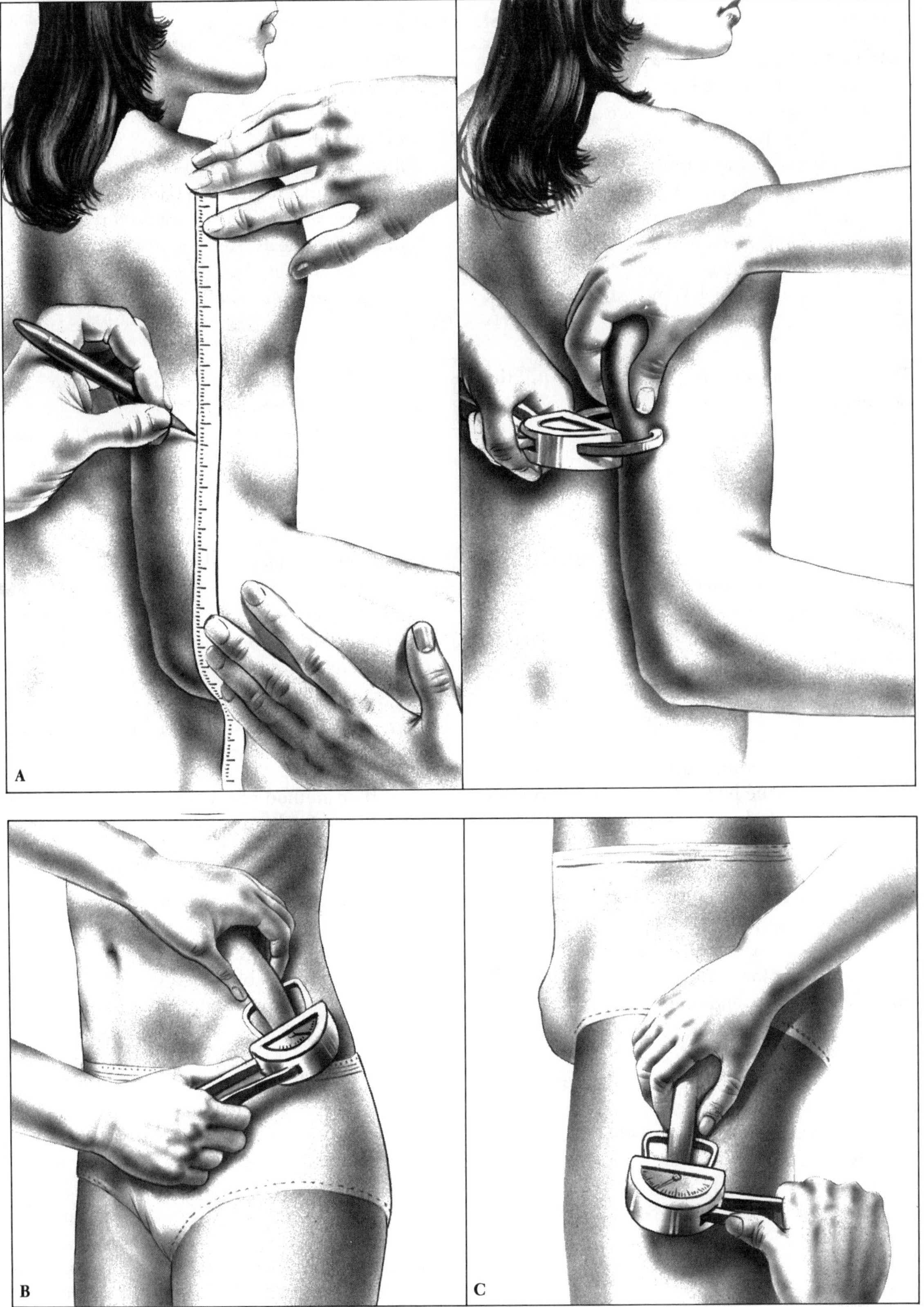

Figure 7-1 Skinfold measurement. (A) Measuring the triceps skinfold. (B) Measuring the suprailiac. (C) Measuring the thigh.

Technique for Skinfold Measurement

1. Grasp the skinfold between the thumb and forefinger. The skinfold should include two thicknesses of skin and subcutaneous fat, but not muscle.
2. Apply the calipers approximately 1 cm below the fingers and at a depth equal to the thickness of the fold.
3. Each fold is taken in the vertical plane while the client is standing except for the subscapular, which is picked up on a slight slant running laterally in the natural fold of the skin.
4. Release the finger slightly so that most of the pressure is on the calipers, not the fingers.
5. Read the dial to the nearest millimeter. Measurement should be made three times, and the average value of the two closest readings should be used as the actual measure (Getchell 1979, pp. 78–79).

The anatomical sites for measuring with the calipers are:

- *Triceps:* the back of the upper arm midway between the shoulder and elbow joints.
- *Subscapula:* the bottom point of the shoulder blade.
- *Thigh:* the front side of the thigh midway between the hip and knee joints.
- *Suprailiac:* just above the top of the hip bone (crest of the ilium) at the middle of the side of the body.

To take the measurement you will need a skinfold caliper. Then you must decide on the measurement sites. All measurements are made on the right side of the body. Because of differences in males and females, measurements are taken at different sites.

Females are measured at suprailiac and triceps areas, males at the thigh and subscapular areas (see Figure 7-1).

The following formulas allow the nurse to calculate body density and then body fat.

Women:
- Skinfold assessment of triceps: Calculate the mean of the three readings.
- Skinfold assessment of suprailiac: Calculate the mean of the three readings.
- Computation for body density (gm/cc): Body density = 1.0764 − (0.00088 × tricep) − (0.00081 × suprailiac)

Men:
- Skinfold assessment of subscapula: Calculate the mean of the three readings.
- Skinfold assessment of thigh: Calculate the mean of the three readings.
- Computation for body density (gm/cc): Body density = 1.1043 − (0.00131 × subscapula) − (0.001327 × thigh)

A good body fat is between 10 and 12% of total body weight for men and between 18 and 20% for women. Over 25% body fat in men and 30% in women is too much fat and indicates obesity. The computation for percentage of body fat (male and female) is as follows:

percentage of body fat =
(4.570/body density − 4.142) × 100

See Figure 7-2.

Another method of calculating body fat without the use of calipers is based on muscularity and height. Tables, such as Tables 7-3 and 7-4, have been developed at Ball State University to estimate ideal weight and body fat.

Clinical Examination

Nutritional status is observed during all phases of physical assessment. Indications of nutritional health may be noted in all body systems but of particular note are the hair, face, eyes, lips, gums, skin, nails, glands, muscular and skeletal systems, and gastrointestinal and nervous systems. The signs of malnutrition, until the late stages, are often nonspecific and must be considered in connection with the total information obtained from the physical assessment and the client history. The overt signs of malnutrition are: dry brittle hair, changes in skin pigment over different parts of the body surface (loss of elasticity), loss of 20–25% of body weight, edema, decreased cardiac output and blood

Women

Skinfold assessment (millimeters)

	Trial 1	Trial 2	Trial 3	Mean
1. Tricip	13.0	16.0	15.0	14.7
2. Suprailiac	7.5	8.0	7.5	7.7

Computation for body density (gm/cc)

Body density

= 1.0764 − (0.00088 × tricep) − (0.00081 × suprailiac)

= 1.0764 − (0.00088 × 14.7) − (0.00081 × 7.7)

= 1.0764 − (.01294) − (.00624)

= 1.057 gm/cc

Computation for percentage of body-fat:

Percentage body fat = (4.570/body density − 4.142)100

= (4.570/ 1.057 − 4.142)100

= .169 × 100

Percentage body fat = 16.9 %

Men

Skinfold assessment (millimeters)

	Trial 1	Trial 2	Trial 3	Mean
1. Subscapula	11.5	11.0	11.0	11.0
2. Thigh	15.0	15.0	—	15.0

Computation for body density (gm/cc):

Body density

= 1.1043 − (0.00131 × subscapula) − (0.001327 × thigh)

= 1.1043 − (0.00131 × 11.0) − (0.001327 × 15.0)

= 1.1043 − (.01441) − (.01991)

= 1.070 gm/cc

Computation for percentage of body fat:

Percentage body fat = (4.570/body density − 4.142)100

= (4.570/ 1.070 − 4.142)100

= (.1290)100

Percentage body fat = 12.9 %

Figure 7-2 Male and female calculations of body density and body fat.

pressure, decreased respirations and a slowdown of the Basal Metabolic Rate, hormonal modifications, malabsorption, diarrhea, and nervous system effects such as apathy or irritability

Table 7-3. Ideal Weights for Women*

Height (inches)	Degree of muscularity: Low	Medium	High
56	78	84	90
57	82	88	94
58	86	92	98
59	90	96	102
60	94	100	106
61	98	104	110
62	102	108	114
63	106	112	118
64	110	116	122
65	114	120	126
66	118	124	130
67	122	128	134
68	126	132	138
69	130	136	142
70	134	140	146
71	138	144	150
72	142	148	154
73	146	152	158
74	150	156	162
75	154	160	166
76	158	164	170

*Based on 18% body fat and degree of muscularity.
From B. Getchell with W. Anderson. *Being Fit: A Personal Guide* (New York: Wiley, 1982), pp. 88–89.

Table 7-4. Ideal Weights for Men

Height (inches)	Degree of muscularity: Low	Medium	High
60	129	135	143
61	132	138	146
62	135	141	149
63	138	144	152
64	141	147	155
65	144	150	158
66	147	153	161
67	150	156	164
68	153	159	167
69	156	162	170
70	159	165	173
71	161	168	176
72	164	171	179
73	167	174	182
74	170	177	185
75	173	180	188
76	176	183	191
77	179	186	194
78	182	189	197
79	185	191	200
80	188	193	203

*Based on 12% body fat and degree of muscularity.
From B. Getchell with W. Anderson. *Being Fit: A Personal Guide* (New York: Wiley, 1982), pp. 88–89.

Technique for Calculating Body Fat

1. Determine muscularity: Measure girth of calf at widest circumference, or measure wrist at smallest circumference.
2. Check Tables 7-5 and 7-6 to see if you have low, medium, or high muscularity.
3. Refer to the ideal weights in Table 7-3 or 7-4. Find your height in inches, and then move across the table to find your degree of muscularity. At that point you will find your ideal weight. Note that these weights are based on optimum percentage of body fat.
4. Calculate your percentage of body fat by using the following formula (Getchell 1982, pp. 86–87):

Women:

$$\frac{\text{existing weight} - (.82 \times \text{ideal weight})}{\text{existing weight}} \times 100 = \%\ \text{fat}$$

Men:

$$\frac{\text{existing weight} - (.88 \times \text{ideal weight})}{\text{existing weight}} \times 100 = \%\ \text{fat}$$

Example:

$$\frac{185 - (.88 \times 165)}{185} = \frac{185 - (145.2)}{185}$$

$$= \frac{39.8}{185}$$

$$= .215$$

$$.215 \times 100 = 21.5\%\ \text{fat}$$

Table 7-5. Calf Girth Measurements

Degree of muscularity (estimate)	Women (inches)	Men (inches)
Low	12½ and below	14 and below
Medium	12½–13½	14–15½
High	13½ and up	15½ and up

From B. Getchell with W. Anderson. *Being Fit: A Personal Guide* (New York: Wiley, 1982), pp. 88–89. Copyright 1982.

Table 7-6. Wrist Girth Measurements

Bone structure (estimate)	Women (inches)	Men (inches)
Low	5¼ and below	6¼ and below
Medium	5½–6	6¼–7
High	6 and up	7 and up

From B. Getchell and W. Anderson. *Being Fit: A Personal Guide* (New York: Wiley, 1982), pp. 88–89. Copyright 1982.

(see Table 7-7). Extreme cases of malnutrition in Africa have been shown by the media.

Degrees of malnutrition can be observed in groups of underserved people in the United States. These people are poorly nourished due to lack of food, unsanitary conditions, inadequate water, lack of education, and other social, geographical, and cultural factors. In the last few years there has been increasing concern for what is referred to as "subclinical" malnutrition. This affects everyone in this country and is a result of extreme processing of food and the addition of chemicals to foods to enhance appearance and increase shelf life.

Dietary Evaluation

With all the published data related to diet, it is relatively easy to calculate the approximate amounts and proportions of fats, carbohydrates, proteins, vitamins, and minerals that should constitute a "healthy" diet. Most people, however, do not read nutritional charts, nor do they know how to define nutritional requirements in terms of actual food consumed. They tend to eat

Table 7-7. Physical Signs and Symptoms of Undernutrition

Organ/tissue	Undernutrition	Good nutrition
Hair	Dry, wirelike Stiff often brittle May exhibit some bleaching of normal color Easily pluckable (pediatric form)	Shiny, lustrous Healthy scalp
Eyes	Thickened, opaque bulbar conjunctivae with angular lesions Increase in vascularity, conjunctival injection Xerosis conjuctivae (the conjunctivae, upon exposure by holding the lids open and having the subject rotate the eyes, appear dull and lusterless and exhibit a striated or roughened surface Bitot's spots—small circumscribed grayish or yellowish dull, dry, foamy superficial lesions of the conjunctiva; seen most often on lateral aspect of conjunctiva and in children; not to be confused with pterygium Xerophthalmia—recorded when bulbar conjunctiva and cornea are dry and lusterless with a decrease in lacrimation; often associated with evidence of infection or, in extreme cases, keratomalacia Keratomalacia (pediatric form shows corneal softening with deformity, either localized, usually central part of lower half of cornea, or total)	Bright, clear, moist
Mouth and tongue Mucous membranes	Lips—angular lesions and scars, indicating cheilosis Tongue—Filiform papillary atrophy (smooth slick), hypertrophy/hyperemia, geographic tongue, fissure/serrations or swelling, red, scarlet, beefy (glossitis), magenta colored (color of alkaline phenolphthalein)	Reddish-pink color to lips, tongue, and mucous membrane Absense of lesions Adequately moist Surface papillae present on tongue
Teeth and gums	Teeth—visible caries Gums—atrophy, recession, inflammation; marginal redness or swelling (marginal redness is a definite red border along dental margin of gum, marginal swelling in a swollen border of gum, which may be spongy or firm); swollen red papillae; bleeding gums, which either bleed spontaneously or bleed upon slight pressure with a swab stick	Teeth straight, bright without crowding, no evidence of caries Gums firm, reddish pink with no evidence of swelling or bleeding
Skin	Follicular hyperkeratosis—rough, dry Xerosis—dry or scaling Hyperpigmentation—seen most frequently on dorsa of hands and lower forearms, particularly where skin hygiene is poor; skin is rough and dry, and often has a grayish cyanotic base	Smooth, slightly moist, good color

(continued on page 140)

Table 7-7. *Continued*

Organ/tissue	Undernutrition	Good nutrition
	Thickened pressure points (other than elbows and knees); look especially at belt area, ischial tuberositis, sacrum, over greater trochanters	
Abdomen and lower extremities	Potbelly (pediatric form only), hepatomegaly Pretibial edema (bilateral) Calf tenderness (adult form only) Absent knee/ankle jerk (adult form) Absent vibratory sense (adult form): test with tuning fork over lateral malleoli; record as positive only if absent bilaterally	Abdomen flat No tenderness, weakness, or swelling of feet and legs
Skeletal (pediatric form only)	Beading of ribs Bossing of skull	Good posture No malformations
Face and neck	Malar pigmentation (adult form)—areas of dark brown pigmentation over malar eminences Nasolabial seborrhea—a definite greasy, yellowish scaling or filiform excrescenses on nasolabial area, which become more pronounced on slight scratching with a fingernail or tongue blade Parotid glands visibly enlarged Thyroid enlarged	Skin of face and neck clear, smooth No thyroid enlargement
Muscles	Flaccid underdeveloped, or wasted in appearance, tender	Well developed, firm

what and when they like or can afford, whether or not the meal has the right nutrients. In the United States, for instance, many students dash off to classes having had no breakfast at all or else a quick meal of coffee and toast. A lunch consists of a hamburger and fries, supplemented with candy or soft drinks. This kind of diet can provide an adequate number of calories to get through the day but inadequate nutrients to nourish all the body systems. A common form of malnutrition in the United States is overconsumption of food, which can create such serious health problems such as obesity and heart disease and contribute to certain forms of diabetes.

Humans differ widely in their caloric requirements depending on size, age, sex, occupation, and so on. The average middle-aged male needs about 2600 calories a day, a woman about 1900, and a 12- to 15-year-old girl or boy from 2500 to 3000. Methods for calculating calorie needs are presented in Tables 7-8 and 7-9. These approximations assume a moderate amount of physical activity. If an individual takes in more calories than are burned, the extra calories are converted to fat and the person gains weight. If one does not take in enough calories, the body begins to convert its own tissue into the calories it needs and weight is lost. Reducing diets based on this principle are often extreme and do not have the necessary vitamins and minerals.

For individuals to meet all their nutritional requirements, they must eat a variety of foods, which nutritionalists have grouped into four

Table 7-8. One Method of Calculating Daily Caloric Needs According to Basal Metabolism and Activity Level

Physical activity	Total calories needed daily
Sedentary to light	$\frac{130}{100}$ × basal caloric need
Moderate	$\frac{150}{100}$ × basal caloric need
Strenuous	$\frac{(175 - 200)}{100}$ × basal caloric need

From H. Y. Hui. *Human Nutrition and Diet Therapy* (Boston: Jones and Bartlett, 1983), p. 295.

Table 7-9. USDA Rule of Thumb for Calculating Daily Caloric Needs

Physical activity	Total calories needed daily*	
	Women	Men
Sedentary	Ideal body weight × 14	Ideal body weight × 16
Moderate	Ideal body weight × 18	Ideal body weight × 21
Strenuous	Ideal body weight × 22	Ideal body weight × 26

*All ideal body weights expressed in pounds.
From H. Y. Hui. *Human Nutrition and Diet Therapy* (Boston: Jones and Bartlett, 1983), p. 296.

broad categories. Nurses need to have knowledge of RDA (Recommended Dietary Allowances) if they are going to adequately assess a client's dietary history. There are several excellent books on nutrition, and, whenever possible, nurses should consult with nutritionists for help in assessment and planning. The following information about the four food groups is brief but will be of assistance in the assessment process.

Food Groups

There are four groups: milk and milk products, meats or meat equivalents, fruits and vegetables, and breads and cereals. Each group contributes a substantial amount of the major nutrients necessary for good health.

1. *Milk and milk products* (see Table 7-10)
   Fluid milk: whole, low fat, skim, fat free
   Dry milk: whole, low fat, skim, fat free
   Other milk: evaporated, condensed
   Milk products: yogurt, cheese, cottage cheese
   Milk alternates: soy milk, powdered soy milk, soy cheese
2. *Meat and meat equivalents*
   Lean meat: beef, veal, lamb, pork, liver
   Variety meat: heart, brain, tongue, kidney
   Fish: shellfish, fresh and saltwater varieties
   Poultry: all fowl (chicken, turkey, guinea hen, duck, goose) and their giblets
   Miscellaneous meats: "turkey ham," hot dogs
   Dry legumes: navy beans, lima beans, lentils, and peanuts
   Nuts: nuts, nut butter
   Peas: all split, dried peas, pinto beans, chick peas, and pigeon peas
   Meat equivalents: eggs, cheese
3. *Fruits and Vegetables* The daily food guides recommend four or more servings of fruits and vegetables each day. See Table 7-11.

Table 7-10. Milk Products That Contribute As Much Protein and Calcium As 1 Cup of Fluid Whole Milk

Milk product	Amount of product containing given amount of nutrient	
	9 g Protein	280 g Calcium
Nonfat milk	1 c	1 c
Cheddar cheese	1⅓ oz	1⅓ oz
Cottage cheese	1⅓ c	⅓ c
Ice cream	1½ c	1½ c
Cream cheese	30 T	9 T

From H. Y. Hui. *Human Nutrition and Diet Therapy* (Boston: Jones and Bartlett, 1983), p. 253.

4. *Cereals and Cereal Products*
   Breads: yeast breads, rolls, quickbreads, biscuits, buns, muffins, pancakes, waffles, crackers
   Breakfast cereals: ready-to-eat types including flaked, rolled, and puffed forms; and cooked types including whole grain and rolled forms
   Other grain foods: macaroni, spaghetti, noodles, flour, rice, cornmeal
   Whole grain products: wholewheat flour and its products, bulgur, dark rye flour, brown rice, whole ground cornmeal

Table 7-12 lists the recommended number of servings from the four food groups. Table 7-13 outlines the nutrient contributions of foods in each of the groups. Tables 7-14 and 7-15 offer suggested meal plans.

Dietary History

A component of the nutritional assessment that is very useful in determining the client's nutritional status is the dietary history. The nurse asks the client to keep a record, usually for 24 hours, of all food eaten and at what times of the day. This is probably the most common way to make

Table 7-11. Foods in the Fruit and Vegetable Group

Varieties rich in vitamin A and carotene

Dark green leafy vegetables: beet greens, broccoli, chard, collards, watercress, kale, mustard greens, spinach, turnip tops, wild greens (dandelion and others)

Orange-colored vegetables: carrots, pumpkins, sweet potatoes, winter squash, yams

Orange-fleshed fruits: apricots, muskmelon, mangoes

Varieties rich in vitamin C

Citrus fruits: grapefruit, oranges, lemons, tangerines; juices of these fruits

Other good and excellent sources: muskmelon, strawberries, broccoli, several tropical fruits (including guavas), raw sweet green and red peppers

Significant sources: tomatoes, tomato juice, white potatoes, dark green leafy vegetables, other raw vegetables and fruits

Other fruits and vegetables

Vegetables: asparagus, lima beans, green beans, beets, cabbage, cauliflower, celery, corn, cucumber, eggplant, kohlrabi, lettuce, okra, onions, green peas, plantain, rutabagas, sauerkraut, summer squash, and turnips

Fruits: apples, avocados, bananas, berries, cherries, dates, figs, grapes, nectarines, peaches, pears, pineapple, plums, prunes, raisins, rhubarb, watermelon; juices and nectars of many fruits

From H. Y. Hui. *Human Nutrition and Diet Therapy* (Boston: Jones and Bartlett, 1983), p. 255.

Table 7-12. Recommended Numbers of Servings from the Four Food Groups

Food group	Serving size	No. of daily servings
Milk and milk products		
Fluid milk	1 c, 8 oz, ½ pt, ¼ qt	Children under 9: 2–3 Children 9–12: ≥3 Teenagers: ≥4 Adults: ≥2 Pregnant women: ≥3 Nursing mothers: ≥4
Calcium equivalent	1 c milk 2 c cottage cheese 1 c pudding 1¾ c ice cream 1½ oz cheddar cheese	
Meat and meat equivalents	2–3 cooked lean meat without bone 3–4 oz raw meat without bone 2 oz luncheon meat (e.g., bologna) ¾ c canned baked beans 1 c cooked dry beans, peas, lentils 2 eggs 2 oz cheddar cheese ½ c cottage cheese 4 T peanut butter	≥2
Fruits and vegetables	Varies by item: ½ c cooked spinach 1 potato 1 orange ½ grapefruit	≥4, including 1 of citrus fruit and another fruit or vegetable that is a good source of vitamin C and 2 of a fair source 1, at least every other day, of a dark green or deep yellow vegetable for vitamin C ≥2 or more of other vegetables and fruits, including potatoes
Bread and cereals	1 slice of bread, 1 oz ready-to-eat cereal ½ to ¾ c cooked cereal, cornmeal, grits, macaroni, noodles, rice, or spaghetti	≥4

From H. Y. Hui. *Human Nutrition and Diet Therapy* (Boston: Jones and Bartlett, 1983), p. 251.

Table 7-13. Approximate Nutrient Contributions of the Different Food Groups

Food group	Major nutrient contributed	Proportional contribution to the American diet
Milk	Protein	⅓
	Calcium	⅔
	Riboflavin	½
Meat	Protein	½
	Thiamin	¼
	Iron	>⅓
	Niacin	>⅓
Fruits and vegetables	Vitamin C	practically all
	Vitamin A and carotene	¾
	Iron	¼
Bread and cereals	Iron, thiamin, niacin, other B vitamins, fiber	>¼
Supplementary foods		
Fats, oils	Calories, fat-soluble vitamins	varies
Sweet products	Fluids, calories, small amount of nutrients	varies
Spices and seasonings	Iodine	varies
Alcohol	Calories	insignificant to ⅓

From H. Y. Hui. *Human Nutrition and Diet Therapy* (Boston: Jones and Bartlett, 1983), p. 258.

Table 7-14. Suggested Meal Plan

Breakfast	Lunch	Dinner
Fruit/juice, ½ c/1 serving	Soup, ½ c	Soup, ½ c
Cereal: hot/6 oz; dry/1 oz	Meat (regular/substitute), 2–3 oz	Meat (regular/substitute), 3–4 oz
Egg (regular or substitute), 1 serving	Vegetable (cooked/salad), ½ c	Fruit/juice, ½ c/1 serving
Meat: 2 strips bacon; 2 sausages; 1 oz regular meat	Potato (regular/substitute), ½ c	Vegetable (cooked/salad), ½ c
Bread, 1–2 slices	Salad dressing, 1 T	Potato (regular/substitute), ½ c
Butter/margarine, 1–3 t	Bread/roll, 1–2 servings	Salad dressing, 1–2 t
Jelly/jam/preserves, 1–3 t	Butter/margarine, 1–3 t	Bread/roll, 1–2 servings
Milk, 1 c	Dessert, 1 serving	Butter/margarine, 1–3 t
Hot beverage (coffee/tea), 1–2 c	Milk, 1 c	Dessert, 1 serving
Cream (regular/substitute), 1–3 t	Hot beverage (coffee/tea), 1–2 c	Milk, 1 c
Sugar, 1–3 t	Cream (regular/substitute), 1–3 t	Hot beverage (coffee/tea), 1–2 c
Salt, pepper	Sugar, 1–3 t	Cream (regular/substitute), 1–3 t
	Salt, pepper	Sugar, 1–3 t
		Salt, pepper

From H. Y. Hui. *Human Nutrition and Diet Therapy* (Boston: Jones and Bartlett, 1983), p. 259.

this assessment. One example of a dietary history format is shown in Table 7-16. Since there are many variations, the nurse should use the one that is most helpful in obtaining the needed information. Information obtained in this assessment can be used by the nurse to develop a teaching plan to meet the client's specific needs. See also Table 7-17. It is helpful to use this or a similar chart when helping clients to plan an adequate diet.

Biochemical Data Evaluation

The final component of nutritional assessment is the biochemical analysis of blood, urine, feces, saliva, and mucus. This analysis is a valuable adjunct to clinical and dietary data. Actual or

Table 7-15. Menu Plan Providing 2,400 kcal and 95 g of Protein

Breakfast	Lunch	Dinner
Orange juice, ½ c	Pea soup, ½ c	Chicken broth, ½ c
Oatmeal, 6 oz	Crackers, 2	Fried chicken, 3 oz
Egg, 1	Ham, 2 oz	Spinach, ½ c
Bread, 2 slices	Lettuce/tomato salad, ½ c	Rice, ½ c
Margarine, 2 t	Noodles, ½ c	Bread, 1 slice
Jelly, 1 t	Toast, 1 slice	Margarine, 1 t
Milk, 1 c	Margarine, 1 t	Milk, 1 c
Coffee, 1 c	Milk, 1 c	Coffee, 1 c
Cream, 1 t	Ice cream, 1 c	Cream substitute, 1 t
Sugar, 2 t	Coffee, 1 c	Sugar, 1 t
Salt, pepper	Sugar, 1 t	Salt, pepper
	Salt, pepper	

From H. Y. Hui. *Human Nutrition and Diet Therapy* (Boston: Jones and Bartlett, 1983), p. 259.

Table 7-16. Dietary History Format

Record of foods eaten and drinks	Amount (cups, tbsps)
Morning	
Food	
Drinks	
Midmorning	
Food	
Drinks	
Noon	
Food	
Drinks	
Afternoon	
Food	
Drinks	
Evening	
Food	
Drinks	
Before bed	
Food	
Drinks	
Vitamin or mineral supplement (list kind and number taken)	

subclinical deficiencies can be determined. Substances analyzed are in three categories: (1) blood components such as proteins, albumin, hemoglobin, and fibrinogen; (2) minerals and specific substances such as cations, hydrogen-ions, adenosine triphosphate, and glutathione; and (3) nutrients and their metabolites such as amino and fatty acids, glycerol, phospholipids, cholesterol, triglycerides, carbohydrates, vitamins, minerals, and hormones. Body wastes to be analyzed include carbon dioxide, water, bilirubin, urea, and creatinine. See Table 7-18.

Physical Fitness Assessment

Physical fitness has taken the country by storm. Health clubs are bustling, aerobic classes are full, and the streets are noticeably busy with walkers, bikers, and joggers. They are on a quest for wellness, fitness, and an improved lifestyle. Fitness is important at all ages. For children,

Table 7-17. Guidelines for Assisting the Client in Dietary Planning

Current dietary patterns		Recommended dietary goals	
42% fat	16% saturated 19% monounsaturated 7% polyunsaturated	10% saturated 10% monounsaturated 10% polyunsaturated	30% fat 12% protein
12% protein			
46% carbohydrates	28% complex carbohydrates and naturally occurring sugars 18% refined and processed sugars	48% complex carbohydrates and naturally occurring sugars 10% refined and processed sugars	58% carbohydrates

From *Dietary Goals for the United States*. U.S. Senate Select Committee on Nutrition and Human Needs. Washington, D.C.: Government Printing Office, December 1977.

Table 7-18. Guidelines for Classification and Interpretation of Group Blood and Urine Data

	Classification category			
	Less than acceptable			
Substance	**Deficient**		**Low**	**Acceptable***
Hemoglobin (g/100 mL)				
6–23 months	< 9.0		9.0–9.9	⩾ 10.0
2–5 years	< 10		10.0–10.9	⩾ 11.0
6–12 years	< 10		10.0–11.4	⩾ 11.5
13–16 years, male	< 12		12.0–12.9	⩾ 13.0
13–16 years, female	< 10		10.0–11.4	⩾ 11.5
>16 years, male	< 12		12.0–13.9	⩾ 14.0
>16 years, female	< 10		10.0–11.9	⩾ 12.0
Pregnant, 2nd trimester	< 9.5		9.5–10.9	⩾ 11.0
Pregnant, 3rd trimester	< 9.0		9.0–10.4	⩾ 10.5
Hematocrit (%)				
6–23 months	< 28		28–30	⩾ 31
2–5 years	< 30		30–33	⩾ 34
6–12 years	< 30		30–35	⩾ 36
13–16 years, male	< 37		37–39	⩾ 40
13–16 years, female	< 31		31–35	⩾ 36
>16 years, male	< 37		37–43	⩾ 44
>16 years, female	< 31		31–37	⩾ 38
Pregnant, 2nd trimester	< 30		30–34	⩾ 35
Pregnant, 3rd trimester	< 30		30–32	⩾ 33
Hemoglobin conc, MCHC (g/100 ml RBC), all ages	—		30	⩾ 30
Serum iron (μg/100 ml)				
0–5 months	—	—	—	—
6–23 months	—	<30	—	⩾ 30
2–5 years	—	<40	—	⩾ 40
6–12 years	—	<50	—	⩾ 50
>12 years, male	—	<60	—	⩾ 60
>12 years, female	—	<40	—	⩾ 40
Transferrin saturation (%)				
0–5 months	—	—	—	—
6–23 months	—	<15	—	⩾ 15
2–12 years	—	<20	—	⩾ 20
>12 years, male	—	<20	—	⩾ 20
>12 years, female	—	<15	—	⩾ 15
Red cell folacin (ng/ml), all ages	<140		140–159	⩾160–650
Serum folacin (ng/ml)	3.0		3.0–5.9	⩾ 6.0
Serum protein (g/100 ml)				
0–11 months	—		<5.0	⩾ 5.0
1–5 years	—		<5.5	⩾ 5.5
6–17 years	—		<6.0	⩾ 6.0
Adult	< 6.0		6.0–6.4	⩾ 6.5
Pregnant, 2nd and 3rd trimester	< 5.5		5.5–5.9	⩾ 6.0
Serum albumin (g/100 ml)				
0–11 months	—		<2.5	⩾ 2.5
1–5 years	—		<3.0	⩾ 3.0
6–17 years	—		<3.5	⩾ 3.5

(continued on page 146)

*Excessively high levels may indicate abnormal clinical status or toxicity.
†May indicate unusual diet or malabsorption.
From *Ten State Nutrition Survey. 1968–1970. I. Historical Development. II. Demographic Data.* U.S. Department of Health, Education and Welfare Publication No. (HSM) 72-8130. Atlanta: Center for Disease Control. 1972, pp. 1-115–1-116.

Table 7-18. *Continued*

Substance	Classification category: Less than acceptable — Deficient	Less than acceptable — Low	Acceptable*
Adult	< 2.8	2.8–3.4	≥ 3.5
Pregnant, 1st trimester	< 3.0	3.0–3.9	≥ 4.0
Pregnant, 2nd and 3rd trimester	< 3.0	3.0–3.4	≥ 3.5
Serum vitamin C (mg/100 ml)			
0–11 months	—	—	—
≥1 years	< 0.1	0.1–0.19	≥ 0.2
Plasma carotene (μg/100 ml)			
0–5 months	—	<10	≥ 10
6–11 months	—	<30	≥ 30
1–17 years	—	<40	≥ 40
Adult	< 20†	20–39	≥ 40
Pregnant, 2nd trimester	—	30–79	≥ 80
Pregnant, 3rd trimester	—	40–79	≥ 80
Plasma vitamin A (μg/100 ml), all ages	< 20	20–29	≥ 30
Urinary thiamin (μg/g creatinine)			
1–3 years	<120	120–175	≥176
4–6 years	< 85	85–120	≥121
7–9 years	< 70	70–180	≥181
10–12 years	< 60	60–180	≥181
13–15 years	< 50	50–150	≥151
Adult	< 27	27–65	≥ 66
Pregnant, 2nd trimester	< 23	23–54	≥ 55
Pregnant, 3rd trimester	< 21	21–49	≥ 50
Urinary riboflavin (μg/g creatinine)			
1–3 years	<150	150–499	≥500
4–6 years	<100	100–299	≥300
7–9 years	< 85	85–269	≥270
10–15 years	< 70	70–199	≥200
Adult	< 27	27–79	≥ 80
Pregnant, 2nd trimester	< 39	39–119	≥120
Pregnant, 3rd trimester	< 30	30–89	≥ 90
Urinary iodine (μg/g creatinine)	< 25	25–49	≥ 50

optimum fitness assists them in normal development and in helping them to be strong enough to meet life's challenges. For the young adult and middle-age client, a fit body helps in prevention of degenerative disorders such as coronary heart disease, obesity, and musculoskeletal disorders. For the older client, maintaining fitness improves quality of life by helping to maintain or improve physical capabilities and also often improves social interactions. Research has demonstrated a link between physical fitness and the improvement in self-attitudes (Ben Leslies & Short 1983, pp. 11–28).

Complete physical fitness assessment can be complex and may require specialized equipment and space. The nurse can do an initial assessment, which will be helpful in making overall plans for client care.

The basic components of health and fitness are cardiovascular function, body composition, strength, and flexibility.

Cardiovascular Function

Cardiovascular function is the most important component in the health-related fitness area. Cardiovascular disease is the leading cause of death among adult populations of most industrialized societies. An alarming aspect of this is the prevalence of heart disease among younger adults. The problem is not confined to adults. In two recent studies of boys and girls ages 7–12, it was noted that 60% exhibited at least one of the

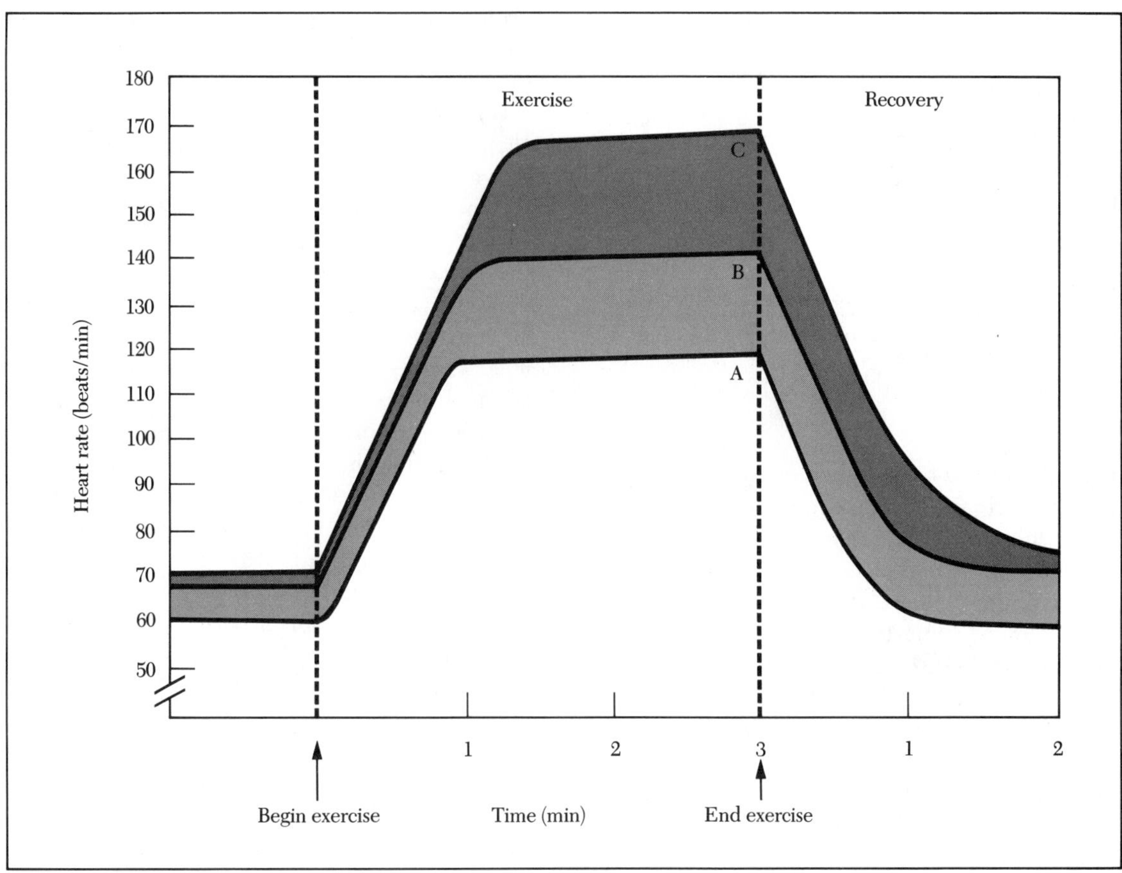

Figure 7-3 Heart rate response to step test. Examples are given for three people, A, B, and C.

risk factors associated with increased coronary heart disease in the adult population (obesity, high serum cholesterol and/or triglycerides, elevated blood pressure, or low work capacity) (Baylor & Dishman 1980, p. 40).

Various laboratory tests, stress tests, and EKG examinations are the most definitive in making an assessment of cardiovascular fitness. Some tests can be easily done by the nurse in carrying out a cardiovascular assessment. The first is the *step test*. This test is an easy-to-use field test, which can give preliminary information on the cardiovascular fitness of the client. It is not stressful for most clients, but caution should be used in testing clients over 40, those who are obese, and those who have a history of cardiovascular problems.

A step 17–18 inches high is needed. The client should be instructed to step up and down on the step, 30 steps per minute for men and 24 steps per minute for women. The following sequence should be used: right foot up, left foot up; right foot down, left foot down. After the client has continued stepping for three minutes (4-count sequence), the pulse is measured. Apical, carotid, or radial pulses may be used. Pulse rates are counted for 30 seconds at the following intervals:

- 1 to 1½ minutes following exercise
- 2 to 2½ minutes following exercise
- 3 to 3½ minutes following exercise

The 30-second pulses are added and the sum is called the recovery index (Getchell 1979, pp. 70–73). See Figure 7-3 and Table 7-19.

Body Composition

Body composition is the relative percentage of fat and fat-free body mass. Body composition is an important correlate to cardiovascular function as far as health-related fitness is concerned. Ex-

Table 7-19. Three-Minute Step-Test Recovery Index

	Cumulated Pulse Rate	
Rating	**Men**	**Women**
Excellent	132 or less	135 or less
Good	150–133	155–136
Average	165–149	170–154
Fair	180–164	190–171
Poor	above 180	above 190

From B. Getchell. *Physical Fitness: A Way of Life*, 2nd ed. (New York: Wiley, 1979).

cess fat is excess baggage and causes the body to have to increase energy expenditure, which in turn causes the circulation to work harder. In addition to increased coronary heart disease among obese persons, there is also greater risk of developing hypertension, diabetes mellitus, gallbladder disease, arthritis, and kidney disease. Methods for assessing body density, fat, and weight were described earlier in this chapter. In addition, body proportions should be considered. If the body is well proportioned, the individual generally feels better about self-image. Norms for determining girth measurements are as follows:

Women

- Bust and hips: same
- Abdomen at waist: 25 to 26 cm < bust and hips
- Thigh: 15 cm < waist
- Calf: 18–20 cm < thigh
- Ankle: 13–15 cm < calf
- Biceps (upper arm): relaxed, 2 × size of wrist

Men

- Chest and hips: same
- Abdomen (at waist): 13–18 cm < chest and hips
- Thigh: 20–25 cm < abdomen
- Calf: 18–20 cm < thigh
- Ankle: 15–18 cm < calf
- Biceps (upper arm) relaxed: 2 × size of wrist (Pender 1982, p. 87)

Strength

Strength, defined as the capacity of a muscle to exert or resist force, is the third component of fitness. Strength is important to the athlete and also to the average individual. Strong muscles protect joints, which in turn protect against strains, sprains, and pulls. Toned muscles help to prevent sagging abdomens, round shoulders, and back pain. Lack of strength can impair the client's ability to carry out even the simplest of activities of daily living.

Bent-knee sit-ups can be used as a test of muscular strength. Clients who have not maintained their fitness level will often find this difficult to do. In females the number of sit-ups is calculated for one minute; for men, the number in two minutes. Clients with cardiovascular disorders or other chronic illness and the elderly must be observed carefully. The nurse may make the judgment that this test would be too distressing for the client and assume that muscle strength is poor. Plans can be made with the client's needs and capabilities in mind to develop a plan that would help to build reasonable muscle strength.

The procedure for assisting the client for bent-knee sit-ups is as follows: have the client lie on his back on a mat or firm support and bend the knees approximately 90° with feet flat on the floor. Hands should be interlocked behind the neck, elbows pointed toward the knees. The nurse can hold the feet while instructing the client to curl the back and raise the trunk until it is perpendicular to the floor. It is important to keep the knees bent during the entire exercise. (See Figure 7-4 and Table 7-20.)

Flexibility

Flexibility refers to the degree to which a joint may move throughout its maximal possible range of motion. Maintenance of the ability to move, bend, and stretch provides good protection to muscle during activity. Flexibility decreases with age and also with a sedentary lifestyle. Poor flexibility may result in misalignment of body structures, crowding of internal organs, and low back pain. Lack of flexibility also makes it difficult for clients to maintain activities of daily living. A quick test of flexibility is to have the client bend forward and, keeping knees straight, touch his toes (see Table 7-21). Poor flexibility is indicated by an inability to reach the toes.

Another test of flexibility measures the client's ability to stretch back and thigh muscles. The procedure for measuring this is as follows: have the client sit on the floor with legs fully extended and feet flat against a box, which has been stabilized against the wall. Instruct the

PLATE 1

THE SKELETAL SYSTEM (front view)

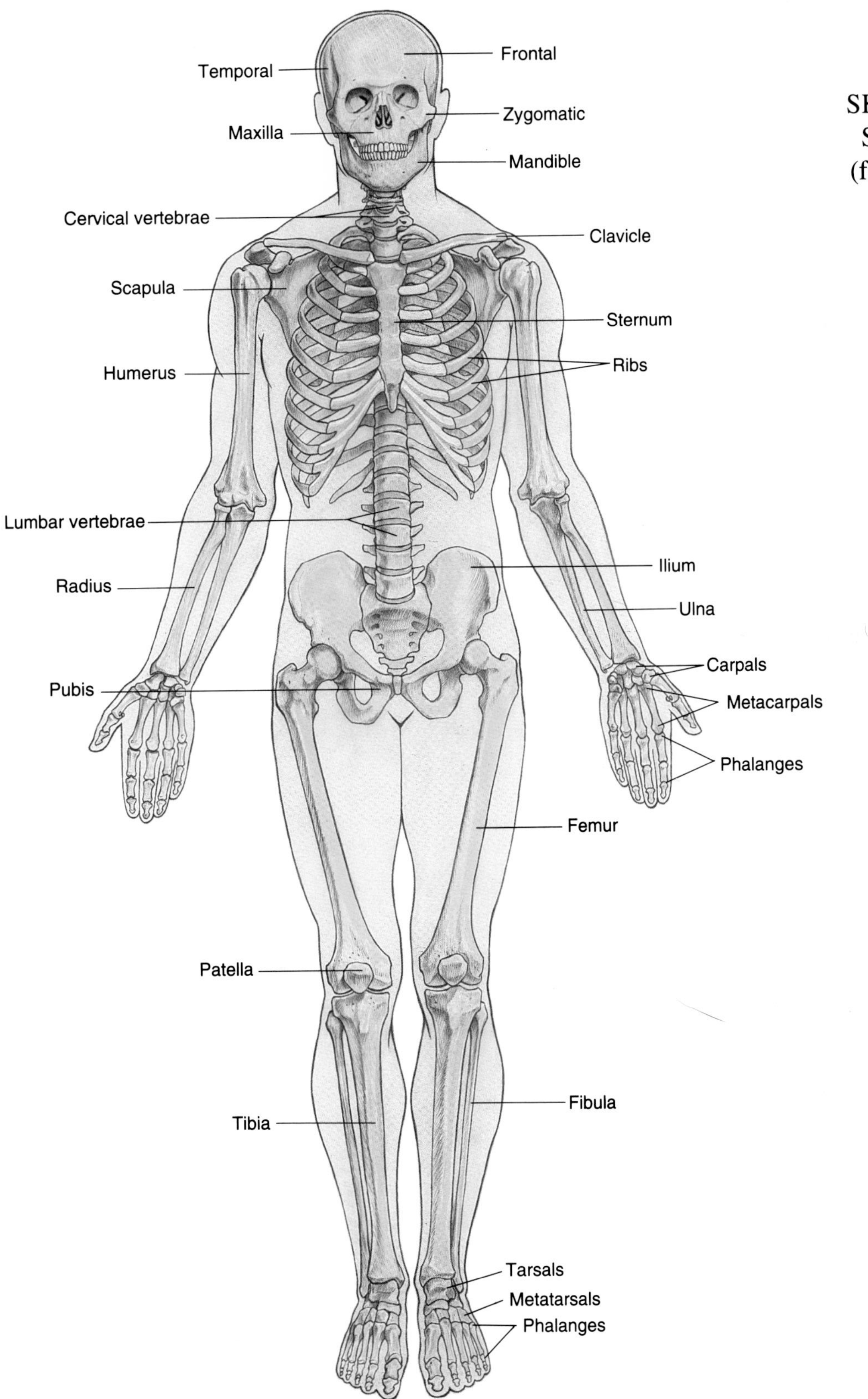

PLATE 2

THE SKELETAL SYSTEM (side and back views)

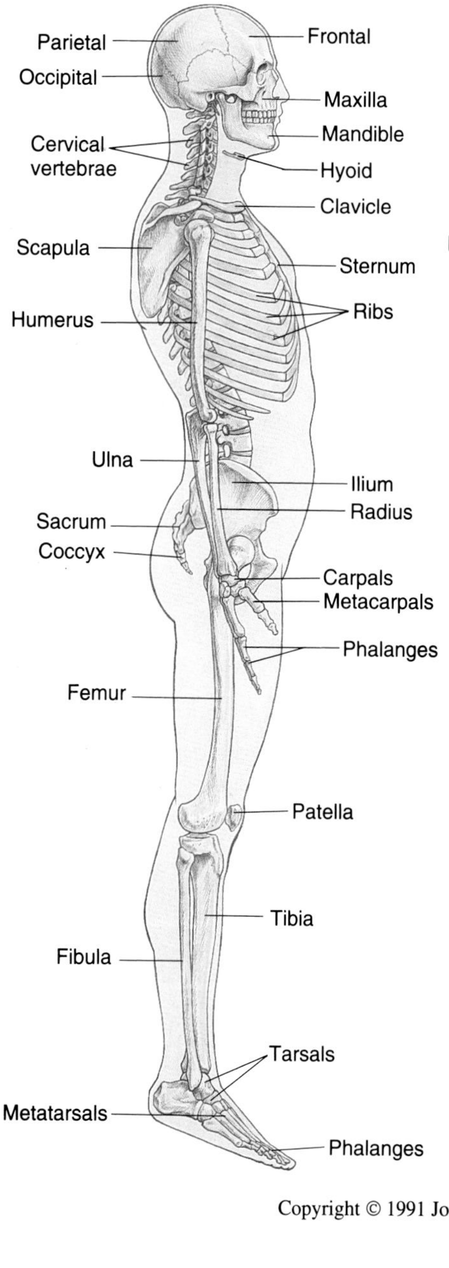

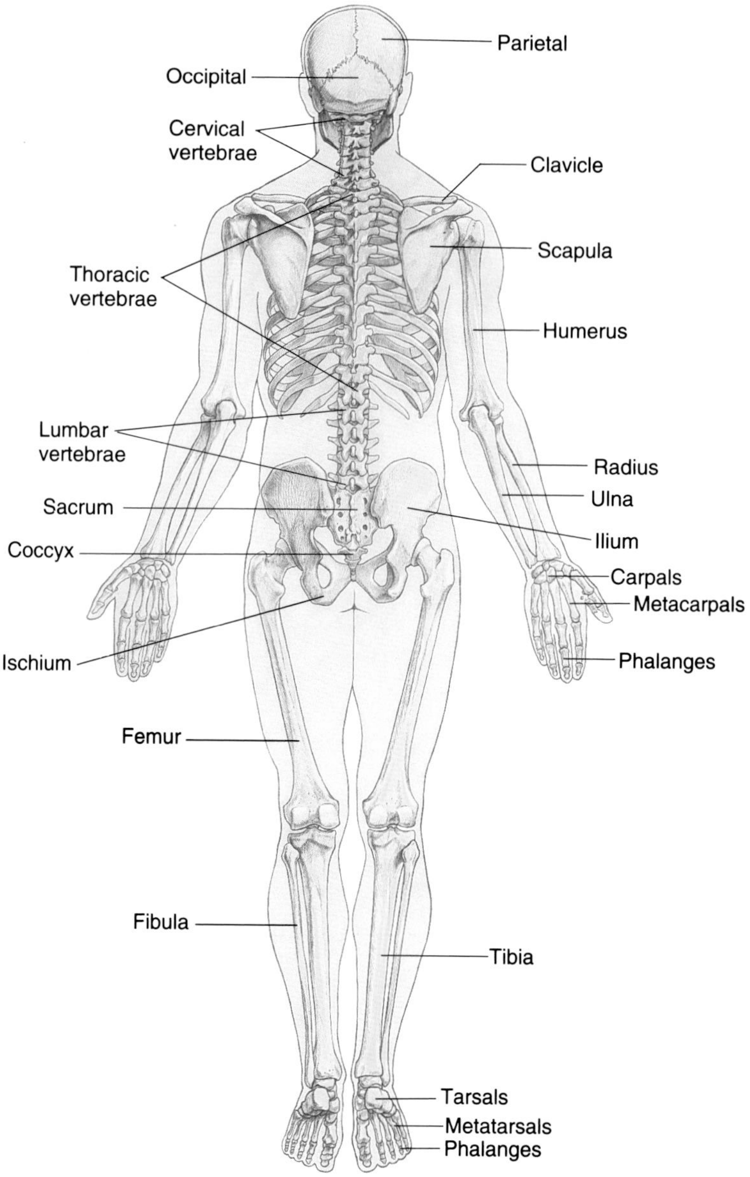

Parietal
Frontal
Occipital
Maxilla
Mandible
Cervical vertebrae
Hyoid
Clavicle
Scapula
Sternum
Humerus
Ribs
Ulna
Ilium
Radius
Sacrum
Coccyx
Carpals
Metacarpals
Phalanges
Femur
Patella
Tibia
Fibula
Tarsals
Metatarsals
Phalanges

Parietal
Occipital
Cervical vertebrae
Clavicle
Scapula
Thoracic vertebrae
Humerus
Lumbar vertebrae
Radius
Ulna
Sacrum
Ilium
Coccyx
Carpals
Metacarpals
Ischium
Phalanges
Femur
Fibula
Tibia
Tarsals
Metatarsals
Phalanges

PLATE 3

THE MUSCULAR SYSTEM (front view)

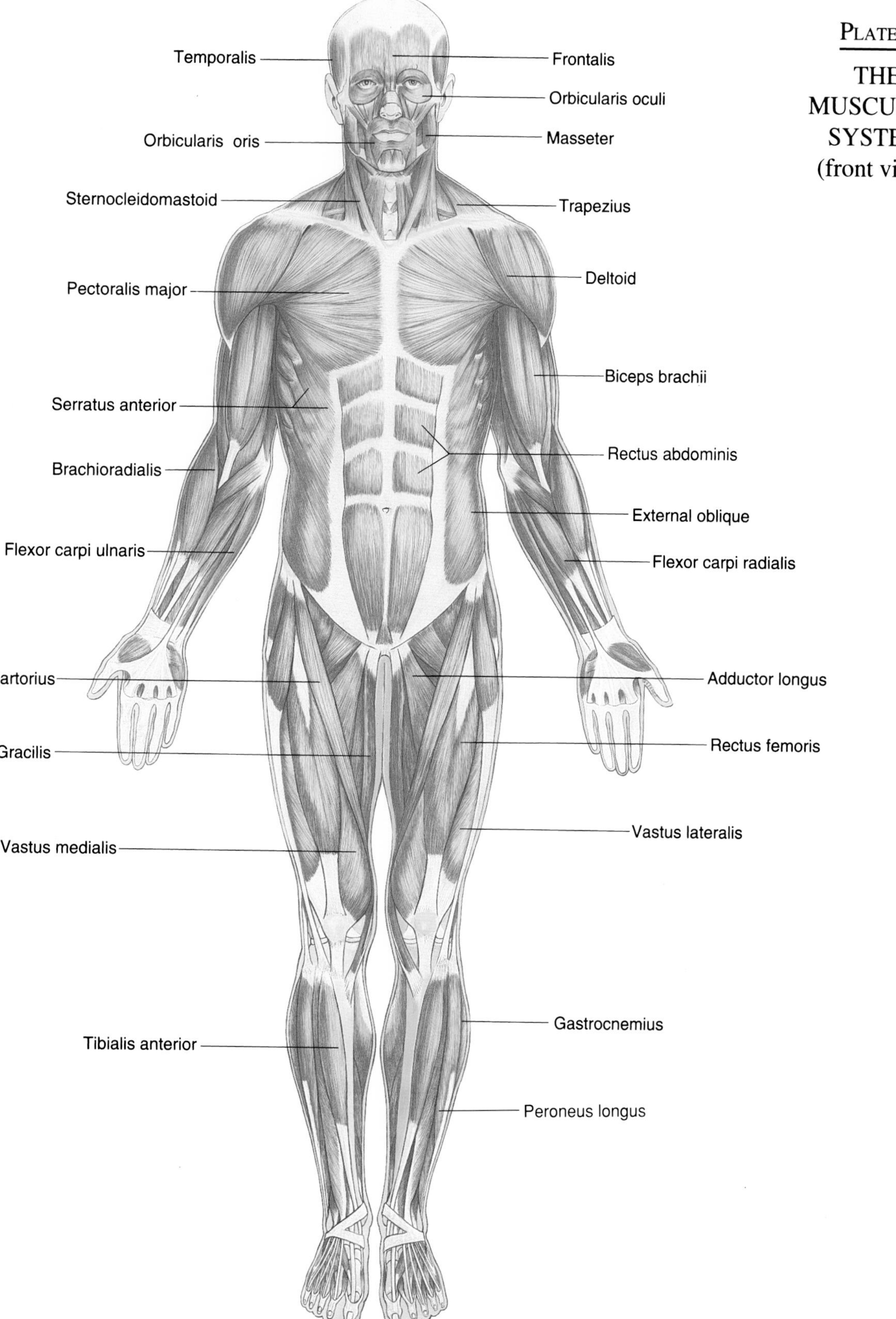
Temporalis
Frontalis
Orbicularis oculi
Orbicularis oris
Masseter
Sternocleidomastoid
Trapezius
Deltoid
Pectoralis major
Biceps brachii
Serratus anterior
Rectus abdominis
Brachioradialis
External oblique
Flexor carpi ulnaris
Flexor carpi radialis
Sartorius
Adductor longus
Gracilis
Rectus femoris
Vastus lateralis
Vastus medialis
Gastrocnemius
Tibialis anterior
Peroneus longus

PLATE 4

THE MUSCULAR SYSTEM (side and back views)

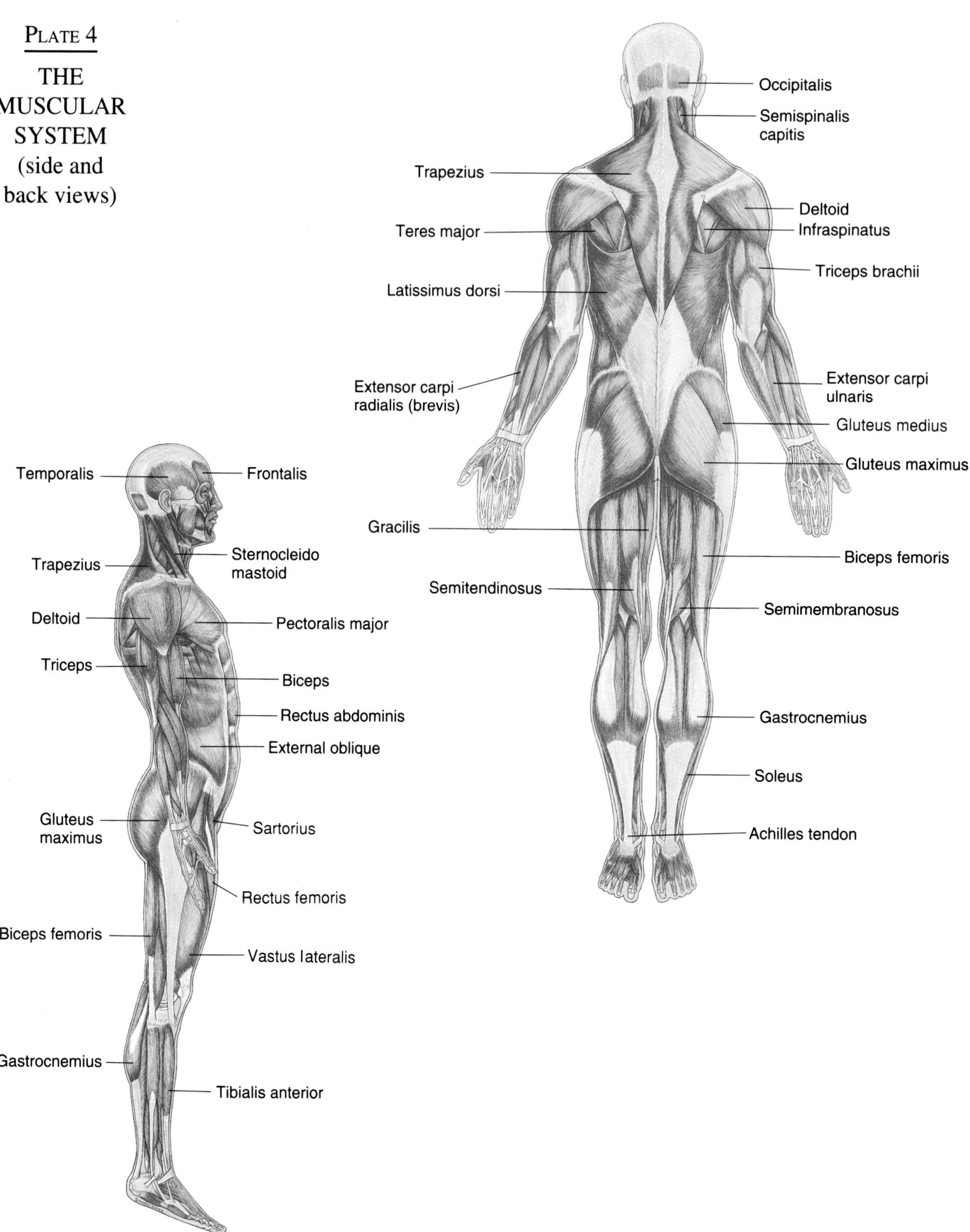

Occipitalis
Semispinalis capitis
Trapezius
Deltoid
Infraspinatus
Teres major
Triceps brachii
Latissimus dorsi
Extensor carpi radialis (brevis)
Extensor carpi ulnaris
Gluteus medius
Gluteus maximus
Gracilis
Biceps femoris
Semitendinosus
Semimembranosus
Gastrocnemius
Soleus
Achilles tendon
Temporalis
Frontalis
Trapezius
Sternocleido mastoid
Deltoid
Pectoralis major
Triceps
Biceps
Rectus abdominis
External oblique
Gluteus maximus
Sartorius
Rectus femoris
Biceps femoris
Vastus lateralis
Gastrocnemius
Tibialis anterior

PLATE 5

THE SKULL and MUSCLES OF THE HEAD

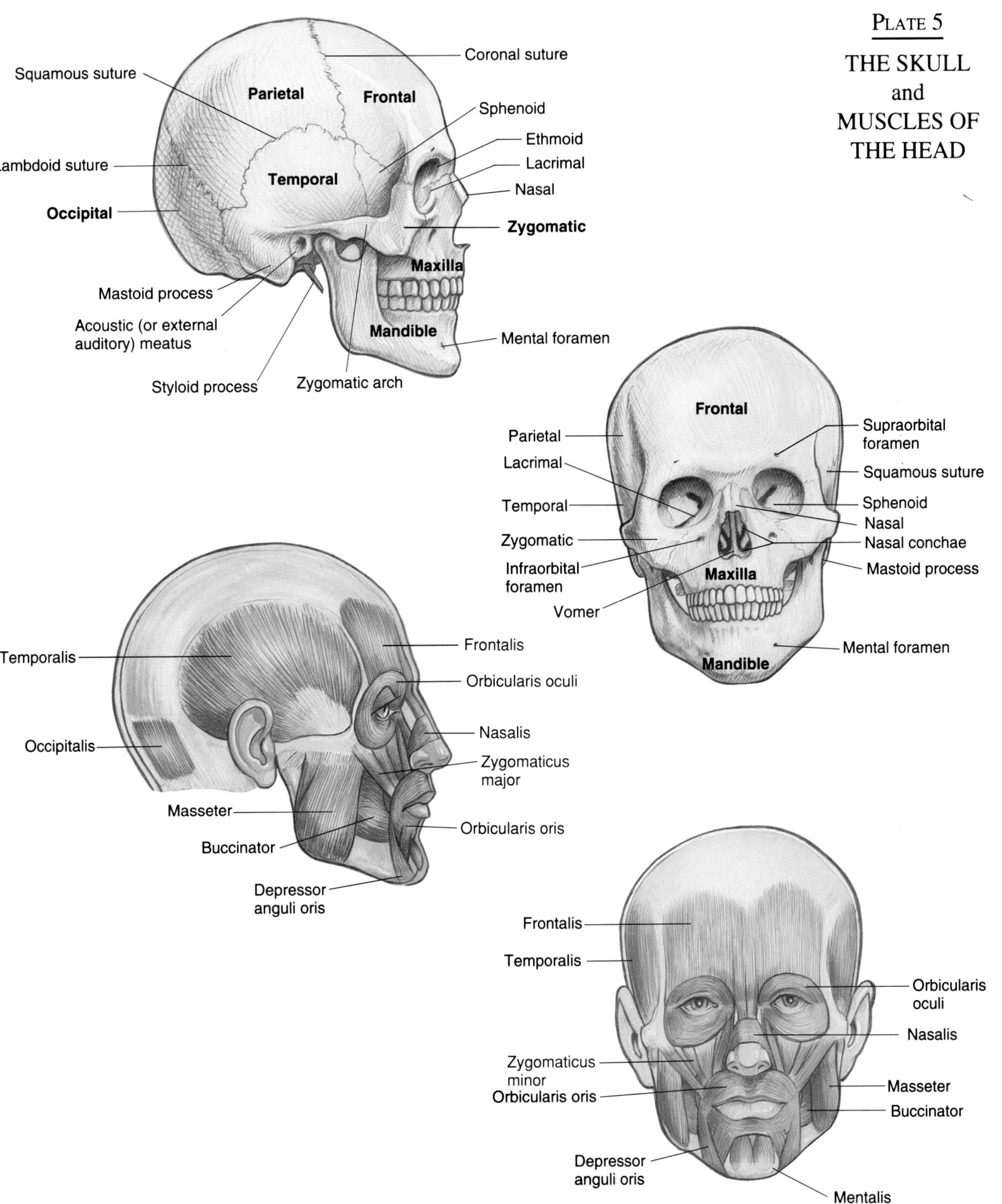

PLATE 6

THE ARTERIAL SYSTEM and THE VENOUS SYSTEM

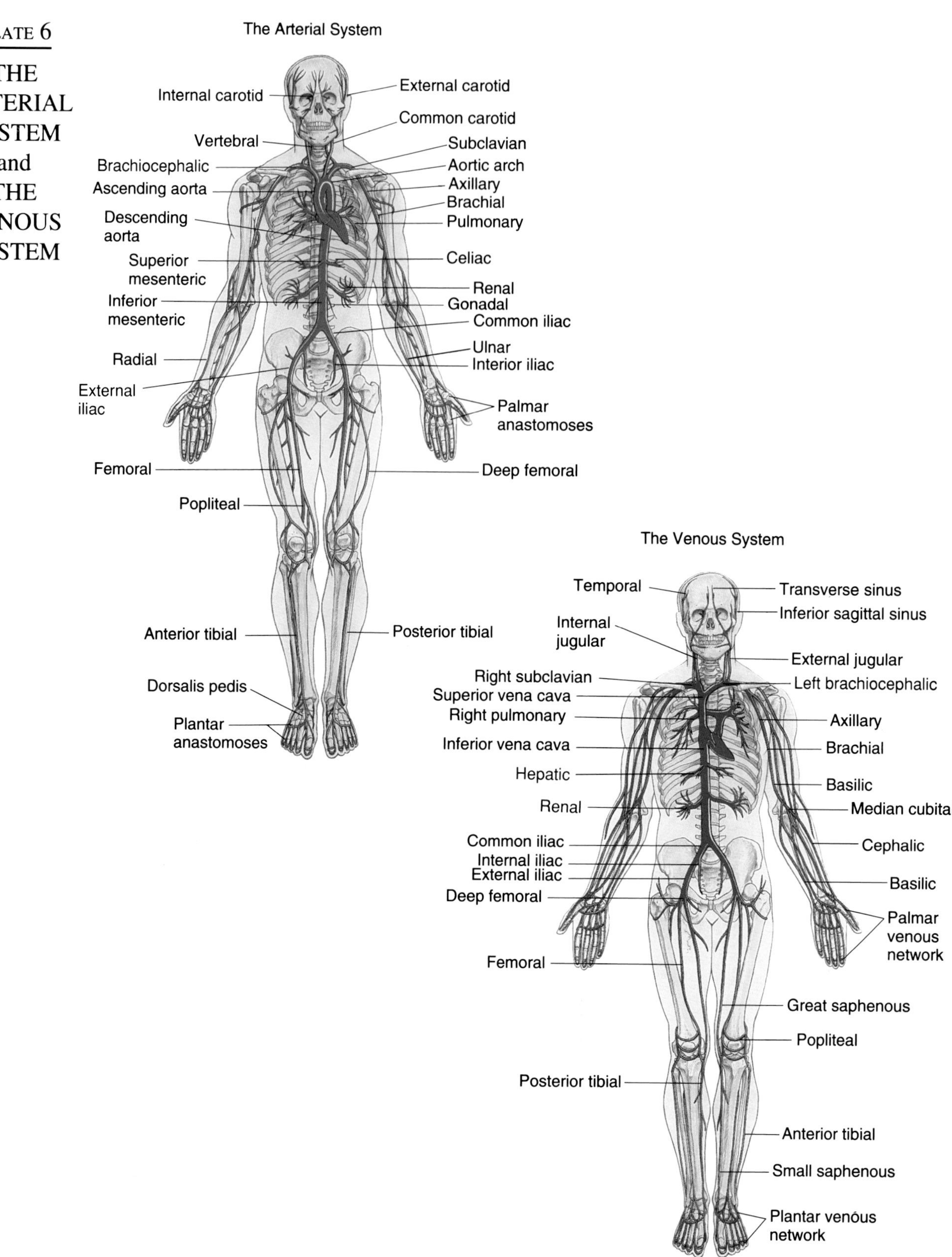
The Arterial System
Internal carotid
External carotid
Common carotid
Vertebral
Subclavian
Brachiocephalic
Aortic arch
Ascending aorta
Axillary
Brachial
Descending aorta
Pulmonary
Superior mesenteric
Celiac
Renal
Inferior mesenteric
Gonadal
Common iliac
Radial
Ulnar
Interior iliac
External iliac
Palmar anastomoses
Femoral
Deep femoral
Popliteal
Anterior tibial
Posterior tibial
Dorsalis pedis
Plantar anastomoses
The Venous System
Temporal
Transverse sinus
Inferior sagittal sinus
Internal jugular
External jugular
Right subclavian
Left brachiocephalic
Superior vena cava
Right pulmonary
Axillary
Inferior vena cava
Brachial
Hepatic
Basilic
Renal
Median cubital
Common iliac
Cephalic
Internal iliac
External iliac
Basilic
Deep femoral
Palmar venous network
Femoral
Great saphenous
Popliteal
Posterior tibial
Anterior tibial
Small saphenous
Plantar venous network

THE ARTERIAL-VENOUS SYSTEM

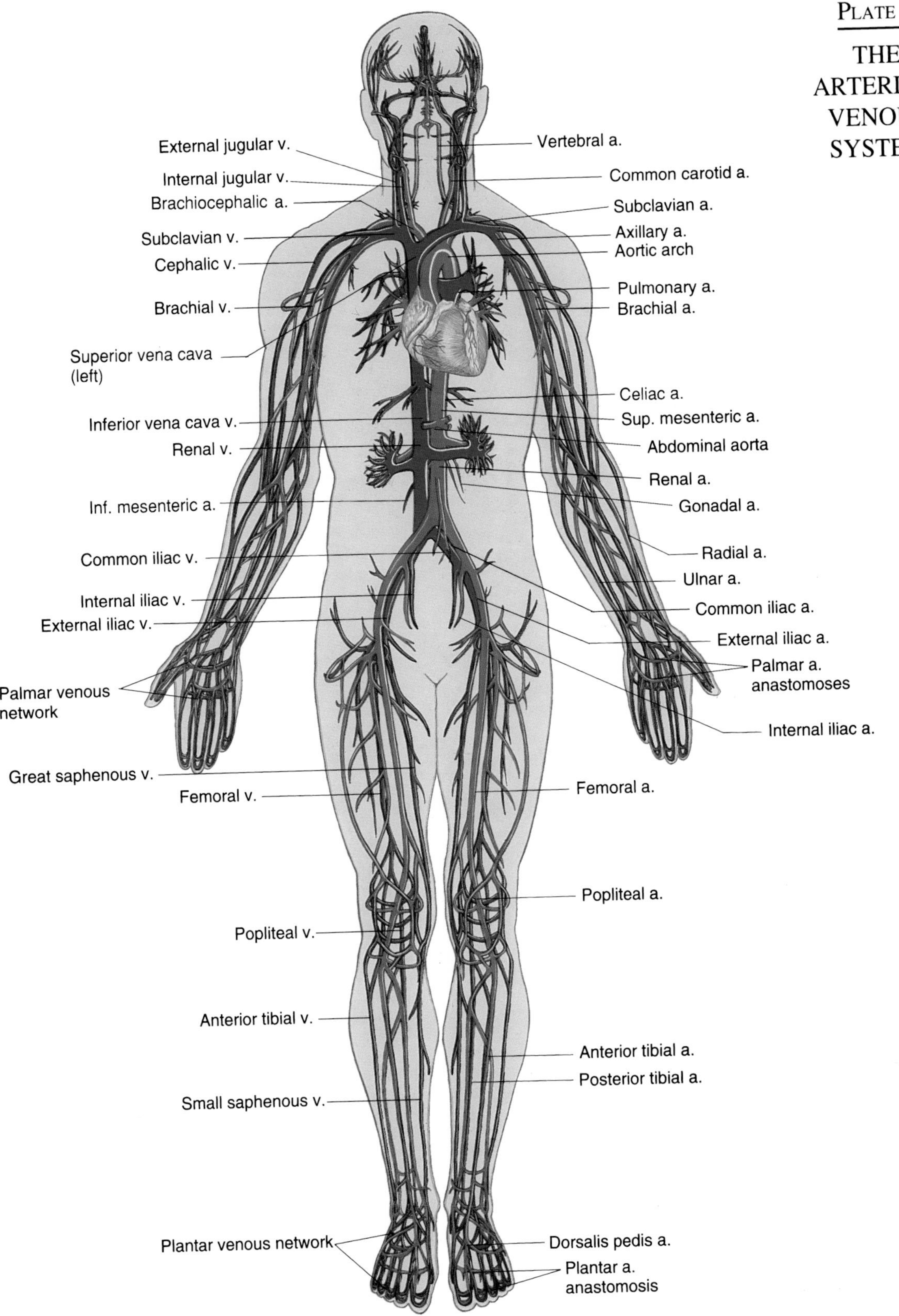
External jugular v.
Internal jugular v.
Brachiocephalic a.
Subclavian v.
Cephalic v.
Brachial v.
Superior vena cava (left)
Inferior vena cava v.
Renal v.
Inf. mesenteric a.
Common iliac v.
Internal iliac v.
External iliac v.
Palmar venous network
Great saphenous v.
Femoral v.
Popliteal v.
Anterior tibial v.
Small saphenous v.
Plantar venous network
Vertebral a.
Common carotid a.
Subclavian a.
Axillary a.
Aortic arch
Pulmonary a.
Brachial a.
Celiac a.
Sup. mesenteric a.
Abdominal aorta
Renal a.
Gonadal a.
Radial a.
Ulnar a.
Common iliac a.
External iliac a.
Palmar a. anastomoses
Internal iliac a.
Femoral a.
Popliteal a.
Anterior tibial a.
Posterior tibial a.
Dorsalis pedis a.
Plantar a. anastomosis

PLATE 8

THE HEART and BLOOD CIRCUITS

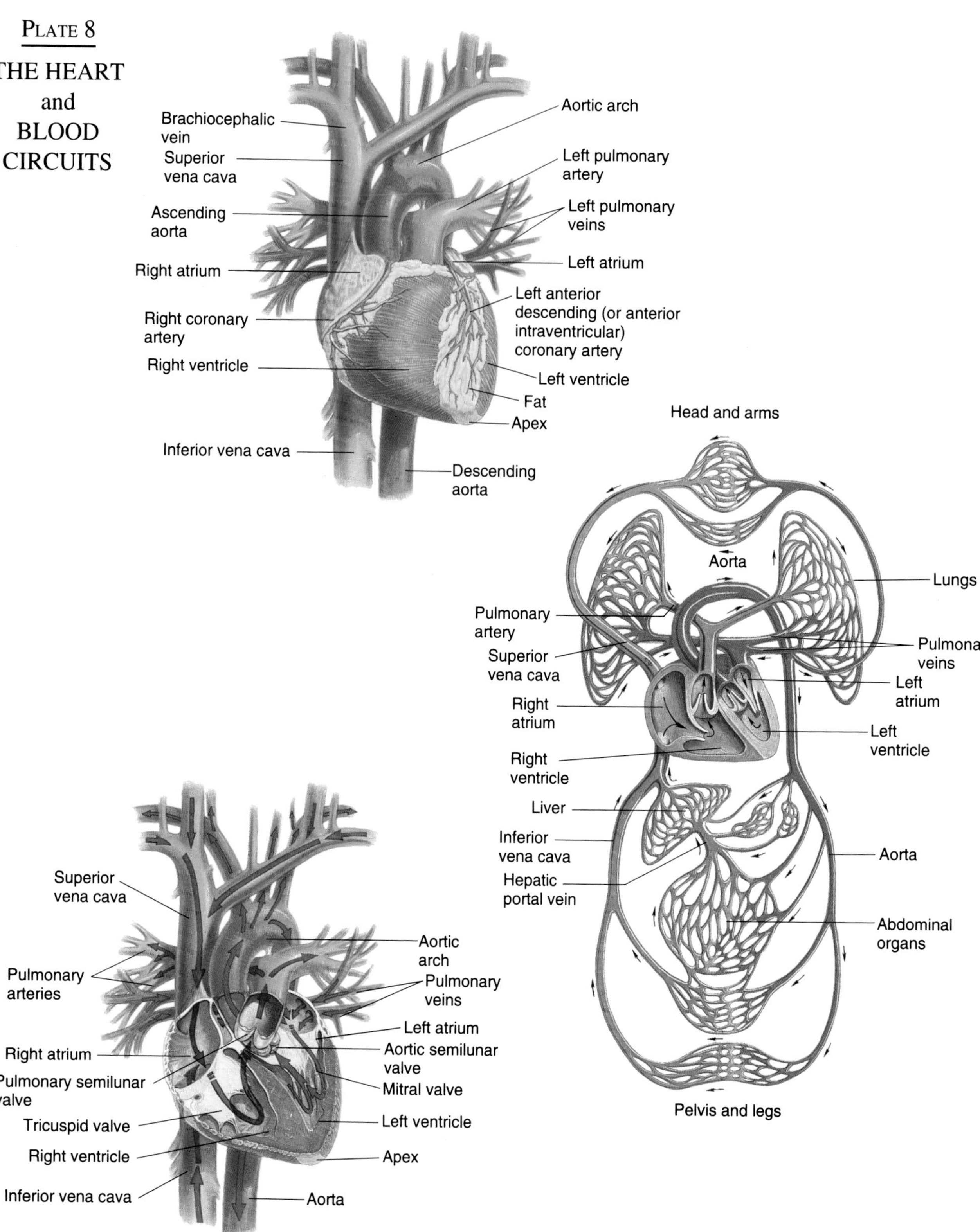

PLATE 9

THE ENDOCRINE SYSTEM

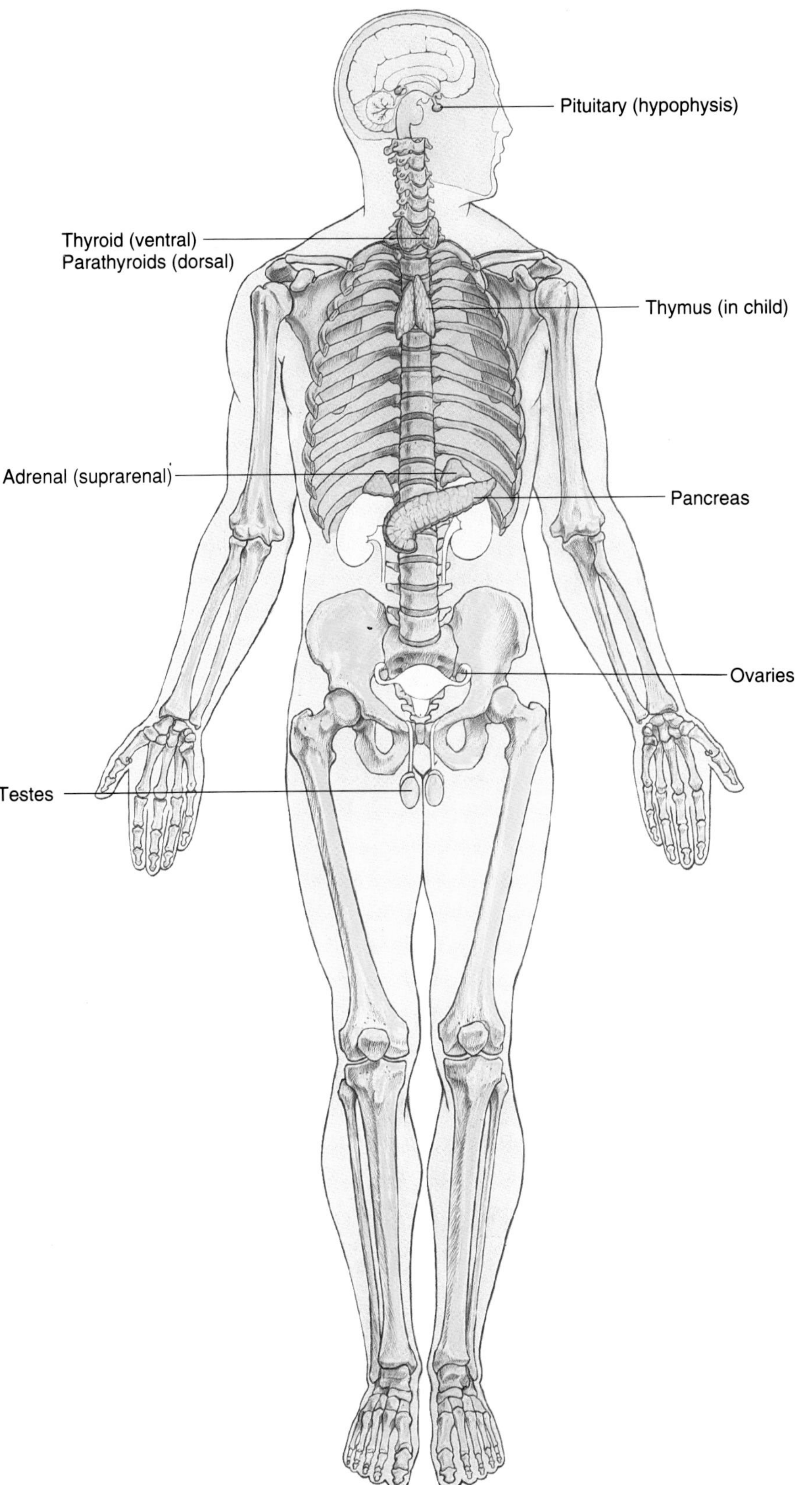

PLATE 10

THE LYMPHATIC SYSTEM

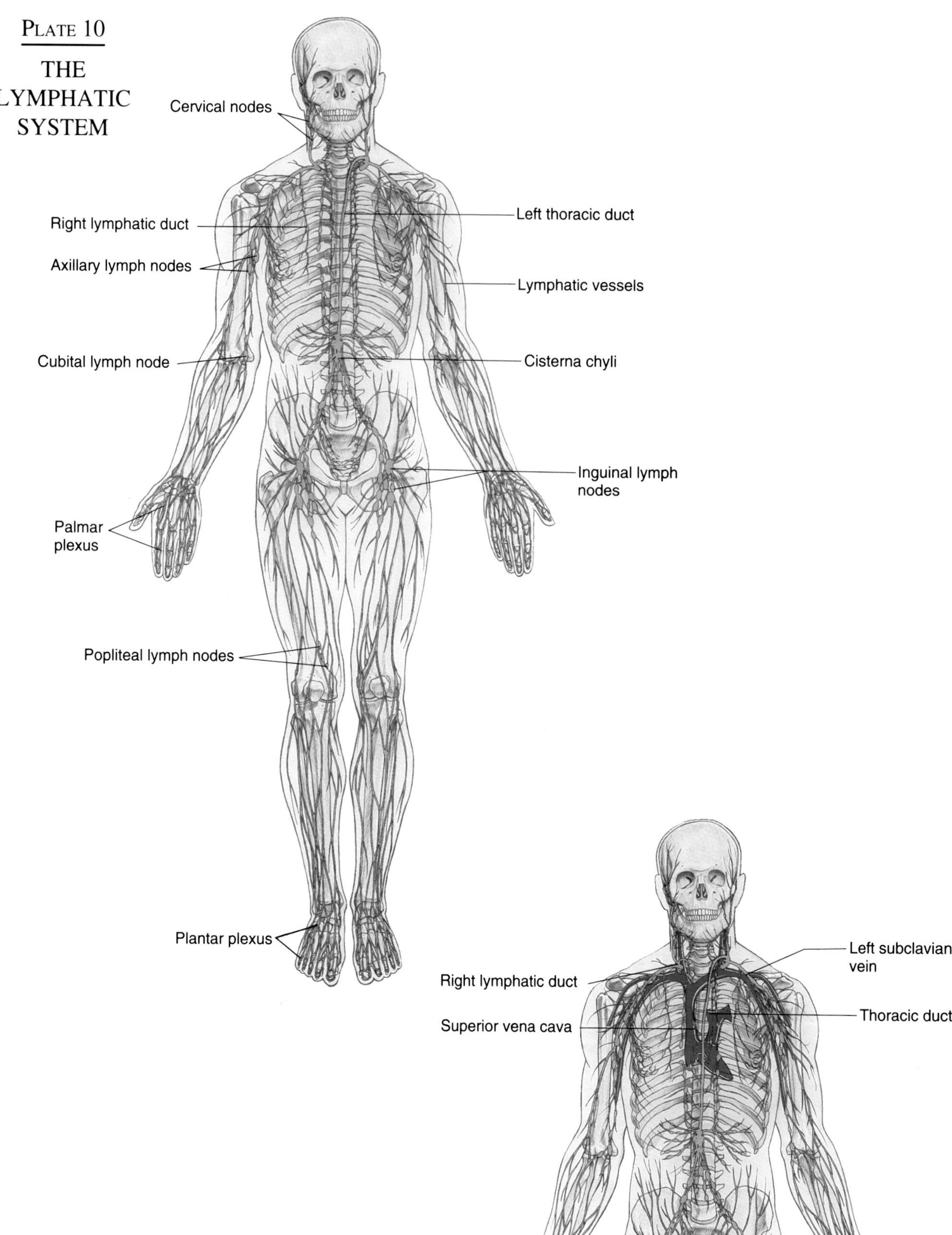
Cervical nodes
Right lymphatic duct
Left thoracic duct
Axillary lymph nodes
Lymphatic vessels
Cubital lymph node
Cisterna chyli
Inguinal lymph nodes
Palmar plexus
Popliteal lymph nodes
Plantar plexus
Left subclavian vein
Right lymphatic duct
Thoracic duct
Superior vena cava

PLATE 11

THE NERVOUS SYSTEM and THE BRAIN (surface and midsagittal views)

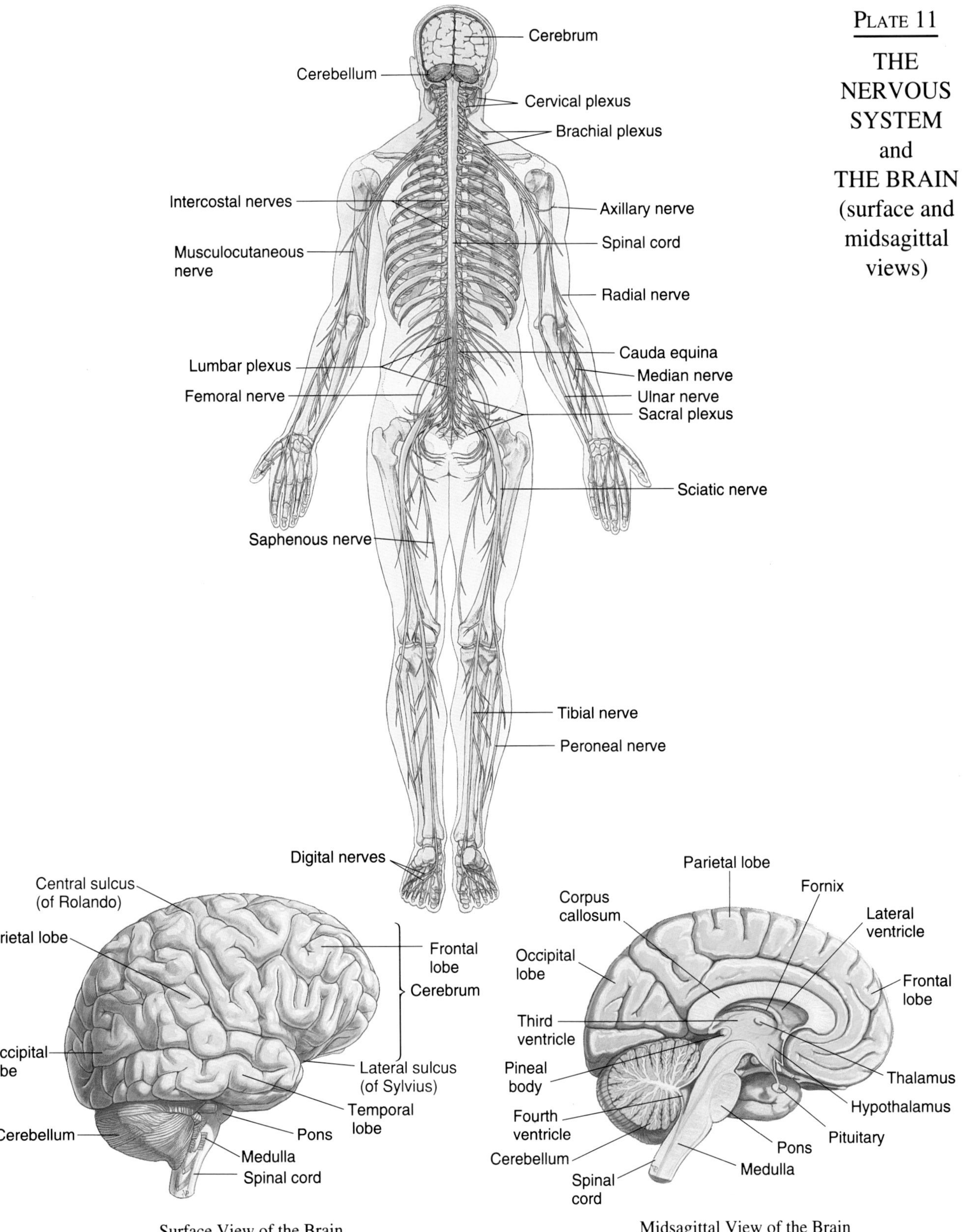

Surface View of the Brain

Midsagittal View of the Brain

Plate 12

THE VISCERA

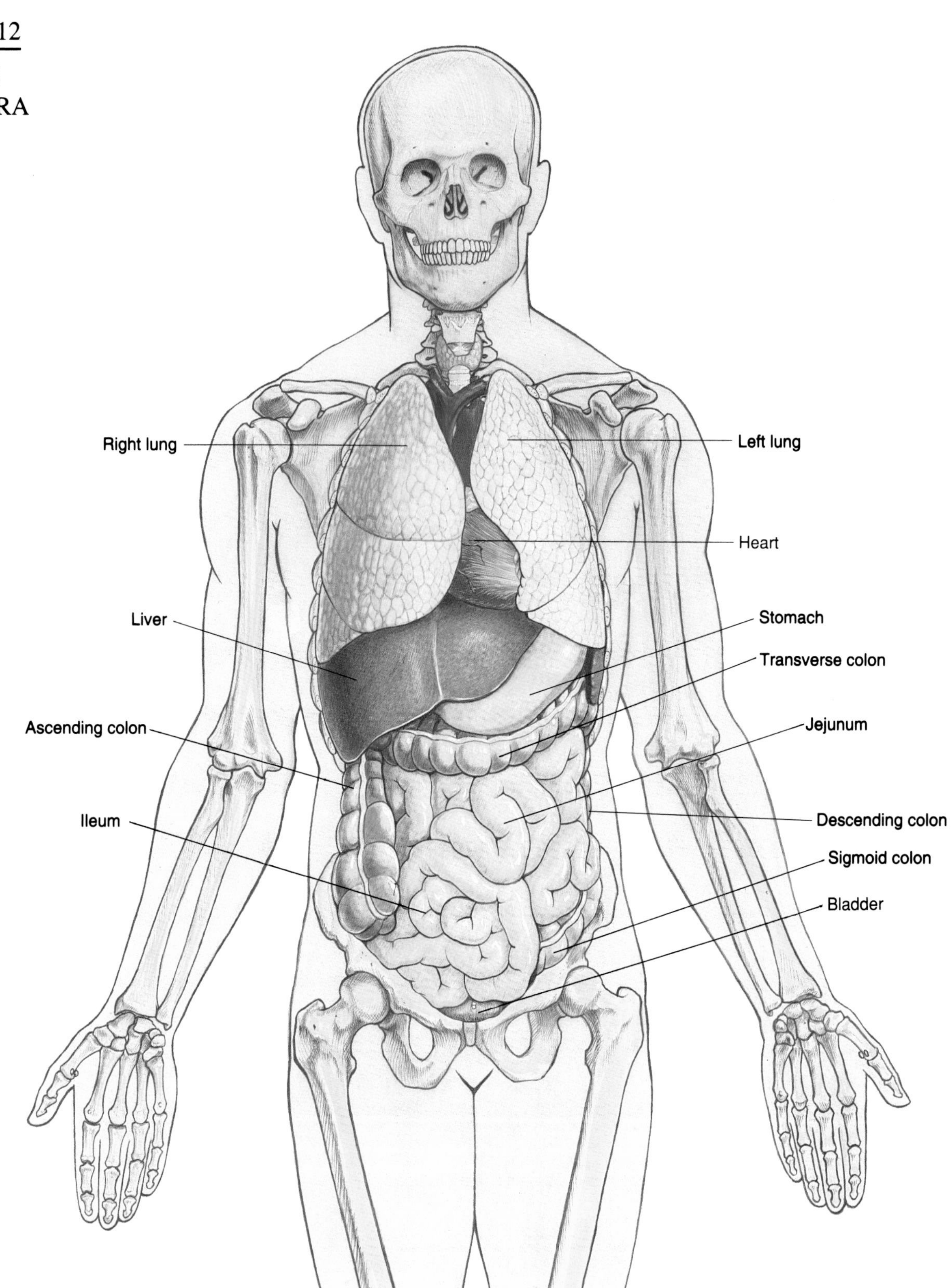

PLATE 13

THE RESPIRATORY SYSTEM

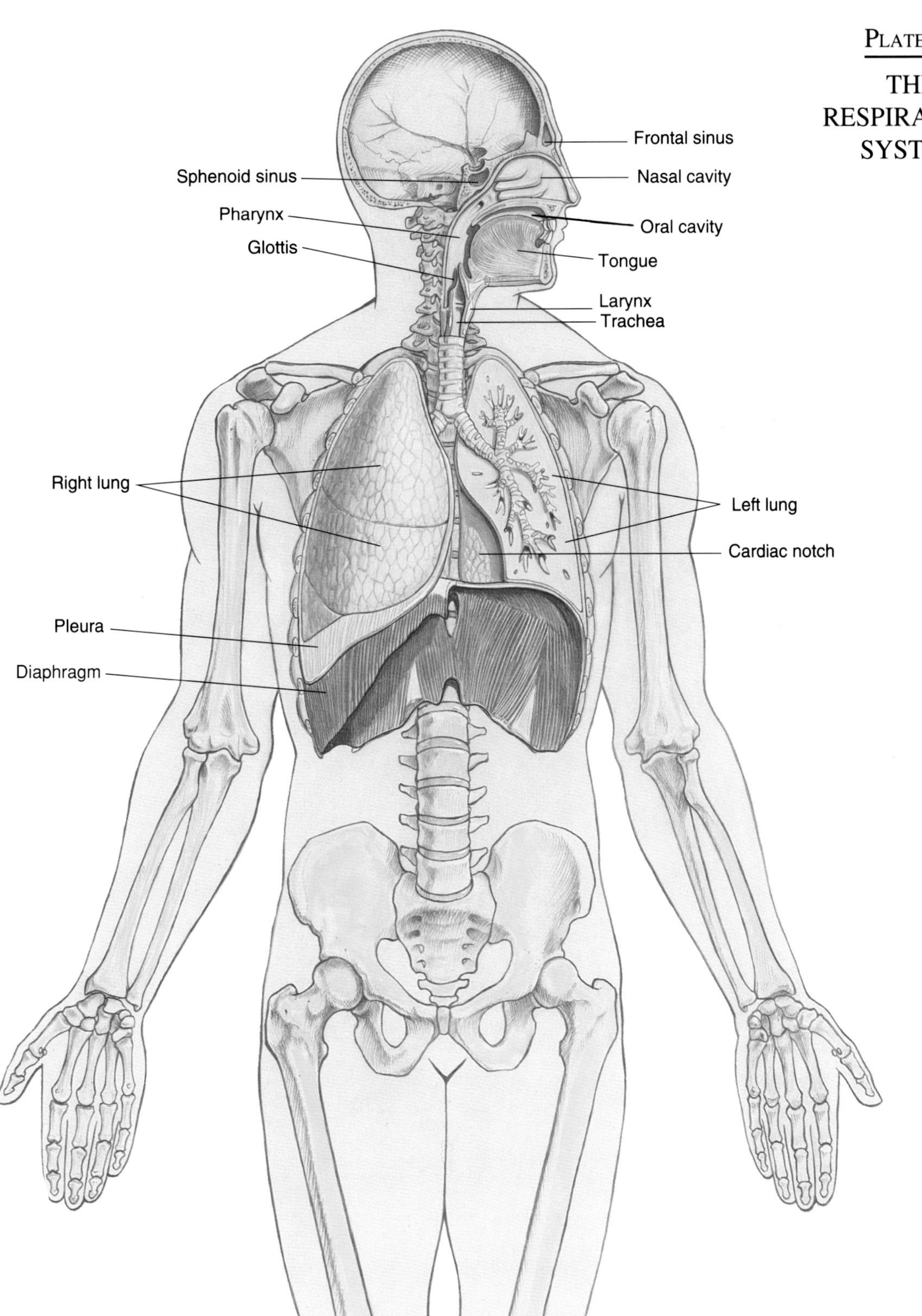

Plate 14

THE DIGESTIVE SYSTEM

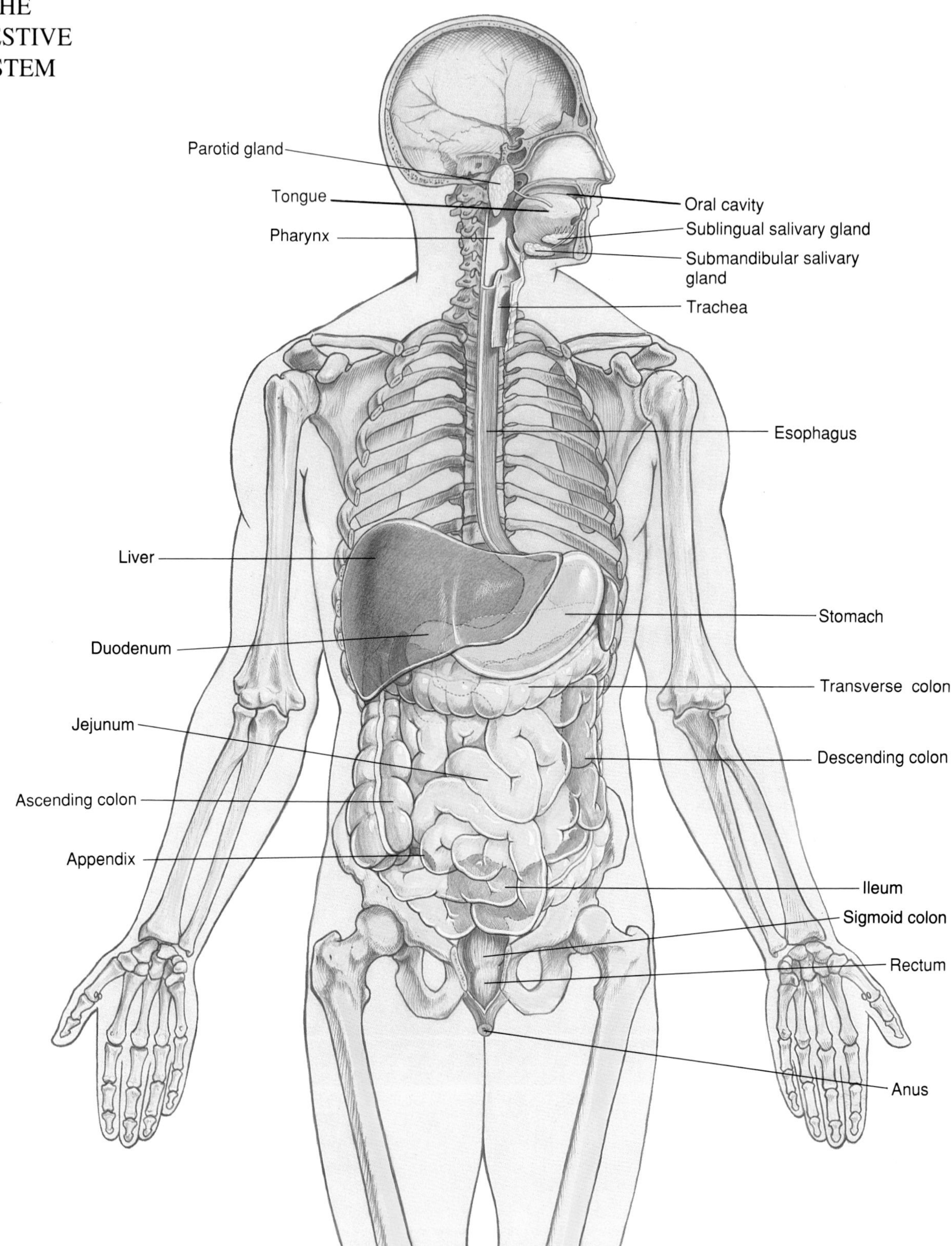

Plate 15

THE URINARY SYSTEM and THE FEMALE AND MALE REPRODUCTIVE SYSTEMS

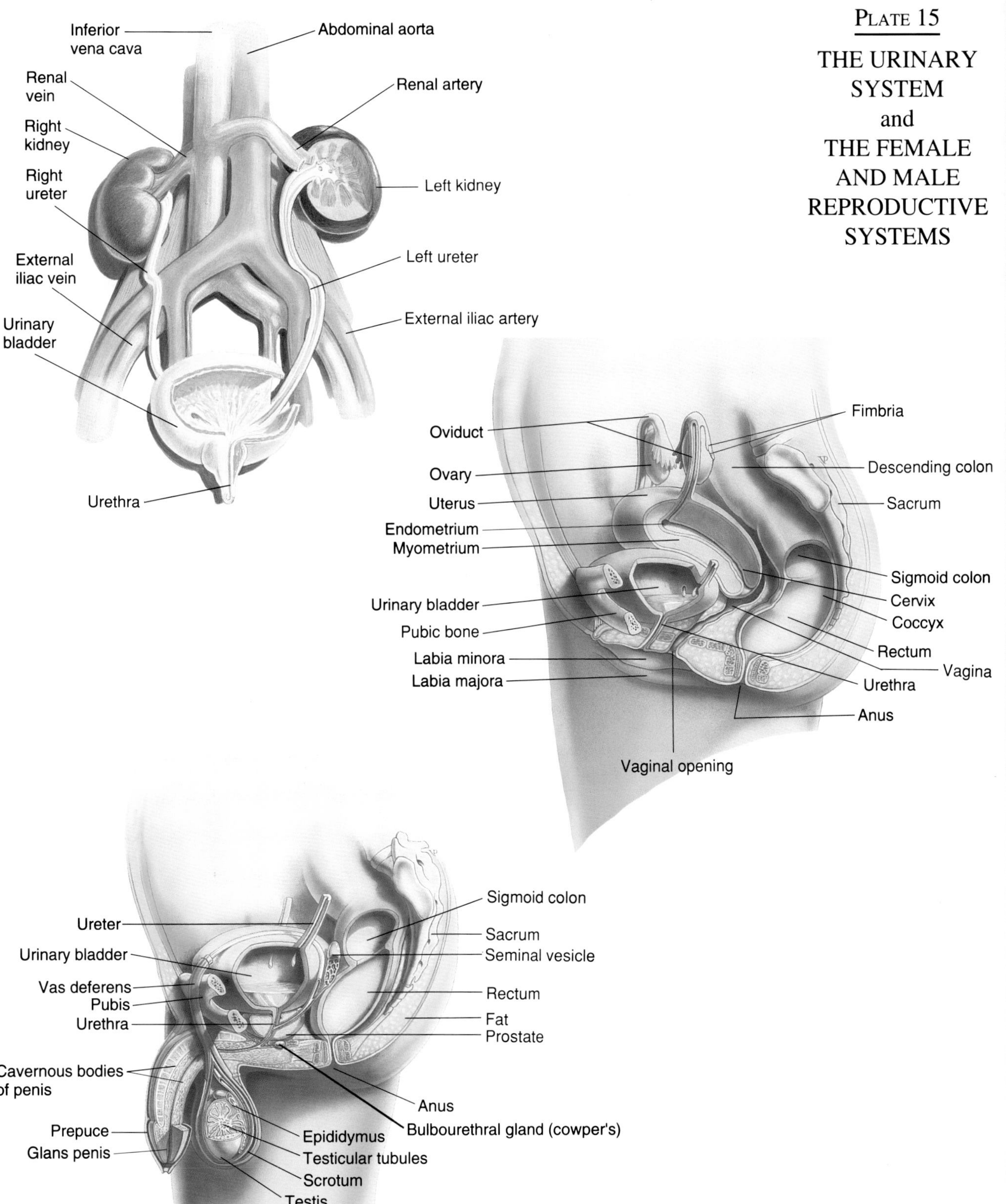

PLATE 16

THE SENSES

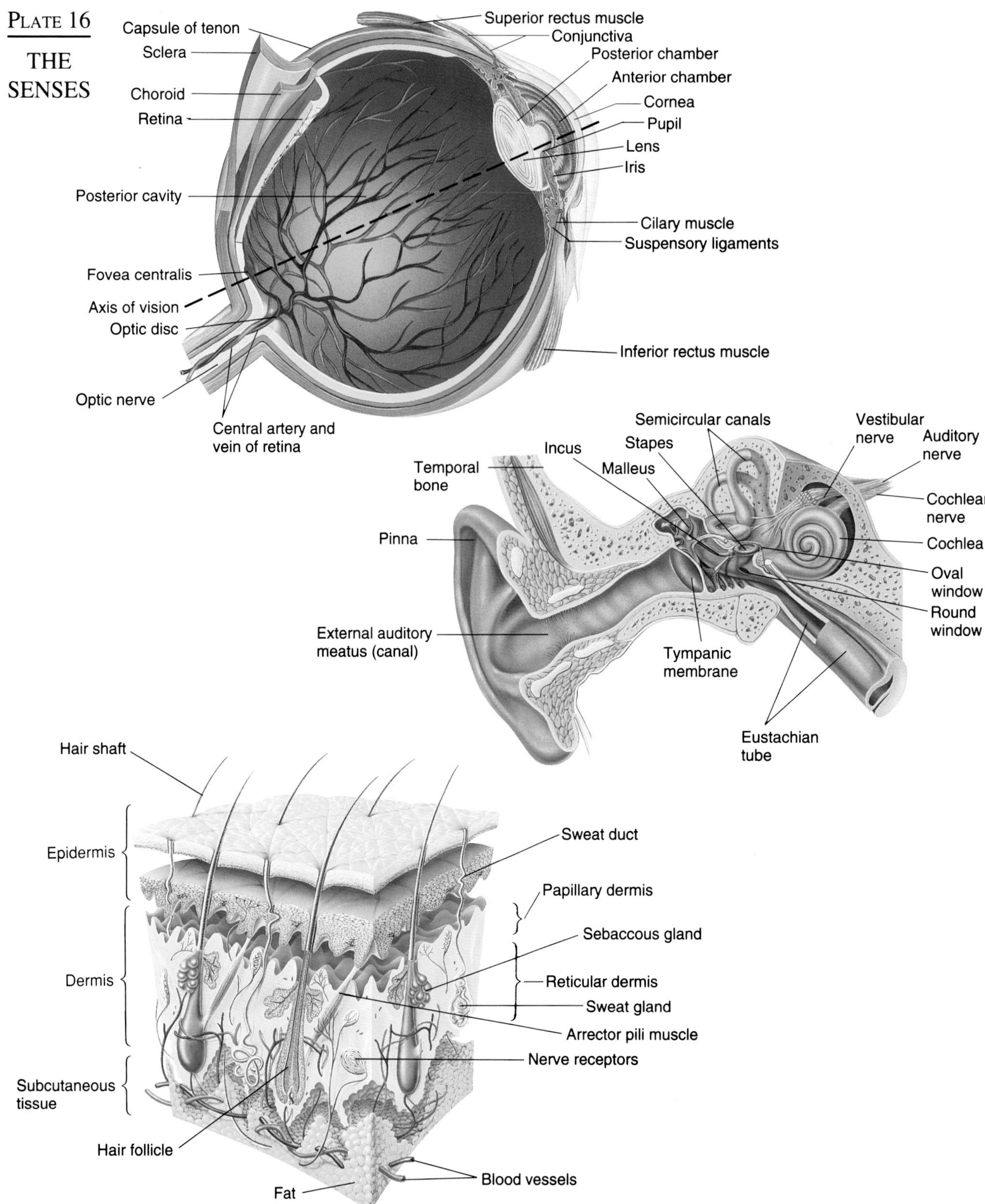
Capsule of tenon
Sclera
Choroid
Retina
Posterior cavity
Fovea centralis
Axis of vision
Optic disc
Optic nerve
Central artery and vein of retina
Superior rectus muscle
Conjunctiva
Posterior chamber
Anterior chamber
Cornea
Pupil
Lens
Iris
Cilary muscle
Suspensory ligaments
Inferior rectus muscle
Semicircular canals
Vestibular nerve
Auditory nerve
Incus
Stapes
Temporal bone
Malleus
Cochlear nerve
Pinna
Cochlea
Oval window
Round window
External auditory meatus (canal)
Tympanic membrane
Eustachian tube
Hair shaft
Epidermis
Dermis
Subcutaneous tissue
Hair follicle
Fat
Sweat duct
Papillary dermis
Sebaccous gland
Reticular dermis
Sweat gland
Arrector pili muscle
Nerve receptors
Blood vessels

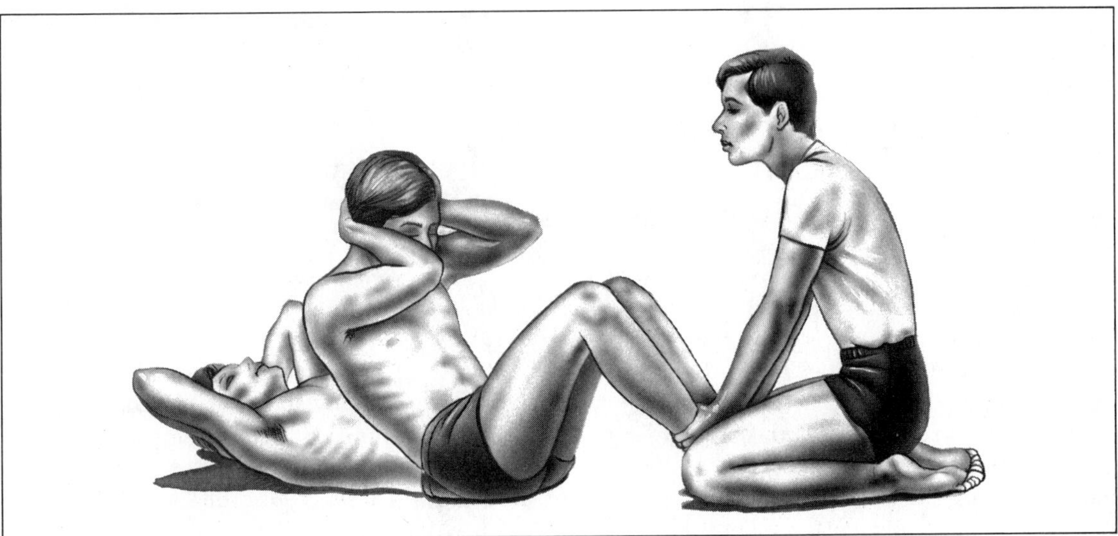

Figure 7-4 Bent-knee sit-ups.

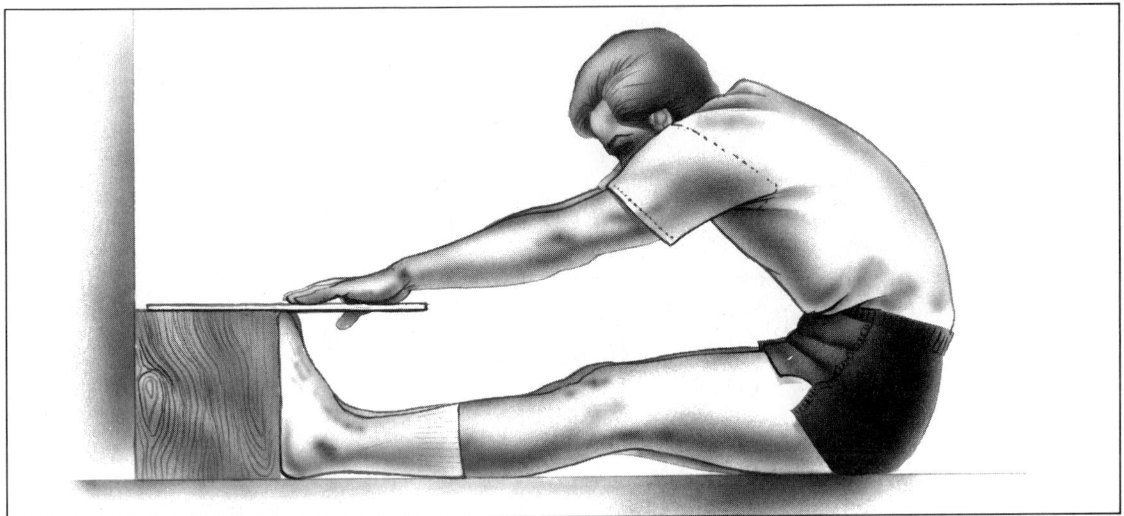

Figure 7-5 Measuring trunk flexion.

Table 7-20. Evaluation of Bent-Knee Sit-Ups

Rating	Women (no. of sit-ups per 1 min.)	Men (no. of sit-ups per 2 min.)
Excellent	33 or up	69 or up
Good	27–32	60–68
Average	20–26	52–59
Low	16–21	42–51
Poor	16 or under	41 or under

Adapted from B. Getchell. *Physical Fitness: A Way of Life*, 2nd ed. (New York: Wiley, 1979), pp. 56–57.

client to extend arms as far forward as possible, stretching from the waist. With a ruler, measure the distance the client can reach beyond the proximal edge of the box. If the client cannot reach the edge, report the distance of the fingertips from the edge as a negative number (see Figure 7-5 and Table 7-21).

Table 7-21. Norms for Trunk Flexion

Range	Women	Men
Normal	+4 to +10 in.	−6 to +8 in.
Average (mean)	+2 in.	+1 in.
Desired	+2 to +6 in.	+1 to +5 in.

From B. Getchell. *Physical Fitness: A Way of Life*, 2nd ed. (New York: Wiley 1979), p. 59.

Summary

There is little doubt that what we eat has a tremendous impact on our health. It is essential that the nurse gather information from each client about eating habits. This assessment initially occurs when the client's history is being gathered. Information obtained at that time will help the nurse to determine if a more in-depth nutritional assessment is needed.

Cardiovascular fitness, body composition, muscular strength, and flexibility are critical components in the overall evaluation of client fitness. The nurse can assess these as separate components in the health evaluation or include them when evaluating various body systems. For example, cardiovascular fitness can be determined while assessing the cardiovascular system. Body composition can be determined while assessing the musculoskeletal system. It is up to the nurse to determine the appropriate time to assess each component.

Discussion Questions/Activities

1. Choose a classmate or family member and have that person keep a food diary for 24 hours.
   a. Review the diary with the individual.
   b. Help to plan a more healthy diet.
2. Discuss your personal diet and exercise program with the class.
3. Using the techniques described, assess a client's cardiovascular status, strength, and flexibility.

CHAPTER 8

Introduction to Physical Assessment

LEARNING OBJECTIVES

1. Recognize that senses can be sharpened to enhance the physical assessment process.
2. Identify general principles of the physical assessment modes of inspection, palpation, percussion, and auscultation.
3. State the areas of the hand best used for the assessment of skin temperature, vibration, and the characteristics of texture, moisture, shape, and consistency.
4. Describe the correct technique used to percuss.
5. Name the various notes produced by percussion.
6. List the components of a general impression.
7. Describe general principles used in the approach to a client to perform a physical assessment.

A complete physical assessment serves as a screening device for detecting abnormalities that are unknown to the client and for identifying signs that may suggest illness or deformity. The findings may serve as support to validate problems suspected from the client's history. The historical information helps you zero in on relevant observations of physical assessment when time is limited for examination.

Cultivating the Senses

Every minute of every day you are gathering data via your sensory system. You see, touch, hear, smell, and taste. It is these senses that are used in the data-gathering process of physical assessment. The sense of taste was skillfully applied in ancient times—to detect glycosuria, for example. A glass catheter was used to obtain a sterile urine specimen, which was then tasted to detect whether a sweetness was present. Today this means of data gathering has been replaced by laboratory tests.

You must recognize that each of your senses can be cultivated. You need only look about you for evidence—the wine taster who has groomed his ability to taste and smell, the musician who has refined his tone and pitch consciousness. The findings gathered by each sense are made meaningful by association to background knowledge; thus, it is practice and experience, coupled with background knowledge, that will lead to the cultivation of your senses for more effective use in physical assessment.

Throughout the process of physical assessment your senses of smell, sight, hearing, and touch are concentrated on the client. Most of the nursing literature overlooks the sense of smell, perhaps because the use of this sense requires some sophistication. There is only one ground rule in using smell in assessment: if you detect a peculiar odor that is out of the limits of the normal, you should investigate it further and seek consultation if in doubt.

Although the whys and the wherefores of specific odors are beyond the scope of this text, a few examples will be helpful:

1. *Skin odors.* The sense of smell can give you clues about the client's hygiene or body functioning. The client may emit a strong body odor or scents of urine or feces. Immediate conclusions might be that the client does not bathe too frequently or too efficiently or, in the case of the odors of urine or feces, that the client is incontinent. It is necessary to investigate further and to validate any assumptions with the client or with a significant other. It may well be that the client practices good hygiene but that he does not use an effective deodorant or that it is the client's clothing that contains the odor. Clothing, especially wool sweaters and suit jackets, become permeated with body odor, and you may need to recommend more frequent cleaning of clothes. Incontinence is not the only cause of urine or fecal odors—the individual may have been holding an infant whose diaper proved insufficient. And, of course, these odors may be quite normal from a younger child who is still learning to control his normal physiologic functioning. More seriously, though, an ammoniacal skin odor may indicate severe renal dysfunction (uremia).
2. *Mouth odors.* Halitosis (bad breath) can result from dental caries or from dyspepsia. Alcohol may be detected on the breath. A sweet, juicy-fruit breath odor may result from the ketoacidosis of diabetic coma or from prolonged use of starvation diets. Foul-smelling sputum may indicate a pharyngeal or lung abscess or bronchiectasis.
3. *Body secretion odors.* Feces that have a foul-smelling, penetrating, pungent odor are commonly found with biliary tract problems (gallbladder or pancreatic dysfunction) and with malabsorption syndrome. A strong ammoniacal odor of the urine may indicate fermentation within the bladder.
4. *Vomitus and pus odors.* Sour-smelling, fermented emesis may indicate food retained in the stomach for a prolonged period or increased gastric acidity. Fecal-smelling vomitus is observed with prolonged vomiting in peritonitis and in intestinal obstruction. The odor of alcohol as well as phenol and other poisons and irritants may be present in vomitus. Purulent material with an odor similar to strong-smelling cheese may be found in abscesses or cysts containing proteolytic bacteria. A nauseating, sweet smell of pus occurs with pseudomonas infections and a pungent, sweet odor (similar to the smell of rotting apples) occurs with gas gangrene.

Techniques of Assessment

Four basic methods are used to systematically guide the uses of the remaining senses of sight, touch, and hearing in physical assessment. They are *inspection, palpation, percussion,* and *auscultation.*

Inspection

Inspection is the visual scrutiny of the client that begins at the first moment of contact. All observations must be conducted with adequate lighting, and as the physical assessment proceeds, each bodily area examined must be adequately exposed. To effectively use the method of inspection, you must train your sense of sight to focus in on detail. The more knowledge and clinical practice you accrue, the more you will improve your ability of inspection.

As you examine the client, you should compare the two sides of his body. Normally, there are slight deviations between the left and right sides of the body, but general symmetry should prevail upon inspection.

The use of the ophthalmoscope with its variety of lenses enhances the examination performed by the naked eye. Additional facilitating instruments include speculums (nasal, vaginal), mirrors (head reflector, pharyngeal), and additional sources of light (penlight). Also, the use of x-rays, electrocardiograms, and other laboratory tests is a common means of extending the process of inspection.

Palpation

Palpation employs your sense of touch. The roughness, smoothness, hardness, softness, moistness, dryness, motility, and configuration of a body surface or of a nodule or mass can be determined by touch. The tactile sense also reveals the temperature of a given part (such as the coolness of an area of arterial insufficiency). Palpation can also inform you of vibrations (such as the presence of a cardiac thrill or of fremitus) and of position.

Because prolonged heavy pressure on the fingertips can dull your tactile sensitivity, light palpation is used for the majority of the examination. It is through light palpation that areas of tenderness may be elicited; these areas should be carefully examined last, in order not to aggravate pain and interfere with the further gathering of pertinent data. The most sensitive area of your hand is the fingertips, but the dorsum of the hand is more sensitive to temperature because the skin is much thinner there. The palmar aspects of the fingers best detect the presence of vibration. (See Figure 8-1.) Other palpation techniques are deep palpation and bimanual palpation. These techniques are described in appropriate portions of the text where their use in the assessment process is necessary.

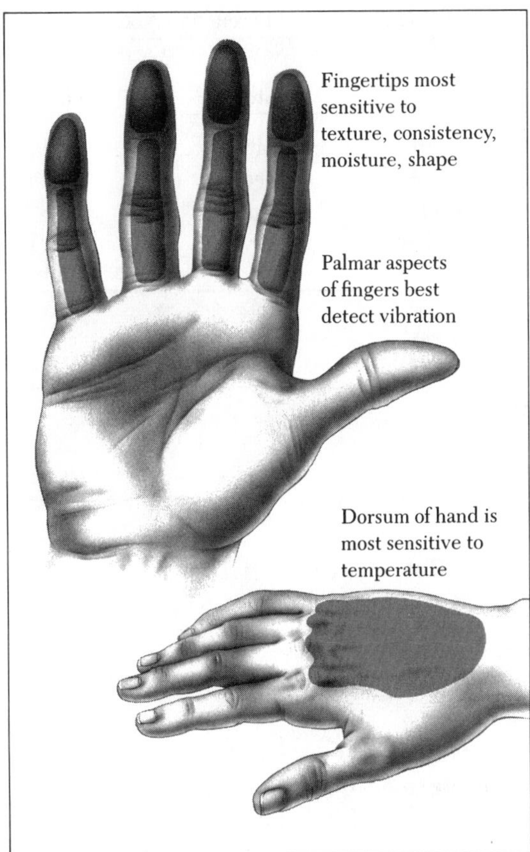

Figure 8-1 Sensitive areas of the hand.

Percussion

Percussion is the striking of a body surface area, noting the "feel" and sounds produced. An evaluation of the underlying structures can be made by interpreting the quality of such stimuli, which vary according to density. There are two basic types of percussion: direct and indirect.

In the direct technique, the body is lightly tapped directly with the fingers or hand. This technique is usually employed when seeking out areas of tenderness. Light percussion may aid not only in identifying areas of tenderness but in differentiating superficial from deep pain. Tapping over an infected sinus will produce pain, as will a blunt but light blow over an infected kidney. A sharp quick blow with a percussion hammer over a tendon will elicit a reflex (the evaluation of reflexes is an essential part of neurologic assessment).

The indirect method is done bimanually. For indirect percussion to be performed properly, the fingernail of the *plexor* should be trimmed short. This protects the *pleximeter* from injury and produces a much better sound quality than using a pad for percussion. Generally, the pleximeter of the left hand (vice versa for those who are left-handed) is placed firmly upon the surface to be percussed. The remaining fingers and the palm of the hand are raised off the area. If the hand or other fingers are allowed to rest on the surface, the sound vibrations will be dampened, much like a drumroll is muffled when a hand is placed on the drumhead. The bull's-eye area of the pleximeter (the distal phalanx) is struck by the tip of the plexor of the right hand. A light tap is best. Some individuals find that using the index and middle fingers together as plexors proves to be the best method for them. Wrist action is the salient feature of any technique for

Table 8-1. Classification of Percussion Notes

	Intensity	Pitch	Duration	Area or organ where percussion sound may occur
Flat	Soft	High	Short	Muscle, bone, thigh
Dull	Medium	Medium	Medium	Liver, spleen
Resonant	Loud	Low	Long	Lung
Hyperresonant	Very loud	Very low	Very long	Emphysematous lung
Tympanic	Loud	High	Medium	Gastric air bubble

Most dense tissue				Least dense tissue
Flat	Dull	Resonant	Hyperresonant	Tympanic

Figure 8-2 The continuum of percussion notes.

producing good quality percussion notes. The elbow and shoulder should not move during the delivery of the necessary brisk, staccato blow—only the wrist should move. Action is much like the wrist action used in spinning a yo-yo.

In order to reach a point at which you can easily and comfortably perform this technique, and to grasp the concept of the changing vibrations and tones that reflect the underlying density of structure, you may want to initially practice percussion techniques on the wall of a room. As you proceed along the wall, you can hear the difference in vibrations and sound as you meet a studboard behind the wall. The more solid the underlying structure, the lesser the vibrations and the shorter the duration of the percussion note. A more solid structure will also have a higher-pitched note upon percussion. Thus, percussion notes can be arranged according to the density that produces them. See Figure 8-2. The classifications of the percussion notes in Table 8-1 are arranged from the most dense to the least dense underlying body structures. Such classification of percussion notes and vibrations will not take on any real significance until you couple this knowledge with actual practice.

The technique of percussion can be used to detect painful body areas, to map out the size of areas of greater density (liver, spleen, tumors, fluid), and to identify the location of the lung bases as well as ascertain diaphragmatic excursion (an indirect measurement of lung inflation). You will need a flexible plastic ruler or a tape measure in centimeters to describe the size of masses and to measure organ sizes percussed. It is also important to realize that the percussion technique is not as helpful with obese individuals, as most general organ structures or masses over a depth of 5 cm go undetected.

Auscultation

Auscultation is the process of listening to sounds produced within the body. Before the advent of the stethoscope, auscultation was done by applying the examiner's ear directly against the client's body; important information went undetected with this method. An adequate stethoscope about 30–35 cm long and about 0.3 cm internal lumen diameter, with both *diaphragm* and *bell* (see Figure 8-3), will enable you to appreciate the method of clinical auscultation. A stethoscope without these qualities will only be good for listening to blood pressure readings. In general, the diaphragm best transmits high-pitched sounds, whereas the bell best transmits low-pitched sounds. Thus, breath sounds, friction rubs, heart sounds, bowel sounds, and crep-

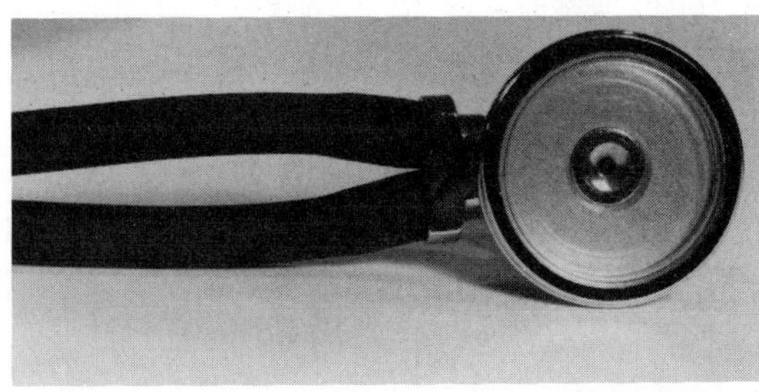

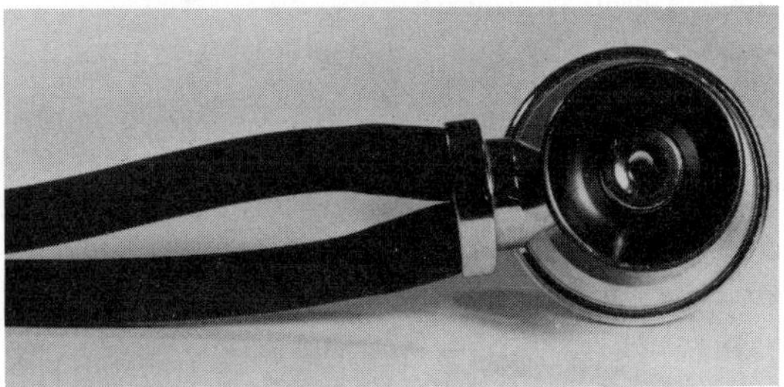

Figure 8-3 Stethoscope with diaphragm (top) and bell (bottom).

itus are best heard with the diaphragm, while bruits (pronounced "bru-ees") of stenotic arteries, heart murmurs, and venous hums are best detected with the bell.

A comfortable and properly fitting stethoscope is paramount. A poorly fitting stethoscope will be as good as a poorly fitting pair of shoes. Because stethoscope earplugs are interchangeable, you should try various sizes to identify your correct size. The soft rubber earplugs are usually considered the most comfortable because of their flexibility, but this is an individual preference. The two metal tubular portions of the stethoscope should be bent slightly with a pair of pliers so that they comfortably fit the angle of your external auditory canals. The metal span tension should be adjusted by manually bending the earpieces closer together or farther apart until the earplugs fit snugly and comfortably. Such fitting of the stethoscope to the individual is necessary for comfortable and efficient use.

Approaching the Client

The practice of washing one's hands before and after performing an assessment should be strictly adhered to and should preferably take place in the client's presence, thus conveying an attitude of cleanliness and protection. You can express thoughtfulness for the client's comfort by using warm water and by making appropriate remarks suggesting your recognition of the discomfort derived from the "cold hands" of an examiner. The same consideration is shown by warming the stethoscope with your hands before applying it to the client's body. A proper physical environment and appropriately applied clothing (examination gown, drapes, and so on) are necessary to provide privacy for the client. The room should be decently soundproof, quiet, warm, properly screened, and well-lighted. Natural light is superior to artificial light for examination and should be used whenever possible.

An unhurried atmosphere accompanied by a warm, personable client-centered approach is best. The examination should not be prolonged, nor should it be performed in such a rush as to sacrifice effectiveness. If a client is seriously ill, attend to the most pertinent portions of the physical assessment first. Provide rest periods if the client becomes fatigued.

At the beginning of the examination you should explain generally what is to be done. Periodically throughout the examination, instruct the client on how to cooperate, and give a step-by-step explanation of your actions. You need to be careful to use language that is understandable to the client and to avoid ill-founded comments of reassurance. Instruct the client at the onset to inform you if he should become tired or experience any pain. In addition, forewarn the client if a specific procedure may be uncomfortable or hurt. Honesty is the best policy for establishing and maintaining a trustful nurse-client relationship. If it is necessary for a client to undergo an uncomfortable or painful procedure, it is helpful to defer it until the end of the physical assessment process.

An effective physical assessment requires that the portion of the client's body being examined be adequately exposed. At the same time, the client must be protected from drafts and overexposure. It is of prime importance that the client's comfort level, physically and psychologically, be monitored carefully throughout the entire health assessment, as well as during the physical examination.

These techniques for securing an effective physical assessment and for providing client comfort during the process are presented for a specific purpose—improving the delivery of health care services provided by nurses. It is not unusual to hear clients speak of past experiences in which they were treated impersonally or were made uncomfortable either psychologically or physiologically. Clients complain that their bodies and their care are fragmented—that health personnel are only interested in body "parts," not in them as a person, as a "whole." Is it any wonder that in order to get attention a psychosomatic individual will complain of body dysfunction or a lonely institutionalized client will use the ploy of pain or illness to get the nurse to his bedside?

Clients reveal that they have often felt like a "number" or one of a group of herded cattle. Some say they have received the impression that they are bothersome and have been hurried through on that account. Others tell of frightening experiences as a child, such as "surprise attacks" with painful procedures or an aggressive, rough-handling examiner. Many clients describe experiences of uncomfortableness, running the gamut from "cold hands" to lack of privacy to no explanations. Need you be reminded that an explanation couched in technical terms is as good as no explanation?

Purposeful planning is imperative in order to avoid reinforcement of such negative feelings and to eliminate such impersonal or uncomfortable experiences for clients in the future. It is trusted that all nurses appreciate the importance of physical and psychologic comfort for the client during health assessment and do place emphasis on its provision.

Developing a General Impression

Your general impression of the client begins to form upon the initial observation. It is representative of your opinion of the client's overall appearance. Despite the inclusion of objective data, the general impression is nevertheless your interpretation of the client as a whole and therefore somewhat subjective. Much of the information discussed in Chapter 5, Mental Health Assessment, is recorded in the general impression, especially if it is within normal range. If the mental health assessment reveals problems requiring nursing prescriptions, the general impression may be of considerable length, or a separate report, under the title "mental health or psychologic assessment," may be warranted. This latter approach is used particularly when a standardized record form limits the space provided for the recording of the general impression (although some standardized record forms have a specific heading and space provided for psychologic assessment). The basic elements usually included in the recording of a general impression are state of consciousness, age, race, sex, development, nutritional state, general state of health, gross abnormalities, striking features, height, weight, and vital signs.

The following discussion of the basic elements provides the rationale for their inclusion and gives examples to aid you in constructing a general impression. By no means are the examples comprehensive, nor is it necessary that all the elements be included in every case. The general impression usually consists of from one to five sentences, so the elements must be stated briefly and succinctly.

State of Consciousness

Terms used to describe the client's conscious state include alert; lethargic; dull; slow or quick to respond; disoriented to person, place, or time; responsive only to pain; and comatose. Evaluation of the state of consciousness is an important determinant of the approach to be taken with the particular client and of other specific nursing prescriptions.

Age

Chronologic age is given, if known. Some pathologies are predominant in certain age categories. Obvious examples would be the diseases of childhood (measles, mumps, chickenpox); Perthes' disease, anorexia nervosa, and acne of adolescence; myocardial infarction and gallbladder dysfunction of middle age; and arthritis, diabetes, peripheral vascular diseases, and depression of old age. Knowing the connections between age and disease not only facilitates diagnostic conclusions but enables you to anticipate possible difficulties and to conduct appropriate preventive health teaching.

You should note whether the client appears to be his stated age or whether he appears older or younger than his chronologic age. Frequently clients who are alcoholics, who are severely debilitated, or who may be harboring a chronic illness appear to be much older than their actual age.

Race

Knowledge of race directs your attention toward investigating possible racial customs—an important constituent of client data that is necessary to considering the client as an individual when planning nursing care. As with age, there are pathologies that are predominantly found in particular races. For example, there is a higher incidence of skin cancer among Whites and a higher incidence of sickle-cell anemia among Blacks.

Sex

A client's sex may make him or her more prone to develop certain diseases. For example, males are more prone to develop gastric ulcers and myocardial infarctions, whereas females are more prone to develop breast carcinoma. Young females are more prone to develop anorexia nervosa, whereas young males are more prone to develop Perthes' disease. Certain pathologies of the gonads are sex-specific, such as epididymitis, prostatitis, and priapism in males, and salpingitis, ovarian cysts, and fibroid uterus in females. Some conditions are genetically sex-linked, such as hemophilia and color blindness, both of which result from a recessive gene carried only on the X chromosome. Such conditions occur primarily in males and are transmitted by normal heterozygous females who carry the recessive gene.

Development

To assess the development of a child, you need to have background knowledge of the normal growth and development phases of the early years of life, because marked changes in both mental and physical abilities occur over a short period of time. A condensed table of age-related developmental abilities and stages is provided in Appendix B. One of the most common screening tools, used with children up to the age of 7, is the Denver Developmental Screening Test (included in Chapter 21). The developmental testing of the child is usually done at the conclusion of the interview and prior to the physical examination. This sequence often aids in establishing a working relationship with the child prior to the physical examination and results in subsequent cooperation. If a sibling is present for health assessment, begin with the older child, who is more likely to cooperate. The older child will generally set a good example for the younger to follow.

For adults, development generally means physical maturation or normal body growth (height, symmetry) and the presence of secondary sex characteristics.

Many developmental abnormalities are results of dysfunction of or damage to the adenohypophysis (anterior lobe of the pituitary gland). The adenohypophysis releases four hormones that stimulate target areas of the body (the target area of each is within parentheses): thyrotropin (thyroid), gonadotropin (sex organs), adrenocorticotropin (adrenal cortex), and somatotropin (general growth). Developmental anomalies can also occur secondary to chronic diseases in childhood, whether nutritional, infectious, cardiac, renal, or metabolic in origin. Some developmental abnormalities in adults are shown in Figures 8-4 through 8-8.

Nutritional State

You may want to note whether the client is well nourished or is either overweight or underweight. Extremes may be described using such terms as malnourished, cachectic (see Figure 8-9), and obese. Often with a rapid weight loss the skin will be loose and sagging, but this phenomenon is also common in the elderly as the result of a lifetime of gravitational pull on the loose tissues of the body.

General State of Health

You should note whether the client appears to be in excellent health, shows any signs of distress, appears chronically, acutely, or gravely ill, or is in no apparent distress.

Gross Abnormalities

Note any gross congenital or acquired defects, such as missing limbs, webbed digits, torticollis, or abnormal curvature of the spine. Describe abnormal positions, such as opisthotonos (seen in severe cases of meningitis and tetanus) or a curled fetallike position (observed in cases of severe withdrawal and sometimes with abdominal pain). Record marked aberrations of body movements, such as athetosis or tics. If the client displays an obvious abnormal gait or speech defect you may record it here, but such signs would

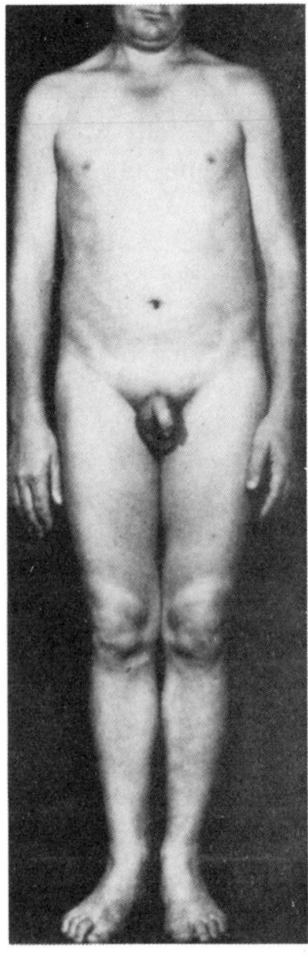

Figure 8-4 Hypopituitarism (chromophobe adenoma). This 33-year-old male lacks a beard and axillary and pubic hair and has lost his libido.

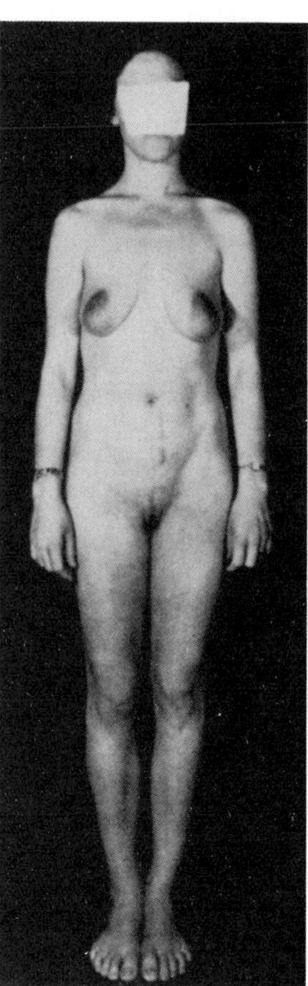

Figure 8-5 Hypopituitarism typical of Sheehan's disease. It is characterized by absence of pubic hair and weight loss.

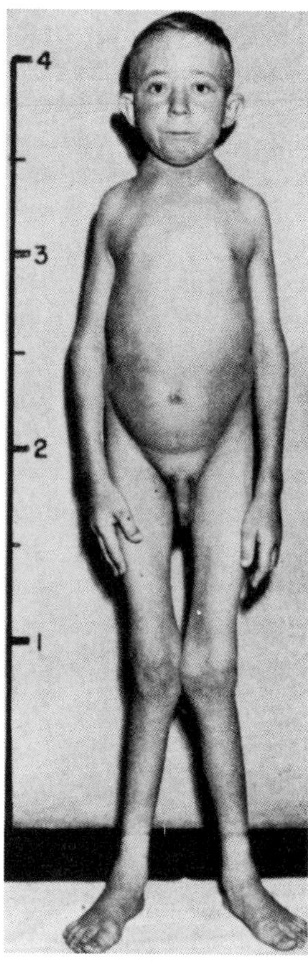

Figure 8-6 Renal dwarfism. This 21-year-old male with chronic renal disease since childhood has stunted growth as a result of severe disturbances in mineral and amino acid metabolism.

warrant further consideration during the portion of the physical examination that focuses on neurologic function.

Striking Features

Striking features run the gamut from physical features to personality characteristics to behavior—whatever seems to "jump out" at you. Endocrine disorders, in particular, produce striking physical changes, as seen in Figures 8-10 through 8-12.

It is often difficult to decide which observations to list under which category. Many of the signs, symptoms, and behaviors discussed so far could be discussed under several; therefore, such categorization is somewhat arbitrary. The important point is that these aspects must be documented somewhere in the general impression.

Height and Weight

The client's height and weight are recorded, and his usual weight is also recorded if he has undergone a marked loss or gain. To assess whether the client's weight is in the normal range, consult height, weight, and body frame tables. Weight standards for men and women are shown in Tables 8-2 and 8-3.

Vital Signs

Vital signs for adults include TPR (temperature, pulse, and respirations) and BP (blood pressure).

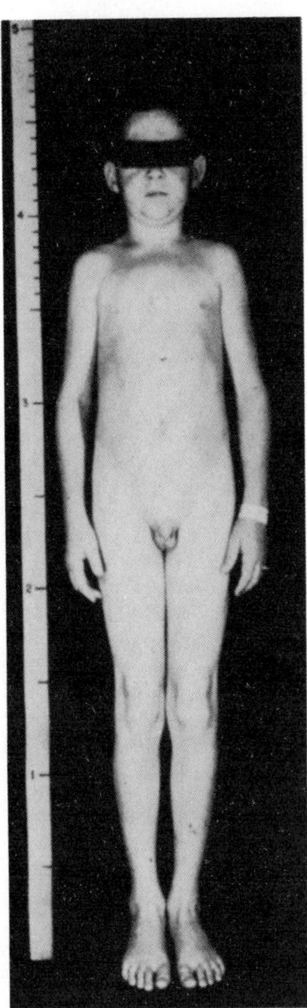

Figure 8-7 Pituitary dwarfism. This 18-year-old male is 54″ tall and weighs 67 pounds. He has no body hair and immature testes.

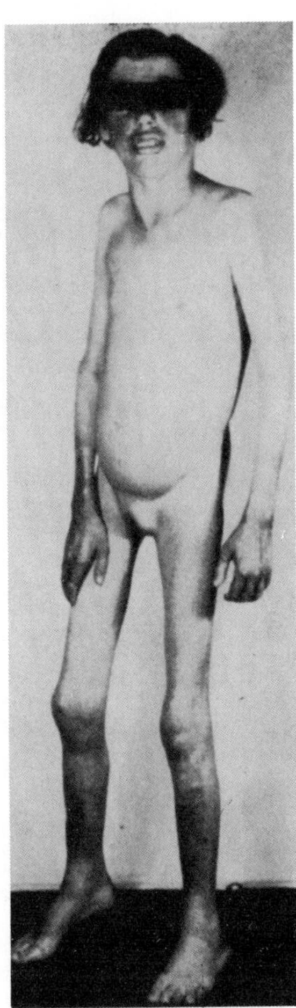

Figure 8-8 Cretinism, which results from hypofunction of the thyroid gland during gestation or infancy, is associated with various degrees of mental retardation. Note the dull expression, thick lips and tongue, potbelly and umbilical hernia, and shortened extremities in relation to trunk from retarded bone growth.

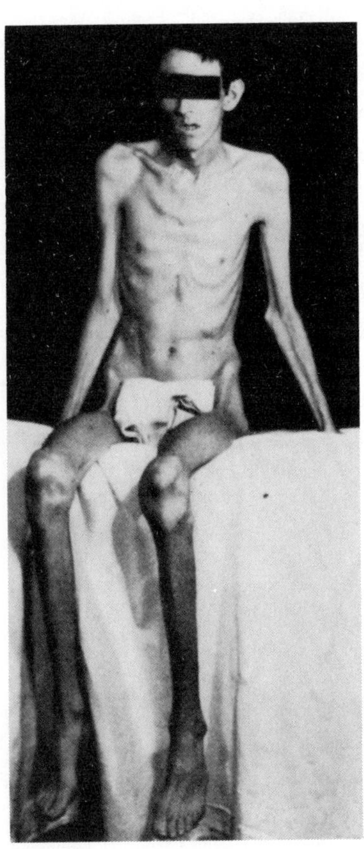

Figure 8-9 Cachexia in a 26-year-old male due to fibrosis of the pituitary.

For infants they would also include head circumference and crown-rump height. In special situations CVP (central venous pressure) would be considered a vital sign.

Vital signs are initially recorded to establish a baseline against which changes can be compared and to identify trends; subsequent recordings should be made as often as you deem necessary. There is no need to wait for a scheduled time to take vital signs should you suspect a change from other observations. It is important that you know the normal range of vital signs according to developmental aspects and that you identify the client's personal variations.

Temperature

The normal range of body temperature in the resting person is 98.6 ± 1 F orally. Axillary temperature registers approximately 1 degree lower than the average oral temperature (97.6 F), whereas rectal temperature is about 1 degree higher than the oral body temperature (99.6 F).

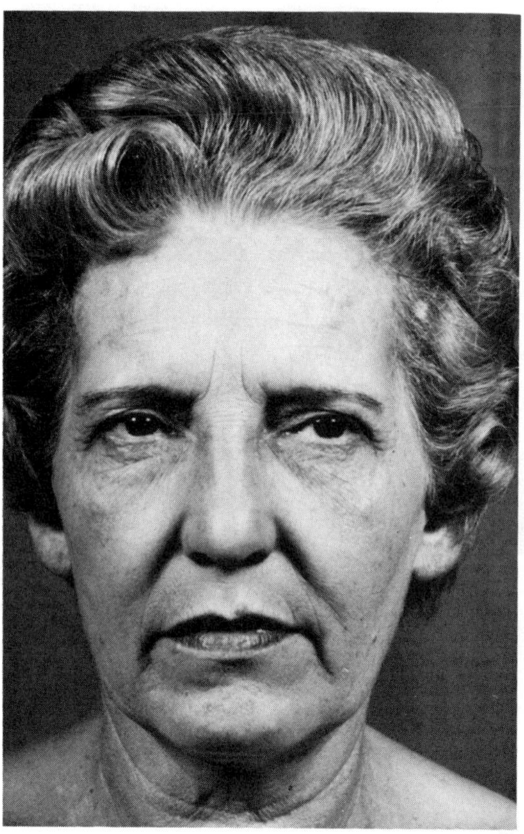

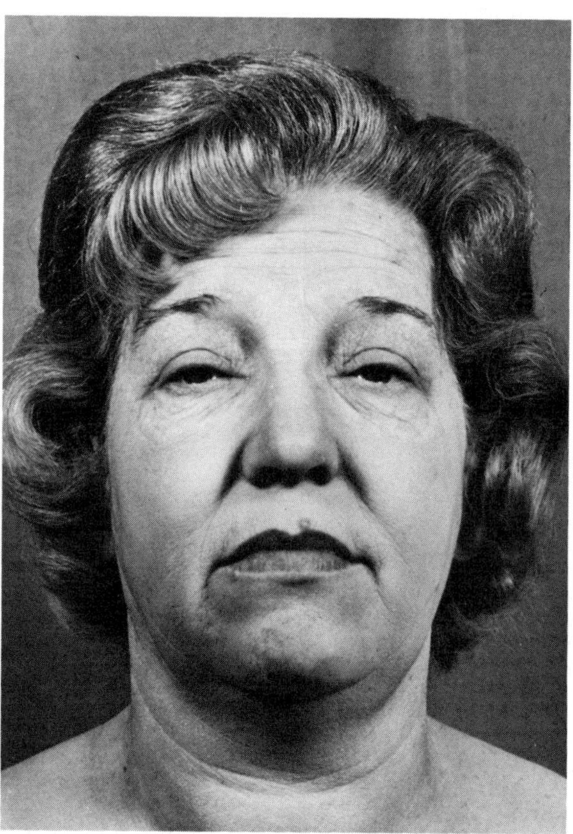

A B

Figure 8-10 (A) Client prior to onset of myxedema. (B) Facies with onset of myxedema (hypothyroidism in adulthood). Note the coarseness of skin, puffy face, and apathetic expression.

Rectal readings are most often taken with children and with adult clients who are mouth-breathers, who are confused, or who are receiving oxygen therapy. It is also necessary to use this method with clients who are unconscious, who have experienced severe trauma (lacerations of the mouth), or who have undergone facial-mandibular surgery (wired fractured jaw, glossectomy).

Each individual has a personal temperature variation. Most commonly, a client's early morning temperature will register 2+ degrees lower than his average temperature, and his temperature in the late afternoon or early evening will register 0.5 to 1 degree higher.

The menstruating female exhibits a well-known temperature pattern. Her body temperature usually drops about 24–36 hours before ovulation. Then, as ovulation occurs, her morning temperature will rise and remain at this high level until just prior to the onset of her menstrual period.

Infants and young children do not have as well-controlled body temperature as adults. The toddler's average rectal temperature is usually 99–100 F (37.2–37.8 C) or higher. Even with minor infections, the infant or young child's temperature may rise to 103–105 F. Yet with a severe infection the infant's temperature may actually be normal or even subnormal.

It is common to witness slight fever a day or two following surgery; pyrexia is also characteristic of vascular, respiratory, and urologic infections and of wound infection. Pyrexia, as well as subnormal temperatures, can also occur from a direct influence on the thermoregulatory centers in the hypothalamus, such as occurs with head injury, cerebrovascular accident, and cere-

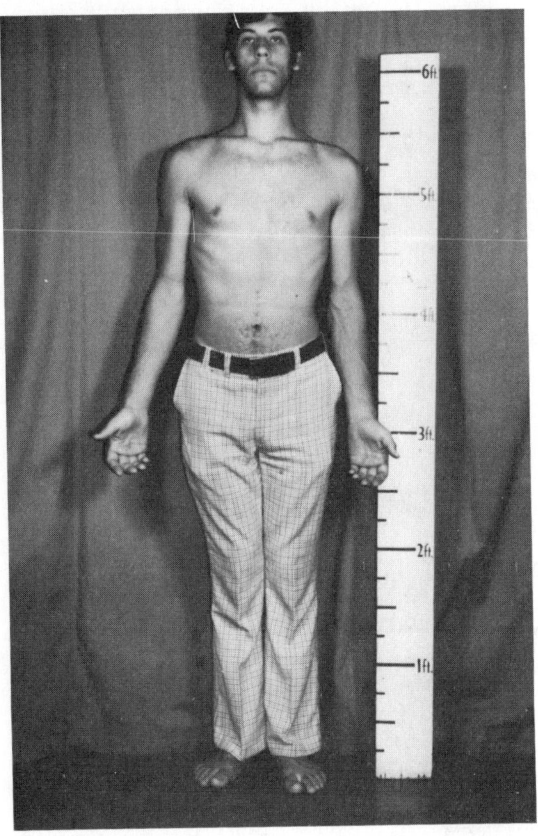

Figure 8-11 Acromegaly. Note the elongation and enlargement of bones, especially of the extremities and jaw, and the soft tissue enlargement of the face, especially of the nose and lips.

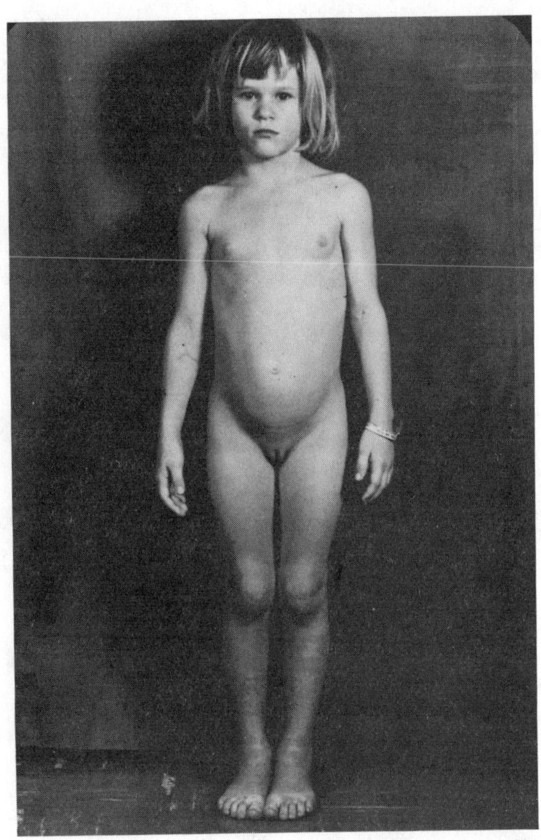

Figure 8-12 Adrenocortical hyperfunction in a preschool girl. Note the breast enlargement.

bral edema or tumor. It is important to keep in mind that anxiety, as well as physical stress, may elevate body temperature.

Clinical thermometers do not record temperatures below 95 F (35 C), so whenever a temperature is recorded in this range, the true temperature should be checked with more sensitive devices. Hypothermia is a particular threat to the elderly, many of whom live in cold conditions because of the high cost of fuel.

Pulse

The pulse recorded with the TPR is the radial pulse in the child and adult and the temporal or apical pulse in the newborn and infant. Pulse is assessed according to rate, rhythm, and quality. The apical pulse is routinely examined in the adult and child during the cardiac portion of the physical assessment. With cardiac arrest, the carotid or femoral pulse is used to determine perfusion.

The pulse rates varies with age, sex, physical exertion, and emotional status. In children it is best to take the pulse for a full minute because there is a greater variation in the pulse rates of infants and children (see Table 8-4). In the adult you can take the pulse for 30 seconds and multiply the result by 2. If you note any irregularity, take the pulse for the entire minute. The normal pulse rate in the resting adult ranges from 60 to 100/min. It is slightly faster in women than in men. Because of arteriosclerotic tendencies with age, the pulse in the elderly client may feel hard and cordlike and may be of a faster rate.

Stimulation of the sympathetic nervous system will increase the heart rate; thus, tachycardia is present in clients experiencing pain,

Table 8-2. Weight According to Frame (Indoor Clothing), Women of Ages 25 and Over*

Height†			Small frame		Medium frame		Large frame	
Feet	Inches	cm	Pounds	Kilograms	Pounds	Kilograms	Pounds	Kilograms
4	10	147.3	92–98	41.7–44.5	96–107	43.5–48.5	104–119	47.2–54.0
4	11	149.9	94–101	42.6–45.8	98–110	44.5–49.9	106–122	48.1–55.3
5	0	152.4	96–104	43.5–47.2	101–113	45.8–51.3	109–125	49.4–56.7
5	1	154.9	99–107	44.9–48.5	104–116	47.2–52.6	112–128	50.8–58.1
5	2	157.5	102–110	46.3–50.0	107–119	48.5–54.0	115–131	52.2–59.4
5	3	160.0	105–113	47.6–51.3	110–122	49.9–55.3	118–134	53.5–60.8
5	4	162.6	108–116	49.0–52.6	113–126	51.3–57.2	121–138	54.9–62.6
5	5	165.1	111–119	50.3–54.0	116–130	52.6–59.0	125–142	56.7–64.4
5	6	167.6	114–123	51.7–55.8	120–135	54.4–61.2	129–146	58.5–66.2
5	7	170.2	118–127	53.5–57.6	124–139	56.2–63.0	133–150	60.3–68.0
5	8	172.7	122–131	55.3–59.4	128–143	58.1–64.9	137–154	62.1–69.9
5	9	175.3	126–135	57.2–61.2	132–147	59.9–66.7	141–158	64.0–71.7
5	10	177.8	130–140	59.0–63.5	136–151	61.7–68.5	145–163	65.8–73.9
5	11	180.3	134–144	60.8–65.3	140–155	63.5–70.3	149–168	67.6–76.2
6	0	182.9	138–148	62.6–67.1	144–159	65.3–72.1	153–173	69.4–78.5

*For women between 18 and 25, subtract 0.5 kg (1 pound) for each year under 25.
†With shoes on—5.1 cm (2-inch) heels
Courtesy of the Metropolitan Life Insurance Company.

Table 8-3. Weight According to Frame (Indoor Clothing), Men of Ages 25 and Over

Height*			Small frame		Medium frame		Large frame	
Feet	Inches	cm	Pounds	Kilograms	Pounds	Kilograms	Pounds	Kilograms
5	2	157.5	112–120	50.8–54.4	118–129	53.5–58.5	126–141	57.2–64.0
5	3	160.0	115–123	52.2–55.8	121–133	54.9–60.3	129–144	58.5–65.3
5	4	162.6	118–126	53.5–57.2	124–136	56.2–61.7	132–148	59.9–67.1
5	5	165.1	121–129	54.9–58.5	127–139	57.6–63.0	135–152	61.2–68.9
5	6	167.6	124–133	56.2–60.3	130–143	59.0–64.9	138–156	62.6–70.8
5	7	170.2	128–137	58.1–62.1	134–147	60.8–66.7	142–161	64.4–73.0
5	8	172.7	132–141	59.9–64.0	138–152	62.6–68.9	147–166	66.7–75.3
5	9	175.3	136–145	61.7–65.8	142–156	64.4–70.8	151–170	68.5–77.1
5	10	177.8	140–150	63.5–68.0	146–160	66.2–72.6	155–174	70.3–78.9
5	11	180.3	144–154	65.3–69.9	150–165	68.0–74.8	159–179	72.1–81.2
6	0	182.9	148–158	67.1–71.7	154–170	69.9–77.1	164–184	74.4–83.4
6	1	185.4	152–162	68.9–73.5	158–175	71.7–79.4	168–189	76.2–85.7
6	2	188.0	156–167	70.8–75.8	162–180	73.5–81.6	173–194	78.5–88.0
6	3	190.5	160–171	72.6–77.6	167–185	75.8–83.9	178–199	80.7–90.3
6	4	193.0	164–175	74.4–79.4	172–190	78.0–86.2	182–204	82.6–92.5

*With shoes on—2.5 cm (1-inch) heels.
Courtesy of Metropolitan Life Insurance Company.

anxiety, anger, or fear. Clients who require greater cardiac output because of situations that have a greater demand for oxygen also display tachycardia. Such situations include exercise, toxic states with high fever, severe anemia, thyrotoxicosis, shock, hypoxia, congenital heart disease, and congestive heart failure. Bradycardia is not unusual in the physically fit athlete, but it can also be indicative of parasympathetic stimulation in digitalis poisoning, syncope, increased

Table 8-4. Pulse Rates per Minute at Rest for Boys and Girls Up to 18 Years

	Boys			Girls		
Age in years	No. of tests	Mean ± σ_m	SD	No. of tests	Mean ± σ_m	SD
0–1	33	135 ± 3.1	18	56	126 ± 2.8	21
1–2	82	105 ± 1.8	16	93	104 ± 1.8	17
2–3	150	93 ± 1.0	12	177	93 ± 0.7	9
3–4	157	87 ± 0.7	9	145	89 ± 0.7	9
4–5	157	84 ± 0.7	8	137	84 ± 0.7	8
5–6	150	79 ± 0.6	7	129	79 ± 0.6	7
6–7	146	76 ± 0.6	8	122	77 ± 0.7	8
7–8	140	75 ± 0.7	8	117	76 ± 0.8	8
8–9	142	73 ± 0.7	9	114	73 ± 0.6	7
9–10	168	70 ± 0.6	7	106	70 ± 0.7	8
10–11	164	67 ± 0.6	7	98	69 ± 0.8	8
11–12	129	67 ± 0.6	7	84	69 ± 0.8	7
12–13	131	66 ± 0.6	7	72	69 ± 0.9	8
13–14	110	65 ± 0.8	8	68	68 ± 0.9	8
14–15	106	62 ± 0.7	7	57	66 ± 1.1	8
15–16	76	61 ± 0.9	8	47	65 ± 1.1	8
16–17	45	61 ± 0.9	6	30	66 ± 1.4	8
17–18	38	60 ± 1.4	8	20	65 ± 1.7	7

Adapted from A. Iliff and V. A. Lee. "Pulse Rate, Respiratory Rate, and Body Temperature of Children Between 2 Months and 18 Years," *Child Development*, 23 (1952): 237. By permission of the Society for Research in Child Development, Inc.

intracranial pressure, myxedema, obstructive jaundice, heart block, and septal defect.

The normal pulse rate is of regular rhythm. However, a state of sinus arrhythmia, in which the pulse rate increases at the peak of respiratory inspiration and decreases upon expiration, is a common nonpathologic phenomenon observed in children and young adults. In such cases, the pulse will beat in regular rhythm when the client holds his breath. Cardiac arrhythmias may be indicated by an irregular pulse rhythm and by a pulse deficit, which occurs when the radial pulse rate is less than the apical pulse rate. Occasionally, a person may experience a premature beat, often described as the heart "skipping a beat." In this case some other pacemaker fires ahead of the sinoatrial node. Frequent PVC's (premature ventricular contractions) can indicate cardiac irritability from such things as digitalis toxicity, potassium imbalance, or hypoxia, or they may represent more serious cardiac arrhythmias. Pairs of beats or triplets aggregated and followed by a pause are termed bigeminal and trigeminal pulses, respectively. Premature contractions are the most common cause of bigeminal or trigeminal pulse irregularities. However, they may be symptomatic of overdigitalization or of partial or 2° heart block.

The quality of the pulse is an important factor. A thready, weak pulse is present in shock and in heart failure. A weak pulse will be found distal to a partial occlusion of an artery and may also occur with cardiac valvular stenosis, myocardial infarction or myocarditis, and pericardial effusion or constrictive pericarditis. These are all conditions in which cardiac output is reduced. A full, strong, bounding pulse (pulsus magnus) accompanies systolic hypertension and may occasionally occur in the normal client during anxiety, excessive physical exertion, or fever. Pulsus alterans, with alternating strong and weak beats, is observed in left ventricular failure, coronary artery disease, and severe arterial hypertension.

Respiration

Normal respirations are effortless, regular, and smooth. Average respirations per minute varies with age. Infants to 2 years of age average 24–34 respirations per minute, children to puberty range from 20 to 26 per minute, and normal adults average 12–18 per minute. Clients with an increased need for oxygenation of the blood, as with exercise or fever, will show an increased rate of respirations. Changes in respirations can also be caused by interference with the respiratory center of the medulla oblongata.

The depth of respirations determines the volume of air moving in and out of the lungs. Extremes of depth vary from shallow breathing to the deep respirations of Kussmaul's breathing. Exact measurement of the depth of respirations requires a spirometer. A decrease in both respiratory rate and depth is seen with metabolic alkalosis, in which the body is attempting to retain carbon dioxide. Conversely, the increase in the rate and depth of respirations seen in metabolic acidosis is the compensatory mechanism that blows off the excess carbon dioxide and neutralizes the excess amounts of hydrogen ions.

When dyspnea is present, it is important to determine how much exertion is necessary to cause it or whether it occurs at rest. You should look for signs of respiratory obstruction as you note the rate and depth of respirations. You should carefully note whether the chest movement is symmetrical with respirations, whether intercostal or sternal retraction is present, and whether there is nasal flaring. Particularly in chronic obstructive pulmonary disease (COPD), there is obvious use of the accessory muscles in the neck for breathing. The client with COPD assumes a characteristic forward position with his hands on his knees or his elbows on the table. This position compresses the abdomen and increases the intrathoracic pressure, thus facilitating expiration. In clients with asthma or emphysema you may observe a bulging of the interspaces caused by trapped air during forced expiration.

Blood Pressure

Blood pressure tests measure vascular pressures. During cardiac systole (contraction of the ventricles of the heart), the maximum pressure of the blood is exerted against the arterial walls by the left ventricle. This is called the *systolic pressure*. The *diastolic pressure* on the walls of the arteries is continually present and reflects blood vessel resistance.

Blood pressure is lowest in the newborn and increases with age. It also increases with exercise and emotional stress and with a gain in weight. Ordinarily, it is at its lowest in the early morning after a night's sleep. A client's blood pressure is also lower when measured in a supine position as compared to a sitting or standing position. The cuff used should cover at least half of the portion of extremity used and not more than two-thirds of the area. Methods for taking blood pressure readings are summarized in Table 8-5.

Blood pressure is taken in all four extremities in clients suspected of having cardiac problems, in those with weak or absent femoral or popliteal pulses, and in children or young adults with hypertension. This last situation could mean coarctation of the aorta (a congenital narrowing). With coarctation the systolic pressure of both arms is surprisingly high, and the systolic pressure of the lower extremities is lower than that of the upper extremities because the femoral arteries are at the lower portion of the aorta and thus below the stenosed segment. Normally, the blood pressure reading for the legs is slightly higher than that for the arms because the larger muscle mass exerts more resistance to arterial compression by the blood pressure cuff. Figure 8-13 shows that the cuff should be placed at the lower third of the leg with the stethoscope over the popliteal artery. There is usually very little if any difference in blood pressure between the two upper extremities; a significant discrepancy could be a result of aortic aneurysm.

Pulse pressure is the difference between systolic and diastolic pressure readings. Normally, it is 25–50 mm Hg. A decrease in pulse pressure may be a sign of heart failure, massive pericardial effusion, aortic stenosis, or mitral stenosis. A widening pulse pressure can be caused by vigorous exercise, fever, increased intracranial pressure, thyrotoxicosis, severe anemia, or severe atherosclerosis of the aorta and large arteries.

Hypertension, as defined by the World Health Organization, is a persistent elevation of blood pressure above 140 mm systolically and 90 mm diastolically (140/90). A pressure below 95/60 is generally considered to be hypotension. However, a hypertensive client may be hypotensive at 150/90.

Essential hypertension is of an unknown etiology. Hypertension can be caused by kidney disease and is usually accompanied by headaches, blurred vision, and renal failure symptomatology. Other causes are coarctation of the aorta, pheochromocytoma, and polycythemia. Associated manifestations of hypertension in-

Table 8-5. Blood Pressure Reading Methods

Palpatory systolic pressure	Auscultatory method	Flush method (for newborns or infants)
1. Place client's arm at heart level.	1. Place client's arm at heart level.	1. Put cuff around ankle or wrist.
2. Avoid clothing constriction.	2. Avoid clothing constriction.	2. Elevate leg or arm.
3. Cuff evenly over brachial artery.	3. Cuff evenly over brachial artery.	3. Squeeze or wrap leg or arm with elastic bandage to occlude blood from the part.
4. Palpate radial pulse.	4. Palpate radial pulse.	4. Inflate to 120–140 mm Hg.
5. Inflate cuff until radial pulse disappears.	5. Inflate cuff until radial pulse disappears.	5. Release squeeze or bandage.
6. Inflate cuff 30 mm Hg more.	6. Inflate cuff 30 mm Hg more.	6. Release cuff.
7. Release pressure of cuff slowly.	7. Place stethoscope over brachial artery in anticubital space.	7. The point of flush return is the mean diastolic-systolic pressure.
8. Read systolic blood pressure at return point of radial pulse.	8. Release cuff pressure.	
	9. The point at which you hear the first sound is systolic pressure. Damping or muffling is diastolic pressure.	
	10. Also record the final sound. Example: 116/80/76.	

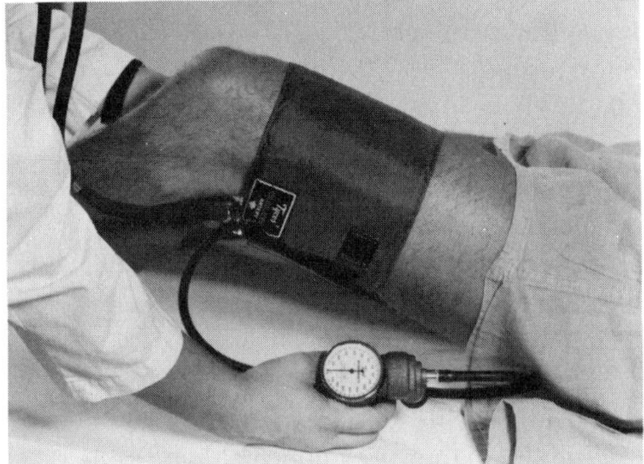

Figure 8-13 Technique for taking blood pressure on the leg.

clude epistaxis, headaches, and irritability. There is a familial tendency for hypertension.

An increased systolic pressure as the result of an increase in cardiac output with a stable diastolic pressure can be found in older clients with atherosclerosis and in clients with anemia, arteriovenous fistula, aortic regurgitation, or hyperthyroidism.

A blood pressure decrease occurs following an acute myocardial infarction, as a result of the diminished cardiac output. Hypotension is also seen with hypovolemia, which can occur in shock from hemorrhage, in burns, in dehydration, and in hypoadrenalism. Oliguria or anuria is an early sign of hypovolemia.

Summary

This chapter introduced you to the basic techniques of physical assessment. It described the four classical methods: inspection, palpation, percussion, and auscultation. Inspection relies primarily on the visual sense, while palpation employs the sense of touch for evaluating such aspects as temperature, contour, surface texture, consistency, and vibration. Percussion requires considerable practice to perfect and is useful in determining density and size of organs and tumors as well as the presence of pain. The sense of hearing is used in auscultation, a technique central in assessing the cardiovascular, respiratory, and gastrointestinal systems.

Also the approach to the client in performing physical assessment, was described as taking into consideration the client's comfort, safety, and age. Then each of the components within the general impression (state of consciousness, age, race, sex, development, nutritional state, general state of health, gross abnormalities,

BIOLOGICAL AND CULTURAL VARIATIONS

Hypertension Among Black Americans

The National Health Survey has determined that 20 to 25 million Americans have either a casual systolic blood pressure of 150 mm Hg or higher or a diastolic blood pressure of 95 mm Hg or higher. However, these high blood pressure levels are twice as frequent among Blacks as among Whites at all ages up to 80 years; hypertension affects 30% of all Black adults, compared to 16% of all White adults. Hypertension is the disease or physiologic disorder diagnosed when an individual consistently has blood pressure readings above 140 mm Hg systolic/90 mm Hg diastolic. Blacks are also more likely to suffer from severe hypertension, the relative rate being 3.3 times higher for Black males than for White males. Mortality rates for Blacks from hypertension and disorders stemming from hypertension (such as cardiac complications, cerebrovascular disease, and uremia) are similarly higher.

The most significant epidemiologic finding concerning hypertension in the United States is the high morbidity and mortality rates of Black Americans. There has been a limited attempt to explain these higher rates. One or several of the factors involved in hypertension might occur to a greater extent among Blacks. Alternatively, it might be that Blacks are more sensitive to one or more of the agents. For example, overweight and obesity are two nutritional conditions that have been found to be highly associated with hypertension. Could this be a factor? As a group, Blacks are more lean than Whites; however, it may be that there are more obese Blacks than Whites. Still, this slight difference in the incidence of obesity would not be enough to explain the great difference in high blood pressure rates. Also, one study has shown that weight is less correlated with blood pressure in Blacks than in Whites (Tyroler, Hyden, & Hames 1975). Thus, more evidence concerning overweight is needed.

Short-term stress can elevate blood pressure quite markedly. It has been proposed that chronic stress might lead to elevated blood pressure. It is possible that Blacks and Whites are subjected to different amounts of life stress and that the higher blood pressure of Black Americans arises from greater life stress. Although this proposition has intuitive appeal, it would be extremely difficult to investigate. For one thing, it is extremely hard to define stress as a variable and measure it. Thus, investigations along these lines have had inconclusive results.

A review of the literature on socioeconomic status and hypertension in the United States shows that the higher the social class, the lower the prevalence, morbidity, and mortality rates (Howard & Holman 1970). Since Blacks as a group are more disadvantaged than Whites, this suggests that the higher Black rates might be due to social class differences. However, studies that have compared Black and White rates in each social class have shown Blacks to still have much higher mortality rates in every class (Howard & Holman 1970). Thus, although social class seems to be an important determinant of blood pressure, the additive effect of race and social class seems to be an even stronger determinant.

There may be certain traits in the genetic composition of the Black population that determine the higher prevalence of hypertension. These traits could involve the metabolism of certain etiological agents, such as sodium or cadmium, or the mechanisms of certain systems, such as the autonomic nervous system. Few studies have investigated these possibilities. Thus, genetic differences and environmental factors interacting with this genetic component may explain the high blood pressure differences.

Obviously the reasons for the higher rate of hypertension among Black Americans remain unclear. This is certainly a question in need of further investigation.

General impression: Mr. J., an apprehensive 18-year-old white male, college freshman, well developed and well nourished. In acute distress — pale, dyspneic, diaphoretic, leaning forward in a sitting position braced by extended arms, and receiving nasal O_2 (4L/min). No apparent speech defects, but his voice is weak and breathless. Mental processes are slowed. TPR 102-110-36. BP sitting left arm: 100/56. Ht: 5'11" Wt: 160 lbs. (normal wt: 175 lbs).

Figure 8-14 Example of a general impression evaluation.

striking features, height, weight, and vital signs) was discussed. Vital signs (temperature, pulse, respiration, and blood pressure) were described carefully and clearly to assist you in understanding their significance in a complete physical assessment.

Discussion Questions/Activities

1. Discuss how you use each of your senses in physical assessment.
2. Of what benefit is your general impression of the client to you or to other health professionals?
3. Why does the initiation of taking vital signs fall into the category of a nursing diagnosis?
4. What would prompt you to take the vital signs of a client and why?
5. Write a general impression of yourself, a classmate, a client (see Figure 8-14 for an example).

Checklist for Developing a General Impression

State of consciousness
Age
Race
Sex
Development
Nutritional state
General state of health
Gross abnormalities
Striking features
Height and weight
Vital signs

CHAPTER 9

Assessment of the Integument

LEARNING OBJECTIVES

1. Review the structure and function of the skin.
2. Describe the techniques and characteristics of the skin used for inspection and palpation.
3. Describe the techniques and characteristics of the hair used for inspection and palpation.
4. Describe the techniques and characteristics of the nails used for inspection and palpation.
5. Recognize biological and cultural variations in assessment of the integument.
6. List the characteristics used to describe skin lesions.
7. Identify primary and secondary skin lesions.

The integument, or covering, of the body is the skin, the body's first line of defense. It protects the body from trauma and infection and aids in temperature regulation. The appendages of the skin are part of the integumentary system: the sweat glands, sebaceous glands, hair, and nails. Inspection and palpation of the client's hands and fingernails is a nonthreatening beginning to physical assessment. Not only can you notice abnormalities in appearance of these bodily parts at this time, but you can assess the client's grasp and the existence of stiffness or bony enlargement of the interphalangeal, metacarpophalangeal, and wrist joints.

Structure and Function of the Skin

Figure 9-1 shows that the skin has three basic layers: the *epidermis*, the *dermis*, and the *subcutaneous tissue*.

Epidermis

The epidermis is avascular. Being devoid of blood vessels, the uppermost layer of the epidermis lacks nutrition and consists of dead keratinized cells. This outermost layer, referred to as

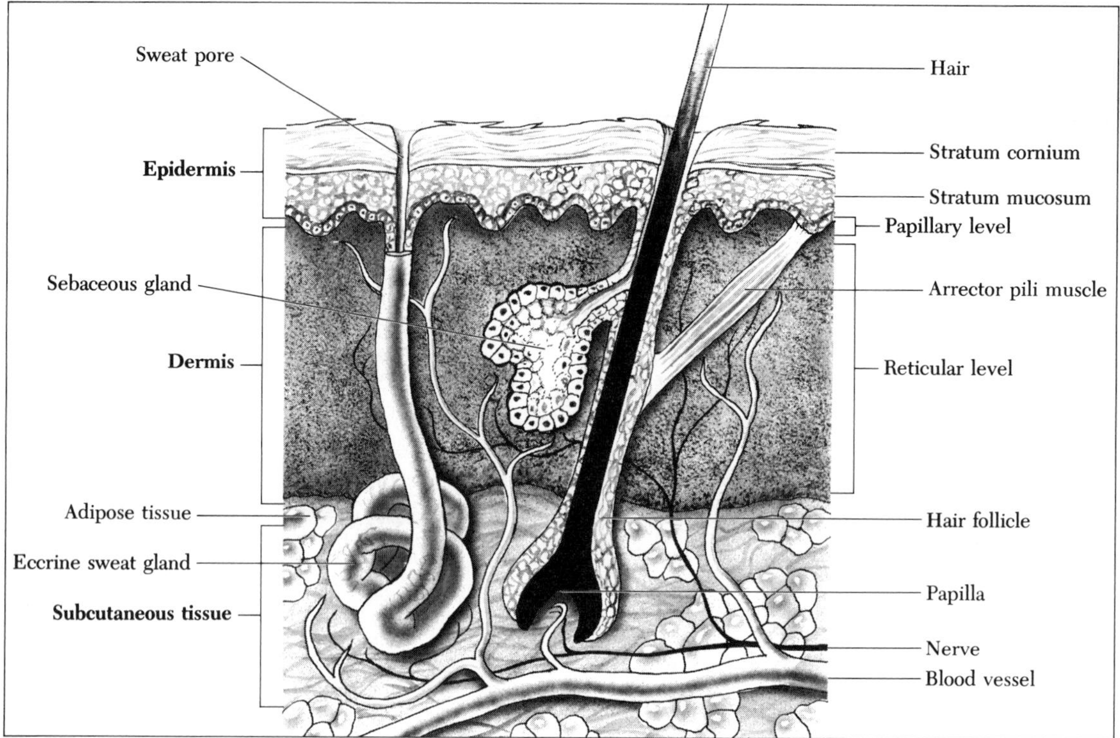

Figure 9-1 Anatomy of the skin.

the horny layer (*stratum cornium*), is continuously being shed, a process called desquamation. Excessive desquamation may be observed in severe dehydration and in dermatologic conditions such as psoriasis and contact dermatitis. The dead keratinized cells may accumulate into plaque formations or into horny, wartlike structures (keratosis). Keratosis is commonly observed in the elderly (see Figure 9-2). Hyperkeratosis at the hair follicles is characteristic of vitamin A deficiency. The keratinized cells pile up around the external hair shaft, producing a sandpaperlike skin, usually on the upper arms and thighs.

The second layer of the epidermis, the *stratum mucosum*, derives nutrition for its keratinocyte and melanocyte cells from the underlying vascular tissues. Both keratin and melanin are formed in the stratum mucosum.

Dermis

The dermis acts as a water and electrolyte storage compartment. The uppermost layer of the dermis, the *papillary level*, consists of dense connective tissue that is molded into the epidermis and that also provides the dermal lining of the hair follicles. The lower *reticular level*, also composed of many connective cells, contains blood vessels, lymphatics, the sensory nerve endings for the skin, the *sweat glands*, the *sebaceous glands*, and the *hair follicles*. The *eccrine sweat glands* are coiled tubules leading to an opening (pore) on the skin surface; their primary function is heat regulation via evaporation. The *apocrine sweat glands*, found primarily in the axillary and genital areas, produce secretions that usually find their way to the skin surface via

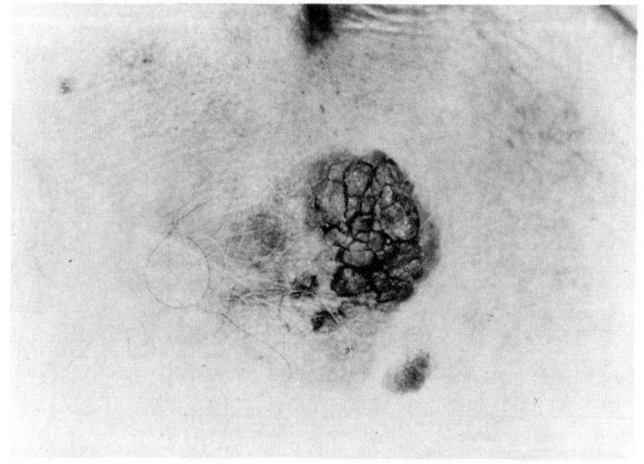

Figure 9-2 Keratosis. These horny plaque formations are commonly observed in the elderly. (See also endsheet plate 1.)

hair follicles. Body odor is the result of bacterial decomposition of apocrine secretions. The sebum-secreting cells of the sebaceous glands are contained in the dermal lining of hair follicles. Sebum, a fatty substance that acts as a protective agent for the skin, enters the distal end of the hair follicle via a connecting duct.

Subcutaneous Tissue

The subcutaneous tissue layer of the skin is the depot for fat storage. Some of the sweat glands and the roots of some hair follicles may extend down into this layer.

Characteristics and Techniques of Examination

Skin

The inspection of the integumentary system begins during the general survey. In fact, a skin disorder may be the most striking feature noted at this time. As each anatomical portion of the body is exposed for inspection during the physical assessment process, you should assess the skin first before proceeding to inspect the part for shape, size, and symmetry. In other words, the assessment process of each bodily area should begin on the outside surface with the skin and move inward, to the muscles, bones, and underlying organs. The integumentary system is often overlooked, thereby losing valuable information about the client's health status. If you consciously place priority on assessment of the integumentary components during each phase of the physical assessment procedure, helpful clues to the state of health of the client will not go unheeded. Inspection and palpation are the chief methods of assessing the integument.

Inspection

Color Lack of skin pigmentation occurs with albinism and vitiligo. The incidence of albinism tends to be high in equatorial areas. Roughly there is one for every 20,000 people in the United States. *Albinism* is an abnormal but nonpathologic depigmentation of the skin, eyes, and hair. Frequently albinos will also show signs of photophobia and nystagmus because the choroid lining of the eye is not adequately protected from light. Most albinos are considered legally blind and cannot get a driver's license. Some

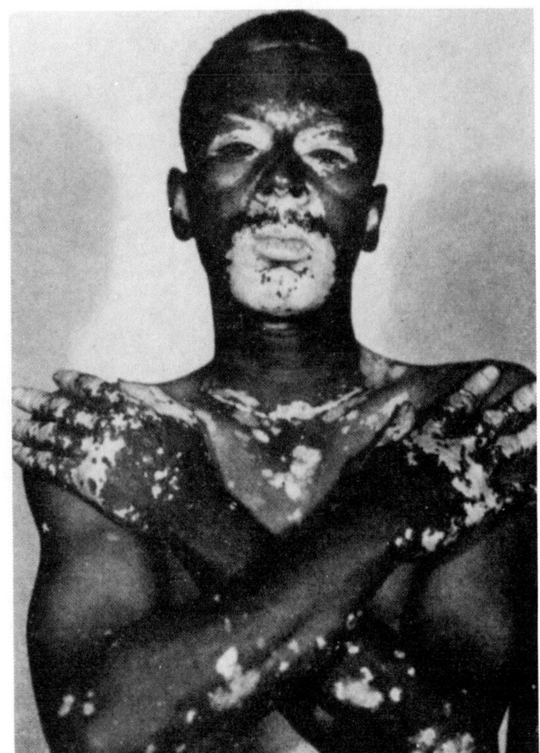

Figure 9-3 Vitiligo. Note symmetrical white patchy distribution.

believe that Noah of the Bible may have been an albino because of descriptions of his white hair and "fire in his eyes." *Vitiligo* is an acquired loss of pigmentation that presents itself as milky white patches of the skin, usually on exposed areas of the body (see Figure 9-3). It is an idiopathic affliction that is most common in tropical zones and among Blacks. Vitiligo of the scalp is accompanied by depigmentation of the hairs of the affected area.

Melanin, hemoglobin, and carotene are the basic pigments in the human body. Racial groups have varied degrees of melanin that account for the differences in skin color (see Table 9-2). The body responds to the irritation of physical agents by increasing pigment deposits. The protective mechanism of increased melanin and the subsequent browning of exposed skin areas is well known and readily apparent in individuals who have repeated and prolonged exposure to the sun or sun lamps, to the heat waves of a stove, boiler, or open-grate fire, to hot-water bottles or heating pads, and to x-ray therapy.

A diffuse or localized melanin hyperpigmentation may be observed during pregnancy. The

BIOLOGICAL AND CULTURAL VARIATIONS

Skin Cancer and Skin Color

Differences in body constitution among population groups are linked to varying rates of cancer mortality. One interesting association is that between skin cancer and skin color. Population groups with dark skins, such as Black Americans, have rather low rates of skin cancer, whereas population groups with lighter skin color have significantly elevated rates. It has been hypothesized that darker skin, with its greater pigmentation, offers protection against the sun's radiation. One study concluded that skin cancer is 45 times as common among Whites as among non-Whites in Hawaii (Allison & Wong 1968). The non-White group was composed of population groups with somewhat darker skin color, such as Koreans, Chinese, Japanese, Hawaiians, and Filipinos. Their darker skin color presumably offered some protection against the damaging effects of the ultraviolet rays of the sun.

face, nipples, areolae, and vulva are affected. A dark line extending from above the umbilicus to the pubic region may appear during the last trimester. This brown line, called the linea nigra, is of no concern; it will gradually fade away after parturition. A bronze tan may be present with Addison's disease (hypoadrenocorticism) and with some pituitary tumors. In these conditions the darker coloring involves the areolae, genitals, and perineum, as with the pregnant female, but it is also more prominent at the pressure and friction points of the body (elbows, buttocks, inner thighs, and axillae). The palmar creases are generally markedly darker and appear as dark brown streaks. It is also fairly common for the exposed areas of the body (face, neck, and arms) to have a darker hue and accompanying black freckles.

A generalized bronze hue is sometimes observed in hyperthyroidism and is characteristic of hemochromatosis, a rare disease that occurs ten times as frequently in males as females and that develops chiefly after the fourth decade of life. Hemochromatosis is accompanied by hepatomegaly, diabetes mellitus, and often cardiac failure.

Mongolian spots—blackish blue areas of the lower back and buttocks—are nonpathologic and are seen particularly in Black, American Indian, and Oriental newborns (Table 9-1). The spots disappear in early childhood.

Jaundice, a yellowing pigmentation, appears first in the posterior portion of the hard palate and the sclerae (when the serum bilirubin is only 2–4 mg per 100 ml). As the bilirubin level rises, jaundice can be observed in the mucous membranes and generally throughout the skin of the rest of the body. Its presence is best detected in natural nonglare daylight rather than in artificial light. A yellow pigmentation of the skin but not of the sclerae or the posterior portion of the hard palate would indicate carotene pigmentation, not jaundice.

One cause of jaundice is the hemolysis of red blood cells. Hemolysis happens in hemolytic disease and in diseases caused by certain pathologic organisms (certain streptococci and staphylococci, tetanus bacilli, and diphtheria bacilli). It can follow severe burns and the intravenous administration of a hypotonic saline solution or of distilled water. All intravenous solutions must be isotonic to the blood; otherwise, the red blood cells expand from the osmotic influx of fluid and eventually rupture, releasing hemoglobin. The liberated hemoglobin is removed from circulation primarily by the liver and the spleen. The iron content is stored, and the non-iron-containing pigment is converted into bilirubin.

Jaundice can also be caused by any condition that results in increased serum bilirubin, such as cirrhosis or biliary obstruction. Jaundice is also commonly observed in infectious mononucleosis; in this disease abnormal liver function tests are found in about 90% of the cases. A normal physiologic jaundice appears the third or fourth day of life in about half of all newborns. It may persist from a week to one month. Jaundice that develops within the first 24 hours after birth or after 2 weeks of age should be regarded with suspicion of pathology.

Appreciable decreases in hemoglobin cause paleness of the skin. Pallor is associated with

Table 9-1. Common Color-Change Abnormalities of the Skin

Terminology	Characteristics	Comments
Albinism	Depigmentation of skin, eyes, and hair	Nonpathologic; photophobia and nystagmus may accompany defective visual acuity. Assess body image concerns.
Vitiligo	Milky white patches usually on exposed areas	Idiopathic; more common in tropical zones and in Blacks. Assess body image concerns. May be familial and may occur in hyperthyroidism, pernicious anemia, diabetes mellitus. May be caused by trauma or autoimmunity.
Mongolian spots	Blackish blue areas of lower back and buttocks	Nonpathologic; disappears in early childhood. Predominantly in Black, American Indian, and Oriental newborns.
Jaundice	Yellow pigmentation of skin, mucous membranes, sclerae	Best observed in natural sunlight. Pathologic state.
Cyanosis	Bluish coloration: lips, earlobes, nailbeds, under tongue	Check for heart, lung abnormalities and type of medications client is taking. Pathologic state.
Carotenemia	Yellow pigmentation of skin—does *not* involve sclerae and mucous membranes; usually on palms, soles, and face	Check for increased carotinoids in diet, signs of diabetes mellitus, myxedema, hypopituitarism.
Erythema	Redness of skin	Assess for sources of irritation, inflammation, infection, heat, chilblain, increased vascularity, exposure to carbon monoxide gas.
Ecchymosis	Black-and-blue marks	Assess for trauma, other signs of bleeding disorder, hepatic dysfunction.
Malignant skin melanoma	Rough uneven surface, irregular notched edges, variegated coloring (red, white, blue, and black appearing lesions)	
Basal cell carcinoma	Generally on sun-exposed areas; central indentation of circumscribed lesion or central ulceration	Early detection enhances prognosis. Referral needed.
Squamous cell carcinoma	Firm lesion that eventually ulcerates	Leukoplakia may precede lesion. Early detection enhances prognosis. Referral needed.

such conditions as chronic disease, anemia, and shock. It is also present in anxiety, fear, and syncope as a result of the peripheral vasoconstriction that occurs with stress. Edema will mask the red hemoglobin tint of the skin. In dark-skinned individuals, pallor is best detected in the nailbeds, palpebral conjunctivae, oral mucosa, and tongue. Intermittent pallor or cyanosis of the extremities may suggest peripheral vascular problems and, particularly if only the fingers and toes are involved, perhaps Raynaud's disease. This condition is due to arteriolar spasm, which is aggravated by emotion or exposure to cold; it is more common in young females, rarely occurring in males.

Cyanosis, a bluish discoloration of the skin, is commonly seen with heart and lung disease and with congenital defects such as atrioseptal heart defects (right to left shunts) and methemoglobinemia. It is most readily detected around the lips, in the earlobes, in the nailbeds, and under the tongue. A similar bluish gray skin color oc-

Table 9-2. Racial or Ethnic Variations of the Integumentary System

Racial or ethnic group	Predominant skin color	Predominant hair color and texture
Black	Light brown to deep brown tones	Black; curly and wooly
Raza and Latino (Mexican or Chicano, Puerto Rican, Cuban, Spanish, Central and South American)	Tan, olive, to dark brown tones	Black or dark brown; wavy, curly or straight
Filipino	Brown tones	Black; coarse, straight or wavy
Chinese	Yellow tones	Black; coarse, straight or wavy
Japanese	Yellow tones	Black or brown-black; coarse, straight or wavy
Vietnamese	Brown tones	Black; coarse, straight or wavy
Eskimo and Aleut	Yellow tones	Black; straight
American Indian	Brown-red tones	Black; straight
Caucasian	Pale pink, tan, olive tones	Black, brown, red, or blond; straight to curly, coarse to very fine

Source: Compiled from *Ethnic nursing care: a multicultural approach*, by M. Orque, B. Bloch, and L. Monrroy (St. Louis: The C. V. Mosby Company, 1983), pp. 102, 139, 169, 197, 263, and 290.

curs from prolonged use of medications containing certain metal salts, such as silver, gold, and bismuth.

Carotenemia produces yellowing of the skin but does not involve the sclerae or mucous membranes. It may be present in myxedema, hypopituitarism, and diabetes mellitus, or it may occur with an excessive intake of food containing carotinoids (carrots, sweet potatoes, corn, squash). Occasionally, carotenemia may be observed during pregnancy. It is typically found on the palms, soles, and face.

Erythema, redness of the skin, can be caused by dilatation of the superficial capillaries as a result of irritation, inflammation, heat, chilblain, fever, or a sympathetic nervous reaction, such as is seen in embarrassment. Transient heat rashes occur in the diaper area of infants. A bright cherry red flush or patches on the face, neck, and chest, accompanied by deep, difficult respirations, are suggestive of carbon monoxide poisoning. Petechiae, ecchymoses, and a fine macular rash can be differentiated from erythema by stretching the skin gently with your thumb and index finger. The red hue of erythema will diminish in color, whereas the color of the others will be accentuated.

Ecchymosis, commonly known as black-and-blue marks, and *petechiae* are purpuric lesions of the skin. Ecchymosis accompanies bleeding disorders such as hemophilia, anemia, leukemia, and hepatic dysfunction and is observed in clients who are taking high doses of anticoagulants. Although ecchymosis is most commonly caused by physical trauma, it is also characteristic of meningococcic, streptococcic, and staphylococcic septicemias. The underlying mechanism is the extravasation of blood into the tissues. At first a deep purple-blue color appears; with time, the color begins to fade to a green-brown and then yellow as the blood is reabsorbed into the vascular system.

It is important to carefully assess and recognize signs of malignancy. Malignancies involving the skin are malignant skin melanoma, basal cell carcinoma, and squamous cell carcinoma. All warrant medical referral (see Table 9-1). Petechiae are tiny reddish purple hemorrhagic spots that occur as a result of capillary bleeding (see Figure 9-4). They are seen in thrombocytopenic purpura (inadequate or defective platelets), hepatic dysfunction, and conditions in which increased capillary permeability is present, such as leukemia and subacute bacterial endocarditis. These small hemorrhagic spots may indicate an increased tendency for bleeding or an embolus to the skin.

Common vascular lesions of the skin are listed and described in Table 9-3. *Spider angiomas* (see Figure 9-5) are arterial in origin. They appear as a fiery red center with radiating legs, most often surrounded by an area of erythema. They are generally found on the face, neck, shoulders, and upper chest. If a glass slide is

Table 9-3. Common Vascular Lesions

Terminology	Characteristics	Comments
Petechiae	Tiny reddish purple spots	Will not blanch. Assess for other signs of bleeding, hepatic dysfunction, subacute bacterial endocarditis.
Spider angioma	Bright red center with radiating legs generally on face, neck, shoulders, upper chest	Will blanch. Assess for liver dysfunction, vitamin B deficiency, and pregnancy.
Venous star	Bluish area most often on legs but may occur on anterior chest	Will not blanch. Assess for sources of increased pressure in superficial veins, e.g. distention, activity, and occupation.
Cherry angioma	Bright red round lesion, may turn brown with age; usually on torso and extremities; usually papular and surrounded by pale halo	Nonpathologic, increase in size and number as aging proceeds in the adult.
Telangiectasia	Dilation of capillaries and thinning of vascular walls. Frequently on face and thighs as erythemic to bluish lines	Check history of alcoholism, polycythemia, and family (Osler-Weber-Rendu disease is hereditary, can affect nose, skin, G.I. & G.U. tract; has hemorrhagic tendency). Will blanch with pressure. Check for signs of bleeding—e.g. Hqb, Hct, urinalysis.

placed over the spider angioma, a pulsation of the central body may be detected; however, a definite blanching will occur. Blanching can also be demonstrated by using the point of a pencil to apply pressure to the spider body. Blanching will not occur with petechiae. Spider angiomas are caused by an excess of 17-ketosteroids. Such an excess occurs with liver dysfunction because it is the liver that metabolizes the 17-ketosteroids. At times spider angiomas may be observed during pregnancy or with vitamin B deficiency. They may also occur in some normal people. A *venous star* (see Figure 9-6) is a bluish area that occasionally may be found on the anterior chest but is most often observed on the legs. It results from increased pressure in a superficial vein (varicose veins). Blanching does not take place with applied pressure. *Cherry angioma* is a nonpathologic lesion that increases in size and number as the individual grows older. It is a bright or ruby red color, may turn brown with age, and is found on the torso and extremities. It is usually papular (raised), is round, and may be surrounded by a pale halo. *Telangiectasia* (essential) is nonpathologic other than an effect it may have on body image. It presents as a small network of dilated superficial venous plexuses generally on the face or thighs. However, a rare

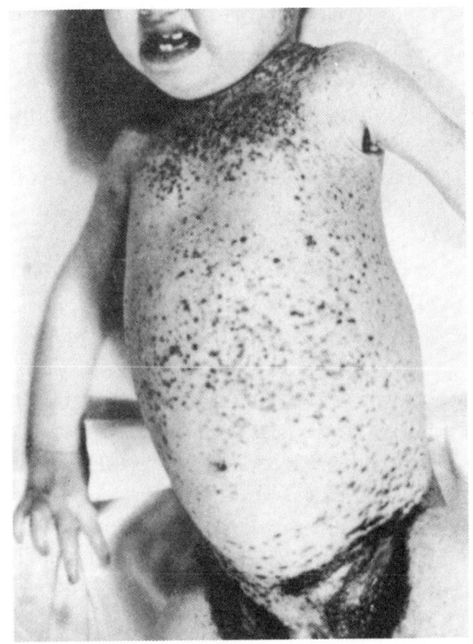

Figure 9-4 Petechiae. These small hemorrhagic spots are caused by capillary bleeding.

hereditary hemorrhagic form (Osler-Weber-Rendu), which becomes progressively severe with age, may cause anemia from continuous bleeding from nose, mouth, stomach, bowel,

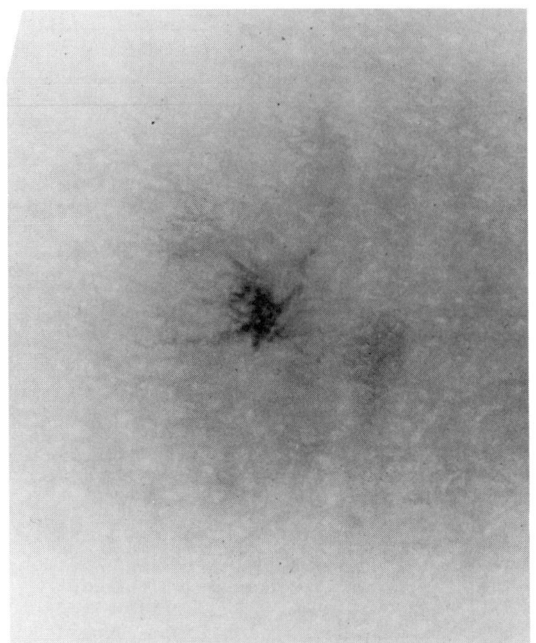

Figure 9-5 Spider angioma, a type of vascular lesion of the skin. (See also endsheet plate 2.)

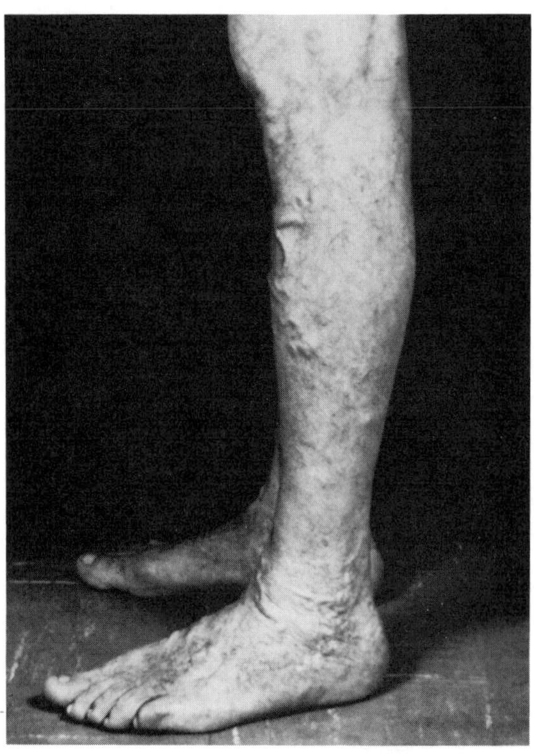

Figure 9-6 Varicose veins with venous star, a result of increased pressure in the vein. (See also endsheet plate 3.)

and urinary lesions. Bleeding can occur with trauma or spontaneously.

Pattern Lesions of the skin at times assume characteristic patterns that may aid in the diagnosis of particular skin diseases. Common patterns include generalized, annular, arciform, iris cluster, zosteriform, polycyclic, and linear (see Figure 9-7). Annular and/or arciform lesions are arranged in circles, arcs, or irregular combinations of the two. Annular and arciform lesions are characteristic of dermatologic reactions to some drugs. This format of lesions is also seen in urticaria and psoriasis. This pattern and/or an iris cluster is characteristic of erythema multiforme (see Figures 9-8 and 9-9). An iris grouping appears as a bull's-eye pattern. Often zosteriform groupings are observed in diseases such as metastatic breast carcinoma, but these lesions, which are arranged in broad bands, are most typical of herpes zoster (see Figures 9-10 and 9-11), and the band follows the line of nerve distribution. A linear or straight-line grouping is seen with lymphangitis and poison ivy lesions.

Location Specific lesions may occur on a particular portion of the body. For instance, acne is commonly present on the face, shoulders, and upper trunk (see Figures 9-12 and 9-13). The moist areas behind the ears, in the axillae, under pendulous breasts, in the umbilicus, in the groin, in the gluteal folds, and of the perianal region are common sites for cutaneous moniliasis (see Figures 9-14 and 9-15). The butterfly lesion characteristic of lupus erythematosus occurs chiefly on the forehead and cheeks (see Figure 9-16). Xanthomas, yellow plaques of lipoid de-

Technique of Inspection of the Skin

1. Adequate lighting and room temperature.
2. Adequate exposure of area being inspected.
3. Equipment: centimeter ruler or tape.
4. Alternate processes: (a) Inspect entire skin surface of body with client disrobed. Or (b) As you proceed with the examination of the various anatomical parts, first examine the skin of the particular area being assessed.
5. Characteristics: color, type, pattern, bodily area, size, abnormalities.

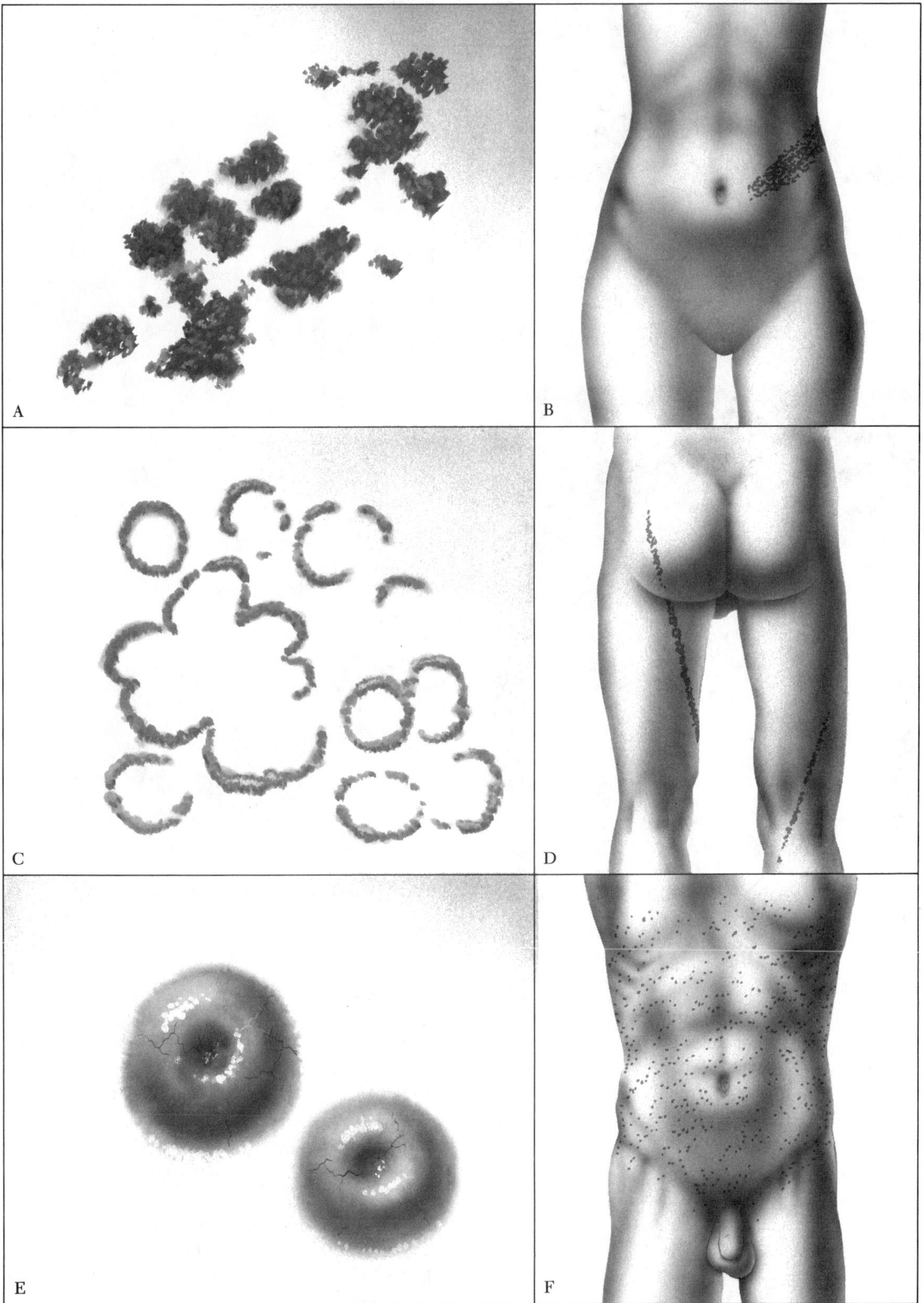

Figure 9-7 Configurations of skin lesions. (A) Grouped. (B) Zosteriform (follows a nerve route). (C) Annular and polycyclic (round). (D) Linear (in a line). (E) Iris cluster (central lesion with ring encircling it). (F) Generalized (diffuse over body or anatomical area).

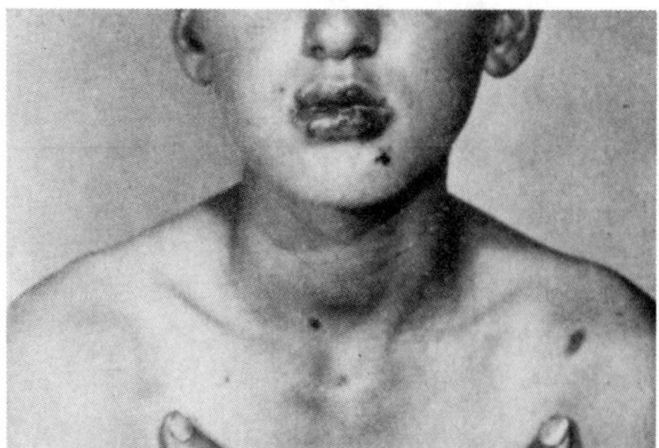

Figure 9-8 Papules of erythema multiforme on skin and lips.

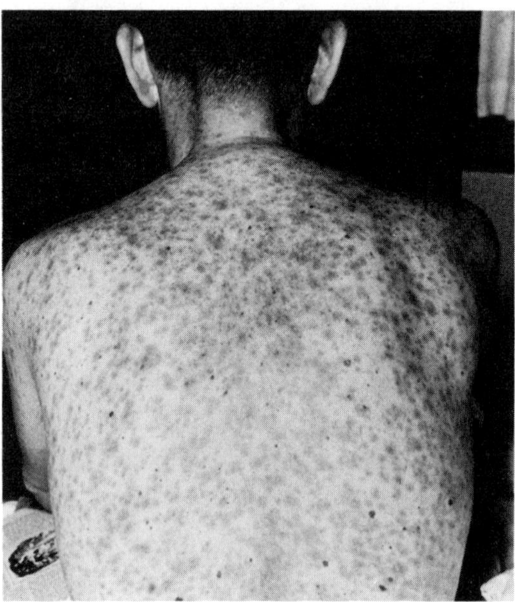

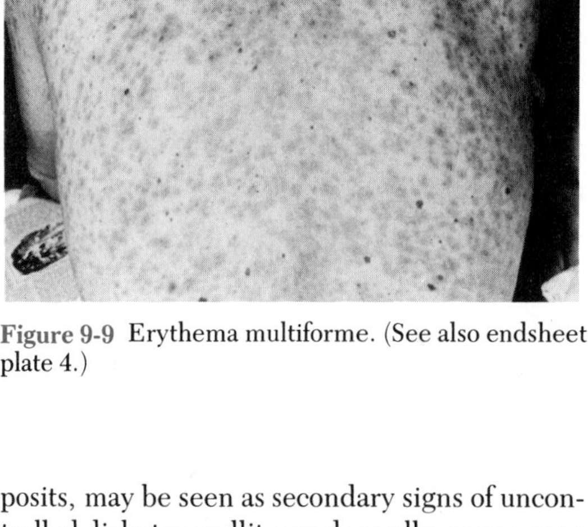

Figure 9-9 Erythema multiforme. (See also endsheet plate 4.)

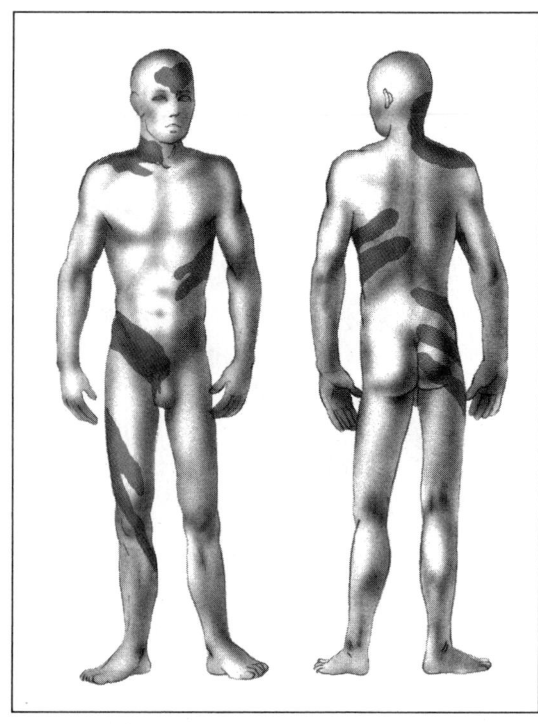

Figure 9-10 Body patterns of herpes zoster.

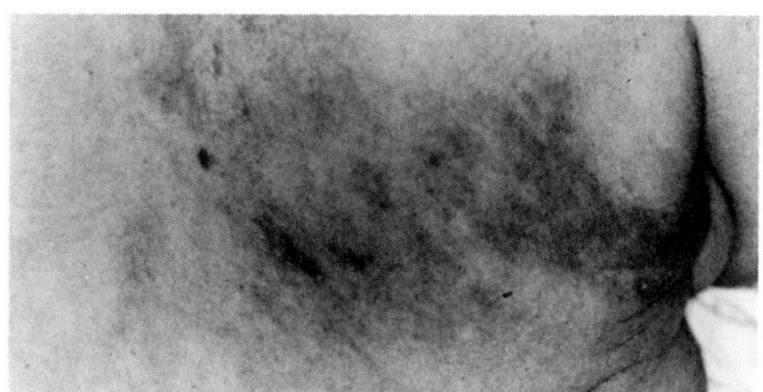

Figure 9-11 Herpes zoster. (See also endsheet plate 5.)

posits, may be seen as secondary signs of uncontrolled diabetes mellitus and usually appear over the hands, about the nasal bridge, and on the eyelids (see Figure 9-17). Intertrigo, a red scaly maceration of the skin in areas of opposing surfaces, is commonly seen on the neck, axillae, and groin of infants because of moisture and constant irritation. Such maceration may be observed in these body areas in obese persons.

When documenting observed lesions, the nurse must be able to use terminology to describe the type of lesion present as well as the pattern and the anatomical location. Characteristics of skin lesions to be documented are:

1. Color—pink, red, yellow, brown, green.
2. Type—macule, papule, wheal, scale, ulcer, scar, and so on.
3. Pattern—annular, linear, clustered, bull's-eye, and so on.
4. Bodily area—generalized, on exposed surfaces, on the extensor surfaces of the joints, in skinfold areas, and so on.
5. Size—if applicable, give width, length, and depth measurements of masses.
6. Mobility—if applicable, give fixed or movable feature of masses.
7. Consistency—if applicable, give stony hard, firm, or soft quality of masses.

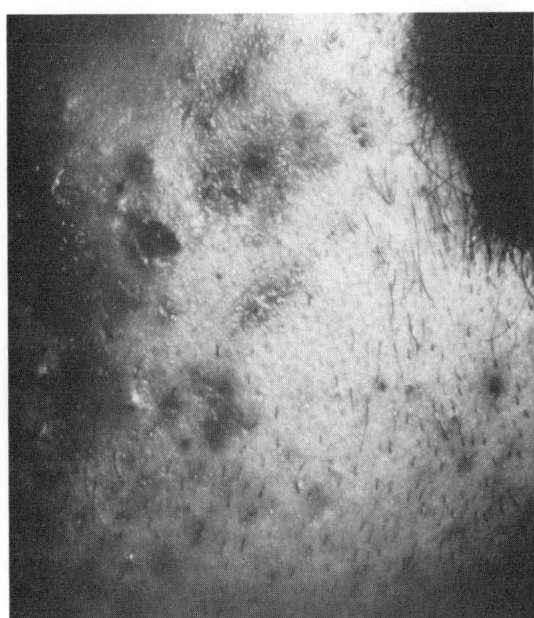

Figure 9-12 Severe acne vulgaris on the face. *Source:* Courtesy H. Gallego, M.D.

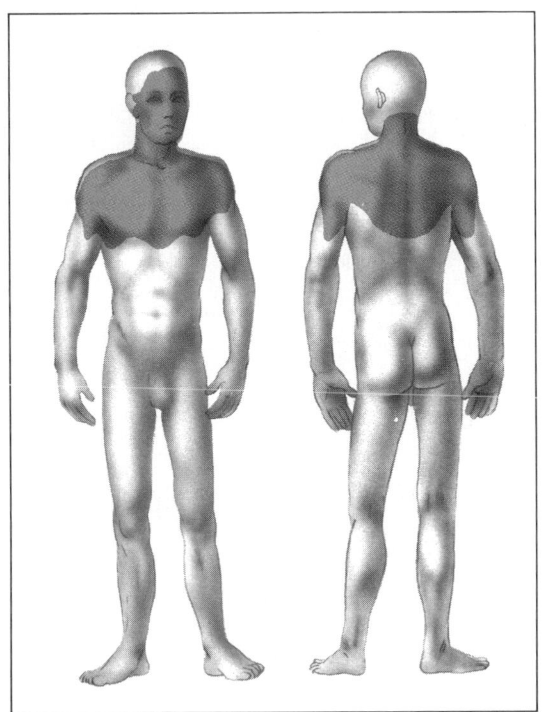

Figure 9-13 Common anatomical areas of acne.

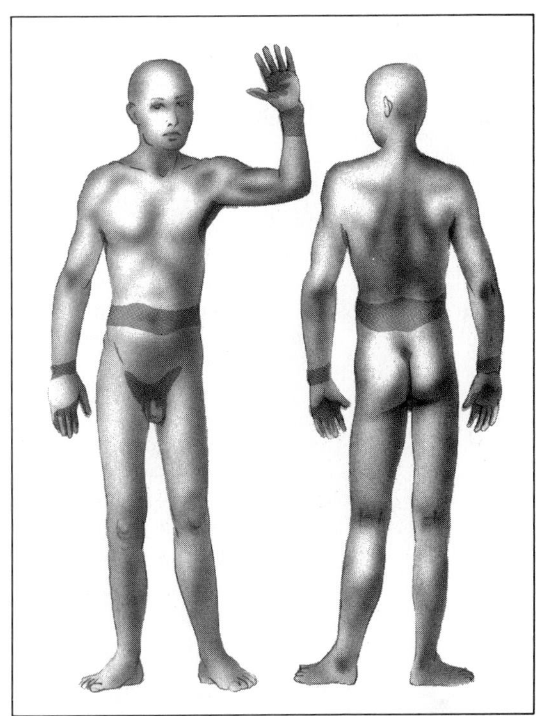

Figure 9-14 Common anatomical areas of scabies lesions.

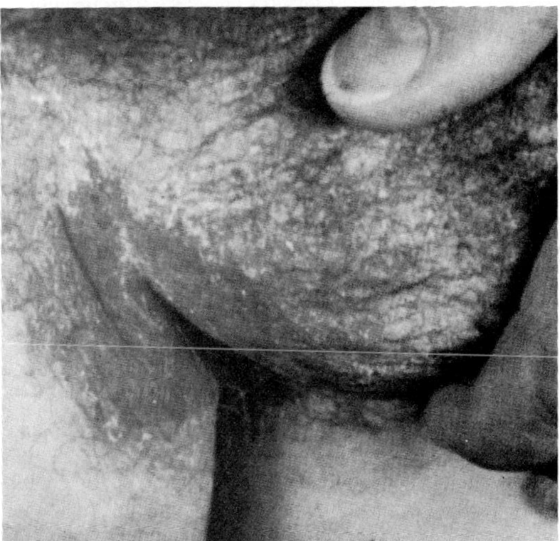

Figure 9-15 Monilial intertrigo, a type of lesion found in moist areas of the body.

Table 9-4 and Figure 9-18 show types of skin lesions divided into two groups: primary lesions and secondary lesions; the latter result from changes that occur because of underlying primary lesions.

Palpation

Temperature Generalized hyperthermia of the skin occurs with sunburn or conditions in which there is an increased metabolic rate, such as fever, hyperthyroidism, and strenuous exercise.

Table 9-4. Primary and Secondary Skin Lesions

Primary lesions		
Type	**Definition**	**Examples**
Macule	A flat, nonpalpable area of change in skin color less than 1 cm in diameter	Measles, scarlet fever, freckle, flat nevus, drug rash
Papule	A solid elevation of skin less than 1 cm in diameter, caused by thickening of the epidermis; definitely palpable	Wart, raised scaly area of psoriasis, pityriasis rosea
Vesicle	An elevation of the skin less than 1 cm in diameter, caused by clear fluid filling the upper layers of skin; palpable	Fever blister, chickenpox, smallpox, poison ivy, second degree burn, herpes simplex (see Figure 1-21), herpes zoster, eczematous dermatitis
Nodule	A solid mass less than 1 cm in diameter, extending deeper into dermis than a papule; moves with skin when palpated (some may extend into subcutaneous tissue; when palpated at this level skin will slide over nodule)	Area of poorly absorbed injection, dermatofibroma, subcutaneous nodule in rheumatic fever (especially with severe carditis and generally near occipital protuberances or over joints)
Plaque	Like a macule or papule but larger than 1 cm in diameter	Vitiligo, mongolian spot, plantar wart, xanthoma, psoriasis, pityriasis rosea, discoid lupus erythematosus
Bulla	Like a vesicle but larger than 1 cm in diameter, palpable	Pemphigus, some lesions in contact dermatitis, burn, sunburn, poison oak, poison ivy, bullous impetigo; on palms and soles with scarlet fever or congenital syphilis
Tumor	Like a nodule but larger than 1 cm in diameter; may be firm or soft	Lipoma, fibroma, carcinoma
Pustule	Like a vesicle or bulla but pus-filled	Acne, impetigo (see Figures 9-20 and 9-21), furuncles (arising from hair follicles), carbuncles (arising from sebaceous glands)
Wheal	A circumscribed elevation of the skin caused by escape of serum into the dermis (the larger the amount of the edema, the paler the wheal on a red to pale color continuum)	Urticaria, insect bite, poison sumac, poison ivy

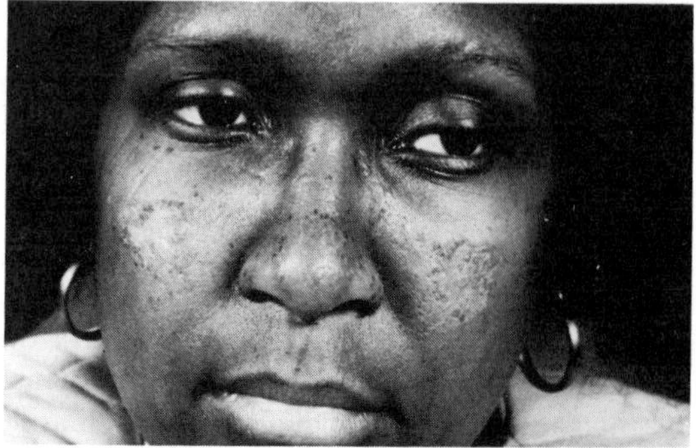

Figure 9-16 Butterfly lesion. (See also endsheet plate 6.)

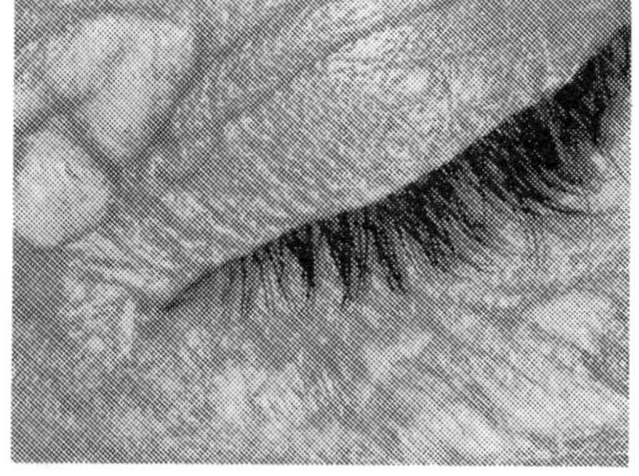

Figure 9-17 Xanthelasma consists of one or more bright yellow, sharply marginated plaques with no epidermal change, usually occurring on the eyelids. All patients with xanthelasma should be investigated for evidence of plasma lipid abnormalities.

Table 9-4. *Continued*

Primary lesions		
Type	**Definition**	**Examples**
Cyst	An encapsulated, fluid-filled area in the dermis or subcutaneous tissue (generally nontender and may transilluminate light)	Sebaceous cyst, epidermoid cyst

Secondary lesions		
Type	**Definition**	**Examples**
Scale	A flake of desquamated dead epithelium	Psoriasis, seborrheic dermatitis, pityriasis rosea, exfoliative dermatitis
Excoriation/ erosion	An absence of superficial epidermis	Superficial scratch, syphilitic chancre
Crust	A dried serum or blood exudate as found on the surface of an abrasion or excoriation or on the site of ruptured blisters	Fever blister, impetigo
Fissure	A crack in the epidermis	Chapping, cracking of lips as seen in severe dehydration or fever
Ulcer	A necrotic loss of epidermis	An open sore seen sometimes on the leg with sickle-cell anemia or on the leg and pressure areas with vascular insufficiency
Scar (cicatrix)	A connective tissue replacing skin damaged to depth of dermis during healing process	Healing site of trauma, wound, or surgery
Keloid	An overproduction of scar tissue that has a red, raised, smooth appearance, contains blood vessels, is sometimes irritable; has high incidence of occurrence in Blacks	Keloid

Localized areas of skin hyperthermia are found at sites of inflammation, such as phlebitis, furuncle, or a localized burn. A localized, hot, painful, indurated area is characteristic of cellulitis. Generalized hypothermia is observed in shock, where there is a general decrease of peripheral blood flow. Localized areas of coolness suggest peripheral vascular disease. Normal skin has a generalized warmth to the touch.

Texture Normal skin is smooth to the touch. Touching the skin surface of an individual with severe hyperthyroidism is like rubbing your hand over a piece of velvet. The skin in hypothyroidism, on the other hand, is quite rough to the touch. A roughness of the skin is also characteristic of hyperkeratosis, of skin reactions to such materials as soap, bubble bath, or wool, and of the irritating and drying effects of cold, wintry winds. The characteristics of roughness and dryness generally seem to go together.

Increased perspiration occurs with a high metabolic rate; thus diaphoresis can be seen in clients with pyrexia or thyrotoxicosis. Increased perspiration also results from stimulation of the nervous system, as in pain and anxiety. Oiliness, particularly of the scalp and face, is common during adolescence. If a preadolescent or adult female demonstrates hyperfunction of the sebaceous glands, with or without the presence of acne, a virilizing hormonal imbalance should be suspected. Seborrhea, common in early childhood, is also caused by hyperfunction of the sebaceous glands (see Figure 9-22).

Testing for skin turgor will reveal the moisture content and mobility of the tissues. Pinch the skin over the inner forearm or over the sternum and note how rapidly it returns to place. Normal skin returns almost immediately. In dehydration it may remain folded for 30 seconds or longer. Poor skin turgor is present with cachexia and also commonly found in elderly clients.

Decreased tissue mobility is noted with edema and in conditions such as scleroderma. Edema can sometimes be detected by inspection, but to determine whether it is pitting

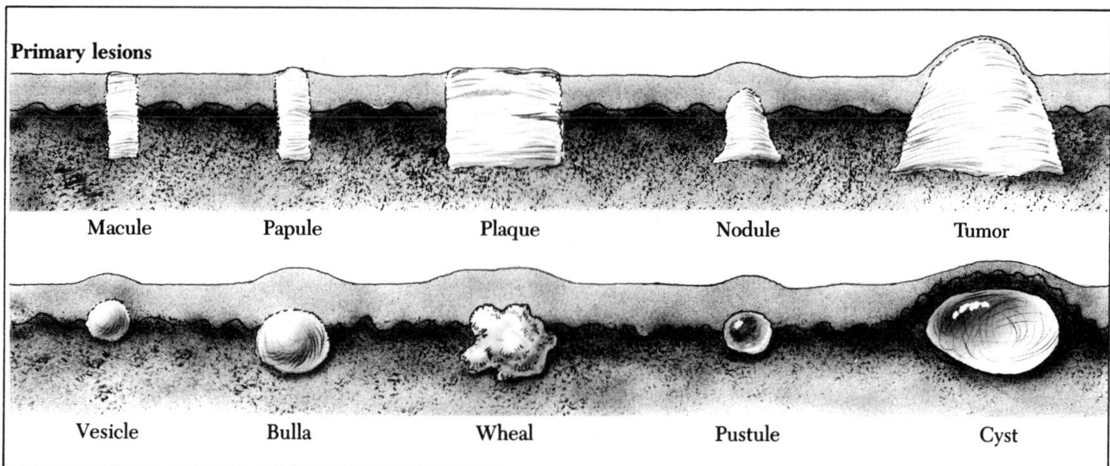

Figure 9-18(A) Primary lesions.

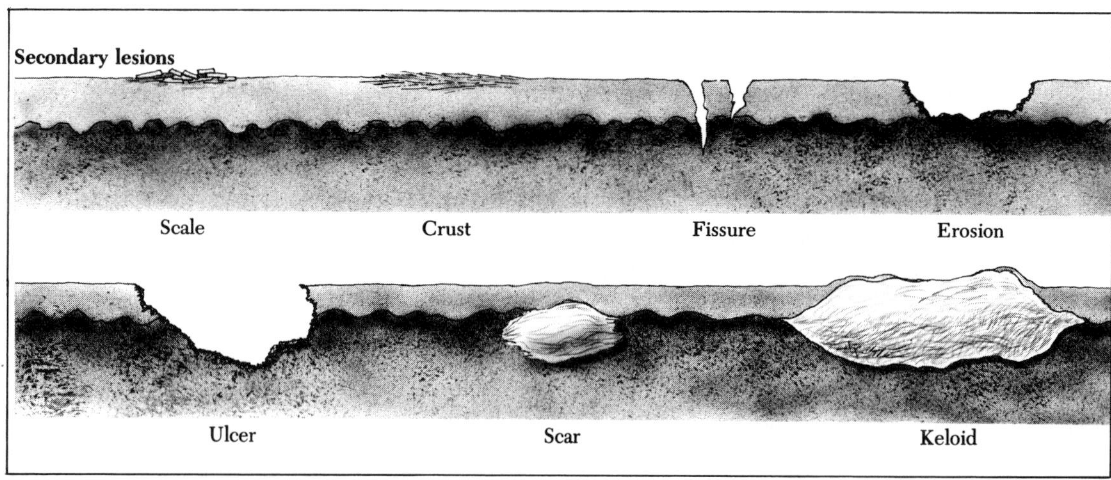

Figure 9-18(B) Secondary lesions.

edema requires palpation. The tissue is firmly pressed for 5–10 seconds; if it does not return rapidly to the normal contour, pitting edema is present (see Figure 9-23). Pitting edema usually occurs first in dependent parts of the body. Thus, if there are no visible signs of edema, the sacrum and tibial aspects of the legs as well as the ankles should be carefully palpated to check for pitting. Two classifications sometimes used for pitting edema are as follows:

Time classification

- 0 No pitting
- 1+ Trace
- 2+ Moderate, disappears in 10–15 seconds
- 3+ Deep, disappears in 1–2 minutes
- 4+ Very deep, disappears in 5 minutes

Extent classification

- 1+ Shallow pit formed by thumb pressure
- 2+ Deep pit formed by thumb pressure
- 3+ Signs of pitting in a dependent part of the body (e.g., limb is 1½ times the normal size)
- 4+ Generalized deep-pitted edema accompanied by ascites (as in severe congestive heart failure)

Edema formation can result from increased hydrostatic pressure within the vascular system (as in hypertension), increased venous pressure (as in congestive heart failure or in obstruction of venous or lymphatic return by tumors or inflammation), increased capillary permeability (as with burns, allergies, insect bites, electrolyte re-

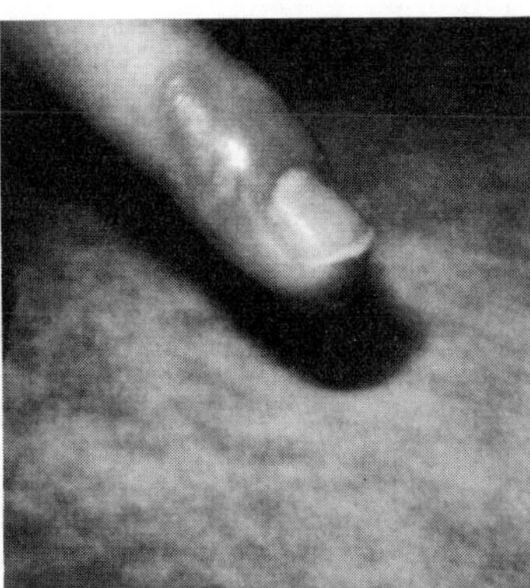

Figure 9-19 Herapetic whitlow, an HSV infection of the fingers, is a recognized hazard among ICU nurses, surgeons, anesthesiologists, and dentists. From Auvenshine/Enriquez: *Comprehensive Maternity Nursing, Second Edition*, © 1990 Boston: Jones and Bartlett Publishers.

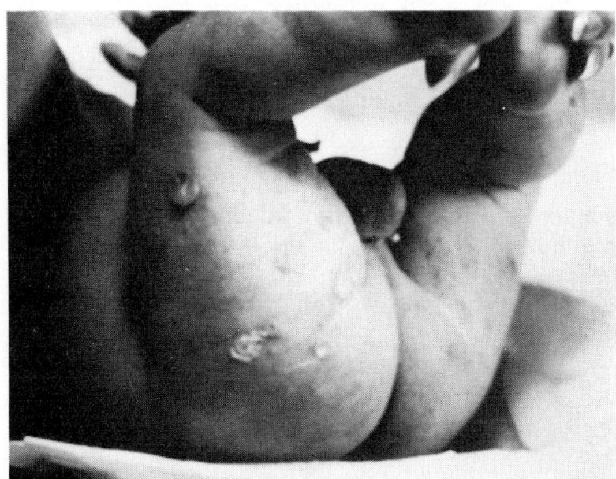

Figure 9-20 Impetigo contagiosa: bullous form. *Source:* Courtesy B. Hoggarth, M.D.

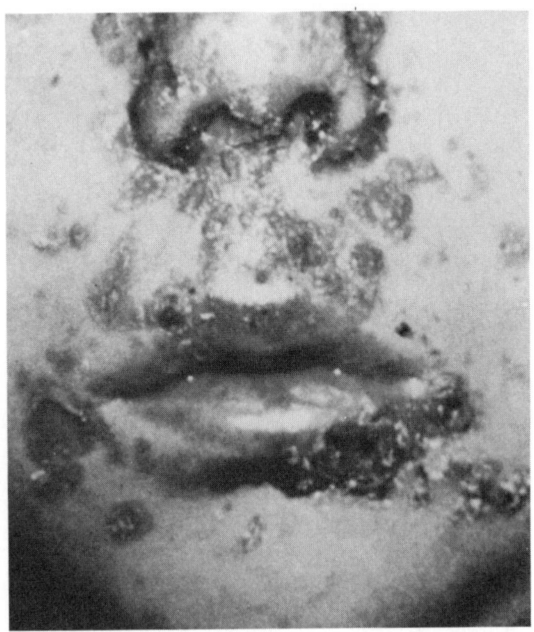

Figure 9-21 Impetigo contagiosa: vesiculopustular form. *Source:* Courtesy B. Hoggarth, M.D.

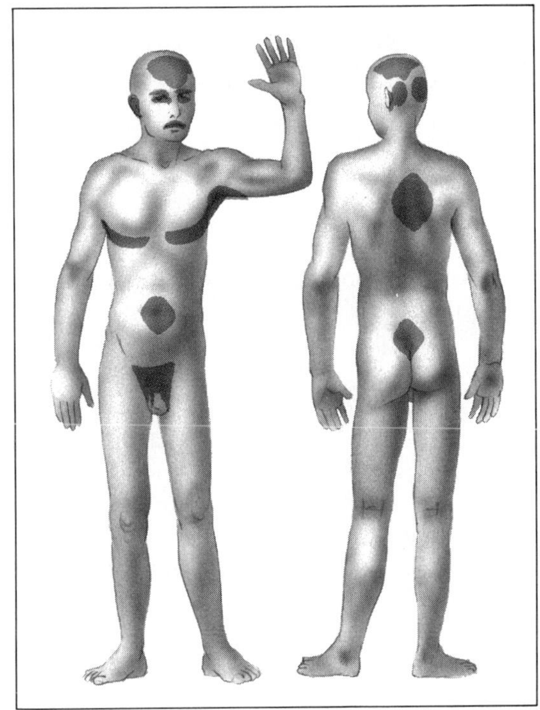

Figure 9-22 Common anatomical locations of seborrheic dermatitis.

tention, hyperaldosteronism, cortisone therapy, and renal shutdown, or just prior to or during the menses), and a decrease in osmotic pressure within the vascular system due to a decrease in serum protein (as in kidney disease or in the hypoproteinemia of starvation or liver disease).

Any skin lesions should be carefully described using the terminology presented earlier in this chapter. Any recently appearing lesion should be regarded with suspicion. In particular, the physical signs of nodule, telangiectasia, and ulceration of sun-exposed areas should be carefully checked by consultation with a physician. Any recent change in the size or color of a wart or mole should also warrant consultation. Any nodular black-gray lesion with irregular margin, and rough, uneven surface, or any lesion that is constantly being irritated or that bleeds needs further evaluation by a physician. Such a lesion could possibly be a basal, or squamous cell carcinoma (see Figures 9-24 to 9-26) or a malignant

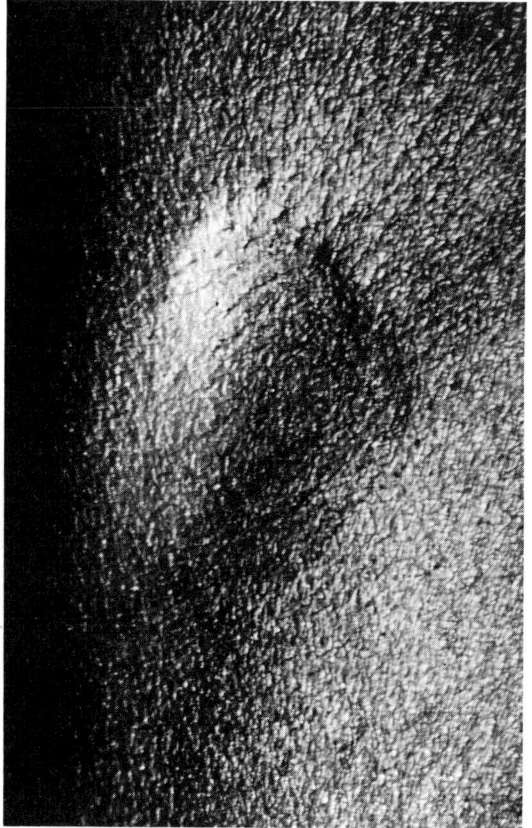

Figure 9-23 Indentation of pitting edema.

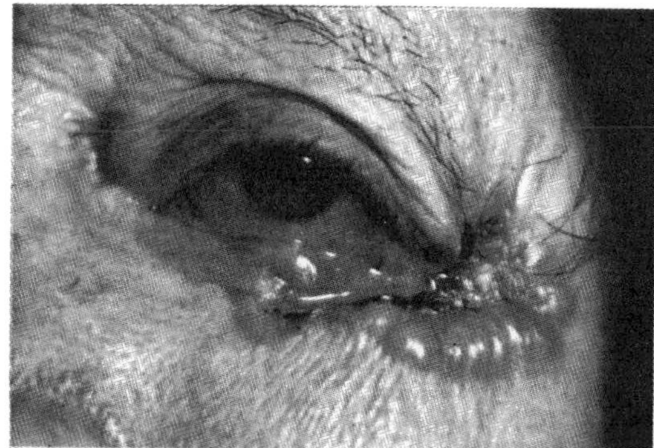

Figure 9-24 Basal cell carcinoma.

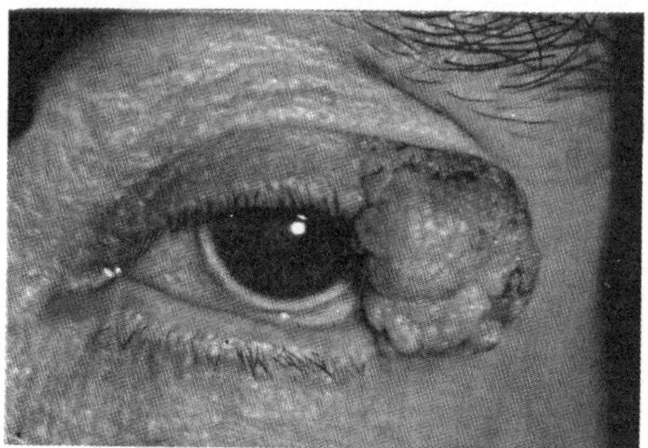

Figure 9-25 Early cancer of lid margin. Also note arcus senilis.

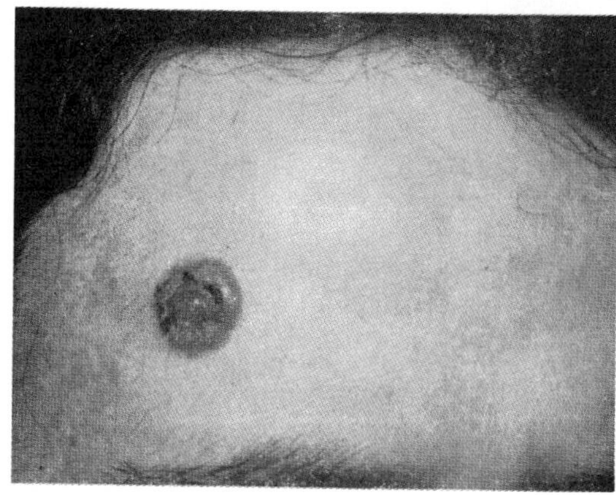

Figure 9-26 Basal cell carcinoma on forehead.

Technique of Palpation of the Skin

1. Use most sensitive area of hand for the particular characteristics
2. Characteristics: temperature (dorsum of hand), texture (fingertips), skin turgor, abnormalities.

melanoma (see Figure 9-27). The assessment and nursing management of insect infestations and viral, bacterial, and fungal skin alterations are in Appendix E.

Hair

Inspection and Palpation

Color and Texture Hair color varies widely, from pale blond to dark black, and it may be changed readily with dyes and rinses. You should inquire about the client's use of such agents, as allergies to them often cause rashes and itching on the scalp, face, ears, and neck. Graying of the hair is a common sign of aging, but it may occur prematurely as a hereditary condition or at birth in albinos. Scalp hair may be fine or coarse. Dry, brittle hair may be seen in hypothyroidism, but it is most frequently caused by overuse of hair dyes and of curling or straightening preparations. In hyperthyroidism the hair has a very fine texture. Hyperfunction of the sebaceous glands causes hair to be oily, particularly close to the scalp. This oiliness is common in both males and females during ado-

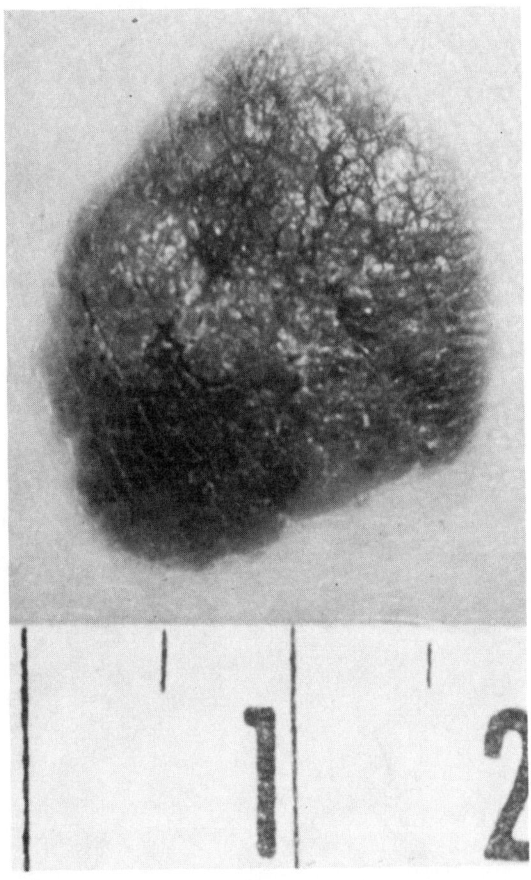

Figure 9-27 Melanoma. (See also endsheet plate 10.)

lescence. Body hair is usually very fine, although hair in the pubic and axillary areas is coarse.

Distribution The newborn baby is covered with lanugo, a downy hair over the entire body. Within a few weeks' time the majority of this hair is lost. Body hair growth begins to develop at puberty in both sexes, but growth patterns differ in males and females. Males normally have more facial and body hair. Both sexes develop axillary and genital hair growth at puberty, but the pubic hair distribution differs. The male pattern resembles a diamond, with the top of the diamond extending to the umbilicus. Female pubic hair is like an inverted triangle, having a straight horizontal plane approximating the level of the pubes. A client with hair distribution more like that of the opposite sex may have endocrine problems. Hirsutism in women and children caused by androgens will assume the distribution pattern of the normal adult male. This condition is observed in clients with masculinizing ovarian tumors, adrenocortical tumors, and Stein-Leventhal syndrome (see Figure 9-28). In hypopituitarism there is a general decrease in or absence of body hair. A total absence of body hair, alopecia totalis, is rare, and the loss of hair may or may not be permanent (see Figure 9-29). Alopecia totalis may result from serious illness, high fever, starvation, or a nervous disease. (See Table 9-5.)

Technique of Inspection and Palpation of the Hair

1. Adequate lighting and exposure.
2. Alternate processes: (a) Inspect and palpate hair of each particular anatomical part of the body as the physical assessment proceeds. Or (b) Inspect and palpate hair of the entire body of the client.
3. Characteristics: color, texture, distribution, abnormalities.

Table 9-5. Other Common Abnormalities of the Integument

Terminology	Characteristics	Comments
Edema	Tissue fluid accumulation, localized or generalized	Check degree of edema and presence of pitting edema.
Diaphoresis	Increased perspiration	Assess for pain, anxiety, fever, high metabolic rate.
Rough, dry skin	Localized or generalized	Assess for exposure to soap, bubble bath, wool, cold, wind, loss of body fluids.
Hirsutism	Increased body hair	Assess for adrenocortical dysfunction, changes in mustache or beard growth and pubic hair pattern.
Alopecia	Decreased or absent body hair	Assess for anxiety, debilitating illness, high fever, starvation, and hypopituitarism.

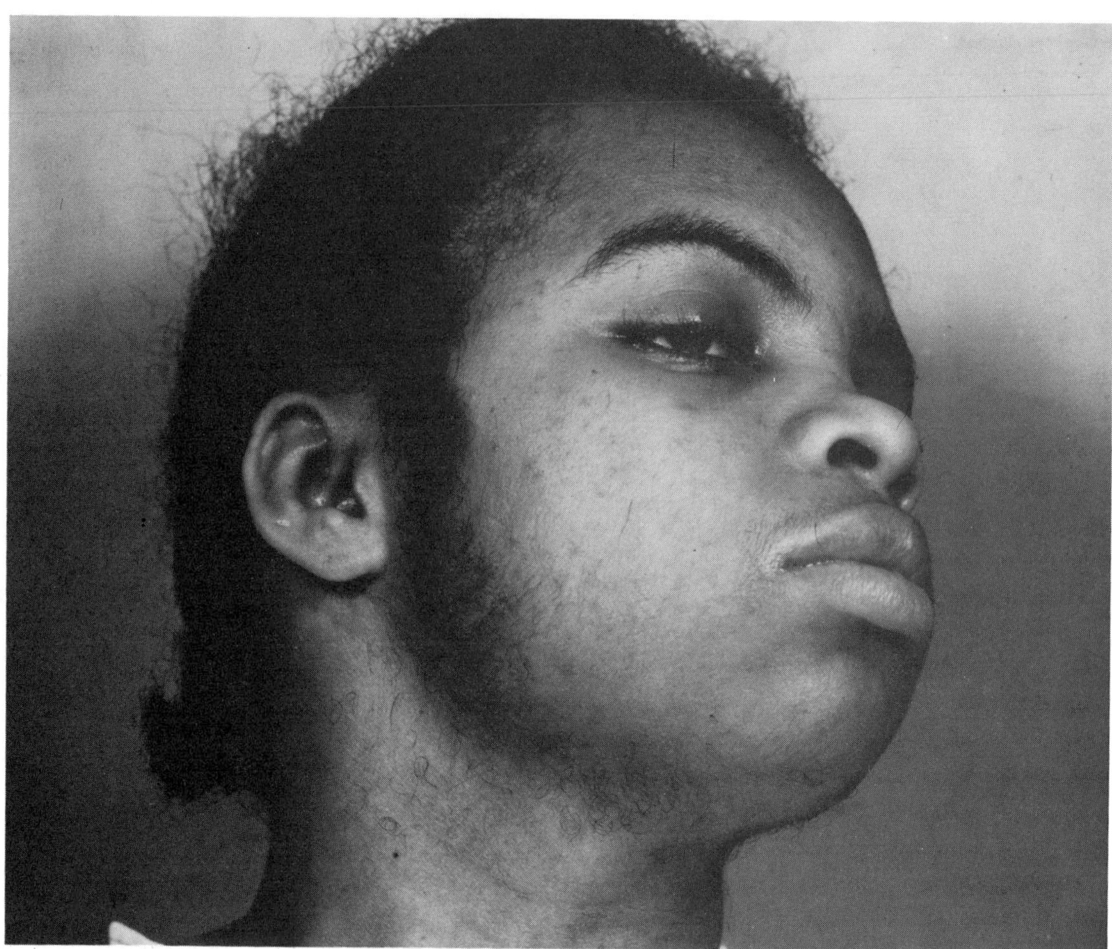

Figure 9-28 Hirsutism in young female. Note beginning mustache and beard growth.

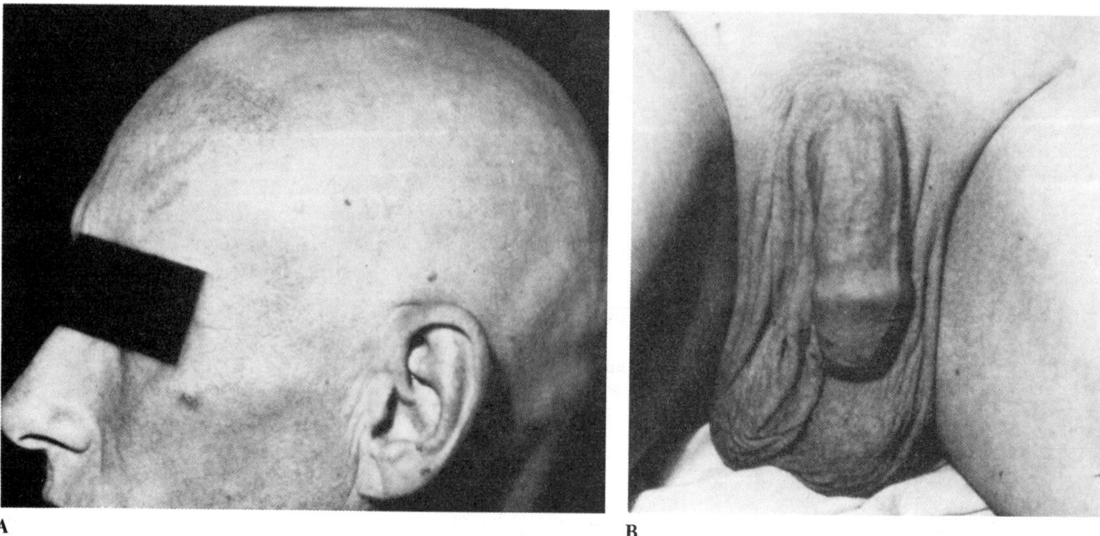

A B

Figure 9-29 Alopecia totalis of (A) the head and (B) the genitals. This rare condition may be permanent in some instances.

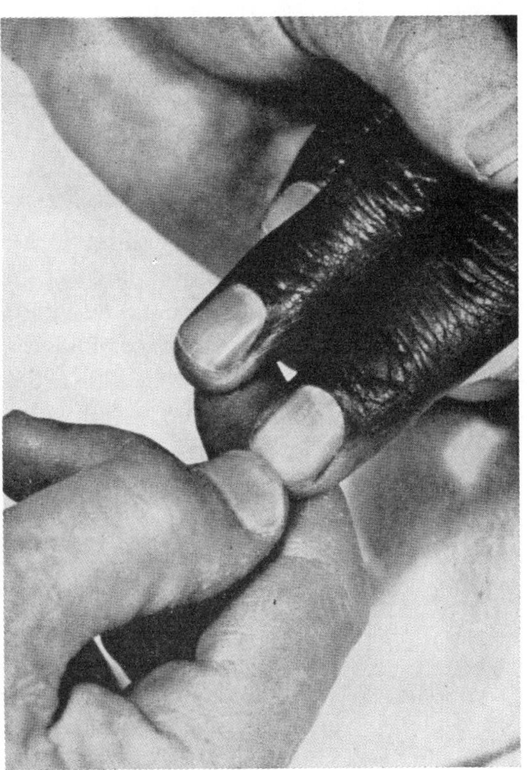

Figure 9-30 Technique for assessing capillary refill.

Nails

Inspection and Palpation

Because the nail plate is translucent, it affords a window to the underlying capillary bed, and the status of circulation to the extremities can be determined. With pressure blanching of the capillary bed beneath the client's fingernail or toenail should occur (see Figure 9-30). Upon release of the pressure, the color should immediately return. The nails are one of the first places of the body where cyanosis is detected.

Figure 9-31 shows Beau's line, a transverse white line or indentation that appears during an acute illness. Beau's line may reflect an earlier systemic disease or may be evidence of local

> **Technique of Inspection and Palpation of the Nails**
>
> 1. Adequate lighting.
> 2. Characteristics: color, texture, nail/nailbed angle, capillary refill, thickness, abnormalities.

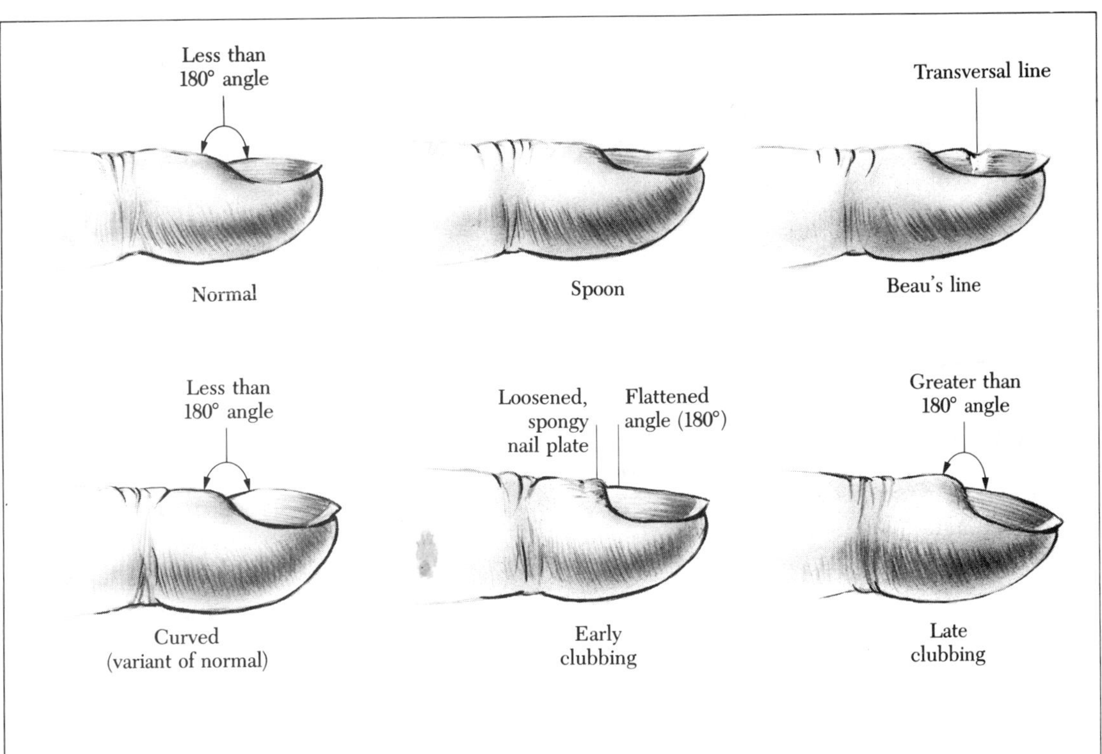

Figure 9-31 Normal and abnormal nails.

trauma. As the nail grows, the line moves toward the distal end of the finger and is eventually trimmed off.

Spoon nails, characterized by a concave profile, may be observed in prolonged iron-deficiency anemia. The normal nail, in contrast, has a relatively straight profile with an angle of less than 180° between nail and nailbed. Curved nails, a variant of the normal, can be differentiated from clubbed nails in that even though they manifest a convex curve and look quite similar to clubbing, the angle between the nail and nailbed is still less than 180°.

In early clubbing the angle between nail and nailbed straightens out to 180°. In late clubbing, the angle increases to greater than 180°. Clubbing of the nails usually occurs first in the thumbs and index fingers and later involves the remaining fingers and the toes. Once the cause is eliminated, the clubbing is reversed. There are several conditions in which clubbing occurs. The most common condition is pulmonary disease, such as emphysema, chronic obstructive lung disease, bronchiectasis, and pulmonary tumor. The second most common condition in which clubbing is observed is cardiovascular disease, including subacute bacterial endocarditis and congenital heart disease with cyanosis. Clubbing may also be present with thyrotoxicosis, cirrhosis, and chronic obstructive jaundice. Clubbing may also be an inherited trait.

Pitting of the nails commonly accompanies psoriasis and fungal diseases of the nails. A ridging hypertrophy of the nails can result from dermatologic conditions, ischemia, direct trauma, and bacterial and fungal infections. Brittle, frayed, or terraced nails are occasionally observed in thyrotoxicosis, malnutrition, iron deficiency, and calcium deficiency, and with x-ray irradiation.

Nails normally grow about 0.1 mm per day. The nails grow more slowly and become thick and yellow when lymphatic circulation is impeded. Splinter hemorrhages, reflected as red or brown streaks, may be nonspecific, although they are commonly observed in subacute bacterial endocarditis and trichinosis.

Summary

The integument is considered to be the body's most important organ. In this chapter the structure and function were presented. The three basic layers were described, with emphasis on appearance and function.

The entire assessment process begins on the outside surface with the skin. Because each area to be assessed has different characteristics, similar and dissimilar methods for examining the skin, hair, and nails were demonstrated.

Discussion Questions/Activities

1. State the aspects of the skin that are assessed and their importance to the assessment of a client's status.
2. Describe the technique used to test skin turgor and the normal finding.
3. Diagram the following patterns of skin lesions: annular grouping; iris cluster/bull's-eye pattern; zosteriform pattern; linear.
4. State the areas of the body where the following skin lesions commonly occur: acne, cutaneous moniliasis; butterfly lesion; xanthomas; intertrigo.
5. Define the following types of skin lesions:
   a. Primary lesions—macule, papule, vesicle, nodule, plaque, bulla, tumor, pustule, wheal, cyst.
   Secondary lesions—scale, excoriation/erosion, crust, fissure, ulcer, scar (cicatrix), keloid.
6. Describe a skin lesion using the criteria presented in the chapter.
7. Perform the techniques used for assessing skin turgor and capillary refill.

Recording of Findings

Normal findings are presented in the first box. The second box contains a recording of abnormal signs and symptoms manifested by a client prior to undergoing an I & D (incision and drainage) of an abscess.

Skin

INSPECTION
Color pink and heavily freckled; clear without excoriations, fissures, scars, or lesions; extremities pink without edema.

PALPATION
Good skin turgor; warm and smooth to touch.

Hair

INSPECTION
Normal distribution, full, and glossy, light brown hair.

PALPATION
Normal texture—soft, flexible.

Nails

INSPECTION
No deformities; no clubbing; no cyanosis.

PALPATION
Good capillary refill.

Skin

INSPECTION
A localized 2 × 3 cm erythematous area left midaxillary region.

PALPATION
Above described left midaxillary region indurated; hot to touch; extremely tender; onset within a 24 hour period.

Hair

INSPECTION
Sparse, gray hair.

PALPATION
Brittle.

Nails

INSPECTION
Bites nails; no clubbing; no cyanosis.

PALPATION
Good capillary refill.

CHAPTER 10

Assessment of the Head and Neck

LEARNING OBJECTIVES

1. Identify the characteristics of the head, face, and neck that are assessed in inspection, palpation, and auscultation.
2. Differentiate between hereditary alopecia and alopecia areata.
3. Describe the procedure for palpating the lymph nodes of the neck.
4. Point out the locations of the lymph nodes of the neck.
5. Describe approaches for palpation of the thyroid gland.
6. Describe the dangers that are inherent in improper palpation of the carotid arteries.

Assessment of the head and neck begins with inspection of gross appearance—that is, size and contour. Palpation is performed simultaneously with a more detailed inspection of specific parts of the head and neck. During the examination of these anatomical areas, you will be evaluating portions of several body systems, including the skin, hair, lymph, endocrine, and cardiovascular systems.

Structure of the Head

The size and shape of the cranium may not be the same in all clients, but identical structures should exist. The regions of the head are identified by the underlying bone structures, as shown in Figure 10-1.

Characteristics and Techniques of Examination

The head is examined by inspection and palpation. Most often inspection and palpation are used simultaneously when assessing the head. Percussion and auscultation are used only infrequently.

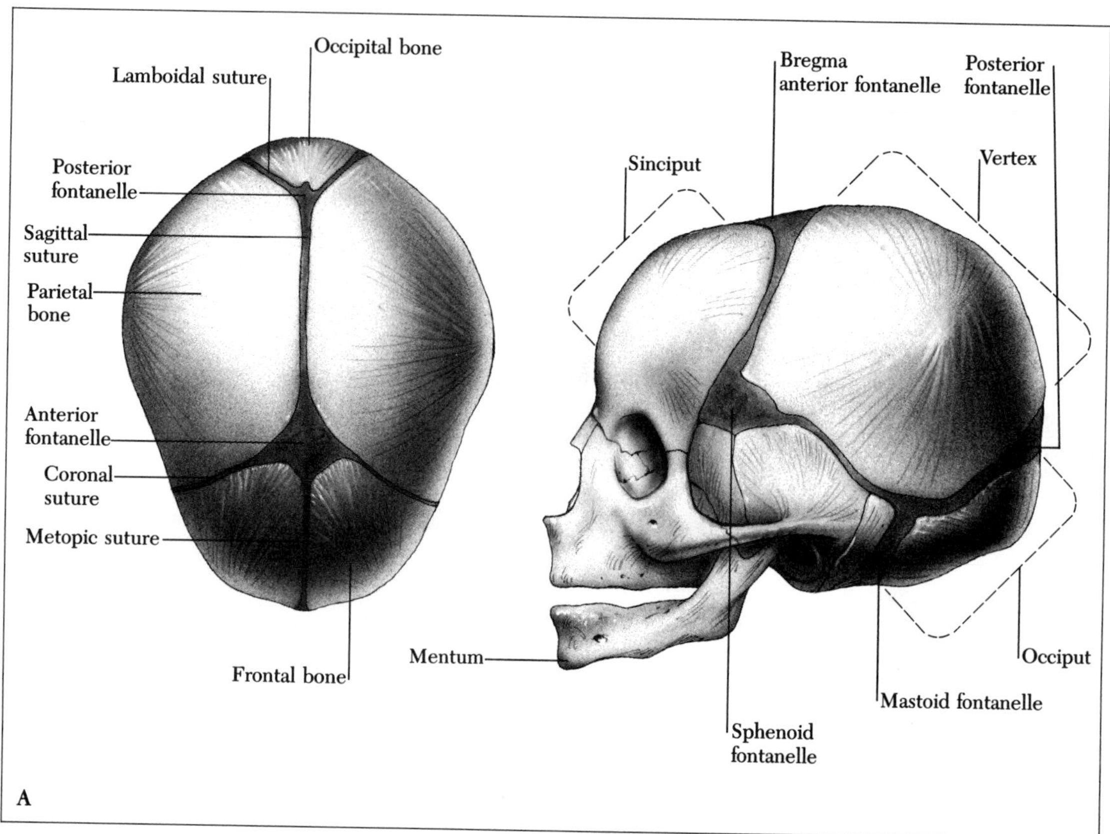

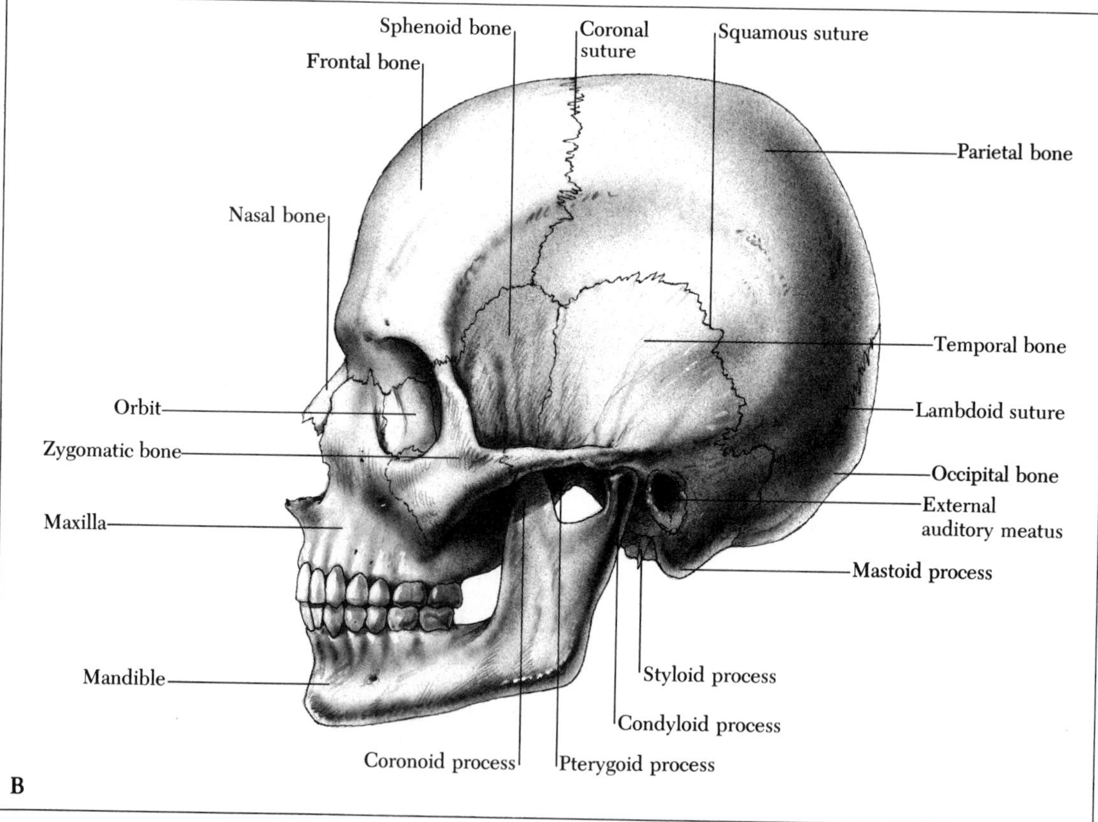

Figure 10-1 (A) Top and side view of an infant head. (B) Regions of an adult head.

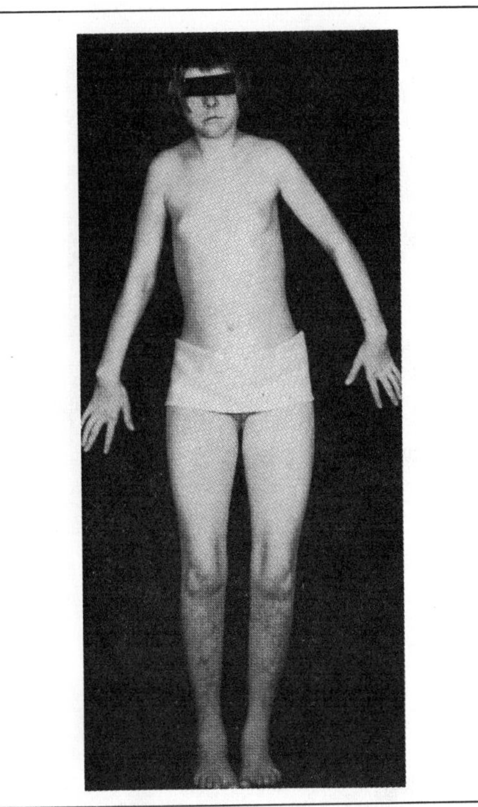

Figure 10-2 A 19-year-old female with microcephalus and mental retardation.

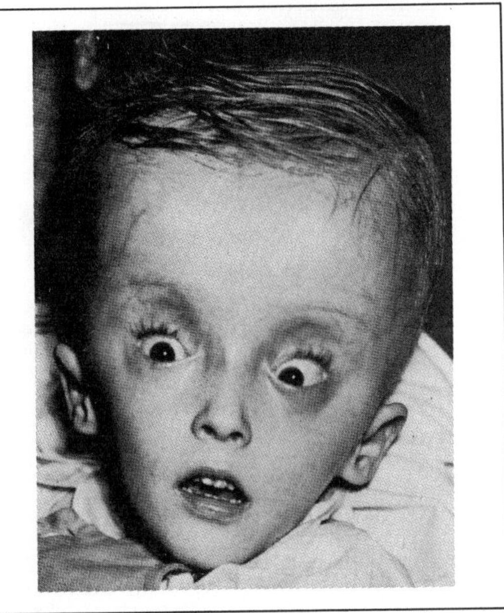

Figure 10-3 Hydrocephalus of severe grade preventing ossification of skull.

Inspection and Palpation of the Head

In a general inspection, note the size and symmetry of the head. The normal skull is usually round, with prominences at the frontal bone and the parietal bone. The *sagittal suture*, which runs from the anterior to the posterior portion of the cranium, is often palpable. There is a definite protuberance of the *occipital bone*, and the prominent *mastoid bones* can be noted behind each ear. Abnormalities in the size and shape of the cranium can be seen in conditions such as microcephalus and hydrocephalus (see Figures 10-2 and 10-3). An early sign of hydrocephalus is dilated scalp veins.

In infants under age 2, head circumference is measured at the level of the eyebrows anteriorly and the protuberance of the occipital base posteriorly. This measurement is then compared with set standards (see Chapter 21). Premature closure of the sutures in the child results in distinctive asymmetry of the head.

The fontanelles are measured next. The *anterior fontanelle* is about 4–6 cm in each dimension at birth and closes by 18 months. Deviations from normal include bulging fontanelles, which occur with increased intracranial pressure, and depressed, sunken fontanelles, which occur with dehydration. A larger than normal fontanelle may be an indication of rickets, hypothyroidism, or osteogenesis imperfecta, as well as of chronic increased intracranial pressure. The *posterior fontanelle* is about 0.5–1 cm at birth and closes by 2 months. Increases in size of this fontanelle may also indicate increased intracranial pressure.

Palpation of the infant's head may reveal certain conditions that are normal until a certain age. For example, cephalhematoma—localized swelling of the scalp in newborns—may persist up to 3 months of age. Caput succedaneum—edema and bruising of the scalp over a portion of the occipitoparietal region—disappears in the newborn after about one week.

In adults, conditions that affect size and shape of the head include acromegaly, a deformity caused by excessive secretion of the growth hormone (see Figure 10-4). In acromegaly, the skull enlarges and thickens. The cranial bones may become so thick that they cause increased intracranial pressure. Vitamin D deficiency (rickets) can cause enlargement of the frontal and parietal bones, and congenital syphilis may also produce enlargement of the frontal bones. Such bulging of the frontal bones is known as "bossing." Trauma or tumors of the skull often create

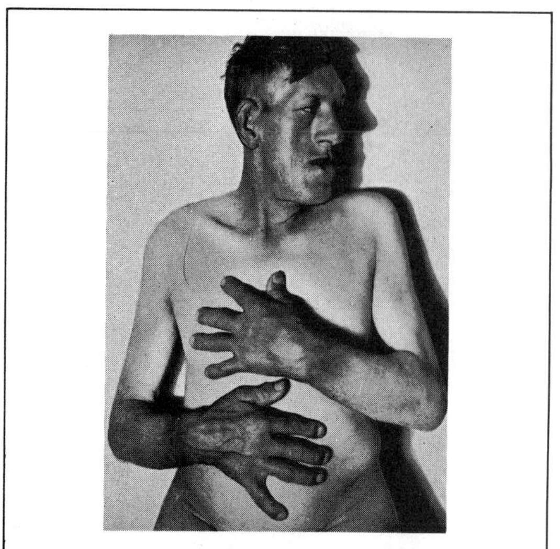
Figure 10-4 Acromegaly.

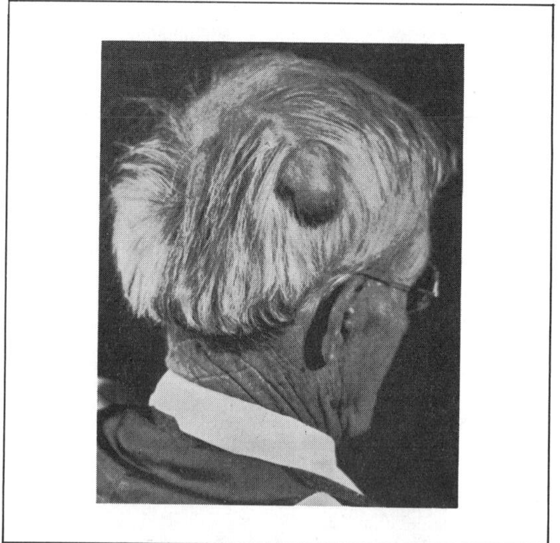
Figure 10-5 Sebaceous cyst of the scalp.

obvious distortions and may be observed or palpated.

Assessment of body hair was discussed in Chapter 9. However, because assessment of scalp hair is usually performed during the examination of the head, it is appropriate to discuss certain characteristics of scalp hair in this chapter.

The condition of the hair and scalp gives important clues about an individual's health. Hair and scalp should be inspected and palpated. Palpation is best accomplished by using the fingertips and a gentle rotating motion. The color, texture, and amount of hair should be noted. In the newborn all the original hair is shed within a few months, and sometimes the new hair is a different color. When examining an adult's hair, remember that hair color is difficult to determine because so many people use hair dyes. Permanents and dyes tend to make the hair dry and brittle. Dry, brittle hair is also a common sign of aging and of myxedema. Fine, soft hair is characteristic of hyperthyroidism.

Flaking or crusts on the scalp may indicate seborrhea, eczema, or an allergic response to hair care products. Sebaceous cysts or wens, which result from the occlusion of glands, are often found in the scalp; they present as smooth, round nodules on the skin (see Figure 10-5).

Alopecia—loss or thinning of hair—is a common condition. The most common type is hereditary alopecia, shown in Figure 10-6, which is manifested in baldness that occurs late in life or prematurely. It is characterized by thinning of the hair and recession of the hairline. Hereditary alopecia is always bilaterally symmetric on the anterior portion of the skull. This differentiates it from toxic alopecia—the rapidly occurring alopecia of severe illness—and alopecia areata.

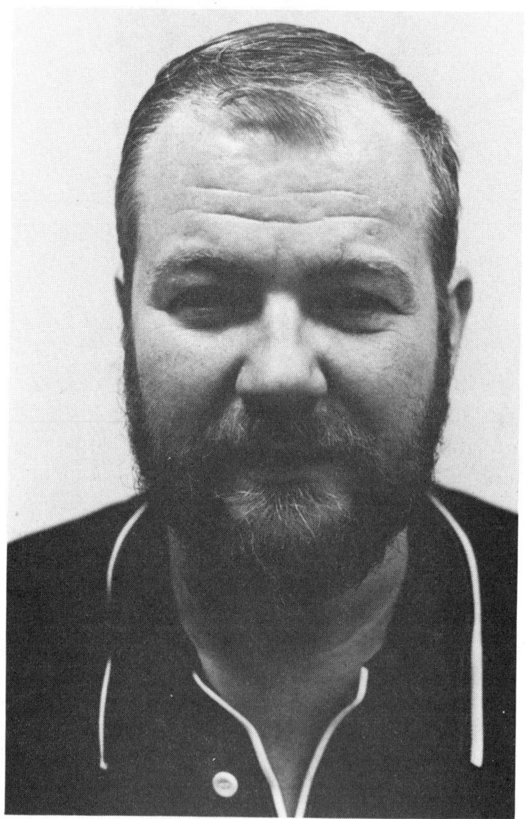
Figure 10-6 Example of hereditary alopecia. Note the symmetry of the receding hairline.

Technique of Inspection and Palpation of the Head

1. Inspection of size and shape of head.
2. Palpation of hair with gentle, rotating motion of fingertips.
3. Inspection and palpation of scalp, noting texture.
4. Abnormalities.

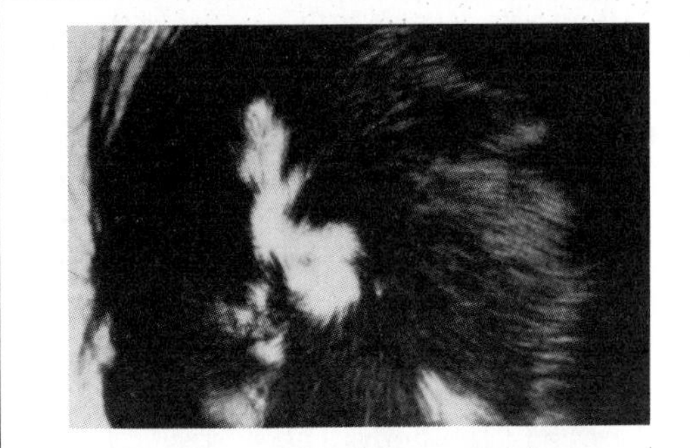

Figure 10-7 Alopecia areata due to secondary syphilis. Note the moth-eaten appearance.

The latter, shown in Figure 10-7, is a patchy loss of hair from the scalp and often from the beard. It is frequently observed in fungus infections and secondary syphilis. In a child, uneven distribution of hair may indicate chromosomal disorders.

Inspection of the Face

You can learn a great deal from careful inspection of the face. Facial expressions may reveal depression, anxiety, hostility, disgust, or embarrassment. It is important to note such manifestations as grimacing, excessive blinking, or continual smiling. Such behavior may indicate illness and may supply information on how the client feels as a person.

There are many physical conditions that can affect the face. Note overall facial symmetry; a cerebrovascular accident or damage to a facial nerve could result in drooping of one side of the face. Drooping eyelids with an accompanying heaviness to the face may indicate myasthenia gravis. Hormonal imbalances may cause puffiness of the entire face, edematous eyelids, thick tongue, the coarse, dry skin of myxedema (thyroid deficiency) (see Figure 10-10) and the startled, anxious appearance of the exophthalmic client with hyperthyroidism (see Figure 10-8). Cushing's syndrome—hyperfunction of the adrenal glands—is accompanied by a characteristic "moonface" and prominent jowls.

Severe debilitating disease such as dehydration, starvation, and fever can produce the cachectic facies, characterized by sunken eyes, hollow cheeks, and dry, roughened skin.

Systemic disease can also produce changes in the face. Atrophy and tightening of the skin occurs in scleroderma (see Figure 10-9). Edema of the face may indicate kidney disease or

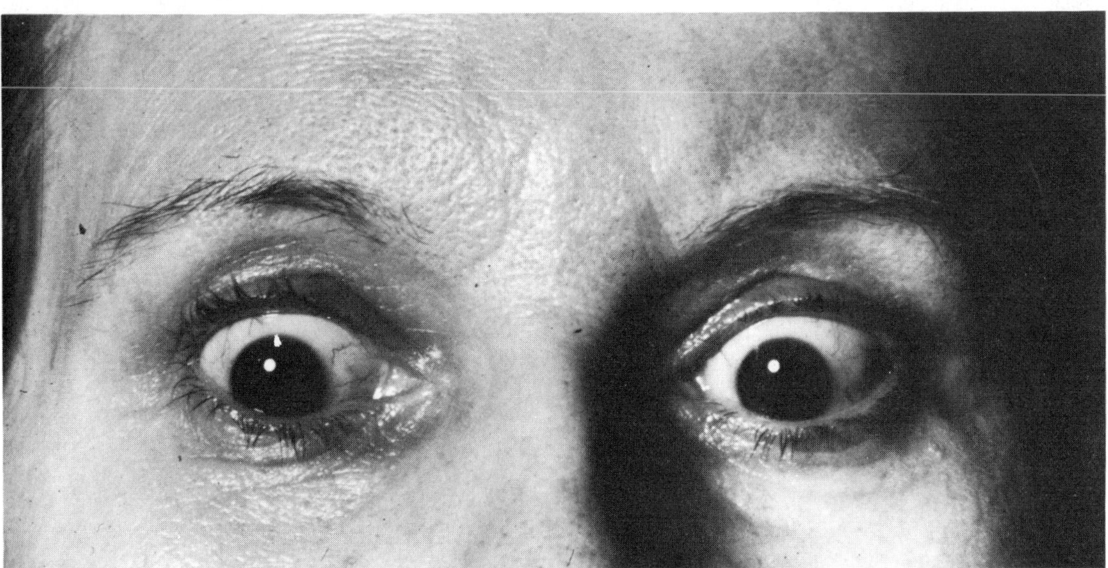

Figure 10-8 Exophthalmos of Grave's disease. Note the staring, startled appearance and wide palpebral fissures.

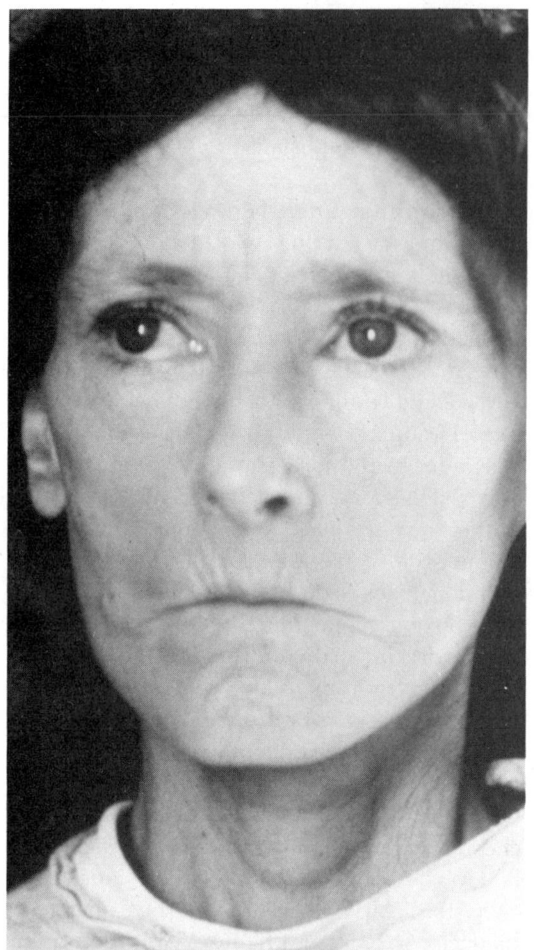

Figure 10-9 Facial changes in scleroderma. Note the drawn, pursed lips. (© Arthritis Foundation 1981.)

Technique of Inspection of the Face

1. Adequate lighting.
2. Facial expression.
3. Facial symmetry.
4. Skin temperature, texture, and color.
5. Abnormalities.

congestive heart failure. The eyelids and surrounding tissues of the eyes are especially prone to edema; orbital edema is often the first sign of fluid retention.

Xanthomas are circumscribed collections of lipids that may occur anywhere on the body but are commonly found on the eyelids, particularly near the inner canthus. They can be flat or elevated, and they vary in size. Occasionally, they are associated with a disease such as cholesteremia or diabetes mellitus, but frequently there is no associated disease process (see Figure 9-17).

Nevi and the lesions of acne may be noted on the face as well as elsewhere on the body. Such changes in facial skin pigmentation as pallor, cyanosis, jaundice, and vitiligo (absence of color) indicate impaired health.

Structure of the Neck

For descriptive purposes the neck is divided into three triangles, as shown in Figure 10-11. The triangle beneath the mandible, termed the *submandibular triangle*, is bordered by the digastric muscles. The middle of the neck is defined by the thyroid cartilage and the *suprasternal notch*. The *anterior cervical triangle* is bounded by the submandibular triangle, laterally by the sternocleidomastoid muscle, and medially by the midline of the body. The *posterior triangle* is situated between the sternocleidomastoid and the trapezius muscle. The *supraclavicular fossa* is between the clavicle and the insertion of the sternocleidomastoid muscle, and the suprasternal notch is immediately above the manubrium of the sternum. The anterior midline structures

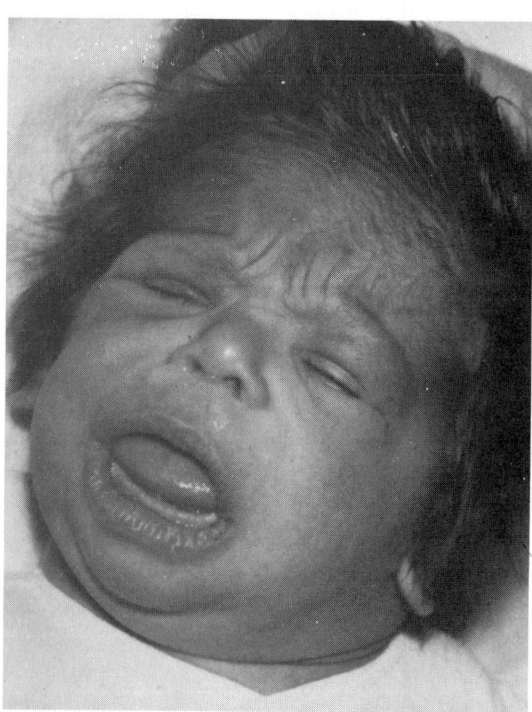

Figure 10-10 The facies of an infant with myxedema.

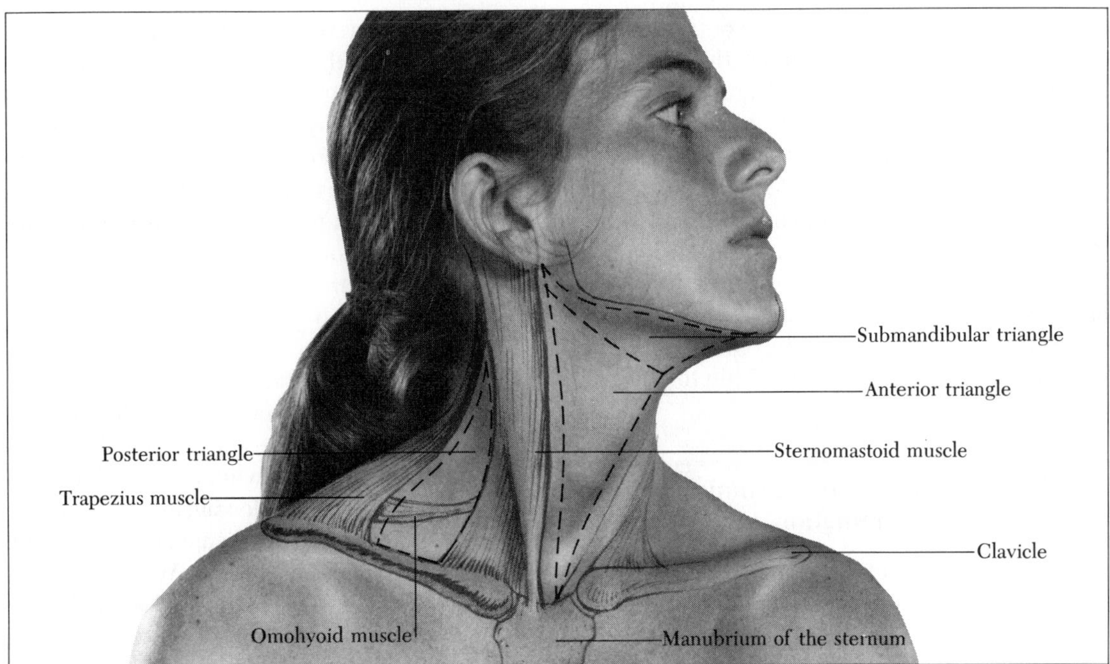

Figure 10-11 Diagram of anterior neck.

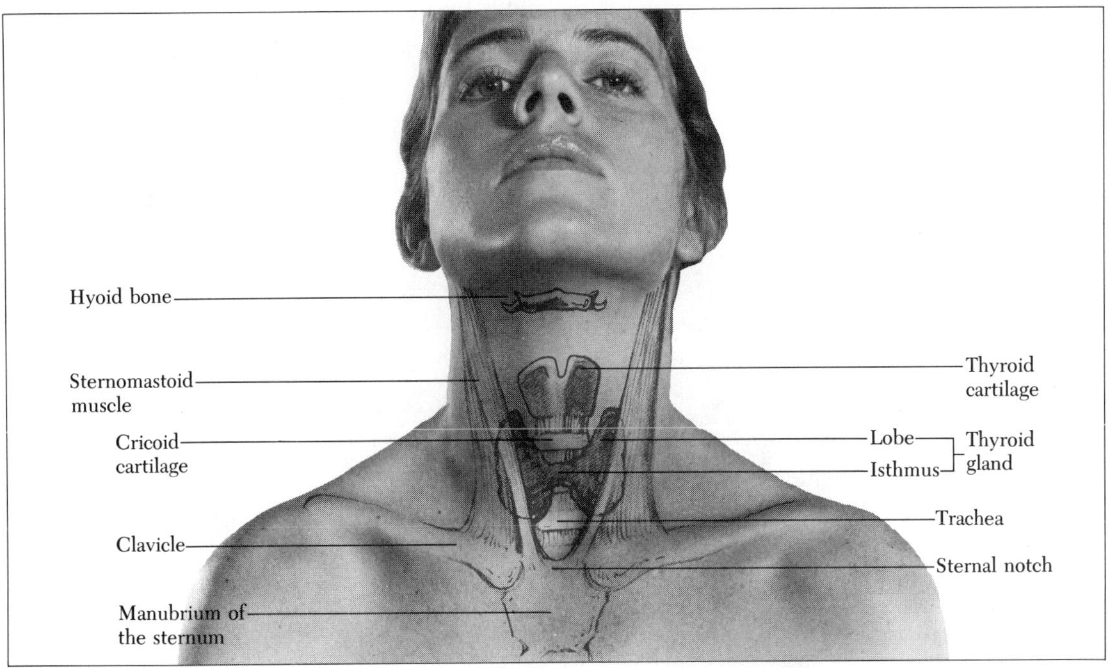

Figure 10-12 Anterior midline structures of the neck.

of the neck are illustrated in Figure 10-12. These structures include the hyoid bone, thyroid cartilage, cricoid cartilage, thyroid gland (lobe and isthmus), trachea, and the sternocleidomastoid muscle.

There are several groups of lymph nodes located in the neck, as illustrated in Figure 10-13. Knowledge of these locations is necessary for thorough assessment of the neck. The lymph nodes function to filter the blood, engulf microorganisms, and produce lymphocytes and monocytes. Careful investigation of the areas of lymph drainage is a valuable diagnostic tool in the detection of acute inflammation, infection, metastatic carcinoma, and systemic diseases.

Figure 10-14 shows the location of the blood vessels of the neck. It is important to know the location of these vessels because the carotid arteries are the major arteries through which blood is circulated to the brain, and the jugular veins are useful indicators of the efficiency of the heart and vascular system. (See Table 10-1.)

Characteristics and Techniques of Examination

The three methods used in assessing the neck are inspection, palpation, and auscultation.

Inspection

Examination of the neck begins with inspection. The position of the head should be noted. If the muscles of the neck are shortened on one side or are in spasm, the head will be tilted to one side. Next note the size and symmetry of the neck. Asymmetry may result from edema, masses, or displacement of the trachea. In normal individuals the thyroid gland is not visible; thus, enlargement of the thyroid gland should be easy to note upon inspection. The thyroid cartilage (Adam's apple) is normally visible and rises upon swallowing. Look for pulsations in the neck region and distention of the veins of the neck. Venous pulsations and distention should not occur when the client is in an upright position.

Palpation and Auscultation

In this section palpation and auscultation are discussed together because the findings from palpation often determine whether auscultation of the area is necessary. Following inspection of the neck, palpate the three triangular areas of the neck for tenderness or masses. While doing so, you should move the client's head and neck through the normal range of motion: rotation (side to side), flexion (chin to chest), hyperextension (tilted backward), and lateral flexion (ear to shoulder). The neck is normally supple, allowing this assessment to be easily performed. If the client has arthritis of the cervical spine, he will turn at the shoulders rather than turn his neck.

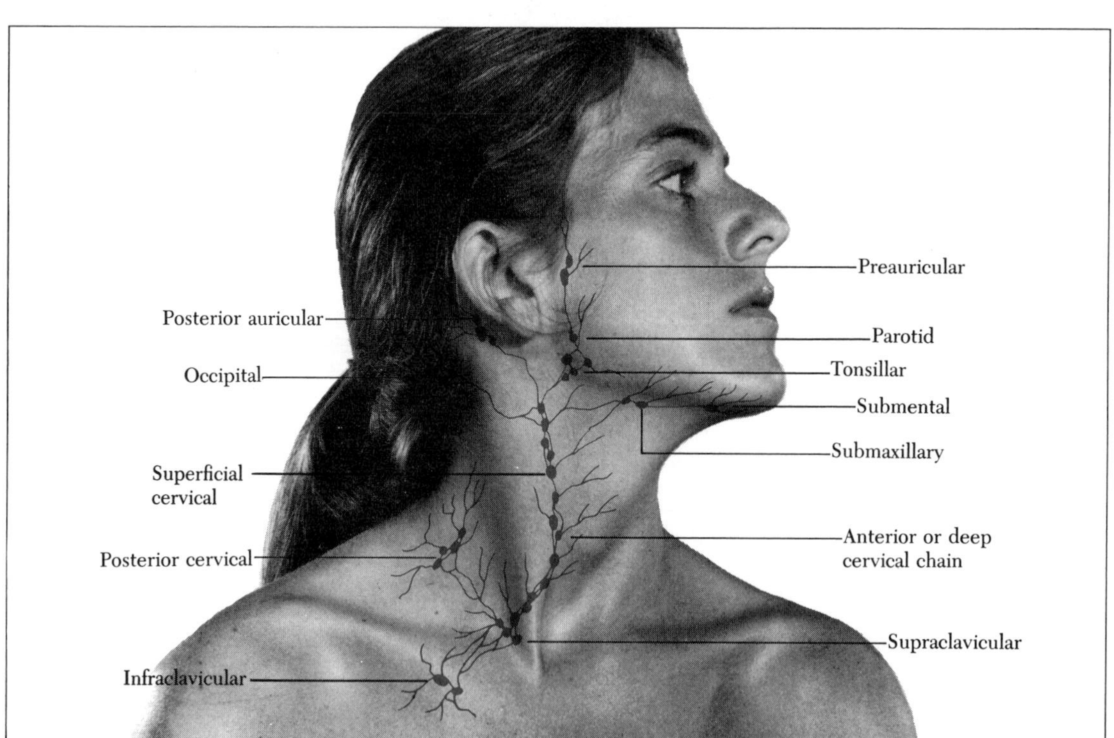

Figure 10-13 Location of the lymph nodes of the neck.

Table 10-1. Common Abnormalities of the Head, Face, and Neck

Terminology	Characteristics	Comments
Microcephalus	Small skull less than two standard deviations below mean for age and sex	Check for history of brain damage; mental retardation common.
Hydrocephalus	Enlarged head caused by blockage of cerebrospinal fluid in ventricular system	Early sign is dilated scalp veins.
Acromegaly	Overgrowth of cartilage and bones; elongation of jaw; enlarged ears, nose, hands, and feet	Increase in hat and glove size. Pressure of thickened cranial bones can cause increased intracranial pressure; excessive growth hormone in the adult.
"Bossing"	Bulging appearance of forehead; enlargement of frontal and parietal bones	Vitamin D deficiency (rickets), congenital syphilis common causes.
Seborrhea (dandruff)	Dry flakes or greasy crusts and scales; pruritus; remissions; exacerbations; accompanies oily skin	Excessive secretion of sebaceous glands. Check seborrheic areas other than scalp, i.e., chin, lateral nasal folds, center of chest and back, axillae, groins.
Wens	Movable, nontender, single, or multiple masses on scalp	Blockage of sebaceous gland of the scalp.
Alopecia areata	Patchy loss of scalp and facial (beard) hair	May accompany fungal infections, secondary syphilis, and chromosomal disorders.
Edema	Generalized facial puffiness, periorbital, moon facies	Check for further signs of trauma, inflammation, nephrotic syndrome, myxedema, congestive heart failure.
Asymmetry	Unilateral ptosis of facial muscles with drooping of eyelid and corner of mouth	Check for signs of local trauma, Bell's palsy (facial nerve damage) and cerebrovascular accident.
Xanthomas	Yellow, raised plaques common on eyelids, nasal bridge, around tendons, i.e. knuckles, large joints	Lipoid deposits. Check for history of diabetes mellitus, hypercholesteremia; check cholesterol blood level.
Lymphadenopathy	Enlarged lymph nodes	Check for additional signs of infection and inflammation. Be aware of potential metastatic disease.
Goiter	Enlarged thyroid gland	Common with iodine deficiency diet and diets of cabbage, turnips, and broccoli; hyperthyroidism; sulfonamides; thiourea drugs.
Carotid bruit	Buzzing sound auscultated over carotid artery	Check for signs of brain ischemia, e.g., syncope, vertigo, headache. Common in carotid stenosis, hyperthyroidism.

Technique of Inspection of the Neck

1. Face the client directly.
2. Have client look straight ahead.
3. Characteristics:
   Size & symmetry of neck
   Position of trachea
   Visibility of thyroid gland
   Visibility of venous pulsation and distention

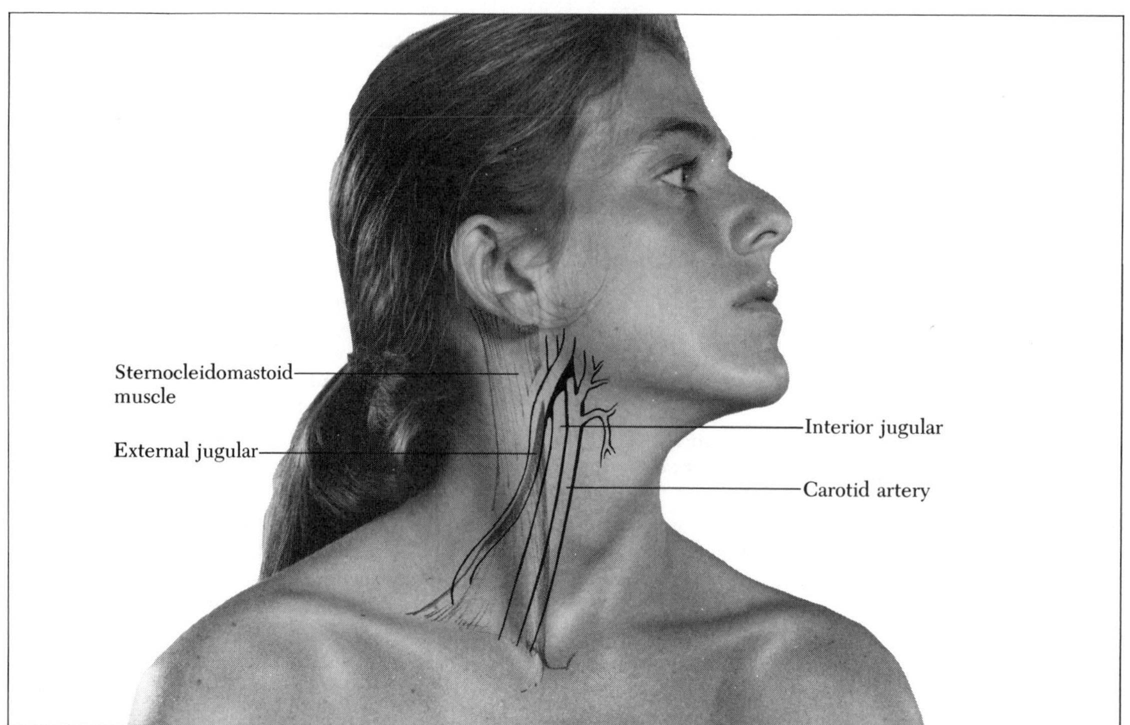

Figure 10-14 Location of blood vessels of the neck.

The lymph glands should be palpated using a gentle to and fro or rotary motion with the fingertips. The nodes are generally palpated beginning with the occipital nodes and then the preauricular and posterior auricular nodes, the parotid gland, the posterior cervical, anterior cervical, submaxillary, submental, tonsillar, and supraclavicular nodes. To best palpate the supraclavicular nodes it is helpful to have the client place his hands on his thighs and move his elbows and shoulders forward. This posture will relax the skin over the supraclavicular areas and provide more direct access to the lymph nodes.

Nodes are not normally palpable in the healthy individual, but enlarged nodes may be found as the result of an old infection. In such cases the history of past illnesses and injuries is helpful in differentiating active from past pathology. In children cervical lymph nodes may be normally palpable until around 12 years of age.

The location of enlarged lymph nodes may give a clue as to the origin of the problem. Occipital node enlargement may be due to scalp infections, whereas posterior auricular lymphadenopathy may indicate ear infection. Enlarged, tender cervical glands should direct your attention to the mouth and pharynx. Enlargement of the anterior cervical nodes may suggest respiratory infection. Submaxillary and submental node enlargement may reflect inflammation of the mouth. Enlarged, tender parotid glands often indicate mumps, a contagious infection. This disease is rarely seen because of the success of widespread vaccination programs.

Enlargement of the lymph nodes can be either local or widespread. Lymphadenopathy can accompany other signs of inflammation. Rapidly enlarging nodes may indicate antibody formation, and they may be quite tender. If the skin overlying the node is inflamed, the node is probably infected. Enlargement of nodes in more than one site may also be due to metastasis, e.g., Hodgkin's disease (see Figure 10-15). Malignant infiltration of the nodes can occur without any accompanying signs of inflammation.

If a mass is detected, it must be palpated to determine its size, location, consistency, mobility, and tenderness. Lymph nodes may be discrete or matted together; they may be extremely hard, moderately hard, soft, or cystic. Nodes that are nontender, hard, and matted together suggest metastatic disease. In acute inflammation the nodes are usually rather soft and tender with enlargement. In chronic infection, as in tuberculosis, the nodes tend to be tender, firm, and matted together.

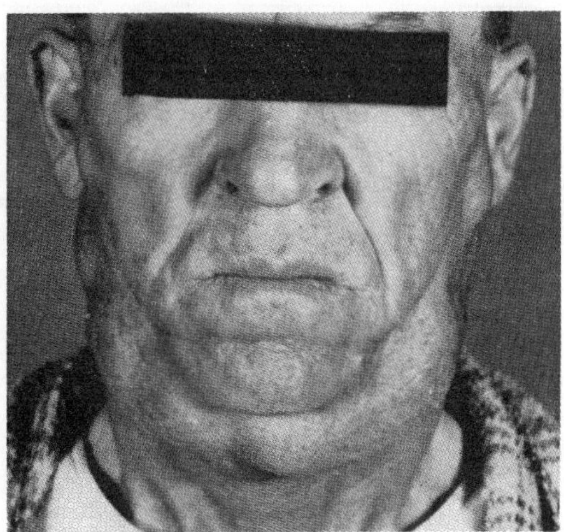

Figure 10-15 Hodgkin's disease manifests as a collar of enlarged lymph nodes. Enlargement of preauricular nodes is also visible.

The thyroid gland can be palpated from in front of the client or from behind. The beginner may find it easier to palpate from behind. Figure 10-16A shows that in this position the client's head is placed on a forward incline, tilted slightly toward the side to be examined, while you use the middle and index fingers of both your hands to locate the thyroid cartilage. The isthmus of the thyroid gland is about 1 cm below this cartilage. For example, if you are palpating the right lobe of the client's thyroid gland, the client's head should be flexed forward and tilted toward the right. This position relaxes the sternocleidomastoid muscle on that side. Use the index and middle fingers of your left hand to displace the thyroid cartilage and the index finger of your right hand to displace the sternocleidomastoid muscle. You can feel the right lateral portion of the thyroid gland with the middle and ring fingers of your right hand. If you instruct the client to swallow, the thyroid will move upward between the examining fingers. Repeat the examination on the client's left side.

Technique of Palpation of the Neck

1. Observe active and passive range of motion: rotation, flexion, hyperextension, and lateral flexion
2. Palpate using fingertips.
3. Characteristics:
   Three triangular areas: submandibular, anterior, and posterior cervical
   Lymph nodes: preauricular, postauricular, occipital, submental, submaxillary, tonsillar, parotid gland, anterior cervical, posterior cervical, supraclavicular, infraclavicular

Technique of Auscultation of Neck

1. Warm stethoscope with hand.
2. Apply bell lightly with edges touching skin.
3. Decision making:
   Auscultate for hum when enlarged thyroid.
   Auscultate for bruit when carotid pulse is weak or absent.

To palpate the thyroid gland from a frontal approach, position your left thumb against the right side of the cartilage and place the second and third fingers of your left hand behind the sternocleidomastoid muscle (see Figure 10-16B). Feel for the lateral lobe with your left thumb as the client swallows. The procedure is reversed to palpate the left lobe. The thyroid should be examined for size, consistency, and the presence of nodules. If the gland is enlarged, place the stethoscope over it and listen for a bruit. A systolic bruit may be heard in thyrotoxicosis because of increased blood flow through the tissues; this bruit will not have a cardiovascular origin. The thyroid may be enlarged in simple goiter, in inflammation, and in the presence of tumors (see Figure 10-17). Thyroid disorders are the most common endocrine disorders in children. Figure 10-18 illustrates a normal thyroid gland, thyroid enlargement, a thyroid nodule, and a multinodular thyroid gland as situated in the anterior, central region of the neck.

Palpation of the carotid arteries should normally reveal bilateral equality. Do not palpate both carotid arteries simultaneously. This will allow full patency of one artery to transport blood and oxygen to the brain. Carotid massage, which may inadvertently occur, may be hazardous in some cases because it lowers pulse rate. If there is weakness or absence of a carotid pulse, listen over the carotids with the bell of the stethoscope. With carotid stenosis a cardiovascular bruit may be detected. You can create an artificial stenosis by placing gentle pressure over the

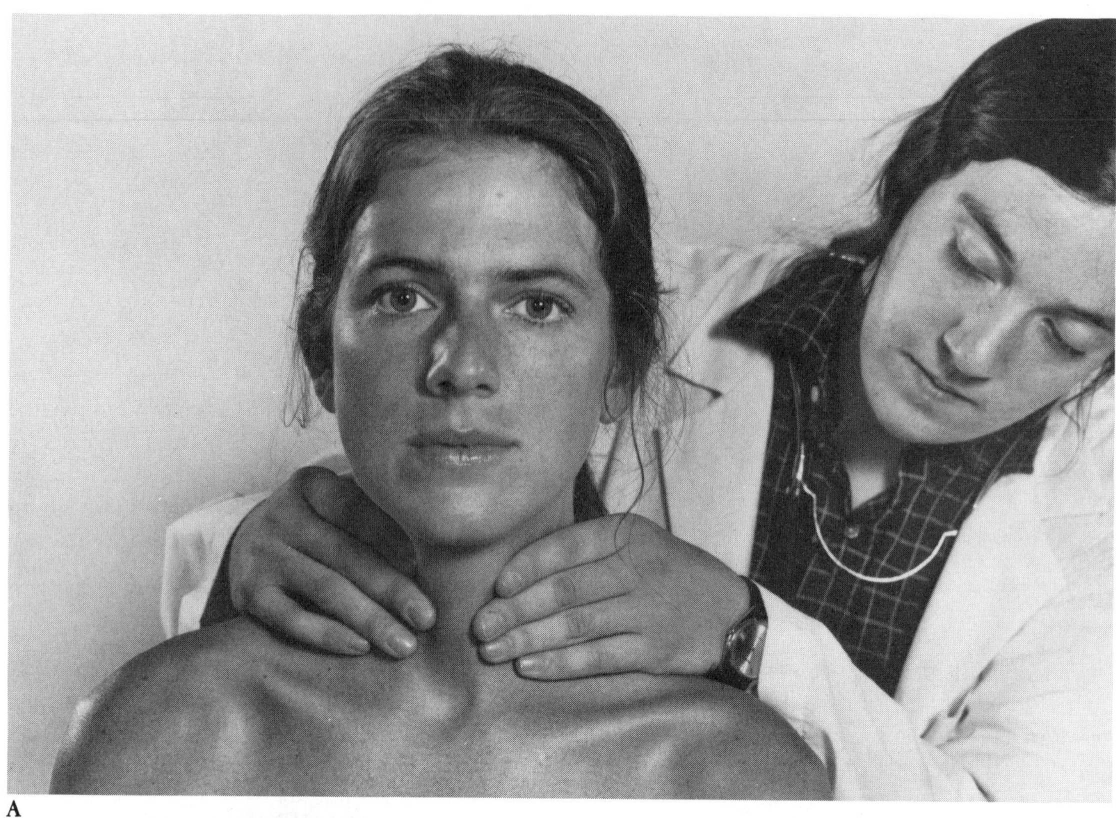

A

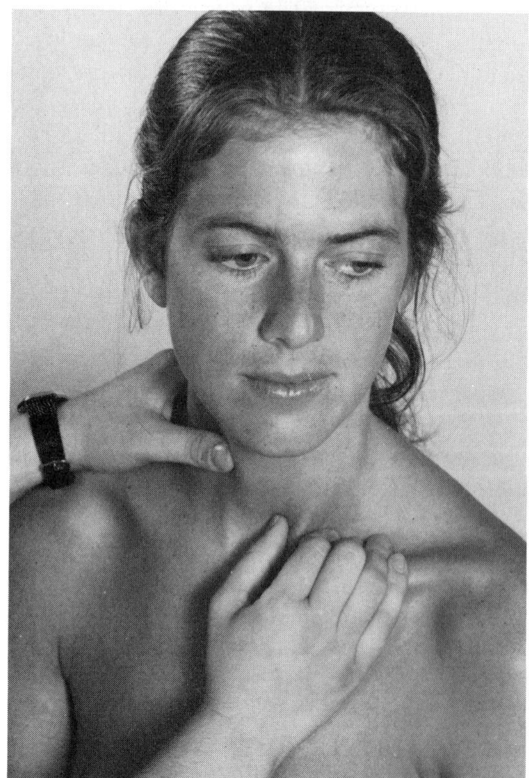

B

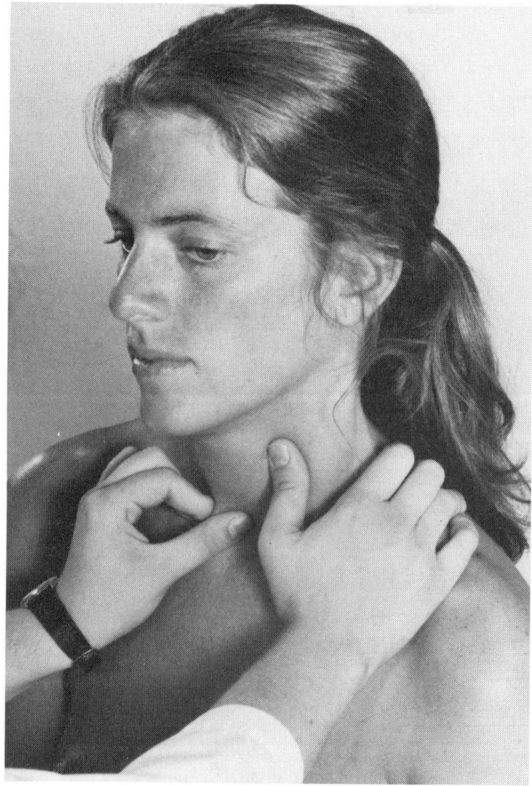

C

Figure 10-16 (A) Palpation of the thyroid from behind. (B) Palpation of thyroid left lobe. (C) Palpation of thyroid right lobe.

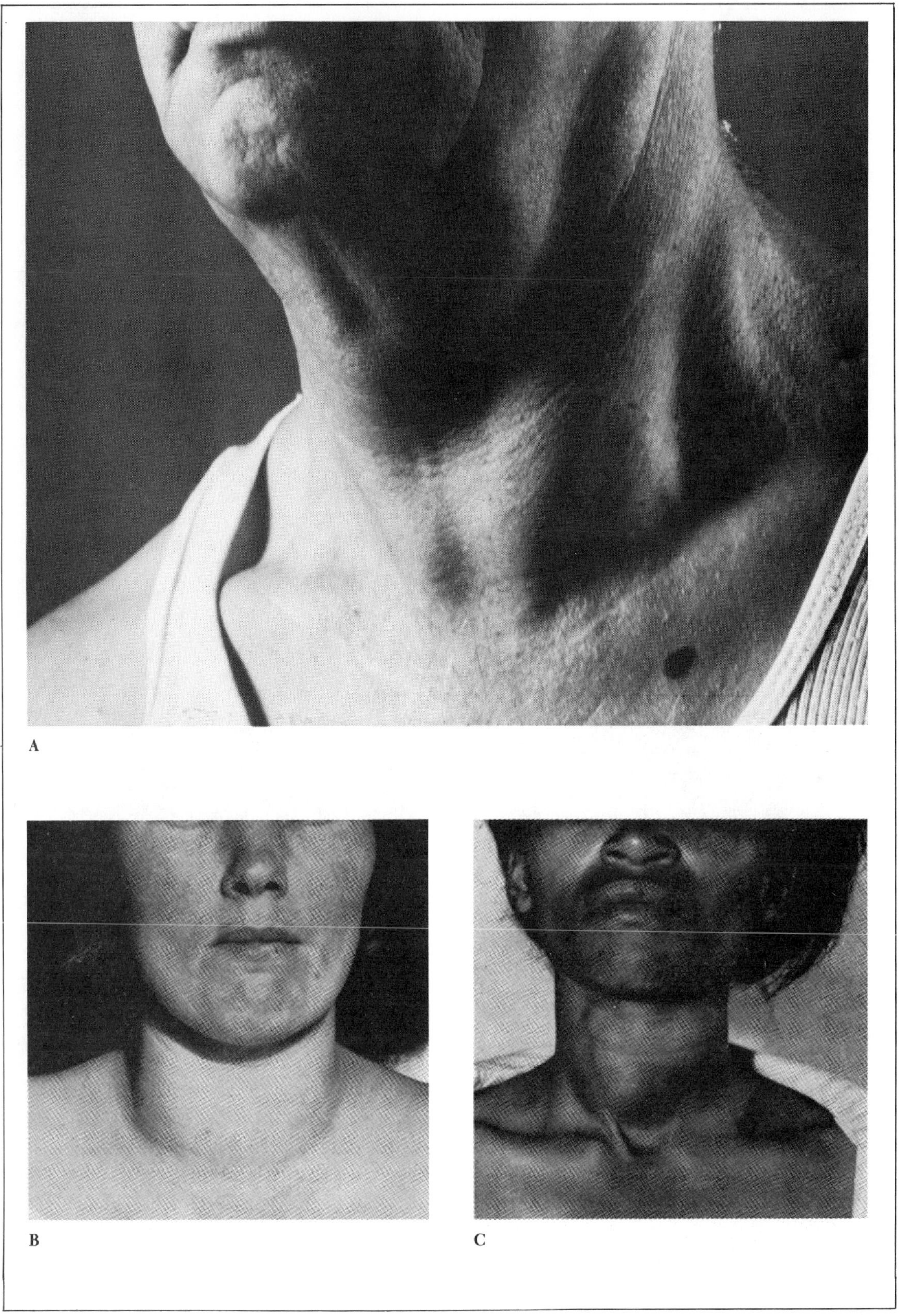

Figure 10-17 Thyroid disorders. (A) Enlarged thyroid. Note swelling at the site of the thyroid isthmus and on either side of the trachea. (B) Diffuse colloid goiter of moderate size. (C) Toxic modular goiter.

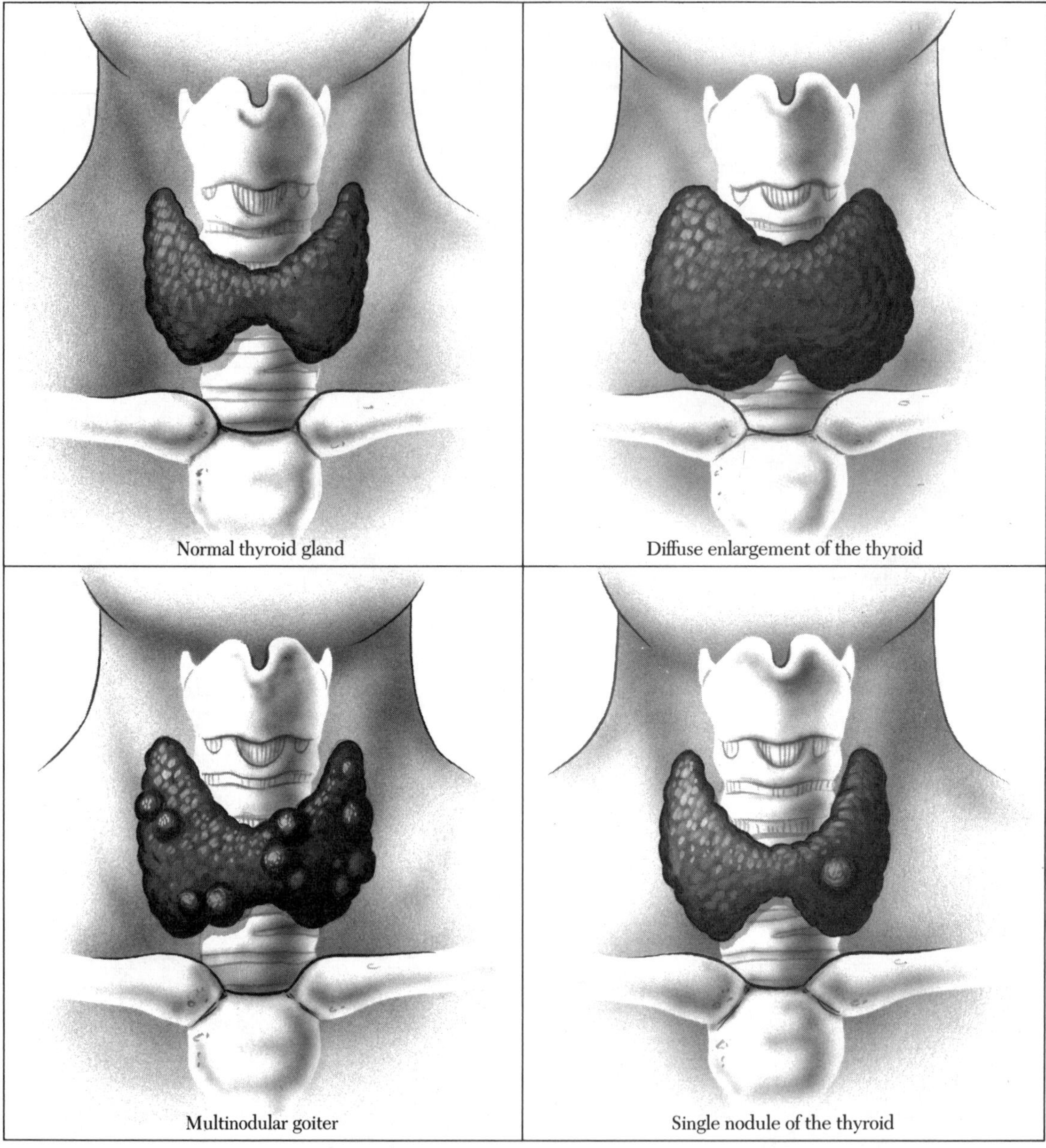

Figure 10-18 Anatomical position of the normal thyroid gland and pathological thyroid findings.

healthy carotid, taking care not to apply so much pressure as to cut off the flow entirely. If you listen above the point of pressure with the bell of the stethoscope, you will be able to hear the artificially produced bruit.

Summary

This chapter described the assessment of the head and neck. The head is examined by inspection and palpation, which are often used simultaneously. Careful inspection of the face can yield much important information about the client's state of health.

Examination of the neck requires three techniques: inspection, palpation, and auscultation. Because many structures must be assessed in this rather small area, the examiner should have a thorough understanding of the anatomy to carry out a comprehensive examination.

Discussion Questions/Activities

1. Why is it important to palpate the client's head during the health examination?

Technique of Palpation of the Thyroid

1. Posterior approach: head slightly forward and tilted toward side being examined; index finger placed high to retract the sternocleidomastoid muscle; middle and ring fingers over the lateral portion of thyroid. Index and middle fingers displace the thyroid cartilage on the contralateral side. Have client swallow as each side is examined.
2. Frontal approach: head slightly tilted toward side being examined; thumb anterior to sternocleidomastoid muscle; two to three middle fingers behind sternocleidomastoid muscle. Thumb and fingers positioned same on opposite side of neck to displace thyroid cartilage.

2. Discuss various changes in the face that might indicate a change in the client's health status.
3. Role-play how you would approach the examination of a client who is wearing a wig.
4. How would you determine whether a client is using hair dye?
5. Demonstrate the normal range of motion of the neck.
6. List the areas of the neck that must be examined for lymph node enlargement.
7. List the aspects of enlarged lymph nodes that must be documented.
8. Demonstrate the technique you would use to palpate the thyroid gland.
9. Discuss the rationale for auscultation of the carotid arteries.
10. Palpate the lymph nodes of the neck in several children and adults. Discuss the differences.
11. Perform a physical assessment of the head, neck, and face of a client, peer, or relative; document your findings.

Recording of Findings

Normal findings are presented in the first box. The second box contains findings of a client in whom a change in the thyroid gland was noted during the health examination.

Head **INSPECTION** Normocephalic, atraumatic; normal hair distribution. Scalp clear. **PALPATION** No lumps; no tenderness.	**Head** **INSPECTION** Normocephalic, atraumatic; normal hair distribution. Scalp clear. **PALPATION** No lumps; no tenderness.
Face **INSPECTION** Symmetrical; no muscular weakness; no involuntary movements; no facial edema; skin pink; no lesions noted.	**Face** **INSPECTION** Symmetrical; no muscular weakness; no involuntary movements; no facial edema; skin pink; no lesions noted
Neck **INSPECTION** Symmetrical; no masses. **PALPATION** Supple with normal range of movement; thyroid nonpalpable; no lymphadenopathy; no venous distention; carotids equal bilaterally and of good quality; trachea midline. **AUSCULTATION** No carotid bruits; no thyroid hum.	**Neck** **INSPECTION** Symmetrical; no masses. **PALPATION** Supple with normal range of movement; thyroid enlarged, 1.5 cm mass with small, extremely hard, nontender, fixed nodules on right lobe; no lymphadenopathy; no venous distention; carotids equal bilaterally and of bounding quality; trachea midline. **AUSCULTATION** No carotid bruits; no thyroid hum.

CHAPTER 11

Assessment of the Eye

LEARNING OBJECTIVES

1. Describe the structure and function of the eye.
2. Identify the structures of the eye that are examined by inspection and palpation.
3. Demonstrate the techniques used for examining the pupils, extraocular muscles, visual fields, and visual acuity.
4. Describe the technique used in conducting the ophthalmic examination.
5. Discuss the relationship between the ophthalmic examination and the client's level of wellness.

The eye is complex and fascinating. Figure 11-1 is a horizontal section of the eyeball, showing its main structures. Assessment of these structures will be considered separately throughout the chapter.

Structure and Function of the Eye

The eye is a sphere almost 1 inch in diameter. The greatest portion of this sphere is recessed in the bony orbit that protects it. Only a small portion of the anterior eye is visible. Figure 11-1 shows that the eyeball is covered by three coats of tissue: the *sclera*, the *choroid*, and the *retina*. The sclera is the outermost coat. The anterior portion of the sclera is referred to as the *cornea*. The cornea lies over the *iris* and is transparent. The rest of the sclera is opaque and has a white appearance on inspection.

The choroid coat, the middle layer, contains a great deal of pigment and a large number of blood vessels. The choroid also provides special structures in its anterior portion. Foremost is the iris, which contains the pigments responsible for eye color. The iris consists of smooth circular and radial muscles arranged to form a round structure with an opening in the middle:

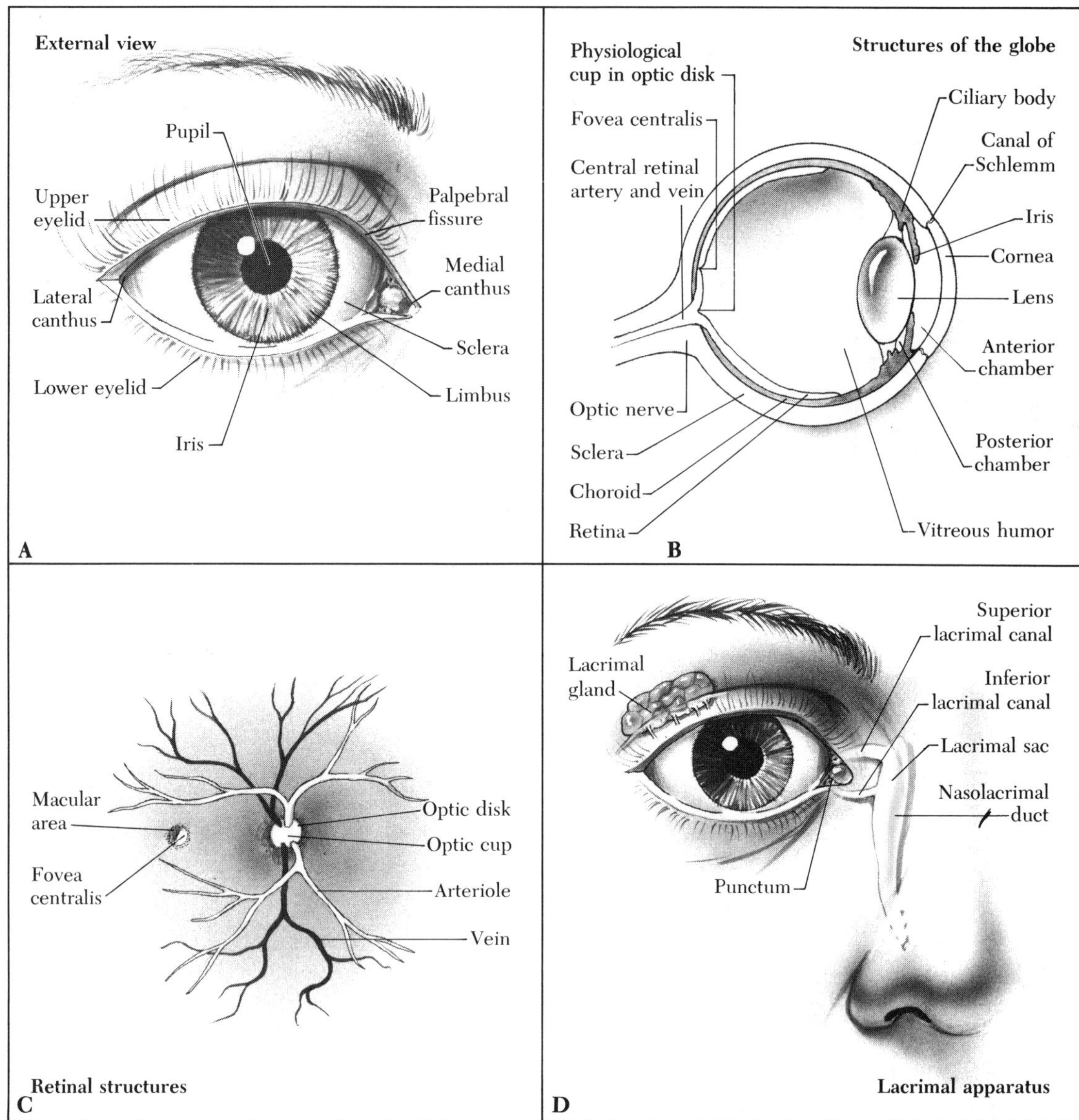

Figure 11-1 The eye. (A) External view. (B) Structures of the globe. (C) Retinal structures. (D) Lacrimal apparatus.

the *pupil.* The involuntary muscles of the iris react to autonomic nervous system stimulation and regulate the size of the pupil. Posterior to the iris the choroid thickens into the *ciliary body,* which is composed of ciliary muscles. These involuntary muscles control the shape of the *lens,* the biconvex body that is part of the refracting mechanism of the eye. The ciliary muscles change the thickness of the lens to accommodate for near and far vision. A circular ligament attached to the ciliary body holds the lens in place.

The retina, the innermost coat of the eye, is composed of nervous tissue that receives the visual images. The *fovea centralis,* a slight depression at the posterior of the eye, marks the point of central vision. The area of the retina immediately surrounding the fovea centralis is called the *macula. Rods* and *cones* are the photoreceptor neurons that constitute the visual receptors of the retina. The rods respond to low-intensity light and shades of gray, while the cones respond to bright light and color. The rods are almost absent from the macula and increase in density toward the periphery of the retina. The cones are most densely concentrated in the fovea centralis. The fact that the rods are more responsive to shades of gray and are located away from the center of the retina can be illustrated by a simple experiment. The next time you are driving at night, tilt your head down so that your eyes will have to move upward to see the road in front of you. This will cause the image of what you are looking at to fall more toward the lower periphery of your retina and to be chiefly received by the rods. You will find that you are much better able to see, even when there is another car approaching you.

The small circular area in the posterior part of the retina is called the *optic disk*. It is here that the *optic nerve* emerges from the eyeball. The arteries and veins that provide the blood supply to the eye also enter and leave at this point.

The anterior compartment of the eye has two subdivisions: (1) the *anterior chamber* between the back of the cornea and the front of the lens, and (2) the *posterior chamber* between the iris and the front of the lens. Aqueous humor, manufactured by the ciliary bodies, fills both of these compartments. It circulates from the posterior chamber to the anterior chamber and then is absorbed into the venous blood through the *canal of Schlemm*, which is located laterally between the junction of the sclera and the cornea.

The posterior compartment of the eye contains vitreous humor, a gelatinlike substance that provides sufficient intraocular pressure to prevent the eyeball from collapsing.

The *lacrimal glands*, which produce tears, are situated in the upper lateral bony orbit. From this site the tears are carried through small ducts to the conjunctiva in order to keep the surface of the eye moist and to wash away particles. Excess tears are gathered by the *puncta*, which can be seen as two small dots at the *medial canthus* of the eye. From the puncta the tears pass through the lacrimal canals into the *nasolacrimal duct*. All the tear ducts are lined with a mucous membrane that is an extension of the mucosa that lines the nose. When this membrane becomes swollen, the nasolacrimal ducts become plugged, causing tears to overflow onto the cheeks instead of draining into the nose as they normally should. Thus, an overflow of tears does not ordinarily occur except when the passageway into the nose is blocked or when tears are overabundant, as with crying or reaction to a foreign particle in the eye.

Characteristics and Techniques of Examination

Inspection and Palpation

As you examine each part of the eye, you will find it less tiring for the client and more systematic to perform inspection and palpation simultaneously. This approach also allows you to complete the examination of one part of the eye before moving to another part.

Lacrimal Apparatus The lacrimal apparatus may be involved with infection, inflammation, and tumors. To examine the system for an enlarged gland, raise the eyelid and look between the upper lid and the eyeball. To check for infection, apply finger pressure to the lacrimal sac at the inside of the lower inner orbital rim. This action will express any mucopurulent drainage from the punctum.

Eyelids The eyelids gain their shape from the tarsal plate, a ridge of thick connective tissue. Figure 11-2 shows that the meibomian (sebaceous) glands lie in vertical columns within the tarsal plates, forming light yellow streaks. These glands open onto the posterior portion of the lid margins.

A *hordeolum* (stye) is an infection of one of the meibomian glands of the eyelid (see Figure 11-3). It may suppurate or may need treatment with an antiseptic and antibiotic. A *chalazion* is a cyst of a meibomian gland that will be seen to bulge through to the surface of the eyelid (see Figure 11-4). Occasionally, it may become infected, but initially it appears as a hard, painless lump. Unlike a hordeolum, it will not subside or rupture on its own. It needs to be surgically removed.

Positional defects of the lids include entropion (inward rolling of the lid) and extropion (outward rolling of the lid) (see Figure 11-5). These defects can often be detected in elderly; the eye may become easily infected or irritated. The defects can be surgically repaired.

Blepharospasm, an involuntary twitching of both eyelids, may occur in elderly clients. It may be an isolated phenomenon due to eyestrain or

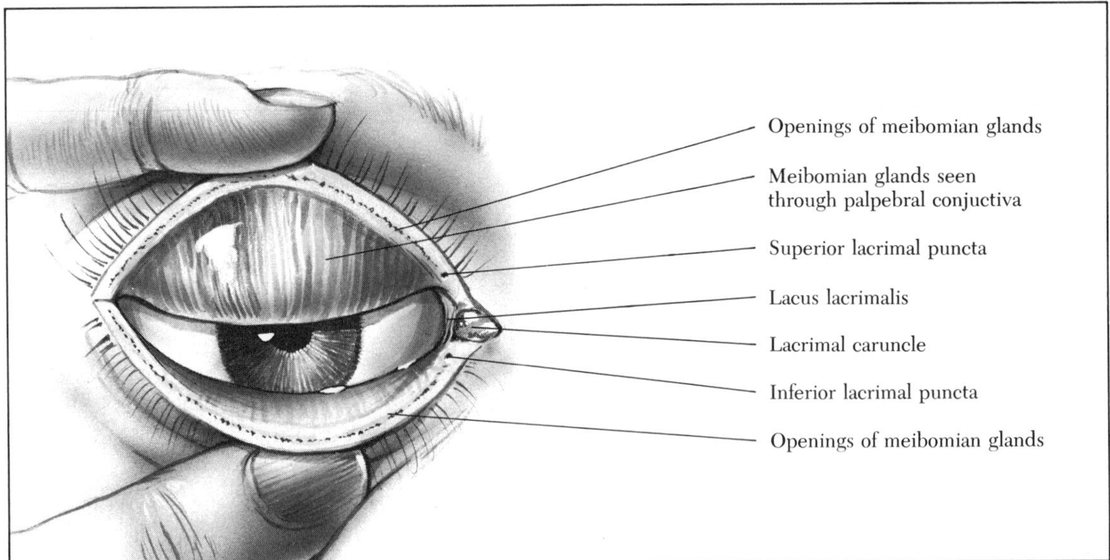

Figure 11-2 Structure of the eyelid.

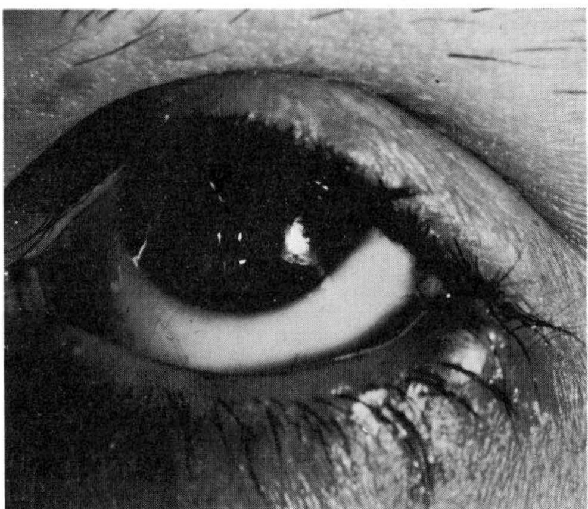

Figure 11-3 Hordeolum (stye).

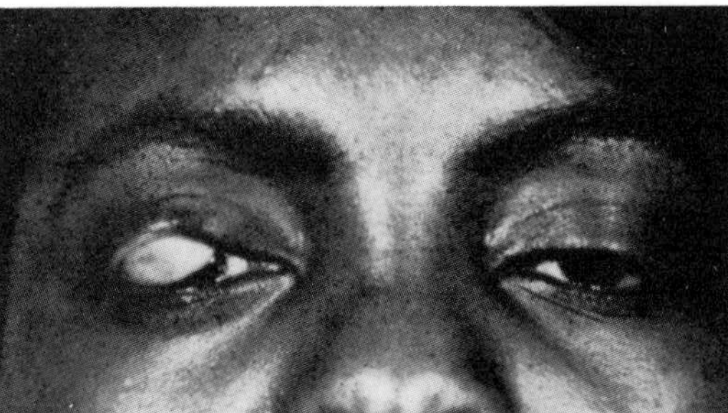

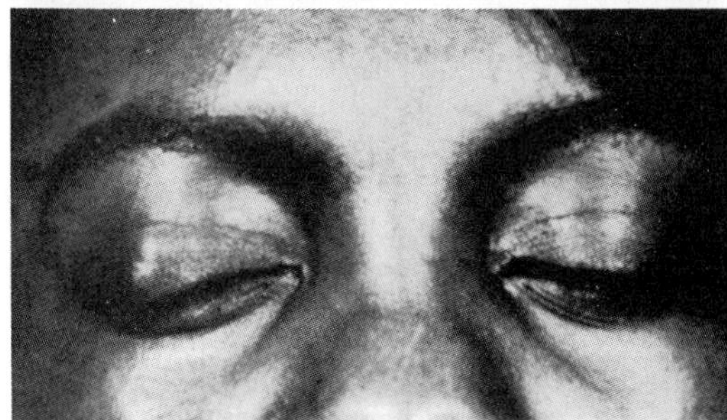

Figure 11-4 Chalazion of right eyelid. Note the small, firm bulge slightly lateral to the midline of the eyelid.

nervous irritability or it may be related to involvement of the facial nerve.

Observe for edema of the eyelid, as this condition often indicates systemic problems such as renal diseases, heart failure, allergy, and thyroid deficiency, as well as direct trauma to the eye. Never press on an injured eyeball. If you determine that the eyeball has been penetrated or has a foreign object embedded in it, stop the examination at once and notify an ophthalmologist.

Under normal conditions, the open eyelids are equally separated. This space between the open eyelids is called the *palpebral fissure*. The lower lid should meet the iris, with the upper lid covering a small fraction of the iris (2–3 mm). When the eyelids are closed, they should meet completely. In clients with exophthalmos, the palpebral fissure is wider than normal, and often the client cannot close the lids completely. Clients with hyperthyroidism may display lid lag. Have the client look downward as you observe his eyes. If a rim of the sclera is seen above the iris as the eye moves downward, lid lag is present (see Figure 11-6).

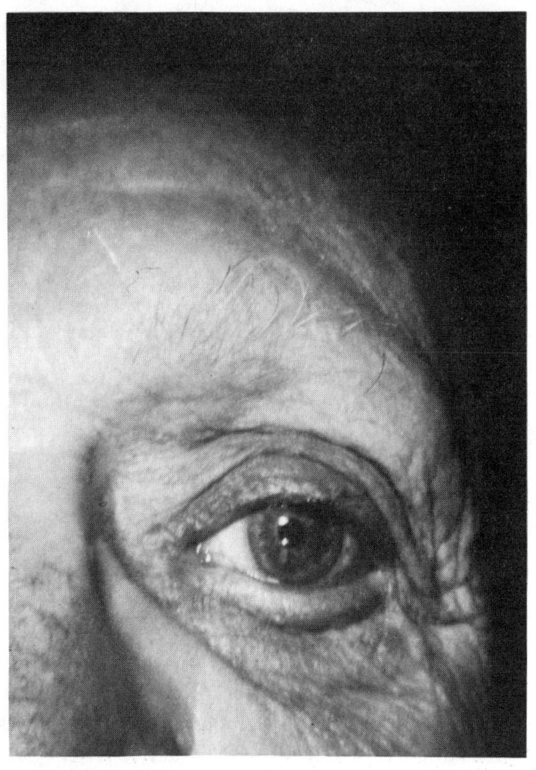
A

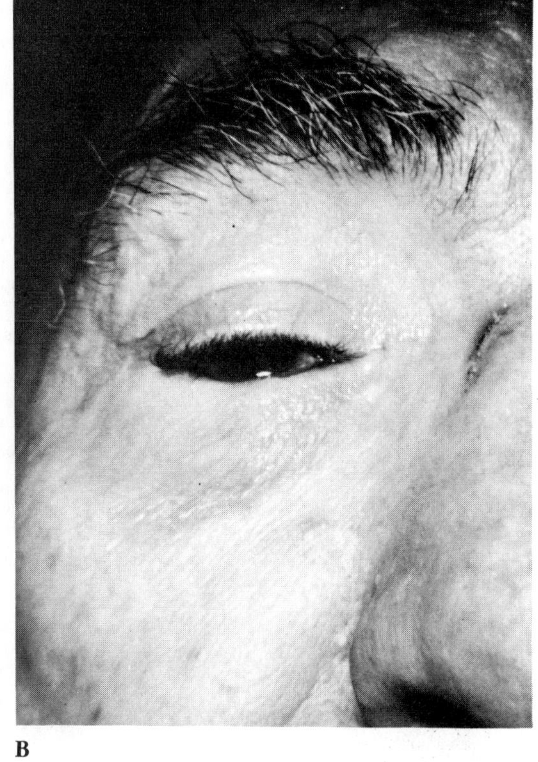
B

Figure 11-5 (A) Extropion of left lower eyelid. (B) Entropion of right lower eyelid.

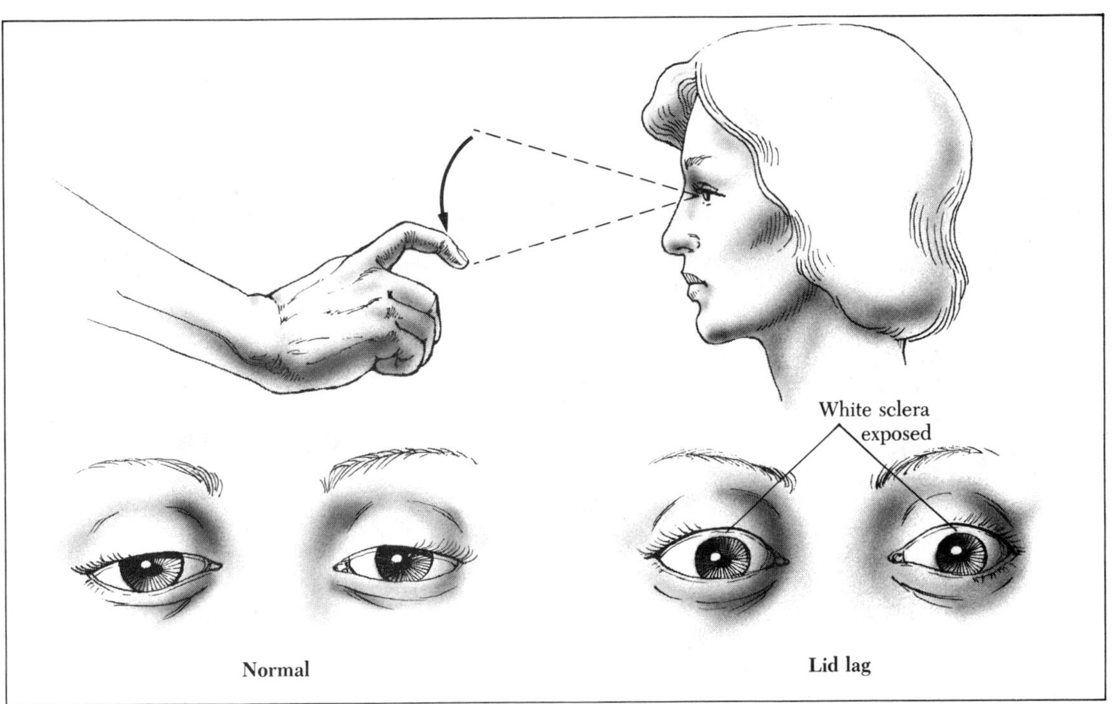

Figure 11-6 Lid lag.

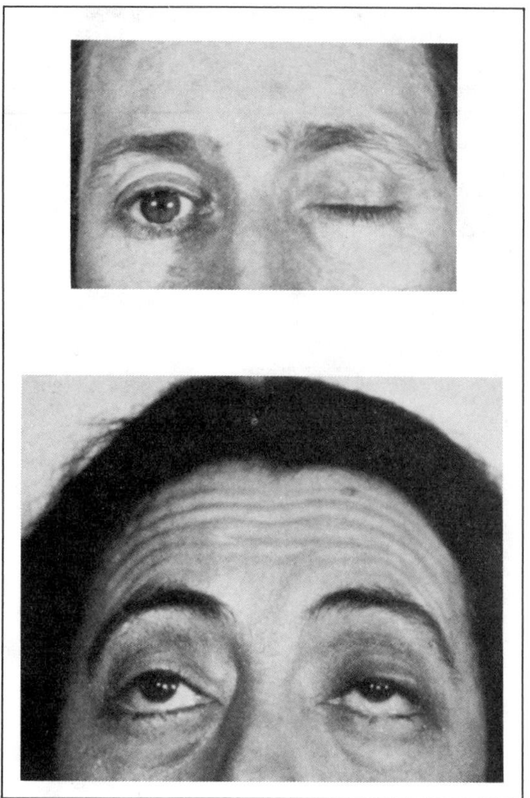

Figure 11-7 Ptosis of left eyelid as a result of oculomotor nerve paralysis.

Ptosis, drooping of the eyelid, can result from muscular weakness, interference with the oculomotor nerve, or interference with the sympathetic nerves that maintain the smooth muscle tone of the eyelid (see Figure 11-7). In Bell's palsy, a disease affecting the 7th cranial nerve, the palpebral fissure is widened and the eyelid will not close. The lower lid sags, and when an attempt is made to close the eyes, the eye on the paralyzed side is seen to roll upward. Partial ptosis may reflect Horner's syndrome, which involves the cervical sympathetic nerves. Marked ptosis of an upper eyelid associated with decreased pupillary light reaction may be an early indication of oculomotor paralysis.

Conjunctiva Examine both the palpebral and the bulbar conjunctiva. To examine the *palpebral conjunctiva*, which lines the underside of the lids, the upper lid must be everted. Figure 11-8 illustrates this technique. With the client looking downward, hold the eyelashes gently forward and upward while placing pressure on the upper tarsal border with an applicator. When the lid is everted, hold the lashes to the brow and inspect the conjunctival surface. The surface of the palpebral conjunctiva is normally pink. To return the lid to its normal position, merely ask

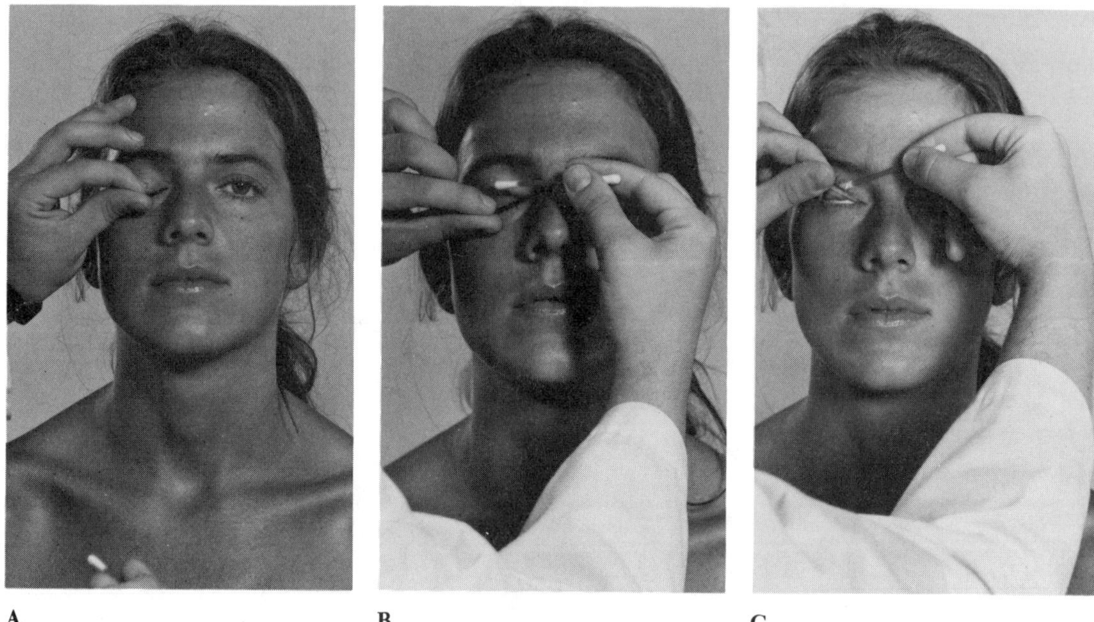

A B C

Figure 11-8 Technique for everting the upper eyelid. (A) Lid pulled down as client looks downward. (B) Pressure applied over tarsal border. (C) Lid gently pulled downward and flipped upward.

the client to look upward. If this does not invert the lid, take hold of the lashes and gently pull forward. The palpebral conjunctiva of anemic clients will generally appear very pale. An erythematous and swollen palpebral conjunctiva indicates irritation or inflammation.

The *bulbar conjunctiva*, which covers the eye up to the limbus (corner of the cornea and sclera), can be observed by separating the lids and having the client look down and to both sides. There are normally many small blood vessels visible on the bulbar conjunctiva. With inflammation (conjunctivitis), the vessels become engorged, and there is redness, swelling, and pain (see Figure 11-9). Not all red eyes are due to conjunctivitis. Individuals who are very tired or who have eyestrain will develop redness of the bulbar conjunctiva. Serious diseases such as iritis, keratitis, and glaucoma can also cause redness and require prompt evaluation and treatment by an ophthalmologist.

Subconjunctival hemorrhage resulting from trauma, increased venous pressure, or hemorrhagic disorders produces a red patch, which is usually in an exposed section of the bulbar conjunctiva (see Figure 11-10). This bright red patch of varying size will most often be reabsorbed in a few days.

A triangular thickening of the bulbar conjunctiva extending from the inner canthus toward the center of the cornea is called a pterygium and is illustrated in Figure 11-11. It may require surgical treatment if vision is impaired.

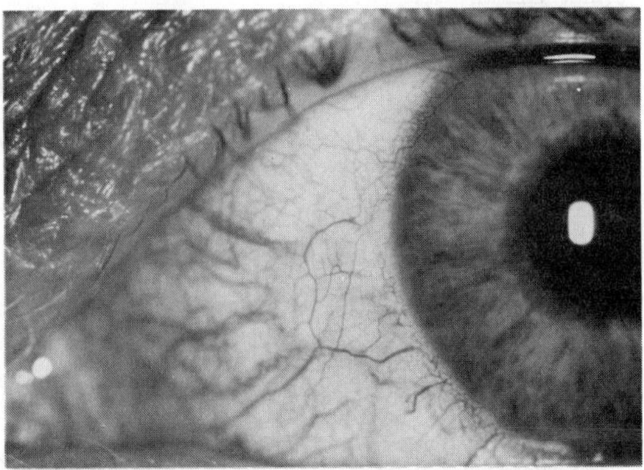

Figure 11-9 Conjunctivitis. (See also endsheet plate 11.)

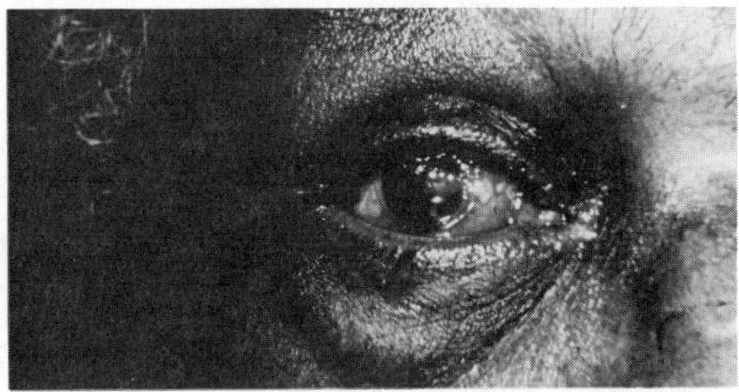

Figure 11-10 Hemorrhage. (See also endsheet plate 12.)

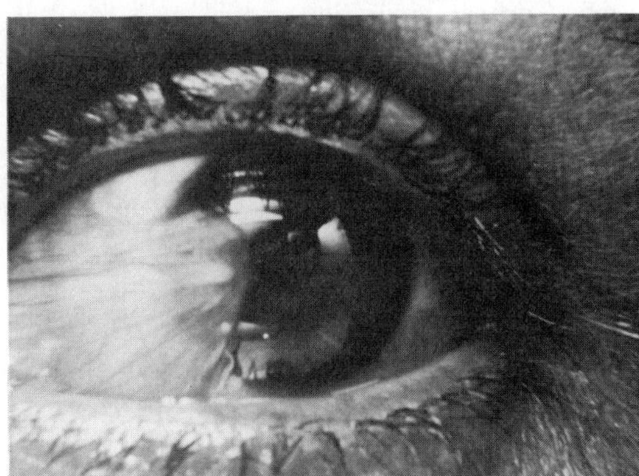

Figure 11-11 Pterygium. (See also endsheet plate 13.)

Sclera Normally the sclera is white. In occasional Blacks it may have a gray-blue hue that is generally recorded as "muddy." In hepatitis the sclerae may become a bright yellow; in obstructive jaundice, greenish yellow; and in pernicious anemia, lemon yellow. Cyanosis and pallor may also be detected by careful observation of the sclerae.

Cornea Note the clearness of the eye. The normal eye has a moist glossiness. A dullness may be noted in nutritional deficiencies (especially avitaminosis A), glaucoma, and hypercholesteremia. The cornea is normally smooth and transparent. Inspect the cornea from an oblique view by shining a penlight on it. Superficial irregularities can be detected in this manner. Any ulceration or opacity is abnormal. Pain, photophobia, and redness of the bulbar conjunctiva accompany active ulcerations. Yellow opacities usually indicate active ulcerations whereas bluish white opacities indicate healed ulcerations. Abrasions are almost impossible to detect with superficial light and need to be stained with fluorescein. Abrasions will stain a brilliant yellow-green color. This staining technique is not part of a routine physical assessment process; when this procedure is warranted, it should be carried out

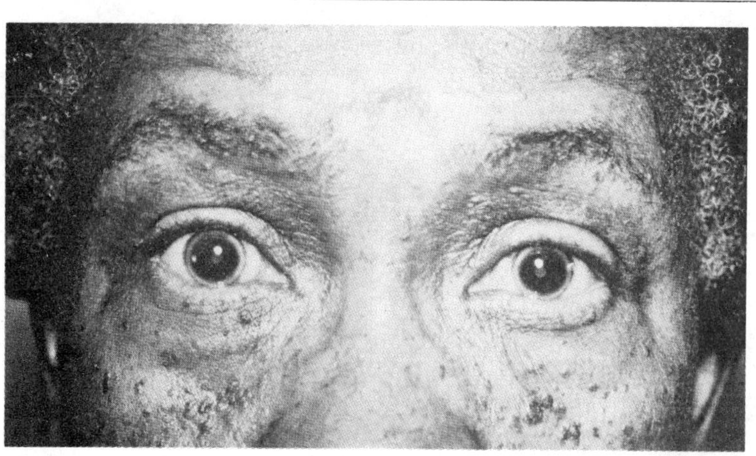

Figure 11-12 Arcus senilis.

only if you have been specially trained in the technique.

Diseases of the cornea are often severe. Trachoma, relatively rare in the United States, causes more blindness in the world than any other condition. Trachoma is a chronic infection of the conjunctiva caused by microorganisms. In the United States, it has a higher incidence among American Indians and Mexican Americans. Corneal ulceration, which can result in corneal perforation, is a major cause of blindness in this country. It can be precipitated by a number of causes, including allergy, diabetes mellitus, and trauma.

In older Caucasians and Blacks, an arch or circle of cloudy white-gray-blue material may be found encircling the periphery of the cornea; this phenomenon is called arcus senilis (see Figure 11-12). It is insignificant unless observed in younger people. Kayser-Fleischer rings—brown-green rings of pigment around the corneal limbus—are of pathologic significance. They occur in Wilson's disease, which manifests serious neurologic and liver degeneration.

The corneal reflex should be tested late in the examination of the eye by touching a wisp of cotton to the center of the cornea and observing for rapid lid closure. Figure 11-13 illustrates this technique. You should approach the client from the side because seeing the cotton wisp near his eye might in itself cause blinking. Test both eyes; they should have equal reaction. Lack of corneal sensitivity indicates injury of the sensory component of the 5th cranial (trigeminal) nerve or failure of lid closure may be due to injury of the motor component of the 7th cranial (facial) nerve.

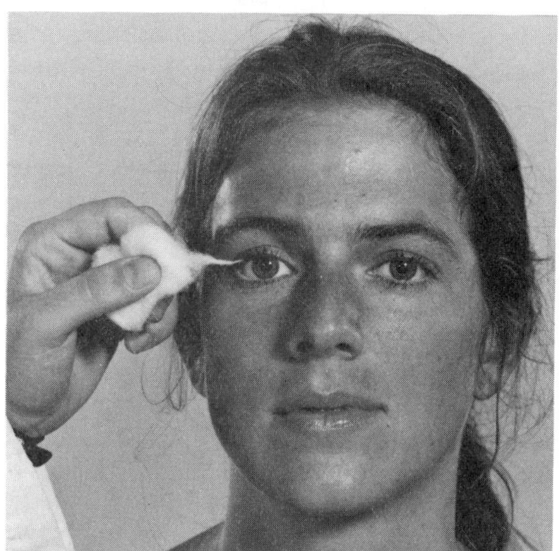

Figure 11-13 Technique for testing corneal reflex.

Pupils Normally the pupils are recorded as PERRLA (pupils equal, round, react to light and accommodation). Inequality in pupil size is called anisocoria. Unequal pupils are always considered abnormal and in need of further investigation. However, there is a nonpathologic condition called Adie's syndrome in which one pupil is dilated. It is observed in young women (see Figure 11-14). In clients with head injury the pupils may be small and unreactive to light, dilated and fixed, or unequal. Drugs, too, have pronounced effects on the pupil. Morphine acts to constrict the pupils, whereas cocaine dilates

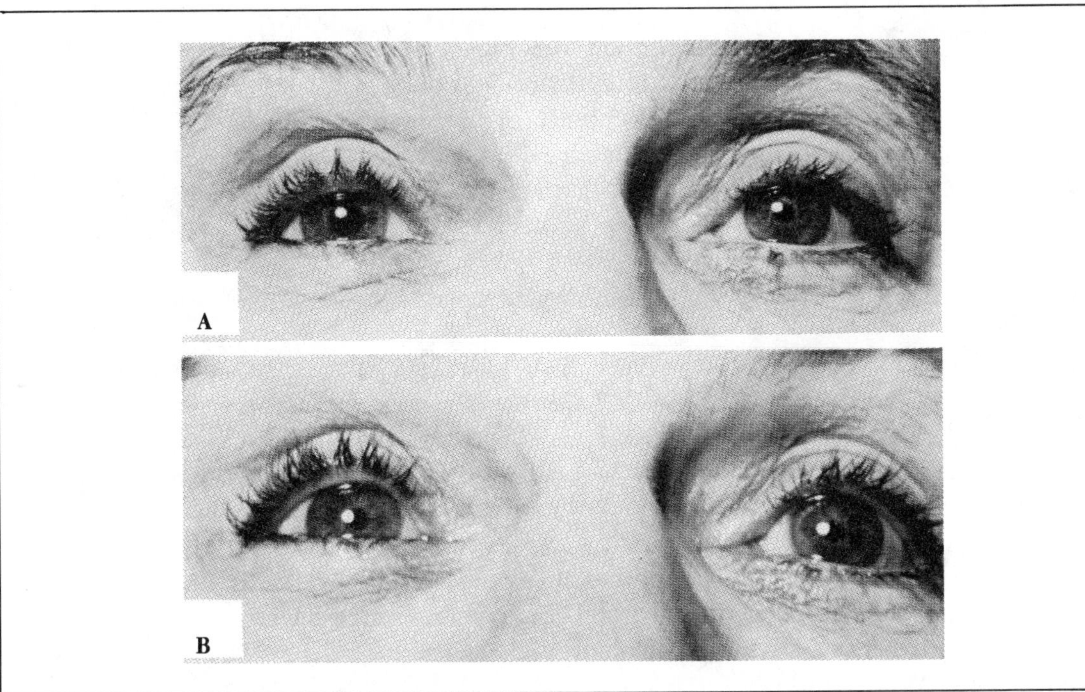

Figure 11-14 Adie's pupil. (A) Unilateral tonic pupil. (B) Constriction following instillation of Mecholyl.

them by stimulating the sympathetic nerve endings. Dilated unreactive pupils are observed in conditions of anoxia or in deep barbiturate poisoning. Cranial tumors can produce dilation or constriction of the pupils, depending on where they are located in the cranium.

To test for direct pupillary reaction, stand on one side of the client and focus a penlight on the pupil. The normal pupillary reaction is constriction. To test for consensual reaction to light, perform the same procedure but observe the opposite pupil—it should also constrict even though no direct light is focused on it. Perform these tests on both eyes. In situations where the optic nerve is diseased, the affected eye will have no direct reaction to light, although it will react consensually if the unaffected eye is stimulated. When the affected eye is stimulated, however, the unaffected eye will not react consensually.

Accommodation is the phenomenon whereby the pupils dilate to bring in more light when looking at a distant object. To test accommodation, have the client look at a distant point and then at your fingers or a pencil held about 15 cm (6 in.) away from and lateral to his face. As the eyes focus on the near object the pupils should narrow. A bright toy held afar and then quickly brought toward a child's eyes will also provoke pupillary contraction. As the eyes focus on a near object both eyes move medially; this phenomenon is normal and is called convergence reaction.

In chronic syphilis the pupils are usually small and irregular and do not dilate in response to mydriatic drugs. The pupils fail to react to light but do accommodate. This phenomenon is referred to as the Argyll Robertson pupil.

The important point in checking for accommodation response is to verify its presence and to determine whether it is equal in both eyes. It is important to recognize that older persons often do not accommodate well and will show a slower, sluggish response. In the infant the accommodation reflex is present by the age of 6 months.

Extraocular Muscles The extrinsic muscles of the eye are those attached to the outside of the eyeball and to the bones of the orbit. They are voluntary muscles responsible for eye movement, and they are innervated by the somatic fibers of the 3rd, 4th, and 6th cranial nerves. Normally these muscles are able to move the eyes in six basic directions. To test whether the extraocular muscles are functioning normally, face the client and ask him to follow a finger or

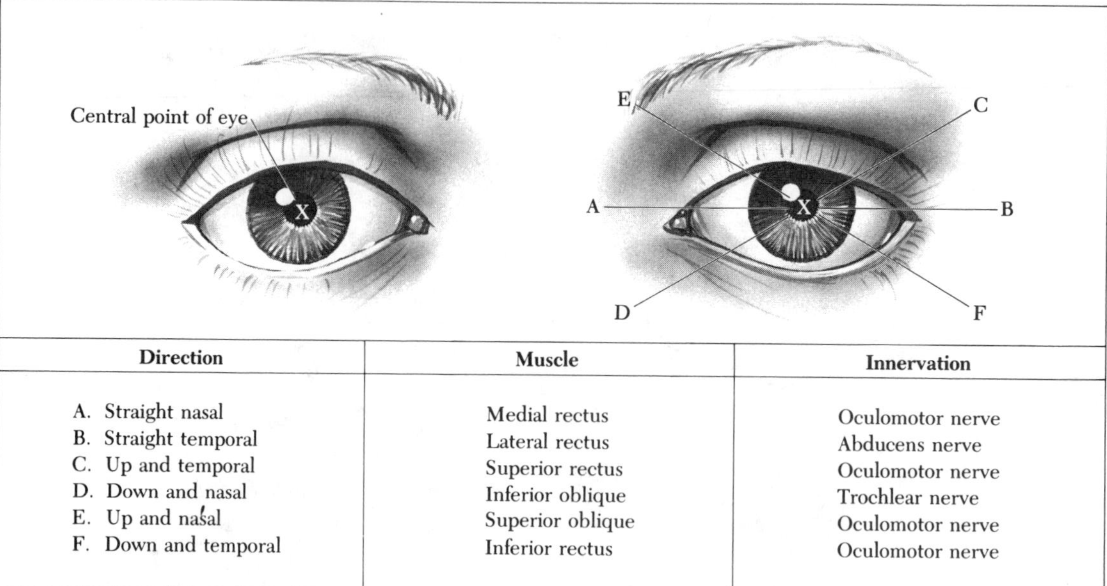

Direction	Muscle	Innervation
A. Straight nasal	Medial rectus	Oculomotor nerve
B. Straight temporal	Lateral rectus	Abducens nerve
C. Up and temporal	Superior rectus	Oculomotor nerve
D. Down and nasal	Inferior oblique	Trochlear nerve
E. Up and nasal	Superior oblique	Oculomotor nerve
F. Down and temporal	Inferior rectus	Oculomotor nerve

Figure 11-15 Cardinal positions of the eye.

moving object as it is moved through the six cardinal positions as illustrated in Figure 11-15. For example, a pencil held at least 30 cm (12 in.) from the client's face is moved from the central point of the eye to the nose and then back to the central starting point; then it is moved to the temporal side of the face, and so on. With a child it is best for you to place a free hand on the top of the child's head so that only the eyes move and not the head.

The eyes should follow the movement smoothly and symmetrically. Inability to move the eye in one of these directions indicates weakness or paralysis of the muscle that corresponds to the particular cardinal position (see Figure 11-16). While performing this test, also observe for nystagmus, an involuntary rhythmic back and forth movement of the eye in a lateral or vertical direction. Although it often occurs in normal persons, it can be the result of a neurologic condition.

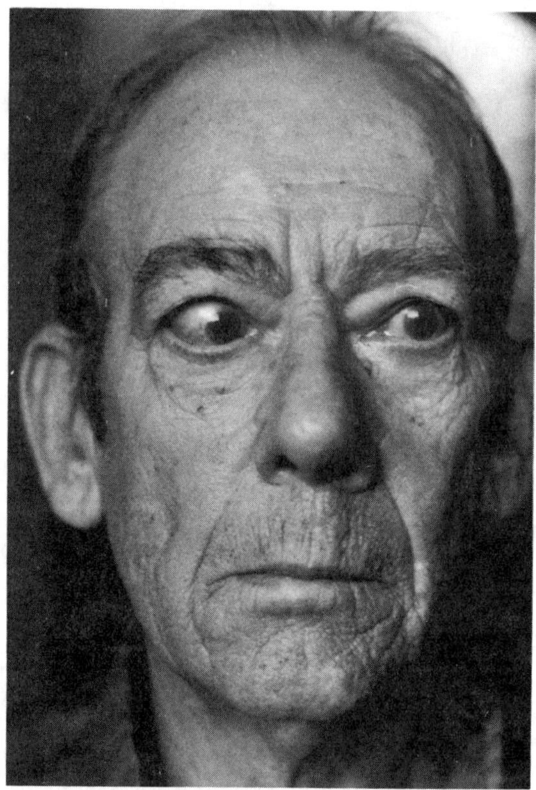

Figure 11-16 Rectus eye muscle.

Intraocular Pressure Palpation of intraocular pressure, shown in Figure 11-17, provides only a crude measurement but may alert you to any abnormality in consistency. Softness is indicative of dehydration. Increased tension would feel similar to the consistency of palpating the tip of your nose. Increased intraocular tension may indicate glaucoma, a serious condition in which unchecked pressure can lead to blindness. If glaucoma is discovered early, it is possible to prevent further damage to the retina by the use of medications or special surgical procedures.

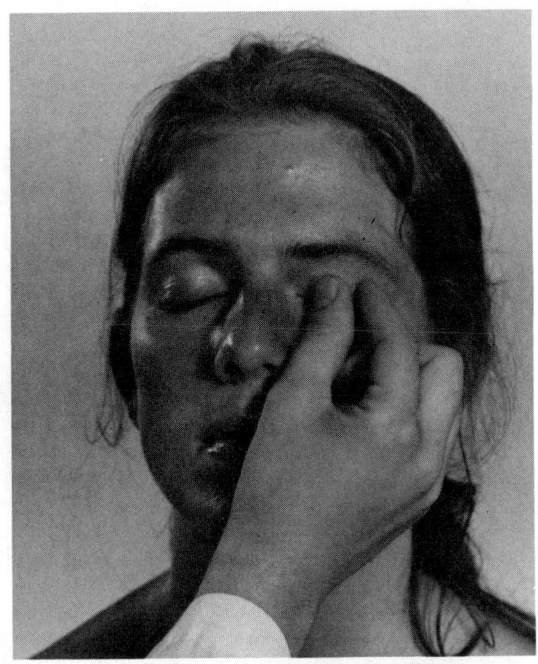

Figure 11-17 Palpation of intraocular pressure.

Since glaucoma has a higher incidence in the middle-aged and elderly population, it is important that routine tonometry, as shown in Figure 11-18, be performed every 2–3 years on all clients over 40 years of age.

Visual Fields

A crude estimate of the peripheral fields of vision can be obtained by a technique called gross confrontation. Figure 11-19 illustrates this procedure. You should be face to face with the client and standing about 2 ft away. With this procedure you are comparing your own field of vision with the client's.

The client's horizontal field of vision is smaller because of interference by the eyebrow, nose, and cheekbone. Therefore, as your fingers move forward from the top of the client's head he should be able to see them at about a 50° angle. The field of vision is about 60° medially and about 70° downward. Any significant reduction of the client's field of vision should be confirmed

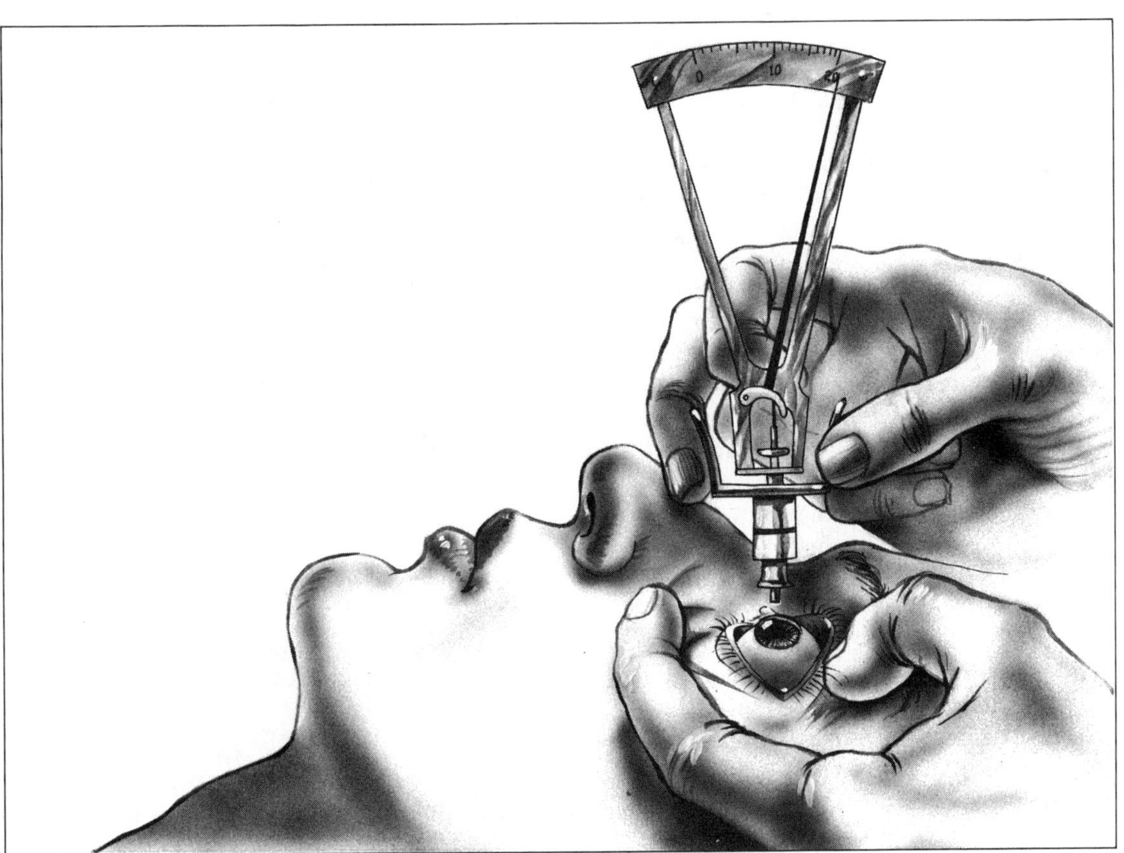

Figure 11-18 Tonometry examination.

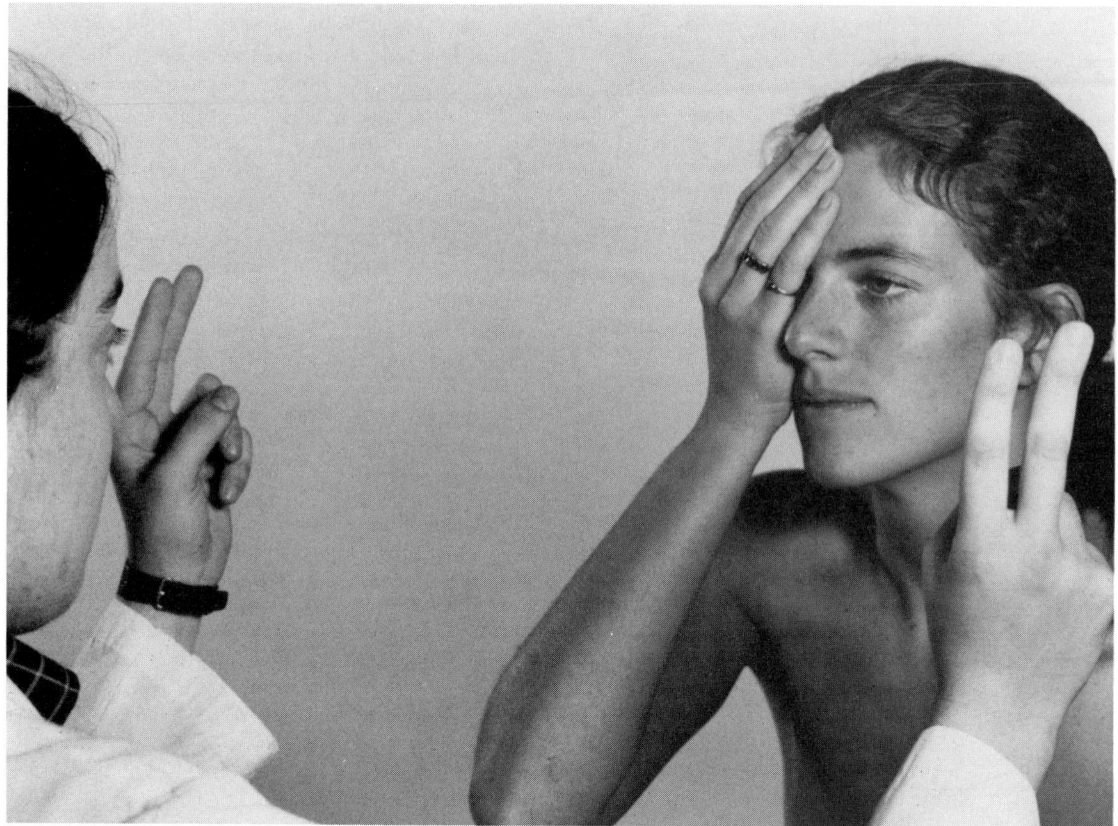

Figure 11-19 Gross confrontation technique.

by an ophthalmologist. Glaucoma is a common serious condition that restricts visual fields.

Visual Acuity

It is crucial that children between the ages of 1 and 6 have annual visual screening, as these years constitute the critical period of development of acute vision. Early detection is imperative to counteract permanent visual defects. Because preschool visual screening in the United States is presently inadequate, parents may want to perform vision screening tests at home with home eye test kits obtained from the National Association for the Prevention of Blindness (16 E. 40th Street, New York, NY). Slight defects must be further assessed by an ophthalmologist.

Testing of visual acuity with the older child and the adult is accomplished by using an eye chart, as shown in Figure 11-20. The client stands 20 feet from the chart and is directed to cover one eye and read the numbers from the top of the chart down. Then he covers the opposite eye and reads the chart again. You then re-

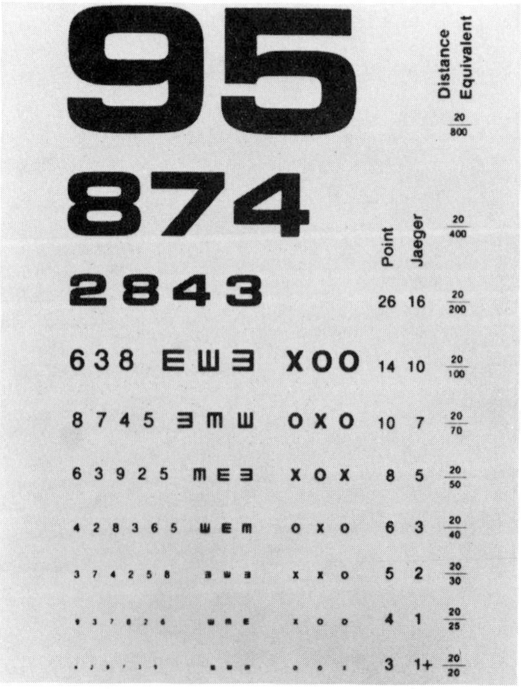

Figure 11-20 Example of an eye chart.

Techniques for Inspection and Palpation of the Eye

1. Adequate lighting.
2. Fullness of eyebrows.
3. Lacrimal apparatus: raise eyelid; check between upper lid and eyeball; apply finger pressure to lacrimal sac.
4. Eyelids: evaluate and observe:
   a. Palpebral fissure.
   b. Position.
   c. Conjunctiva:
      (1) palpebral: gently evert upper lid.
      (2) bulbar: separate lids; have client look down and to both sides.
   d. Sclera.
   e. Cornea: use oblique lighting.
   f. Pupils—equal, round.
   g. Pupillary reaction to light: bring penlight from lateral side to focus on pupil.
   h. Consensual reaction: note response of the pupil of one eye as light is focused on the opposite eye.
   i. Accommodation: tell client to look at distant spot then at finger 15 cm away from and lateral to face.
   j. Convergence: have client follow your finger as it is moved inward to 2–3 inches from the tip of the client's nose.
5. Extraocular muscles: face client directly; have client follow finger or pencil through six cardinal positions.
6. Intraocular pressure: have client close eyes; place tip of thumb and index finger lightly on eyelid; palpate gently for consistency.
7. Visual fields: face client directly at 2 ft away; ask client to cover one eye. Cover your opposite eye; have client fix gaze on your uncovered eye; place outstretched arm equidistant between client and you. If client is unable to see your fingers at this point, move your wriggling fingers toward the nose. Repeat same procedure, moving hand from the superior, inferior, and medial periphery of the visual field of the eye being assessed. Repeat the procedure for the opposite eye.

cord the last line of which the client can read at least 50% of the numbers. This recording is a fraction. The numerator expresses the distance to the chart (20 feet), and the denominator, listed by each line on the chart, represents the distance at which the average eye can read that particular line of the chart. Therefore, a recording of 20/40 means that the client is 20 feet away from the chart and can read the line that the average eye can read at 40 feet. A recording of 20/200 indicates that at 20 feet the client can read only the largest number of the chart. This number can be seen at 200 feet by a person with normal vision. Any recording greater than 20/40 is referred for ophthalmologic assessment

For young preschoolers and people who cannot read, a chart such as this one where the letter "E" is arranged in different positions and of various sizes can be used. In this situation the client merely points to the direction in which the legs of the "E" are facing.

The results of the visual acuity testing are recorded for each eye and for both eyes: for example, OD (right eye) 20/30; OS (left eye) 20/20; and OU (both eyes) 20/20. If the client customarily wears glasses for distance, they should be worn for the test. Reading glasses often blur distant vision. Always record whether corrective lenses were worn during the examination. Table 11-1 describes the range of visual acuity, lists symptoms of visual conditions, and provides corrective methods.

Ophthalmoscopic Examination

The ophthalmoscopic examination of the eye requires a great deal of practice, so the beginner should not become discouraged.

Careful examination of the interior eye will assist in detecting not only eye diseases but systemic disease as well. Several structures are examined through the ophthalmoscope—the lens, retina, optic disk, arteries, veins, and macula.

Conducting the Examination The posterior eye (fundus) is best examined when the pupil is dilated, but dilation is not done routinely during health assessment unless the client's history or other physical findings indicate that a more thorough examination is needed. If so, refer the

Table 11-1. Types of Visual Acuity

Condition	Interpretation	Signs and symptoms	Treatment
Emmetropia 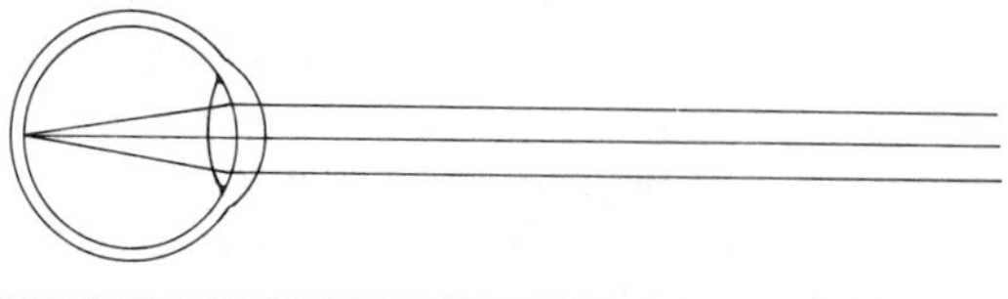	Ideal eye	None: light is focused on retina easily by accommodation	None
Hypermetropia (Hyperopia) 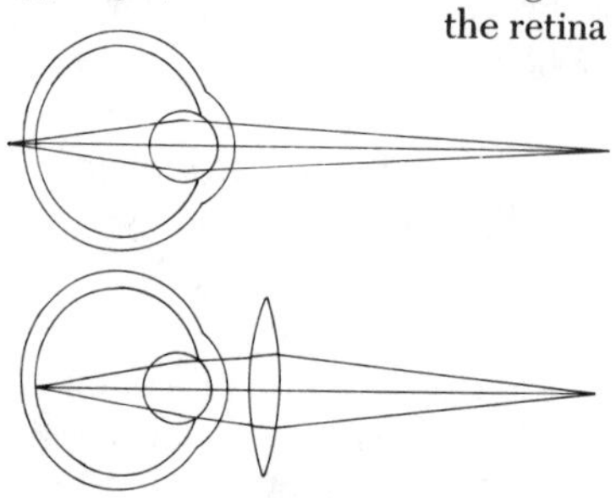	Far-sighted eye; light is brought to focus behind the retina	Eyestrain; may be blurring of vision, headache, nausea	Convex lens
Myopia 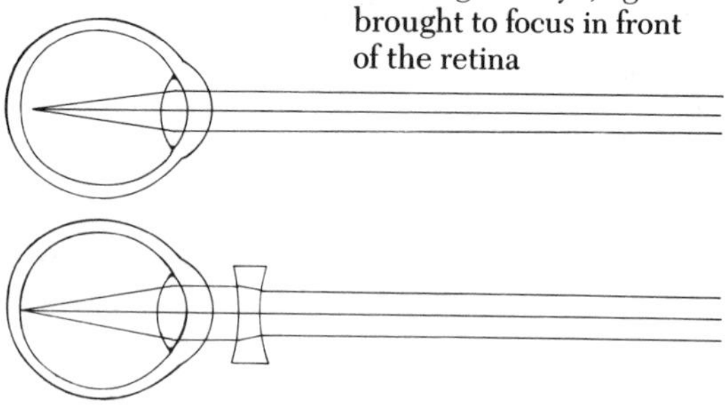	Near-sighted eye; light is brought to focus in front of the retina	Defective vision; eyestrain not as frequent as noticed in hyperopia	Concave lens
Astigmatism 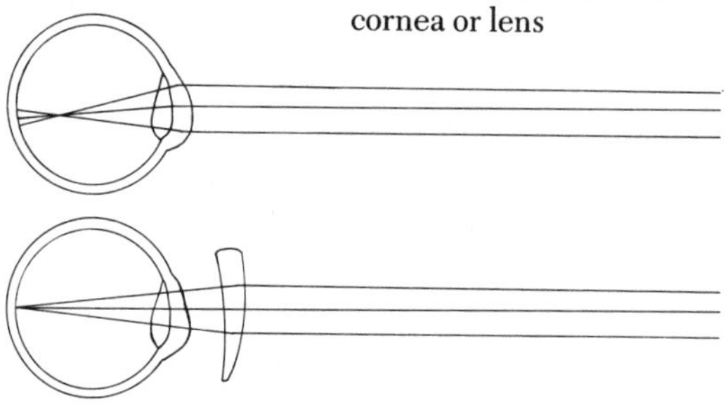	Abnormal curvature of cornea or lens	Defective vision; images do not focus properly on retina (irregular astigmatism may follow corneal injury or ulcer)	Corrective lenses (cylindrical, thick); glasses worn continuously in high degrees; in lower degrees only for work causing eyestrain
Presbyopia	"Old sighted" eye; physiologic process in which lens begin to lose elasticity and ciliary muscles begin to weaken, resulting in gradual loss of accommodation; usually affects persons past the age of 45	Inability to read without holding reading material over 30 cm away from the eye	Glasses for near work; bifocals (distant correction plus magnifying lenses at the bottom for near vision)

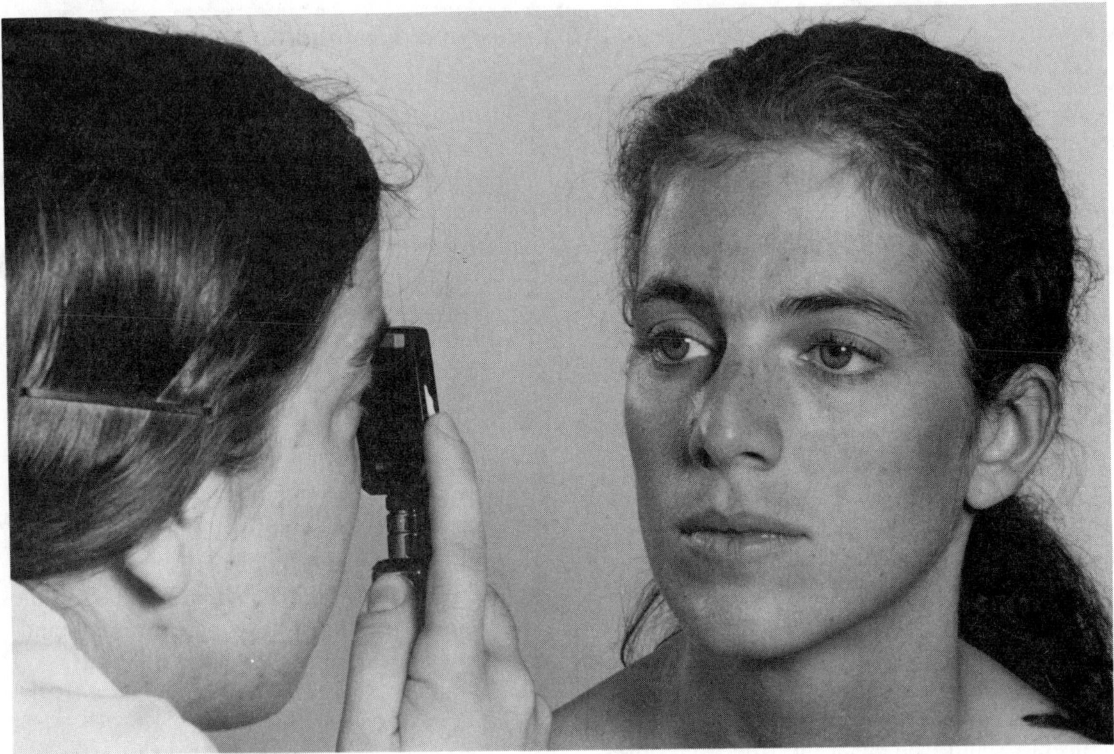

Figure 11-21 Same-eyes examination technique.

client to be examined by a physician or an ophthalmologist, whichever is more appropriate with regard to your findings.

For optimum viewing of the eyegrounds (fundus), the room should be darkened. Begin by facing the client either in a sitting or standing position. As Figure 11-21 illustrates, the hand holding the ophthalmoscope, your examining eye, and the client's eye to be examined should all be on the same side of the body. In other words, your *right* hand holds the ophthalmoscope while your *right* eye examines the client's *right* eye. Failure to use this procedure will result in an uncomfortable collision with the client's nose. If you can use only one examining eye, you can avoid collision by examining the client's opposite eye while he is in the supine position. This approach is illustrated in Figure 11-22. In this position the client's opposite eye can be approached from the head of the examining table; this upside-down approach will place your nose lateral to the client's head. Most practitioners who wear glasses or contact lenses do not remove them while performing the examination.

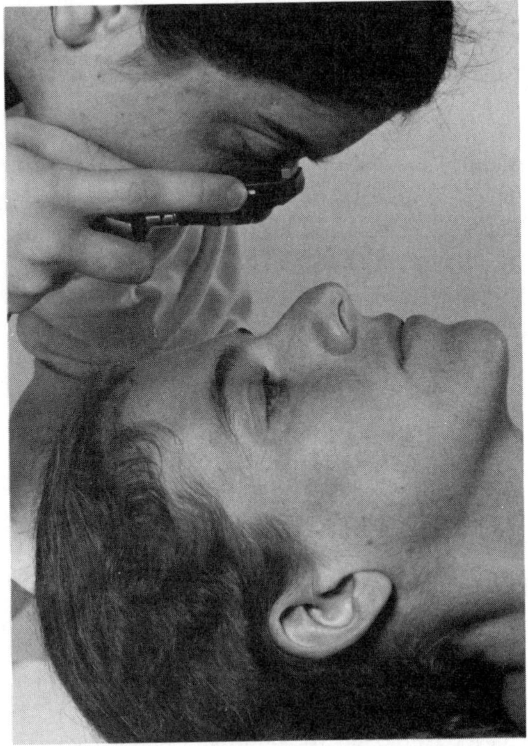

Figure 11-22 Inverse head-of-bed approach.

Technique for the Ophthalmoscopic Examination

1. Darken room.
2. Face client, sitting or standing.
3. Holding ophthalmoscope in right hand, use your right eye to examine client's right eye. Repeat for left eye, using left hand and left eye to client's left eye.
4. Place index finger on focus wheel.
5. Hold ophthalmoscope firmly against your brow.
6. Position viewing aperture in front of your eye.
7. Hold client's upper eyelid open with thumb of your "free" hand.
8. Direct beam of light into client's pupil from distance of 30 cm and find red reflex.
9. Move closer with red reflex toward the client's pupil until client's and your foreheads are almost touching.
10. Note characteristics of retina, disk, and vessels.

You should place your index finger on the lens wheel to allow for focusing and brace the head of the ophthalmoscope solidly against your brow, with the viewing aperture positioned in front of your eye. Begin the examination by directing the beam of light into the client's pupil from a distance of about 30 cm; a red reflex from the healthy fundus will be seen to fill the eye. The red reflex should be clear and free from opacities. Then begin to move closer following this reflex until both your foreheads are almost touching.

Blinking of the client's eye can interfere with the examination. You can control this reflex by slightly elevating the upper lid of the client's eye with the thumb of your free hand. The remainder of your free hand can be rested upon the client's head and will serve to steady it. Movement will cause the beam of examining light to move out of alignment with the client's pupil. The lens, controlled by the lens wheel, should be set at zero and then adjusted to the setting that provides the best viewing. Minus numbers (red) focus further away; plus numbers (black) focus nearer. The red reflex must be kept in focus until your forehead is practically touching that of the client. If you lose it, move back and begin again.

Absence of the red reflex indicates poor positioning of the ophthalmoscope or an abnormality of light transmission through the lens. If there are diffuse dense opacities in the client's eye, a dull red or black reflex will be observed. Black spots showing against the red reflex are produced by opacities in the lens or vitreous humor. The dark spots, when visualized, can be clearly focused by moving the ophthalmoscope back and forth. Once they are focused, ask the client to look slightly upward. Spots on the cornea or anterior lens will move upward, whereas vitreous opacities will remain stationary.

In order to recognize abnormalities of the eyegrounds, you must have a clear understanding of the appearance of the normal fundus.

Examination of the fundus begins with the location and assessment of the optic disk. To visualize the disk, direct the light of the ophthalmoscope from about 15° temporal to the straight-ahead gaze of the client. The disk is situated more nasally on the retina and normally appears round or vertically oval with flat discrete edges. It is a creamy yellow or pinkish-yellow color and is about 1.5 mm in diameter. The diameter, referred to as DD (disk diameter), is a unit of measure used to document the location and diameter of lesions (distance in disk diameters from the optic disk margin). Abnormal findings are also located according to the hour sign on the face of a clock. A sample recording would be: dark red spot ¼ DD in size, 1½ DD away @ 3:00. Most disks have a funnel-shaped depression in the temporal side that presents as a white or pale yellow area; it does not extend completely to the disk margin. This is referred to as the physiologic depression, or physiologic cup.

Vessels can be seen emerging from the cup and extending to the periphery of the retina. Arteries are bright red and reflect a narrow white streak of light. They are smaller than veins; the normal artery-vein ratio is about 2:3. Veins lack the central white reflex stripe and are larger and darker red than arteries (see Figure 11-23). Usually at the proximal end of veins a slight pulsation can be visualized; this pulsation is normal and helps to differentiate veins from arteries—retinal arteries do not pulsate.

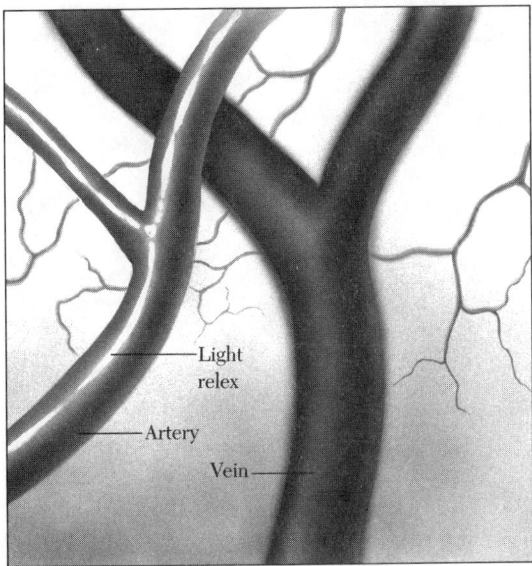

Figure 11-23 Normal retinal artery and vein.

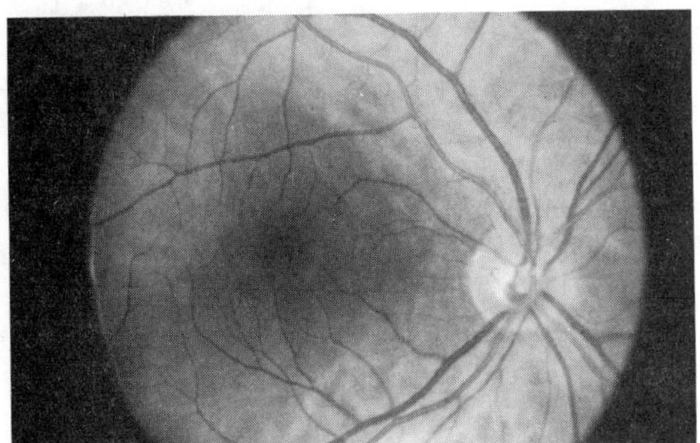

Figure 11-24 Caucasian fundus. (See also endsheet plate 14.)

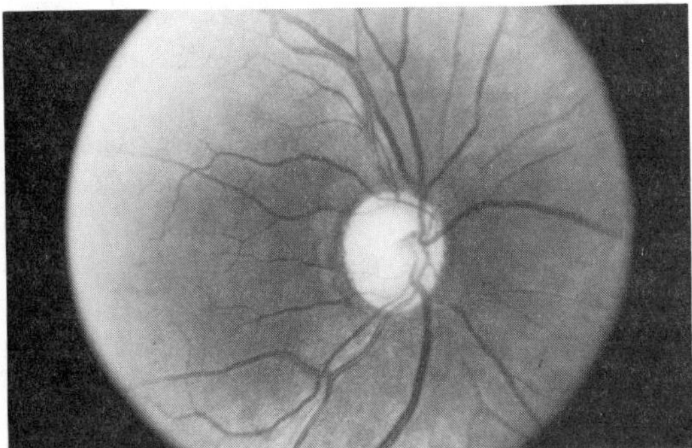

Figure 11-25 Black fundus. (See also endsheet plate 15.)

The arteriovenous decussations (where the arteries and veins cross) should be carefully observed for any indentation (nicking) or displacement (humping). These do not normally exist in the healthy individual.

If you have difficulty finding the optic disk, follow a vessel. The vessel will become larger as it approaches the optic disk, and will eventually meet and enter the disk.

The entire fundus should be examined by having the client rotate the eye so that different areas can be explored. The macula should be examined last, as it is the point most sensitive to light. The macula is a small area about 1 DD wide and approximately 2–3 DD temporal to the disk and in the same horizontal plane. It is a slightly deeper red color than the surrounding fundus. It is avascular, and the bright spot in the middle represents reflected light from the fovea centralis.

The pigmentation of the fundus can vary and still remain within normal limits. Generally, the darker the skin, the darker the fundus and vice versa. Figure 11-24 shows a normal Caucasian fundus, while Figure 11-25 shows a normal Black fundus, which has a darker blue tint.

The optic nerve fibers are myelinated up to the point where they emerge into the retina. In some individuals the myelination of these fibers continues beyond the lamina cribrosa, producing a striking appearance. This is a normal variation in which semiopaque white brushes project from about the disk, partially or completely obscuring the retinal vessels and disk margin.

Interpreting Findings The red reflex provides information about the condition of the transparent portions of the eye. Small cataracts, corneal scars, and opacities will produce a shadow in the red reflex. Hemorrhage and extensive cataracts may completely block out the reflex. The major abnormalities affecting the optic disk are papilledema, optic atrophy, and "glaucomatous cup."

Papilledema (choked disk) is a serious condition in which either unilateral or bilateral swelling and elevation of the nerve head is seen, with the retinal vessels bending sharply over its edge. Signs of papilledema are blurred margins of the optic disk, filling in of the physiologic depression, full retinal veins, and absence of venous pulsations. Many disease states produce papilledema; the most common are increased intracranial pressure (from brain tumor, hydrocephalus, meningitis, or subarachnoid hemorrhage) and severe hypertension. The presence of papilledema, illustrated in Figure 11-26, is often the first sign of a serious condition.

Optic atrophy results from partial or com-

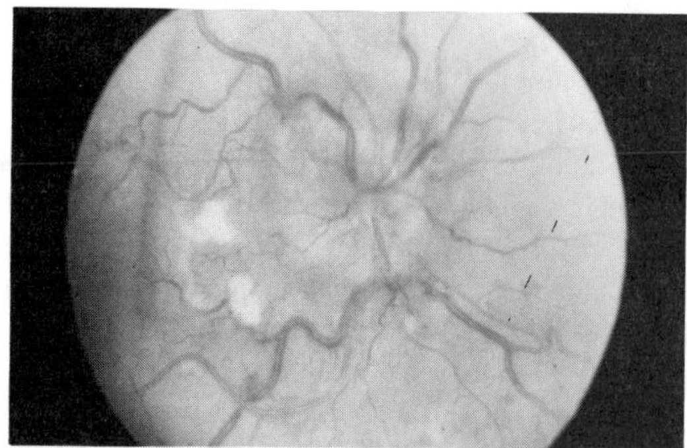

Figure 11-26 Papilledema. (See also endsheet plate 16.)

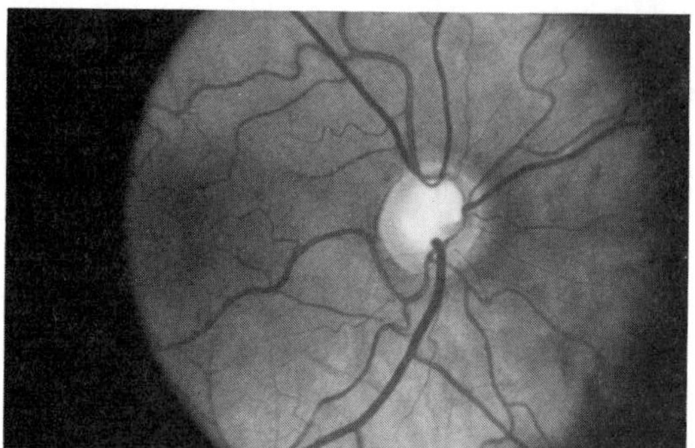

Figure 11-27 Glaucomatous cup. (See also endsheet plate 17.)

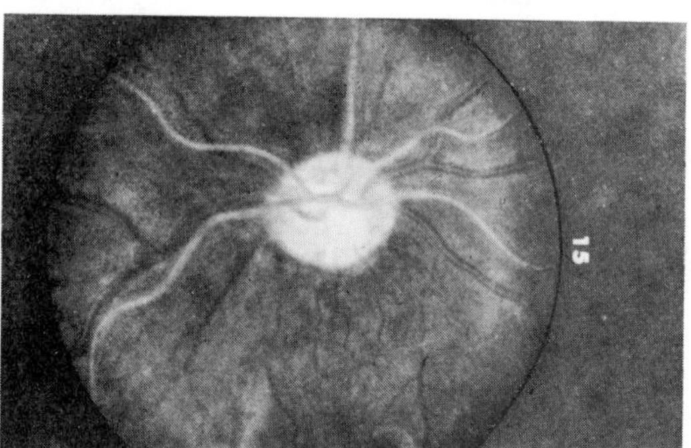

Figure 11-28 Copper-wire arteries. (See also endsheet plate 18.)

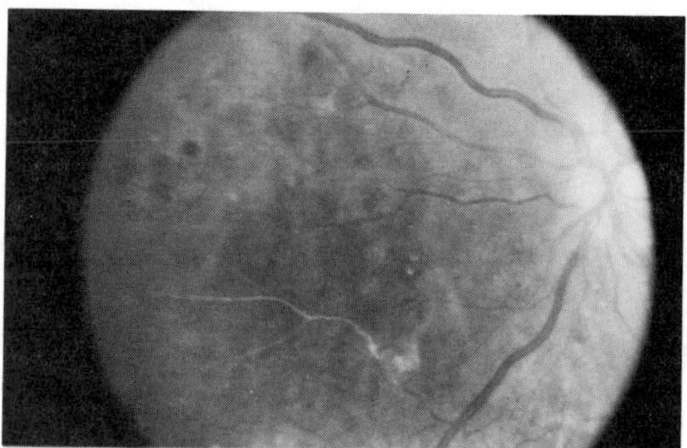

Figure 11-29 Silver-wire arteries. (See also endsheet plate 19.)

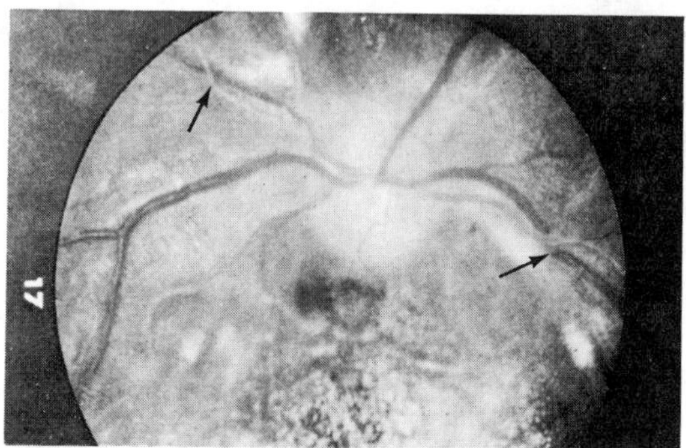

Figure 11-30 AV nicking. (See also endsheet plate 20.)

plete compression (death) of the optic nerve and can cause blindness. It is presented as pallor or a chalky whiteness of the disk. This condition can be caused by severe papilledema, glaucoma, or tumors of the brain. Nerve degeneration occurs in conditions such as multiple sclerosis and in rare cases may be hereditary. Optic atrophy is frequently observed in tabes dorsalis.

"Glaucomatous cup," as shown in Figure 11-27, is a diagnostic sign of glaucoma. The cup may be deep and is bluish white, with the vessels disappearing behind the edge of the cup.

The small retinal vessels are most sensitive to disease processes. The walls of the arterioles are transparent when viewed by the ophthalmoscope; what is seen is a column of blood. In arteriosclerosis, usually occurring with hypertension, the lumens of the vessels are narrowed because of fibrous tissue replacement. The light reflection becomes brighter. In moderate disease the arteries may be a burnished copper color (*copper-wire arteries*) (see Figure 11-28). Later, in far advanced arteriosclerosis, they will appear as widened white strips (*silver-wire arteries*) (see Figure 11-29). Also, the arteries will disappear sooner than the veins, as both project out toward the periphery of the fundus. When the arteries become thick and stiff, they will cause deflection of a vein as they cross it. This condition is referred to as arteriovenous (AV) notching or nicking (see Figure 11-30). With AV nicking a portion of the vein on either side of the overlying artery is not visible.

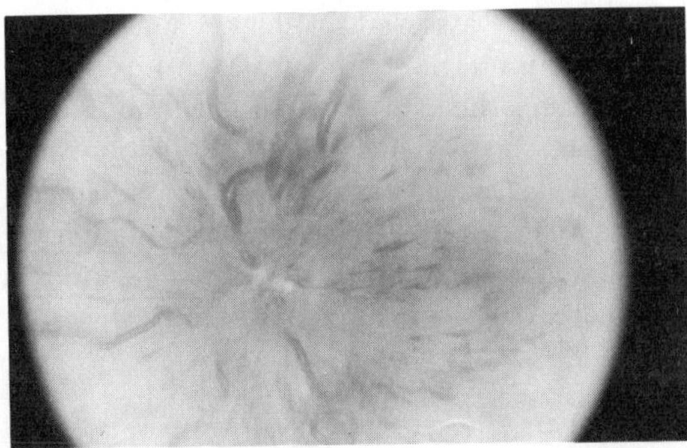

Figure 11-31 Tortuous vein distention. (See also endsheet plate 21.)

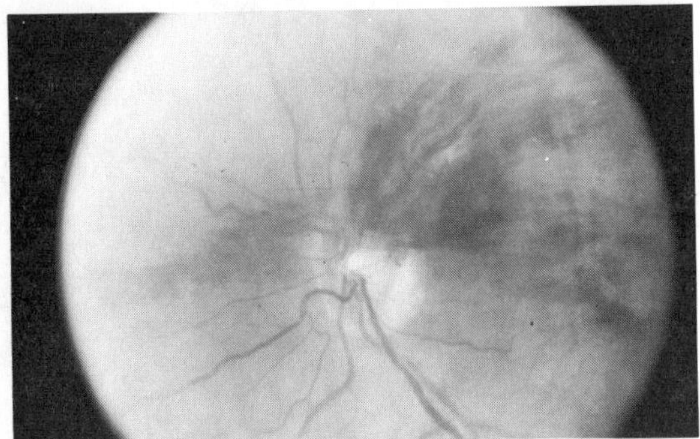

Figure 11-32 Blotchy hemorrhage. (See also endsheet plate 22.)

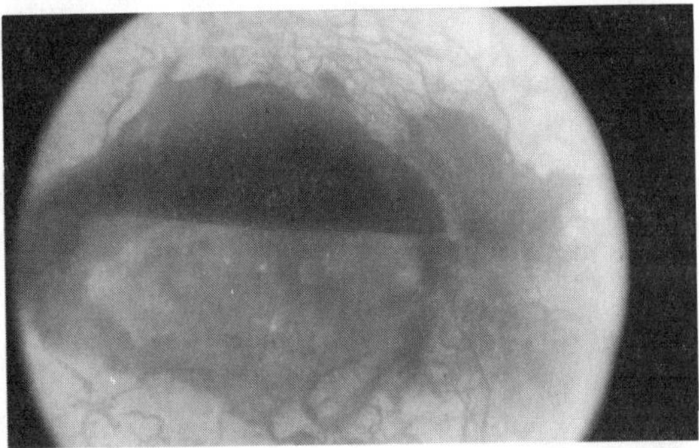

Figure 11-33 Blotchy hemorrhage. (See also endsheet plate 23.)

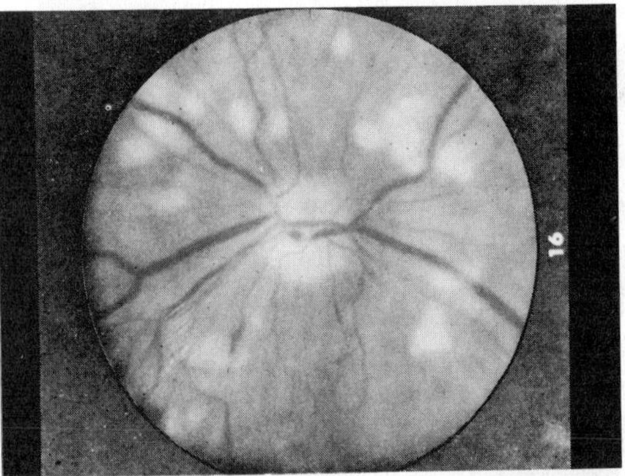

Figure 11-34 Cotton-wool patches. (See also endsheet plate 24.)

Tortuous and engorged veins are often observed in atherosclerosis, diabetes mellitus, multiple myeloma, polycythemia, and leukemia. Venous distention can occur in congenital heart disease, diabetes mellitus, and leukemia (see Figure 11-31).

Hemorrhages and exudates are always pathognomonic. The shape of the hemorrhage indicates the depth at which it occurs in the retina. Superficial hemorrhages are flame shaped, and deeper ones are more round and blotchy. See Figures 11-32 and 11-33 for examples of blotchy hemorrhages. Small, rounded hemorrhages are seen in diabetes mellitus, whereas flame-shaped hemorrhages are seen in hypertension. The presence of microaneurysms, tiny discrete red dots with smooth edges, is often suggestive of diabetes mellitus, where they occur chiefly about the macula. They may be difficult to distinguish from small hemorrhages, but it is helpful to know that hemorrhages usually have irregular and slightly blurred edges.

Exudates, which occur in many systemic diseases including diabetes mellitus and hypertension, are dense, grayish localized retinal infiltrates. There are two types: "soft" and "hard." The soft exudates, often referred to as "cotton-wool patches" (see Figure 11-34), are gray to white fluffy, indistinct areas. Soft exudates are arteriolar microinfarctions. They are often accompanied by microaneurysms. Cotton-wool patches occur in hypertension, subacute bacterial endocarditis, and lupus erythematosus, and with papilledema regardless of its cause. Hard exudates, illustrated in Figure 11-35, are numerous small whitish-yellow spots with distinct edges and smooth solid-looking surfaces. Hard exudates are thought to be intraretinal lipoid or colloid deposits in old deep hemorrhages.

Drusen, often seen in older clients, are benign degenerative hyaline deposits in the fundus. They are either gray or yellowish spots and are almost always symmetrically located in both eyes. Drusen are distributed in a haphazard formation, whereas hard exudates usually form cir-

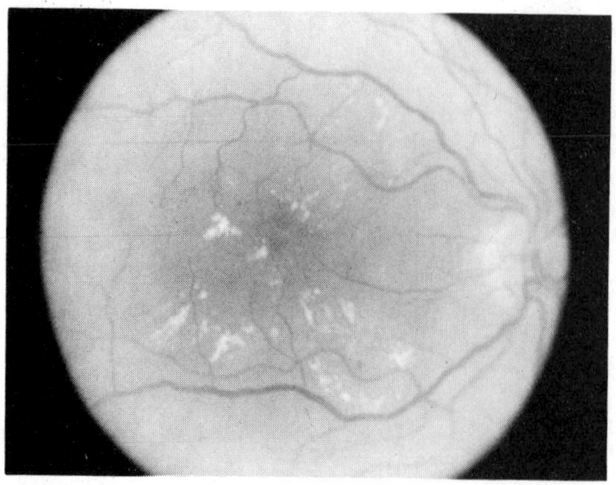

Figure 11-35 Hard exudates. (See also endsheet plate 25.)

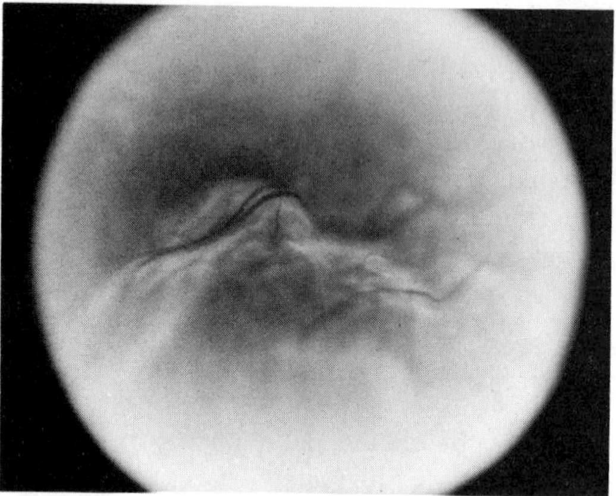

Figure 11-36 Detached retina. (See also endsheet plate 26.)

cular or linear patterns, but, even so, it is difficult to differentiate the two. Drusen are not pathognomonic, nor do they affect vision.

Moderate retinal detachment may appear as an area out of focus in comparison to the remainder of the fundus. As the retina becomes more widely separated, it presents as a wrinkled gray sheet (see Figure 11-36). Retinal detachment is usually idiopathic, although underlying tumors or postretinal hemorrhage may be causes.

Summary

This chapter described assessment of the eye. Because the eye is a complex organ, each part of the eye is examined separately in a systematic manner. Inspection and palpation are the initial techniques used and are carried out simultaneously. The lacrimal apparatus, eyelids, conjunctiva, and cornea are inspected and palpated. The pupils are assessed for light reaction, size, and accommodation. Special techniques are used to check the extraocular muscles and intraocular pressure. Visual field examination and testing of visual acuity are part of the assessment process. The ophthalmoscope examination is used to assess landmarks within the eye and reveals many types of health conditions.

Discussion Questions/Activities

1. In the following diagram, identify the components of the eye.

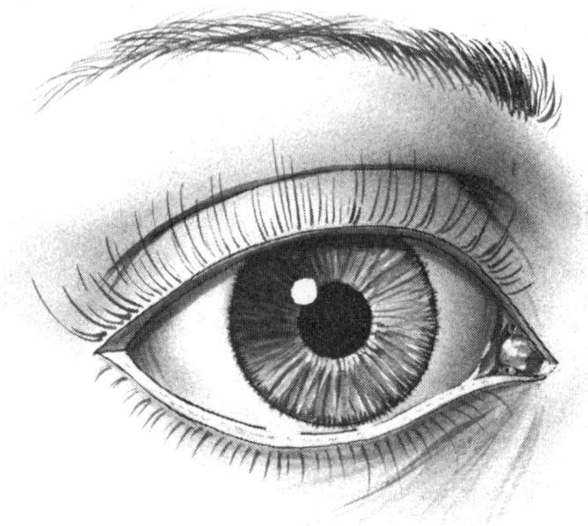

2. Describe the procedure for examining the external eye.
3. Discuss common abnormalities found in the following areas: eyelids, conjunctiva, sclera, cornea.
4. Demonstrate how you would test for direct pupillary reaction and for consensual reaction to light.
5. Demonstrate the technique you would use to test for accommodation and for extraocular muscle movement.
6. Demonstrate the use of the Snellen Chart for testing visual acuity.
7. Demonstrate the technique used to assess peripheral vision.
8. Demonstrate the technique for using the ophthalmoscope.
9. Describe how you would locate the following: red reflex, optic disk, macula.
10. Discuss what is meant by the following terms: AV nicking, cotton-wool patches, exudates, flame-shaped hemorrhage, glaucomatous cup.
11. What means would you use to test the vision of a preschool child?

Recording of Findings

Normal findings are presented in the first box. The second box contains recordings for a client who was later medically diagnosed as being hypertensive.

Eye	Eye
INSPECTION Eyes moist and glossy. Eyebrows full; lashes present; no orbital edema; equal separation of palpebral fissures; no lid lag; no ptosis; conjunctiva pink without bulbar injection; sclerae white; cornea clear; PERRLA/ consensual reaction; EOM's intact; no nystagmus; no strabismus; visual fields normal by gross confrontation; OD 20/20, OS 20/20, OU 20/20 without corrective lenses. Fundoscopy: red reflex clear; disk well demarcated, pinkish yellow color; A/V 2:3; no AV nicking; no hemorrhages; no exudates. **PALPATION** Ocular tension—soft on palpation.	**INSPECTION** Dull appearance. Eyebrows full; lashes present; no orbital edema; equal separation of palpebral fissures; no lid lag; no ptosis; conjunctiva pink without bulbar injection; sclerae white; cornea clear; PERRLA/ consensual reaction; EOM's intact; no nystagmus; no strabismus; visual fields normal by gross confrontation; OD 20/20, OS 20/20, OU 20/20 without corrective lenses. Fundoscopy: red reflex clear; blurred disk edges; narrowed copper-wire arteries; AV nicking; flame-shaped hemorrhages ½ DD away at 4:00; diffuse cotton-wool patches. **PALPATION** Ocular tension—soft on palpation.

CHAPTER 12

Assessment of the Ear, Nose, Mouth, and Pharynx

LEARNING OBJECTIVES

1. Review the structure and function of the ear, nose, mouth, and pharynx.
2. List the characteristics of the ear, nose, mouth, and pharynx that are noted during inspection.
3. Describe the technique of using the otoscope in the examination of the auditory canal and tympanic membrane.
4. Explain the Weber and Rinne tests and the normal finding of each.
5. Discuss the techniques of palpation and transillumination in assessing the maxillary and frontal sinuses.
6. Recognize the normal findings regarding the ear, nose, lips, gums, buccal mucosa, teeth, tongue, palate, and oropharynx.

This chapter describes assessment of the ears, nose and mouth, and pharynx. The structure and function of each anatomical area is discussed, followed by an explanation of the special techniques needed in assessing the area. The oto-ophthalmoscope is used to facilitate examination of these structures.

The authors have found it most effective to carry out this examination by first assessing the ears, followed by nose and mouth, and finally the pharynx. Others may prefer to follow a different sequence, such as nose, mouth, pharynx, and ears. The main thing to keep in mind is that the examination should be performed systematically.

Structure and Function of the Ear

The ear consists of three parts: the external ear, the middle ear, and the inner ear (see Figure 12-1). The external ear has two parts: the flap on the side of the head called the *auricle*, or *pinna*, and the *external auditory canal*, a tube leading from the auditory meatus (opening) to the temporal bone. The auditory canal in children is horizontal, but in adults it is angulated inward, forward, and then downward (see Figure 12-2). Its length is about 3 cm. The external ear is sepa-

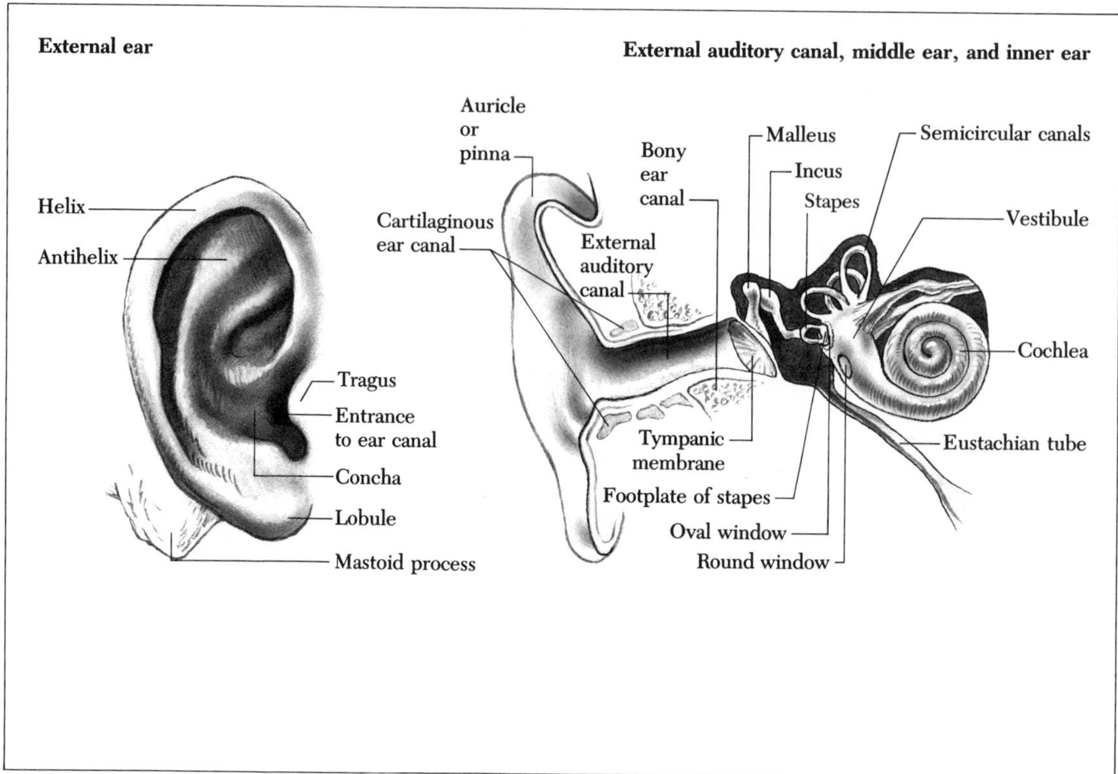

Figure 12-1 Diagram of the ear.

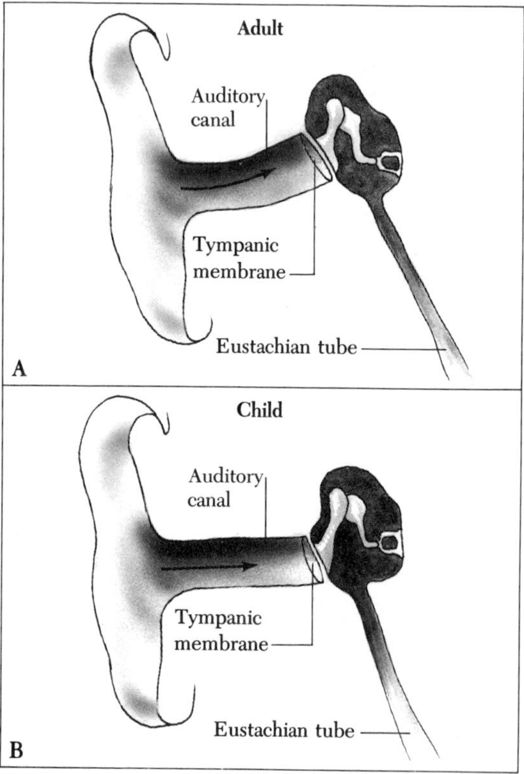

Figure 12-2 Differences in the auditory canals of (A) an adult and (B) a child.

rated from the middle ear by the *tympanic membrane* (eardrum).

The middle ear contains three auditory ossicles (bones): the *malleus* (hammer), the *incus* (anvil), and the *stapes* (stirrup). There are four openings into the middle ear: one from the external canal—the opening covered by the tympanic membrane, in which the handle of the malleus is embedded; two from the internal ear—the *oval window*, into which the stapes fits, and the *round window*, which has a membrane covering; and one from the *eustachian tube*—the opening that extends from the middle ear to the nasopharynx. The eustachian tube is important in the equalization of pressure between the inner and outer surfaces of the tympanic membrane.

The inner ear consists of a bony labyrinth with a membranous labyrinth inside. The bony labyrinth contains the *vestibule*, the *cochlea*, and the *semicircular canals*. The membranous labyrinth consists of the *utricle* and *saccule*, two sacs that are inside the vestibule and that line the cochlear duct (of the cochlea) and the endolymphatic duct (of the semicircular canals). Within the walls of the utricle and saccule are macula utriculi and macula sacculi, respectively; these are sensory epithelium whose function is to conduct impulses to the brain that allow for a sense of position of the head. Within the cochlea is the hearing sense organ, the *organ of Corti.* It is from here that impulses are conducted to the brain, producing the sensation of hearing. The semicircular canals contain receptors that function as organs for the sense of equilibrium.

For hearing to occur, the auditory area of the cerebral cortex must be stimulated. The process of hearing begins when sound waves are picked up by the pinna and are channeled into the auditory canal, where they strike the tympanic membrane, setting up vibrations. When the membrane vibrates, the malleus vibrates, establishing a chain reaction in the incus and stapes, with the latter vibrating against the oval window. It is at this point that the sound waves begin to move through conduction of fluid. The transmission of the impulses continues through the cochlear duct, the organ of Corti, and the cochlear nerve (a division of the 8th cranial nerve) to the brain stem; through the medulla, pons, midbrain, and thalamus; and finally to the auditory area of the temporal lobe.

In examining the ear you are able to view only the external portion, the auditory canal, and the tympanic membrane. Conditions involving the middle ear cannot be visualized but may be reflected by the tympanic membrane.

Characteristics and Techniques of Examination

Inspection and Palpation

Note the position of the ears on the head. The helix should be in line with the eyebrows. Low-set ears often reflect mental retardation, usually that resulting from congenital defects. This condition can be seen in children with Down's syndrome. Observe the external ear and palpate it for lesions or nodules, particularly tophi (see Figure 12-3). Tophi are hard, pale, nontender collections of urate crystals; they are usually associated with gout. The cartilage of the ear should be stiff but not rigid. "Cauliflower ears," thickened and gnarled, are evidence of repeated trauma and are commonly seen in prize-fighters. Very large ears are said to be observed in pernicious anemia.

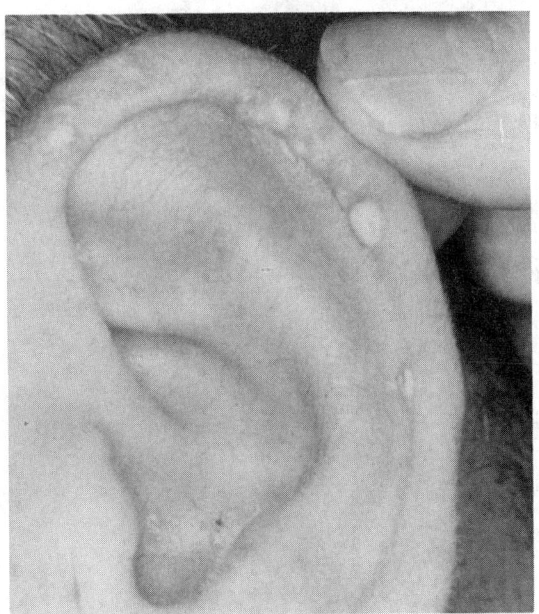

Figure 12-3 Gouty tophi of the ear. (© Arthritis Foundation 1981.)

Palpate the antrum of the mastoid bone for tenderness. Mastoiditis is no longer commonly seen because of the use of antibiotics, but tenderness in the mastoid process area is often associated with acute otitis media (middle ear infection) (see Figure 12-4).

To visualize the canal, you may have to remove cerumen (earwax) (see Figure 12-5). This can be accomplished with gentle and careful use of a cotton-tipped applicator or with irrigation using warm water, mineral oil, or a commercial preparation (e.g., Cerumenex) designed specifically for this purpose. Examine the canal and the tympanic membrane with the otoscope. Speculums for the otoscope come in various sizes; choose the one that is the largest size that will fit the canal. The speculum dilates and straightens the ear canal.

Technique for examination is illustrated in Figure 12-6. During examination of the auditory canal, the position of the client's head is very important; it should be tipped sideways toward the opposite shoulder to facilitate examination. Instruct the client to hold his head very still. To examine the right ear, grasp the auricle between your left thumb and forefinger. Because the adult ear canal angulates, it is necessary to pull upward ("up" for "grownups") and outward on the auricle to view the tympanic membrane. Then gently insert the speculum into the canal

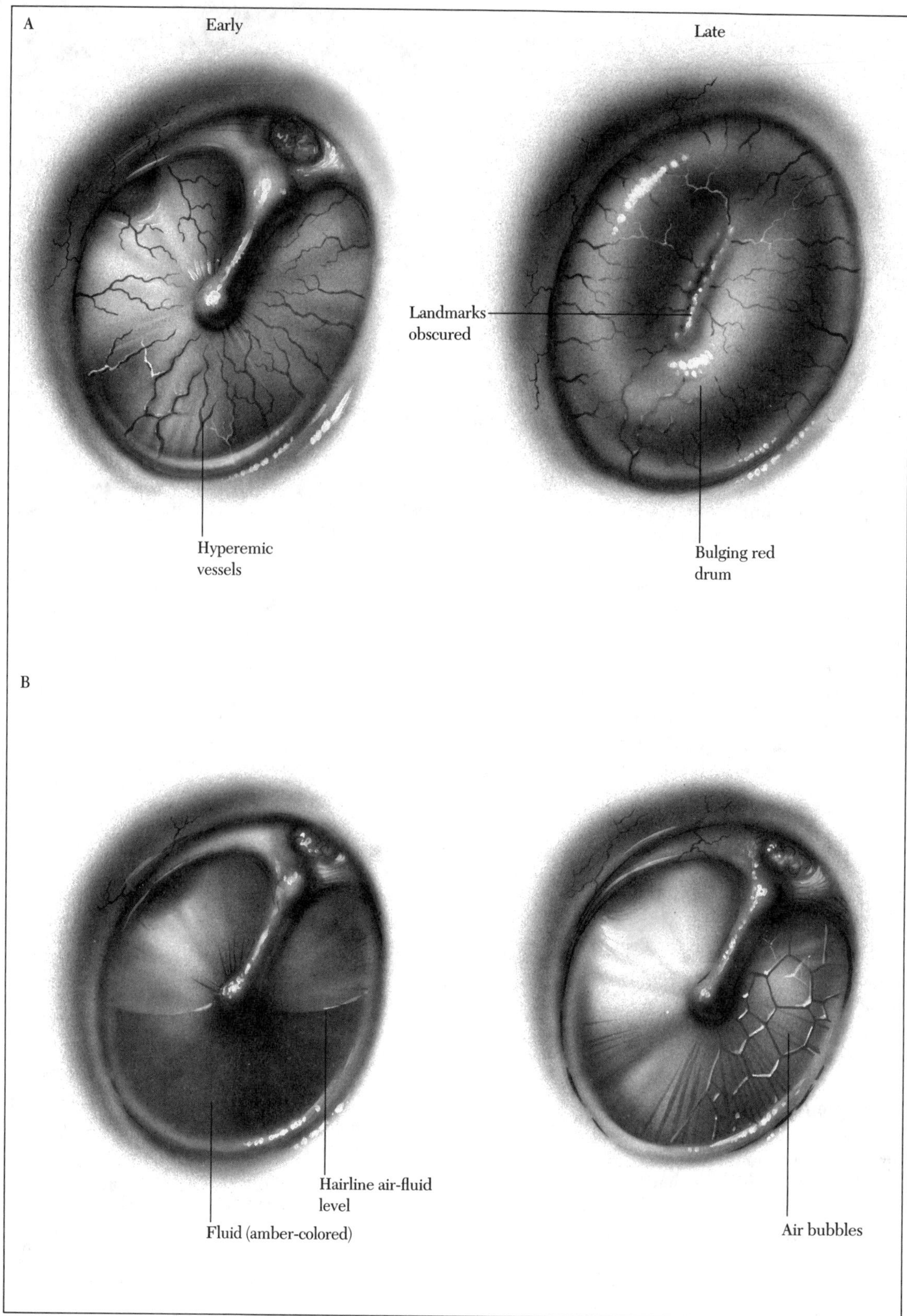

Figure 12-4 (A) Acute purulent otitis media. (B) Serous otitis media.

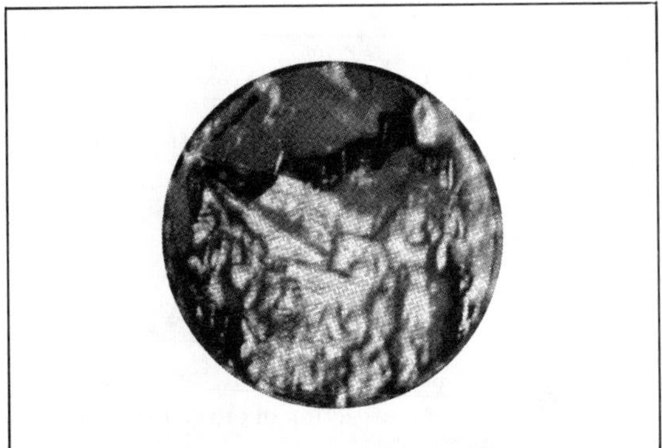

Figure 12-5 Otoscopic view revealing excessive cerumen.

with your right hand. About halfway to the tympanic membrane pressure from the speculum can be quite painful, so gentleness is important. Never insert the speculum into the auditory canal without following its progress with your eye. Examine the external canal for erythema, swelling, patency, amount of cerumen, discharge of any type, and foreign bodies.

After examining the auditory canal, carefully inspect the tympanic membrane. The normal eardrum is a pearly gray color. There are three landmarks on the drum (see Figure 12-7): (1) the annulus, which forms the outer border of the drum and is a paler color than the remainder of the membrane; (2) the malleus, which angles downward posteriorly from the annulus to a point at the center of the tympanic membrane; and (3) the light reflex, which is a bright cone-shaped reflection of light in the lower anterior aspect of the tympanic membrane. It is located

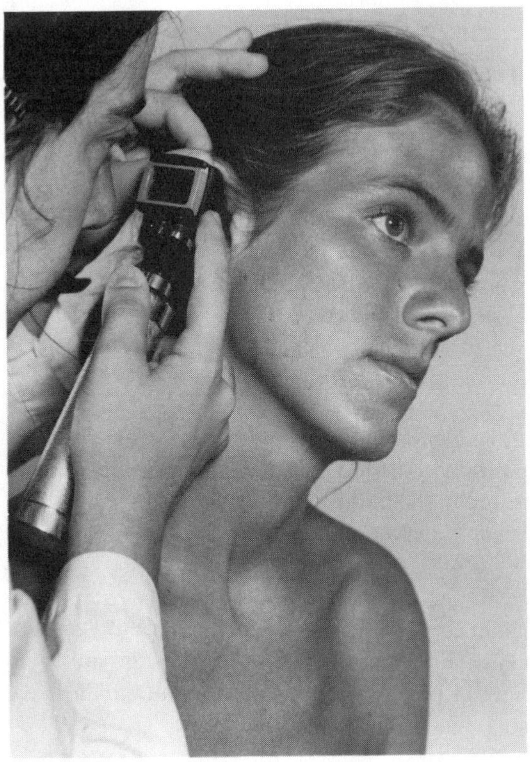

Figure 12-6 Examination of the auditory canal and tympanic membrane.

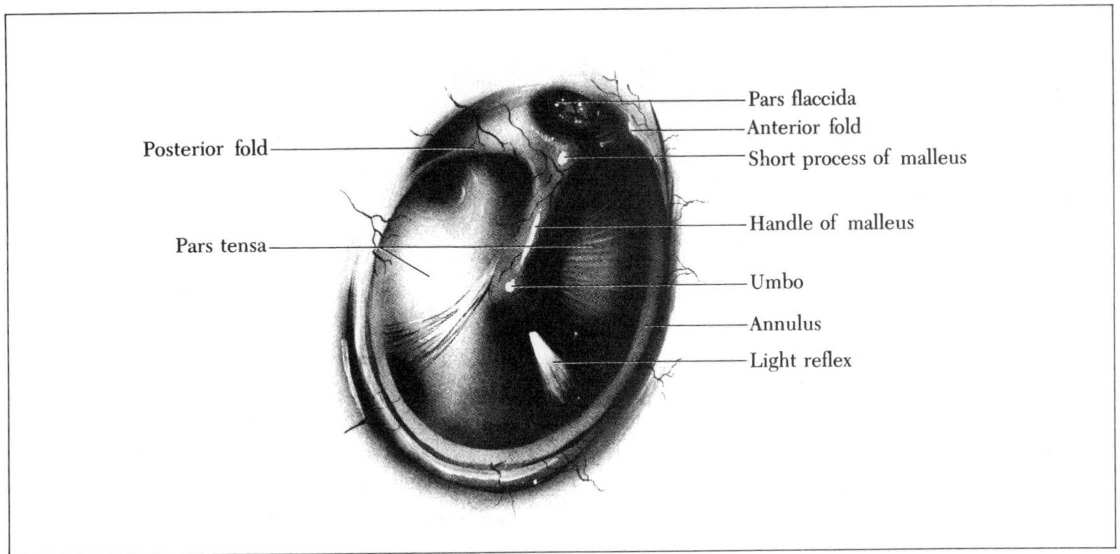

Figure 12-7 Diagram of the right eardrum.

Table 12-1. Pathologic Manifestations of the Tympanic Membrane

Manifestation	Cause	Condition
Yellow or amber	Serum or pus	Acute or chronic otitis media
Blue	Blood behind drum	Skull injury
Bright red	Inflammation	Acute otitis media
Bubbles behind drum	Serous fluid	Serous otitis media
Absent light reflex	Bulging of drum	Suppurative otitis media
White thick drum	Scarring of drum	Untreated infection
Chalky granulated nodule	Inflammation	Chronic inflammatory process
Malleus very prominent	Retraction of drum	Obstruction of eustachian tube
Dark areas	Perforation	Rupture of drum

at 5 o'clock in the right ear and at the 7 o'clock position in the left ear. In disease, changes in the color of the membrane and in the landmarks become very significant (see Table 12-1 and Figure 12-4).

To test the mobility of the drum, instruct the client to pinch his nose closed and blow against closed lips. A normal drum will bulge outward. Do not perform this test with clients who have an obvious ear disease.

Hearing Loss

Hearing loss may be classified in several ways. *Conduction deafness* refers to the hearing loss that occurs when there is interference with the functioning of the structures in the middle ear. The most common causes of middle ear deafness are otitis media, otosclerosis, and rupture of the tympanic membrane. Hereditary otosclerosis is the most frequent cause of progressive conduction deafness; it is the factor responsible for 50% of deafness in adults.

Sensorineural deafness results from disease occurring anywhere from the organ of Corti to the brain. Nerve deafness has many causes: heredity; rubella in the pregnant mother; chronic middle ear infection in childhood spreading to the inner ear; and exposure to loud noises, such as gunfire, dynamite blasting, and working with heavy equipment. Teenagers and others who listen to loud amplified music may develop a form of nerve deafness referred to as "rock and roll" deafness.

Central deafness occurs from damage to the auditory pathways or auditory center; this may happen with a cerebrovascular accident. *Functional deafness* refers to cases in which there is no organic basis for the loss of hearing.

Hearing loss can be determined by testing with a tuning fork (Figure 12-8). The Rinne test detects conduction deafness. To perform the Rinne test, use a number 512 fork, strike the tuning fork, and place the handle to the mastoid process, as shown in Figure 12-9A and B. Ask the client to indicate when he can no longer hear the sound. When this point is reached, immediately place the vibrating head of the tuning fork near to the external ear, as shown in Figure 12-9B. Normally, sound transmitted through air is heard better than sound transmitted through bone, so the client should continue to hear the sound. If so, the test is referred to as being positive. Recording of a positive Rinne test usually

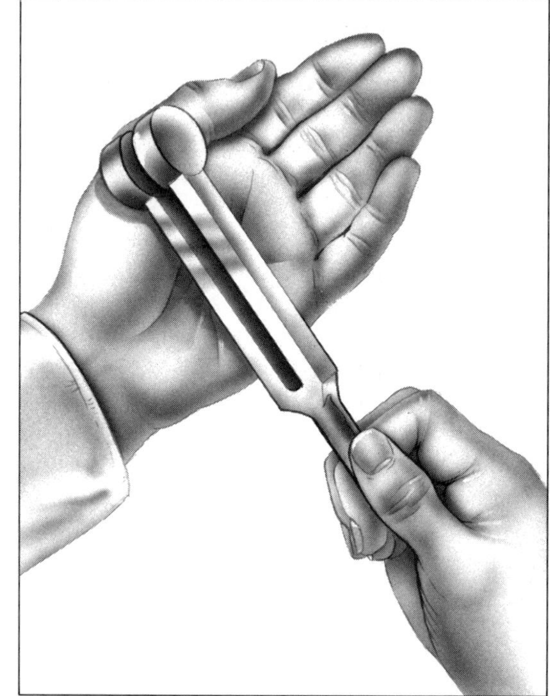

Figure 12-8 Technique for using a tuning fork in the Rinne test. The ends of the tuning fork are pinched and the fork is tapped against the heel of the hand.

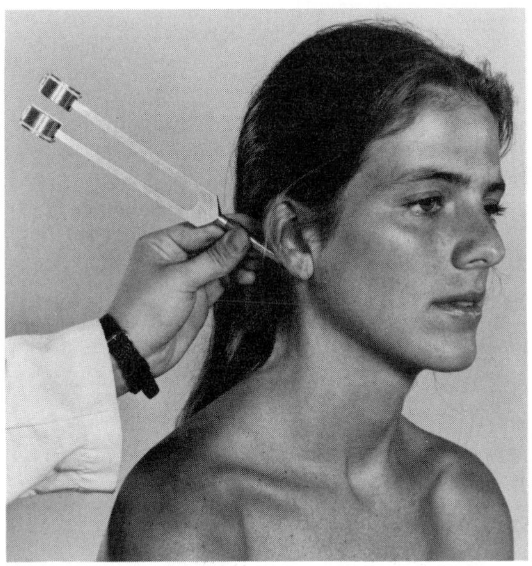
A

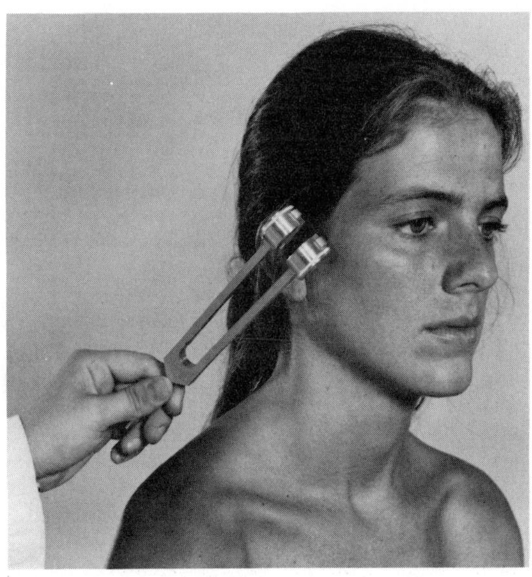
B

Figure 12-9 The Rinne test. (A) The tuning fork is placed on the mastoid process and the client is asked to indicate when she can no longer hear the sound. (B) The tuning fork is placed next to the external ear as soon as the client says she cannot hear the bone-conducted sound.

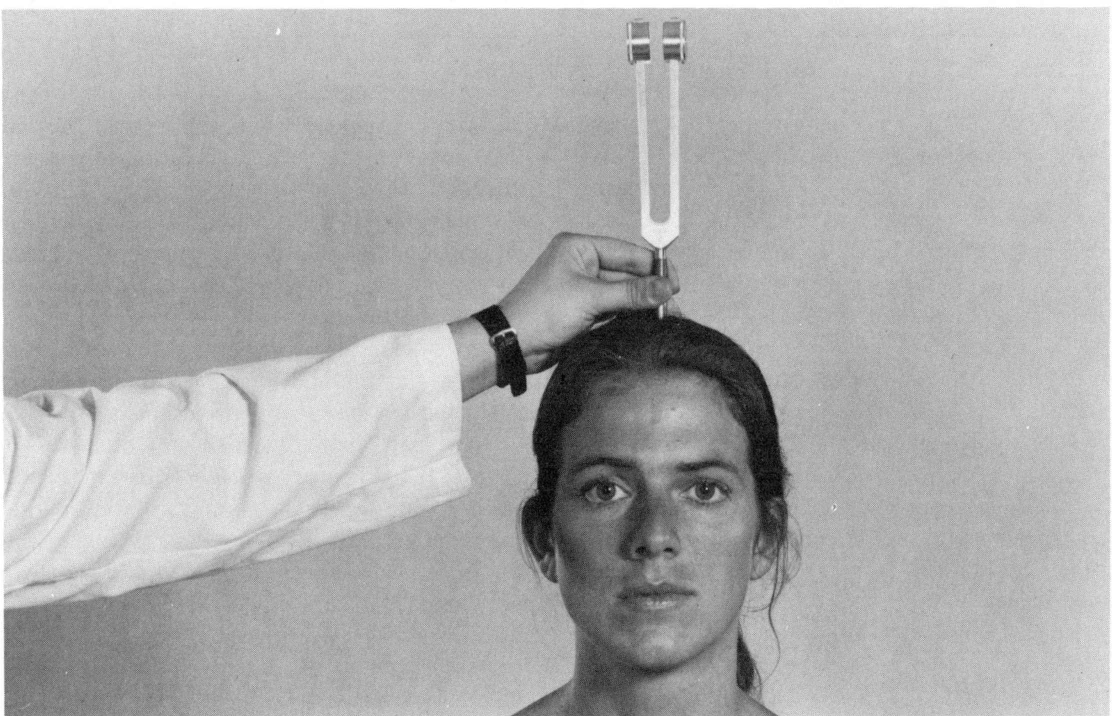

Figure 12-10 The Weber test.

takes the following form: "AC > BC" (air conduction is greater than bone conduction). If the Rinne test is negative (the sound cannot be heard when the fork is brought before the ear), bone conduction is greater than air conduction; this means that a conduction defect exists.

The Weber test is used to detect conduction deafness or sensorineural deafness. The tuning fork is struck and then placed in the center of the forehead or in the middle top anterior portion of the skull, as illustrated in Figure 12-10. Ask the client whether he hears the sound better in one

Table 12-2. Common Causes and Clinical Findings of Hearing Losses

	Conduction loss	Sensorineural loss
Site of damage	External or middle ear	Inner ear or nerve (from the organ of Corti to the brain)
Etiology of dysfunction	Excessive cerumen, ruptured tympanic membrane, otosclerosis, otitis media	Exposure to loud noise—e.g., loud music, dynamite, jackhammer, gunshots, heredity, rubella in pregnant mother, chronic middle ear infection spreading to inner ear
Weber test Normal finding: does *not* lateralize	Lateralizes to affected ear because bone vibrations are detected better than normal without the distraction of environmental noise; you can simulate an external or middle ear conduction loss by occluding one ear with your finger and you will experience the vibrations lateralizing to your occluded ear; in an absolutely quiet room a normal finding of no lateralization will result	Lateralizes to unaffected ear because bone vibrations are not conducted to brain due to inner ear or nerve damage
Rinne test Normal finding: $AC > BC$	Air conduction of the vibrations is blocked; therefore, bone conduction will bypass the external and middle ear and last longer ($BC > AC$)	Air conduction of the vibrations are longer than bone ($AC > BC$); therefore, the normal finding prevails, but hearing is diminished by both routes

ear or the other. The normal client will hear the sound equally in both ears; some clients may respond that they hear the sound "all over" the head. With pathology the client will readily answer that he hears the sound better in one ear than in the other. Thus, any hemming or hawing by the client denotes the absence of pathology. Recording of a normal testing is: "Weber test—no lateralization."

If the client has conduction hearing loss in one ear, he will hear the sound better in that ear. This is because normal noise in the room tends to obscure hearing in the normal ear. The ear with conduction loss will not hear the room noise and thus has a better chance to hear the bone-conducted sound. If the client has sensorineural loss, he will hear the sound better with the normal ear. A sensorineural loss manifests a positive Rinne ($AC > BC$) and an abnormal Weber (lateralizes to the good ear) (see Table 12-2).

Two gross tests of hearing are the whispered or spoken voice test and the watch tick test. For the former, approach the client from the side so that he cannot read your lips. Direct your whispered voice toward the ear being tested. The client's other ear should be prevented from picking up the sound. To muffle the sound for the other ear, lightly rub the palm of your hand over it or place a finger in the external auditory canal and gently wiggle it during the testing. (As with the testing of the eyes, the testing of the ears should be done one at a time.) The client with normal hearing acuity should be able to hear your whispered voice at a distance of 2 feet from the ear in a quiet room. The watch tick test is simply an evaluation of the client's ability to hear a watch ticking as it moves away from his ear. Because this method tests only high frequency sounds, it is a poor test to use exclusively.

In young children, carefully observe responses to loud noises, whispers, and watch ticking and note the ability to make verbal sounds. Cooperation with the Rinne and Weber testing can be elicited from children as young as 2 years old. Younger infants can be tested with an automated sensor called the crib-o-gram, which can test several newborns at one time. It records the physical movements before, during, and after a sound is presented through a nearby microphone. Hearing loss is detected through analysis of the recordings.

If you discover evidence of hearing loss as a result of the gross tests or tuning fork tests, you should refer the client to an audiologist for further quantitative measurements. Because audiologists do not have a medical background, the

Technique for Inspection and Palpation of the Ear

1. Note position and size.
2. Palpate for lesions or nodules.
3. Palpate antrum of mastoid bone for tenderness.
4. If necessary, gently remove cerumen.
5. Choose speculum of appropriate size.
6. Tip client's head sideways (toward opposite side being examined).
7. Ask client to hold very still.
8. Grasp auricle of ear being examined between thumb and forefinger.
9. Adult—pull auricle upward and outward.
10. Gently insert speculum (follow progress with eye).
11. Examine external canal.
12. Examine tympanic membrane.
13. Test for hearing loss:
    Rinne test—strike tuning fork and place handle to mastoid process; when vibration stops hold tuning fork before pinna (repeat for other ear).
    Weber test—strike tuning fork and place in center of forehead or middle top anterior skull.
    Gross tests: whispered voice, watch tick

client should be referred to a physician if diagnosis and treatment of ear disease are required. If a specialist seems warranted, refer the client to an otologist (a physician with advanced education in this field).

Two common pathologic conditions that require medical attention and treatment are otitis externa and otitis media.

Otitis externa, infection of the external ear, is most frequently seen in children and young adults. It often occurs secondarily to getting the ears wet, as with frequent swimming or hair-washing. It may also be due to staphylococcal or Pseudomonas infection. In these infections the ear canal is swollen and discharges purulent material. If pulling gently on the tragus elicits pain, the diagnosis is almost always external otitis.

The most common ear infection in childhood is probably simple otitis media. In this condition the tympanic membrane will be erythematous, and there will be pain in and about the ear; this pain can be quite severe. If the condition becomes subacute, persistent purulent drainage may result. The tympanic membrane can rupture, with a resultant chronic otitis media. The chronically infected ear is characterized by persistent or recurring purulent drainage, with or without pain, and by differing degrees of hearing loss, usually of the conduction type.

Trauma and rupture of the eardrum occur most often as a result of accident. People who clean their ears with Q-tips or with sharp objects (such as hairpins) covered with tissue may inadvertently puncture the eardrum. This is as common in adults as in young children.

Structure and Function of the Nose

Figure 12-11 shows that there are two nasal chambers, called *nares*. They open externally through the nostril (*anterior nares*) and posteriorly through the *nasopharynx* (via the *posterior nares*). The nasal chambers are lined with respiratory mucosa except anteriorly, where there is epithelium (skin) containing sebaceous glands and multiple coarse nasal hairs. These hairs are very important in the filtering of the entering air. The two nasal chambers are separated by the *nasal septum*, which is composed of cartilage and bone. The olfactory hair cells—the receptors for the sense of smell—are located in the superior portion, which is lined with neuroepithelium. This highly vascular membrane is continuous with the external skin and the internal mucous membrane lining the sinuses.

Figure 12-12 shows the superior-posterior portion of the nose, which contains the *inferior, middle,* and *superior turbinates*. These bones increase the mucous membrane surface of the nasal passages and slightly obstruct the current of air flowing through them. The mucous membranes also serve to moisten and warm the inhaled air. The cleft between these bones is referred to as a *meatus*. Each meatus is named after the adjacent turbinate.

The paranasal sinuses, shown in Figure 12-11, are air-filled cavities within the bones of the skull; they are lined with mucous membrane. Only the frontal and maxillary sinuses can be easily examined. The *maxillary sinuses* are located on either side of the nose in the maxillary

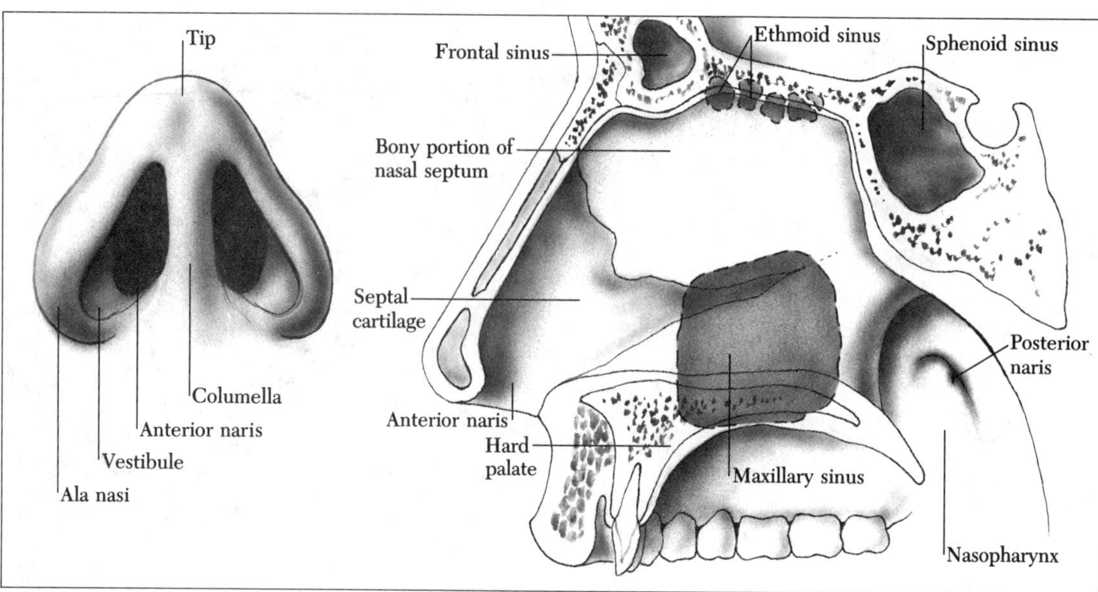

Figure 12-11 Cross-section of the nose.

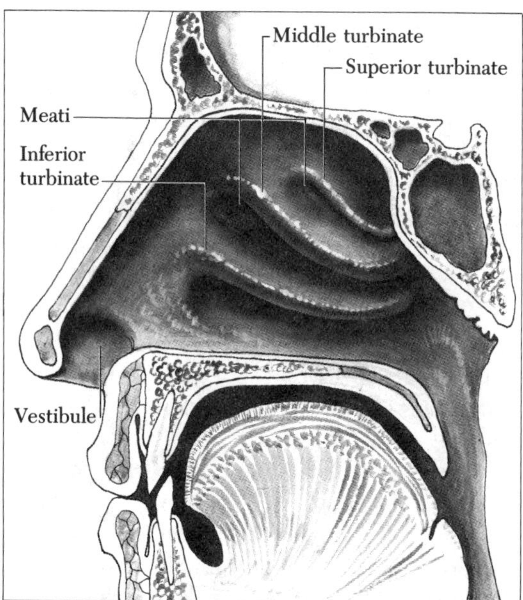

Figure 12-12 Cross-section of the nose showing turbinates and meati.

bones. The *frontal sinuses* are located in the lower forehead between and above the eyes. The *ethmoid sinus* is between the eyes over the roof of the nose. The *sphenoid sinus* is posterior to the ethmoid and maxillary sinuses. One of the functions of the sinuses is to give timbre and resonance to the voice.

Characteristics and Techniques of Examination

Inspection

Simple inspection of the external nose is usually adequate unless injury has occurred. In that case, light palpation will elicit the location of pain and tenderness. The nose is examined by using an illuminated nasal speculum (see Figure 12-13). The large, short speculum on the otoscope can be used. To obtain adequate visualization, lift up the tip of the nose and introduce the speculum. Inspect the mucous membrane for changes from the normal red color. Rhinitis, inflammation of the mucous membrane of the nose, produces a definite erythematous and edematous mucosa. In allergy, however, the mucosa is bluish gray.

Note the presence and character of any discharge. Discharge is common in rhinitis and sinusitis. Severe chronic rhinitis is characterized by thick greenish discharge with an offensive odor.

In most adults the septum is not completely straight; it usually deviates toward one of the passages. Perforation of the septum may result from continuous use of cocaine, continuous nose picking, syphilis, or nasal-septal surgery. The anterior septum is a common site of epistaxis,

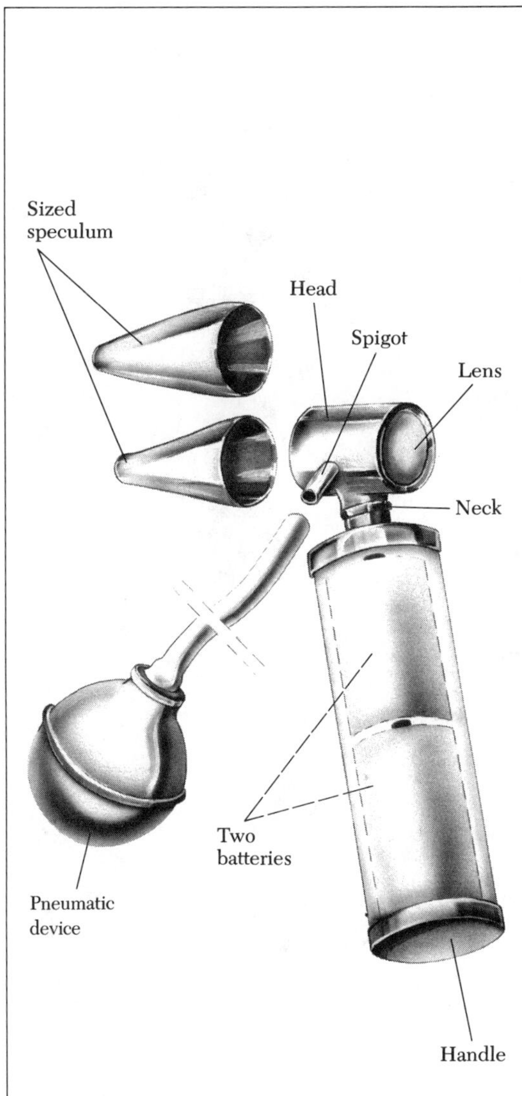

Figure 12-13 The large speculum of an otoscope can be used as a nasal speculum.

which can be easily controlled. Bleeding from the posterior nares is frequently profuse and is more difficult to control.

In the superior-posterior area look for the large inferior turbinate, which is ordinarily easy to see. The middle turbinate can be viewed most of the time unless there is swelling of the mucosa, a common condition in certain climates. Never attempt to push the speculum past a swollen turbinate. The posterior turbinate is rarely seen because of its position. Purulent drainage from the middle meatus, the cleftlike area between the anterior and middle turbinates, indicates sinusitis.

Nasal polyps appear as smooth, mobile, pale tumors. Nasal obstruction will occur as they become larger. Carcinomas of the mucosa are unusual; such growths are gray-white and relatively insensitive.

Palpation

The maxillary and frontal sinuses, shown in Figure 12-14A, are palpated and percussed lightly with the fingertips, as demonstrated in Figure 12-14B. Normally they are nontender; pain usually indicates sinusitis. The ethmoid sinus can only be examined by intranasal inspection.

Transillumination

Figure 12-14C shows how transillumination of the maxillary sinuses is accomplished by placing a very bright light into the mouth and closing the lips. Normally the air-containing sinuses light up symmetrically. If one or the other contains fluid, it will be darker than the other. Figure 12-14D shows how to transilluminate the frontal

Technique of Inspection and Palpation of the Nose

1. Carry out a visual inspection.
2. Lightly palpate if indicated.
3. Put large, short speculum on otoscope.
4. Lift tip of nose and insert speculum in nares (repeat with other nares).
5. Inspect mucous membrane for:
   Color
   Discharge
6. Inspect septum.
7. Look for large inferior turbinate and middle turbinate.
8. Palpate and percuss sinuses:
   Frontal
   Maxillary
9. Transilluminate
   Maxillary sinuses—place bright lighted attachment on handle of oto-ophthalmoscope into mouth and have client close mouth.
   Frontal sinuses—press very bright light under superior orbital ridge.

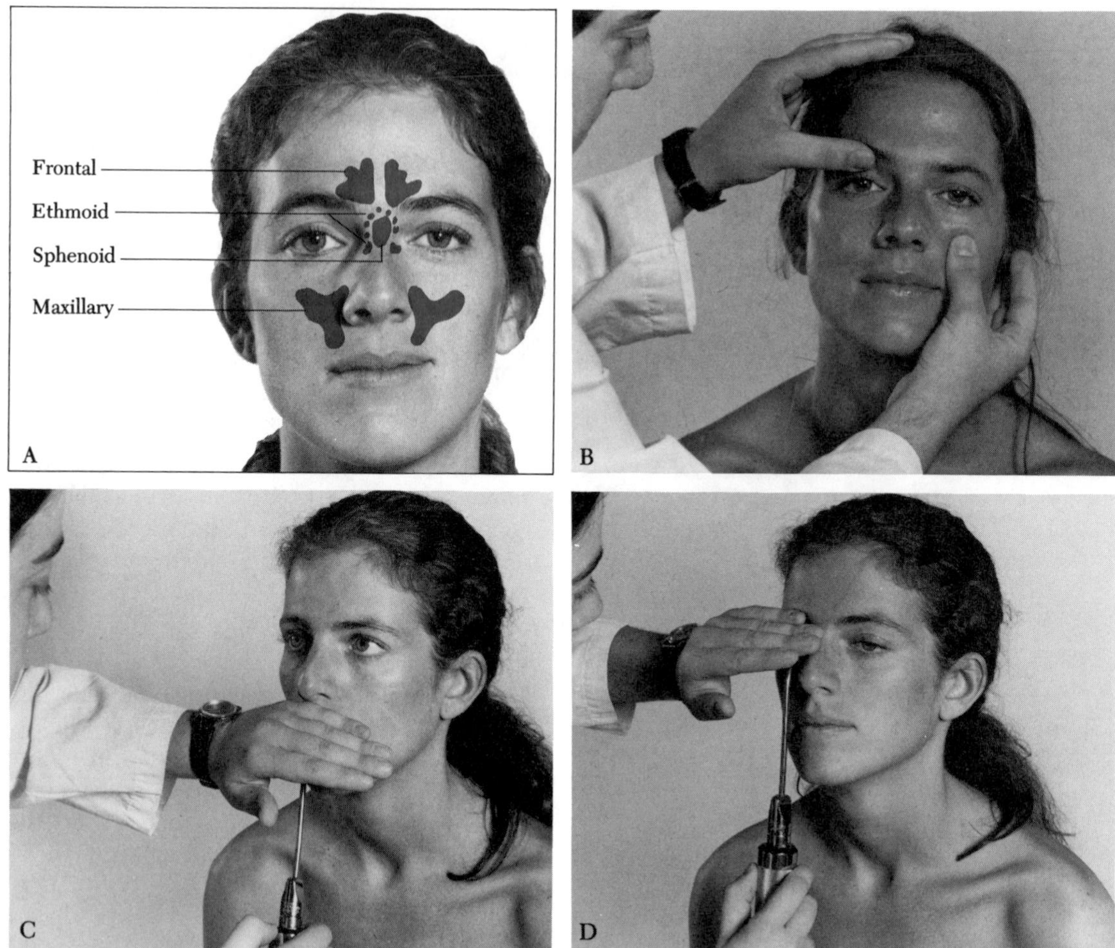

Figure 12-14 Palpation and transillumination of the sinuses. (A) Sites of sinuses. (B) Palpation is done with the left thumb on the right frontal sinus and the right thumb on the left maxillary sinus. (C) Transillumination of the maxillary sinuses. (D) Transillumination of the frontal sinus.

sinuses by pressing the lighted attachment on the oto-ophthalmoscope handle under the superior orbital ridge.

Structure and Function of the Mouth and Pharynx

Figure 12-15 depicts the buccal cavity, which is made up of the cheeks, the tongue and its muscles, the hard and soft palates, and the teeth. Its entire surface is lined with mucous membrane. The floor of the mouth consists of the tongue and underlying muscles. The rough elevations on the tongue are called *papillae*. Beneath the tongue is a tissue fold, the *frenulum*, that connects the tongue to the floor of the mouth. On either side of the frenulum, presenting as small elevated dark dots, are the *submaxillary glands*. The ducts of the *parotid glands* open into the *buccal mucosa* at a point opposite the upper second molar. The *hard palate*, anteriorly, is composed of bone; the *soft palate*, posteriorly, is composed of muscle in the shape of an arch on either side. These arches are known as the *palatine arches*. The inferior portion of the arch is called the *anterior tonsillar pillar*. The arches lead to the *oropharynx*, at which point they become the fauces, which is where the tonsils are located. Posterior to the arch is the *posterior tonsillar pillar*. The *uvula* projects downward from the middle of the soft palate.

Children may be born with teeth or may not have any tooth eruption until about 16 months of age. The average child at 1 year of age generally has six teeth; at 18 months, twelve teeth; at 2 years, sixteen teeth; and at 2½ years, twenty teeth. The first set of teeth (deciduous teeth) are

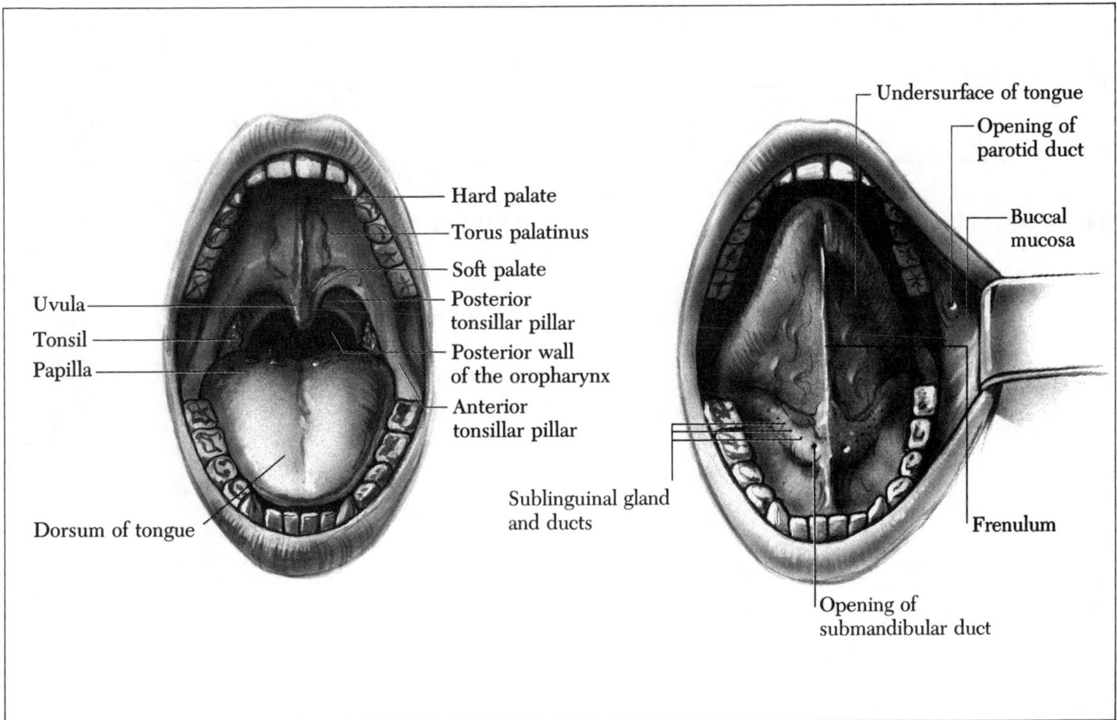

Figure 12-15 The buccal cavity.

temporary; they are shed and replaced by a second set of permanent teeth. The approximate ages for specific tooth eruption are presented in Table 12-3. The thirty-two permanent teeth, sixteen in each jaw, are identified in Figure 12-16.

The throat, or pharynx, is lined with mucous membrane and extends from the base of the skull to the esophagus. It has three divisions: (1) the nasopharynx, located behind the nose, (2) the oropharynx, posterior to the mouth, and (3) the laryngopharynx, which is posterior to the larynx. The *adenoids* are located on the roof of the nasopharynx, and the *tonsils* are on either side of the oropharynx. These organs are responsible for guarding the body from organisms entering the mouth and throat.

Characteristics and Techniques of Examination

Lips

Examination of the mouth and pharynx begins with inspection of the lips. First note the color of the lips. Circumoral pallor or pale mucosa is seen in anemic states. Cyanotic lips accompany hypoxic states. Cherry red lips are characteristic of acidotic states and of aspirin or carbon monoxide poisoning. The lips should be inspected for any signs of inflammation or the presence of any lesions, such as pustules, ulcers, fissures, or desquamation. Herpes simplex, commonly known as "cold sores" or "fever blisters," is seen in a majority of the population. Such lesions can occur on both the lips and the face; they appear as clear vesicles.

Cheilitis, inflammation of the lip, can be caused by poor oral hygiene, by overexposure to sunlight or wind, or by the chemicals in lipsticks and other creams and cosmetics. It is also manifested in seborrheic dermatitis of the lips and in hypertrophy of the mucous glands and their ducts. *Cheilosis* is frequently seen in vitamin B complex deficiency, especially riboflavin, and with monilial and other infections. This condition is characterized by reddened lips and cracks or fissures in the corner of the mouth that are generally very painful. Most tumors of oral cancer occur on the lips, primarily on the lower lip.

The lips are symmetrical. Small degrees of asymmetry are difficult to see. Asymmetry may be accentuated by asking the client to smile or

Table 12-3. Approximate Age of Tooth Eruption

Deciduous teeth		Permanent teeth	
Name	Erupt (age in months)	Name	Erupt (age in years)
Lower central incisors	5–9	First molars	6–7
Upper central incisors	8–12	Central incisors	7–8
Upper lateral incisors	10–12	Lateral incisors	7–8
Lower lateral incisors	12–15	First premolars	9–10
Anterior (first) molars	12–15	Second premolars	9–10
Canines	18–24	Canines	12–14
Posterior (second) molars	24–30	Second molars	12–15
		Third molars	17–25

From Clayton L. Thomas (ed.), *Taber's Cyclopedic Medical Dictionary*, 14th ed. (Philadelphia: F. A. Davis, 1981), p. 1429.

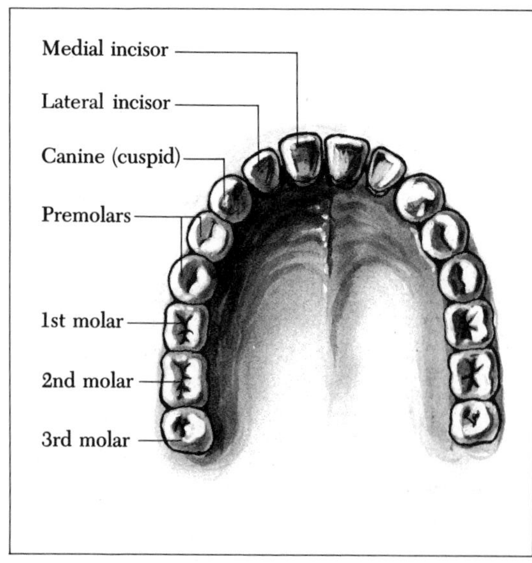

Figure 12-16 The permanent teeth.

by having him clench his teeth with his lips open. A drooping to one side may indicate paralysis of the facial or trigeminal nerve.

After examining the lips, proceed to the remainder of the mouth and pharynx, keeping in mind that the mouth is full of bacteria. Use a tongue blade and bright light, as well as gloves if inflammation is present. The tongue blade is used to retract the lips, cheeks, and tongue for proper visualization of all structures.

Gums

Inspect the gums. In the healthy individual they are pink and firm. *Gingivitis*, inflammation of the gums, may result from poor dental hygiene or may indicate the presence of a systemic disease. This condition is manifested by red, swollen, and bleeding gums. Vitamin C deficiency

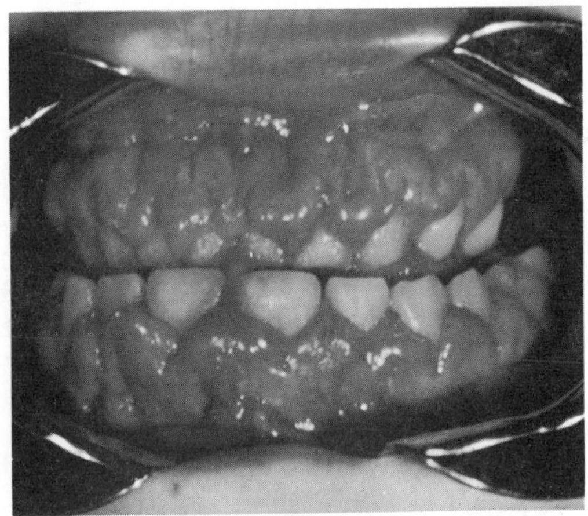

Figure 12-17 Hyperplasia of the gums in acute monocytic leukemia.

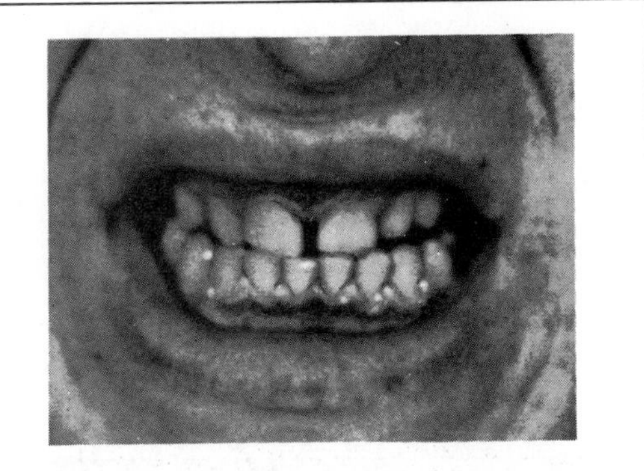

Figure 12-18 Lead line.

also causes reddened and hemorrhagic gums (see Figure 12-17).

Periodontitis, a serious inflammation of the periodontium caused by residual food, bacteria, and calcium deposits (tartar) can, if unchecked, spread inflammation to the bone in which the teeth are rooted, causing loosening and loss of the teeth.

Gingival bleeding is present in leukemia, as is ulceration of other structures of the mouth such as the buccal mucosa, the soft palate, the pharynx, or the tonsils. A dark line along the gingival margin is characteristic of both lead and bismuth poisoning (see Figure 12-18). However, a melanotic line may be normally found in the Black client.

Note the amount of salivation. It is minute in infants under 3 months of age and in clients receiving atropine. Excessive salivation—drooling—is observed during the teething process in children and with stomatitis (inflammation of the mouth). Saliva may collect in the mouth as a result of pseudobulbar palsy, the dysphagia that occurs with 9th or 10th cranial nerve injury (the glossopharyngeal and vagus nerves).

Mucous Membrane

Examine the mucous membrane lining the mouth. The membrane lining the cheeks is normally pink and clear of lesions. In anemia the mucosa may be pale. Koplik's spots, small bluish-white spots within the lower lip and scattered about the mucosa at the level of the lower teeth, are visible early in measles and are pathognomonic of that disease. Red spots over the buccal mucosa and the palate are frequently an early sign of German measles. Petechiae may be evident in leukemia and in subacute bacterial endocarditis. Leukoplakia (see Figure 12-19), a patchy white lesion on the mucous membrane of the cheeks, gums, or tongue, is usually raised and has well-defined borders. It can be caused by chronic irritation (as from smoking), poor nutrition, or syphilis. These lesions can be precancerous. Leukoplakia is distinguishable from monilial infection in that the lesions cannot be peeled away. In Addison's disease the oral mucosa undergoes pigment changes manifested by irregular spots or brown blotches.

Teeth

Inspect the teeth for caries and type of occlusion, and compare the number with the average number for the client's age. The condition of the teeth is a good indicator of the general health of

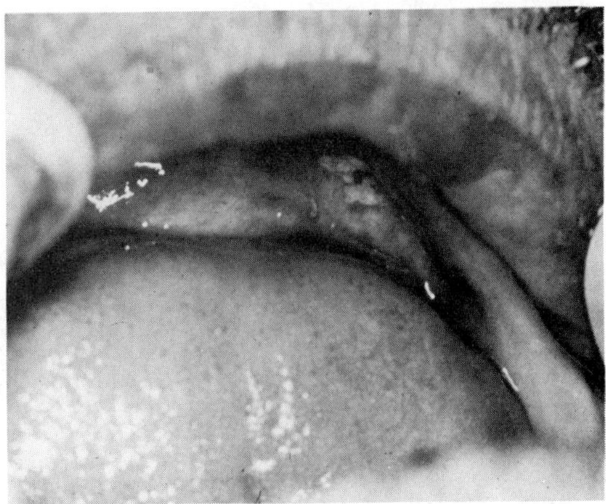

Figure 12-19 Leukoplakia under tongue. (See also endsheet plate 27.)

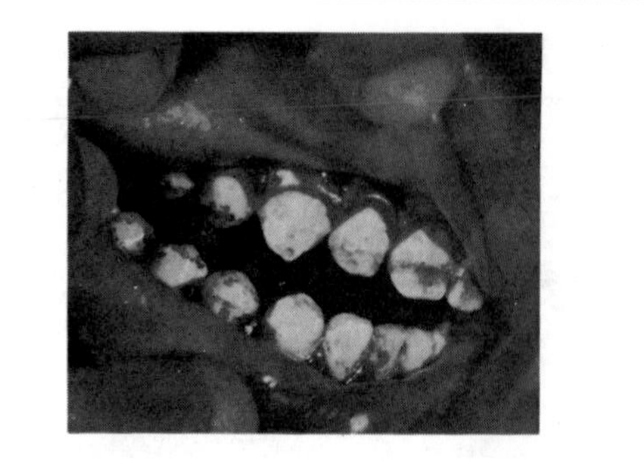

Figure 12-20 Mottled enamel due to fluoride in water.

the client. Yellow-brown teeth may be seen in infants and in women in the last trimester of pregnancy who have been given tetracycline (this discoloration may persist for several years following cessation of the drug). Green, brown, or blue discoloration may be seen in erythroblastosis fetalis. Pitting, white spotting, or brown staining can be the result of excessive fluoride ingestion (see Figure 12-20). Defects of the enamel range from deep grooves or grooves around the surface of the crown to absent incisal edges or occlusal surfaces. These defects are associated with gastrointestinal disturbances or with deficiencies of calcium, phosphorus, or vitamins A and B. Pegged lateral incisors and notched central incisors (Hutchinson's teeth) are a sign of congential syphilis (see Figure 12-21).

In young children malocclusion can cause severe earaches. Improper occlusion may indicate neoplasms, although malocclusion of the permanent teeth in older children may be caused by persistent thumb-sucking.

Delay in the appearance of deciduous teeth may indicate such conditions as rickets, cretinism, congenital syphilis, or Down's syndrome.

Tongue

Inspect the tongue for color, texture, deviation, size, symmetry, and lesions. Thorough examination of the tongue requires palpation as well as

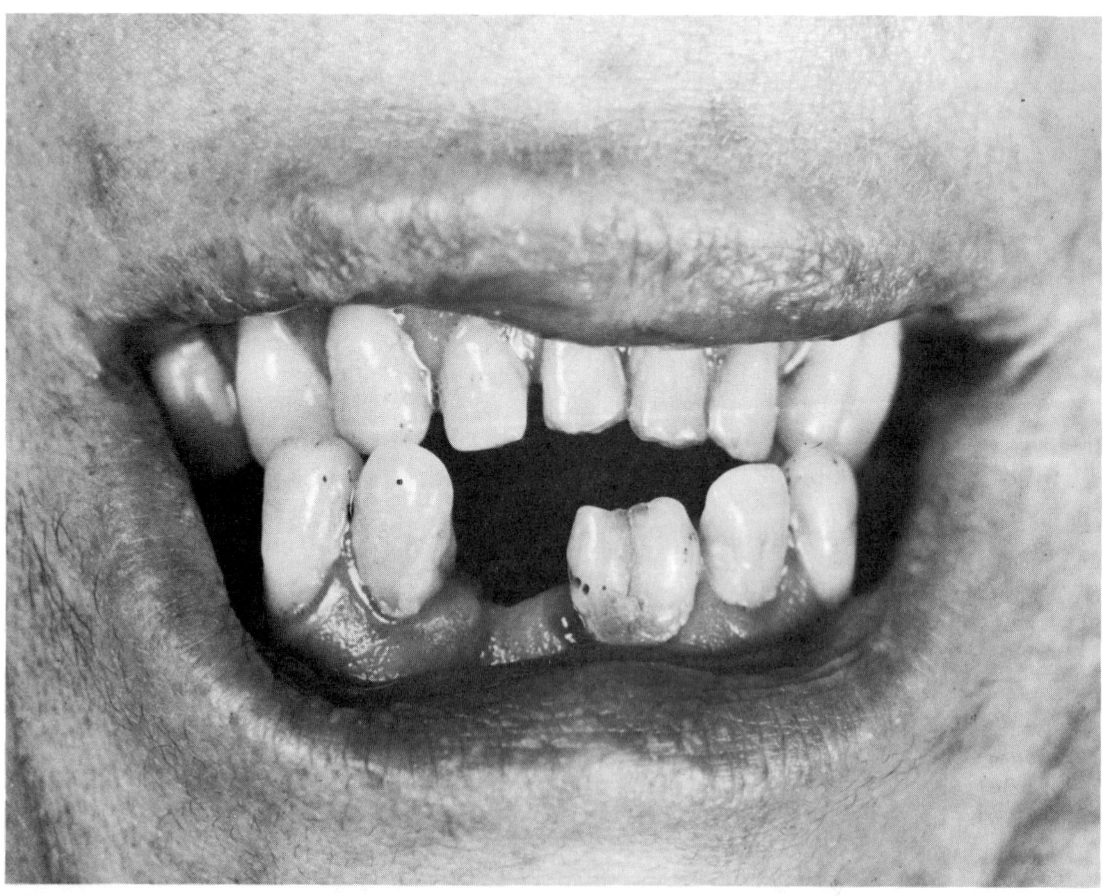

Figure 12-21 Hutchinson's teeth. Note notching of the central incisors and pegged lateral incisors.

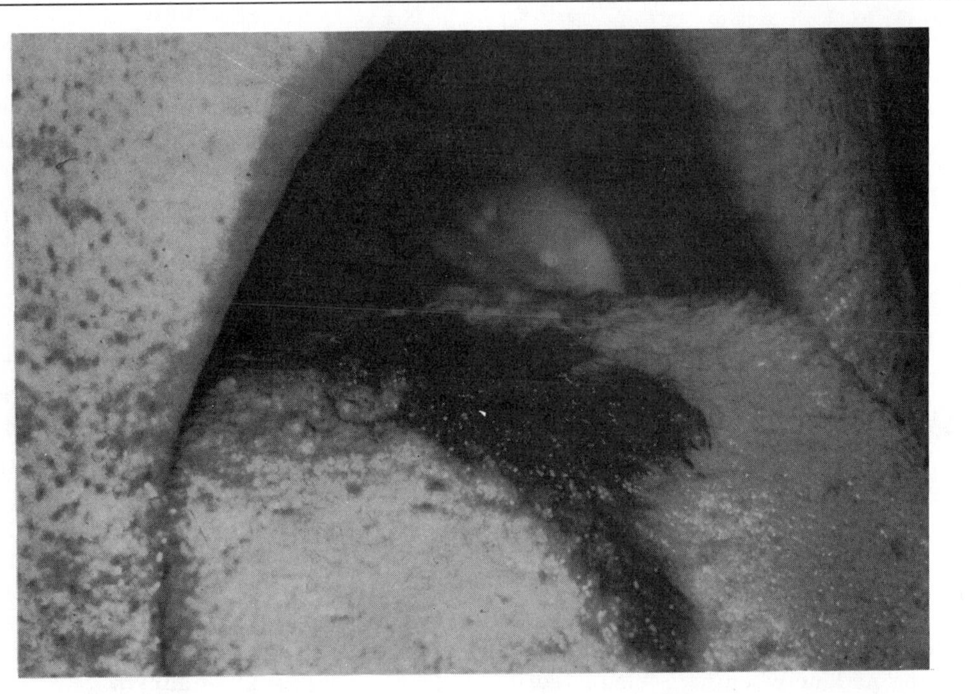

Figure 12-22 Hairy tongue. From Prior, John & Silberstein, Jack S. *Physical Diagnosis* (CV Mosby Co.: St. Louis 4ed., 1973 p. 146)

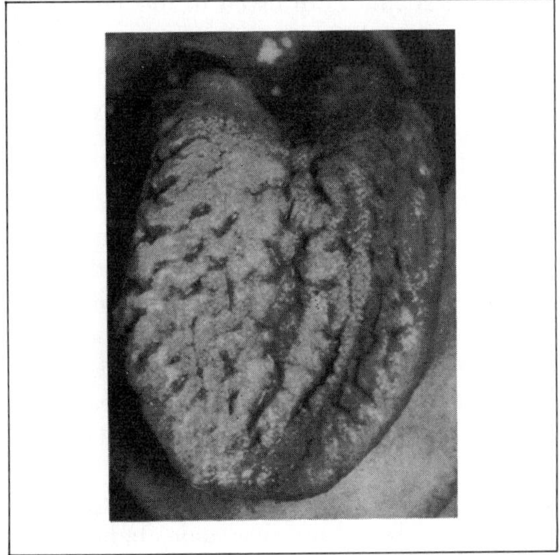

Figure 12-23 Scrotal tongue.

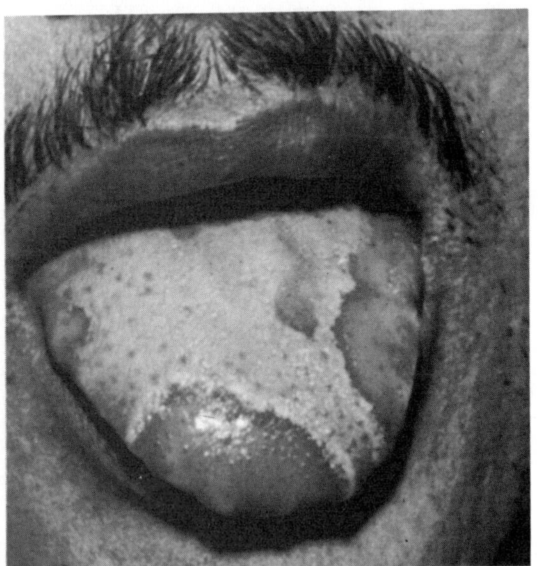

Figure 12-24 Geographic tongue.

inspection, since some diseases of the tongue have no surface manifestations and need to be felt in order to be detected. The tongue normally has a whitish coating through which the papillae show. A sore, red tongue and diminished or absent papillae occur with pernicious anemia and with riboflavin and niacin deficiencies. A red, beefy tongue is characteristic of pernicious anemia. A black, hairy tongue can occur following the use of antibiotics (see Figure 12-22). Deep fissures can indicate dehydration or malnutrition. Congenital fissures run horizontally across the tongue, whereas the fissures observed in dehydration are vertical (see Figures 12-23 and 12-24).

The client should be able to move his tongue

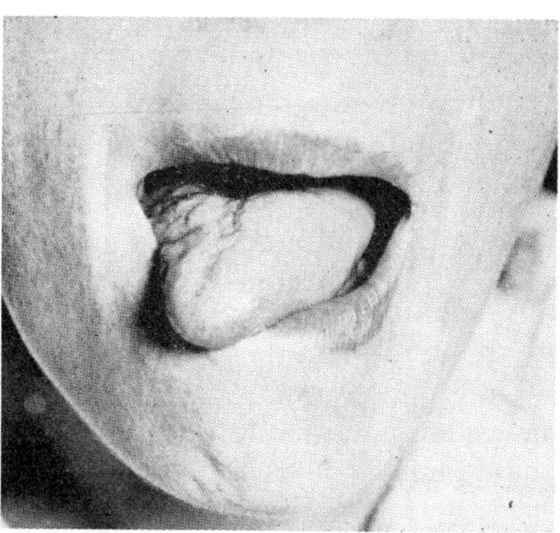

Figure 12-25 Deviation and atrophy of tongue due to paralysis of the hypoglossal nerve.

from side to side, and his tongue should protrude in the midline when he is instructed to stick it out as far as possible. Deviation to one side may indicate hypoglossal nerve damage (see Figure 12-25). Normally there are no fasciculations or tremors. Fine tremor may be present in hyperthyroidism, and gross tremor is observed in cerebral palsy. A small tongue may be seen in malnutrition and in paralysis of the hypoglossal nerve. A large tongue may be an early sign of hypothryoidism or acrom galy. The tongue may also appear large in clients with mental retardation. Asymmetry of the tongue may be due to nodules or growths or to neoplasms or bacterial or fungal diseases. Wear a glove to palpate such lesions.

An area commonly missed in the examination of the mouth is the floor beneath the tongue. Ask the client to raise the tip of his tongue toward the roof of his mouth. The frenulum is normally loose and pliable. In adults, inability to extend the tongue may be the result of a neoplasm; in children, it may be due to a shortened frenulum. In the latter condition, speech defects may be noted, particularly in the pronunciation of the letters *d, t, th, n,* and *l.* Correction of this condition, commonly known as being "tongue-tied," consists of a small incisional loosening of the frenulum; this minor surgery is usually performed in the emergency room.

Palpate the sublingual glands. These glands are normally firm and uniform.

Palate

Tilt the client's head slightly back in order to see the palate. Congenital cleft palate is readily observable in the neonate. The soft palate is normally pink and has fine vessels under the mucosa. The hard palate is whiter, more irregular, and has rugae running transversely. The hard palate is also a good area in which to detect jaundice. Many adults have a bony protuberance in the midline of the palate; this projection is termed a *torus palatinus.*

Note whether there is any deviation of the uvula. When the client is asked to say "aah," his uvula should rise in the midline. If it does not, there may be impairment of the 9th or 10th cranial nerve. Such failure may also be an early sign of poliomyelitis or diphtheria. The presence of pus or large amounts of mucus on the posterior wall of the pharynx is generally evidence of inflammation of the nasopharynx or of the sinuses.

Oropharynx

In order to inspect the oropharynx and the tonsils, which are located on either side of the oropharynx, the tongue blade must be inserted deeply. It should be pressed to the side of the tongue to avoid the gag reflex. (Testing of the gag reflex is not usually performed during a routine examination unless there are suspicious signs of abnormality, such as hoarseness, dysphagia, or uvular deviation.) All lymphoid tissues, including the tonsils, are enlarged in the young child. Acute tonsillitis presents as red, swollen tonsils. A white tonsillar membrane is found in diphtheria, infectious mononucleosis, leukemia, and beta streptococcal infection.

Acute pharyngitis, a viral or bacterial infection, causes a bright fiery red pharyngeal membrane. The tonsils also become swollen and flecks of exudate are visible. In streptococcal sore throat, the pharynx is diffusely reddened, and the tonsils and tonsillar nodes beneath the angles of the mandible are enlarged. The uvula is edematous, and an exudate covers the tonsils and the pharynx. Streptococcal infection may also be asymptomatic; therefore, routine pharyngeal culturing is performed during seasons of highest incidence and in geographic areas of risk. Following examination of the oropharynx and tonsillar areas, the gag reflex can be elicited if necessary by pressing on the posterior tongue with the tongue blade. Absence of the gag reflex

Technique for Examination of Mouth and Pharynx

1. Inspect lips.
2. Use bright light, gloves, and tongue blade to examine:
   Gums
   Mucous membrane
   Teeth
   Tongue:
   color size
   texture symmetry
   deviation lesions
   Palate and uvular reflex
   Oropharynx
   Tonsils—insert tongue blade deeply to each side. (Try not to elicit gag reflex, unless a problem is suspected.)

may indicate a problem with the glossopharyngeal or vagus nerve.

Summary

In this chapter assessment of the ear, nose, mouth, and pharynx was described.

Examination of the ear involves assessing the external portion, the auditory canal, and the tympanic membrane. The otoscope is used to inspect internal structures. There are several tests that can be used in determining hearing loss.

The techniques used for examining the nose are inspection, palpation, and transillumination of the sinuses. Examination of the mouth, including the lips, gums, teeth, and tongue, and of the palate and oropharynx consists mainly of inspection and palpation (see Table 12-4 for a summary of abnormalities).

Table 12-4. Common Abnormalities of the Nose, Mouth, and Pharynx

Terminology	Characteristics	Comments
Nose		
Rhinitis	Erythema and edema of mucosa	Note thick, greenish, odorous discharge for chronic condition. Note bluish gray mucosa in allergic rhinitis.
Perforation of septum	Difficulty breathing, dryness of mucosa, epistaxis	Note hole in septum; look for habits including nose picking and/or cocaine use. History of venereal disease. History of nasal-septal surgery.
Sinusitis	Inflammation, drainage, pain over sinuses, fever, chills, headache	Check for causative agent: virus, bacterium, allergy. Presence of polyps, deviated septum, dental abscess in maxillary bone, or general debility.
Polyps	Smooth, mobile, pale tumors; bleed easily	Should be removed if possibility they will become malignant. Nasal obstruction as they grow larger.
Lips		
Herpes simplex	Cluster of clear vesicles on lips that rupture, ulcerate, and become crusted	Caused by invasion of virus, herpes simplex type 1 or 2.
Cheilitis or cheilosis	Red, cracked, dry, bleeding lips; painful cracks, fissures in corner of mouth	Check for poor oral hygiene, overexposure to sunlight, wind, or chemicals. Vitamin B complex deficiency, monilial infection, seborrheic dermatitis.

Continued on page 236

Table 12-4 *Continued*

Terminology	Characteristics	Comments
Gums		
Gingivitus	Red, swollen, bleeding	Note poor dental hygiene; check for systemic disease, Vitamin C deficiency.
	Dark line along gingival margin	Check for lead or bismuth poisoning.
Peridontitis	Red, swollen peridontium (tissues surrounding the tooth)	Note dental hygiene, calcium deposits. Be aware that teeth will be lost.
Excessive salivation	Drooling	Check for inflammation of mouth, 9th or 10th cranial nerve injury.
Mucous membranes		
Anemia	Pale mucosa	Assess for development of mouth lesions or ulcers.
Koplik's spots	Small bluish white spots on lower lip and mucosa of lower teeth	Check for measles, since these spots are diagnostic before rash appears.
Petechiae	Small, purplish hemorrhagic spots	Check for leukemia, subacute bacterial endocarditis.
Leukoplakia	Patchy, raised, white lesion on cheeks, gums, or tongue; has well-defined borders	Check for chronic irritation, poor nutrition or syphilis. These lesions can be precancerous. Lesion cannot be peeled away as a monilial infection can.
Teeth		
Dental caries	Brown, gray, to gray-orange areas on tooth surfaces; size of area varies	Note dental hygiene. Some have a familial predisposition to caries. Check nutritional status.
Discoloration	Yellow-brown	Check for use of tetracycline.
	Green-brown	Often seen in clients who had hemolytic disease as newborns.
	Pitting, white spotting, or brown	Excessive fluoride ingestion; dental plaque.
Defects in enamel	Deep grooves, absent edges of incisors or occlusal surfaces	Note history of gastrointestinal problems, deficiency of calcium, phosphorus, or vitamins A and B.
Hutchinson's teeth	Pegged lateral incisors Notched central incisors	Congenital syphilis.
Tongue		
Alteration in color	Red, sore, beefy papillae, decreased or absent	Check for pernicious anemia. Riboflavin and/or niacin deficiencies.
	Black, hairy	Note use of antibiotics.
	Bright red, dorsal surface resembles map	Geographic tongue (nonpathologic)
Alterations in contour	Deep vertical fissures	Check for dehydration, malnutrition
	Deep horizontal fissures	Congenital defect (scrotal tongue)
Positional deviation	Tremors, fasciculations	Fine tremors may be present in hyperthyroidism. Gross tremors in cerebral palsy.
	Tongue doesn't protrude to midline or can't move from side to side	Possible hypoglossal nerve involvement
Asymmetry	Small tongue	Note malnutrition, paralysis of hypoglossal nerve.
	Large tongue	Hypothyroidism, acromegaly, mental retardation. Note nodules, growths—neoplasm, fungus, bacteria.

Table 12-4. *Continued*

Terminology	Characteristics	Comments
Palate		
Torus palatinus	Bony protuberence in midline of palate	Nonpathologic.
Cleft palate	Fissure, which is bilateral or unilateral, forming a passageway between mouth and nose	Congenital anomaly.
Deviation of uvula	Uvula does not rise in midline	Check for 9th, 10th cranial nerve involvement. Can be early sign of polio or diphtheria.
Oropharynx		
Acute tonsillitis	Red, swollen tonsils with yellowish exudate. Chills, including temperature, headache, pains and aches in back and extremities, pain when swallowing	Check for beta-hemolytic streptococcus, carditis, nephritis.
Infectious mononucleosis	White tonsillar membrane	Check for cervical, axillary, and inguinal lymphadenopathy or splenomegaly.
Acute pharyngitis	Bright, fiery red pharyngeal membrane, tonsils swollen with exudate; edematous uvula, white exudate covering tongue and tonsils; malaise, fever, dysphagia	Streptococcal infection.

Discussion Questions/Activities

1. Discuss the anatomy and physiology of the conduction of sound.
2. Describe the difference between the external auditory canal of the adult and of the child. How would this difference affect examination of the ear?
3. What is the light reflex and where is it located?
4. Describe various manifestations of pathology that are reflected by the tympanic membrane.
5. Demonstrate the Rinne and Weber tests.
6. Demonstrate the technique for examining the ear.
7. Demonstrate the procedure for examining the nares.
8. Why is it often difficult to view the middle and superior turbinates?
9. Which paranasal sinuses can be examined easily? What is the procedure for this examination?
10. Describe some common abnormalities that may be found when examining the lips, buccal mucosa, and tongue.
11. Discuss the rationale for having a client with dentures remove them during examination of the mouth.
12. What structures are examined in the oropharynx?

Recording of Findings

Normal findings are presented in the first box. Abnormal findings are presented in the second box.

Ear

INSPECTION
Normal positioning, no deformities.

PALPATION
No masses, lesions or tenderness; no cerumen or discharge; no redness or swelling of ear canal; eardrum pearly gray color, no perforation; light reflex present.

PERCUSSION
Watch ticking heard bilaterally; Weber test—no lateralization; Rinne: $AC > BC$.

Nose

INSPECTION AND PALPATION
No tenderness or deformity; patent bilaterally, no perforations or deviation of septum; can identify alcohol; no redness, swelling, or discharge.

PERCUSSION
Sinuses not tender. Frontal and maxillary sinuses transilluminate.

Mouth

INSPECTION
Lips normal, no cracks or fissures; buccal mucosa pink; soft and hard palate clear—no ulcers, sores, or lacerations; tongue normal—no cracks, fissures, or edema, protrudes in midline, no tremor; teeth in good condition, no caries or missing teeth.

PALPATION
No nodules, no tenderness.

Pharynx

INSPECTION
Mucosa pink; uvula rises in midline on phonation; tonsils present without inflammation; gag reflex present.

Ear

INSPECTION
Normal positioning, no deformities.

PALPATION
No masses or lesions; left ear: pinna painful to touch, canal reddened, eardrum yellow; light reflex absent; right ear normal color, no perforation, light reflex present.

PERCUSSION
Watch ticking heard bilaterally; Weber lateralizes to left ear; Rinne: $BC > AC$.

Nose

INSPECTION AND PALPATION
No deformity; mucosa reddened and swollen with moderate amount of clear drainage; patent bilaterally; no perforations of septum; unable to identify alcohol and soap.

PERCUSSION
Frontal and maxillary sinuses tender on light percussion and do not transilluminate.

Mouth

INSPECTION
Lips dry and cracked; buccal mucosa pale; soft and hard palate clear—no ulcers, sores, or lacerations; tongue midline without cracks, fissures, tremors, or edema; multiple dental caries; lower lateral incisors absent.

PALPATION
No nodules; no tenderness.

Pharynx

INSPECTION
Mucosa red; uvular reflex present; tonsils enlarged and reddened; gag reflex present.

CHAPTER 13

Assessment of the Thorax and Lungs

LEARNING OBJECTIVES

1. Review the structure and function of the thorax and lungs.
2. Compare the shape of the thorax of the adult to that of the child.
3. State the characteristics of respirations that are noted on inspection.
4. Recognize the landmarks of the thorax used in documentation of physical findings.
5. Describe the norm and technique of assessing fremitus.
6. Describe the techniques of percussion and auscultation of the lung fields.
7. Identify the various percussion notes and breath sounds and the locations where they are normally heard on the thorax.
8. Explain the technique of determining the diaphragmatic excursion.

This chapter considers the assessment of the thorax and lungs. Assessment begins with noting the gross appearance of the thorax—its size and shape. Next, progressing from the outside, the skin is examined; then the muscles and bones are assessed, followed by examination of the lungs.

Structure and Function of the Thorax

The thorax is a bony cage defined by the sternum, the costal cartilages, the ribs, and the bodies of the thoracic vertebrae. In the normal client it is cone-shaped—narrow at the top and wide at the bottom. The thorax supports the bones of the shoulder and upper extremities and contains the lungs, heart, and upper portions of the major blood vessels.

The *sternum*, located at the anterior medial chest, is a flat narrow bone about 15 cm long. It is divided into three parts: the upper part, or *manubrium*; the middle part, or *body*; and the lower part, or *xiphoid process* (see Figure 13-1). The upper seven costal cartilages are attached to the manubrium and body. The xiphoid process has no attached ribs but does provide for the attachment of some of the abdominal muscles.

The thorax contains 24 ribs, with 12 on each

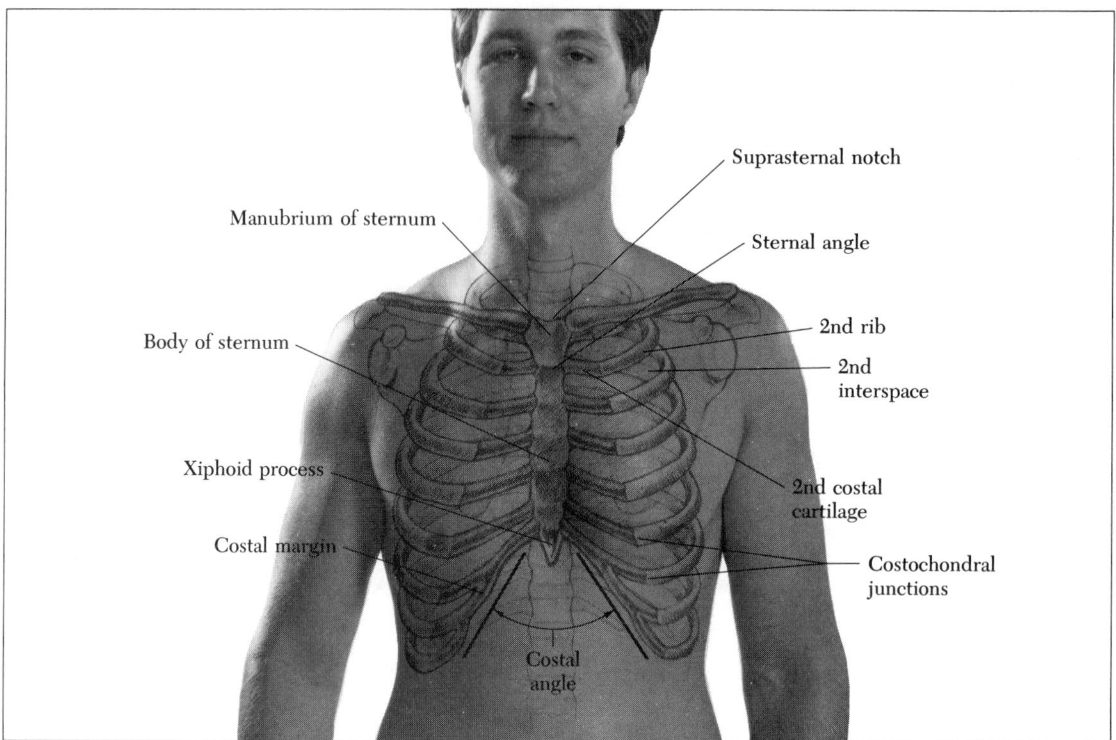

Figure 13-1 Anatomy of the chest.

side of the thoracic cavity. All the ribs are attached to the vertebral column. The first 7 pairs, which are connected to the sternum by means of the costal cartilages, are called true ribs. Of the remaining five pairs, called the false ribs, the upper three are attached to the costal cartilage of the next rib above. The two lowest ribs are termed floating, or vertebral, ribs. The spaces between the ribs are the *intercostal spaces.*

Structure of the Lungs

The lungs are elastic conelike sacs that fill up the pleural section of the thoracic cavity. The base of the lungs extends to the diaphragm. The apices rise slightly above the clavicles. Both lungs lie against the rib cage anteriorly and posteriorly. Figure 13-2 illustrates the *trachea,* which brings air to the lungs and divides at the *hilum* into the right and left main *bronchi.* These further divide into *bronchioles* and finally terminate in the *alveoli,* where the major part of respiration occurs—the diffusion of oxygen and carbon dioxide.

The *mediastinum* is the mass of tissues in the center of the thoracic cavity dividing the lungs and containing the esophagus, trachea, and large vessels of the heart.

Figure 13-3 shows that the left lung is divided into two lobes, upper and lower, while the right lung is divided into three: upper, middle, and lower. The lungs are covered by the *pleura,* a smooth membrane. The lining of the thorax is the *parietal pleura,* the lung coverings the *visceral pleura.* The potential space between the two is referred to as the pleural space.

In order to locate findings in the thorax, you must understand the placement of the ribs. On the anterior chest an important landmark is the *manubriosternal junction,* referred to as the *angle of Louis.* This ridge lies next to the second rib. From this point you can identify the second intercostal space and count the other spaces as necessary in order to identify the location of other structures within the thoracic cavity. This is also the area wherein the trachea bifurcates

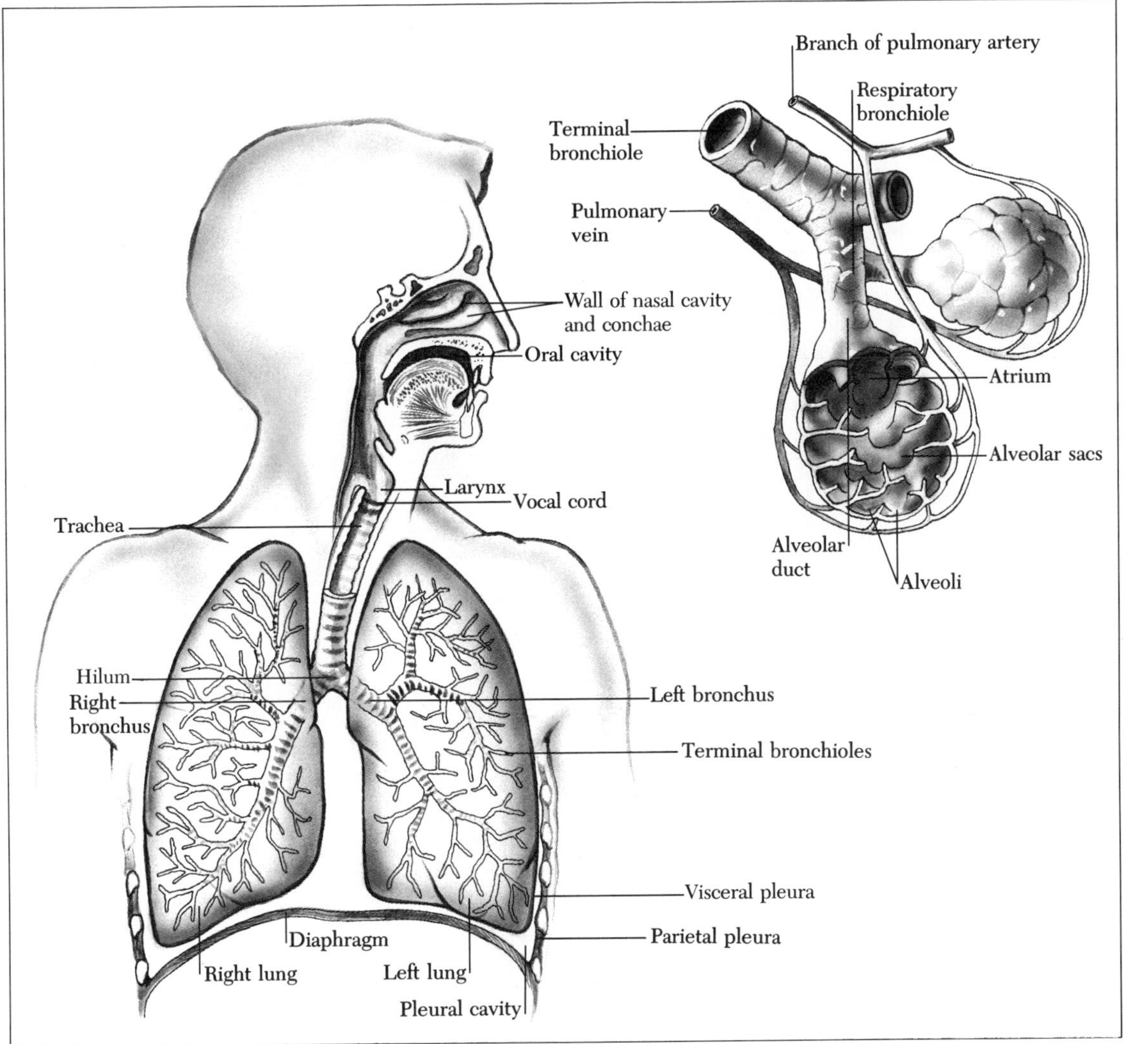

Figure 13-2 Structure of the lung, with detail of alveoli.

and where the fifth thoracic vertebra is located, as well as the upper portions of the right and left atria. On the posterior portion of the chest wall the seventh cervical vertebra is at the base of the neck and is the most prominent spinous process. Just below this is the first thoracic vertebra, which is often as evident as the seventh cervical.

The scapulae lie approximately between the second and eighth ribs and are about 4 cm from the midspinal line.

Certain anatomic landmarks illustrated in Figure 13-4 are helpful in describing physical findings. On the lateral chest they are the *anterior axillary line* (AAL), the *midaxillary line* (MAL), and the *posterior axillary line* (PAL). On the anterior chest these are the *midsternal line* (MSL), the *midclavicular line* (MCL), the *intercostal spaces* (ICS), the *ribs*, the *suprasternal notch*, the *precordium*, and the *epigastric area*. On the posterior thorax the *midvertebral line*, the *midscapular line*, and the spinal vertebrae serve as helpful landmarks.

Characteristics and Techniques of Examination

Inspection

The assessment of the thorax is carried out using the technique of inspection. Palpation of the thorax occurs during the assessment of the lungs.

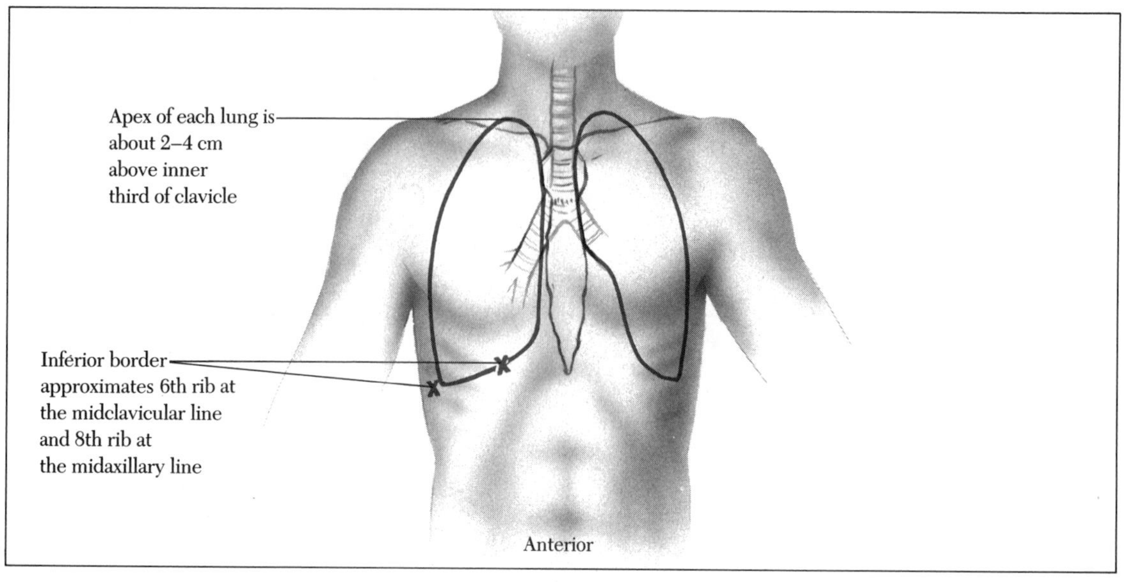
Apex of each lung is about 2–4 cm above inner third of clavicle
Inferior border approximates 6th rib at the midclavicular line and 8th rib at the midaxillary line
Anterior

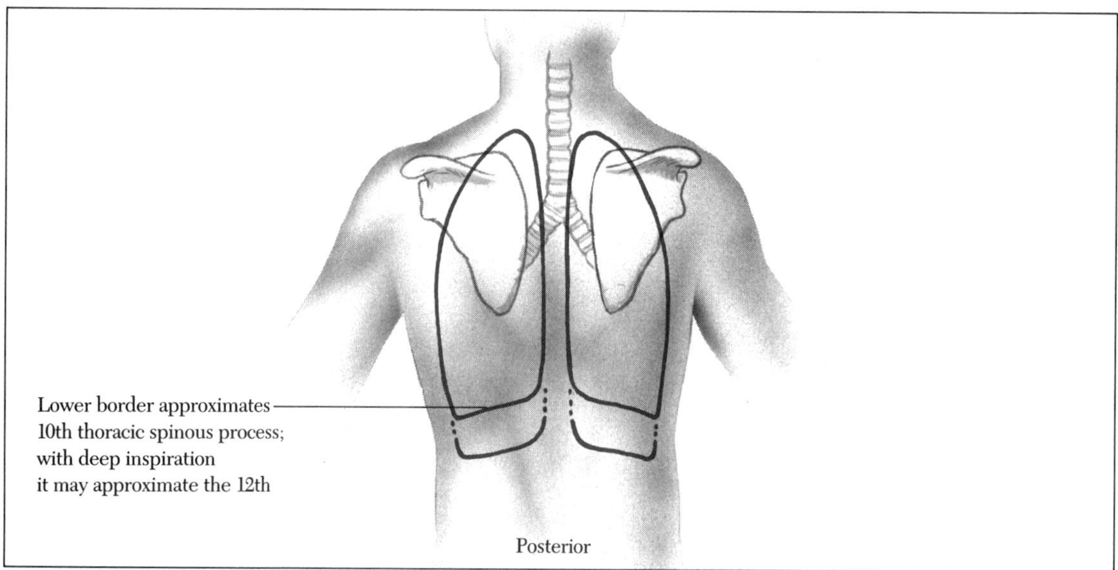
Lower border approximates 10th thoracic spinous process; with deep inspiration it may approximate the 12th
Posterior

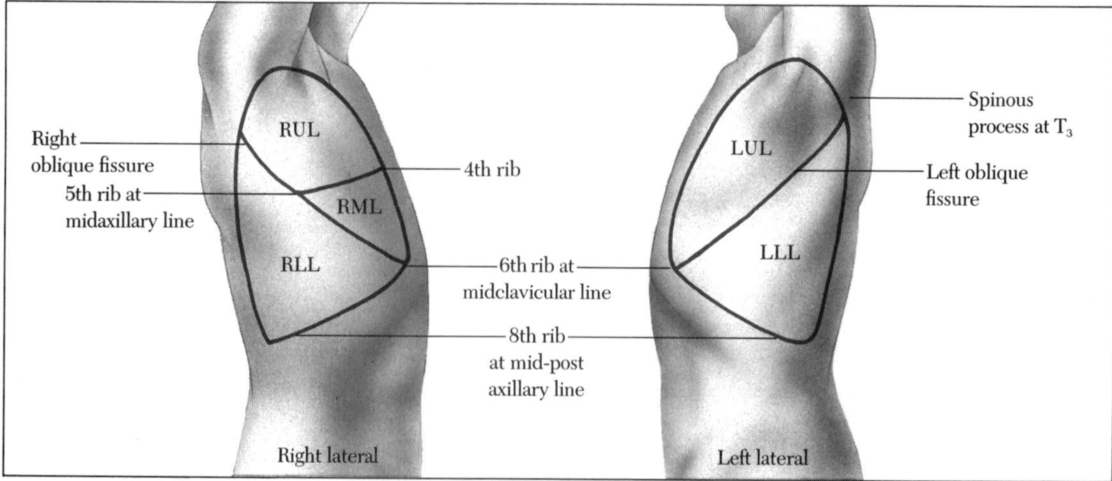
Right oblique fissure
5th rib at midaxillary line
RUL
RML
RLL
4th rib
6th rib at midclavicular line
8th rib at mid-post axillary line
LUL
LLL
Spinous process at T_3
Left oblique fissure
Right lateral
Left lateral

Figure 13-3 Position of the lungs and ribs.

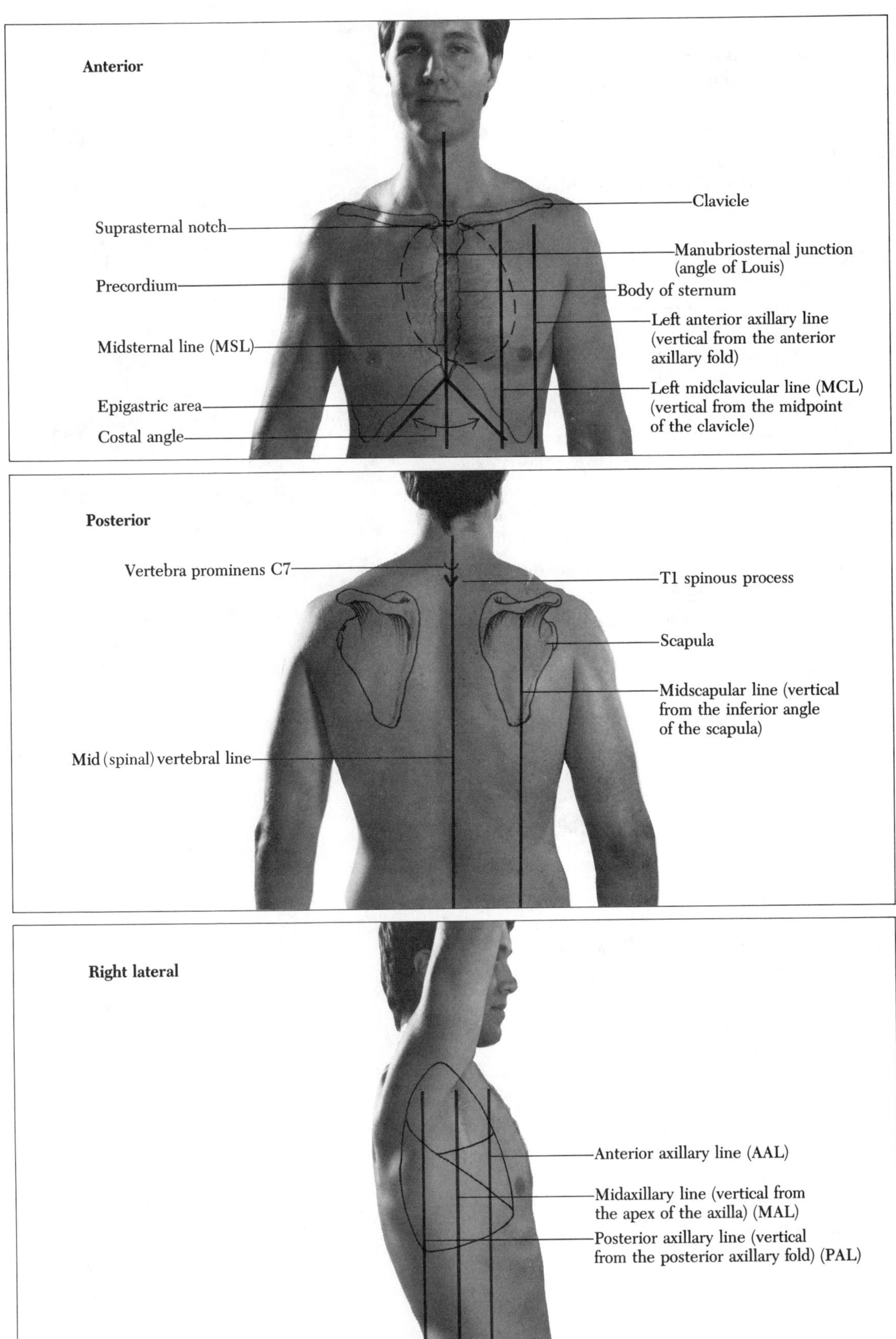

Figure 13-4 Topographic landmarks for physical assessment of the chest and respiratory system.

In order for the chest to be adequately inspected, the client must be stripped to the waist and lighting must be good. The chest may be examined with the client in the supine or in the sitting position. If the client cannot sit up, be sure that his body is straight and is as flat as can be tolerated. Whether in the sitting or supine position, the client's back must be straight. In our discussion, the examination and accompanying diagrams will refer to the client in the upright position.

Examine the skin of the chest. Males generally have more body hair than females. In the male the hair growth is less abundant on the posterior aspect of the thorax in comparison to the anterior chest. In females that amount of hair growth on the anterior and posterior thorax is essentially the same. Acne lesions, seborrheic keratosis, and cafe au lait spots more often occur on the posterior aspect of the thorax. Dilation of superficial veins on the anterior chest wall is characteristic of superior vena cava obstruction.

Observe the anteroposterior (AP) diameter of the client's chest from a lateral position. The AP diameter of the adult thorax should be less than the transverse diameter. Alterations in the AP diameter will be seen in conditions such as emphysema, where the client exhibits the classic barrel chest (see Figure 13-5). The shape of the normal adult thorax is elliptic; the infant's is cylindric. In the child a persistent round chest after the age of 6 suggests a chronic pulmonary disease such as asthma. With the child, at least until 2 years of age, the chest circumference should be measured at the level of the nipple line. The measurement should be approximately the same (± 2 cm) as the child's head size.

Next check for symmetry of the thorax. Minor degrees of asymmetry are not serious. The shoulders should be at one level, but in many clients one shoulder may be slightly lower than the other, which can be perfectly normal. Very often the handedness of the client will result in greater muscular development on one side. Asymmetry is also common with scoliosis, an abnormal condition.

When the lower sternum is markedly depressed, with the ribs flared outward, the condition is called *pectus excavatum*, or funnel chest (see Figure 13-6). When the sternum protrudes markedly, the chest takes on the configuration of a pigeon and is thus referred to as a

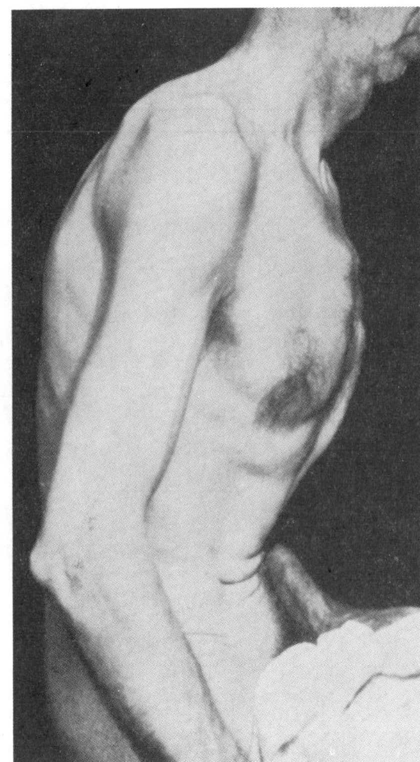

Figure 13-5 Barrel chest of emphysema. Note the increase in anterior-posterior diameter.

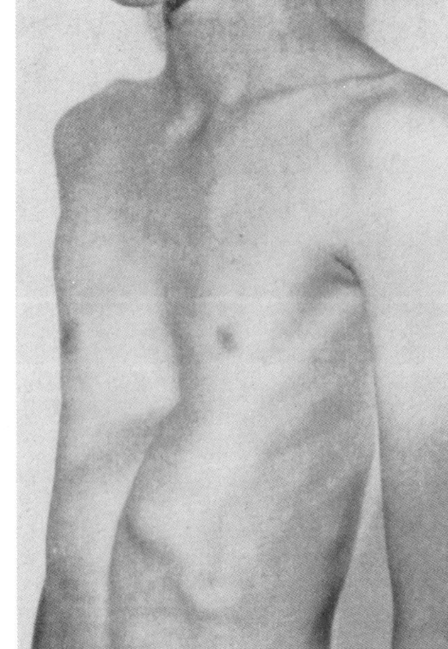

Figure 13-6 Funnel chest. Note the deep depression of the lower sternum and the outward flare of the lower ribs.

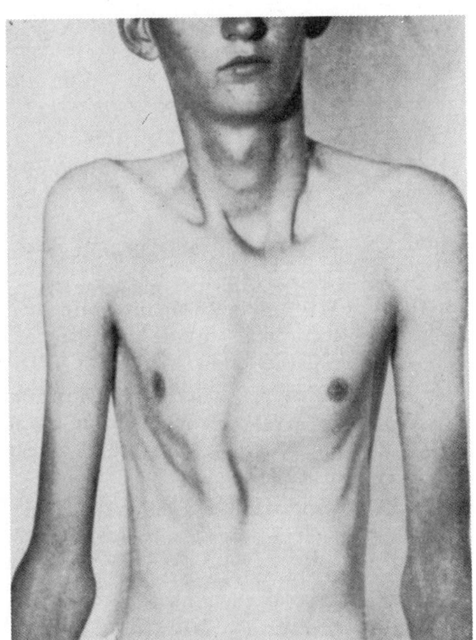

Figure 13-7 Pigeon breast as a result of rickets. Note the bilateral depression of the lower chest portion and the protrusion of the sternum.

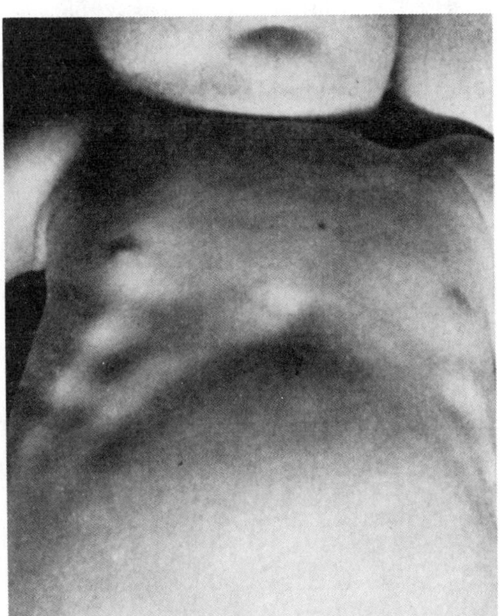

Figure 13-8 Rachitic rosary. Note the series of prominences corresponding to the costochondral junctions.

pigeon breast (see Figure 13-7). This is termed *pectus carinatum*.

Retraction of the ribs and intercostal spaces may indicate a collapsed lung or fractured ribs. Bulging of the chest wall is suggestive of a greatly enlarged heart or of an aortic aneurysm.

Long-standing vitamin deficiencies such as rickets cause prominence of the costochondral junctions. This condition is referred to as rachitic rosary because of the prominent knobs that form at these angles (see Figure 13-8).

Observe the posterior chest for the location of the scapulae and the spine. The spine should be straight with a slight concavity at the thoracic area.

Examine the rate, depth, and type of respiration. The respiratory rate varies with age and activity. Inspiration is active, whereas expiration is passive. Respiration is usually diaphragmatic in males and costal in females. Clients with reduced compliance of the lungs, as in heart disease, tuberculosis, and atelectasis (collapsed lung tissue), tend to have rapid, shallow breathing. The accessory muscles of the neck should be observed; they become strained in such diseases as emphysema and asthma, where the act of breathing becomes an effort.

The following terms are used when recording types of breathing patterns. *Dyspnea* refers to a difficulty in breathing characterized by air hunger or a desire for air. *Stridor* is the term used to characterize the high-pitched crowing sounds that occur with difficult inspiration; it is observed in children with croup and in aspiration of a foreign object. *Tachypnea* describes increase in the respiratory rate; *hyperpnea*, increase in the rate and depth of respiration. *Hyperventilation* is an increase in both rate and depth. Hyperventilation can be caused by central nervous system lesions (in the medulla oblongata), metabolic acidosis, and anxiety states. *Cheyne-Stokes respirations*—periods of hyperpnea and apnea (cessation of breathing)—are characteristic of clients with severe cerebral

Technique for Inspection of the Thorax and Lungs

1. Provide adequate lighting and a warm room.
2. Bare the client to the waist.
3. Have client sit with back straight.
4. Characteristics: Symmetry, skin, AP diameter, scapulae, spine, respirations, abnormalities.

Table 13-1. Common Abnormalities of the Thorax and Lungs

Terminology	Characteristics	Comments
Thorax		
Barrel chest	Increased AP diameter; chest has no apparent movement during respiration	Seen with chronic pulmonary disease.
Funnel chest	Lower sternum depressed; ribs flare outward	Rickets, congenital abnormality.
Retraction of ribs and intercostal spaces	Abdominal, intercostal, or supraclavicular muscles draw back during inspiration	May be due to tumor, foreign body, secretions, chronic lung disease, collapsed lung or fractured ribs.
Bulging of chest wall	Intercostal spaces protrude further forward than ribs on expiration	Possibly due to enlarged heart, aortic aneurysm, pleural effusion, tension pneumothorax, chronic pulmonary disease.
Rachitic rosary	Prominent costochondral junctions; knobs form at angles	Long-standing vitamin deficiency such as rickets.
Lungs		
Dyspnea	Difficulty breathing; air hunger	Normal when due to vigorous work or athletic activity. Results from insufficient oxygenation of lungs (i.e., circulatory disturbances, low Hgb, acidosis, lesions in respiratory center). May also be a subjective feeling.
Stridor	High-pitched crowing sounds on inspiration	Obstruction of air passage (i.e., aspiration of foreign object). Croup.
Tachypnea	Increased respiratory rate (40 or more breaths per minute)	May occur in hysteria, neurasthenia. May cause excess loss of CO_2 if prolonged.
Hyperpnea	Increase in both rate and depth of respiration	May be normal following exercise. Can be caused by pain, drugs, hysteria, or high altitude.
Hyperventilation	Increase in rate and depth of respiration	Anxiety, metabolic acidosis. Central nervous system lesions.
Cheyne-Stokes respirations	Periods of hyperpnea and apnea	Signs of severe cerebral hemorrhage or impending death.
Kussmaul's breathing	Extreme rate and depth	Metabolic acidosis, diabetic acidosis, or renal disease.
Decreased respiratory movement	Inspiration is barely noticeable	Chest trauma, pain, pleurisy consolidation, fibrosis, atelectasis, pneumothorax, COPD.
Asymmetrical respiratory movement	On palpation, nurse's hands move unequally since two lungs don't expand symmetrically	Fractured ribs, pleurisy, fibrosis, arthritis of spine, pneumonectomy.

hemorrhage as well as of those nearing death. *Kussmaul's breathing* (extreme rate and depth of breathing) is so labored that it is readily noticed from across a room. It is characteristic of metabolic acidosis and is observed in diabetic acidosis and renal disease. The anxious client may complain of apprehension, shortness of breath, and a sense of suffocation. Sighing respirations often pinpoint the neurotic client; this kind of breathing may be described as overbreathing accompanied by a deep inspiration and a long sighing expiration. (See Table 13-1.)

Palpation

With few exceptions, palpation is conducted using the palmar aspects of both hands. The palpation technique will inform you of the texture of the skin and will reveal any pulsations, masses, crepitus, or tenderness.

To determine whether both sides of the res-

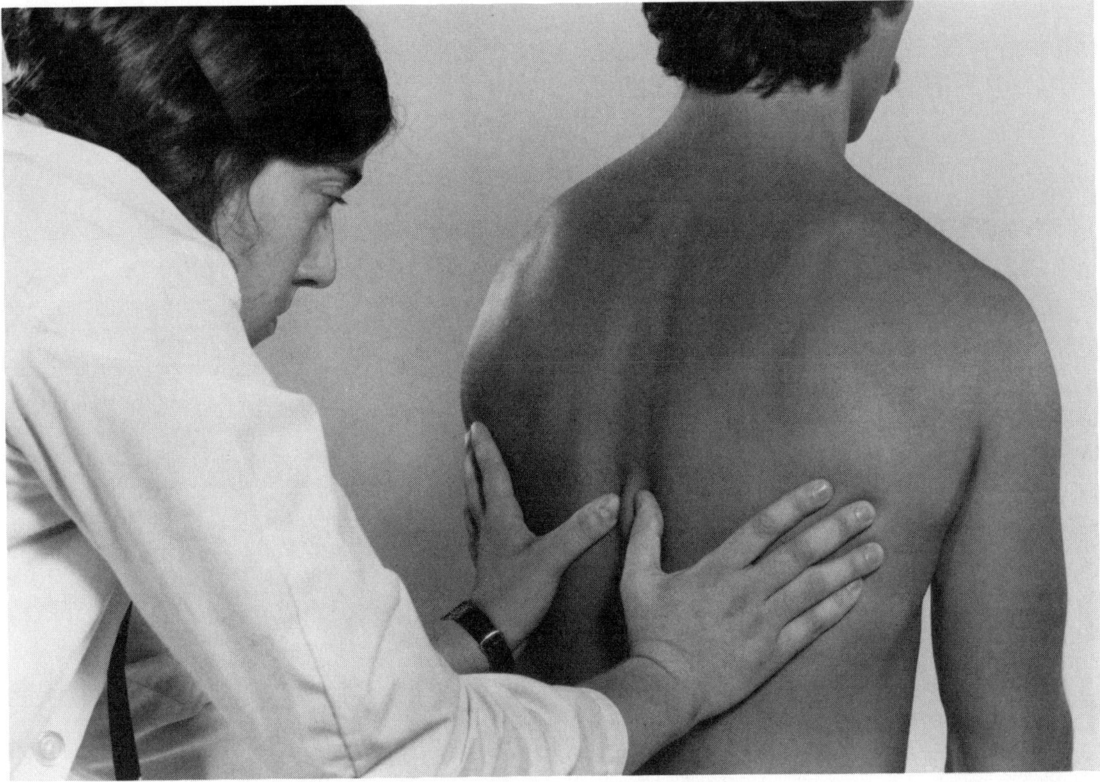

Figure 13-9 Technique for determining respiratory expansion.

piratory system expand equally, stand behind the client and place your hands over the lower posterolateral aspect of the thorax with your thumbs adjacent and near the spine, as illustrated in Figure 13-9. During deep inspiration your thumbs should move apart at the same time and should be equal in the distance of their movement. Fractured ribs, pleurisy, pulmonary fibrosis, and arthritis of the spine can all produce uneven or reduced chest expansion. In severe emphysema there is little expansion because air is trapped in the lungs, leaving them more or less always expanded with little room for additional movement.

Palpate the entire thorax for pain, swelling, or crepitation. Pain, swelling, or abnormal movement may be indicative of fractured ribs or pleurisy. With pleurisy the pain becomes distinctively more severe upon deep inspiration. Pain in the intercostal spaces may be caused by a neuritis of the intercostal nerves and by myositis (irritation of a muscle). Crepitation, a coarse, crackling sensation of the skin that results from air escaping from the respiratory system and entering the subcutaneous tissues, may be observed in pneumothorax and sometimes in the tissues surrounding a tracheostomy.

The normal spoken voice produces palpable vibrations called *vocal fremitus*, or tactile fremitus. Figure 13-10 illustrates how fremitus is detected with the ulnar aspect of the hands (A) or with the palmar aspects of the fingers (B). The hands are placed on the corresponding sides of the posterior chest wall, and the client is asked to repeat words that normally set up increased vibrations, such as "ninety-nine," "blue moon," or "one-two-three." Fremitus is present in the normal lung. Fremitus is easy to palpate on the chest of the crying baby. Transmission of the tactile vibrations should be compared on both sides of the chest; that is, vibrations felt over the left lung field should be compared to those felt over the right lung field. The lateral aspects of the thorax, particularly the anterior thoracic area overlying the middle lobe of the right lung, should also be palpated. Low-pitched voices, generally found in males, will be more palpable. Fremitus also is more intense at the back of the neck, between the scapulae, and in the first and second intercostal spaces. Increased vocal fremitus occurs when there is consolidation of the lung, as in pneumonia. Decreased or absent fremitus may be found in the obstruction of a bronchus or in pneumothorax.

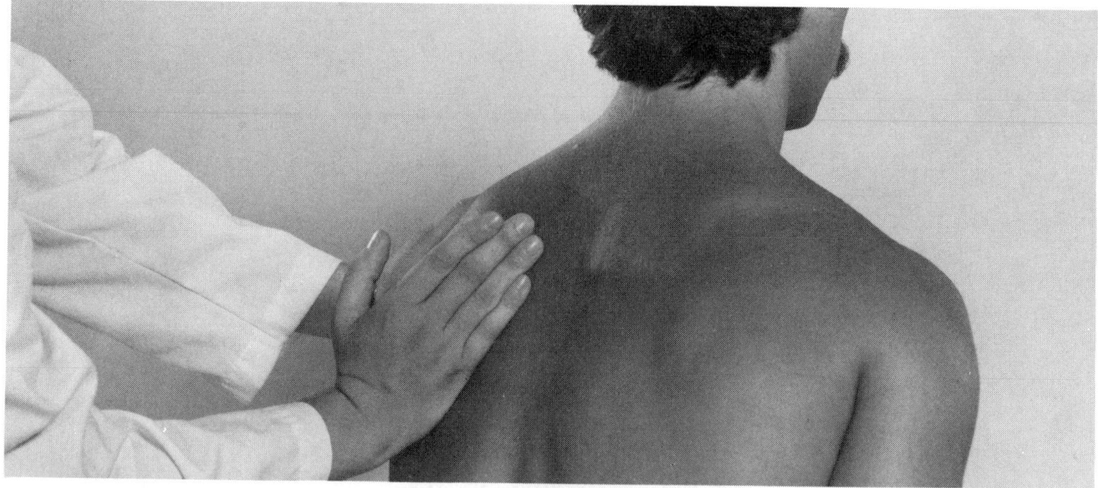

A

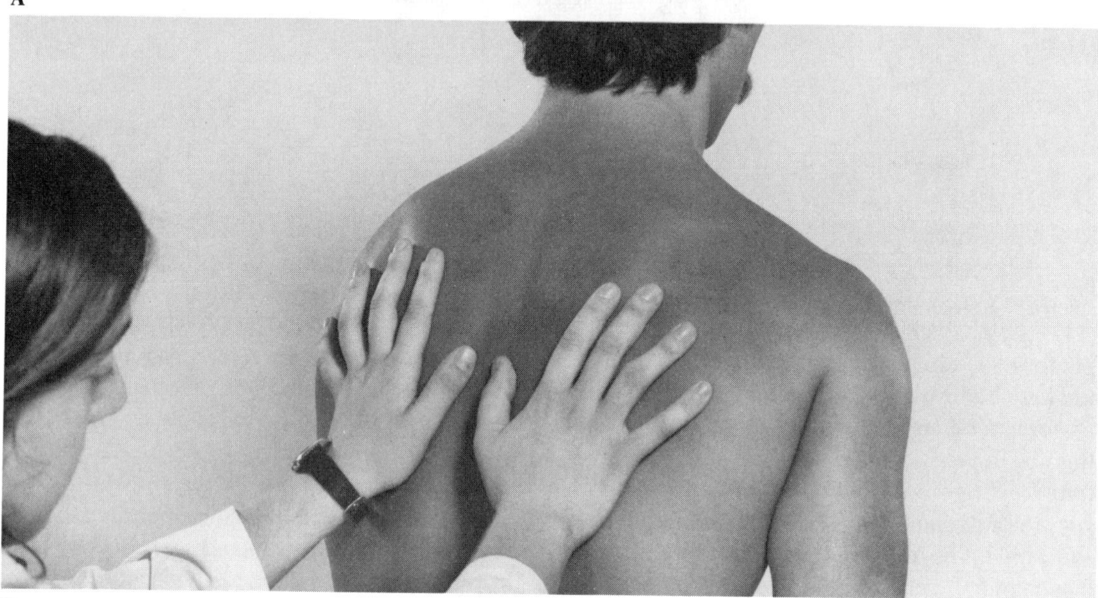

B

Figure 13-10 Palpation technique for fremitus. (A) Ulnar. (B) Palmar.

Palpation of the trachea should be performed to determine movement and possible presence of deviation. On inspiration the trachea stretches downward. A deviation to one side may be seen in tension pneumothorax or in mediastinal shift resulting from a pneumonectomy.

Percussion

Percussion should be attempted in the intercostal spaces rather than on the ribs, as percussion on the ribs will elicit dullness. Percussion of the lungs should be carried out in a systematic manner on the anterior, lateral, and posterior walls of the chest. On the anterior wall, begin percussion above the clavicles in the supraclavicular space and continue down to the diaphragm; as with palpating for fremitus, compare one side of the chest to the other. Figure 13-11 illustrates this procedure. Percussion of the lateral chest wall should begin in the axilla and work down a few inches at a time to about the level of the tenth rib. Similarly, the posterior chest should be percussed on both sides beginning at the apices of the lungs, percussing left side and then the right, each time moving downward toward the diaphragm. In percussing the posterior wall it is helpful to have the client lean forward with arms folded at the waist and the head flexed.

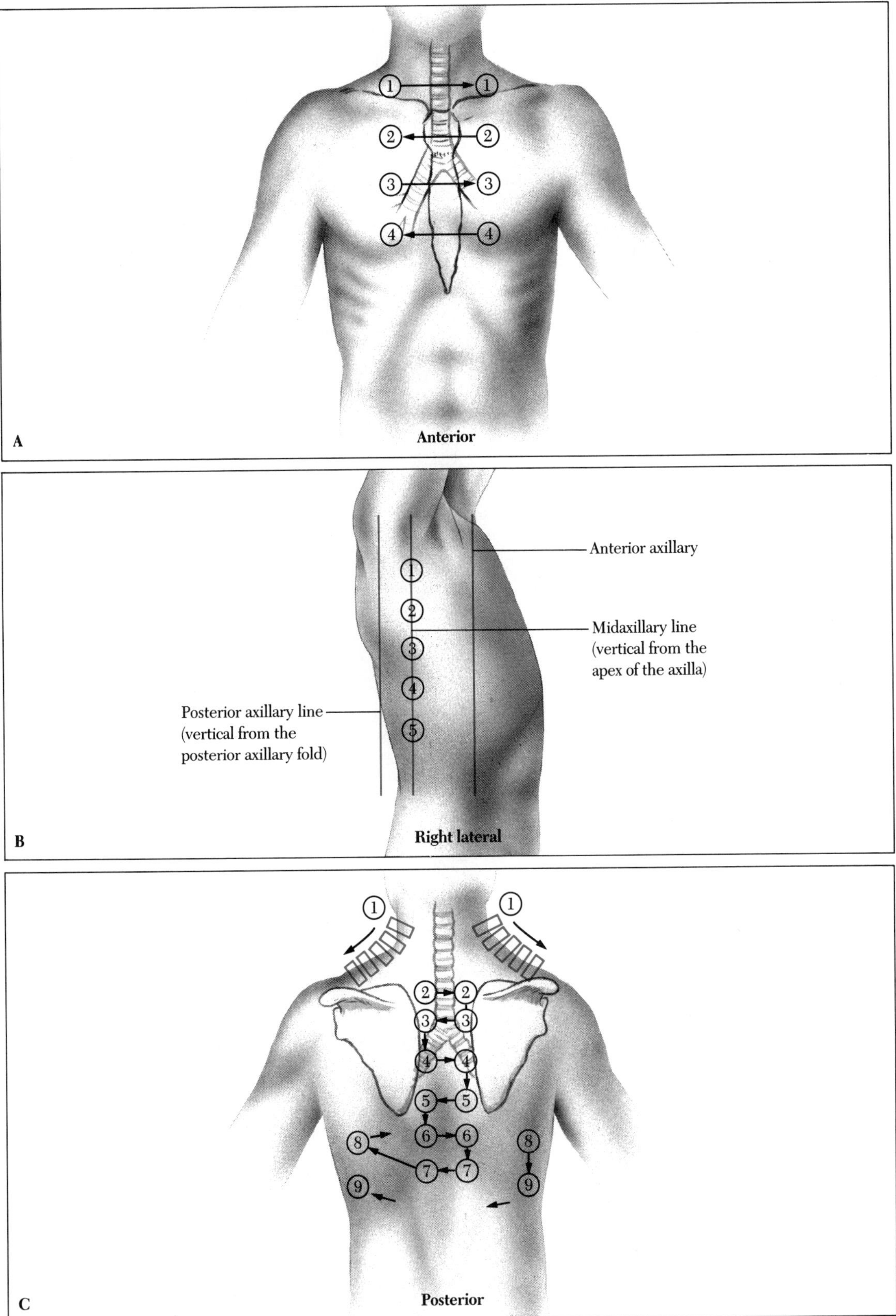

Figure 13-11 Method of thoracic percussion. (A) Percussion of anterior thorax. (B) Right lateral percussion. (C) Percussion of posterior thorax.

Table 13-2. Description of Percussion Notes

Note	Intensity	Pitch	Duration	Quality	Normal location
Flatness	Soft	High	Short	Extreme dullness	Thigh
Dullness	Soft	High	Moderate	Thudlike	Liver
Resonance	Moderate to loud	Low	Long	Hollow	Peripheral lung
Hyperresonance	Very loud	Very low	Very long	Booming	Child's lung
Tympany	Loud	High	Moderate	Musical, drumlike	Air-filled stomach

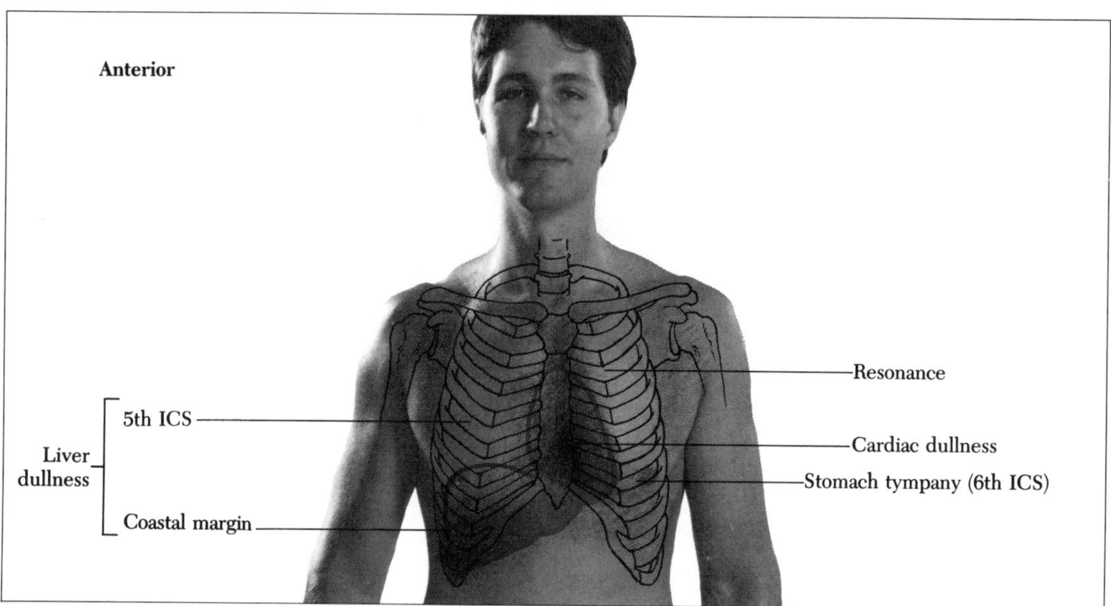

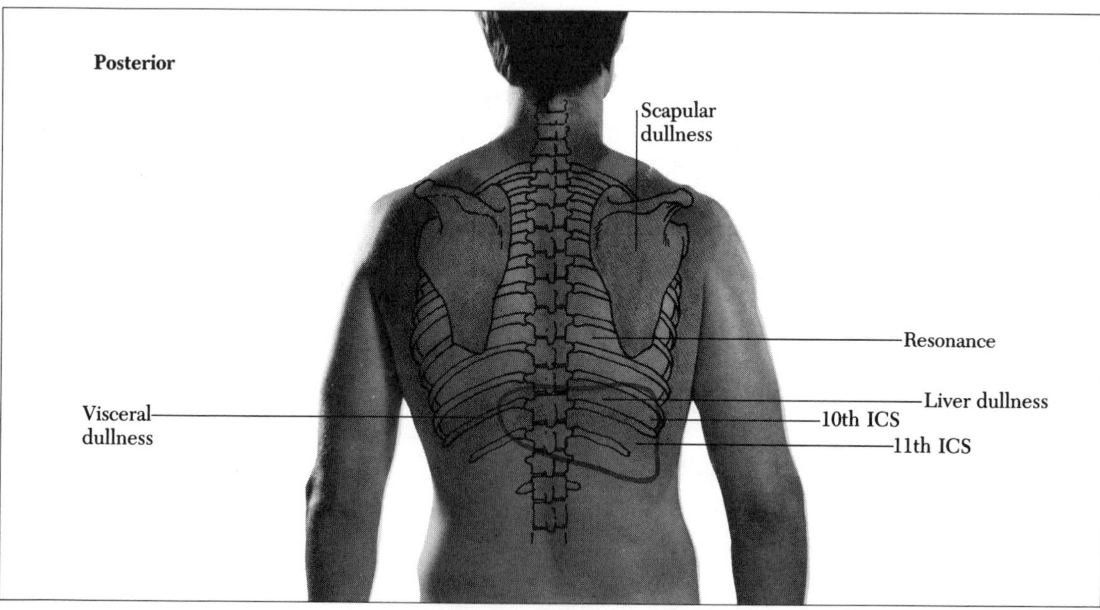

Figure 13-12 Normal percussion notes on the anterior and posterior chest.

Technique for Palpation of the Thorax and Lungs

1. Gently palpate the bones of the thorax.
2. Palpate the equal expansion of the lungs.
3. Use palmar and/or ulnar aspects of your hands.
4. Have client say "99" or "blue moon."
5. Compare side to side.

Table 13-2 and Figure 13-12 illustrate the percussion notes of a normal chest. The percussion notes heard over the normal lung should be resonant. The sound is loudest where the chest wall is thinnest. Because the chest wall is thinner in children, the percussion notes over their lung fields are more resonant than those of adults. Hyperresonance is the percussion sound heard over a hyperinflated lung, as in emphysema. Because there is little difference between resonance and hyperresonance, other clues may be needed to confirm hyperresonance. For example, a suspected hyperresonant percussion note may be more credible if there are accompanying signs of emphysema, such as a lowered diaphragm level below the tenth rib and a barrel chest. Dullness is percussed over solid organs such as the heart, liver, and spleen. On the posterior chest wall dullness is encountered over the scapulae and the heavy shoulder muscles, as well as areas of consolidation. The client with pneumonia will exhibit dullness over the affected lung. Pleural fluid, pleural thickening, fibrosis, tumors, and an area of atelectasis (collapsed lung tissue) will sound dull in relation to surrounding normal lung tissue. On the lower left anterior chest wall tympany may be elicited, because of the presence of a gastric air bubble.

The lowest point in the normal lung where resonance can be detected is at the diaphragm, which is at about the level of the eighth to the tenth rib (see Figure 13-3). This border changes during inspiration (diaphragm moves downward, expanding the area for resonant percussion) and during expiration (diaphragm moves upward). As the lungs expand and deflate, the area of underlying lung tissue with the accompanying percussion resonance does the same. To determine the degree of *diaphragmatic excursion*, illustrated in Figure 13-13, ask the client to take a deep breath and hold it. Meanwhile, percuss down one side of the posterior thorax until

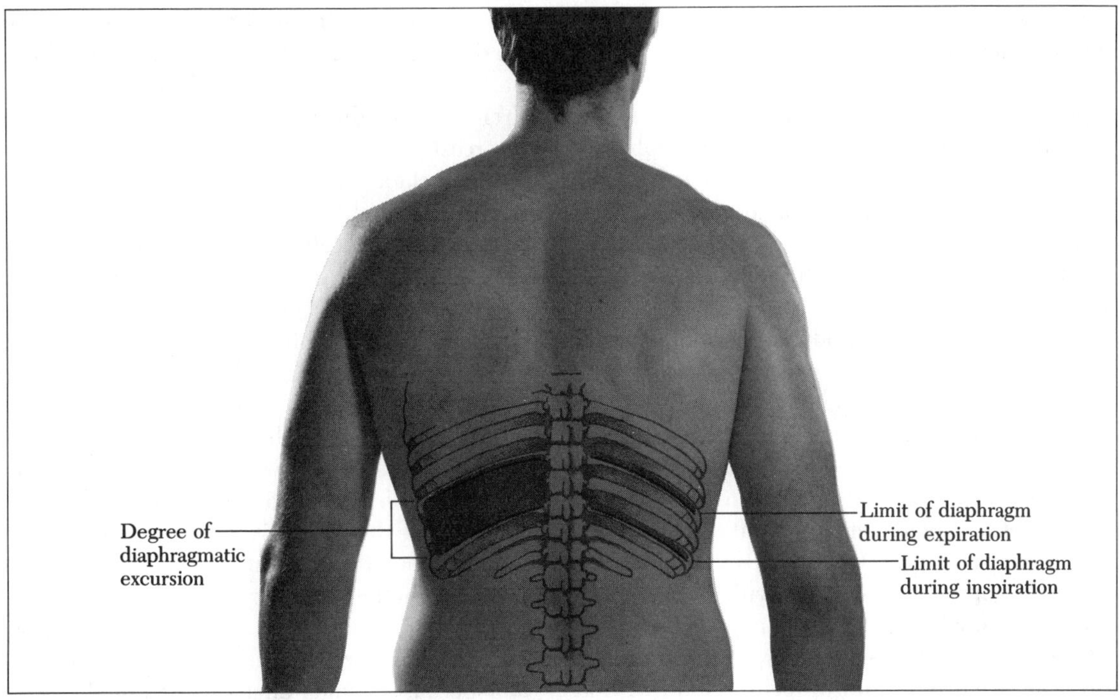

Figure 13-13 Method of determining diaphragmatic excursion.

Technique for Percussion of Lung Fields

1. Percussion done in the intercostal spaces.
2. For percussion of posterior wall have client flex neck and lean slightly forward with arms folded at waist.
3. Percuss anterior, posterior, and lateral walls of the chest.
4. Proceed side to side on the anterior and posterior aspects at 2–3 inch intervals.
5. Proceed from axilla downward at 2–3 inch intervals to about the 10th rib for assessment of lateral aspects.
6. Decision making: Employ techniques of bronchophony, egophony, and whispered pectoriloquy over area(s) of abnormal percussion notes (see section "Other Techniques" later in this chapter).

Technique for Determining Diaphragmatic Excursion

1. Have the client take a deep breath and hold it.
2. Percuss downward from area of resonance.
3. Mark the level of dullness.
4. Ask client to let out his breath and hold before taking a second breath.
5. Percuss from about 5–6 inches above the marked level of dullness.
6. Mark the new level of dullness and measure the distance upward from the first level of dullness.
7. Observe client for pallor and vertigo during procedure.

dullness is found; this level of dullness identifies the lower lung base and the level of the diaphragm. Note this level, then ask the client to let out his breath and hold it before taking a second breath. Repeat the percussion of the side to the border of dullness, which will normally be higher, since the lungs will have become shorter and the diaphragm will have moved up in the normal respiratory system. Measure the distance from the first level of dullness up to the second level of dullness; this is the diaphragmatic excursion. Repeat the same procedure on the other side of the posterior thorax. The diaphragmatic excursion of both left and right sides should be essentially equal. The normal diaphragmatic excursion is about 1–2 rib spaces in children and 3–6 cm in adults. An athlete will ordinarily have a diaphragmatic excursion in the upper end of the normal range.

Diaphragmatic excursion is decreased in the hyperinflated condition of emphysema. Emphysematous effects are often seen in the elderly because of age-related enlargement of the alveoli and bronchial ducts. Upward displacement of the diaphragm is associated with atelectasis, intra-abdominal masses, pregnancy, severe obesity, and ascites. It may be decreased if there is pleural effusion or pneumothorax. Phrenic nerve paralysis causes the diaphragm to move upward, and its motion may be paradoxical during respiration. When performing this procedure, carefully observe the client so that he does not become hypoxic.

Auscultation

The diaphragm of the stethoscope should be used to auscultate breath sounds in adults. It is better to use a small diaphragm or bell with children because their chests are smaller and the intercostal spaces are narrower. Make certain that the client's head is in the midline position during auscultation. This is especially important with children because a slight turn of the head may narrow their flexible bronchi and decrease the breath sounds, suggesting possible pathology when none actually exists.

When auscultating the lungs, instruct the client to breathe normally through an open mouth. Place the diaphragm of the stethoscope firmly upon the chest wall and listen to the anterior chest from slightly above the clavicles to the base of the lungs. Auscultation of the left lung is difficult on the anterior wall because the sounds from the heart interfere.

Listen from under the axilla to the base of the lungs on both sides of the chest. This is important because sounds emanating from the right middle lobe can best be heard on the right lateral side of the chest.

Auscultate on the posterior chest wall from above the scapulae (this will include the apices of the lungs). Compare both sides of the chest as you auscultate first the left side and then the right side before moving down a couple of inches each time toward the base of the lungs.

Always place the stethoscope firmly against the chest wall. Without firm placement, chest hair may rub against the diaphragm, mimicking fine rales. If chest hair interferes with auscultation, moisten the hair with a wet washcloth; this will cause the hair to adhere to the chest, and there will be less movement of the hair directly on the diaphragm of your stethoscope. Avoid blowing or breathing on the stethoscope while auscultating, as this, too, will produce abnormal sounds.

The sounds heard by auscultation of the lungs are the result of the movement of air through the trachea, bronchi, and alveoli. Normal breath sounds are of three variations: vesicular breath sounds, bronchial sounds, and bronchovesicular sounds. You should listen over normal lung fields to begin to understand and identify these sounds.

Vesicular breath sounds, heard over most of the normal lung, result from air swirling through the bronchioles and alveoli. They are soft, low-pitched sounds often described as gentle sighing or as like a "breeze in the trees." They are basically an inspiratory sound because they reflect the passage of air into the alveoli. The best example of this sound can be heard at the base of the lungs. With vesicular breathing the inspiratory phase is longer than the expiratory phase. Inspiration is usually higher pitched and louder than expiration. At times expiration may be inaudible. The sound is usually diagrammed as follows: ^

Bronchial sounds are moderately high-pitched sounds that result from turbulence of air as it passes through the bronchi. To understand how bronchial respirations sound, listen near the manubrium. These sounds are much louder than vesicular sounds and are characterized by a short inspiratory phase and a long expiratory phase:

/\

Tracheal sounds are loud and raspy. Listen directly over your trachea just below the larynx. They have a loud, long inspiratory phase, a pause, and then a loud, long expiratory phase. Tracheal sounds are *never* heard over *normal* lung fields. /\

Bronchovesicular sounds are a mixture of the other two types. Normally, these sounds can be heard over the bronchi on each side of the sternum at the level of the first and second intercostal spaces; they are also heard posteriorly between the scapulae. The inspiratory and expiratory phases in bronchovesicular breathing are approximately equal and do not have a pause between inspiration and expiration: ^

The various normal breath sounds and their location on the neck and on the thorax can be seen in Figure 13-14.

In the adult bronchovesicular sounds are not heard in any areas of the normal lung other than those mentioned above. In the child the lung sounds are normally louder because of the thinness of the chest wall; therefore, the sound quality affords little diagnostic value.

The most common cause of changes in breath sounds is the presence of fluid in the lungs. Thus, bronchovesicular sounds heard at the base and the periphery of the lungs are present in such conditions as pneumonia and pleurisy.

Sounds not usually heard over the normal lung fields are referred to as *adventitious* (extraneous) *sounds*, such as *crackles* (rales and rhonchi), *wheezes*, and *rubs*. Adventitious sounds are signs and symptoms of a variety of lung disorders, as shown in Table 13-3.

Rales (pronouned "rahls") or *crackles* are produced by movement of air into fluid-containing tissue. They are always considered abnormal, although transient fine rales may be detected in clients who have been underventilating, such as bedridden elderly clients. A cough or a few deep breaths will expand the lung bases and eliminate these adventitious noises. Persistent smokers often have rales that disappear after coughing. Rales that disappear after coughing usually have no significance.

In some instances having the client cough at the end of expiration will loosen pulmonary exudates and produce inspiratory rales. This maneuver will elicit the rales that are an early sign of fluid accumulation.

Rales are classified in many ways, but the simplest and best is according to the sound pitch. In this approach rales are termed fine, medium, or coarse:

1. *Fine rales* are best heard at the end of inspiration and reflect the passing of air through

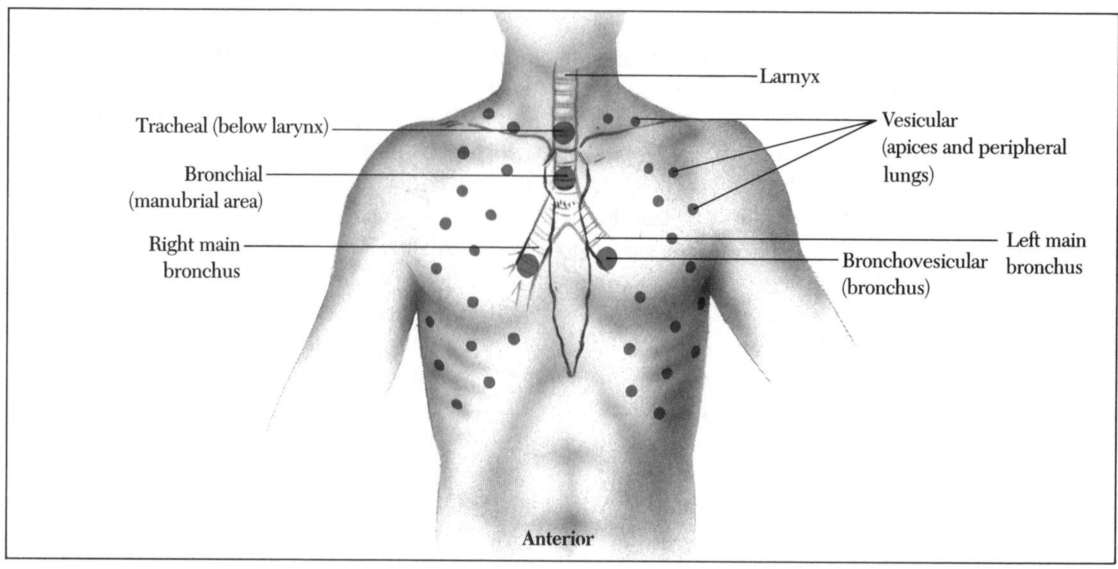

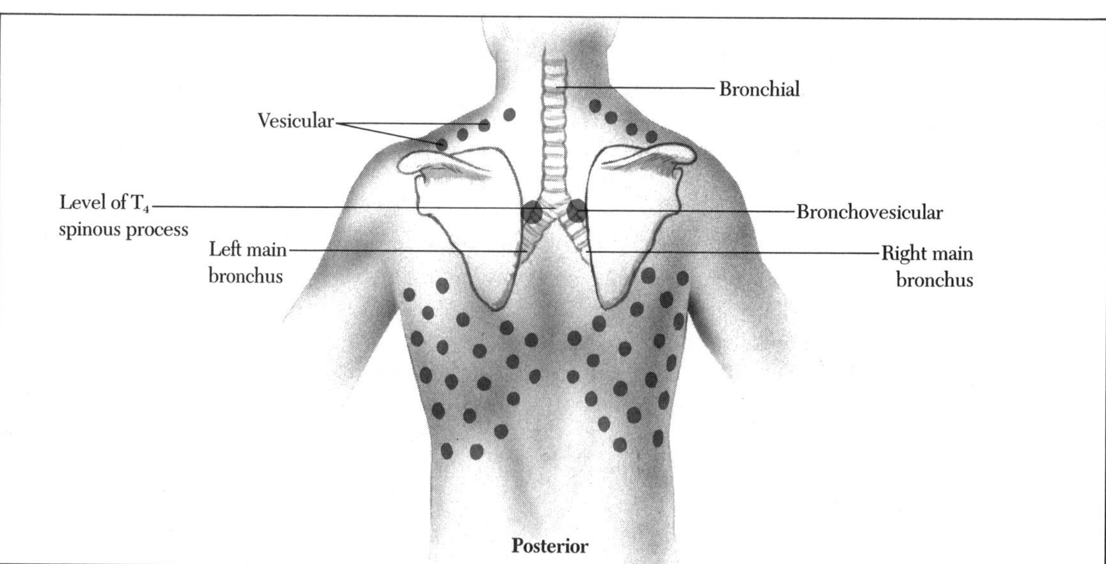

Figure 13-14 Locations of normal breath sounds of the neck and thorax (all small circles are vesicular).

Table 13-3. Signs and Symptoms of Lung Disorders

Process	Inspection	Palpation	Percussion	Auscultation
Pneumonia	Coryza symptoms; pyrexia, chills; productive cough; rapid, shallow, grunting respirations (dyspnea); pleuritic pain (splinting of chest); occasional cyanosis	Limited motion of chest on affected side; increased fremitus when consolidation fully established	Dullness; decreased diaphragmatic excursion	Early: decreased breath sounds Later: bronchial sounds; bronchophony; whispered pectoriloquy; fine crepitant rales; occasional pleural friction rub

Table 13-3. *Continued*

Process	Inspection	Palpation	Percussion	Auscultation
Chronic obstructive lung disease	Increased respiratory rate; pursed lip breathing; increased AP diameter (barrel chest); use of accessory muscles and intercostal retraction; leaning forward to assist breathing; cyanosis or hyperemia (depends on type); increased JVP	Decreased fremitus; diminished chest expansion; possible crepitus; rhonchal fremitus	Decreased diaphragmatic excursion; hyperresonance; lowered hepatic dullness	Decreased breath sounds; prolonged expirations; rales, wheezes, or rhonchi; in some instances no adventitious sounds present
Bronchitis	Cough with sputum production; sore throat; fever; malaise; occasional dyspnea with use of accessory muscles	Normal fremitus	Resonance	May have prolonged expirations with vesicular breath sounds; wheezes, rales, and rhonchi may be heard
Pleural effusion	Pain; dyspnea; pallor	Prominence of interspaces; tracheal deviation from side of effusion; decreased fremitus	Increasing dullness with the increase in amount of fluid	Decreased breath sounds; egophony and whispered pectoriloquy
Neoplasm	Asymptomatic or mild cough; fever; chills; sputum	Mass may be palpated if on chest wall; absent fremitus	Dull over area of lesion	Decreased breath sounds if airway is occluded; egophony and whispered pectoriloquy if airway is not occluded; often fine rales and localized wheezes; occasional pleural friction rub
Atelectasis	Increased respiratory rate; increased pulse; often cyanosis	Tracheal shift to side of involvement; decreased fremitus; decreased chest expansion on affected side	Dullness	Diminished breath sounds; occasional rales
Pulmonary edema	Increased respiratory rate; cyanosis; sitting upright; use of accessory muscles; apprehension	Increased fremitus	Dullness	Bronchovesicular breath sounds, often obscured later by rales, rhonchi, and wheezing

Continued on page 250

Table 13-3. *Continued*

Process	Inspection	Palpation	Percussion	Auscultation
Pneumothorax	Pain; dyspnea and cyanosis; apprehension; increased respiratory rate	Possible tracheal shift to side of pneumothorax; absent fremitus on affected side	Hyperresonance; decreased diaphragmatic excursion on affected side	Absent breath sounds on affected side
Emphysema	Dyspnea; wheezing; cough with sputum; increased use of accessory muscles of the neck; exhaustion	Normal fremitus or decreased; occasional palpable rhonchi	Hyperresonance; decreased diaphragmatic excursion	Vesicular or bronchovesicular sounds; wheezes/ rhonchi throughout chest

Technique for Auscultation of the Lungs

1. Warm stethoscope with hands.
2. Check that client's head is in midline position.
3. Ask client to breathe through open mouth and take slightly deeper than normal breaths.
4. Diaphragm of stethoscope placed firmly on chest.
5. Proceed at 2–3 inch intervals side to side on anterior and posterior aspects of chest.
6. Proceed at 2–3 inch intervals from axillae to lung bases.
7. Decision making: Employ bronchophony, egophony, and whispered pectoriloquy techniques if abnormal ausculatory sounds are detected.

fluid in the intricate alveoli of the lungs. The sound of a fine rale can be simulated by holding several pieces of your hair close to your ear and rolling them back and forth between your thumb and index finger.

2. *Medium rales* occur with the presence of increased fluid in the bronchi, as would exist in congestive heart failure with pulmonary edema and in bronchial inflammation (bronchiolitis, bronchitis). They sound like the fizz of a carbonated beverage, a bit louder than fine rales.
3. *Coarse rales* are produced by air passing through fluid-filled bronchi and the trachea. They are fairly continuous throughout inspiration and expiration and have a gurgling bubbly quality; the coarsest are characterized by the "death rattle."

Wheezes (musical rales), or rhonchi, occur when air passes through narrowed trachea, bronchi, and bronchioles. They occur in both phases of respiration but are more prominent during expiration, when there is more resistance. To accentuate these adventitious sounds, instruct the client to take a deep breath and then to force it out hard. A wheeze or sibilant rhonchus is a high-pitched sound generally heard on inspiration and expiration as the air passes through partially collapsed or obstructed airways, whereas a sonorous (snoring) rhonchus is a low-pitched sound heard on expiration. Wheezes are characteristic of chronic bronchitis, cystic fibrosis, asthma, and foreign body aspiration.

Pleural friction rub is caused by the rubbing together of the visceral and parietal pleurae. Normally, these two structures glide easily over one another. In cases where there is inflammation of the pleura, as in pleurisy, the roughened inflamed edges rub together, producing a characteristic grating sound. You can imitate this sound by placing the palm of your hand over your ear and then scratching the dorsum with the fingernails of your other hand. A pleural friction rub is best heard in the lower anterior and lateral portions of the chest, as these are the areas of greatest thoracic movement. The rub is heard during both phases of respiration and increases in intensity during inspiration and with

BIOLOGICAL AND CULTURAL VARIATIONS

Tuberculosis Among Black Americans and Native Americans

Tuberculosis is an infectious disease caused by the bacillus *Mycobacterium tuberculosis*. As a communicable disease, it is usually contracted through inhaling airborne respiratory droplets from an individual with an active case. Because the tubercle bacilli are usually contacted in this way, pulmonary tuberculosis is the most frequent form of the infection, as opposed to renal, intestinal, or bone and joint forms of the disease.

At the turn of the century, tuberculosis was the second leading cause of death in the United States, accounting for 11.3% of all deaths. By 1972, however, it was no longer ranked among the twenty leading causes of death. In that year, the age-adjusted death rate from tuberculosis among White Americans was 1.7 per 100,000. The decline in morbidity and mortality rates from tuberculosis is attributed to a number of changes, including improvements in public health and sanitation measures after the turn of the century, and general improvement in the economic status and lifestyle of most Americans, and the onset of specific chemotherapy measures in 1946.

However, there are some population groups in the United States that continue to suffer from relatively high rates of tuberculosis morbidity and mortality. Most notable are Native Americans and Black Americans. In 1972, records from Indian health service agencies and hospitals showed the age-adjusted death rate from tuberculosis among Native Americans to be 9.1 per 100,000, which is over five times the death rate of White Americans (U.S. Congress American Indian Policy Review Commission 1976). Alaskan Natives appear to be particularly at risk. In the same year, the tuberculosis mortality rate for Black Americans was also much higher than that of White Americans. The rate for nonwhite Americans (of which over 90% are Black Americans) was 5.9 per 100,000 (U.S. Congress American Indian Policy Review Commission 1976). Tuberculosis morbidity rates were also remarkably higher among Indians and Blacks. The proportion of individuals with active cases of tuberculosis in these population groups was 94.3 per 100,000 Indians, 151.4 per 100,000 Alaskan Natives, 50.3 per 100,000 nonwhite Americans, and 10.8 per 100,000 White Americans.

Environmental differences appear to be the cause of these higher tuberculosis rates. Native Americans and Black Americans have lower average income and socioeconomic status than White Americans and thus have less adequate medical care, housing, sanitation facilities, and nutritious food. There is a greater probability that individuals from these population groups will live in crowded, poorly ventilated homes with poor sanitation facilities, such as on reservations or in ghettoes in urban centers. Ghettoes and slum areas have long been high-risk environments that allow the rapid spread of tuberculosis. For example, in 1945 the TB death rate for Black Americans in cities of over a million people was almost twice that of Black Americans in cities of 100,000–200,000 people (Pettigrew & Pettigrew 1974). The poor also tend to have inadequate diets and poor nutritional status, which leads to decreased disease resistance and increased rates of infection. For example, vitamin deficiencies, anemia, and protein deficiencies continue to be major health problems among Native Americans (U.S. Congress American Indian Policy Review Commission 1976).

It had long been hypothesized that Black Americans and Native Americans had decreased resistance to tuberculosis because of genetic and constitutional differences. It is true that Blacks have a high incidence of a disease type that tends to present as acute tuberculosis pneumonia or to involve the mid-lung (Williams 1975). However, it is now clear that environmental differences offer the real explanation. If economic opportunities and living conditions continue to improve among Black and Native Americans, tuberculosis rates will probably continue to decrease and approach the rate for White Americans.

Special Assessment Techniques of the Lungs

1. *Bronchophony:* Place diaphragm of stethoscope over abnormal area of lung field. Ask client to softly repeat "1-2-3." **Normal finding: "1-2-3" sounds muffled.** Presence of bronchophony is pathologic. Finding in bronchophony is clearly transmitted "1-2-3."
2. *Egophony:* Place diaphragm of stethoscope over abnormal area of lung field. Ask client to say "eeeeeee." **Normal finding: "eeeeee" sound maintained.** Presence of egophony is pathological and is reflected by the change of "eeeeee" to an "aaaaayyh" sound.
3. *Whispered Pectoriloquy:* With the diaphragm of the stethoscope over an abnormal area of the lung, ask the client to whisper "1-2-3." **The normal finding is a muffled, whispered "1-2-3."** The pathological presence of whispered pectoriloquy is reflected by sharp/distinct, clear transmission of the whispered "1-2-3."

deep breaths. The sound also usually increases if the stethoscope is placed more firmly against the chest wall. This rub can be differentiated from a pericardial friction rub by asking the client to hold his breath. If the sound is still heard it is a pericardial friction rub rather than a pleural friction rub. Pleural friction rub may be heard in such conditions as pneumonia, pulmonary embolus, emphysema, lung abscess, and tuberculosis.

Other Techniques

If abnormal percussion notes or abnormal lung sounds are discovered, you can perform three additional techniques: bronchophony, whispered pectoriloquy, and egophony. Although these techniques are not performed routinely in a screening examination, they can be used for further investigation of an abnormality discovered in the lung examination. The underlying scientific principle of these techniques is that fluid or consolidation will transmit the vibrations of the spoken or whispered voice through the lungs to the chest wall.

Both bronchophony and whispered pectoriloquy will aid in the detection of consolidation. In testing for bronchophony the client is asked to softly repeat the words "one-two-three" several times. In testing for whispered pectoriloquy, the client is asked to whisper so that the vocal cords are not used. Normally you can hear the client's spoken word over a bronchus, but if you hear it clearly during these procedures through your stethoscope in the periphery of the lung, an abnormal condition is indicated. The client's whispered voice should be heard faintly and indistinctly through the chest wall. If the whispered words become distinguishable throughout the chest wall, abnormality exists.

Egophony is a form of bronchophony that utilizes the principle that fluid favors higher pitches and that it will alter the pattern of the spoken word. Ask the client to repeat the sound "eeee." If egophony is present, it will sound like "aaaa" through your stethoscope. This change of sound denotes abnormality.

These abnormal sounds will be heard in varying degrees depending on the amount of consolidation and fluid present.

Table 13-4 addresses assessment regarding oxygen supply and demand.

Summary

This chapter provided information about the structure and function of the thorax and lungs. The chest has certain landmarks that are helpful in describing physical findings. The thorax and lungs are examined beginning with inspection, then palpation, followed by percussion and auscultation. Percussion should be carried out in a systematic manner on the anterior, lateral, and posterior walls of the chest. Auscultation involves listening to breath sounds; all variations, both normal and abnormal, were discussed, as were a number of additional techniques not performed routinely in a screening examination.

Discussion Questions/Activities

1. Compare the characteristics of the adult thoracic cage to that of the young child.

Table 13-4. Assessing Problems of Oxygen Supply and Demand

Component of respiration	**Conditions for healthy lungs**	**Conditions that alter function**	**Nursing assessment**
Ventilation	Normal chest anatomy	Scoliosis Kyphosis	Inspection Structural deformity Tracheal deviation Use of accessory muscles Retractions Effect of position on breathing Depth of ventilation Length of expiration Abdominal distention Wounds, incisions Restrictive dressing Rate and pattern of ventilation Level of consciousness Neurological examination Palpation Symmetry of chest excursion Crepitus Tactile fremitus Ausculation Breath sounds Adventitious sounds Voice sounds
	Intact and compliant chest wall	Flail chest Barrel chest	
	Functioning respiratory muscles receiving appropriate neuro-transmissions	Spinal cord injury Guillain-Barré syndrome Muscle relaxants Status epilepticus Tetanus	
	Intact pleural membranes with negative intrapleural pressure	Pneumothorax Pleural effusion	
	Open and intact upper airways	Aspiration Laryngeal edema Bronchospasm	
	Compliant lung tissue	Atelectasis Fibrosis	
	Appropriate conscious control	Anxiety Plain on inspiration	
	Functioning chemical and neurological systems	Cerebral anoxia High fever Barbiturates, opiates Anesthesia Acid-base imbalance Increased intracranial pressure	
Diffusion	Adequate O_2 and tension	High altitudes	Inspection Dyspnea Cough Sputum Vital signs Digit clubbing Cyanosis (a late sign) Palpation Tactile fremitus Ausculation Breath sounds Adventitious sounds Voice sounds
	Thin, health alveolar-capillary membrane	Thick alveolar-capillary membrane: fibrosis exudate	
	Adequate alveolar-capillary surface area	Lobectomy Chronic obstructive pulmonary disease	
	Adequate perfusion	Increased dead space	
	Adequate ventilation	Increased shunting	
Oxygen transport to the tissues	Adequate red-blood-cell count and hemoglobin levels	CO Poisoning Anemia Abnormal RBCs Left shift in oxyhemoglobin	Inspection Color of membranes, nailbeds, skin Capillary refill Restlessness Edema Bruising Palpation Peripheral pulses Skin turgor, temperature Ausculation Apical pulse Blood pressure Breath sounds
	Appropriate blood volume	Hemorrhage Dehydration	
	Adequate cardiac output	Cor pulmonale Shock	
	Appropriate hemostasis	Abnormal bleeding and/or clotting	
	Unimpeded blood flow	Thrombosis	

Source: Nielsen, L. 1980. Assessing patient's respiratory problems. *American Journal of Nursing* 80, no. 12 (December 1980):2194–2195.

2. Discuss some possible causes for unequal expansion of the lungs.
3. Describe what is meant by the term fremitus. How is fremitus detected?
4. Describe various percussion notes that can be heard over the thorax and why.
5. What is meant by the term diaphragmatic excursion? Demonstrate the procedure for determining the degree of diaphragmatic excursion.
6. Describe the three variations of normal breath sounds heard over the lung fields.
7. Name and describe the three categories of sounds heard in the lungs due to pathology and/or fluid.

Recording of Findings

Normal findings are presented in the first box. The second box contains findings for an individual who has been medically diagnosed as having chronic obstructive lung disease.

Lungs	**Lungs**
INSPECTION Symmetrical expansion; AP diameter less than anterior side-to-side diameter.	**INSPECTION** Increased AP diameter; sits forward with hands on knees; marked retraction of ICS; dyspnea at rest.
PALPATION No tenderness, pulsations, or crepitus; expansion equal bilaterally; fremitus present.	**PALPATION** Expansion decreased, fremitus present.
PERCUSSION Lung fields resonant; diaphragmatic excursion 4 cm bilaterally.	**PERCUSSION** Right lung and left upper lobe hyperresonant; dullness over left lower lobe; diaphragmatic excursion 1 cm bilaterally.
AUSCULTATION Vesicular breath sounds present; no crackles, wheezes, or rubs.	**AUSCULTATION** Normal vesicular sounds in right lung and left upper lobe; tracheal breath sounds noted in left lower lobe; inspiratory and expiratory wheezing; egophony in left lower lobe.

CHAPTER 14

Assessment of the Cardiovascular System

LEARNING OBJECTIVES

1. Identify the locations for palpation of the peripheral pulses.
2. State the various categories of pulse amplitude.
3. Review the structure and function of the heart.
4. Identify the areas on the anterior chest inspected and palpated in assessing heart function.
5. Describe the techniques of percussion and auscultation of the heart.
6. Explain the normal heart sounds.
7. Describe the technique for measuring jugular venous distention.

Assessment of the cardiovascular system requires mastery of a number of special abilities and techniques. For example, the nurse must learn to categorize pulse amplitude and to distinguish the various types and qualities of heart sounds and interpret their meaning and significance. In this chapter the necessary techniques to assess the cardiovascular system will be described in detail as well as the basic structures of the cardiovascular system.

Assessment of Peripheral Pulses

Palpation of the peripheral pulses is an ancient and time-honored practice. The pulses are an index of the heart's action. With each ventricular contraction the blood is ejected into the aorta and the pressure of this is transmitted as a wave. This wave causes expansion and elongation of the arteries, which results in palpable and visible pulses.

The peripheral pulses (temporal, carotid, brachial, radial, femoral, popliteal, posterior tibial, and dorsal pedal) are routinely assessed during the physical assessment process. They should always be assessed in clients with peripheral vascular disease (atherosclerosis, arteriosclerosis, diabetes mellitus, alcoholism, Raynaud's disease, Buerger's disease, aneurysm), femoral bypass surgery, and vein ligations (see Figure 14-1).

The following is a standardized scale used to categorize pulse amplitude:

0 Absent pulse
1+ Weak, thready pulse; may fade in and out and is obliterated with light pressure
2+ Normal; easily palpable; not easily obliterated by pressure
3+ Bounding; easily palpable; not obliterated with pressure

Figure 14-2 illustrates a record of peripheral pulse amplitudes using the standardized 0–3+ scale. In a normal recording, 2+/3+, the numerator 2+ indicates normal pulse on a scale with 3+ as the maximum pulse amplitude.

The carotids should be palpated one at a time low in the neck and far away from the bifurcation of the carotid artery into the external and internal carotid branches. The scientific rationale for this approach is that: (1) pressure on both carotids simultaneously may produce vertigo or syncope as a result of cerebral hypoxia (this is especially true in the elderly and in those clients with generalized vascular disease or local carotid artery pathology); and (2) because the carotid sinus is located in the neck just above the bifurcation of the common carotid artery, pressure on or massage of this area can slow the heart rate. In certain situations this slowing of the heart action could be dangerous. In Figure 14-3 the examiner is pointing out the location of the carotid sinus.

Pulses		L	R
Carotid	C	2+	2+
Brachial	B	2+	2+
Radial	R	2+	2+
Femoral	F	2+	1+
Popliteal	P	2+	0
Posterior tibial	PT	2+	0
Dorsal pedal	DP	2+	0

Figure 14-2 Peripheral pulse amplitudes for a client diagnosed for right femoral partial occlusion.

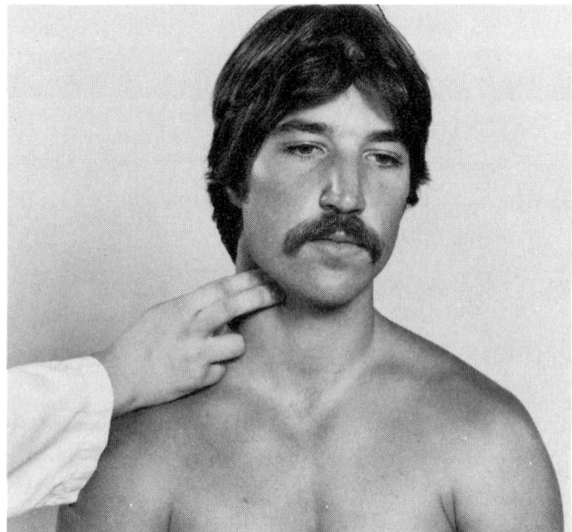

Figure 14-3 Location of the carotid sinus.

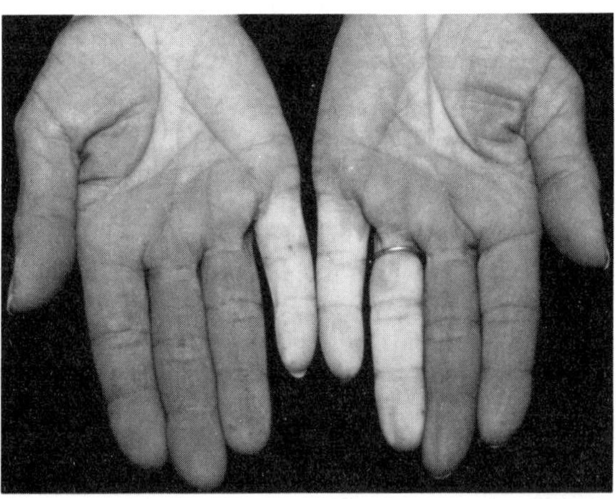

Figure 14-1 Marked pallor of digits due to vasospasm (Raynaud's phenomenon).

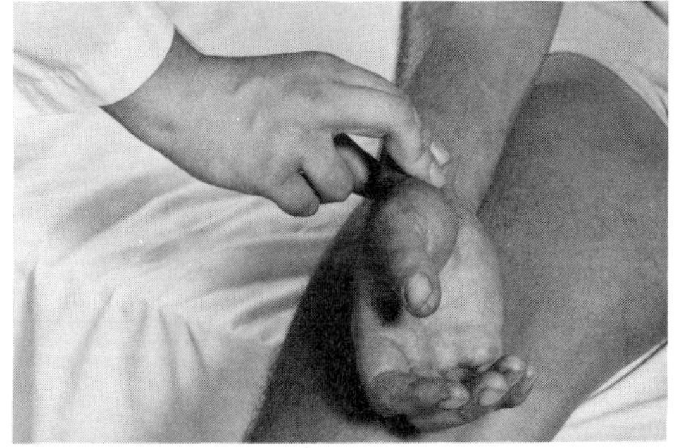

Figure 14-4 Palpation of the radial artery.

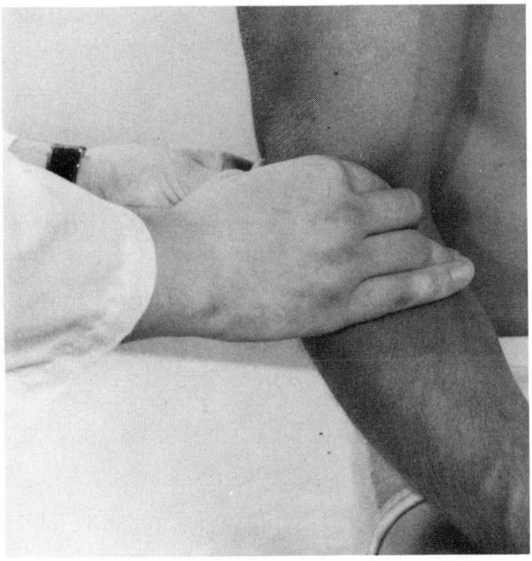

Figure 14-5 Palpation of the brachial artery.

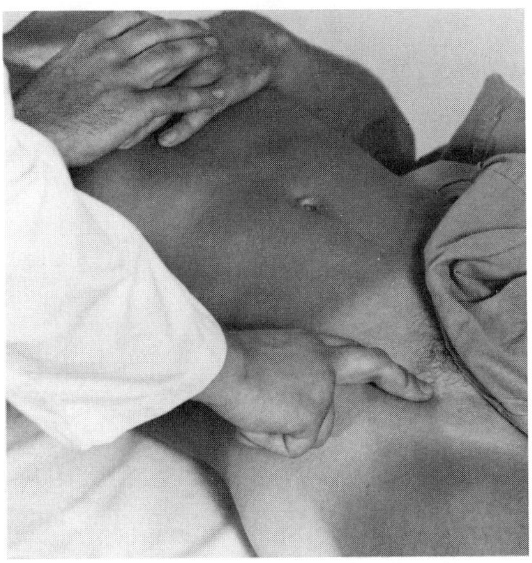

Figure 14-6 Palpation of the femoral artery.

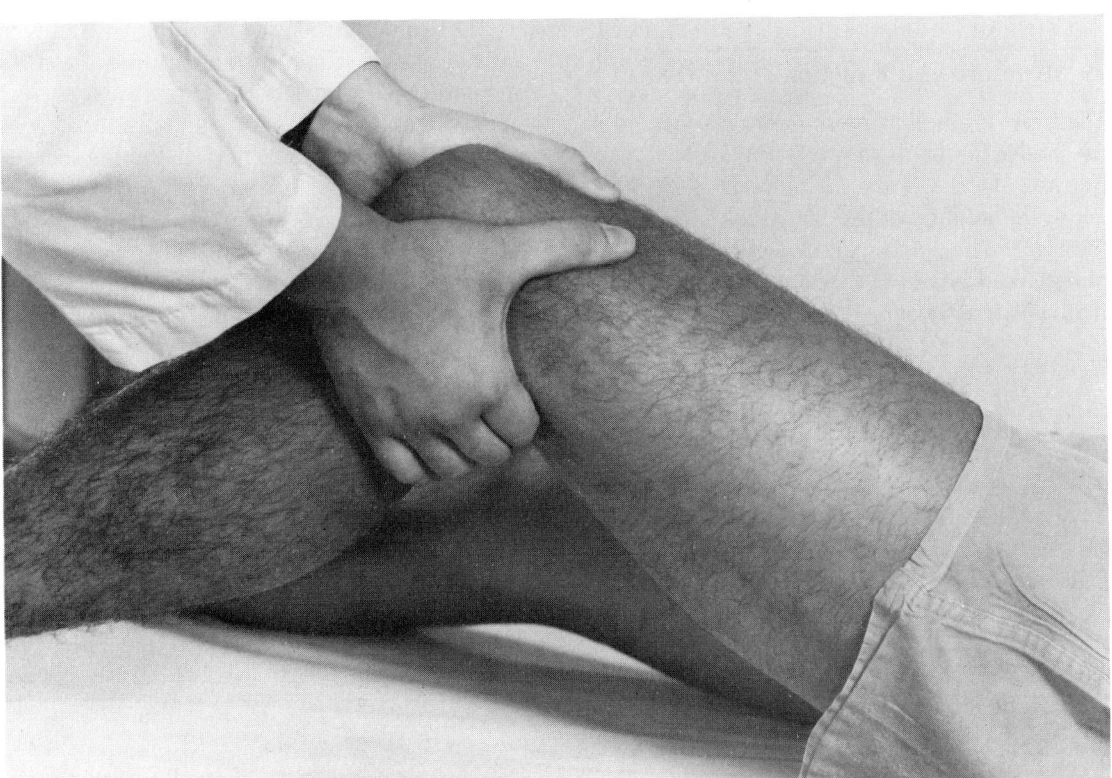

Figure 14-7 Palpation of the popliteal artery.

The palpation of the peripheral pulses, illustrated in Figures 14-4 through 14-9, is performed to detect the existence of arterial insufficiency. Particularly in the elderly, the absence of a posterior tibial pulse (Figure 14-8) or of a dorsal pedal pulse (Figure 14-9) may be normal, but it can also indicate arterial obstructive disease. It is not uncommon to find a 1+ posterior tibial

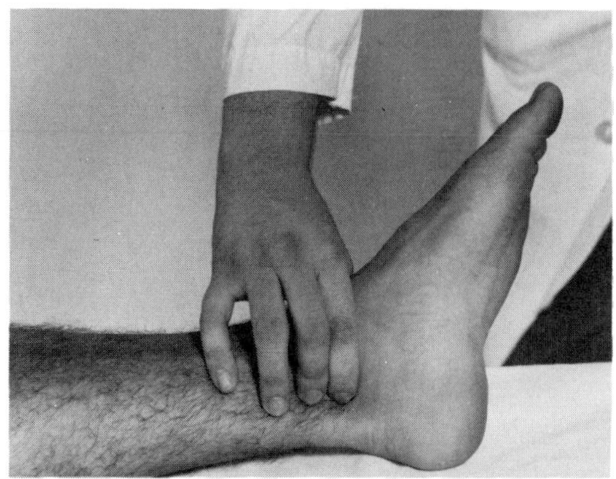
Figure 14-8 Palpation of the posterior tibial artery.

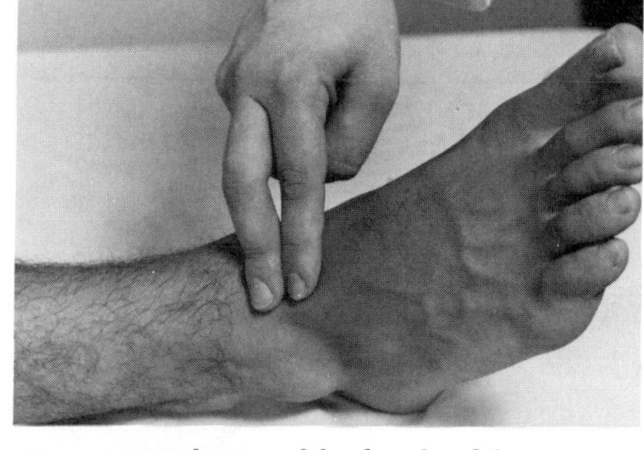
Figure 14-9 Palpation of the dorsal pedal artery.

and/or dorsalis pedis pulse(s) in a normal person. Common abnormalities of rate, rhythm, and intensity in the arterial pulses are noted in Table 14-1.

Structure and Function of the Heart

The heart is a hollow muscular organ located in the mediastinum, as shown in Figure 14-10. Approximately two-thirds of the heart lies to the left of the midline of the body and one-third to the right. The apex is located close to the diaphragm and points to the left. The apical heart rate can be determined by placing the stethoscope directly over the heart at its apex, which is normally at the fifth or sixth intercostal space, close to the left midclavicular line. The base of the heart lies below the second rib on either side of the sternum.

The strong fibrous sac encasing and protecting the heart is called the pericardium. Between the pericardium and the heart is a small amount of serous fluid, which provides for easy, low-friction movement. The pericardium is secured to the diaphragm, sternum, pleura, esophagus, and aorta. The heart is composed of three layers. The epicardium is a thin, smooth lining that covers the outside of the myocardium and interfaces with the pericardium. The myocardium is a spe-

Table 14-1. Common Abnormalities of the Arterial Pulses

Terminology	Characteristics	Comment
Weak pulse	Slow rise and prolonged peak, diminished pulse pressure	Congestive heart failure, aortic stenosis, shock
Bounding pulse	Pulse reaches higher in intensity than normal, then disappears quickly	Best detected when arm held aloft; may be due to anxiety, exercise, fever, anemia, hyperthyroidism; aortic regurgitation
Pulsus alternans	Regular rhythm with alternating weak and strong pulsations	Left-sided heart failure
Bigeminy	Two regular beats followed by a longer pause	Myocarditis, valvular disease; premature ventricular contractions
Pulsus paradoxus	Abnormal fall (8mm Hg) in systolic blood pressure on inspiration	Obstructive lung disease, adherent pericarditis
Diminished femoral pulse	Determined in relation to radial pulse	Blood takes longer to reach lower extremities due to obstructed flow through aorta (i.e., coarctation of aorta, occlusive aortic disease)
Posterior tibial or dorsal pedal	Weak or absent	Can be normal, but may indicate arterial obstructive disease

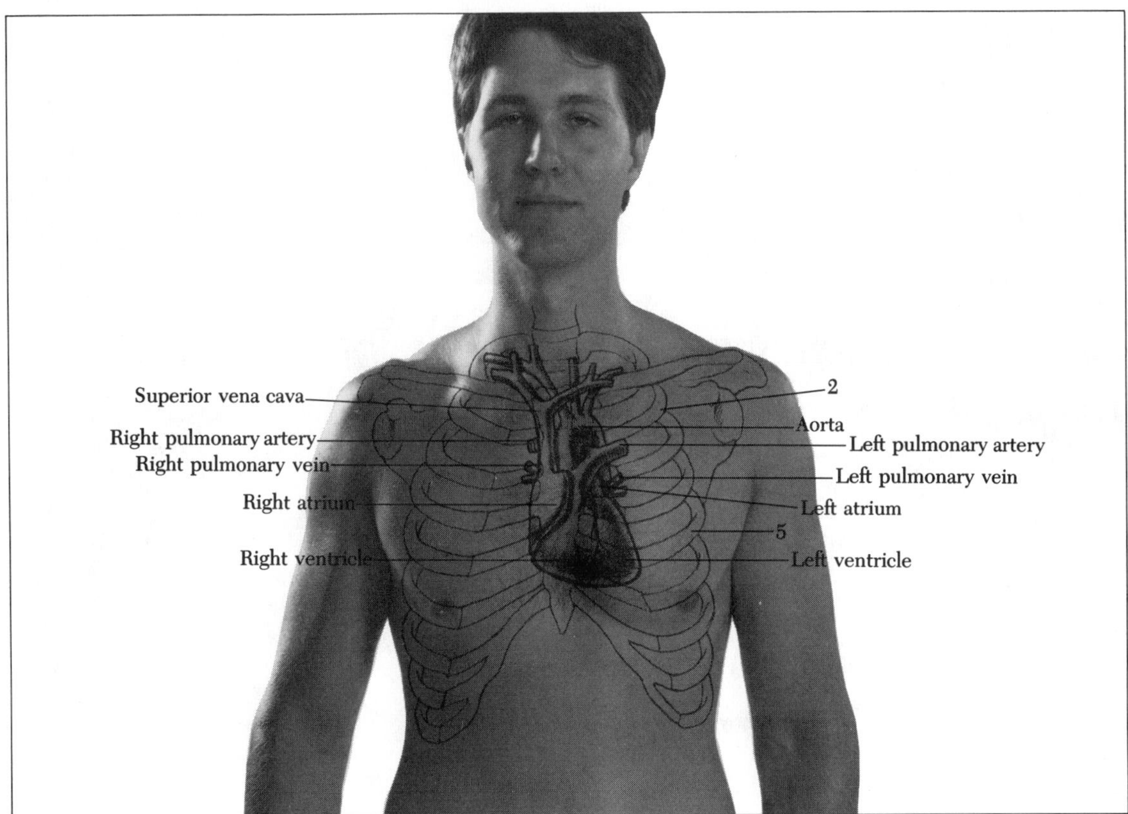

Figure 14-10 Location of the heart and great vessels.

cialized muscular layer of the heart. The endocardium is a thin, delicate lining that lines the chambers of the heart and the heart valves.

Most of the anterior surface of the heart consists of the *right ventricle*. The *left ventricle* lies to the left and behind the right ventricle and forms the left cardiac border. The *left atrium* is situated posteriorly except for a small atrial appendage that makes up the left cardiac border. This appendage is located between the *left pulmonary artery* and the left ventricle and cannot usually be identified on physical examination. The right margin of the heart is formed by the *right atrium*; this portion of the heart is also not usually identifiable on physical examination.

The *superior* and *inferior vena cava* carry venous blood from the upper and lower parts of the body and empty into the right atrium. The *pulmonary artery* is located in the superior portion of the right ventricle. It bifurcates into the right and left branches and carries blood to the lungs. Oxygenated blood is returned through the pulmonary veins, which empty into the left atrium. The *aorta* curves upward from the left ventricle to the level of the sternal angle and then arches back and down behind the heart.

The heart valves, shown in Figure 14-11, are devices that permit flow of blood through the heart in one direction only. The *tricuspid valve*, between the right atrium and the right ventricle, consists of three flaps of endocardium and is anchored to the right ventricle by cordlike structures called chordae tendinae. The *mitral valve*, between the left atrium and the left ventricle, is similar to the tricuspid valve in structure except it has only two flaps and is sometimes referred to as the "bicuspid" valve because of this. The construction of both these valves is such that blood is allowed to flow into the ventricles but is prevented from flowing back out of the ventricles into the atria.

The *aortic valve* and the *pulmonary valve* are located in the left and right ventricles, respectively, and allow the blood to flow from the ventricles into the aorta and the pulmonary artery. The aortic and pulmonary valves are called the

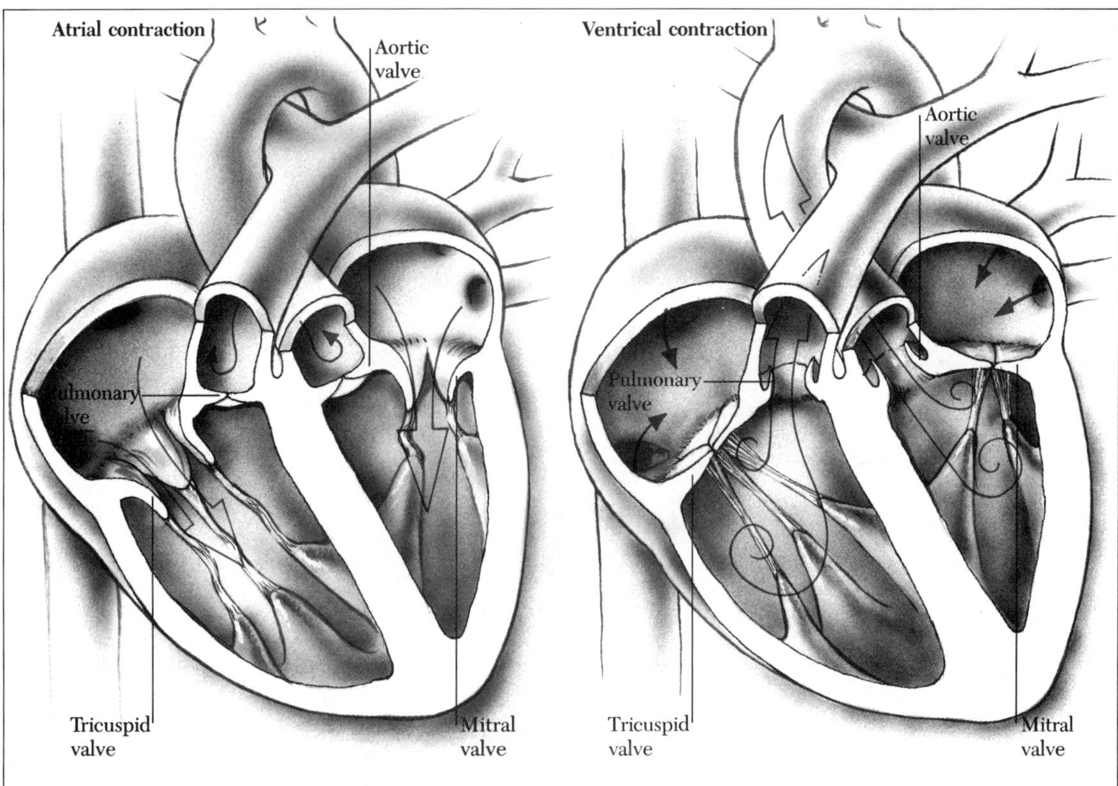

Figure 14-11 Schematic diagram of the heart.

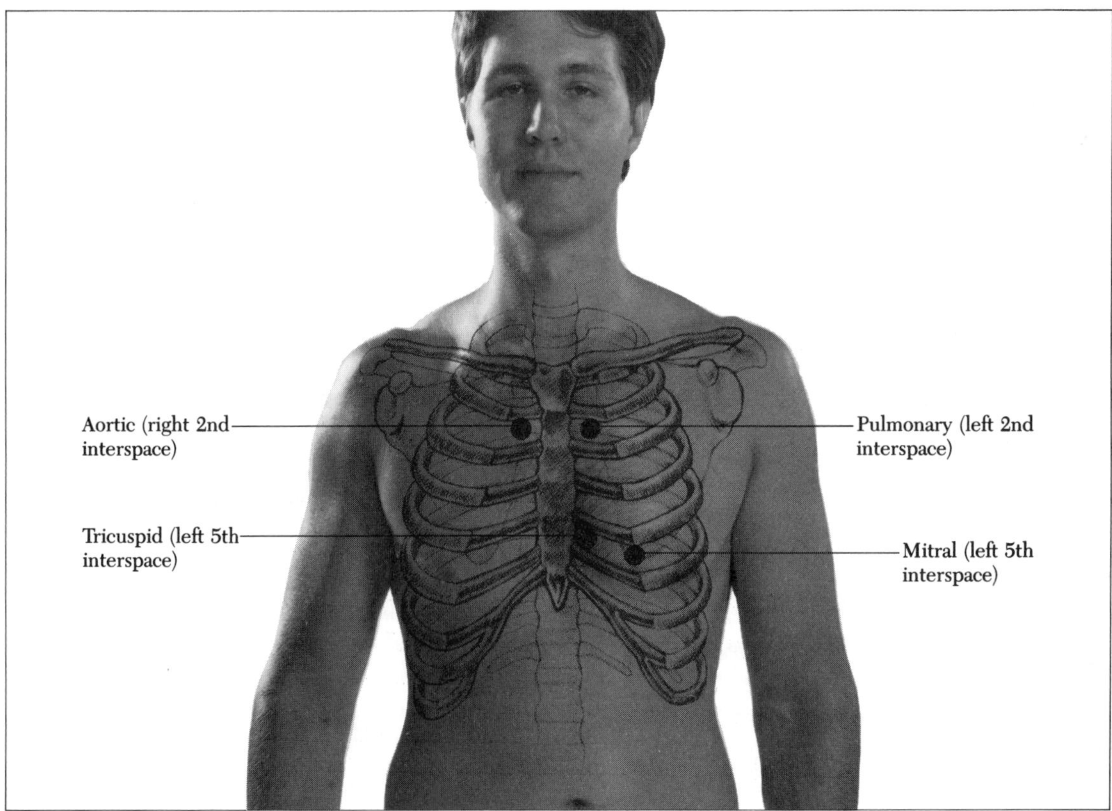

Figure 14-12 Palpatory and auscultatory projections of the heart valves.

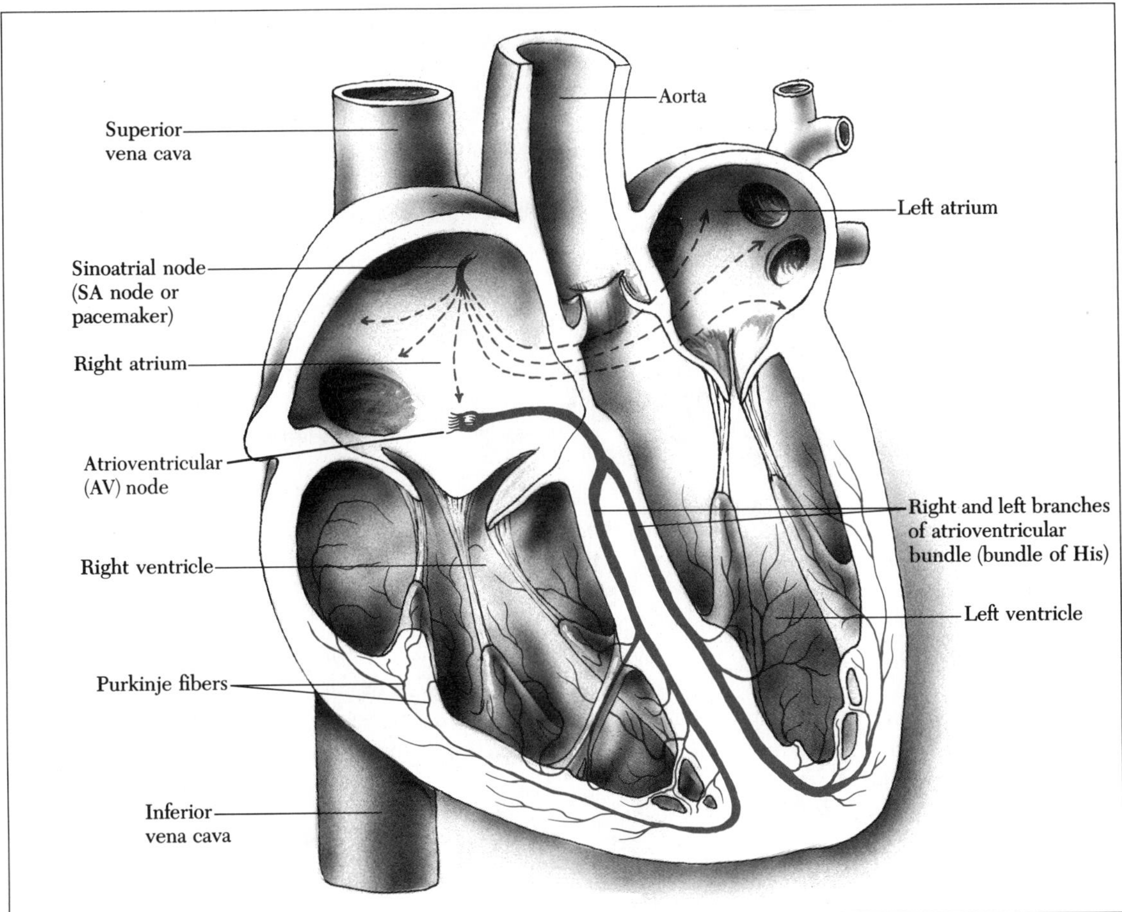

Figure 14-13 Conduction system of the heart.

semilunar valves because they consist of half-moon-shaped flaps growing from the pulmonary artery and the aorta. The valves prevent the blood from retrograde flow back into the ventricles. Figure 14-12 locates the palpatory and auscultatory projections of the heart valves.

The Conduction System

The heart has a specialized system for generating impulses that cause contraction of the heart and for conducting these impulses throughout the heart muscle (see Figure 14-13). The adult human heart generally beats about 70–80 beats per minute. The impulse for these contractions begins in the *sinoatrial (SA) node*, which is located in the posterior part of the right atrium below the opening of the superior vena cava. The SA node is called the pacemaker of the heart because under normal circumstances it initiates each heartbeat. The excitation waves generated by the SA node cause the atria to contract. The impulse is then sent to the *atrioventricular (AV) node*, which is located at the lower part of the right atrium just above the tricuspid valve. At the AV node the impulse is delayed slightly. From there the impulse passes through the *bundle of His* and the *Purkinje fibers* to the ventricles, causing them to contract. These impulses generate electrical currents that can be recorded by the electrocardiograph (ECG).

The following terms are used to describe the ECG waves illustrated in Figure 14-14:

- *P wave*—represents electrical activity of the impulse from the SA node and its spread through the atria.
- *PR interval*—represents the time for the original impulse to pass from the SA node through the atria and the AV node to the ventricles.
- *QRS complex*—represents the spread of the impulses through the bundle of His and the Purkinje fibers and the ventricular contraction.
- *ST segment*—represents the period between

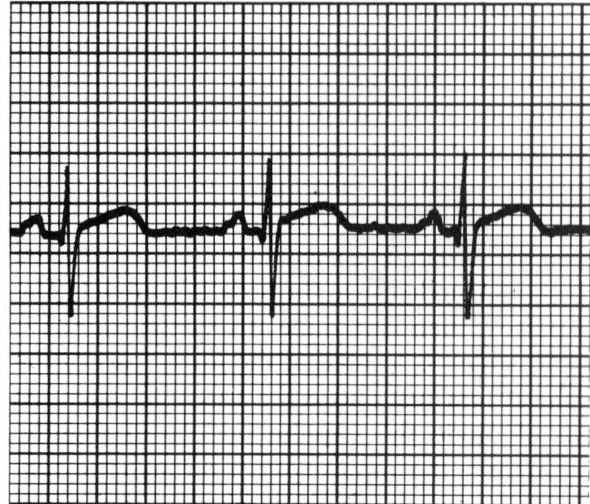

Figure 14-14 The ECG.

completion of the ventricular contraction and the recovery of the ventricular muscle.

- *T wave*—represents the recovery phase of the ventricular muscle.

The Cardiac Cycle

The *cardiac cycle*, or complete heartbeat, has two phases: systole and diastole. *Systole* is the phase in which blood is ejected from the contracting ventricles of the heart out through the aorta and the pulmonary artery. It is the shortest phase of the two and constitutes one-third of the cardiac cycle. At the beginning of systole the atrioventricular valves (tricuspid and mitral valves) close concomitantly with a pressure build-up in the ventricular walls. When this pressure exceeds the pressure in the aorta, the semilunar valves open. At the end of ventricular contraction the blood flows backward, closing the semilunar valves.

It is during *diastole* that repolarization of the ventricular muscle and cycle occurs. There is a rapid decrease in ventricular pressure, causing it to be less than the atrial pressure. The atrioventricular valves open, and the increased pressure of the atria causes blood to rush into the ventricles. At the closing of this ventricular-filling phase, atrial contraction causes the last bit of blood to be emptied into the ventricles. The semilunar valves are closed during this phase. Diastole is longer than systole and constitutes two-thirds of the cardiac cycle.

Heart Sounds

The heart makes typical sounds during the cardiac cycle; their relationship to the ECG is illustrated in Figure 14-15. When heard through a stethoscope they sound like "lub-dub" (S_1—S_2). The first heart sound occurs at the beginning of ventricular systole and reflects the closing of the mitral and tricuspid valves. This sound is referred to as S_1 (the first heart sound). The second heart sound (S_2) represents the beginning of ventricular diastole and is caused by the closure of the aortic and pulmonary valves. A third sound, S_3, may occur soon after the second sound, and a fourth heart sound, S_4, may be heard immediately preceding S_1. These third and fourth heart sounds are so spaced that they resemble the sound of a galloping horse when they are present.

S_3 is also called a protodiastolic gallop or ventricular gallop, as it occurs in the early phase of diastole and represents ventricular filling. It is usually best heard at the apex with the client positioned on the left side; it is often accompanied by a precordial heave. An S_3 sound may be heard when there is overdistention of the ventricles (as in ventricular hypertrophy or ventricular aneurysm). The reason for this can be seen in the following example. If you were to compare the intensity of the sound made when pouring water into a glass with that made when pouring water into a large rain barrel, you would find that the filling sound of the large rain barrel would be louder. Similarly, with right ventricular hypertrophy the intensity of an S_3 is likely to increase during normal inspiration, whereas with left ventricular hypertrophy S_3 intensity remains unaffected by inspiration. Ventricular hypertrophy can be grossly identified by percussion, as we shall see later, but it is verified by a chest x-ray. An excessive volume or rapid flow of blood may also accentuate the ventricular filling sound, thus making possible the detection of an S_3 heart sound. A pathologic S_3 heart sound will be accompanied by a poor or barely audible S_1 heart sound.

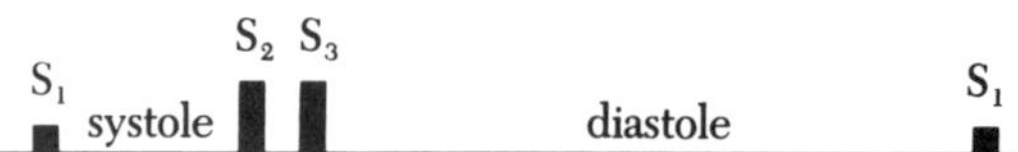

A physiologic S_3 will have an accompanying loud S_1 heart sound.

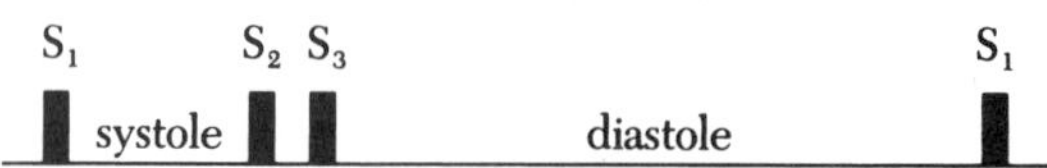

Also, a physiologic S_3 will disappear within 20–30 seconds after the client sits up.

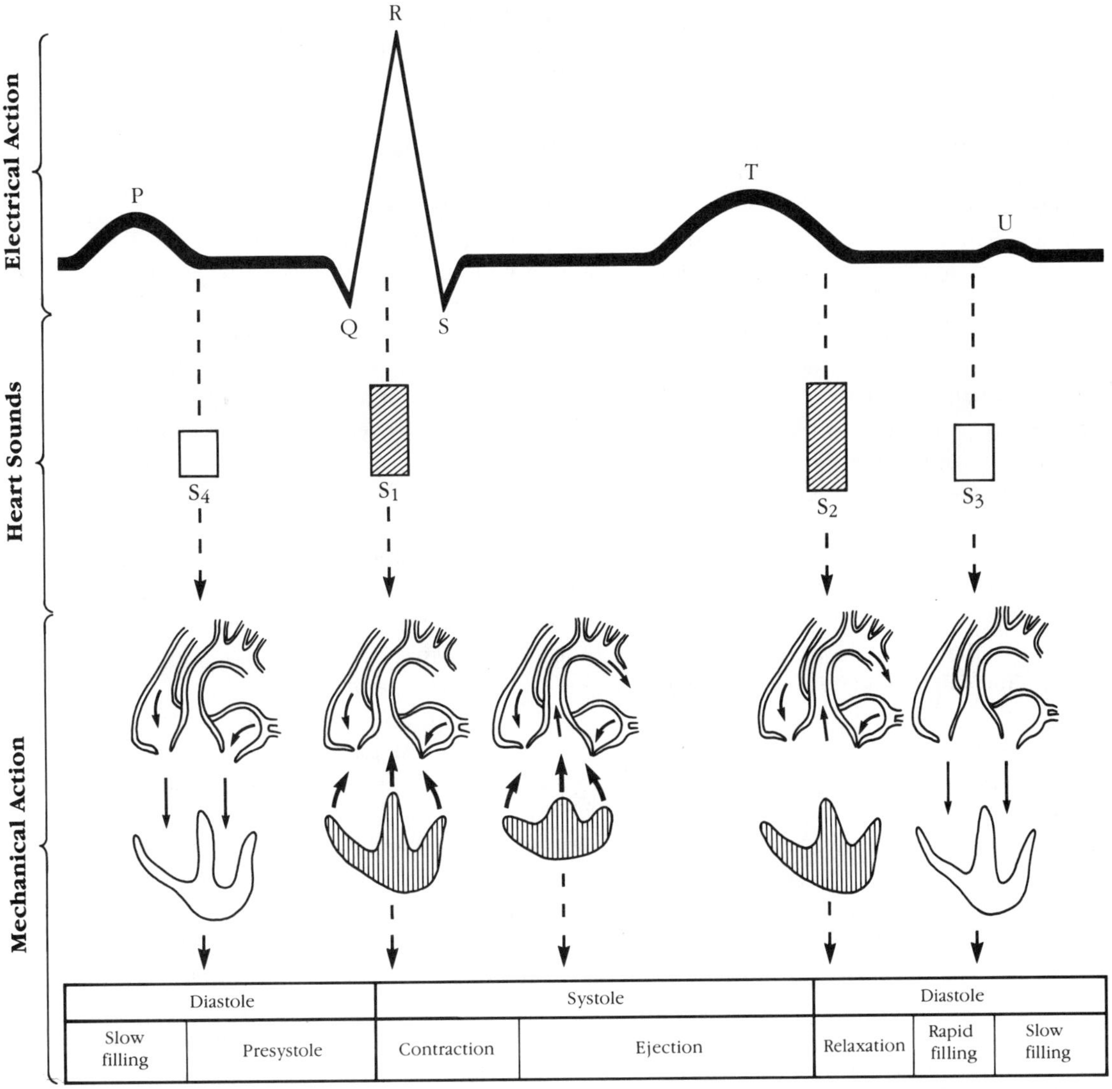

Diastole		Systole		Diastole		
Slow filling	Presystole	Contraction	Ejection	Relaxation	Rapid filling	Slow filling

Figure 14-15 The electrical sequence of heart activation and contraction. From Servonsky/Opas: *Nursing Management of Children*, © 1987 Boston: Jones and Bartlett Publishers.

S_4 is also called a presystolic or atrial gallop, as it occurs just prior to S_1 and systole.

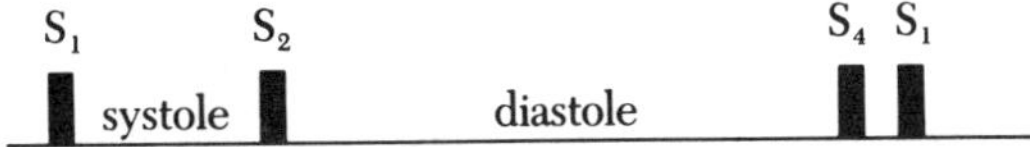

S_4 represents an atrial sound. S_4 may be heard in clients with hypertension and in clients who have had a myocardial infarction. With the scarred, stiff ventricle there is a loss of compliance. Therefore, the atrium is emptying into an area of higher pressure. Retrograde pressure builds, resulting in higher pressure against the atrial wall. The atrium will then contract with more energy, according to Starling's law: the more stretch of the fiber, the stronger the recoil. This force generates the S_4 sound and is sometimes referred to as an atrial kick. An S_4 will also occur with an excessive blood volume or with a rapid blood flow. S_4 is a presystolic sound.

A quadruple rhythm of the heart sounds occurs when both protodiastolic and presystolic sounds are heard. This pattern is called a summation gallop. As we have noted, both S_3 and S_4 heart sounds are louder with increased blood volume. Therefore, it should not be surprising that an edematous client may exhibit these sounds one day and, upon administration of a diuretic, not exhibit them the next day.

S_3 and S_4 heart sounds are normal in children,

BIOLOGICAL AND CULTURAL VARIATIONS

Sickle-Cell Anemia Among Black Americans

Approximately 3 out of every 1,000 Black infants in the United States are born with the genetic condition called sickle-cell anemia. These children have inherited two hemoglobin-S genes. As homozygotes, they are only capable of manufacturing a form of hemoglobin that causes red blood cells to assume a sickled shape. The sickled cells clog arterioles and capillaries, obstructing blood flow and oxygen transport to the tissues. Children and adolescents with sickle-cell anemia experience periodic crises of terrific pain in the limbs and abdomen, resulting from tissue hypoxia. Tissue hypoxia may also produce brain damage, bone deformities, and retinal lesions. Another symptom is an enlarged spleen, for the spleen becomes clogged with red blood cells that it is attempting to destroy. The child's resistance to infections decreases because of spleen dysfunction. Massive destruction of red blood cells causes anemia and a jaundiced appearance.

Roughly 1 in 8–10 Black Americans carries at least one gene for sickle-cell hemoglobin. Individuals with one hemoglobin-S gene (heterozygotes) are said to have the sickle trait, a condition that normally causes no health problems to the carrier. Although these 2 million heterozygotic Americans do not have anemia, they can pass sickle-cell anemia on to their offspring if they mate with another heterozygote. The probability is one in four that two heterozygotic parents will produce a child with sickle-cell anemia. Genetic counseling and screening programs have been set up to offer information to Black Americans. However, there are controversial aspects to these programs.

Until recently, with the development of new medical treatments, the average life expectancy for a person with sickle-cell anemia was 20 years. Very few patients lived beyond age 40. The highest death rate occurred during the first 6 years of life. Now patients may expect to live longer, but there are still no cures for the disease and its periodic crises.

In the United States, the frequency of the sickle-cell gene among Black Americans is approximately 5%. However, in certain populations in Africa, the frequency of the gene rises to as high as 30%. One might expect a high morbidity and mortality rate from sickle-cell anemia in these populations. How could such a lethal gene have risen to such a high frequency?

The reason for the high frequency of the sickle-cell gene in Africa and the moderately high frequency in the United States seems to stem from a heterozygote advantage for the gene in Africa. Black Americans are the descendants of mainly West and Central African populations, who were forced to migrate to the United States as slaves approximately 200 years ago. When they migrated, they brought the gene in high frequencies. While the frequency has fallen to more moderate levels in the United States over the years, in West and Central Africa the sickle-cell gene has persisted at higher levels because of the advantage it offers heterozygotes in surviving attacks of malaria. In Africa, malaria is transmitted by the bite of the *Anopheles gambiae* mosquito, which harbors the parasite *Plasmodium falciparum* in its salivary glands. Attacks of falciparum malaria are particularly serious in young children, for they have not yet built up active immunities to the disease. When untreated, malaria kills about 25% of these young children. However, young children who are heterozygotes for the sickle-cell gene have a much lower death rate. The variant form of the hemoglobin on the red blood cell apparently gives them an advantage in weathering attacks of the disease. Children who are homozygotes for the sickle-cell gene would presumably also have such an immunity to malaria, but they succumb to sickle-cell disease instead. Thus, the heterozygotes are at a greater survival advantage than either of the homozygotes. In this way, the frequency of the sickle-cell gene has risen and still persists in Black American population groups. With the absence of the malarial pressure in the United States, it is expected that the frequency will continue to fall in future generations.

in thin people, and in young adults. They are not normal in people over 30 years of age. S_3 and S_4 heart sounds may accompany hyperdynamic circulation; thus, they may be observed in the pregnant client and in the client with such illnesses as hyperthyroidism, Cushing's disease, and pheochromocytoma.

Splitting of Heart Sounds

The heart valves do not close simultaneously. During auscultation physiologic splitting of the heart sounds is often heard, particularly the splitting of S_2. The mitral valve (M_1) closes before the tricuspid valve (T_1) and the aortic valve (A_2) closes before the pulmonary valve (P_2). Thus, there are actually two components to the heart sounds, but they are so close together that they are difficult to hear. Hearing the normal physiologic splitting takes concentration, time, and practice in listening.

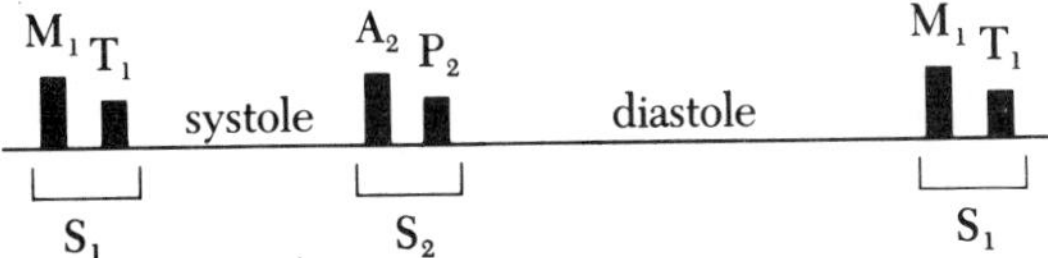

Splitting of the first heart sound is usually faint; if it can be heard at all, it is best heard somewhere between the apex and the sternum. When the split is heard, the mitral component (M_1) is usually louder than the tricuspid component (T_1). The widening of the S_1 split can be heard on expiration.

Splitting of the second heart sound is best heard on inspiration, over the pulmonary valve area or around the third or fourth left intercostal space near the sternum. In the adult the aortic valve closure (A_2) is louder than the pulmonary valve closure (P_2). Therefore, the relationship of A_2 to P_2 in the adult is $A_2 > P_2$. But $A_2 > P_2$ in the child is indicative of hypertension. In healthy children and young adults the intensity of the aortic and pulmonary valve closure should be of equal intensity ($A_2 = P_2$). In the adult $A_2 < P_2$ may signify pulmonary hypertension.

There are three main types of pathologic splitting:

1. *Wide splitting*—An abnormal degree of splitting on inspiration that occurs with conditions such as right bundle block and atrial septal defect, in which contraction or emptying of the right side of the heart is delayed, causing delay in pulmonary valve closure.
2. *Fixed splitting*—In this type of splitting there is little or no change in the degree of splitting during either phase of respiration. Such splitting can be detected in atrial septal defect and pulmonary stenosis.
3. *Paradoxical splitting*—In this type the splitting of S_2 widens during expiration and disappears during inspiration. This type of splitting can be heard in left bundle branch block.

Extra Heart Sounds During Systole

Early systolic *ejection clicks* are related to the sudden opening of the aortic and pulmonary valves. Aortic ejection clicks are heard over the base of the heart as well as at the apex, although they are often louder at the apex. They occur in such conditions as stenosis of the aortic valve, aortic regurgitation, coarctation of the aorta, aneurysms of the ascending aorta, and hypertension with dilatation of the aorta. Pulmonary ejection clicks are best heard in the left second intercostal space. They are heard in stenosis of the pulmonary valve, in pulmonary hypertension, and in situations where the pulmonary artery is dilated.

Middle and late systolic ejection clicks are often not pathognomonic. However, in some cases they are found in conjunction with a late systolic murmur; this usually indicates cardiac pathology.

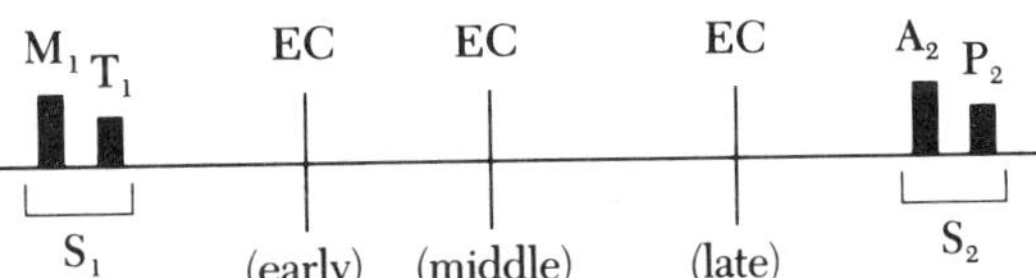

Extra Heart Sounds During Diastole

Opening snaps are heard during diastole. Under normal conditions the opening of the mitral valve is not audible. The clicking, high-pitched sound of an opening snap is heard in mitral stenosis, tricuspid stenosis, and atrial tumors. Opening snaps are best heard at Erb's point, with the client in the left lateral position.

OS

S_1 systole S_2 diastole S_1

All of these extra heart sounds are difficult to hear and to identify—even for the cardiologist. (See Table 14-2.)

Heart Murmurs

Cardiac *murmurs* are abnormal sounds produced by the blood as it flows through altered or deficient valves or produced by vibrations of the heart itself or in the walls of the pulmonary artery or the aorta. They are heard best over the valve from which they originate (see Table 14-3).

Murmurs can be caused by either regurgitation or stenosis. A valve that does not close properly, allowing blood to flow backward across it, is described as *regurgitant.* (The terms regurgitation and insufficiency are synonyms. In this text the term regurgitation will be used.) *Stenosis* refers to a valve or lumen that has become smaller because of pathologic changes.

The features that must be carefully studied and used to describe a murmur are location, timing, quality/pitch, and intensity.

Location The exact location of the murmur should be described according to the specific anatomic landmarks. Some murmurs may be confined to a small area and may be heard directly over the valve area. Others may be more diffuse and heard over the entire precordium. Certain ones can also be heard radiating to the neck region or axillary region.

Timing Murmurs are described as either systolic or diastolic:

S_1 ——— systole ——— S_2 ——— diastole ——— S_1

Systolic murmurs are referred to as being early, middle, or late. For example, mid-systolic murmurs are caused by the flow of blood through stenotic aortic or pulmonary valves. They can be described as crescendo-decrescendo because they are usually separate from the first and second heart sounds. A visual representation of the sound would look something like this:

This type of murmur can also be caused by increased flow of blood through competent valves, as in anemia or hyperthyroidism. It can also occur when blood flow through a normal valve empties into an enlarged aorta or pulmonary artery.

Some murmurs may persist throughout the entire systolic period, in which case they are termed pansystolic or holosystolic murmurs. Pansystolic murmurs are produced by flow of blood from a high-pressure chamber (left or right ventricle) to a low-pressure chamber (left or right atrium). For example, pansystolic murmurs may be heard in mitral and tricuspid regurgitation and in ventricular septal defect. This type of murmur would be visualized as follows:

Diastolic murmurs may occur in various parts of diastole and are described as being early diastolic, mid-diastolic, or presystolic. Early diastolic murmurs start with the second sound. In mid-diastolic murmurs there is a short pause after the second sound. Presystolic murmurs occur late in diastole but are caused by an atrial contraction. Diastolic murmurs are produced by mitral or tricuspid stenosis, since these valves should be open during diastole, or by aortic or pulmonary valve regurgitation, since these valves should be closed during diastole.

A murmur is described as continuous if it is heard both in systole and diastole and is of the same quality during both phases.

Quality and Pitch The quality of a murmur may be described as blowing, harsh, musical, or rumbling. The pitch of a murmur is dependent on the velocity of blood flow. When the velocity is great, the pitch is high; when the velocity is slow, the pitch is low. Murmurs are described as being high-pitched, medium, or low-pitched. Differences in quality and pitch are extremely important in diagnosis (see Table 14-4).

Table 14-2. Extra Heart Sounds

Terminology	Characteristics	Comments
Third heart sounds in adults (normal in children and young adults)	Best heard in lateral position with bell of stethoscope while client is exhaling. Occurs about 0.10 sec after aortic component of second sound and is of very low frequency.	Caused by sudden distention of ventricular wall when blood flows into ventricle from atrium during period of rapid ventricular filling. May be heard in anemia, hyperthyroidism, ventricular septal defect, mitral regurgitation, constrictive pericarditis.
Fourth heart sound (not always abnormal)	Precedes first heart sound, low frequency, heard best at apex, near xiphoid or in substernal notch.	Often associated with hypertension, aortic insufficiency, aortic stenosis.
Ejection click	Heard best at base of heart. High pitched, caused by sudden dilation of aorta and pulmonary artery.	Must be differentiated from split S_1. Usually associated with pulmonary hypertension, pulmonary valve stenosis, idiopathic dilation of pulmonary artery.
Midsystolic click	Heard best over apex. Sharp clicking sound heard in mid to late systole, often moving with respirations. Click closer to S_1 in inspiration and closer to S_2 in expiration.	Floppy mitral valve. Mitral prolapse associated with women more than men and causes increased risk of bacterial endocarditis.
Gallop rhythms	Best heard a little below apex but may be heard over entire precordial area. A dull, low-pitched sequential sound from the intensification of S_3 or S_4.	Not always a sign of heart failure. May occur with rapid heart rate. Aortic stenosis, aortic insufficiency.
Protodiastolic gallop	Intensification of S_3—has rhythm and accent of word *Ken-tuck-y.*	Position client on left side. Often accompanied by precardial heave. Ventricular hypertrophy.
Presystolic gallop	Intensification of S_4—has rhythm and accent of word *Ten-nes-see.*	Myocardial infarction, excessive blood volume or rapid blood flow.
Summation gallop	Presence of S_3 and S_4 sounds—occurs when heart rate becomes rapid.	Seen in hyperdynamic circulation (e.g., hyperthyroidism, Cushing's disease).
Fixed split	Split of S_1 or S_2—little or no variation with respirations.	Atrial septal defect. Pulmonary stenosis.
Widened split S_2	Split of S_2 varies with respirations but is more than 0.01 sec on inspiration and less than 0.04 sec on expiration.	Increased pulmonary blood flow (atrial septal defects). Decreased pulmonary pressure (pulmonary stenosis). Mitral insufficiency.
Paradoxical split	Split of S_2 becomes wider and more pronounced on expiration and decreases on inspiration.	LBBB (left bundle branch block), aortic stenosis, hypertension.
Adventitious sounds:		
Pericardial friction rub	Scratchy, high-pitched sound heard throughout cardiac cycle. Best heard with client sitting upward and forward at 3ICS to the left of sternum.	Inflammation of pericardium (e.g., rheumatic pericarditis).
Venous hum	Turbulent blood flow in internal jugular vein. Continuous, low-pitched humming or roaring sound. Best heard with client sitting up. Listen above medial one-third of clavicle especially on the right. Sound may radiate to 1st and 2nd ICS.	Anemia, thyrotoxicosis.

Table 14-3 Valvular Problems and Resultant Heart Murmurs

Terminology	Characteristics	Comments
Aortic stenosis	*Location:* Best heard in 2nd right interspace, radiates into neck and down left sternal border. Frequently heard at apex. *Quality:* Harsh. *Pitch:* Medium, usually that of a whispered *R*, to high. *Intensity:* Reached in late systole. Thrill may be palpated over the precordium, best felt in aortic area and apex. Associated with diminished S_2; early ejection click; a thrusting, sustained apical impulse; slowly rising carotid pulse; contour and narrow pulse pressure.	Congenital or acquired disease. May result from rheumatic endocarditis or atherosclerosis. Symptoms include extreme weakness, fatigue, debilitation, venous hypertension, edema, hepatomegaly, and ascites.
Pulmonic stenosis	*Location:* Best heard at pulmonic area (L 2ICS) and L 3ICS. Radiates toward left shoulder and upward toward neck. *Quality:* Often harsh. *Pitch:* Medium to high. *Intensity:* Variable; thrill may be palpated in pulmonic area. Associated with a widely split S_2 and a diminished to absent pulmonic component of S_2, early ejection click, and right ventricular hypertrophy (left parasternal lift).	Usually a congenital defect. Frequently associated with other congenital heart lesions such as ventricular septal or atrial septal defect.
Mitral stenosis	*Location:* Best heard at apex—not widely transmitted—frequently heard in area no larger than bell of stethoscope. Client should be in left lateral position and bell of stethoscope should be pressed lightly to skin. *Quality:* Rumbling. *Pitch:* Low. *Intensity:* Variable, soft. Can be accentuated with exercise. Associated with opening snap and an accentuated S_1 in the mitral area.	Ventricular filling murmur produced by obstruction to flow of blood across mitral valve during ventricular diastole. Most commonly seen in women under 45. Results from rheumatic endocarditis. Symptoms include fatigue, SOB, cough, bronchitis, orthopnea, PND, cyanosis, and pulmonary edema.
Mitral regurgitation	*Location:* Best heard at apex—transmitted to the left axilla and may be heard in the back on the left side. *Quality:* Soft, blowing. *Pitch:* High. *Intensity:* Variable but often loud; may be associated with an apical thrill. Does not increase with inspiration. May be preceded by a click. Decreased S_1 and an S_3, a thrusting sustained apical impulse displaced downward and to the left.	Majority of those affected are men. Rheumatic fever is principal cause. May be congenital anomaly or developed secondary to bacterial endocarditis or aortic valvular disease. Many clients never develop cardiac symptoms, but most feel fatigue followed by dyspnea on exertion and cough.

Table 14-3. *Continued*

Terminology	Characteristics	Comments
Tricuspid regurgitation	*Location:* Tricuspid area. *Quality:* Blowing. *Pitch:* High. *Intensity:* Variable; increases with respiration associated with left parasternal lift and systolic pulsations in the jugular venous pulse. Hepatojugular reflex can be elicited. Systolic thrill may be palpated over right ventricle.	Organic tricuspid regurgitation is rare but functional. Tricuspid insufficiency due to dilation of right ventricle is not uncommon. Due to value impairment, blood leaks back into right atrium as well as being pushed forward into pulmonary circulation, causing venous engorgement and right heart failure. A slate-colored complexion is sometimes seen.
Aortic regurgitation	*Location:* Best heard at L 3ICS—at left sternal margin with client leaning forward and in forced expiration. Diaphragm of stethoscope should be used. Sound distinctive and rarely identified incorrectly. *Quality:* Blowing. *Pitch:* High. *Intensity:* Variable, faint. Occurs during any phase of diastole. Associated with aortic diastolic murmur, S_3, wide pulse pressure, and a sustained thrusting apical impulse displaced inferiorly and laterally.	Occurs most often in men. May be congenital or acquired. Rheumatic endocarditis principal cause. Syphilis may be an etiologic factor. Symptoms include sinus tachycardia, dyspnea on exertion, angina, and symptoms related to pulmonary congestion.

Table 14-4. Examples of the Quality and Pitch of Murmurs

Type of murmur	Quality	Pitch
Aortic and pulmonary stenosis	Usually harsh	Medium-high
Mitral and tricuspid regurgitation	Blowing	High
Ventricular septal defect	Usually harsh	High
Mitral stenosis	Rumbling	Low
Aortic regurgitation	Blowing	High

When the client is standing, blood pools in the extremities, so there are fewer dynamics in the heart. Thus, murmurs and sounds tend to disappear. It has been said that many individuals with low-grade murmurs have passed military physicals because they are generally examined while standing. One of the few murmurs that become louder and longer when the individual stands up (the heart gets smaller) is that of aortic regurgitation.

Intensity A six-point grading system is used to describe the loudness of a murmur (see Table 14-5).

Grade I murmurs are frequently encountered in persons who do not have organic heart disease. Grade III murmurs or louder seldom occur in a normal heart. Low-grade murmurs are commonly heard in the elderly, who have valves with ragged edges or that are stiff to open merely from the wear and tear of aging. If a low-grade murmur remains as such for years, it is probably of little or no significance. However, a murmur that increases in intensity over the years is an indication of progressive valvular disease.

It is difficult to determine significant murmurs in a child. Children may have murmurs without having organic pathology, or they may not demonstrate murmurs despite the existence of severe heart disease. The detection of a heart murmur warrants consultation with a physician for further evaluation. In particular, a murmur

BIOLOGICAL AND CULTURAL VARIATIONS

G6PD Deficiency in Mediterranean Peoples

Americans who are descended from Mediterranean peoples such as Italians, Greeks, Armenians, Sephardic Jews, and other Middle Easterners have a relatively high frequency of certain genetic disorders, such as familial Mediterranean fever and glucose-6-phosphate dehydrogenase (G6PD) deficiency. The symptoms of familial Mediterranean fever, which are similar to those of brucellosis include chills and fever, severe headache, and abdominal and joint pain.

G6PD deficiency is a genetic deficiency of glucose-6-phosphate dehydrogenase, an enzyme that normally acts to maintain levels of reduced glutathione in the red blood cells (Katz & Schall 1979). Individuals with G6PD deficiency have lowered levels of reduced glutathione in their red blood cells, which under normal conditions causes them no significant problems. However, if the G6PD-deficient person takes the antimalarial compound primaquine or eats some raw fava beans, his reduced glutathione levels will be lowered even further, producing a hemolytic anemic crisis. Red blood cells will undergo massive destruction within a few hours or a few days of the fava bean consumption (favism) or primaquine ingestion (primaquine sensitivity). Death may occur in as many as one in twelve cases. The hemolytic crisis may also be triggered by any of a number of bacterial or viral infections.

Like the hemoglobin abnormalities of the sickle-cell trait, G6PD deficiency seems to act as a buffer against morbidity and mortality from malaria—persons with G6PD deficiency living in malarial belts in the Mediterranean have a lower incidence rate of malaria. Apparently, the malarial parasites cannot thrive in the G6PD-deficient red blood cells, presumably because of the low levels of reduced glutathione. Such a survival advantage against malarial mortality explains the high rates of G6PD deficiency in Mediterranean population groups.

Table 14-5. Grading System of Heart Murmurs

Grade	Loudness of murmur
I	Is difficult to hear; experienced examiner and quiet environment are needed
II	Is not readily heard upon laying stethoscope on chest; examiner must listen closely to hear
III	Requires no effort to hear and is readily heard when stethoscope is placed on chest
IV	Is accompanied by a thrill; loud enough that there is no question of its presence
V	Can be heard with stethoscope held an inch away from chest; thrill present
VI	Does not require use of stethoscope to hear; thrill present

that radiates or occurs during diastole is considered indicative of heart disease until otherwise disproved.

Adventitious Sounds

In addition to heart murmurs, adventitious heart sounds include pericardial friction rub and venous hum. *Pericardial friction rub* is caused by the rubbing together of the two layers of the pericardium. Such rubbing occurs when the surfaces become roughened as the result of an inflammatory process. Inflammation and a resultant pericardial friction rub may be heard in rheumatic pericarditis or following a myocardial infarction. A pericardial friction rub can be differentiated from a pleural friction rub in that it is unaffected by respirations. If the client is instructed to hold his breath, a pericardial friction rub will continue to be heard, whereas a pleural friction rub will cease. The intensity of the pericardial friction rub varies with position and is often best heard when the client is sitting upright and leaning forward. Often pressure over the liver or right upper quadrant of the abdomen will accentuate the rub, as will pressure with the stethoscope on the chest wall.

Venous hum is created by turbulence of blood flow in the internal jugular vein. This increased blood flow can occur in such conditions as anemia and thyrotoxicosis. Venous hum is a continuous low-pitched hum that can be heard in the neck and upper part of the chest just above the

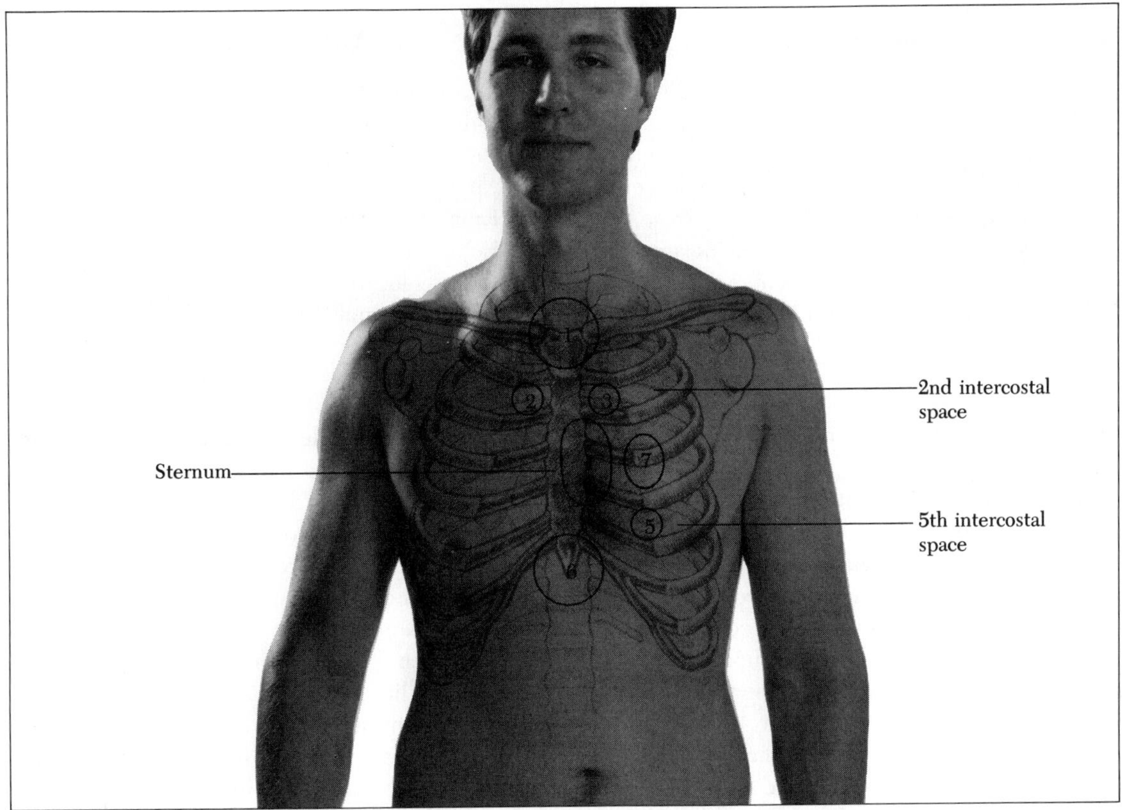

Figure 14-16 Specific areas for inspection and palpation of the anterior chest.

clavicle in the angle between the insertion of the sternocleidomastoid muscle and the clavicle. Sometimes it can also be heard at the base of the heart. It is most commonly heard on the right side, although it can be heard on either side. The most effective position for detection of venous hum on the right side is for the client to be sitting up with his head turned to the left and tilted upward. The position of the head should be reversed when listening for a hum on the left side.

Characteristics and Techniques of Examination

Inspection and Palpation

Inspection and palpation are best accomplished with the client lying supine or with the head of the bed elevated approximately 45 degrees. The entire precordium should be observed and palpated for symmetry and pulsations. The observations must be made in an orderly fashion. Tangential lighting helps in detecting pulsations. The palmar surface of the hand is most sensitive to vibrations, and the fingertips are most sensitive to pulsations.

Initially the *sternoclavicular area*, labeled 1 in Figure 14-16, is examined for the presence of pulsations. Few or no pulsations are normally visualized in this area. Pulsations detected here may be reflective of a dissecting aortic aneurysm, an aneurysm due to arteriosclerosis or syphilis, and Tetrology of Fallot. Occasionally pulsations may be seen in elderly clients with a tortuous innominate artery.

Then examine the *aortic area* (second intercostal space to the right of the sternum), labeled 2 in Figure 14-16. Observe this area for pulsations. Pulsations here may be due to dilatation of the aorta caused by an aneurysm or perhaps aortic regurgitation. Palpate the area to check for thrills. A *thrill* is a murmur that can be palpated; it feels something like the sensation of placing a hand on the throat of a purring cat. A systolic thrill felt in the aortic area may be the result of aortic stenosis and may radiate to the right side of the neck. A diastolic thrill at the apex of the heart may accompany mitral stenosis and may radiate to the left axilla. Patent ductus

Techniques for Inspection and Palpation of Anterior Chest

1. Adequate lighting, warm room, privacy.
2. Client exposed to the waist.
3. Client in supine or semifowler position.
4. Use of tangential lighting best to detect pulsations.
5. Inspect and palpate the following areas on the anterior chest with palmar surfaces and then the fingertips of your hand:
   Sternoclavicular area
   Aortic area
   Pulmonary area
   Right ventricular area
   Apical area
   Epigastric area
   Ectopic area
6. Identify location of the PMI.
7. Note abnormalities.

arteriosus may produce a continuous thrill at the base of the heart.

Next inspect and palpate the *pulmonary area* (second intercostal space to the left of the sternum), labeled 3 in Figure 14-16. In instances where the pulmonary artery is compromised, abnormal pulsations can be detected. In pulmonary hypertension and mitral stenosis, the pulsations are slow and forceful, whereas in atrial septal defect they are more vigorous. A systolic thrill due to pulmonary stenosis may be palpated in this area and can radiate to the left side of the neck. A slight thrill may be palpated in normal children and thin, nervous adults; the thrill can be accentuated by such conditions as fever, anemia, and pregnancy.

Next inspect and palpate the *right ventricular area* (anterior precordium), labeled 4 in Figure 14-16. This area encompasses the lower half of the sternum and the intercostal spaces to the left and the right of the sternum. Pulsations in this area are usually associated with right ventricular hypertrophy. Some of the conditions that result in right ventricular hypertrophy include cor pulmonale, pulmonary hypertension, repeated pulmonary emboli, and mitral stenosis. A thrill in this area suggests ventricular septal defect or tricuspid regurgitation.

In the *apical area*, labeled 5 in Figure 14-16, observe and palpate for the apical impulse. This is sometimes referred to as the PMI (point of maximum impulse or of maximum intensity). By age 7 and in adults the apical impulse is normally located at the fifth or sixth left intercostal space at the midclavicular line or slightly medial to it. Prior to age 7 the PMI is at the third or fourth left intercostal space just to the left of the midclavicular line. Particular attention should be given to the size, location, and character of the impulse. The impulse is felt as a slight tap and is normally 2 cm or less in diameter. It begins about the time of the first heart sound and lasts through the first third of systole. If you cannot find it, ask the client to turn to the left side or to sit up and lean forward. In left ventricular hypertrophy the apical impulse may be displaced to the left and may be very forceful and sustained. Such a forceful pressure is called a cardiac heave, lift, or thrust. Any disease that shifts the mediastinum may also displace the PMI. Occasionally, the apical impulse may be increased in amplitude and duration from noncardiac causes. This situation may sometimes be observed in pregnant women or in clients who are thin or have anemia or hyperthyroidism—situations in which the blood flow is dynamic. A thrill palpated in the apical area may be due to mitral regurgitation (systolic thrill) or mitral stenosis; the latter produces a diastolic thrill that may radiate to the left axilla.

Next, examine the *epigastric area*, labeled 6 in Figure 14-16. Pulsations in this area occur occasionally in normal individuals, usually following strenuous exercise. Large bounding pulsations may be due to aortic aneurysms or aortic regurgitation. Fever, anemia, and thyrotoxicosis may also produce pulsations in the epigastric area. It may be difficult to view pulsations in the epigastric area in a client with an emphysemic chest. In such a case, place your hand on the epigastric area and slide your fingers up under the rib cage. Pulsations of right ventricular hypertrophy will be felt on the fingertips, and aortic events will be reflected on the palm of your hand.

Lastly, examine the *ectopic area*, labeled 7 in Figure 14-16, located in the left midclavicular line between the pulmonic and apical areas. A systolic pulsation may be observed during an anginal attack or an acute myocardial infarction.

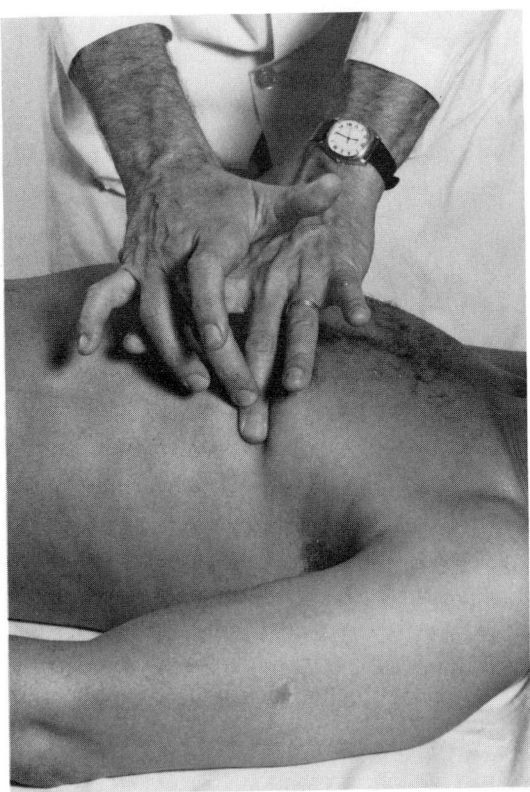

Figure 14-17 Percussing the contour of the left cardiac border.

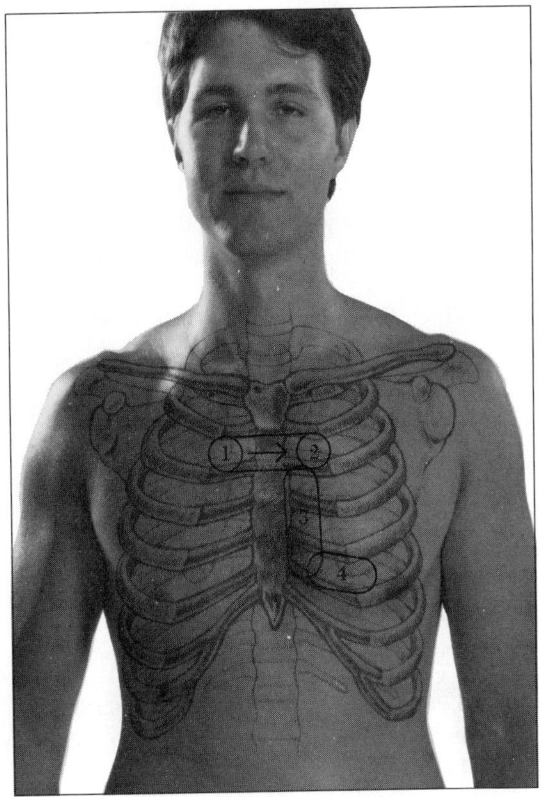

Figure 14-18 Method of cardiac auscultation.

This pulsation will disappear within 2–3 weeks. Clients, who develop a ventricular aneurysm following a myocardial infarction will manifest a persistent pulsation in the ectopic area.

The size of the pulsation is determined and measured. Also the location and time in the cardiac cycle (systole, diastole, or both) are documented.

Percussion

Although specialized procedures such as x-ray and fluoroscopy are much more accurate in determining the size of the heart, a gross estimate of the contour of the left cardiac border is possible by percussion. Because the right cardiac border lies underneath the sternum, under normal conditions it is difficult to detect. To percuss the left cardiac border, begin laterally with the pleximeter finger either parallel or perpendicular to the intercostal spaces. Percuss toward the midline in the fifth, fourth, and third interspaces, as shown in Figure 14-17. Usually the left border dullness will be detected about the midclavicular line or slightly medial to it. If the left cardiac border dullness occurs prior to reaching the left midclavicular line, the distance from the midclavicular line should be measured and recorded. A sample documentation would read: "LCBD (left cardiac border dullness) 2 cm lateral to left of MCL at the 5th ICS." Another technique is to measure from the left cardiac border dullness to the midsternal line. In the adult the distance ranges from approximately 9 cm to 12 cm. A sample recording of this type measurement would read: "LCBD to MSL at the 6th ICS is 11 cm."

Lateral displacement of the left cardiac border can sometimes be detected in such conditions as left ventricular hypertrophy, cirrhosis, and pregnancy. Absence or decrease in dullness is suggestive of emphysema. The use of percussion is not diagnostic in itself but is helpful because results can be immediately correlated with other clinical findings at the time of the examination.

Auscultation

To become proficient in the technique of auscultation, you will need years of practice and a thorough knowledge of the origins of normal and ab-

Technique for Auscultation of Heart

1. Quiet, warm room.
2. Client's chest exposed.
3. Client in supine position.
4. If hairy chest, wet hair with a washcloth.
5. Warm stethoscope with hands.
6. Place diaphragm of stethoscope firmly at apex.
7. Inch stethoscope toward sternum.
8. Proceed up left sternal border to pulmonary area.
9. Inch across at 2nd ICS level to aortic area on client's right side.
10. Next place the bell on the aortic area so all sides of the bell rim are lightly touching the skin.
11. Inch across to the pulmonic area.
12. Inch down the left sternal border.
13. Inch over to the apical area.
14. At each area assess the following: S_1, S_2, splitting, A_2:P_2 relationship, presence of extra heart sounds and/or adventitious sounds.
15. Repeat process with client in the left lateral position.
16. Repeat process with the client leaning forward in a sitting position.

Technique for Percussion of Anterior Chest

1. Client preferably in supine position.
2. Percuss from the left MAL toward the MSL in the 4th or 5th ICS.
3. Measure from point of first detection of dull percussion note (LCBD) to the MSL.

normal cardiac sounds. Because heart sounds are generally low pitched, you must perform auscultation in a quiet room in order to improve your ability to hear the sounds. You must perform auscultation in an unhurried manner, concentrating on what you hear. First examine the client in the supine position, then in the left lateral position, and finally leaning forward in the sitting position.

The heart should be examined in each of the four valve areas and over the precordial area. Listening should be done systematically. Begin at the apex and inch the stethoscope over to and up the left sternal border to the pulmonary area and the aortic area, or begin in the aortic area and inch the stethoscope across to the pulmonary area, then down the left sternum and across to the apex of the heart (see Figure 14-18). Whichever system you choose, stick to it to maintain thoroughness; do not hopscotch about the chest with the stethoscope.

Auscultation is carried out first with the diaphragm and then with the bell of the stethoscope. The diaphragm should be held firmly against the skin. If the client has a hairy chest, it may be wise to wet the chest with a washcloth in order to make the hair lie more smoothly. Otherwise, hair under the diaphragm may sound like fine rales of the lungs. The diaphragm is better at picking up high-pitched sounds, whereas the bell is better at detecting low-pitched sounds. The bell should be placed lightly on the chest; firm placement will stretch the skin tight, causing the skin to act as a diaphragm, in which case low pitches may go undetected. Auscultation is the best technique for accurately determining the rate and rhythm of the heart. Further, some alterations are heard more readily by auscultation.

The first heart sound (S_1) is loudest at the apex in the normal individual. If you have difficulty differentiating the first from the second heart sound, palpate the carotid pulse. The first heart sound and the beat of the carotid pulse will be simultaneous. Another technique is to listen to the length of the systole and diastole. Systole is normally shorter than diastole; thus, there is only a short pause between S_1 and S_2. The pause following S_2 will be longer (diastole) before S_1 reappears. S_1 should be listened to for intensity, variations in intensity, and splitting. S_2, which is loudest at the base of the heart (at the aortic and pulmonary areas), should be auscultated for these same components.

The degree of splitting and its relationship to inspiration and expiration are important to note. You must also listen for systolic clicks, third or fourth heart sounds, and diastolic opening snaps. Then concentrate your attention on listening for murmurs, during both systole and diastole.

Since murmurs often radiate to other areas, listen up into the neck region and over into the left axillary region. For example, murmurs in the aortic area may radiate to the neck and down the left sternal border. Murmurs in the mitral area are often best heard after exercise when the client is in the left lateral position. Murmurs in the aortic area are best heard when the client is sitting and on expiration. A third heart sound is usually best detected when the client is in the left lateral position.

Auscultation may also reveal previously undetected arrythmias and can supplement what is learned from an electrocardiogram. Arrhythmias are classified according to heart rate and the type of rhythm, as illustrated in Table 14-7.

A summary of normal and abnormal heart sounds is presented in Table 14-6.

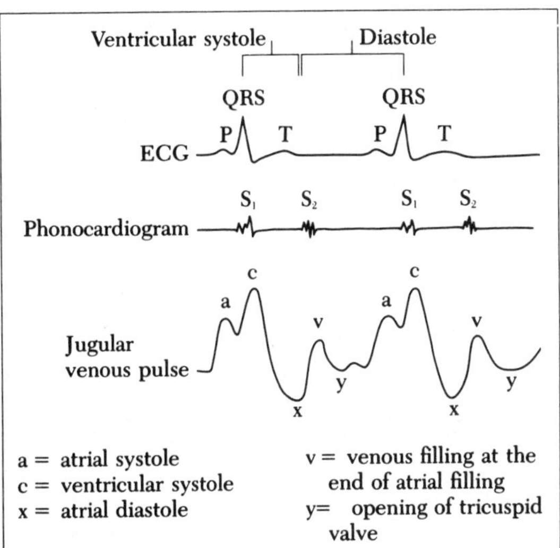

Figure 14-19 Relationship of jugular venous waves to heart sounds.

Measurement of Jugular Venous Pulse

It is important to inspect the jugular veins, since alterations in pressure or pulse waves indicate the presence of pathology. The internal and external jugular veins, illustrated in Figure 10-14 on page 202, terminate at the subclavian vein and return blood from the head to the right atrium. The internal jugular vein is situated deep in the sternocleidomastoid muscle and can be traced as arising from the supraclavicular fossa. The external jugular arises from beneath the clavicle lateral to the internal jugular and crosses it diagonally over the sternocleidomastoid. The jugular venous pulse and pressure reflect the blood volume of the area; thus, they are an indirect indication of the ability of the right atrium to receive blood, as well as of left ventricular contractility. The internal jugular vein provides the more accurate data, as the external jugular may be abnormal because of obstruction or kinking at the base of the neck. If the internal jugular cannot be visualized, use the external jugular to measure the pulse, with the understanding that it will not be as accurate.

Two facets of the pulse must be considered: the venous pulsations and the venous pressure. In most normal adults in the supine position, venous pulsations can be seen at the base of the neck. These pulsations are described in terms of a, c, and v waves and x and y troughs, as seen in Figure 14-19. Analysis of these waves reveals important information about the cardiac cycle and the function of the right atrium. The a wave is caused by right atrial contraction, which occurs just before the first heart sound. Identify it by palpating the carotid artery. The a wave will immediately precede the carotid pulsation. Abnormally large waves occur when the right atrium contracts very forcefully. These types of waves may be present in conditions of tricuspid stenosis, pulmonary stenosis, right ventricular hypertrophy, and pulmonary hypertension. Absence of an a wave will occur during atrial fibrillation because the atria contract in a disorganized pattern.

The c wave is very small and is rarely seen. It begins at the end of the first heart sound and is sometimes said to be a reflected wave from the carotid artery. The v wave occurs in late systole as blood from the periphery enters the right atrium. Large v waves are transmitted with tricuspid regurgitation. Atrial fibrillation often accompanies this pattern.

The x and y troughs are downward waves, or "negative" waves. The x wave is produced by atrial diastole and follows the c wave. The y wave occurs when the triscupid valve opens and blood flows from the right atrium into the right ventricle. Large x and y deflections are seen in chronic pericarditis, pericardial effusion, and severe right heart failure.

The external jugular veins are often distended with the client in the supine position; they will collapse with inspiration and fill with expiration. In the healthy individual, this distention disappears when the head of the bed is elevated 45

Table 14-6. Summary of Normal and Abnormal Heart Sounds

Heart sound	Auscultatory site	Location on chest	Timing	Auscultatory sounds	Physiology	Characteristic of heart sounds
S_1	Mitral (apical) area	Fifth left intercostal space just medial to the midclavicular line; in children under 2 years, fourth left interspace in or just lateral to the left midclavicular line	Presystolic	*Lub*-dub	Mitral and tricuspid valves close simultaneously.	S_1 is heard the loudest at the apex but can be heard over the entire precordium. Carotid pulse follows immediately. Intensity increases when valve leaflets are made rigid by calcium deposits as in rheumatic heart disease. First sound increases in intensity in rheumatic fever. Lasts approximately 0.10 seconds. Best heard with diaphragm chest piece as a low-frequency sound.
Split S_1	Mitral (apical) area Tricuspid area	Fifth left intercostal space just medial to the midclavicular line; in children under 2 years, fourth left interspace in or just lateral to the left midclavicular line Fifth left intercostal space, close to the sternum	Presystolic	*T-lub*-dub	Closure of mitral and tricuspid valves occurs at different times. Tricuspid valve closes slightly after mitral valve.	The dominant component of S_1 is the closure of the mitral valve. This closure is louder than tricuspid closure; therefore, the split S_1 is not easily heard. Closure of the mitral and tricuspid valves are separated by more than 0.02 sec when the split S_1 is audible. True S_1 splitting is heard not at the apex but closer to the xiphoid in the tricuspid area. Varies in intensity depending on PR interval, such as a wandering atrial pacemaker or heart block. Heard with the diaphragm chest piece and is unaffected by respiration.
S_2	Aortic area	Second right interspace close to the sternum	Postsystolic	lub-*dub*	Closure of aortic and pulmonic valves is almost simultaneous.	S_2 is heard louder than S_1. S_2 is higher-pitched, shorter, and "snappier" than S_1. A_2 P_2 separation normally 0.02 to 0.06 sec with inspiration. A single S_2 is heard in alterations where (1) S_2 is single, (2) S_1 is inaudible, or (3) the two sounds are fused. Examples include tetralogy of Fallot, pulmonary atresia, and ventricular septal defect with pulmonary hypertension. Best heard with the diaphragm chest piece.

Split S_2 (physiologic)	A_2—Aortic area P_2—Pulmonic area	Second right interspace close to the sternum Second intercostal space, just to the left of the sternum	Postsystolic	lub-*T-dub*-lub-dub	Closure of aortic and pulmonic valves is asynchronous. Aortic valve closes first, followed by closure of pulmonic valve. Inspiration delays pulmonic valve closure.	During expiration, A_2 and P_2 are heard as one sound, due to the scant interval between them. The splitting of A_2 and P_2 is evident at the height of the inspiratory phase during quiet respiration. This splitting during inspiration is due to an increased venous return to the right heart secondary to the decrease in intrathoracic pressure. Thus, right ventricular systole is lengthened, and the closure of the pulmonic valve is delayed. Normal physiological splitting of S_2 is heard in all normal children (with increasing age, the chest size increases and the pulmonic sound softens). Best heard with the diaphragm chest piece.
Split S_2 (fixed and persistent)	A_2—Aortic area P_2—Pulmonic area	Second right interspace close to the sternum Second intercostal space, just to the left of the sternum	Postsystolic	lub-*T-dub*	Closure of aortic and pulmonic valves is asynchronous. The pulmonic valve closes after the aortic valve during inspiration and expiration.	Persistent splitting occurs during both inspiration and expiration, with A_2 and P_2 being more widely split on inspiration. The splitting becomes fixed when the degree of splitting remains unchanged during respiration. In the child and adolescent, persistent splitting can be a normal occurrence.
S_3 (ventricular gallop)	Mitral (apical) area Right ventricular areas	Fifth left intercostal space just medial to the midclavicular line; in children under 2 years, fourth left interspace in or just lateral to the left midclavicular line Lower left sternal border, at the xiphoid process over the epigastrium, or at the left midprecordium	Early diastolic	Ken-*tuc*-ky	Results from premature rapid filling of ventricles that have limited elasticity.	S_3 occurs about 0.12 to 0.16 sec after S_2. Represents a normal physiologic finding in children and young adults. The descriptive term *gallop* is used because it has the acoustical effect of the canter of a galloping horse. Heard as a faint low-pitched sound with the bell chest piece. It is best heard at the apex and occasionally at the left lower sternal border at the beginning of respiration.

(continued on page 302)

Table 14-6. *Continued*

Heart sound	Auscultatory site	Location on chest	Timing	Auscultatory sounds	Physiology	Characteristic of heart sounds
S_4 (atrial gallop)	Mitral (apical) area	Fifth left intercostal space just medial to the midclavicular line; in children under 2 years, fourth left interspace in or just lateral to the left midclavicular line	Late diastolic or presystolic	*Ten*-nes-see	At the end of the diastolic period, the atrial contribution to a stiff or overfilled ventricle results in the fourth heart sound.	Heard as a soft, brief sound. Best heard with the child lying in the supine position. Is louder on inspiration. Only heard with the bell of the stethoscope.

From Servonsky/Opas: Nursing Management of Children, © 1987 Boston: Jones and Bartlett Publishers.

degrees. This is the point at which measurement should be made, because veins that are distended more than 2–3 cm at this angle (45 degrees) are a sign of pathology. Figure 14-20 illustrates the technique for measuring jugular venous distention.

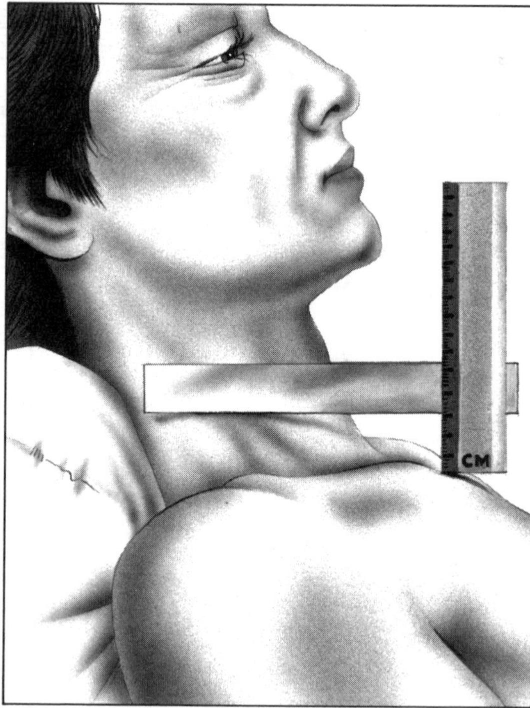

Figure 14-20 Technique for measuring jugular venous distention (JVD = 3 cm).

Technique for Measuring Jugular Venous Distention

1. Adequate lighting.
2. Provide for good exposure of neck and upper chest.
3. Position client in semifowler position (45 degrees).
4. Place metric ruler perpendicular to sternal line (Angle of Louis).
5. Draw an imaginary line from the top of the distention of the internal jugular vein on a level horizontal plane to the metric ruler and read the measurement at this imaginary line point of contact on the ruler.

Table 14-7. Classification of Arrhythmias

	Rhythm		
Heart rate	Regular	Rhythmically or accidentally irregular	Absolutely irregular
	A.	D.	G.
200	Supraventricular tachycardias	Supraventricular tachycardias with ventricular premature contractions	Atrial fibrillation untreated
175	1. Sinus tachycardia 2. Atrial tachycardia 3. Atrial flutter 4. Atrial tachycardia with block		
150	5. Nodal tachycardia	Atrial flutter	Atrial flutter
125	Ventricular tachycardias		
	B.	E.	H.
100	Sinus rhythm Atrial flutter with 3:1 or 4:1 block	Sinus arrhythmia Ventricular premature contractions	Atrial fibrillation with partial block (digitalis, sclerosis)
75	Sinus or atrial tachycardia with 2:1 block	Atrial premature contraction Partial heart block (Wenckenbach's phenomenon)	Atrial flutter Sinus arrhythmia of the aged
50			
	C.	F.	I.
25	Sinus bradycardia Complete heart block Partial heart block with 2:1 or 3:1 block	Partial or complete heart block with ventricular premature contractions	Partial or complete heart block with ventricular premature contractions.

From Abe Ravin, *Auscultation of the Heart*, 2nd ed. (Chicago: Yearbook Medical Publishers, Inc., 1967).

To determine the venous pressure, measure and record the highest point of oscillation of the internal jugular venous blood or the level of the external jugular venous distention. Then measure (in centimeters) the vertical distance between either of these points and the sternal angle; this is the venous pressure. In severe congestive heart failure, distention of both the internal and external jugular veins may be seen extending to the angle of the jaw.

A phenomenon called the hepatojugular reflux can be elicited in right heart failure. With the client seated at a 45 degree angle, use the palm of your hand to apply firm pressure over the upper right quadrant of the abdomen. This pressure constitutes a venous dam. Apply the pressure for 30–45 seconds. When you release the pressure, the dammed venous blood will return rapidly to the heart. In the client with right heart failure, the large rapid return of blood will not be able to be handled by the heart and will back up into the jugular veins, causing increased jugular venous pressure. A positive hepatojugular reflux may be a first sign of impending right-sided heart failure. In the normal individual, this manipulation will not cause the venous pressure to rise, as the healthy heart will be able to accommodate the increased blood return.

Summary

This chapter provided discussion of assessment of the arterial pulses and detailed information on the structure and function of the heart. The chambers, valves, conduction system, cardiac cycle, and heart sounds must be thoroughly understood before assessment of the heart can proceed.

Inspection and palpation, best carried out with the client in the supine position, are the initial techniques used. Percussion is used to help determine heart size. Auscultation of the heart is a difficult technique and takes years of practice and a thorough knowledge of cardiac sounds. Examination of the internal and external jugular veins provides valuable information about heart functioning.

Discussion Questions/Activities

1. Assess peripheral pulses of an adolescent and an older adult. Note any differences.
2. Discuss the location and function of the heart valves.
3. Discuss the electrical conduction of the heart and its relation to the ECG.
4. Describe the relationship of the heart sounds to the cardiac cycle.
5. Describe what is meant by splitting of the heart sounds. Give examples of pathologic splitting.
6. State the criteria used to determine a physiologic S_3.
7. State the criteria used to determine a normal S_1 and S_2.
8. Discuss the origin of common heart murmurs. Describe the location, timing, quality and pitch, and intensity of these murmurs.
9. Demonstrate the procedure for performing cardiac auscultation.
10. Demonstrate the method for measuring the jugular venous pressure.

Recording of Findings

Normal findings are presented in the first box. Abnormal findings of aortic regurgitation are presented in the second box.

Heart	Heart
INSPECTION AND PALPATION Apical impulse left at 5th ICS at MCL—no pulsations, heaves, or thrills. **PERCUSSION** LCBD → MSL at the 5th ICS = 10 cm **AUSCULTATION** Rate 78/regular. A_2 = P_2; S_2 split on inspiration—no murmurs, gallops, or rubs; carotids equal bilaterally; JVP not elevated.	**INSPECTION AND PALPATION** Apical impulse at left 7th ICS 3½ cm lateral to MCL—no pulsations or thrills, cardiac lift present. **PERCUSSION** LCBD → MCL at the 5th ICS = 15 cm **AUSCULTATION** Rate 96/regular; S_1 accentuated at base of heart; S_3 present; high-pitched blowing diastolic murmur heard at L 3ICS near sternum $\bar{c}$ pt. in sitting position and leaning forward. ↑ intensity $\bar{c}$ forced expiration. Does not radiate to neck or axilla.

CHAPTER 15

Assessment of the Breast

LEARNING OBJECTIVES

1. Review the structure and function of the breast.
2. List the characteristics of the breast that are noted during inspection.
3. Describe palpation of the breast and pertinent lymph nodes.
4. State the characteristics that are to be documented when a mass is detected in the breast.
5. Recognize how carcinoma of the breast is diagnosed.
6. Identify the common site of carcinoma of the breast in both men and women.

There is a high incidence of disease in the breast; it is therefore a very important routine part of the assessment of health status. The breast is the second most common site of carcinoma in women (the first is the lung). Men can also develop breast carcinoma, although the incidence is low (1–5% of cases). As a nurse you play a vital role in screening for early detection of breast carcinoma and in health teaching. Clients need to know the why, when, and how of self-breast examination and the importance of following up on any abnormalities. In this chapter you will become more familiar with the structure and function of the breast and the lymph nodes that drain the breast areas. The techniques of breast and lymph node assessment and the pertinent characteristics to be noted are discussed.

Structure and Function of the Breast

During the prenatal period, estrogen from the mother crosses the placenta. This estrogen may produce hypertrophy of the breasts of the newborn, a not uncommon condition. The hypertrophy may be either unilateral or bilateral and may be present for as long as 1 to 2 months. In addition, milky secretions may also be observed, but

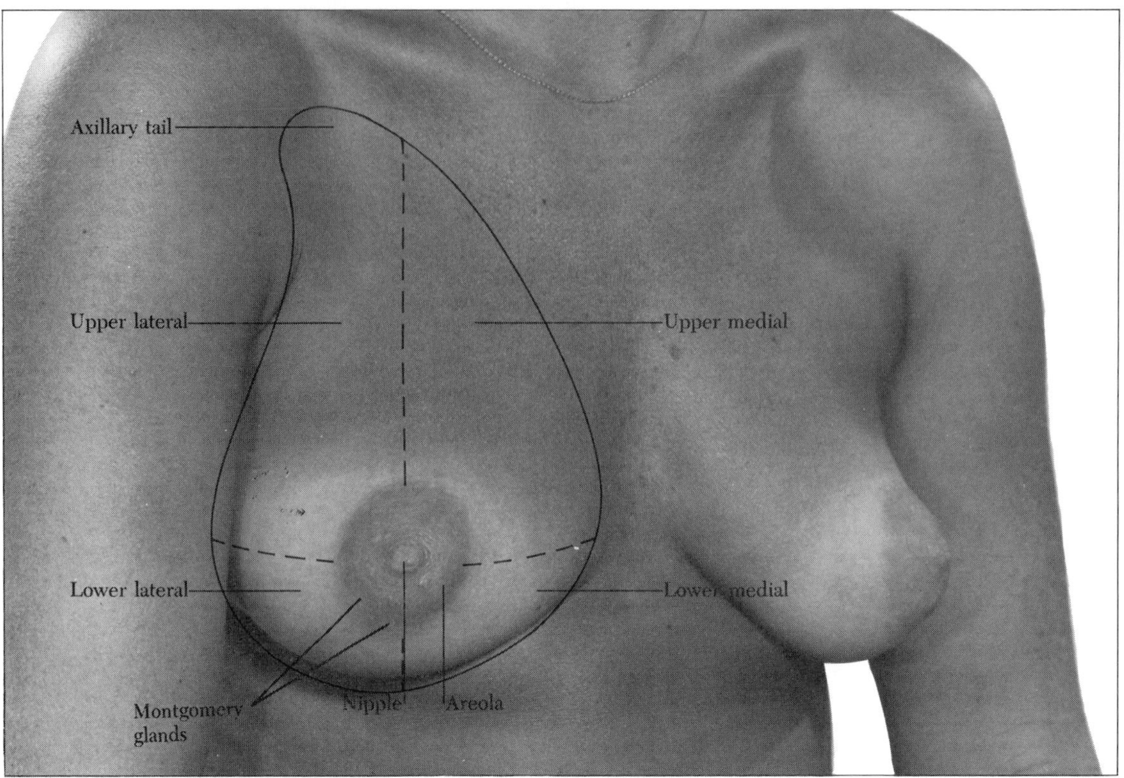

Figure 15-1 Anatomical divisions of the breast.

they are of no significance unless accompanied by signs of inflammation.

Female breast development normally begins about 8–14 years of age; it is quite often asymmetrical with one breast developing before the other. Tenderness of the breasts during early development is common. The male may have some tender breast hypertrophy in adolescence that may last for a couple of years, but there should be no signs of inflammation.

The breast tissue is a circular area with an extension projecting to the axilla; this extension is called an *axillary tail*. Figure 15-1 shows how the breast is anatomically divided into four quadrants (*upper* and *lower medial quadrants* and *upper* and *lower lateral quadrants*) and the axillary tail. The areolae of the female breasts contain Montgomery's glands (sebaceous glands). With lactation, they secrete a lipoid substance to protect the nipple during breast-feeding. Prominence of Montgomery's glands may occur from edema of the breast.

The breast is affected by many diseases, but probably the most dreaded is cancer. The breast is the second most common site of carcinoma in females, and breast cancer *does* occur in males. As a matter of fact, 2–5 out of 100 cases of breast cancer involve men. The most common site of breast cancer in the female is the upper lateral quadrant; in the male it is directly under the areola. Early detection is of prime importance to successful treatment. Most breast tumors are discovered accidentally by the client, frequently during bathing. Therefore, routine, systematic self-examination should prove all the more reliable for detection. There is a higher incidence of breast cancer among daughters and sisters of women who have had breast carcinoma, but *all* clients, regardless of family history, should be taught the self-breast-examination procedure, along with the rationale as to why regular self-examination is necessary. Provide the client with an explanatory pamphlet to reinforce your teaching of the procedure. Copies of this pamphlet are available for distribution to clients from your local branch of the American Cancer Society.

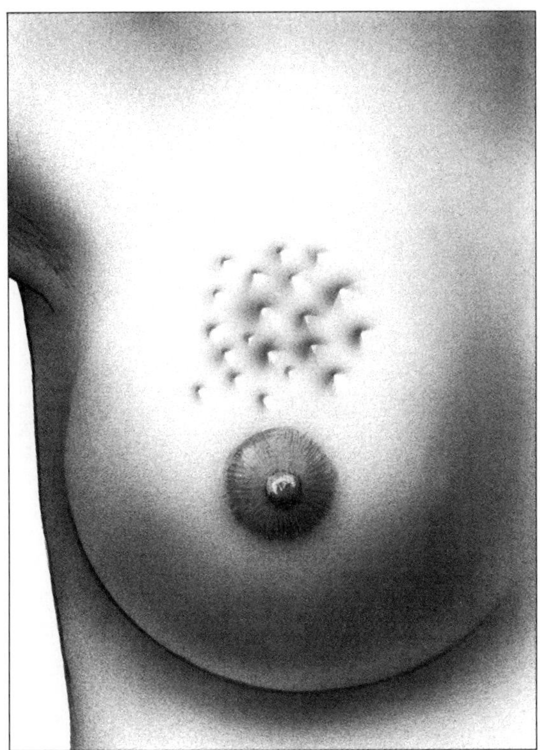

Figure 15-2 Peau d'orange. Note the rough, pitted appearance.

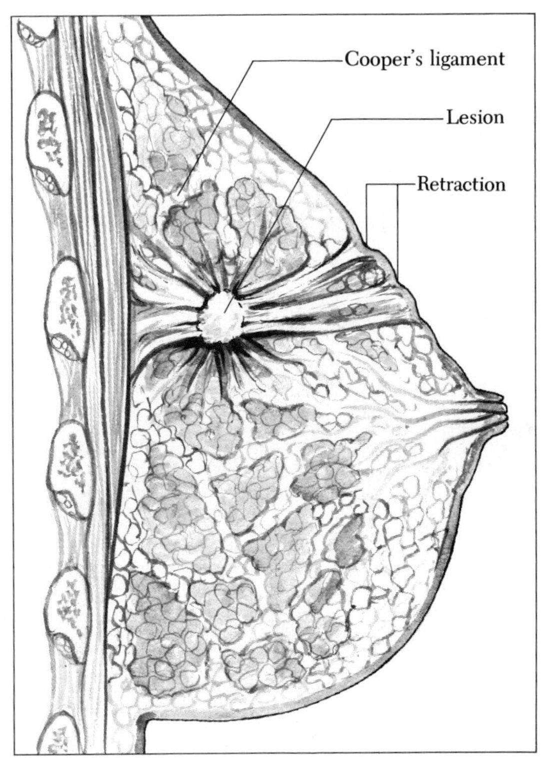

Figure 15-3 Cross-section showing breast retraction.

Characteristics and Techniques of Examination

In assessing the breasts, follow the same sequence of steps for both male and female clients. It is ideal to perform the breast examination in the menstruating female immediately following each menstrual period. This is because many women have some degree of edema and tenderness about mid-cycle or just prior to the onset of the menstrual period. The nonmenstruating (such as menopausal) female with breast development is instructed to establish a specific day each month to perform self-breast examination so that the procedure will not be overlooked. She should choose a day that will be easy for her to remember, such as the first or last day of each month.

Inspection

The assessment of the client's breasts should be performed with the client in both the sitting and supine positions. Examine the skin of the breasts for any lesions, increased vascular patterns, color changes, edema, or irregularities of the surface, such as dimpling, retraction, or the "pig skin" or "orange peel" (peau d'orange) appearance that results from the lymphatic edema of carcinoma of the breast (see Figure 15-2). Retraction can be the result of scarring following inflammation or trauma, but most often it is an indication of malignancy. Figure 15-3 shows how the presence of a lesion can cause abnormal traction of the suspensory ligaments (Cooper's ligaments), creating retraction.

Figure 15-4 shows how retraction can be accentuated by several activities that pull on the suspensory ligaments of the breasts. Instruct the client to perform these activities during breast examination. Inspect the breasts as the client forcibly presses her hands on her hips (A), as she raises her arms overhead (B), and while her hands are pushed together in front of her (C). Each woman should become familiar with the shape and feel of her own breasts. Inspect the axillary and clavicular areas for any erythema or

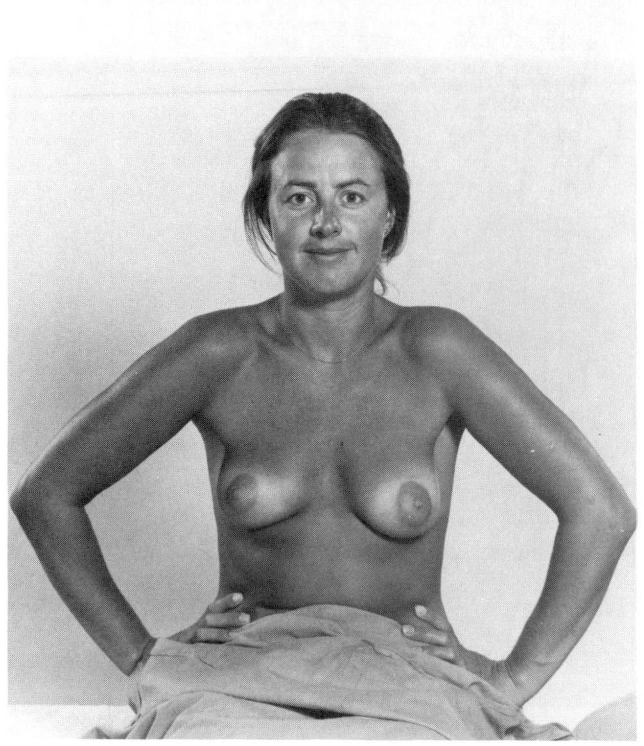

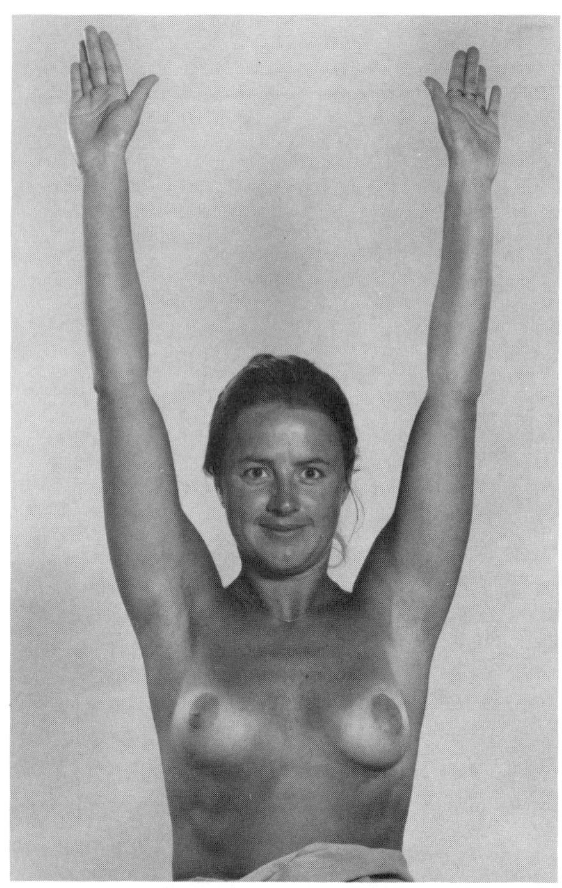

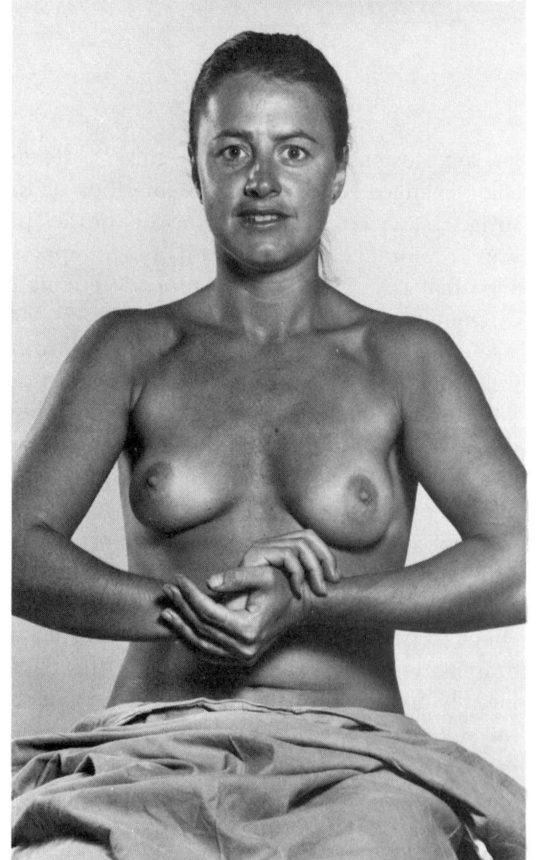

Figure 15-4 Method of breast inspection. (A) While client presents her hands on her hips. (B) With client's arms raised overhead. (C) With client's hands pushed together in front of her.

bulging, as they are the chief regions of lymphatic drainage for the breasts.

The areolae are a darker color in brunettes as opposed to the light pinkish hue in blondes. Clients who are pregnant and those taking oral contraceptives will have darker areolae. Deep brown areolae are characteristic of adrenogenital syndrome.

Both sexes may demonstrate polymastia (multiple breasts) or polythelia (multiple nipples). Multiple nipples are of no significance. They are similar in appearance to moles and are generally small; upon close inspection a minute nipple and areola can usually be seen. They are mostly present in the mammary line of the thorax and abdomen, analogous to the mammary line of animals having polymastia as a norm, such as cats and dogs. Infrequently in the human, polymastia

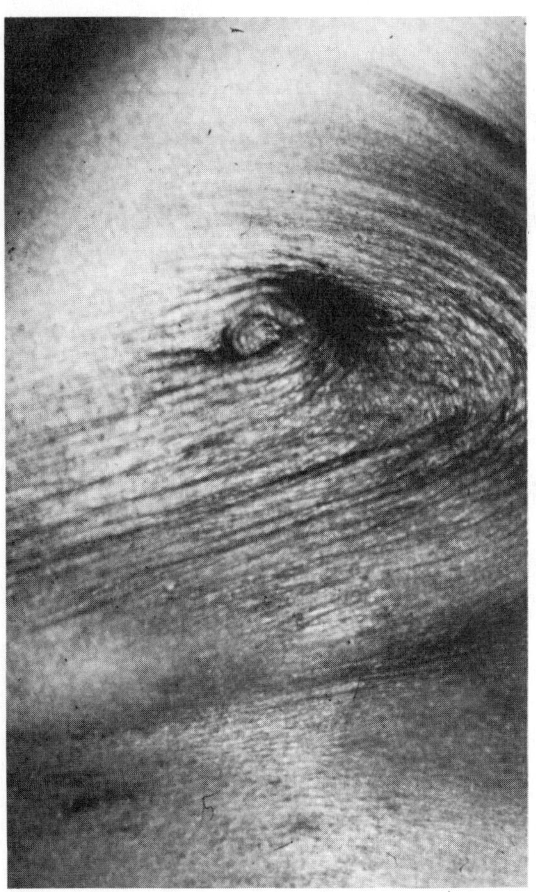

Figure 15-5 Inverted nipple of the right breast.

and polythelia have been known to occur in the axillae and on the shoulder, flank, groin, or thigh.

Clients should be made aware of the fact that there is a slight asymmetry of the breasts. This is most noticeable in the sitting position. Although the left breast is generally larger than the right, the nipples should be symmetrically placed within the breasts. Underlying skin retraction will oftentimes cause the nipple to turn toward the involved area, so that the nipple points to the lesion.

Note whether the nipples are inverted (see Figure 15-5) or erect. Inverted nipples may be congenital, but any recent inversion of a nipple is a significant finding and could be the result of inflammation or abscess, as well as of a malignancy. Inspect the nipples for any scaling, crusting, or fissures (cracks). Bilateral involvement is usually observed in dermatologic conditions. Paget's disease, a slow-developing intraductal carcinoma, is usually unilateral and begins as scaling and erythema, which eventually progresses into ulceration.

Have clients with pendulous and large breasts lean forward while you inspect the breasts.

Palpation

Gently compress the nipples or use a stripping action to check for discharge. Any discharge is significant and requires consultation and further investigation. Discharge may be present in either benign or malignant conditions. Cytology of the discharge and/or a breast tissue biopsy is indicated. With chronic cystic mastitis the secretions may range from a clear yellow to a green or blue color. Surprisingly, bloody discharge is observed in only about 1% of the cases of breast cancer. Although a sanguineous or dark brown drainage may occur in Paget's disease, it can also be present in acute mastitis, in benign intraductal papilloma, or with a breast abscess.

If the client complains of tenderness or a mass in one breast, you should palpate that breast last. Mastodynia, pain in the breasts, most generally

Technique for Inspection of the Breast

1. Provide adequate lighting, warm room, and privacy.
2. Client is exposed to the waist.
3. Client is sitting, preferably before a mirror.
4. Explain each step (health teaching).
5. Note characteristics: contour and size, skin, nipples, areolae, axillary and clavicular lymph node areas, abnormalities (lesions, color changes, increased vascular patterns, edema, dimpling, retraction).
6. Ask client to raise arms overhead: inspect.
7. Ask client to press hands on hips: inspect.
8. Ask client to push palms of hands together: inspect.
9. Ask client with large or pendulous breasts to stand and lean forward as you hold her hands in yours: inspect the suspending breasts.

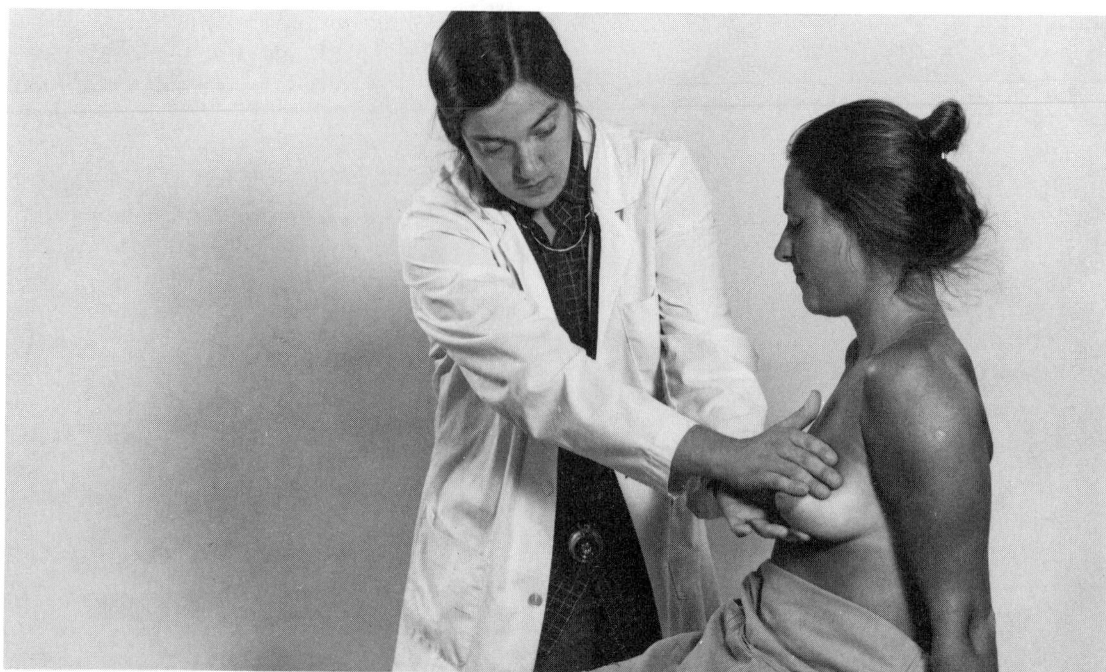

Figure 15-6 Bimanual palpation of the breast with client in sitting position.

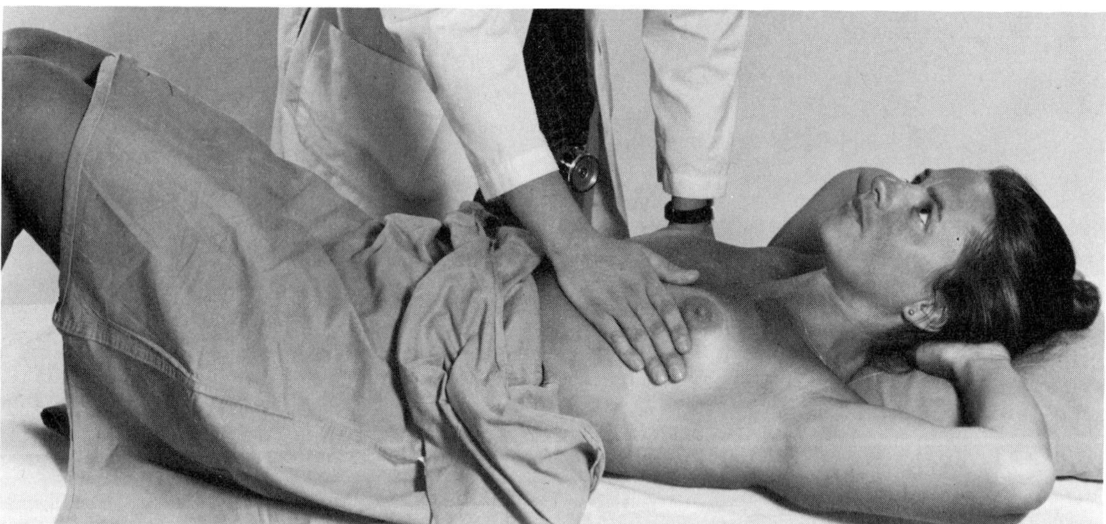

Figure 15-7 The supine position for breast palpation.

accompanies benign disease, but malignancy cannot be ruled out. As mentioned previously, the breasts may normally be tender or painful just prior to and during menstruation. Pain that occurs at a time that it never has before should be considered abnormal.

Upon palpation the younger client's breasts will be soft and of an even consistency, whereas the older female's breasts may be more coarse or nodular. In the menopausal female, atrophy of the breasts will be noted, with accompanying sagging of the nipples below the fourth intercostal space. In the climacteric male, the breast tissue may normally appear fuller and may sag.

Palpation of the female breasts should be performed both in the sitting position, as shown in Figure 15-6 and in the supine position, as shown in Figure 15-7. The supine position provides the most accurate information. In the sitting position palpation of the breasts, the axillary region, and

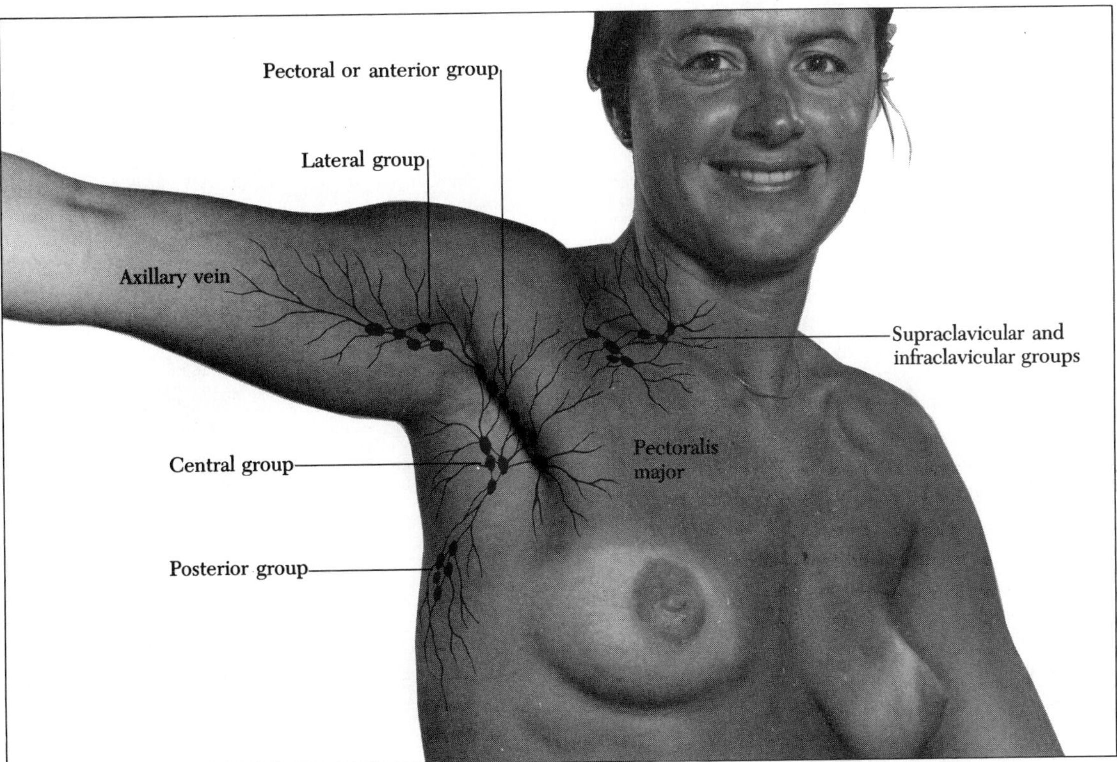

Figure 15-8 Location of the lymph nodes.

the clavicular region should be performed first with the client's arms down at the sides and then with her arms raised overhead. The axillary and clavicular regions contain the lymph nodes responsible for draining the breast area. It is important to palpate all of these lymph node groups. Figure 15-8 illustrates their anatomical location. A bimanual technique, particularly with large breasts, may prove beneficial in detecting small, deep-seated masses. In the supine position a small pillow or folded towel placed under the shoulder of the side being palpated helps in spreading the breast tissue more symmetrically over the chest wall. The arm on the side being palpated should be extended over the head. As with the sitting position, the axillary and clavicular nodes should also be examined, first with the arms raised and then with the arms at the client's sides.

Palpation should begin in the upper lateral quadrant. Using a gentle to and fro rotary motion with the palmar aspects of the fingers, move from the periphery to the areola. Figure 15-9 shows how palpation should move clockwise about the periphery of the breast, each time proceeding in to the areola. A tracing of the sequence would look like a wheel with spokes.

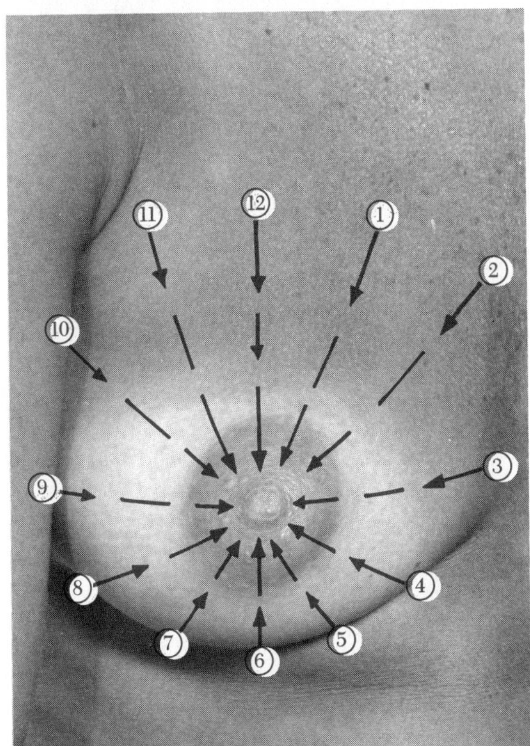

Figure 15-9 Sequence of palpation of the breast. Palpation begins on the upper lateral quadrant (arrow) and proceeds in a clockwise direction around the periphery of the breast and moves inward toward the areola. Locations of masses are documented in the o'clock axis (circles).

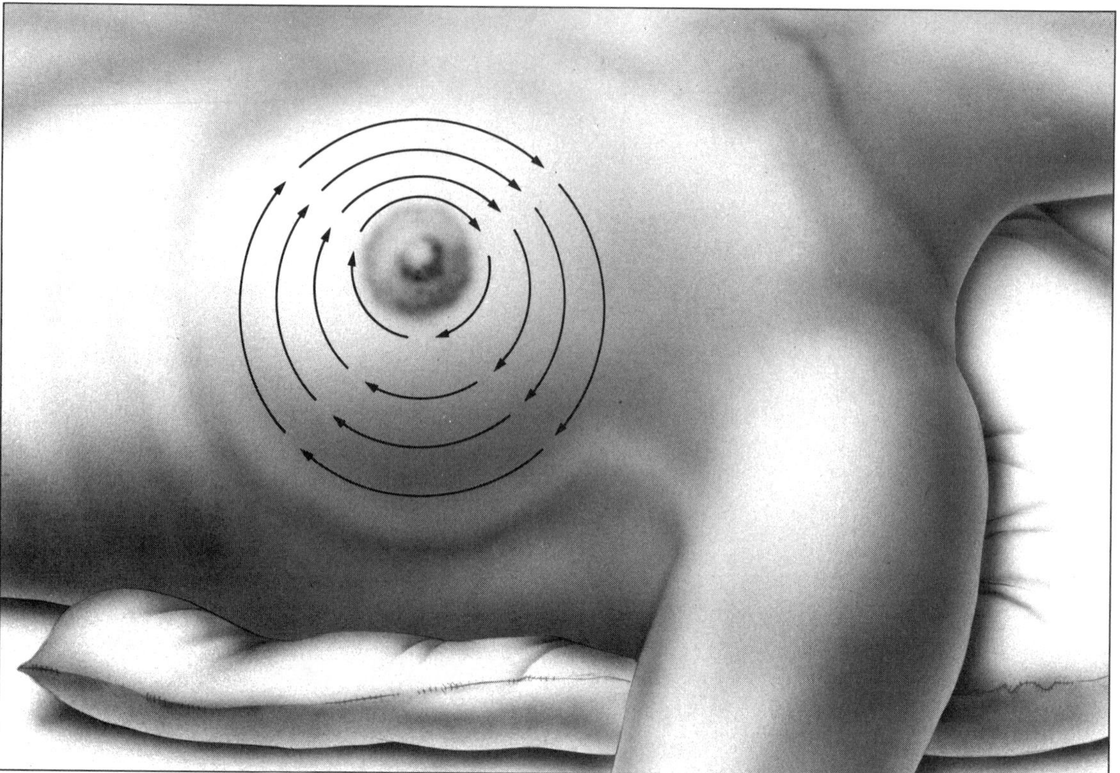

Figure 15-10 Spiral technique recommended for clients to use in palpating the breast. Performed in both sitting and supine positions.

After light palpation, examine the breast again with deep palpation. Start at the top of the upper lateral quadrant and feel in a clockwise motion full circle. Then move one inch toward nipple and repeat. Repeat at least twice more. Then palpate nipple area last. This is called the spiral technique and is recommended for clients to use by the American Cancer Society (see Figure 15–10). Careful palpation of the areolar area, the axillary region, and the clavicular region is especially important in the male, as there is early metastasis of breast carcinoma to the lymphatics because of the paucity of breast tissue.

Should a mass be detected, the following characteristics should be described in the consultation report:

1. *Location*—Cite distance from the nipple, in the schema of a clock, and indicate whether the client's arms were at the sides or extended overhead, as these positions may change the location. For example: "Located at 3:00 axis of left breast 1 cm from the areolar border with arms extended overhead." (See Figure 15-11.)

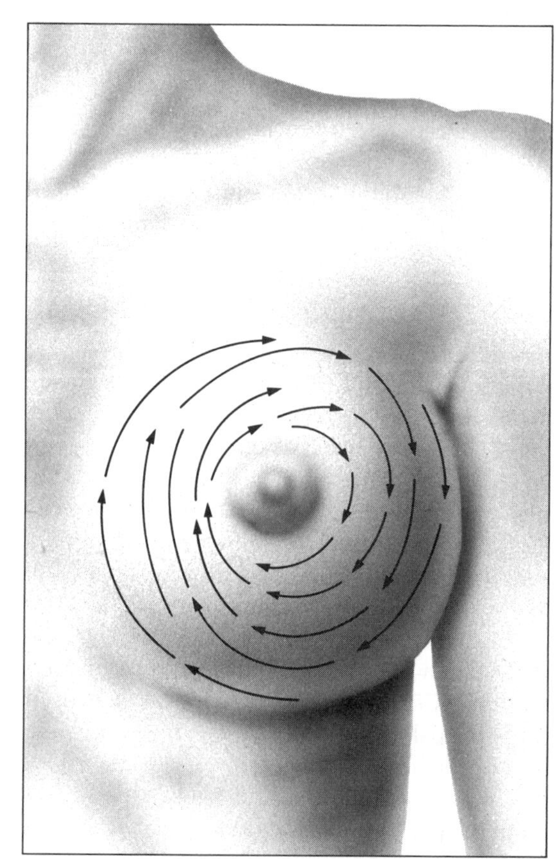

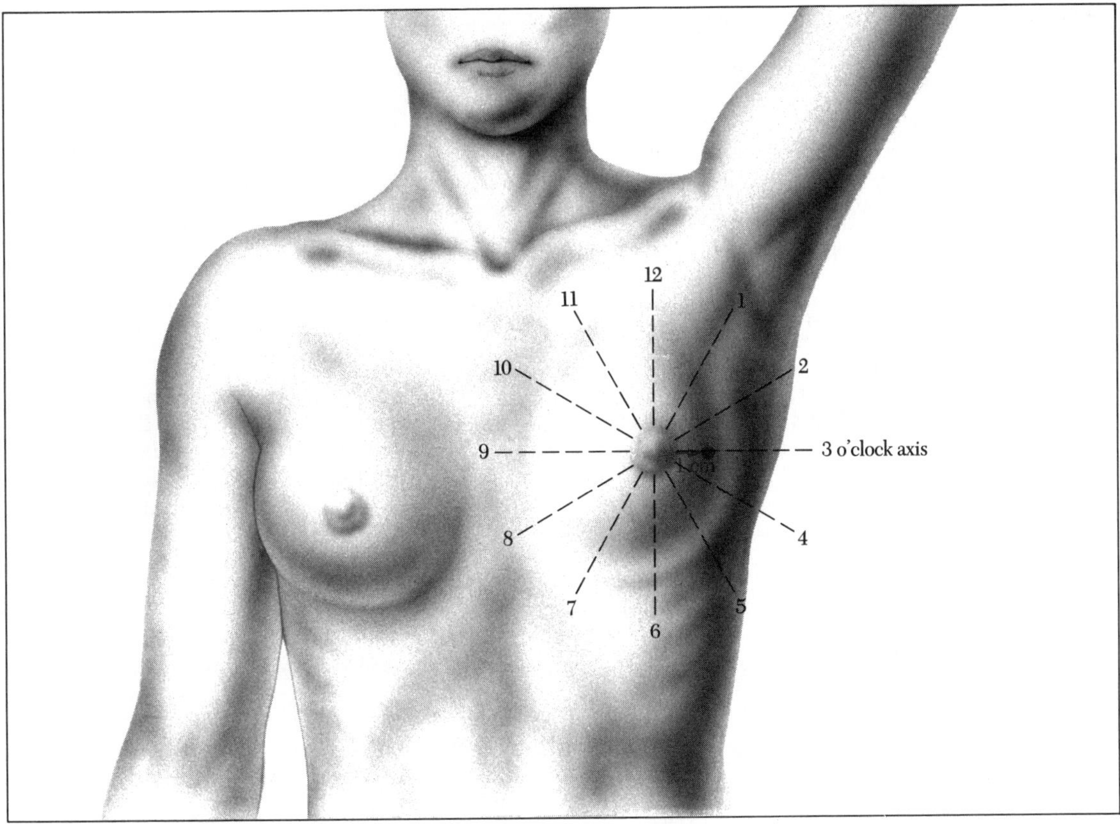

Figure 15-11 Clock axes of left breast and location of mass at the 3 o'clock axis of the left breast, 1 cm from the areolar border with arm extended overhead.

Technique for Palpation of the Breast

1. Client in sitting position.
2. Use palmar aspects of your fingers to knead breast tissue.
3. Palpate axillary and clavicular lymph nodes with a cupped hand, first with client's arm raised and supported at the wrist with your hand and then with client's arm at the side.
4. Begin palpation of breast with the axillary tail and upper lateral quadrant.
5. Lightly palpate from periphery to nipple, like spokes of a wheel.
6. Repeat palpation of breast using deep palpation performed in a spiral technique. Palpate the nipples last.
7. Compress nipple between thumb and forefinger. Note any discharge.
8. Perform bimanual palpation of each breast particularly when client's breasts are large.
9. Place client in lying position.
10. Place small pillow or folded towel under shoulder of side to be inspected and palpated.
11. Ask client to extend arm overhead on side being examined.
12. Repeat inspection of each breast.
13. Repeat above palpation steps (2–7) for each breast.
14. Transfer small pillow or towel to the opposite side when inspecting and palpating the remaining breast.

Table 15-1. General Characteristics of Benign and Malignant Lesions*

Characteristics	Benign	Malignant
Surface	Smooth and regular	Uneven
Discreteness	Well-defined margins	Discrete in early stage, irregular borders
Consistency	Soft	Generally firm to hard
Mobility	Easily movable	Fixed as progresses to invasion of underlying tissues
Tenderness	Usually tender	Generally nontender
Transillumination	May or may not, if cyst, usually will	No
Retraction	Rarely	Often present
Incidence	Young women, men over 50 yrs old	1 out of 10–15 women; most common in middle aged and elderly; 1–5% of cases of breast carcinoma in men
Lymph node involvement	Rarely	Most common site (females): upper outer quadrant; variable involvement Most common site (males): under areola with early metastasis to axillary lymph

*Note well that these are general characteristics and are *not* diagnostic of either benign or malignant lesions. Carcinoma of the breast is diagnosed only by biopsy.

2. *Size*—State three dimensions, if possible (length, width, and thickness). If unable to determine discrete margins, record this also.
3. *Surface*—Indicate whether smooth and regular or irregular contour.
4. *Discreteness*—Note whether margins are difficult to determine or if easily detected (a discrete mass).
5. *Consistency*—Indicate whether soft, firm, or stony hard.
6. *Mobility*—Note whether mass is movable or firmly or moderately fixed.
7. *Tenderness*—Note whether mass is painful or nontender.
8. *Transillumination*—Note whether transillumination is present. Most often a fluid-filled cyst will transilluminate.

The *only means* to *diagnose* breast carcinoma is by a *biopsy*. There are general characteristics that are ascribed to benign and malignant lesions, but these are *not* diagnostic in themselves. The key word to be remembered is "usually." *Usually* the signs delineated in Table 15-1 are found with the occurrence of benign and malignant lesions.

Common abnormalities occurring in the breasts of women and men are listed in Table 15-2. Of particular importance is Paget's disease of the breast, a malignancy, which begins as an innocent allergiclike scaling appearance but is deadly and warrants referral. This innocent beginning progresses into erythema and eventually a seeping ulceration of the breast tissue with resultant necrotic tissue.

Summary

This chapter discussed assessment of the breast. The techniques used in examination of the breast are inspection and palpation. Breast examination in both males and females should be careful and systematic. Any masses should be palpated and described in detail. Characteristics of benign and malignant lesions and common abnormalities of the breasts were discussed.

Discussion Questions/Activities

1. Where is the most common site of breast carcinoma in the female? in the male?
2. When should breast examination be performed?
3. What factors are considered when inspecting the breasts? when palpating the breast?
4. Demonstrate the procedure for breast examination.
5. Draw a diagram illustrating the lymph drainage system for the thorax and breast.

Table 15-2. Common Abnormalities of the Breast

Terminology	Characteristics	Comment
Nipple discharge	Clear	May be caused by oral contraceptives, phenothiazines, digitalis, diuretics, steroids.
	Clear or bloody from single duct	Most likely single or multiple large-duct papillomas or duct ectasia.
	Clear or gray from multiple ducts	Most likely duct ectasia.
Nipple excoriation	Scaly crusting about the nipple, usually bilateral	Has client used creams or other medications? History of eczema or allergic dermatitis? Scrape tissue for evaluation; biopsy may be warranted.
Paget's disease of the breast	Scaling nipple to erythema to ulceration	Usually unilateral—malignancy requires referral.
Cyst	Palpable mass, usually discrete, usually transilluminates	May be aspirated in physician's office. Light green or pale amber fluid usually discarded. Otherwise sent for pathologic examination. Aspirate is smeared on 2 or 3 slides and fixed as for Pap smears.
Inflammation	Irregular contour, fixed mass of firm consistency, moderate to marked tenderness	Antibiotic therapy required.
Juvenile mastitis	Red, firm tender mass beneath nipple; usually unilateral involvement	Occurs in both sexes 20–30 yrs old. Runs course of a few weeks.
Chronic cystic mastitis	Bilateral diffuse, multiple nodules; usually tender thick tissue clear to yellow, green or blue nipple discharge	Referral warranted to rule out breast carcinoma.
Acute mastitis	Usually single quadrant involved; red, hot, tender, edematous; seldom axillary lymphadenopathy	Occurs particularly during lactation; in males usually from trauma. Usual cause is pyogenic infection.
Inflammatory breast carcinoma	Signs similar to acute mastitis except *entire* breast swollen; early lymph node involvement	Needs referral.
Gynecomastia	Smooth, firm, movable mass; unilateral or bilateral, often tender	Frequently occurs with normal puberty (usually unilateral). Encountered in leukemia, lymphoma, pulmonary carcinoma, chorioepithelioma of testes, cirrhosis, Cushing's, thyrotoxicosis. Medications: digitalis, spironolactone, estrogens, phenothiazines.

6. List some abnormalities that may be found on breast examination and some variances within the normal range.
7. What characteristics would you record if you discovered a breast mass in a client? What would your plan of action be for that client?
8. Describe the characteristics usually ascribed to benign and to malignant lesions.
9. Identify the characteristics of some common abnormalities of the breasts listed in the text.

Recording of Findings

Normal findings for breast assessment are presented in the first box. The second box contains a recording of a female client referred by a nurse to a consulting physician.

Female Breast

INSPECTION
Symmetrical; everted nipples; regular, smooth contour; no lesions; no dimpling; no retraction.

PALPATION
Normal consistency for age and parity; no discharge; no masses; no lymphadenopathy.

Male Breast

INSPECTION
No breast tissue; everted nipples; no dimpling; no lesions; no retraction. (Climacteric male: sagging breast tissue—normal for age.)

PALPATION
No discharge; no masses; no lymph node enlargement—axillary, supraclavicular, infraclavicular.

Female Breast

INSPECTION
Symmetrical; everted nipples; regular, smooth contour; no lesions; no dimpling; no retraction.

PALPATION
Normal consistency; no discharge; no lymphadenopathy. Soft, nontender, mobile mass with discrete smooth margins, approx. 1 × 2 × ½ cm in size; 3 cm away from areolar border at 4:00, axis with arms at sides; transilluminates.

CHAPTER 16

Assessment of the Abdomen

LEARNING OBJECTIVES

1. Recognize the four quadrant and nine divisional areas of the abdomen and the abdominal contents of each.
2. State the characteristics of the abdomen that are noted in inspection.
3. Explain the rationale for change in the systematic approach to examination of the abdomen—that is, inspection, auscultation, percussion, and palpation.
4. State the criterion for determining absence of bowel sounds.
5. Identify the norms of size of the abdominal viscera.
6. Recognize the significance of costovertebral (CVA) tenderness.
7. Describe the techniques for detection of hernias.
8. Identify the location of the inguinal and femoral lymph nodes.

The abdomen contains a number of organs and structures that should be assessed during the course of an examination. These structures include the liver, stomach, spleen, kidneys, gallbladder, pancreas, intestines, and sigmoid colon. In this chapter we will describe these basic structures and the methods used to examine them.

Structure of the Abdomen

To assist in identifying areas for examination, the abdomen can be divided into sections by imaginary lines. The most common format is to divide it into four segments (see Figure 16-1): a vertical line is drawn from the xiphoid process to the symphysis pubis; a horizontal line crosses the abdomen through the umbilicus.

In another division, shown in Figure 16-2, nine regions are identified. Vertical lines are drawn through the midpoint of the right and left inguinal ligaments (Poupart's ligaments); the top horizontal line crosses the abdomen at the level of the ninth rib and the lower line at the level of the iliac crests.

In this text reference will be made to the format using the four segments. Figure 16-3 illustrates the placement of the organs of the body

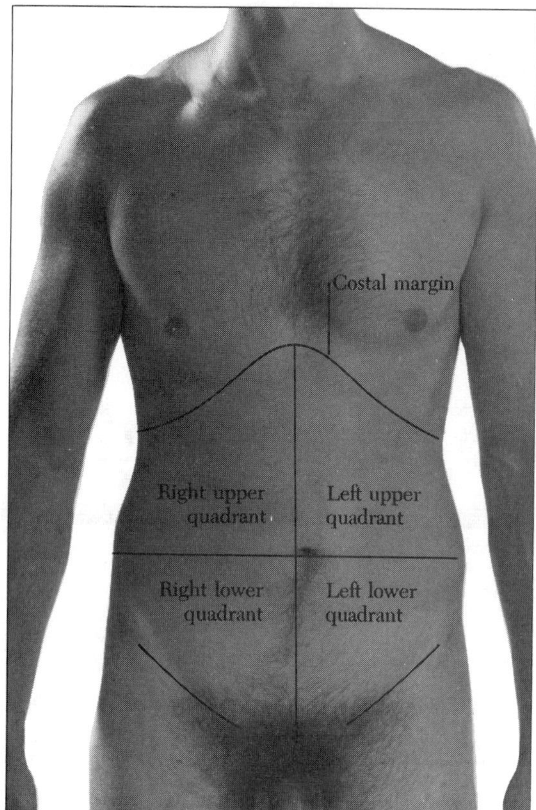

Figure 16-1 Four divisions of the abdomen.

within each of the four quadrants. A complete list of these organs is provided in Table 16-1.

Table 16-1. Abdominal Contents Within the Four Quadrants of the Abdomen

Quadrant	Contents
Right upper	Liver Gallbladder Duodenum Pancreas Right kidney and right adrenal gland Hepatic flexure of the colon
Left upper	Stomach Spleen Left kidney and left adrenal gland Pancreas Splenic flexure of the colon
Right lower	Cecum Appendix Right ovary and tube (female) Bladder (if distended) Uterus (female—if enlarged) Right spermatic cord (male) Right ureter
Left lower	Sigmoid colon Left ovary and tube (female) Bladder (if distended) Uterus (female—if enlarged) Left spermatic cord (male) Left ureter
Midline of lower abdomen	Bladder Uterus (female)

Characteristics and Techniques of Examination

In preparing the client for examination of the abdomen it is important to remember that this is a very sensitive area. Even clients without pain become tense and anxious when their abdomen is examined. Because the abdomen should be relaxed during the examination, it may be necessary to spend a few minutes reassuring the client. Explain that you will be gentle and unhurried and that you will not perform any painful procedures.

Place the client in the supine position with a small pillow to elevate his head; his arms should be relaxed at the sides or folded across his chest. Relaxation can often be encouraged by having the client take some deep breaths and let them out slowly; it is also helpful to have the client's knees slightly flexed, with a small pillow underneath the popliteal area for support.

All clothing should be removed and suitable draping applied so that the area from the sternum to the pubis is exposed. You can best examine the abdomen from the client's right side.

The usual sequence of inspection, palpation, percussion, and auscultation is modified in the examination of the abdomen. Auscultation comes immediately after inspection because auscultatory findings may be markedly different following percussion and palpation.

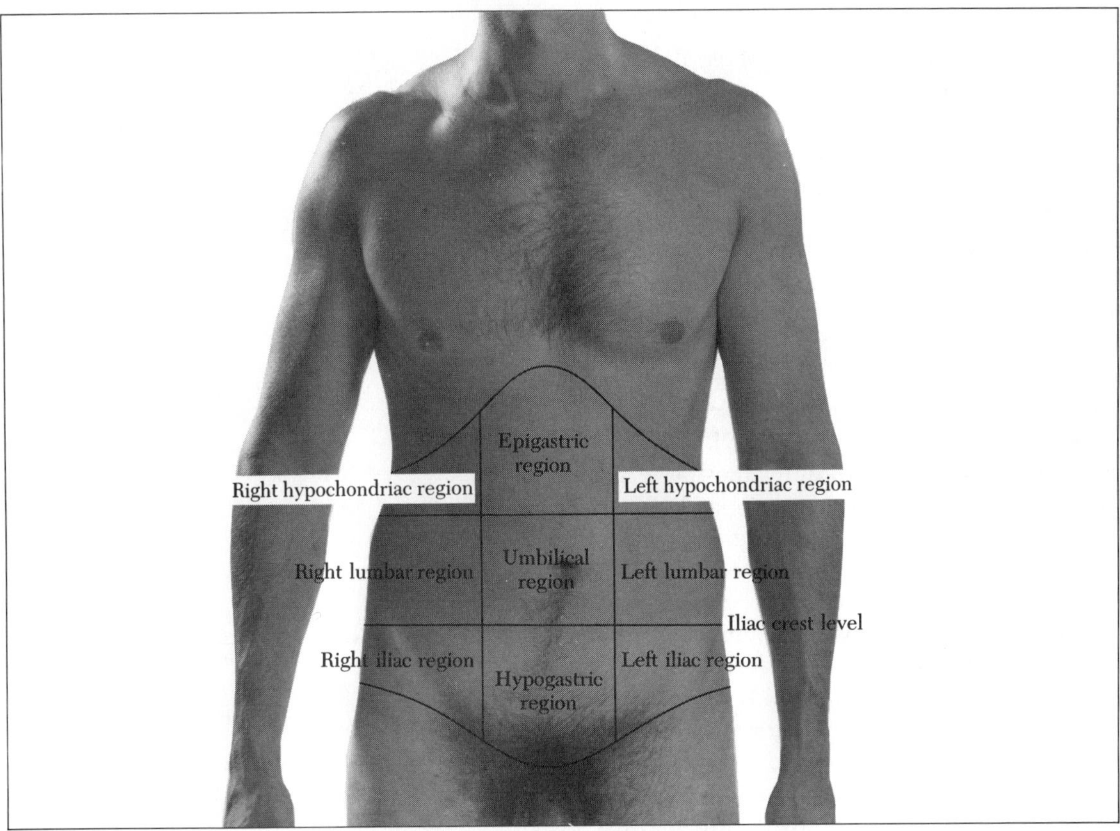

Figure 16-2 Nine divisions of the abdomen.

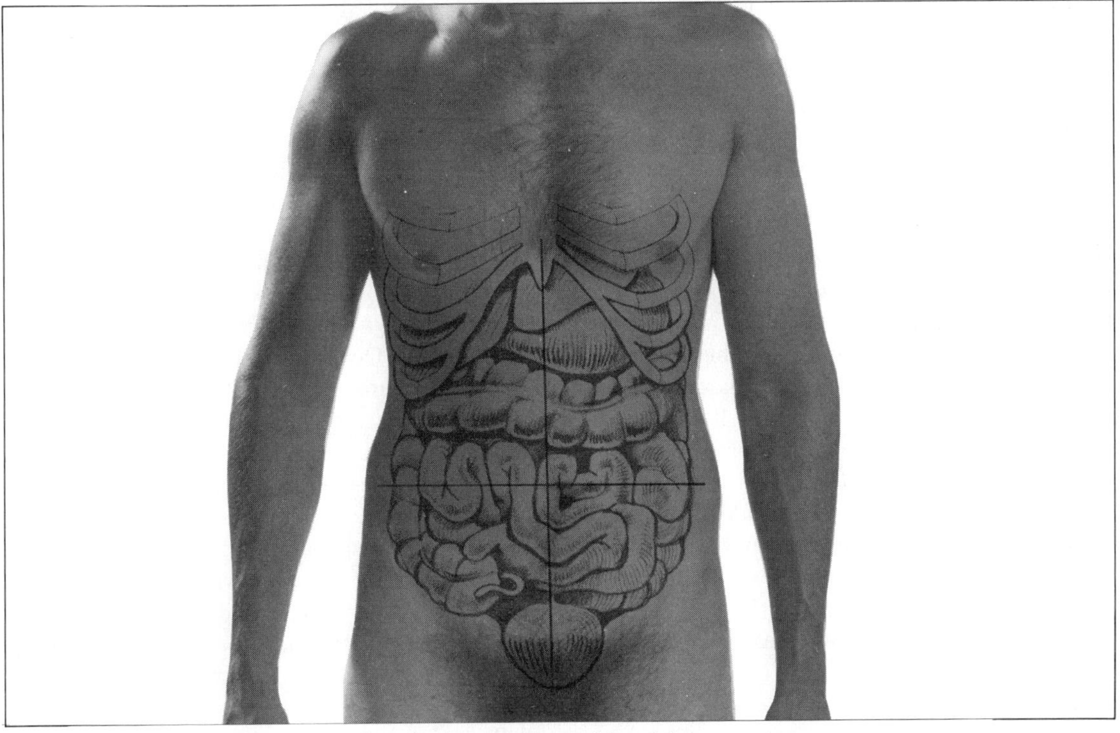

Figure 16-3 Placement of organs within the four divisions of the abdomen.

Inspection

Inspect the condition of the skin of the abdomen first. Note color, lesions, and visible veins and peristalsis as well as distended veins.

Striae are often seen on the lower abdomen following pregnancy or rapid weight gain. Recent striae are pink or blue; older striae are silvery streaks. Clients with Cushing's disease have characteristic pigmented striae on the abdominal wall. A hyperpigmented line extending from the umbilicus to the symphysis (linea nigra) denotes previous pregnancy. Lesions of tinea corporis and scabies are often found on the abdomen.

Scars or burns are easily observed. The color of scars indicates how recently they have occurred. They are pink for approximately 6 to 8 months and then turn white. Overgrowth of scar tissue (keloid) may be seen. Dotted scars over the abdomen and the thighs may reflect insulin injection sites in clients with diabetes mellitus.

Many gastrointestinal disorders are manifested by changes in the skin. Multiple small nodules may be the first indicator of carcinoma. Cutaneous angiomas (spider nevi) can be seen on the upper abdomen and chest of clients with cirrhosis; clients with ulcerative colitis may exhibit erythema nodosum (tender nodules in or under the skin). Localized ecchymosis in the flank may reflect abdominal or retroperitoneal hemorrhage.

To check for symmetry of the abdomen look not only from the side but from the foot of the examining table. The abdomen is normally symmetrical. The contour of the abdomen can be described as flat, round, or scaphoid as illustrated in Figure 16-4. The flat abdomen is usually seen in young, well-developed, or athletic individuals. The rounded abdomen is characteristic of varying degrees of obesity, but it also is characteristic of young children. The abdomen of children under age 4 is always large, but an increase may be due to tumor, ascites, or congenital defect. Babies who cry a lot often swallow air, which causes distention. The scaphoid abdomen is seen in very thin individuals of any age. In a child a scaphoid abdomen is not normal and is usually the result of severe malnutrition and dehydration.

Asymmetry of the abdomen can result from a variety of causes. It may be due to hernia, bowel obstruction, tumor, or spinal curvature. In the upper abdomen changes may represent involvement of such structures as the liver, pancreas, spleen, stomach, or transverse colon. Asymmetry of the lower abdomen may result from bladder distention, pregnancy, or masses in the ovaries, uterus, or colon.

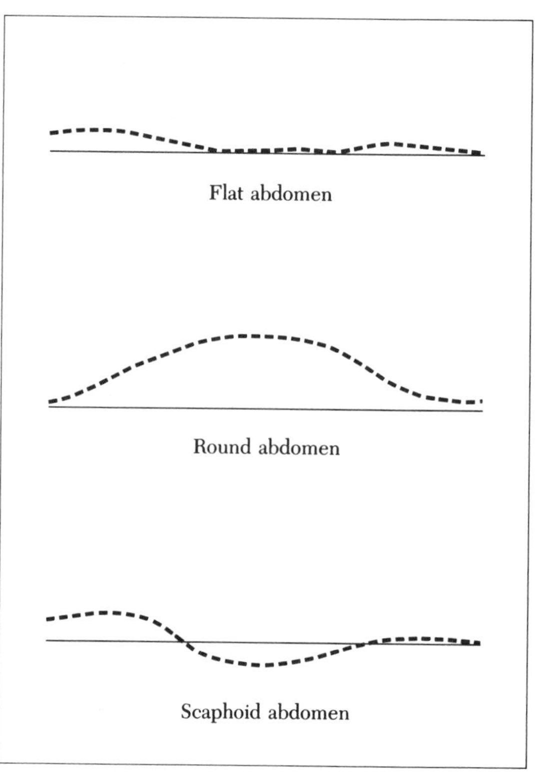

Contours of the abdomen.

Generalized symmetrical fullness can be caused by ascites, obesity, or gas distention. The characteristic picture of ascites is of a tense, distended abdomen with tightly stretched skin and bulging flanks. If the ascites is extreme, the umbilicus becomes everted. When the abdomen has the shape of a dome with the intestinal loops displayed as visible ridges, it is usually due to intestinal obstruction or distention. A mass in the epigastrium with left-to-right visible peristalsis may indicate pyloric obstruction (stenosis) and may be accompanied by projectile vomiting. To best visualize peristalsis, direct a light over the abdomen, with your eyes at the level of the abdomen for inspection. Dancing shadows will be observed when excessive peristalsis exists. Visible peristalsis is considered an abnormal sign, and obstruction must be ruled out. A tumor of the liver may be seen as a mass in the right upper quadrant that moves with respirations.

The umbilicus of the newborn should be inspected for proper healing. Normally, the cord

BIOLOGICAL AND CULTURAL VARIATIONS

Lactose Intolerance Among Orientals, Native Americans, and Black Americans

Lactose, or milk sugar, is a simple carbohydrate that is present in milk and that provides a major energy source for infants and young children. However, during childhood and adolescence in many population groups, levels of lactase, the enzyme that breaks down lactose, decrease markedly and individuals lose the ability to break down lactose after consuming a large quantity of milk. The resulting syndrome is called lactose intolerance. Symptoms are similar to those of fermentive diarrhea and include cramps, gas, belching, and a watery explosive diarrhea (McElroy & Townsend 1979). Lactose intolerance is common among Orientals (about 95% are intolerant), Black Americans (about 75%), and Native Americans (about 60%). It is present in some White American groups, with levels as high as 24% in Mediterranean peoples and Middle Easterners.

Various anthropologists and nutritionists have noted an interesting correspondence between the incidence of lactose intolerance and the history of dairying and milk consumption in population groups. Groups such as Orientals and Black Americans, who did not practice dairying, have a high incidence of lactose intolerance. An interesting exception among African peoples are the Bahima of Uganda, a traditional herding people who are remarkably lactose tolerant. On the other hand, White Americans, who are the descendants of northern and western Europeans who practiced dairying, have a markedly low incidence of lactose intolerance.

One explanation for the correspondence between milk consumption and lactose tolerance is that individuals who continue to consume lactose throughout life maintain lactase production and therefore continue to efficiently digest milk. However, experiments in which people's milk consumption was raised or lowered showed that experience had little effect on lactose metabolism. More recent explanations for this phenomenon are genetic. Researchers suggest that dairying populations maintained higher frequencies of genes responsible for lactose metabolism. Such genes in these populations would have allowed better nutritional status in individuals who possessed them; they may have suffered less from diseases such as rickets and osteomalacia and may have reproduced more than individuals not possessing such genes.

falls off after 7–14 days. Failure to heal creates the potential for the development of ventral and umbilical hernias or defects in the abdominal wall, such as extrophy of the bladder or diastasis recti. Umbilical hernias can be seen as protrusions in the umbilical area when the child cries. In the adult, rising to a sitting position without use of the arms will accentuate an umbilical hernia; coughing, too, will foster protrusion of a weak abdominal wall. Inguinal hernias are most often detected as a mass in the scrotum in males but sometimes can be observed as a mass in the groin.

Note the presence of distended or dilated abdominal veins, which may indicate obstruction of the portal circulation or of the inferior vena cava. Above the umbilicus blood flow in the veins is upward; below the umbilicus the flow is downward. Reversal of the blood flow is indicative of inferior vena cava obstruction or portal hypertension. To determine the direction of flow, compress the vein with the tips of both index fingers. Move the fingers apart to milk the vein. Then remove one finger at a time, observing the direction of flow. The vein will fill fastest in the direction of blood flow.

In premature babies and many infants, veins are easily seen and may normally be observed until puberty. They are especially noticeable in malnourished children. In adults, however, observable veins may accompany portal hypertension, ascites, and portal or hepatic obstruction.

A slight pulsation may be noted in the midepigastric area, particularly in very thin clients. This is the pulsation of the abdominal aorta. Vigorous pulsations may indicate the presence of

Technique for Inspection of the Abdomen

1. Adequate lighting, warm room, and adequate exposure.
2. Instruct client to inform you of any discomfort.
3. Position client in supine position with arms at side or folded across chest.
4. Have client flex knees and take some deep breaths and let them out slowly in order to relax abdominal muscles.
5. Characteristics: contour, symmetry, symmetrical fullness (distention), skin, visible veins, visible peristalsis, hernias (have client raise head and shoulders off bed without using arms, and cough or "bear down"), blood flow (compress vein with tips of index fingers; move fingers apart to milk the vein; remove one finger at a time and observe direction of flow).

masses lying over the aorta or conditions such as aortic regurgitation or right ventricular hypertrophy.

Note the distribution of hair. In the normal female pubic hair growth is triangular with the base at the symphysis pubis. In males it is diamond-shaped with hair often growing to the umbilicus.

Auscultation

Following inspection of the abdomen, perform auscultation of the area. The sounds you listen for in the abdomen are those of peristalsis and of vascular abnormalities. The bell of the stethoscope should be placed lightly on the abdomen in all four quadrants; in the epigastrium; above, below, and on both sides of the umbilicus; and over the liver. (Recall that the bell picks up low-pitched sounds.) Next repeat the sequence but use the diaphragm of the stethoscope firmly placed upon the abdomen.

Bowel Sounds The sounds of peristalsis vary in intensity, frequency, and pitch. They may be rumbling, like the sounds of a bowling alley, or bubbly and gurgling. The intensity and frequency often depend on the phase of digestion that is occurring at the time. For example, when the client is hungry and has not had a meal in some time, the sounds are quite loud. About 5–6 hours after a meal they may be persistent and continuous over the area of the ileocecal valve. Sounds can be heard better in thin clients. To differentiate normal from abnormal sounds, you must listen to many normal abdomens in order to establish a baseline.

Significant bowel-sound abnormalities are the absence of sound, weak and infrequent sounds, and a rushing high-pitched sound. Listen for these conditions in all areas of the abdomen. *Bowel sounds must be unheard for one full minute in each of the abdominal quadrants before recording that bowel sounds are indeed absent.*

Lack of sounds occurs in such serious conditions as paralytic ileus, late obstruction, and peritonitis. Weak and infrequent sounds often indicate that the bowel is becoming increasingly immobile as a result of these conditions. High-pitched tinkling sounds are indicative of bowel obstruction. When obstructed, the bowel fills with air and the peristalsis occurring in the tensely distended bowel produces the high-pitched tinkling sound. In developing obstruction the peristalsis above the point of pathology becomes increased. Other conditions in which the bowel is hyperactive are gastroenteritis, severe diarrhea, and intestinal hemorrhage. Borborygmi sounds are present in these conditions. Pain usually accompanies peristalsis in both the hyperactive bowel and the tensely distended bowel of abdominal obstruction. It is therefore important to note whether the client presents any manifestations of pain.

Blood Flow Blood flow through dilated or constricted blood vessels results in a turbulence that can be detected by auscultation. Bruits may be heard over a diseased aorta and over renal, femoral, hepatic, and splenic arteries. Listen in the midepigastric area above the umbilicus for aortic bruits, which are often caused by aneurysms and aortic stenosis. Renal artery bruits can also be detected in this area but may be detected in the flank areas or posteriorly over the kidney areas and at the costovertebral angles. Femoral bruits should be listened for in the groin regions. Bruits originating from diseased hepatic or splenic arteries are best heard in the right and

Table 16-2. Common Auscultatory Abnormalities of the Abdomen

Terminology	Characteristics	Comments
Bruit	Soft high-pitched sound heard over a blood vessel; heard in same area even if client's position changes; may be continuous or heard only during systole	Caused by turbulent blood flow resulting from atherosclerotic plaques, aneurysms, or congenital bands (e.g., abdominal aorta aneurysm). Renal artery stenosis, iliac artery and femoral artery stenosis.
Venous hum	Continuous soft humming sound over liver or upper abdomen	Caused by increase in collateral circulation of portal and systemic venous system or dilated preumbilical circulation. Heard with liver disease with portal hypertension. Portal or splenic vein thrombosis.
Friction rub	Rough grating sound	Occurs with irritation of the peritoneal surface of an organ. Splenic infarction. Primary or metastatic tumor of liver. Peritonitis.

Technique for Auscultation of the Abdomen

1. Client in supine position.
2. Quiet, warm room.
3. Warm stethoscope with hands.
4. Place bell of stethoscope lightly and listen to bowel sounds in all four abdominal quadrants.
5. Then repeat with diaphragm of stethoscope in all four quadrants.
6. Auscultate the blood flow using the bell at the following areas:
   Midepigastric area and over lower liver area
   Medial hypochrondriac areas
   Flank areas (posteriorly over the kidneys)
   Groins
7. Decision making: If bruit detected, move client into various positions. Sound must persist to be significant.
8. Auscultate over lower area of liver and over splenic area for detection of friction rubs.

left hypochondrium (the abdominal area that lies beneath the ribs on either side of the epigastrium). Sometimes bruits may be transmitted heart murmurs. To differentiate them, palpate the carotid artery while auscultating the abdomen. If the sound is a transmitted murmur, it will occur simultaneously with the beat of the carotid pulse. Localized bruits will occur slightly later than the carotid pulse. To be considered significant an abdominal bruit must be heard as the client is moved into various positions.

A venous sound representing portal obstruction may be heard with liver or splenic disease. This sound is softer than a bruit; it occurs continuously and has a humming quality. Such a venous hum is best heard in the upper epigastric area and over the liver.

Friction Rubs Peritoneal friction rubs are produced in the abdomen, particularly over the liver and spleen. They usually occur when there is an abscess or tumor of these organs. The friction rub is usually accentuated with deep respirations (see Table 16-2).

Percussion

Light percussion of the abdomen is performed to determine enlargement of an organ, the presence of masses, or abdominal distention. A dull percussion note will be heard over the area of a dense abdominal organ, such as the liver or spleen, and over a solid tumor or fluid. With gaseous distention tympany will be elicited throughout the abdominal area. Tympany is the normal percussion note present throughout the abdomen except for areas over the liver, spleen, and pubic symphysis bone (see Figure 16-5).

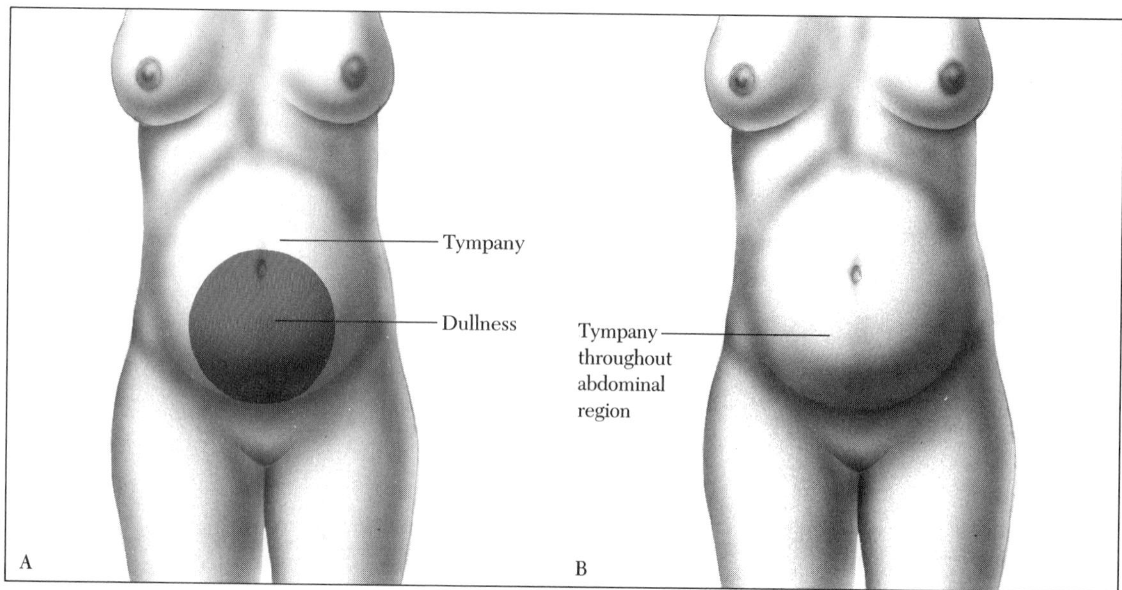

Figure 16-5 (A) Percussion dullness over pelvic tumor. (B) Generalized tympany due to gaseous distention of abdomen.

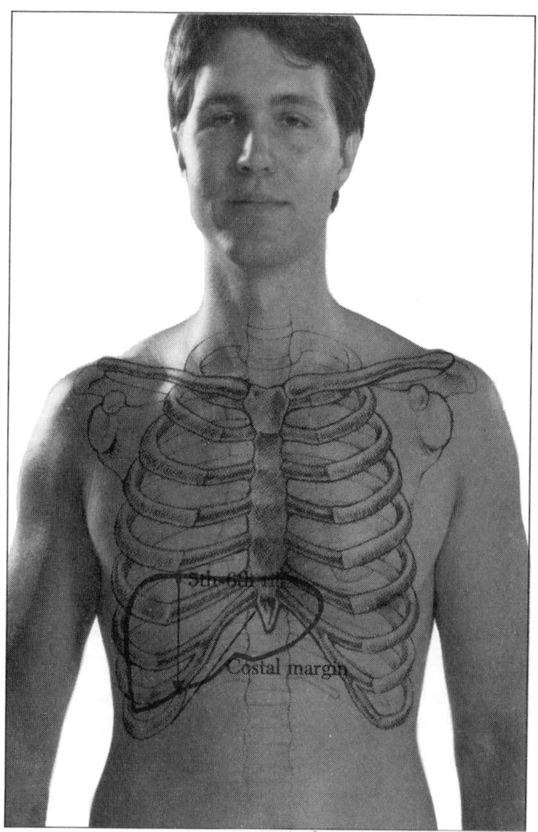

Figure 16-6 In measuring vertical span of liver dullness, measure slightly medial to the right MCL.

Liver Begin percussion down the right midclavicular line. Resonance over the lung will be detected until about the fifth to seventh intercostal space, where liver dullness begins. Continue percussion downward until the lower edge of liver dullness is heard. The normal lower level is at the costal margin. The vertical span of liver dullness represents the size of the liver; in the adult this is normally about 6–12 cm. Figure 16-6 illustrates how to measure the vertical span of liver dullness. In the child the liver and splenic percussion dullness will be well within the costal margin. Below the costal margin normal tympany should be heard. Since the liver moves downward on inspiration, ask the client to inhale, and percuss downward again. Upon inspiration, there should be an increase of about 2–4 cm from the previous lower edge of liver dullness. In clients with emphysema the lower level of liver dullness may be anywhere from 2 cm to 6 cm below the right costal margin. This is because continued lung inflation has displaced the liver. Barring liver problems, the span of liver dullness (liver size) should be within the normal range. In the alcoholic with cirrhosis, the liver can be enlarged, but in an advanced stage of cirrhosis the liver becomes necrotic and atrophied. In severe hepatitis the liver also decreases in size after initial hepatomegaly.

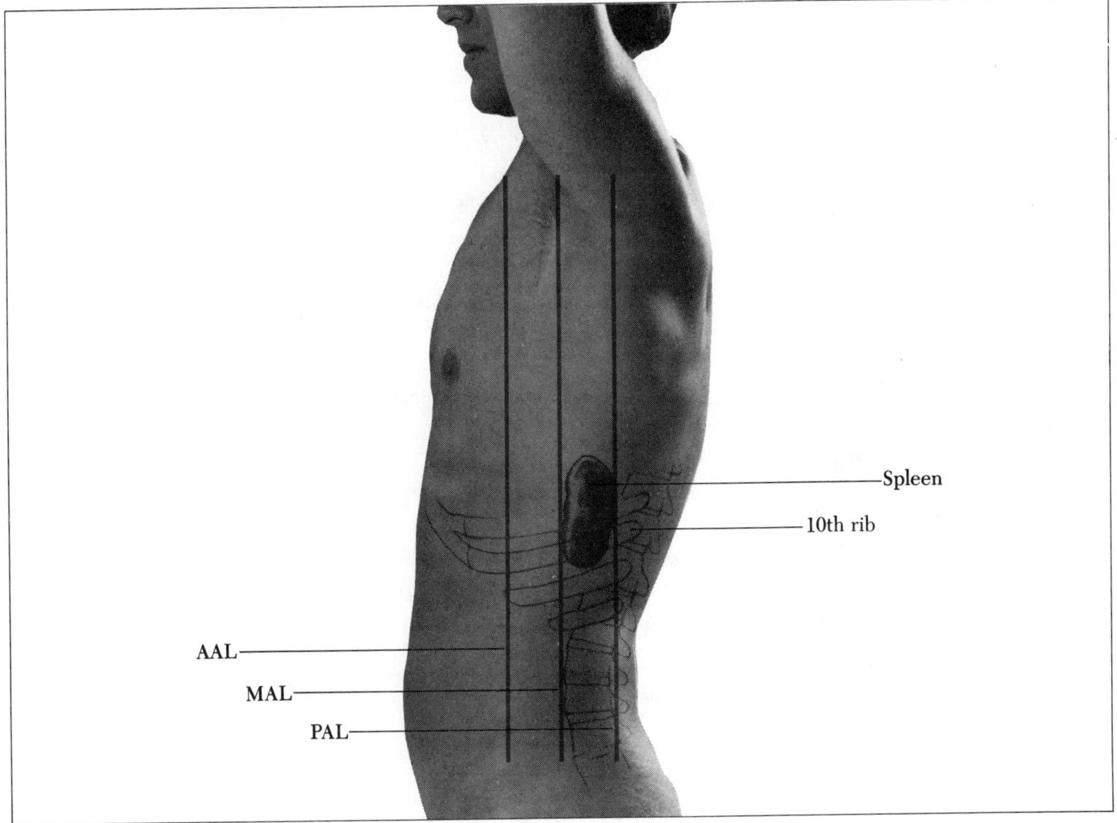

Figure 16-7 Location of the spleen.

Spleen The spleen lies slightly posterior to the left midaxillary line, between the eighth and eleventh intercostal spaces, as shown in Figure 16-7. Therefore, as you percuss downward in this area, you will hear lung resonance before reaching splenic dullness. Below the spleen the characteristic tympanic note of the abdomen will be elicited. The vertical span of splenic dullness is approximately 6–8 cm in the adult. Another procedure, which is particularly useful with children, is to percuss the lowest left intercostal space at the point between the left anterior axillary line and the midclavicular line. Percussion at this location is normally tympanic even when the client takes a deep breath. Modest splenic enlargement will produce a dull percussion note at this site upon deep inspiration. Therefore, the absence of tympany at this site is a significant finding. The tympany of the "gastric bubble" over the stomach is elicited at the sixth or seventh intercostal space at the left midclavicular line. Size of the gastric bubble is variable. Abdominal distention and increase in the size of the gastric bubble may be due to gastric dilatation.

Dullness in this area may also indicate enlargement of the left lobe of the liver. Dullness over other areas of the abdomen suggests the presence of tumor masses or fluid. In the pelvic area you may elicit the dull percussion notes of a distended urinary bladder.

Ascites Fluid in the peritoneal cavity (ascites) can be detected by two techniques: shifting dullness and fluid wave. Figure 16-8 illustrates the technique of shifting dullness. When the client is lying supine, fluid in the abdomen, influenced by gravity, moves to the dependent flank areas. With the client supine begin percussion at the umbilicus and proceed toward the nearest flank. From the area of the umbilicus tympany will be elicited until the area overlying the fluid is reached; at this point dullness will be heard. Mark the point where the dullness is first heard (A). Then have the client turn onto his side so

BIOLOGICAL AND CULTURAL VARIATIONS

Diabetes and Gallbladder Disease Among Native Americans

Epidemiologists and physicians have noted an alarming rise in the frequency of diabetes among various Indian tribes in the United States (West 1974). Whereas prior to 1940 diabetes seemed to be extremely rare or nonexistent among Native Americans in the Midwest, Southwest, and Alaska, in more recent years diabetes rates have equalled or surpassed those of White Americans. For example, in 1954 there were 94 known cases of diabetes among a Pima Indian population of about 6,000. By 1961, the number of diabetics had risen to 283 out of a population of approximately 7,000.

Between 1963 and 1967, the records of forty-six Public Health Service hospitals serving Indian communities and reservations showed the percentage of admissions due to diabetes to be 2.2%. The comparable figure for non-Indian hospitals throughout the United States was between 1.0% and 1.5% (Niswander 1968). The 2.2% admission rate was of course an average of a range of values for different tribes. In some Native American groups the occurrence of diabetes is extremely high. Among the Cherokee Indians of North Carolina, for example, the admission rate for diabetes was 10%. It is estimated that the prevalence rate for diabetes among Cherokee Indians over age 30 in 1964 exceeded 25%, which is the highest rate for any population group reported up to that time.

The reason for this epidemic of diabetes is not clear. As is the case in many chronic diseases, the etiology is probably a combination of genetic and environmental factors. There is probably an underlying genetic propensity for the disease among Native Americans that has been triggered by changing dietary practices and increasing rates of obesity. Neel has proposed the "thrifty gene" hypothesis, which points to the aboriginal lifestyle of the Native Americans. He hypothesizes that during the many centuries in which Indian groups lived a migrating, hunting-and-gathering way of life, marked by periods of feast and famine, a thrifty gene rose in frequency in many population groups. This gene might have affected carbohydrate metabolism and storage so that in times of feast carbohydrates would have been efficiently stored to serve energy needs in times of famine. In modern times, marked by an excessive supply of carbohydrates and calories, the thrifty gene leads to problems in carbohydrate metabolism, which in turn lead to diabetes (Niswander 1968). The thrifty gene hypothesis has never been proven, nor has the exact physiological mechanism been precisely stated. There are, of course, problems with generalizing the varied experiences and cultures of Native Americans. However, it may be that the high incidence rates of diabetes are due to some combination of genetic factors and modern dietary patterns and practices.

Another metabolic disease that exists in high frequency in many Native American population groups is gallbladder disease. For example, among Pima Indians the prevalence rate of gallbladder disease among adult males is 37.5% and among adult females is 67.6% (Burch, Comess, & Bennett 1968). Again, the factors contributing to these high rates are not known. Burch, Comess, and Bennett point to the potential contribution of diet, obesity, and diabetes. The rates of gallbladder disease are highly correlated with the diabetes incidence rates. Tribes that had high admission rates for diabetes also had high rates of gallbladder disease (Niswander 1968). It can be concluded that diabetes and gallbladder disease among Native Americans are important health problems for which mechanisms and contributing factors are very possibly related.

Technique for Percussion of the Abdomen

1. Have client remain in comfortable position.
2. Percuss entire abdomen lightly in all four quadrants.
3. *Liver*
   a. Percuss down right MCL to liver dullness and to lower edge of liver dullness.
   b. Measure span of liver dullness vertically at the right MCL.
   c. Ask client to inhale and percuss downward again.
4. *Spleen*
   a. Percuss downward behind the left MAL between 8th and 11th ICS.
   b. Measure the vertical span of splenic dullness.
   c. Percuss lowest left ICS at point between left AAL and the MCL. Note presence or absence of tympany.
5. Percuss gastric air bubble.
6. Decision making: Employ techniques for detection of shifting dullness and fluid wave in the presence of abdominal distention.
   a. Technique of shifting dullness
      1. Client supine.
      2. Begin percussion at umbilicus and move toward nearest flank.
      3. Mark point of dullness.
      4. Have client turn onto side.
      5. Repeat percussion from umbilicus downward.
      6. Note whether level of dullness has shifted.
   b. Technique for measuring fluid wave
      1. Place palm of one hand on client's flank.
      2. Have third person or client place ulnar edge of hand firmly into middle of client's abdomen.
      3. Examiner strikes opposite flank with free hand.

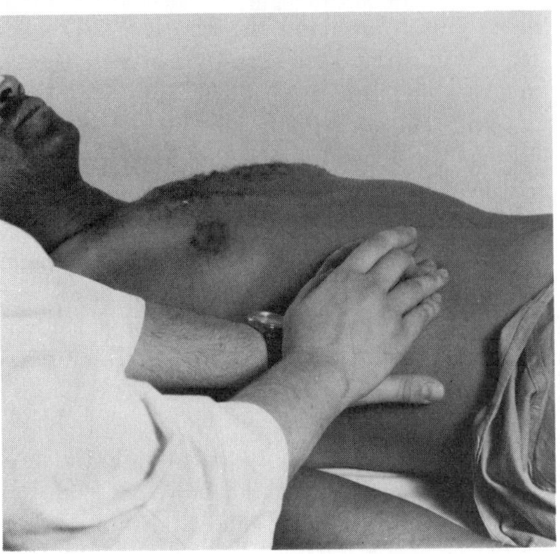

A

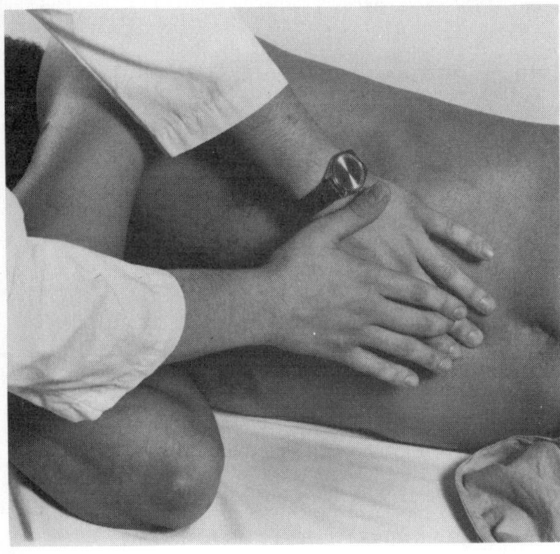

B

Figure 16-8 Technique of shifting dullness. (A) With patient supine, percuss from umbilicus to flank until dullness is heard. (B) Repeat percussion with client on side.

that he is facing you (B). Repeat percussion from the umbilicus downward. In the presence of ascites (see Figure 16-9), the fluid that previously rested in the opposite flank area will gravitate downward, and the level (point) of dullness will move closer (shift) to the midline.

With an appreciable amount of fluid in the abdominal cavity, a fluid wave can be elicited. The technique for producing a fluid wave is illustrated in Figure 16-10. In order to perform this technique place the palm of one hand on the client's flank. Have the client or a third person

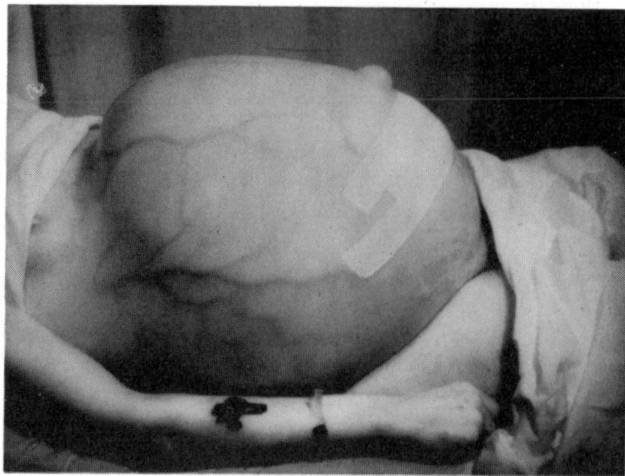

Figure 16-9 Severe ascites. Note the characteristic distended veins and the commonly occurring umbilical hernia.

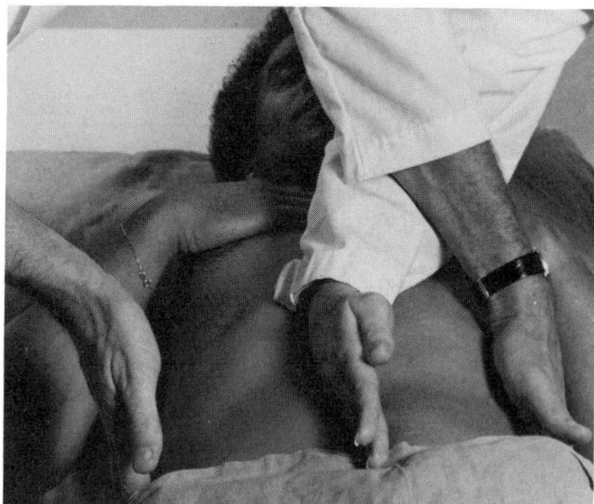

Figure 16-10 Production of fluid wave.

press the ulnar edge of his hand firmly into the middle of the abdomen. Then strike the opposite flank with your free hand. With ascites, the blow will be transmitted by the fluid moving across the abdomen and will be felt against the palm of the hand pressed on the opposite flank.

Palpation

In order for palpation of the abdomen to be effective, the client should be as comfortable and relaxed as possible. If the client is nervous or fearful, the muscles of the abdomen will tense, interfering with the examination and falsely suggesting involuntary rigidity of the muscle wall, a cardinal sign of peritoneal inflammation. The normal abdomen is soft upon palpation and free of tenderness or pain.

Palpate the entire abdomen lightly to detect the presence of pain or masses. If pain is detected, determine whether it is constant or intermittent by increasing pressure over the area. Pain resulting from inflammation does not usually change with increased pressure, whereas pain resulting from involvement of a viscus is generally reduced when pressure is applied.

When pain is presented, test for rebound tenderness by gently and slowly pressing the examining hand deep into the abdomen and then quickly releasing the hand. As the peritoneum snaps back, the client with rebound tenderness will cry out in pain. Immediately inquire where the pain is felt, as it may be in a location different from that where the pressure was applied. An inflamed appendix (as well as inflammation of the peritoneal lining) will cause rebound tenderness. See Table 16-3 for characteristics of common disease conditions of the abdomen.

Following light palpation of the abdomen, perform deep palpation of the abdominal organs.

Liver To palpate the liver, place your right hand just below the lower right costal margin, with your fingers pointing toward the client's right shoulder. Then push the fingers deeply into the abdomen with a constant pressure and simultaneously push up under the rib cage. This technique is illustrated in Figure 16-11. Ask the client to take a deep breath; this will cause the liver to descend. The normal-sized liver may be felt sliding over the fingertips. Usually, though, the normal liver is nonpalpable. With chronic emphysema the liver can be palpated even though it is not enlarged, because the flattened diaphragm forces the liver downward. In the cirrhotic liver a nodular texture is often noted upon palpation. After palpating the hepatic area continue deep palpation to the iliac crest.

Spleen The spleen may be palpable in the normal infant and young child; however, with the older child and adult the spleen must be considerably enlarged before it can be palpated. To palpate the spleen, stand at the right side as the client lies supine. Place your left hand under the client's left flank at the level of the eleventh and twelfth ribs; push your right hand gently under the left anterior costal margin. Instruct the client to take a deep breath. When enlarged, the spleen will be palpated as a firm, superficial mass that slips from under the ribs against the fingers of your right hand. Figure 16-12 illustrates the technique for palpation. A grossly enlarged

Table 16-3. Common Disease Conditions of the Abdomen

Terminology	Characteristics	Comments
Appendicitis	Fever, malaise, abdominal pain and either constipation or diarrhea. Discomfort begins in periumbilical area. Pain localizes in RLQ at McBurney's point. Finger pressure at this area will elicit *rebound tenderness*. If appendix retrocecal, pain may be in flank or pelvic area.	Can occur at any age, although characteristically a disease of the young. Cause of abdominal sepsis in the elderly. If appendix perforates into free peritoneal space, peritonitis will occur with symptoms of pallor, a *quiet* abdomen, and shock.
Pyloric obstruction (stenosis)	Excessive projectile vomiting of sour and fermented undigested food. Obstinate constipation. Bulging of epigastric area. Left to right visible peristalsis. Palpation-splashing fremitus. Percussion—(↑) area of gastric bubble. Auscultation—splashing sounds often audible at some distance.	May be due to narrowing of pyloric orifice or hypertrophy and hyperplasia of mucosa and submucosa.
Paralytic ileus	Weak, infrequent tinkling sound as ileus progresses. Silent abdomen when ileus becomes adynamic. Abdomen tense.	Acute intestinal obstruction—failure of progression of intestinal contents due to inadequacy of intestinal muscular activity.
Gastroenteritis	Abdominal cramps, vomiting, diarrhea. Bowel sounds—high pitched and tinkling. Borborygmi sounds may be present.	Inflammation of the stomach and intestinal tract affects the small bowel predominantly.
Acute peritonitis	Chills, fever, abdominal pain. Severe abdominal tenderness, resulting in difficulty with respiration and body position. Vomiting, constipation. Bowel sounds—weak, infrequent, and then absent.	Rupture of an intra-abdominal viscus, such as appendix or stomach. Infection from an inflamed adjacent organ or septicemia.
Acute cholecystitis	Tenderness of a palpably enlarged gallbladder on inspiration (Murphy's sign). Client unable to take full, deep breath when examiner's fingers are deep beneath right costal arch below hepatic margin.	Almost always caused by gallstones. Other causes may be bacteria or chemical irritants.
Acute pancreatitis	Intense, boring epigastric or left upper quadrant pain, with nausea, vomiting and severe prostration. Paralytic ileus develops characterized by abdominal distention, absence of bowel sounds. There is a rigid boardlike abdomen with rebound tenderness if peritoneal contamination occurs.	Most common pathologic factor is excessive alcohol consumption.
Acute diverticulitis	Similar to appendicitis but involving lower left quadrant, cramping pain and dyschezia (painful defecation).	Diverticula of bowel develop over time. If they become inflamed or obstructed, diverticulitis results.

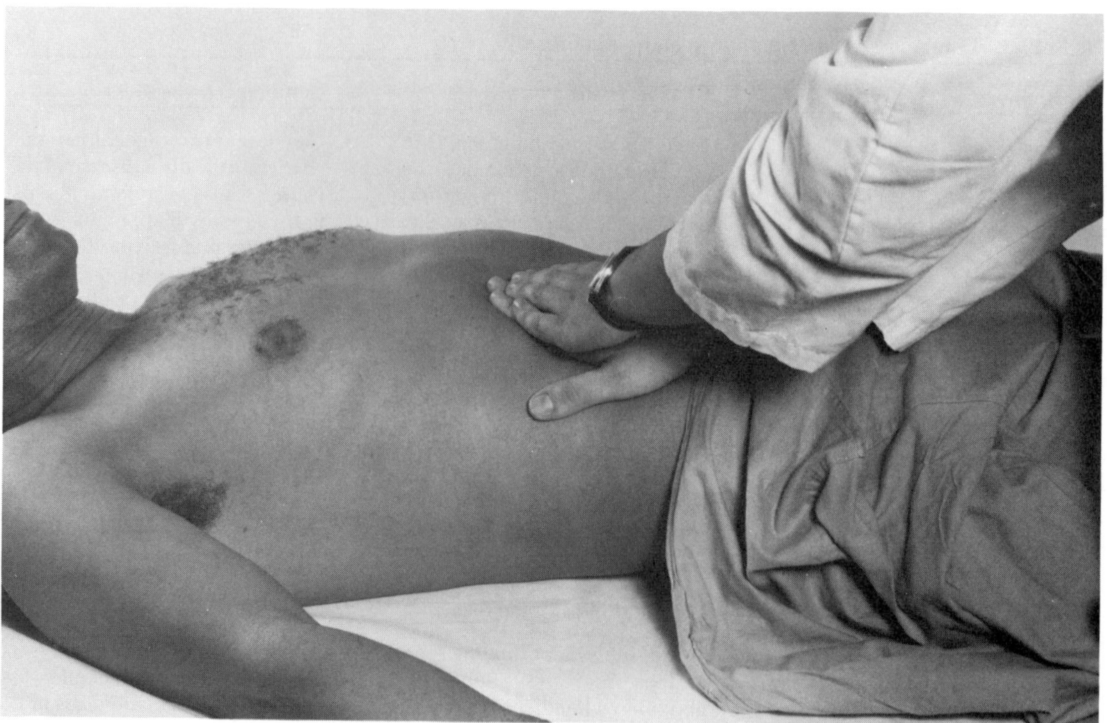

Figure 16-11 Palpation of the liver.

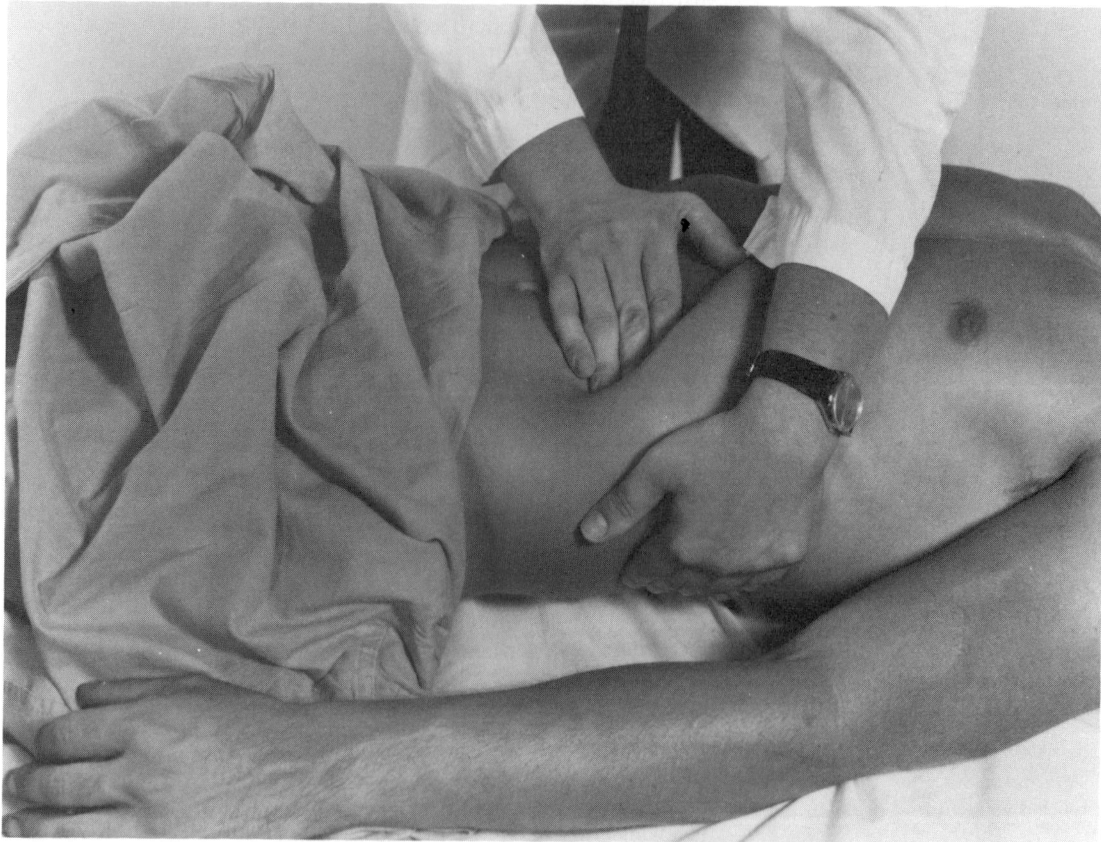

Figure 16-12 Palpation of the spleen.

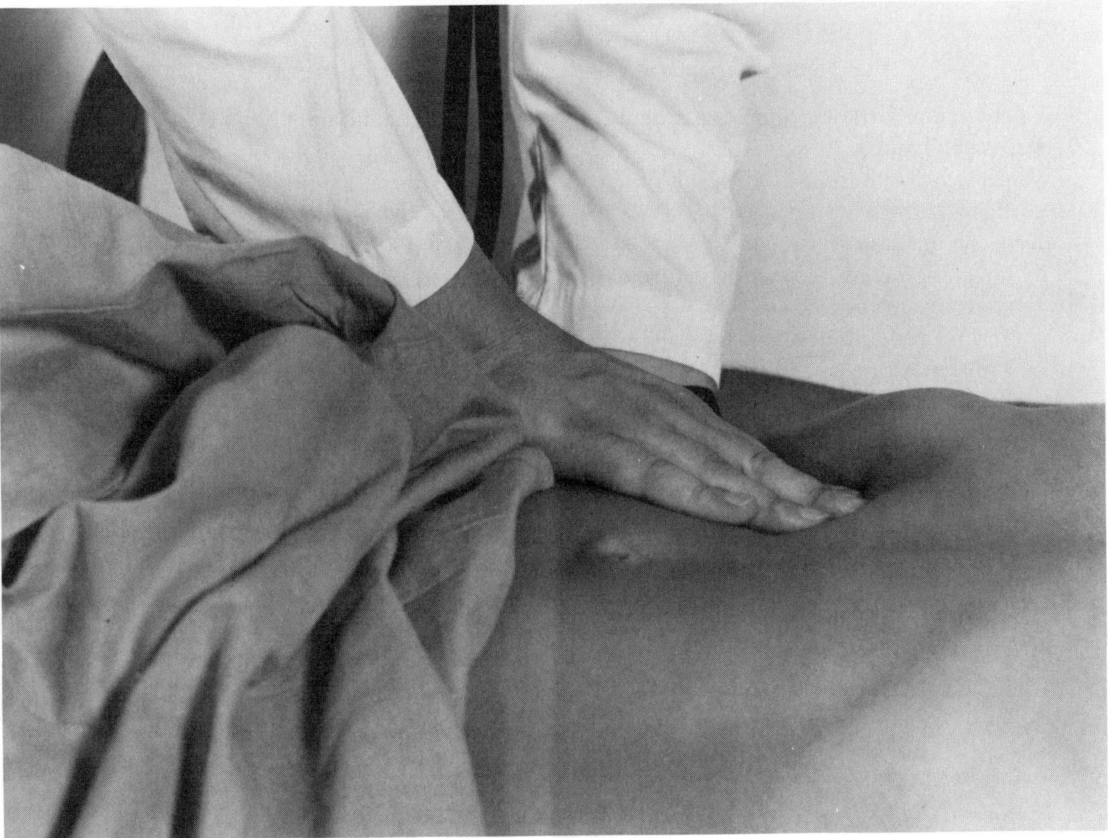

Figure 16-13 Palpation of the kidney.

spleen will be able to be visualized as asymmetry with the entire left side of the abdomen raised. If further investigation is desired because of the suspicion of splenomegaly, it is useful to have the client turn to the right side. Place your hands as previously described and again ask the client to take a deep breath. This technique forces the spleen to move anteriorly.

The spleen enlarges in several contagious diseases, systemic infections, and blood dyscrasias. These include infectious mononucleosis, septicemia, sickle-cell anemia, and hemolytic jaundice. Bacterial endocarditis is an infection that is accompanied by splenic enlargement. Although not often seen in this country, malaria and schistosomiasis, endemic in other countries, lead to splenic enlargement. Extremely large spleens are encountered in leukemia, Hodgkin's disease, and lymphosarcoma.

The spleen is a highly vascular organ; if enlargement is detected, it must be palpated very gently.

Kidneys The kidneys are located deep in the abdomen on the posterior abdominal wall. The right kidney is lower than the left and is easier to palpate. Both kidneys are usually difficult to palpate because of their location, but occasionally they may be felt in children and in adults with scaphoid abdomens.

To palpate the left kidney, place your right hand on the anterior abdomen in the midclavicular line lateral to the umbilicus; place your left hand under the client's left flank. Instruct the client to take a deep breath while you apply pressure with the examining hand. You may feel the right pole of the kidney between your hands as the client inhales. Although it is difficult to feel the left kidney, you can attempt palpation by following the same procedure only on the left side of the abdomen. Figure 16-13 illustrates palpation of the right kidney.

Enlarged kidneys may be palpated in hydronephrosis. Large kidneys with palpable cysts are found in polycystic kidney disease. In children,

Technique for Palpation of the Abdomen

1. Client in comfortable, relaxed position.
2. Use warm hands.
3. Palpate entire abdomen lightly with fingertips.
4. Decision making:
   a. If pain detected, increase pressure of fingertips over area.
   b. Test for rebound tenderness by gently and slowly pressing examining hand deeply into abdomen and then quickly releasing.
5. Begin deep palpation of abdominal organs:
   a. *Liver*
   (1). Place right hand below lower right costal margin and point fingers toward client's right shoulder.
   (2). Push fingers deeply into abdomen while pushing up under rib cage.
   (3). Ask client to take deep breath.
   (4). Continue deep palpation to iliac crest.
   b. *Spleen*
   (1). Stand at right side of supine client.
   (2). Place left hand under client's left flank at level of 11th and 12th ribs.
   (3). Push right hand gently under left anterior costal margin.
   (4). Decision making: if suspicious of splenomegaly, have client lie on right side and repeat technique described above.
   (5). Remember to palpate gently.
   c. *Kidneys*
   (1). Right—place right hand on anterior abdomen in MCL next to umbilicus. Place left hand under client's left flank. Ask client to take deep breath while applying pressure with examining hand.
   (2). Left—difficult to feel left kidney but palpation can be tried using same technique described above.
   (3). CVA tenderness—strike CVA with heel of hand or closed fist on left and right sides.
   d. *Hernias*
   (1). Ventral—often can be seen. Palpate incisional site. Ask client to cough.
   (2). Umbilical—push index finger into navel. Also ask client to cough to assist visualization.
   (3). Inguinal—have client stand with leg on side being examined slightly flexed. For indirect hernias, place index finger into loose skin on scrotum and advance finger to external inguinal ring. Ask client to bear down. For direct hernias, press palmar aspect of hand over inguinal area. Ask client to bear down or cough.
   e. *Lymph Nodes and Pulses*
   (1). Using rotary motion of fingertips, palpate inguinal and femoral nodes on both sides of body.
   (2). Using tips of fingers, locate and evaluate femoral pulse on both sides of body.
   (3). Decision making—If femoral pulses weak, delayed, or absent, take BP in leg.

Wilms' tumor, a rapidly developing sarcoma of the kidneys, presents as a large abdominal mass. In hypernephroma, the most common neoplasm in adults, a large abdominal mass may be felt.

To detect the presence of tenderness of the kidneys, strike the costovertebral angle (CVA) with the heel of your hand or a closed fist on both the left and the right sides (see Figure 16-14). CVA tenderness is often due to an infectious process in the kidney. The normal kidneys are nontender.

Should a mass or nodule be palpated, describe the location, approximate size, consistency, and degree of tenderness to the consulting physician. Occasionally, feces may be mistaken for a tumor upon abdominal palpation. Every mass in the abdomen must be verified before the client can be described as free of disease.

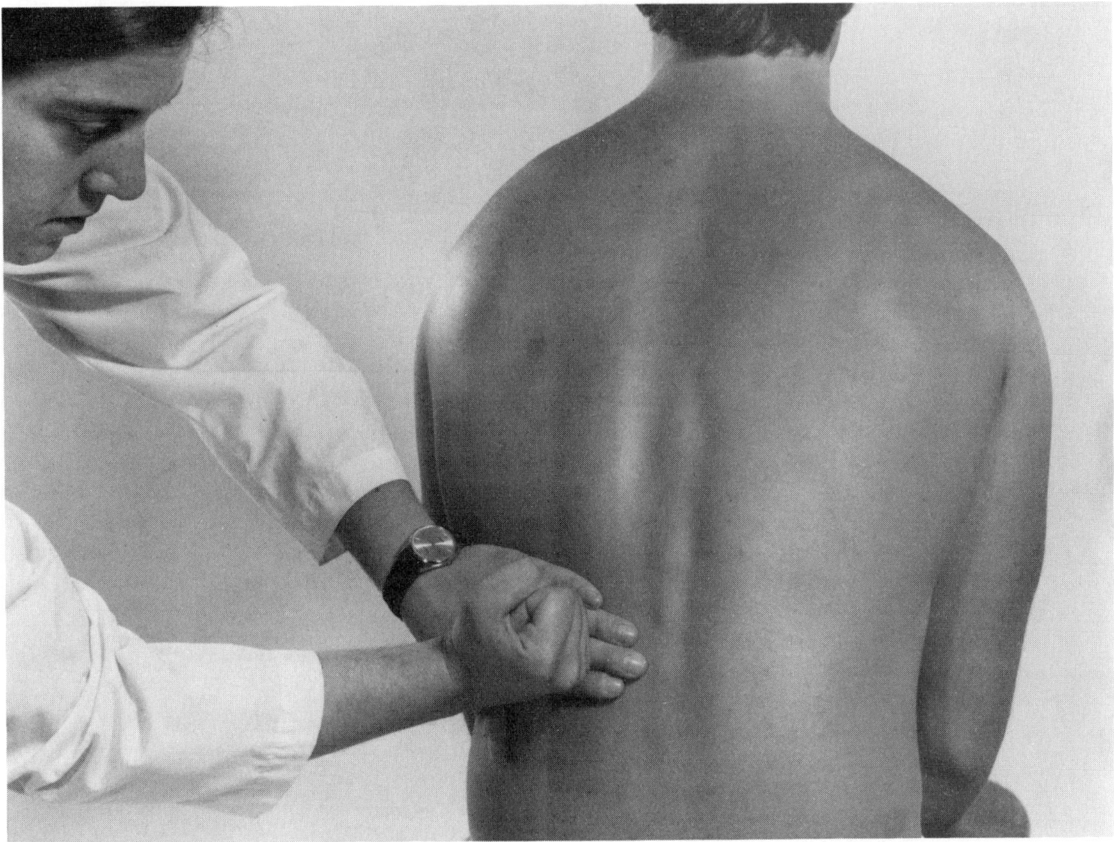

Figure 16-14 Blunt percussion for CVA tenderness.

Hernias Next, palpate the abdomen for the presence of hernias. The three most common types of hernias are ventral, umbilical, and inguinal.

Ventral (incisional) *hernias* usually occur at the site of a surgical incision that has not healed properly or where scar tissue is not as strong as normal tissue. This type of hernia can often be seen as well as palpated. It usually appears as a soft mass on the abdominal wall. Coughing generally causes it to bulge outward (see Figure 16-15A).

Umbilical hernias are most generally congenital and are best visualized when the client coughs. When you push your index finger into the navel, a ring of fascia will be detected around a soft center. They may occur with pregnancy, ascites, and obesity. (See Figure 16-15B.)

Inguinal hernias, most often seen in males, may be direct or indirect. An indirect hernia follows the spermatic cord through both the internal and external rings and through the inguinal canal. Occasionally, one becomes very large and descends into the scrotum (see Figure 16-15C). To palpate an indirect inguinal hernia, it is best to have the client stand with his ipsilateral (same side as being examined) leg slightly flexed. Place an index finger into the loose skin low on the side of the scrotum and advance it up to the external inguinal ring. Figure 16-16 illustrates this technique. If possible, advance the finger through the inguinal ring. Instruct the client to strain or "bear down." An indirect hernia will be felt as a small soft mass that presses against the fingertip.

Direct hernias pass through the weak muscular wall and into the external inguinal ring. They may be visualized or can be palpated by pressing the palmar aspects of the hand over the inguinal area and having the client cough or bear down.

Diastasis recti is the separation of the two abdominal rectus muscles that is congenital or acquired through conditions that weaken these muscles, e.g. obesity, pregnancy. It manifests by

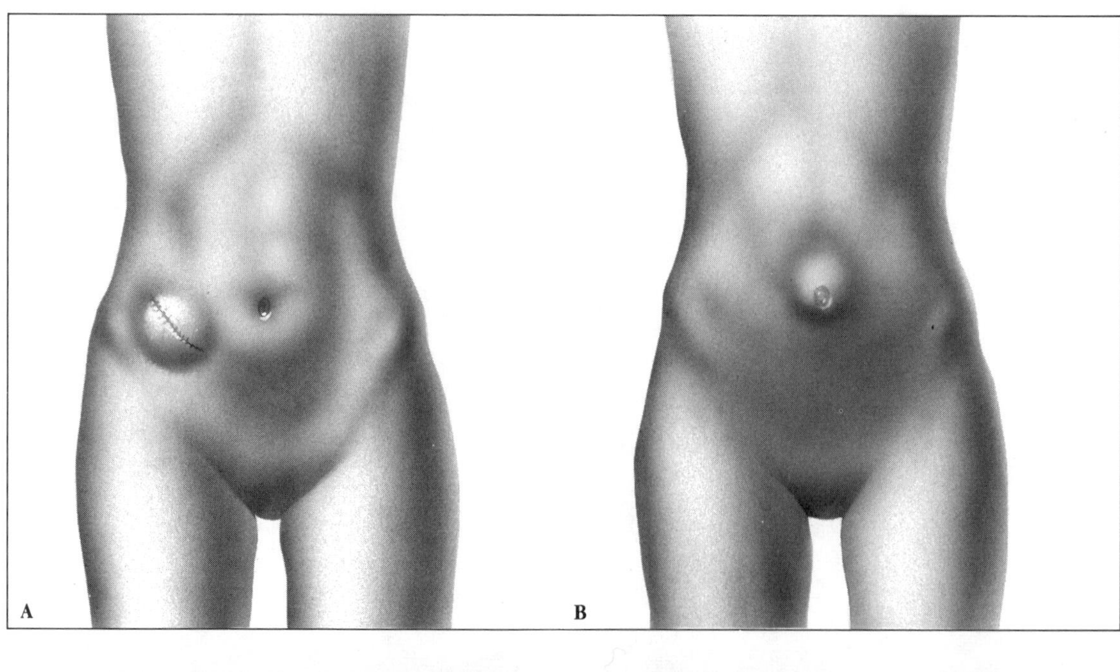

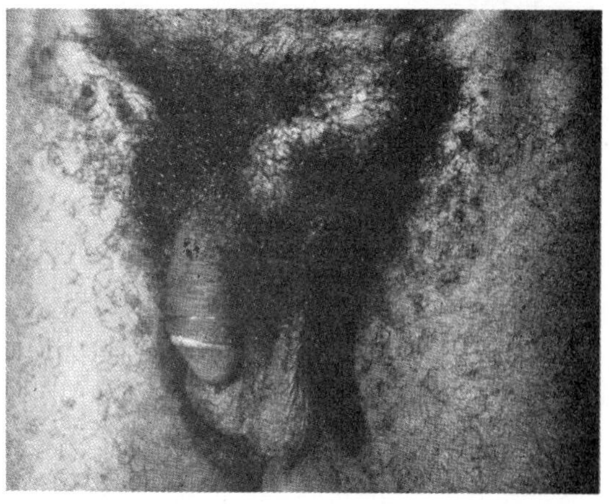

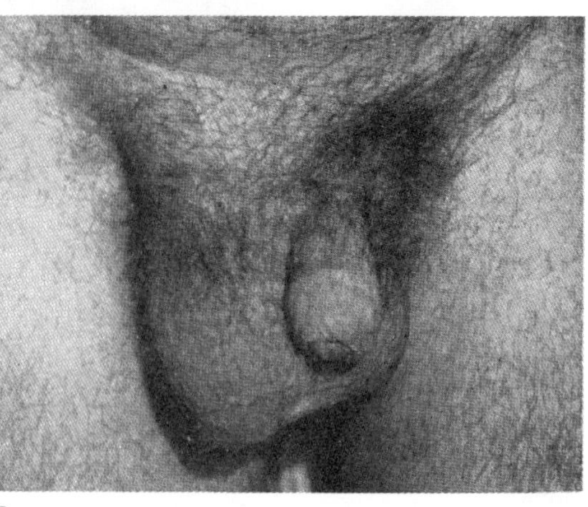

Figure 16-15 Hernias. (A) Ventral incisional hernia. (B) Umbilical hernia. Periumbilical bulging is seen in a child with umbilical hernia. In an adult, bulging radiates upward from the umbilicus. (C) Direct inguinal hernia. (D) Indirect inguinal hernia.

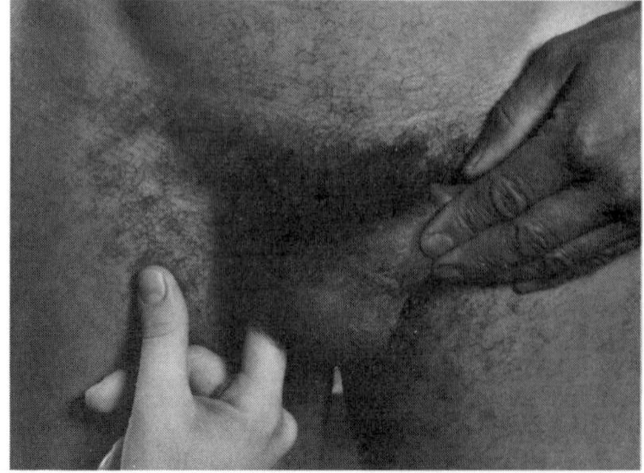

Figure 16-16 Examination technique for indirect inguinal hernia.

a protuberant midline abdominal ridge when the client raises his head and shoulders when in a supine position (see Figure 16-17).

Lymph Nodes and Pulses Palpate the groin areas to determine the status of the lymph nodes and the femoral pulses. Figure 16-18 illustrates the position of the *inguinal lymph nodes*, which drain the lower abdomen, buttocks, and genital area. The *femoral lymph nodes*, also shown in Figure 16-18, drain the lower extremities. The

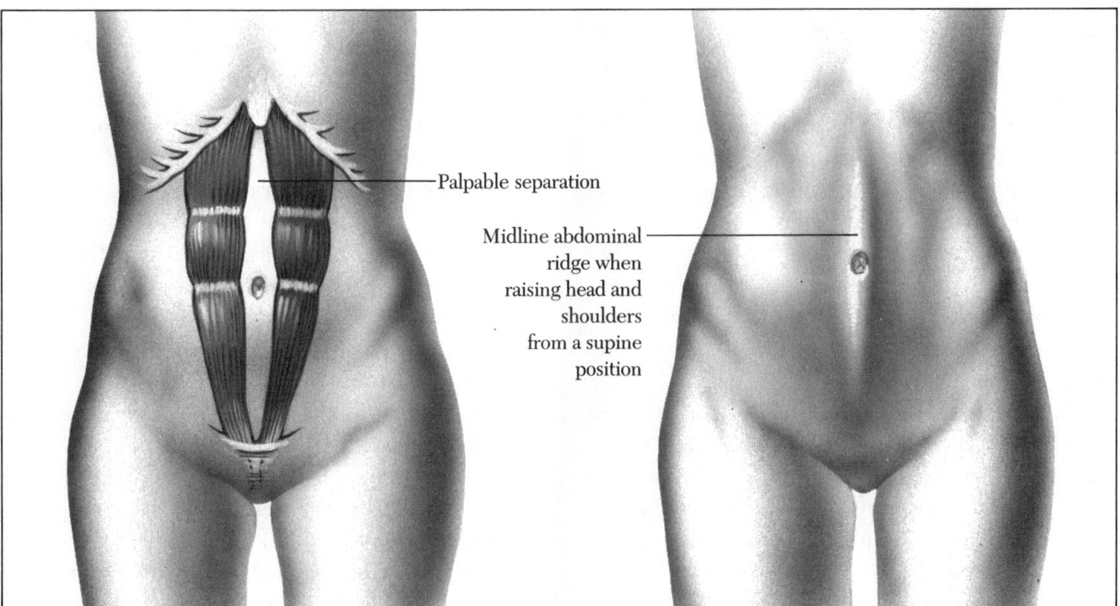

Figure 16-17 Diastasis recti.

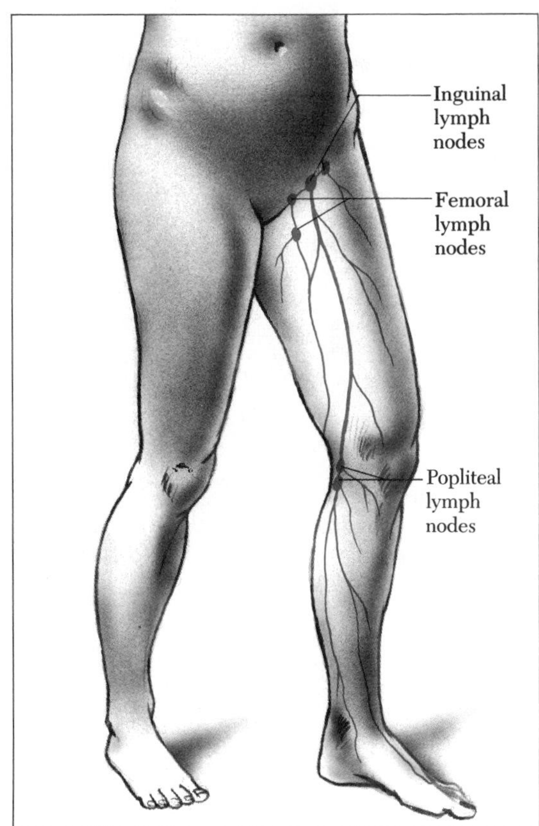

Figure 16-18 Location of inguinal and femoral lymph nodes.

lymph nodes are examined by using a rotary motion of the fingertips. It is not uncommon to find nontender lymph enlargement in the groins; if not accompanied by other signs and symptoms, such enlargement is not significant. This is a common finding in the elderly.

Lymphadenopathy accompanies acute infections and systemic diseases, and enlarged, tender nodes may be present with inflammation of the thighs, legs, or feet. The femoral pulse is located bilaterally with the tips of several fingers as shown in Figure 14-6 (page 281). A weak, delayed, or absent femoral pulse is found with coarctation of the aorta; this warrants that the blood pressure be taken in the leg as well as the arm. With coarctation of the aorta the leg blood pressure will be lower than the arm pressure reading. Weak or absent femoral pulse may also be detected in vascular insufficiency of the lower extremities due to advanced atherosclerosis.

Summary

This chapter discussed the structure and location of the various organs in the abdomen and the various techniques used in assessment of the organs. Assessment of the abdomen is best accomplished with the client in a supine or side lying position. In contrast to the other areas of the body, initial inspection is not followed by palpation but by auscultation and percussion. The sounds listened for on auscultation are those of peristalsis and of vascular abnormalities.

Percussion is performed to determine whether there is enlargement of an organ, presence of masses, or abdominal distention. Specific sounds heard at differing locations were described in the chapter.

Palpation, the last technique performed in assessment of the abdomen, is performed to examine the liver, spleen, kidneys, hernias, and lymph nodes. Emphasis is placed on the importance of making the client as comfortable and as relaxed as possible.

Discussion Questions/Activities

1. List the abdominal contents within each of the four abdominal quadrants and the midline area of the lower abdomen.
2. Give the rationale for the following sequence of approach to the assessment of the abdomen: inspection, auscultation, percussion, palpation.
3. State the criterion for documenting "absence of bowel sounds."
4. What areas of the abdomen would be auscultated to assess whether bruits, venous hums, and peritoneal friction rubs are present?
5. Demonstrate the techniques for palpating the liver, spleen, and kidneys.
6. Demonstrate the method for determining the size of the liver and spleen by the percussion technique.
7. Describe the techniques used for detecting the various hernias.

Recording of Findings

Normal findings are presented in the first box. Findings for a client complaining of being "constantly tired" are presented in the second box.

Abdomen	Abdomen
INSPECTION Abdomen flat; no scars; no venous engorgement; no lesions; no visible pulsations; symmetrical; no flank fullness.	**INSPECTION** Abdomen round, asymmetrical—right upper quadrant; flank fullness with some pitting edema; 3 cm McBurney's scar in right lower quadrant; no lesions, no visible pulsations.
AUSCULTATION Bowel sounds present in all four quadrants; no bruits.	**AUSCULTATION** Bowel sounds present in all four quadrants; no bruits.
PERCUSSION Tympany in all four quadrants; gastric air bubble; liver 9 cm at right MCL; lower edge of liver dullness at costal margin; splenic dullness 6 cm at left MAL.	**PERCUSSION** Decreased tympany in all four quadrants; liver 15 cm at right MCL; gastric air bubble; spleen 7 cm; 2 cm shifting dullness present.
PALPATION No masses; no tenderness; liver, spleen, kidneys nonpalpable.	**PALPATION** Liver palpated at 5 cm below RCM—smooth contour; spleen and kidneys nonpalpable; no tenderness or masses.

CHAPTER 17

Assessment of the Musculoskeletal System

LEARNING OBJECTIVES

1. Review the structure and function of the musculoskeletal system.
2. Recognize the characteristics noted in inspection and palpation of the muscles, bones, and joints.
3. Interpret muscle movement in order to categorize the grade of muscle strength.
4. Define the abnormal curvatures of the spine, such as kyphosis, lordosis, and lateral scoliosis.
5. List the joints that are routinely inspected and palpated.
6. Describe range of motion of the various joints of the body.
7. Describe the technique to detect effusion of the knee.

In assessing the musculoskeletal system three specific structures should be examined: the muscles, bones, and joints. It is important that the anatomic area being examined be fully exposed and free from any kind of restriction of movement from clothing or appliances. Merely rolling up a pantleg is not sufficient for thoroughly examining the leg. The anatomic area being assessed must be accessible to the main techniques to be used, inspection and palpation.

The comprehensiveness of the examination of the musculoskeletal system will vary from client to client. A client with questionable musculoskeletal history would warrant a detailed, systematic physical assessment of this system. You would need to proceed carefully, placing emphasis on identifying existing deformities and on determining the status of specific muscles and joints. The most valuable adjunct assessment modality for evaluating the musculoskeletal system is x-ray.

Certain observations of the musculoskeletal system are mentioned elsewhere in this text. For example, inspection of the cranium is more appropriately done during the assessment of the head. Similarly, a cursory inspection of spinal curvature is easily accomplished during examination of the posterior thorax.

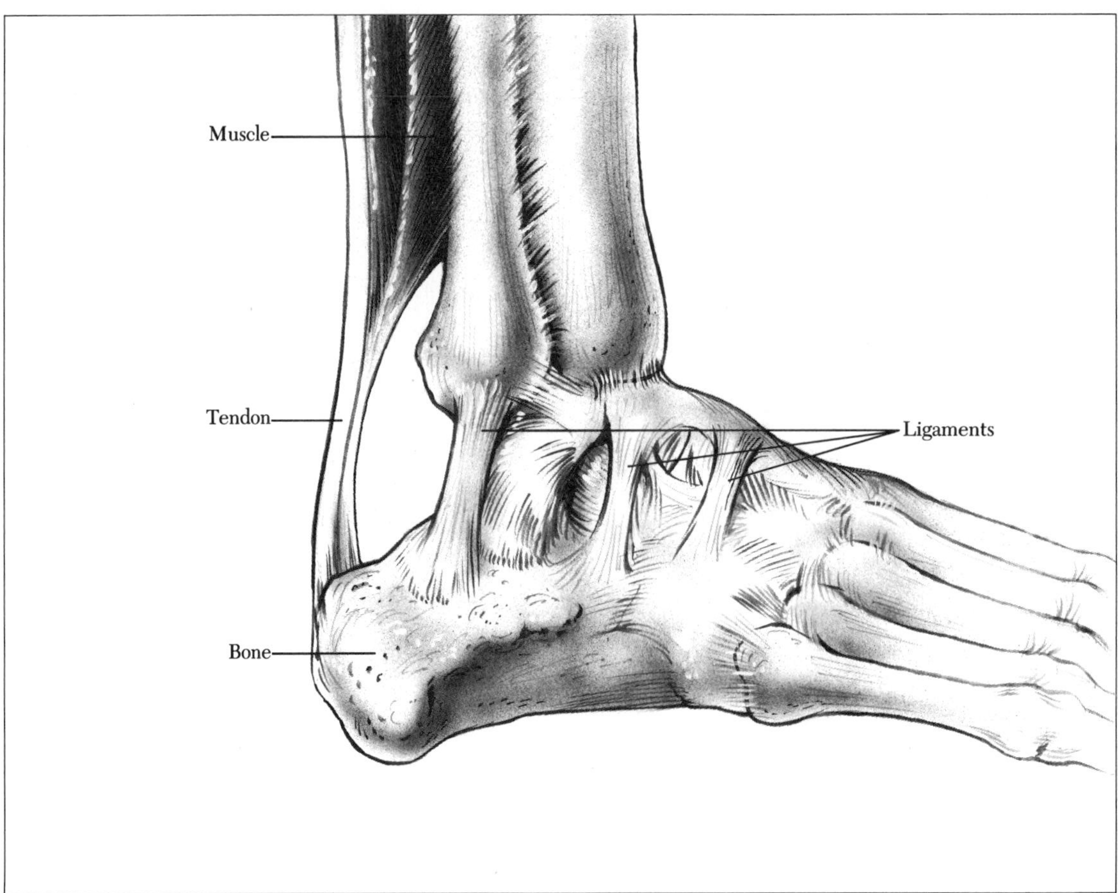

Figure 17-1 The relation of muscle to bones, tendons, and ligaments.

Structure and Function of the Musculoskeletal System

Muscles, Tendons, and Ligaments

Muscle fibers are grouped together to form fascicular bundles, which in turn are surrounded by connective tissue. The muscle mass consists of groups of these bundles. The skeletal muscles, which are characteristically composed of cross-striated muscle fibers, move parts of the body and are used in both voluntary and reflex movements. They are the major focus in this chapter.

Muscular tissue is specialized for contractility. The point of attachment of the muscle to the bone is called the *origin*. The freely movable end is called the *insertion*. *Tendons* are fibrous connective tissues that attach muscles to the skeletal structure. *Ligaments* are bands of strong fibrous connective tissue that connect cartilage together, that connect the articular ends of the bones, and that serve as support or attachment for fascia or muscles (see Figure 17-1).

Bones

The skeletal system forms the solid structure around which the body is built. The bones provide surfaces for the attachment of muscles, tendons, and ligaments. Some of the bones form cagelike configurations to house and protect internal structures and organs. Examples are the cranium, which contains the brain, and the vertebral column, which protects the spinal cord. Many bones act as passive levers for moving various parts of the body.

Bone growth occurs in circumference and in length. Growth in diameter is due primarily to the activity of the osteoblastic cells. Longitudinal growth results from activity of the epiphyseal cartilage cells, at the end of the long bone shafts, which are eventually replaced by osteoblasts. Growth in bone length continues until the epi-

BIOLOGICAL AND CULTURAL VARIATIONS

Bone Density and Disorders Among White Americans

Certain differences in body constitution among population groups are associated with different disease rates. It has been shown, for example, that Black Americans have greater body density than White Americans. This difference is due to a number of differences in body constitution between the two population groups. Black Americans have less average subcutaneous fat than Whites and smaller fatfold thicknesses at various sites on the body such as the arms, legs, and torso. Since fat is less dense than muscle mass, this difference contributes to the lesser body density of White Americans. Black Americans also have longer leg length in relation to sitting height, which includes length of the head and torso. A third reason for the greater body density of Black Americans is that they have denser bones. Black Americans have a greater skeletal mass than White Americans and also tend to lose less bone in the later decades of life, when bone resorption becomes a significant problem for other population groups.

The increased bone density of Black Americans may account for their remarkably low frequency of certain bone disorders that present health problems for White Americans. The rate of occurrence of congenital dislocation of the hip during infancy and Legg-Calvé-Perthes disease during childhood is 50 times greater for Whites than for Blacks (Damon 1977). There are also significant differences in bone disease patterns during old age. Among elderly females, the rate of traumatic fractures is 50 times greater among White Americans than among Blacks, and osteoporosis affects 5 times as many elderly White females as Black.

physes are closed; this happens at about 18–20 years of age.

Joints

The articulation or point of juncture between two bones is called a *joint*. Joints are classified as synarthrodial, or immovable (as in cranial sutures); amphiarthrodial, or slightly movable (symphysis pubis); and diarthrodial, or freely movable, which provides the greatest range of movement (wrist, elbow, hip).

Bursae, closed sacs lined by synovial membrane, are found in some regions. The synovial membrane secretes fluid that prevents friction between the surfaces that glide over each other within the bursa. The most important bursae are located at the shoulder, the elbow, the knee, the hip, and the heel.

Characteristics and Techniques of Examination

Muscles

The muscular portion of the musculoskeletal system is examined by assessing symmetry, muscle size, muscle tone, and muscular strength. As each of these components is assessed systematically, the corresponding muscles on each side of the body should be compared. The muscle strength of an elderly client or that of a child cannot be compared with that of an athlete, nor is it easily compared to a scale of norm. Each individual has his own normal range of muscle strength; thus, he serves as his own scale by self-comparison.

Inspection

In assessing the muscle size, it is usual to compare the arms, thighs, and calves. If there appears to be a discrepancy, obtain the size measurements with a tape measure. Any signs of atrophy or muscular hypertrophy should be noted. Observe for contractures or shortening of muscles and tendons, as these may result in skeletal atrophy or deformity. Diminished muscle mass can be associated with disuse or can be the result of neuromuscular disease such as poliomyelitis, diseases of the brain or spinal cord, peripheral neuropathy, or peripheral nerve injury. Atrophy of the muscle may also be due to primary muscle disease such as muscular dystrophies and myotonia. Muscular dystrophies manifest as muscular weakness; yet there is the appearance of hypertrophied muscles. This is because muscle tissue has been replaced by fibrous tissue.

The small tender nodules often palpated in the periscapular, back, and gluteal muscles are called fibrocytic nodules. Tumors of the muscle are rare.

Myositis ossificans, found in the quadriceps muscles and in back and arm muscles, is so typical among football linemen that it is referred to as "blockers' node."

Congenital anomalies of muscles occur most frequently in the sternocleidomastoid and the pectoralis major muscles. Portions of these muscles may be absent. Enlargement of muscles or groups of muscles is found in congenital hypertrophy and in pseudohypertrophic muscular dystrophy.

Inspect the fine muscles of each hand for wasting. The hands as well as all muscles should be inspected for signs of tremors or fasciculations. *Fasciculations* are involuntary twitchings of isolated bundles of muscle fibers and often occur with damage to neurons in the spinal cord (lower motor neuron damage). To examine for tremors, have the client stretch his arms out in front of him. Fine tremors can be made more easily visible by placing a sheet of paper on top of the client's hands. If tremors do exist, determine whether they are resting tremors or intention tremors. A *resting tremor* is accentuated by rest and diminishes upon movement; it is the characteristic tremor of Parkinson's disease. An *intention tremor* is accentuated by voluntary movement and is found in cerebellar disease and multiple sclerosis. Tics and certain other gross involuntary movements become exaggerated when the client is under stress and usually disappear when the client is sleeping. These movements suggest disturbance of the extrapyramidal motor areas, in particular the basal ganglia. Some involuntary movements may be of an emotional origin or may be due to muscle fatigue.

Palpation

To determine muscle tone, palpate the muscles at rest. The tone and consistency of the muscles should be documented as being normal, flaccid, or spastic. During the performance of active and passive ranges of motion, the muscles should be assessed as to whether they are flaccid, rigid, or smooth moving. Flaccid, easily movable muscles are present in lower motor neuron disease, whereas spastic muscles (which demonstrate initial resistance and then suddenly give) are found in pyramidal disease—cerebrovascular accident, or upper motor neuron damage in the cerebrum or brain stem. Typically, with pyramidal disease the tone in the flexor muscles of the arms increases whereas in the legs the tone of the extensors increases.

To assess muscle strength or power, have the client squeeze your finger with each hand; then compare the pressure of the two grasps. When testing strength of hand grip, cross your arms so that the client grasps your *left* index finger with his *left* hand, and vice versa. In this way you can easily identify which hand grasp may be weaker by associating the weakness with your own body side. Otherwise, it is easy to mix up the client's left and right sides, as they are opposite your own left and right sides.

Ask the client to flex and extend the major joints actively without resistance. The client should move his limbs horizontally without the influence of gravity; that is, he should move his arms while they are resting on a table and abduct his legs while supine in bed. Compare the distal strength of each limb to the proximal strength, as well as the strength of the muscles as the client moves the major joints against applied resistance; observe neck flexion, extension, and rotation and shoulder abduction and adduction, elbow flexion and extension, wrist flexion and extension, hip flexion and extension, knee flexion and extension, and ankle plantar flexion and dorsiflexion. For examples of measuring

Technique for Inspection and Palpation of the Muscles

1. Examine both sides of the body.
2. Compare muscle size of arms, thighs, and calves. Measure with tape if discrepancy noted.
3. Examine for tremors: Have client stretch arms in front. To detect fine tremors, place sheet of paper on top of client's hands.
4. Palpate muscles at rest.
5. Note condition of muscles when client does active and passive range of motion.
6. Assess client's muscle strength.

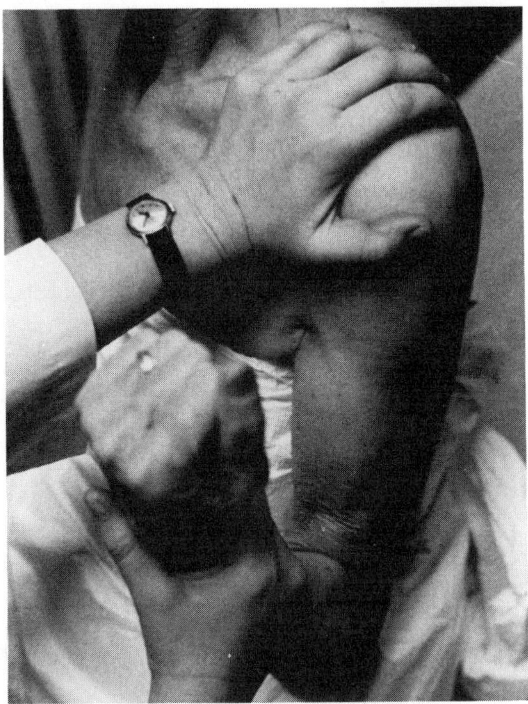

Figure 17-2 Testing muscle strength, left biceps. Ask the client to bend her elbow and resist attempts to straighten it. Place your left hand on the client's shoulder. With your right hand, grasp the client's wrist and attempt to straighten the arm. The degree of resistance is then assessed. If you release the client's wrist suddenly, her fist should not strike the hand on her shoulder. Such an overshooting response occurs in cerebellar disease.

strength against resistance, see Figures 17-2 and 17-3. The normal individual has equal strength in all areas—on both sides and on the proximal and distal portions of the body.

A pattern of weakness may aid in determining whether there is dysfunction of a single peripheral nerve or of an entire nerve root. Muscle weakness or paralysis indicates neurologic disturbance or a lesion along the pyramidal pathway in the cerebrum, within the brain stem and spinal cord, in the peripheral nerves, at the neuromuscular junctions, or in the muscle tissues themselves. Table 17-1 presents the various scales used to document the grading of muscle strength.

Bones

Inspection

In gross examination of the skeletal system, keep in mind not only the normal structure and form of the body but the deformities that can occur as well. Limb deformities include such conditions as clubfoot (talipes varus and valgus), toe-walking deformities (talipes equinus) (see Figure 17-5) flatfoot (pes planus), abnormal hollowness of the sole of the foot (pes cavus), and congenital amputation—the absence of a limb or portion thereof. Knee deformities include genu varum (bowlegs) and genu valgum (knock knees). Another deformity of the skeletal system is Spren-

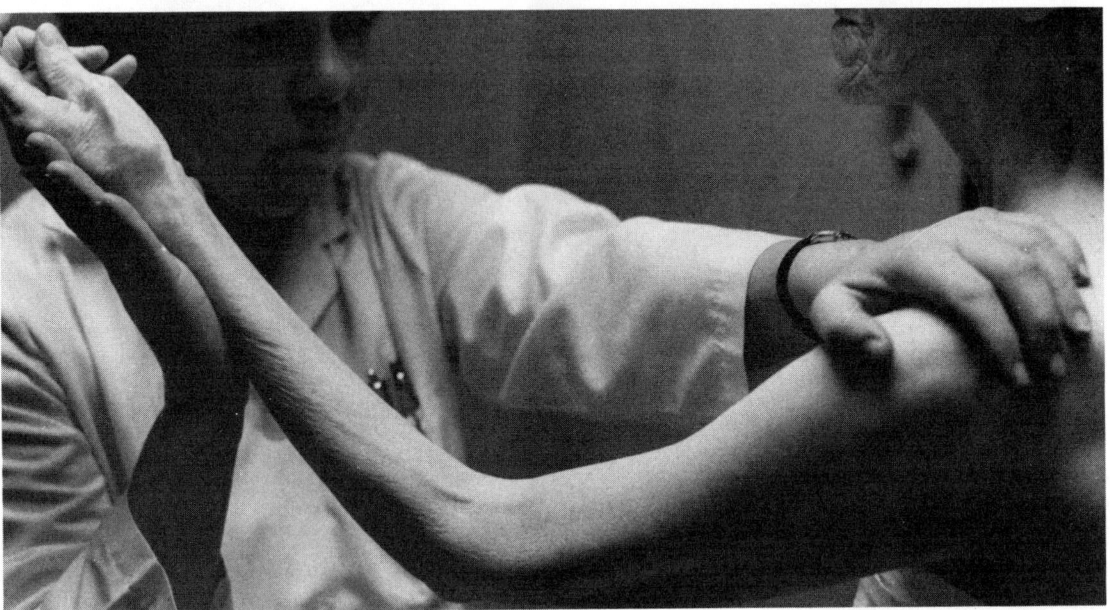

Figure 17-3 Testing muscle strength, left triceps. Ask the client to hold her left arm bent at the elbow. Place your left hand on the client's shoulder. Support the client's wrist with your right hand and ask the client to straighten her elbow against the resistance of your right hand.

Table 17-1. Scales for Grading Muscle Strength

Letter scale	Percent scale	Number scale	Interpretation
Normal (N)	100%	5	Normal power
Good (G)	75%	4	Muscle can make full normal movement but not against resistance
Fair (F)	50%	3	Muscle cannot move against resistance nor make full normal movement but can make normal movement against gravity
Poor (P)	25%	2	Full muscle movement possible with force of gravity eliminated
Trace (T)	10%	1	No movement of limb or joint, but contraction is visible or palpable
Zero (0)	0%	0	Total paralysis

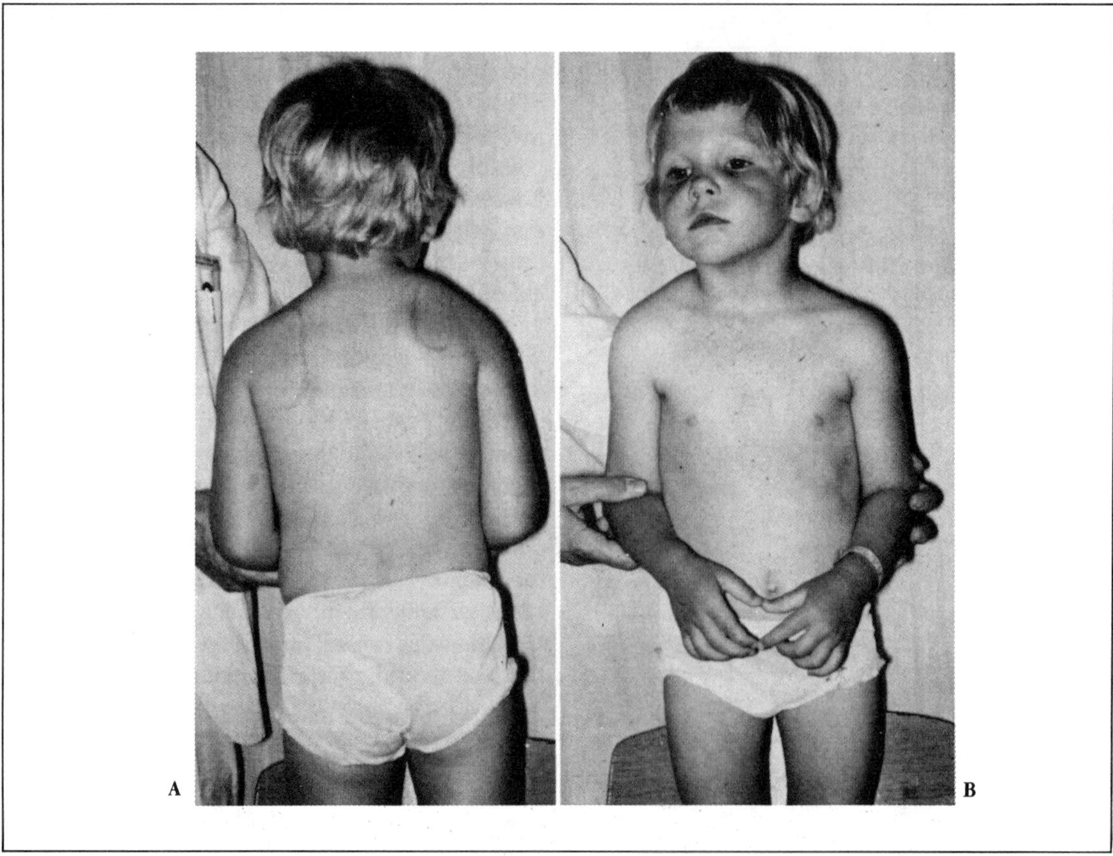

Figure 17-4 (A) Congenital elevation of the scapula (Sprengel's deformity). (B) Same patient from front demonstrating asymmetry of the shoulder girdles and short neck.

gel's deformity, a congenital elevation of the scapula (Figure 17-4). A skeletal deformity that follows a Colles' fracture of the wrist is sometimes referred to as a "silver fork" deformity. Two common hip deformities are those of dislocation of the hip and of hip fracture. Adduction of the leg and internal rotation with hip and knee flexion are characteristic on the side of hip dislocation. A fractured hip results in external rotation and leg abduction of the affected side (see Figure 17-6). Arthritis causes skeletal deformity of the joints (see Figures 17-7 through 17-10 and Table 17-2).

The normal spinal column is curved poste-

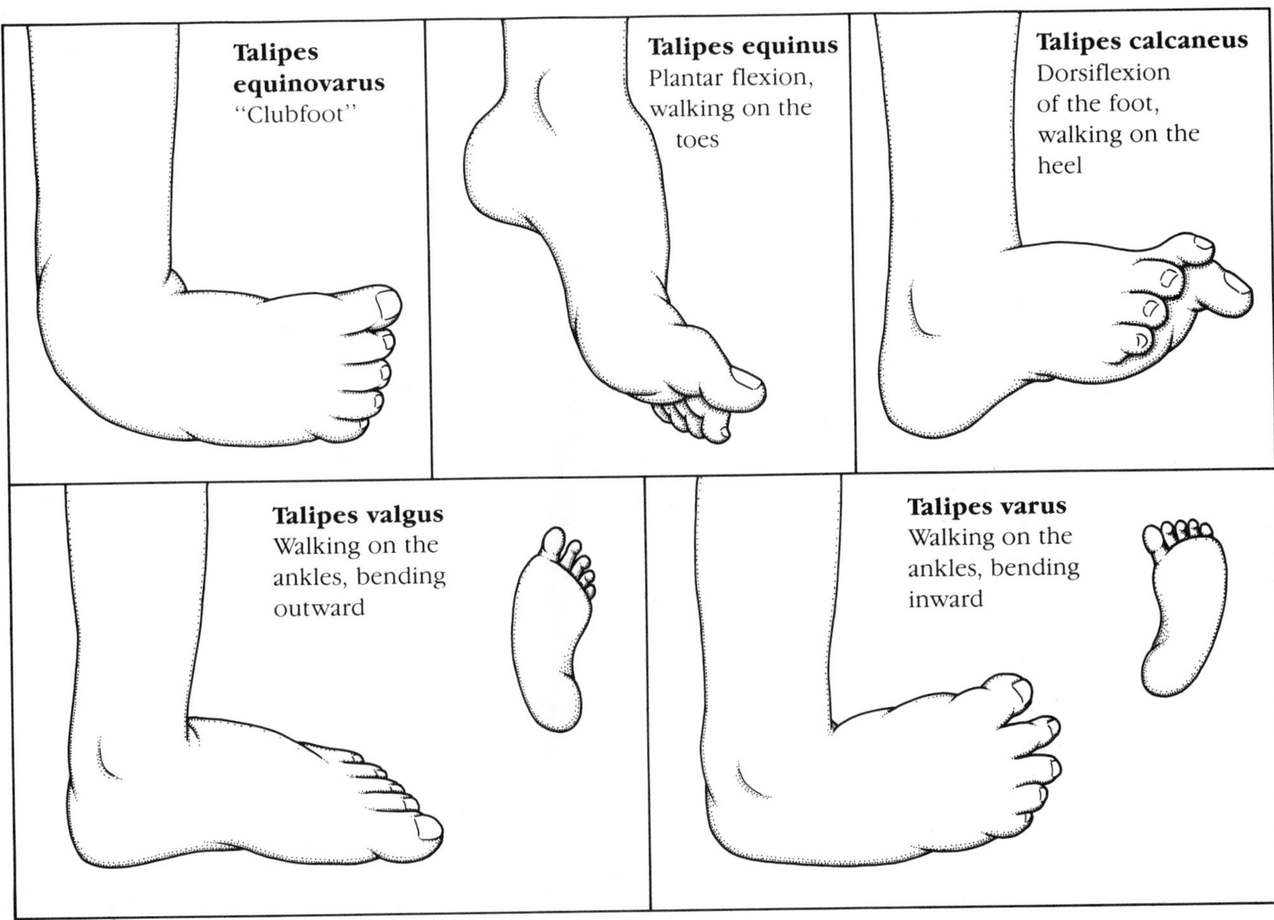

Figure 17-5 Variations of congenital clubfoot.
From Servonsky/Opas: *Nursing Management of Children*, © 1987 Boston: Jones and Bartlett Publishers.

riorly in the thoracic region and anteriorly in the cervical and lumbar regions. From a posterior view, the normal spinal column is straight. Observe the client from the side to note any abnormality in the cervical, thoracic, or lumbar curvature. Observe the client from behind for any abnormality in lateral curvature. Sometimes posture will simulate a mild scoliosis, so instruct the client to straighten up and hold back his shoulders; also observe the spinal curvature as the client bends over from the waist. Scoliosis which occurs from unequal leg length will disappear in this position. Structural scoliosis will be exaggerated in this position. Movements such as twisting the shoulder side to side, bending to each side, and bending backward will tend to exaggerate spinal deformities and aid in their detection. The common spinal curvature abnormalities (see Figure 17-11) are kyphosis (humpback), lordosis (swayback), and scoliosis (lateral S curve). Nutritional deficiencies can influence skeletal structure. The disease of rickets (see Figure 17-12), caused by vitamin D deficiency or by renal insufficiency, is manifested in skeletal malformation.

Legg-Calvé-Perthes disease will also cause skeletal disorders. This condition generally has its onset in children between the age of 3 and 12. It occurs four times more often in boys than in girls. The signs of this skeletal problem are intermittent and include a protective limp, limited movement of the hip joint, and atrophy of the thigh muscles due to disuse. Any child who displays such signs should be referred to a physician.

Palpation

As you examine each anatomic area, palpate all bones to detect tenderness. Bone pain is often the only symptom of osseous disease. Acute pain accompanies fractures and osteomyelitis.

Table 17-2. Juvenile Rheumatoid Arthritis

Subgroup	Behavioral assessment	Diagnostic criteria
Polyarticular: seropositive	Large and small joints are affected—warm, tender, and swollen; morning stiffness; may have mild fever, anemia, malaise; progression to severe, crippling arthritis common; 80% female.	Positive rheumatoid factor (RF) Positive antinuclear antibodies (ANA) Human lymphocyte antigen (HLA) DR4
Polyarticular: seronegative	Large and small joints affected—warm, tender, and swollen; morning stiffness; progression to severe arthritis unusual; 90% female.	Negative RF Negative ANA
Pauciarticular: type I	Large joints, such as knees, ankles, and elbows, commonly affected; iridocyclitis common; crippling arthritis rare; young age of onset; 80% female.	Negative RF Positive ANA HLA DR5 HLA DR8
Pauciarticular: type II	Large joints commonly affected as in type I, plus sacroiliac and hip; iridocyclitis rare; may develop ankylosing spondilitis or bowel disease; onset late childhood; 90% male.	Negative RF Negative ANA HLA B27
Systemic-onset	High fever; fleeting macular rash; hepatosplenomegaly; lymphadenopathy; pericarditis; pleuritis, abdominal pain; multiple small and large joints affected; outlook variable, with severe arthritis in 25%.	Negative RF Negative ANA

From Servonsky/Opas: *Nursing Management of Children*, © 1987 Boston: Jones and Bartlett Publishers.

When examining the musculoskeletal system, you should also be alert to the signs and symptoms of fractures, including pain with acute tenderness over the site of the fracture, edema and bruising, deformity and possible shortening of a part, and limitation of movement. The elderly, whose bones tend to become more porous and brittle with decreasing circulatory nutrition, are particularly prone to fractures. The tumbling preschooler is also prone to fractures, especially of the clavicle, as are school-age and college students who are active in sports.

Chronic bone pain is present in such conditions as osteoporosis, neoplasms, hyperparathyroidism, Legg-Calvé-Perthes disease, and Paget's disease.

Joints

Disease within or outside of a joint can cause limitation of joint movement. The disease process is within the joint if joint movement is uniformly restricted in all directions. Limitation of movement in only one direction is usually the result of bony or soft tissue block outside the joint.

Technique for Inspection and Palpation of the Bones

1. Observe client from front, side, and back.
2. Ask client to straighten and hold back shoulders.
3. Ask client to bend over at the waist.
4. Palpate all bones for tenderness, pain.

A joint is considered unstable if motion can be carried through a greater than normal range. Excessive motion ordinarily occurs in only one direction and results from injury to a specific ligament or ligaments, as in a sprain. Joints should be carefully palpated at the points of attachment of the various ligaments to pinpoint identification of the injured ligament, because the point of maximum tenderness indicates the site of injury. Massive instability of a joint, permitting grotesque motion, is characteristic of neurologic diseases. This type of condition can be seen in the Charcot's joints associated with tabes dorsalis and occasionally with diabetic neu-

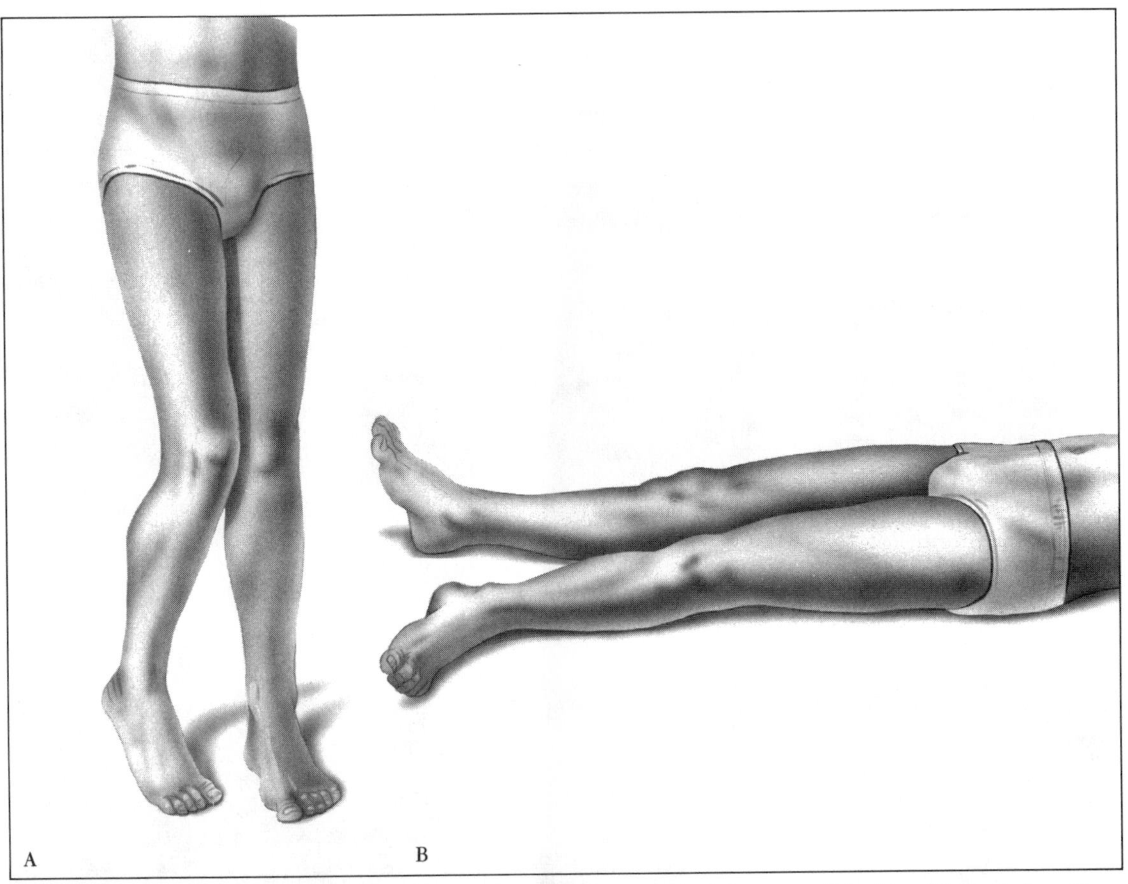

Figure 17-6 Hip deformities. (A) Characteristic position of traumatic dislocation of the hip. (B) Typical position assumed in fracture of the left hip.

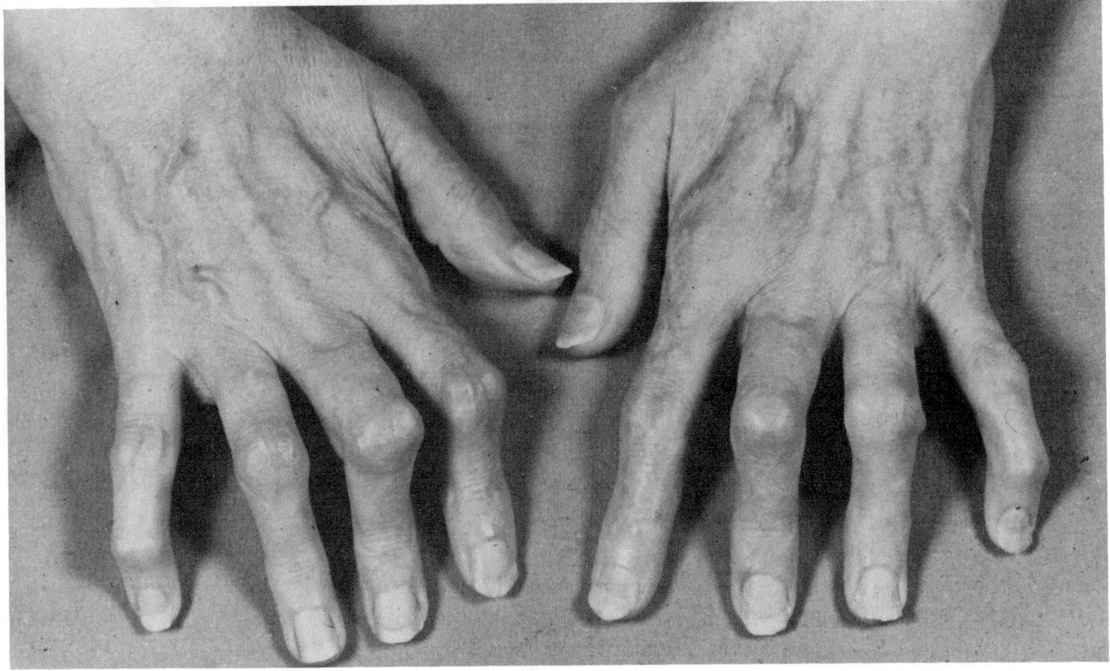

Figure 17-7 Arthritic hands. Note distortion and swelling, particularly the proximal interphalangeal joints.

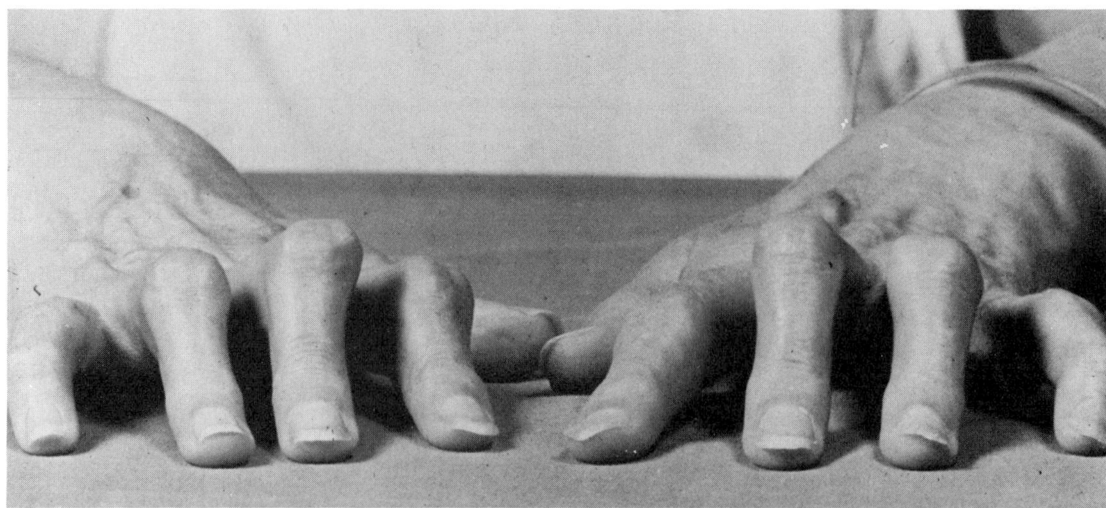

Figure 17-8 Arthritic hands. Note retraction of fingers.

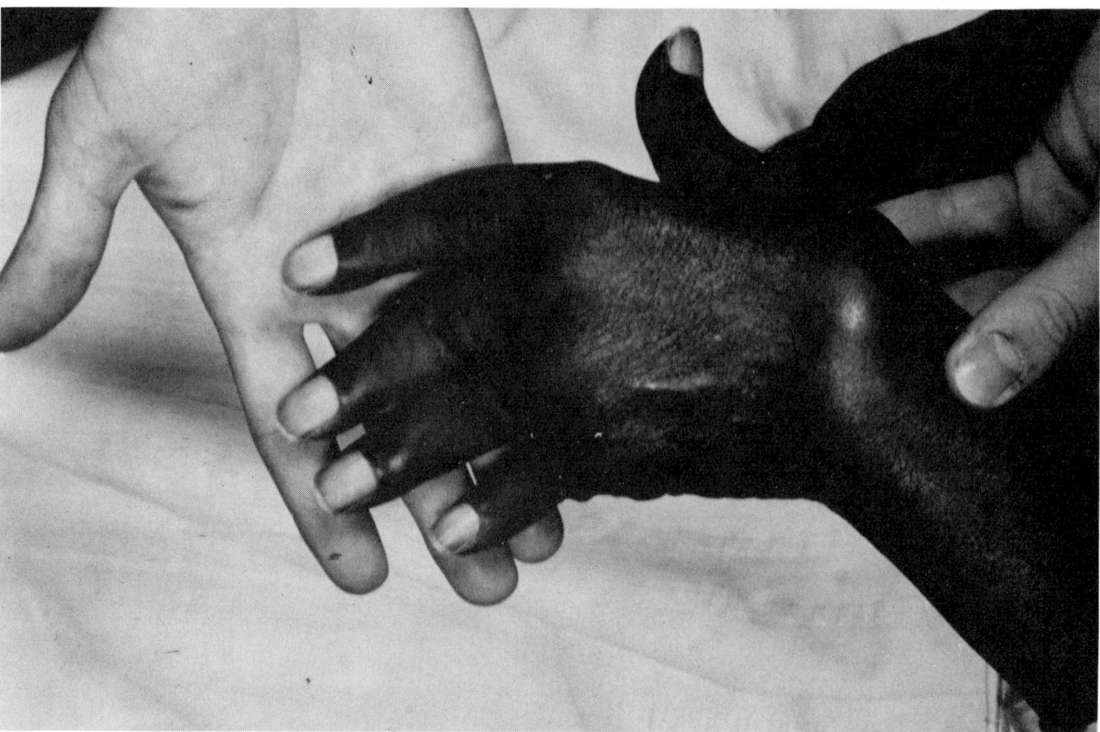

Figure 17-9 Arthritic hand. Note the characteristic ulnar deviation.

ropathy. Note the unusual alignment (in Figure 17-13) as the client supports himself on such joints. Hyperflexibility of joints is a hereditary trait, and people with this condition are referred to as double jointed or loose jointed. There is a rare condition in which clients exhibit generalized hyperflexibility called the Ehlers-Danlos syndrome.

Swelling of a joint may be caused by fluid within the joint or within an overlying bursa.

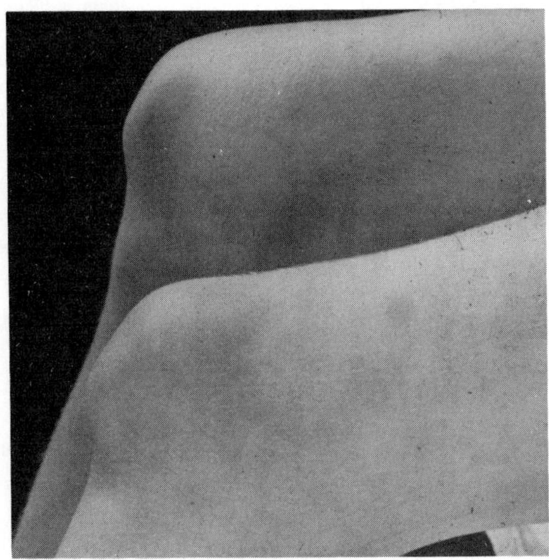

Figure 17-10 Nodular appearance of arthritic knees.

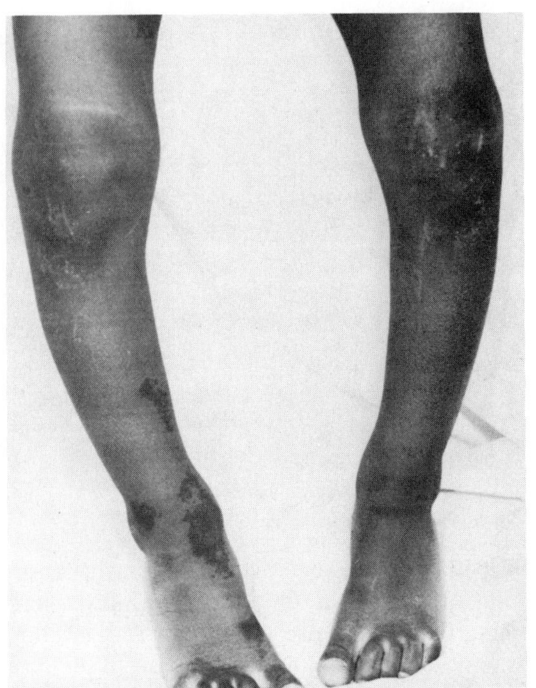

Figure 17-12 Rickets disease. Note bowing of legs.

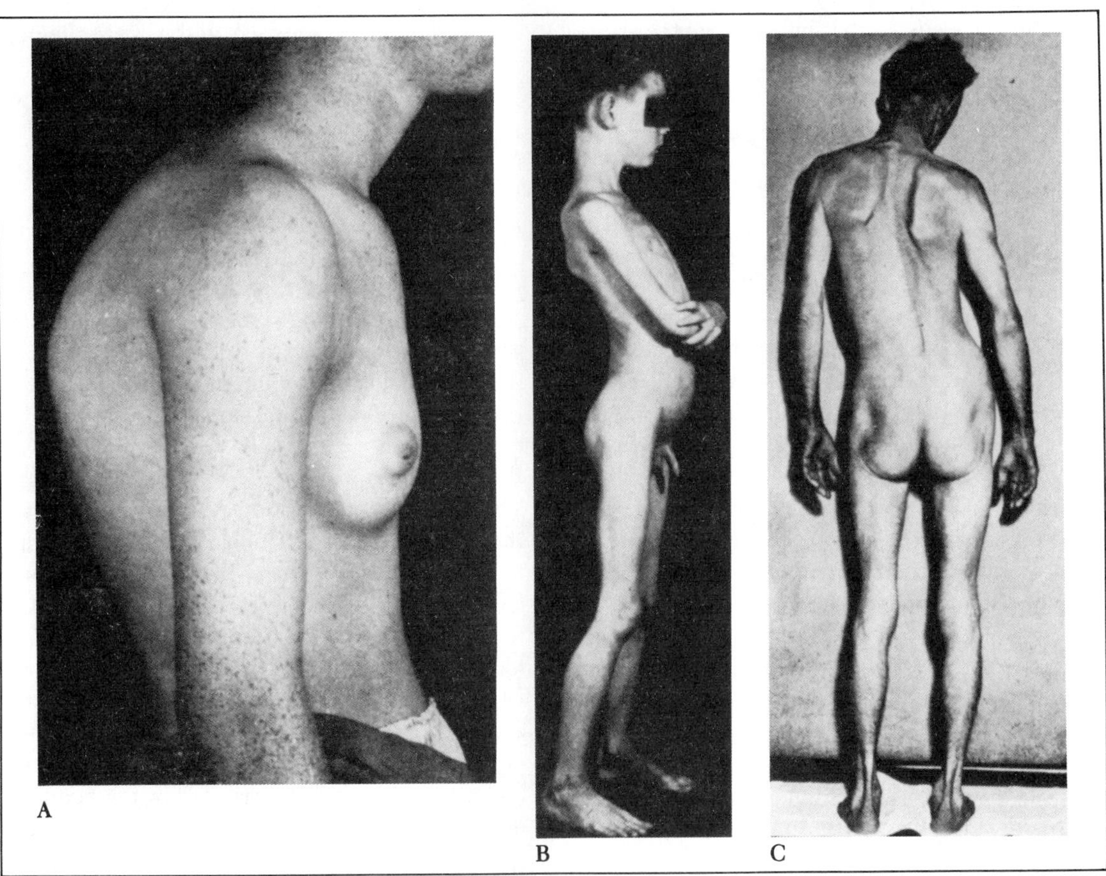

Figure 17-11 Spinal deviations. (A) Kyphoses. (B) Lordosis. (C) Scoliosis.

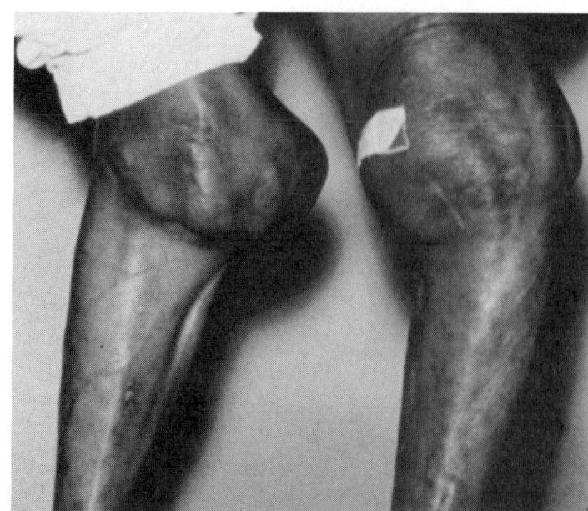

Figure 17-13 Charcot's joints in a patient with tabes dorsalis.

Palpation will reveal swelling over the entire joint area when the fluid exists within the joint and a smaller sharply localized area of swelling when the fluid is in a bursa. A rise in the local skin temperature about a joint suggests inflammation. Crepitus is a crackling that can be heard, or it may be palpated as a grating sensation, or both, when the joint is moved through its range of motion. It occurs with roughening of the articular surfaces and also is found in stenosing tenosynovitis. Crepitation may be heard on movement of a complete fracture in which the bone is completely severed; it is heard on movement of the ends of the broken bone at the fracture site.

The knee joint is a site of frequent traumatic and medical disorders throughout life because it is vulnerable, particularly for athletes. Swelling of the knee within several hours following an injury usually implies inflammatory effusion. Swelling minutes after trauma suggests a laceration of tissues with blood in the joint. The client with a locked knee (limitation of complete extension) usually relates a history of something slipping in the knee accompanied by pain in the lateral or medial region and the inability to extend the joint. Also in the area of the knee, three types of discrete masses can be noted:

1. Popliteal cysts, found in the posterolateral and posteromedial aspect. These cysts occur in children and adults and are often termed Baker's cyst.
2. Cysts of the lateral semilunar cartilage, which are in close proximity to the lateral joint compartment.
3. Synoviomata, which are neoplasms arising from normal or abnormal synovial elements.

All joints should be assessed for tenderness, bogginess, swelling, thickening, crepitation, and nodules.

Inspection and Palpation

The following joints (see Figure 17-14) are routinely inspected and palpated:

1. *Temporomandibular joints*—inspect, palpate, and listen for crepitation as client opens and closes his mouth (see Figure 17-15).
2. *Neck*—inspect and note suppleness of movement.
3. *Interphalangeal, intermetacarpal, and carpal bones and joints*—inspect and palpate.
4. *Elbows*—inspect and, with the elbow mildly flexed, palpate the groove on either side of the olecranon process with close attention to the epitrochlear lymph nodes at the medial, inner aspects of the elbow.
5. *Shoulders*—inspect and palpate sternoclavicular joint, acromioclavicular joint, and the head of the humerus.
6. *Hips*—inspect length of legs as well as alignment and palpate areas for tenderness.
7. *Patellar areas*—inspect and palpate the popliteal space, and then have the client sit to palpate both sides of each patella and the suprapatellar pouch (see Figure 17-16).
8. *Ankles and feet*—inspect and palpate for tenderness.
9. *Vertebral column and thoracic cage*—Inspect, noting any difference in the height of the scapulae and the iliac crests. Inspect for straightness of the spine from the back as the client bends forward to touch his toes. Next palpate along the spinous processes and ribs for tenderness or muscle spasm.

Range of Joint Motion

The range of joint motion is a pertinent part of the assessment of the musculoskeletal system. Ask the client to actively put his body through various movements as you note the extent of movement and the smoothness and ease of performance. Normally you should observe smoothness and little effort exerted on the part of the client. Figures 17-17 through 17-24 show the normal range of motion for each joint. Positive characteristics may be disrupted by joint damage or deformity, muscular dysfunction, or neurologic problems. Next, passively manipulate the client's joints through range of motion. Record any resistance or limitation in movement.

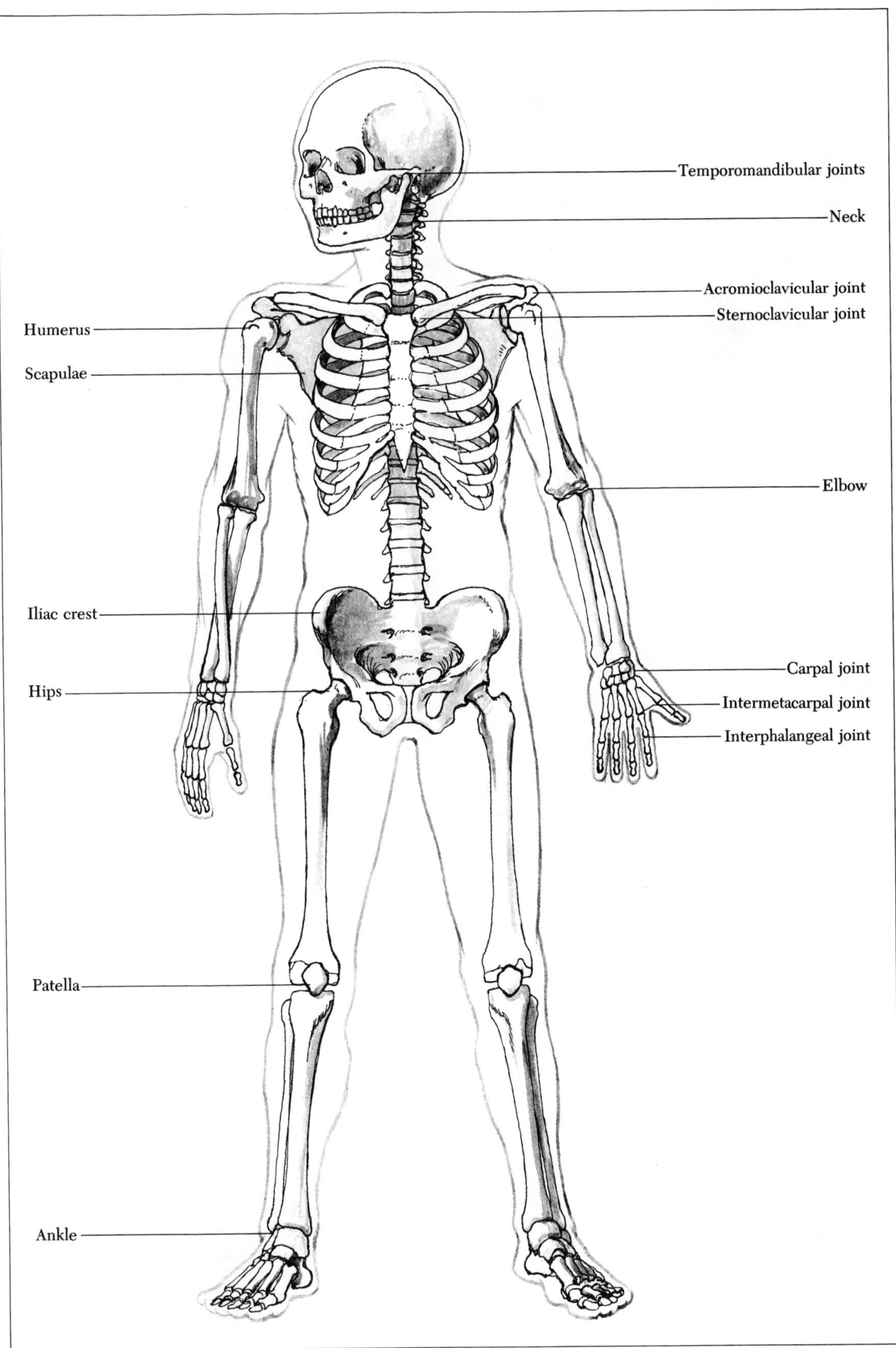

Figure 17-14 The major joints of the body.

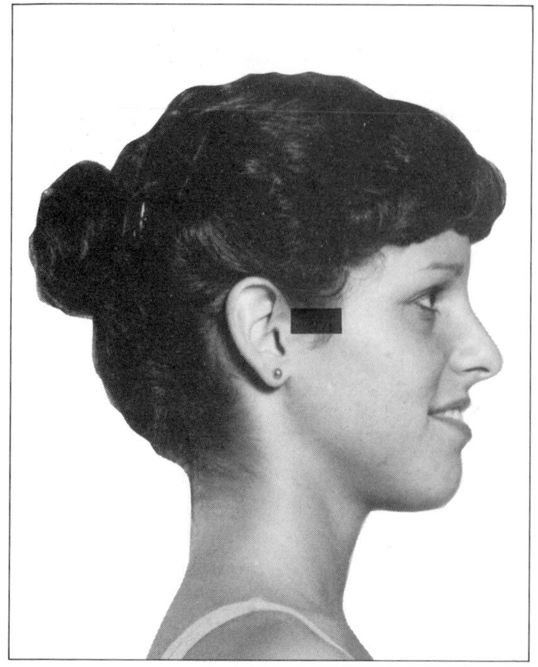

Figure 17-15 Location of the temporomandibular joint.

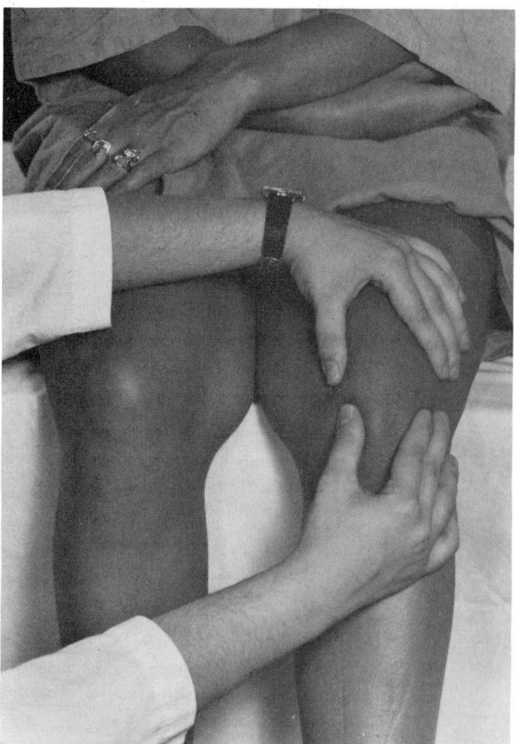

Figure 17-16 Palpation of the knee. With the client seated and her leg allowed to hang loosely, palpate the articulation between the thumb and index finger of your right hand. To test for effusion, apply compression above the patella with your left hand. If fluid is present, it is forced down and causes a bulge below and on either side of the patella.

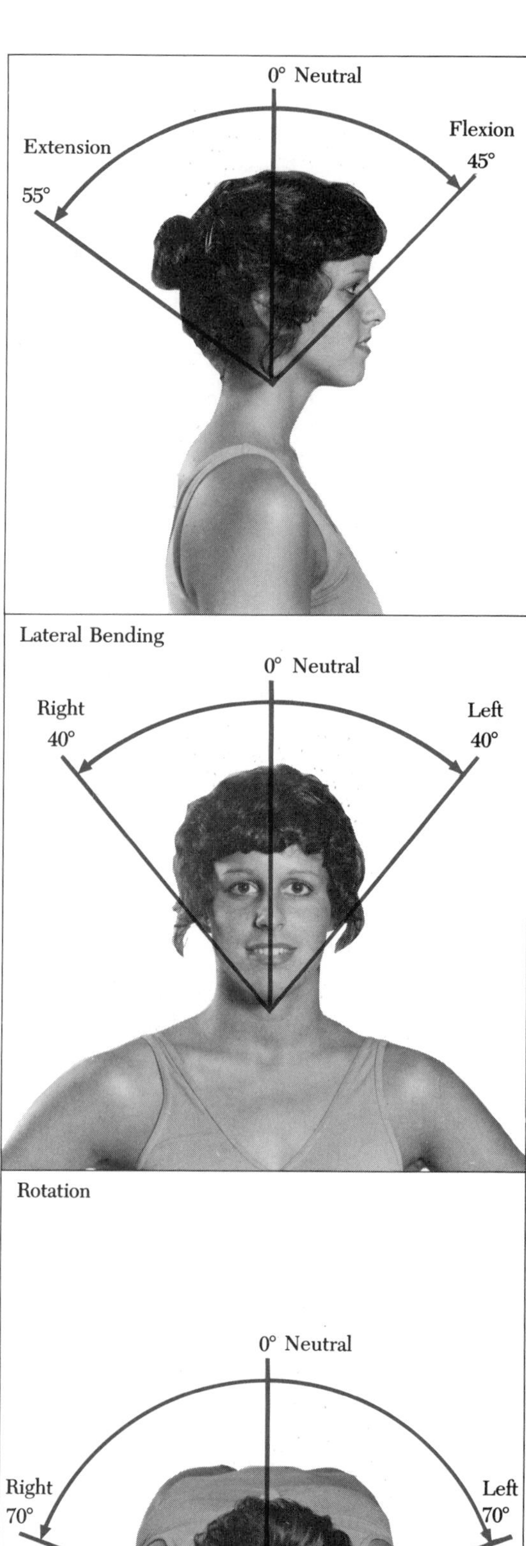

Figure 17-17 Range of motion of the neck.

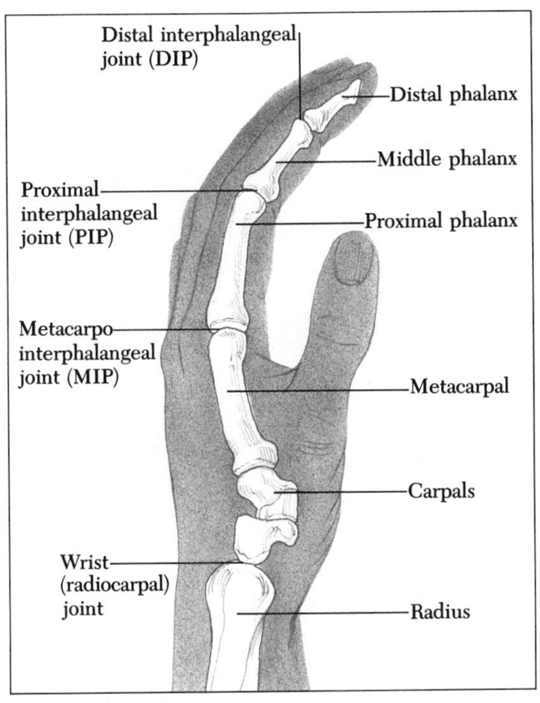

A

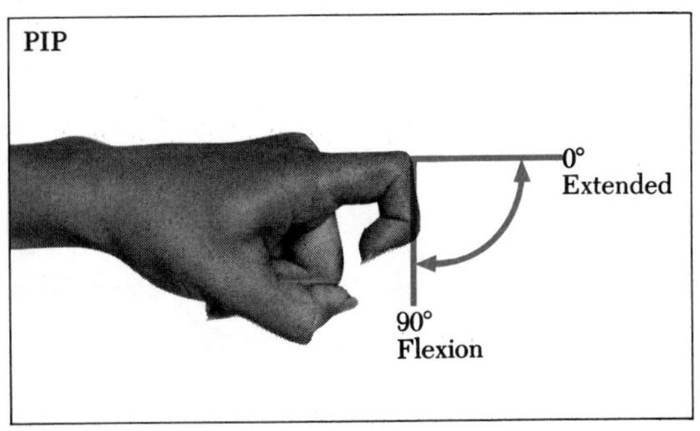

D

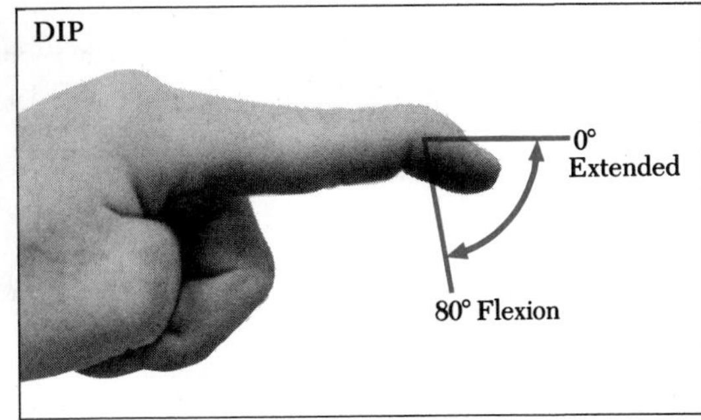

E

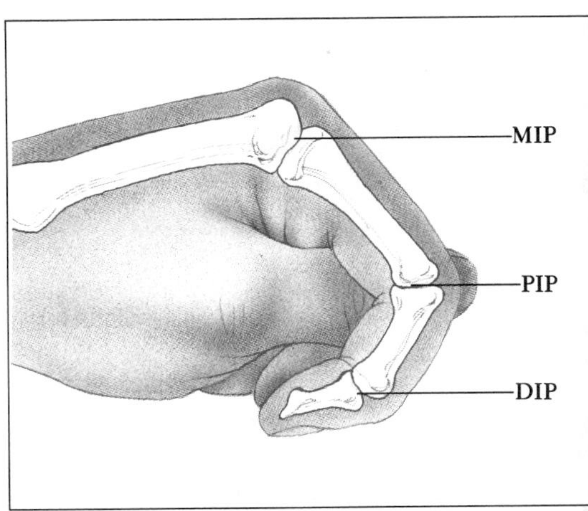

B

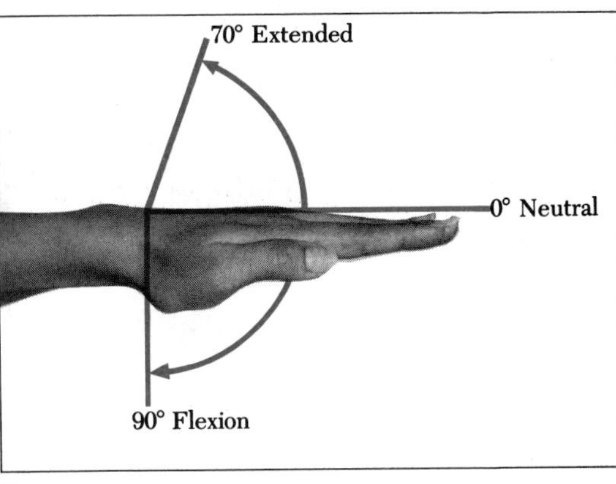

F

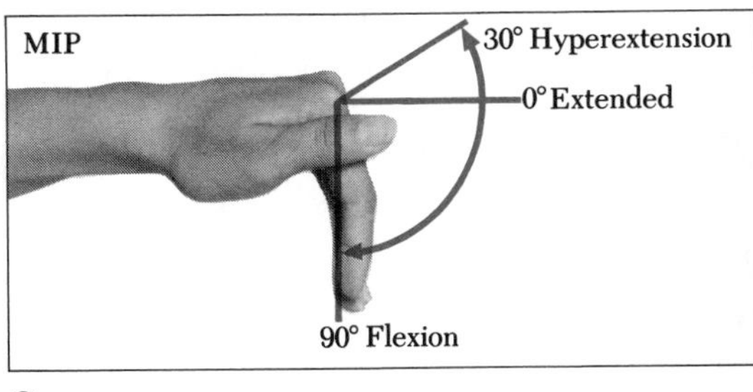

C

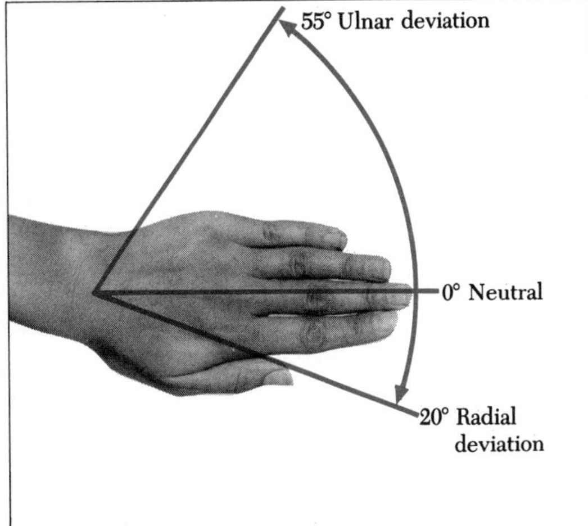

G

Figure 17-18 Location and range of motion of the interphalangeal, intermetacarpal, and carpal joints and bones. (A) Basic joints of the hand. (B) Normal fist. (C, D, E) Range of movement of finger joints. (F, G) Range of wrist motion.

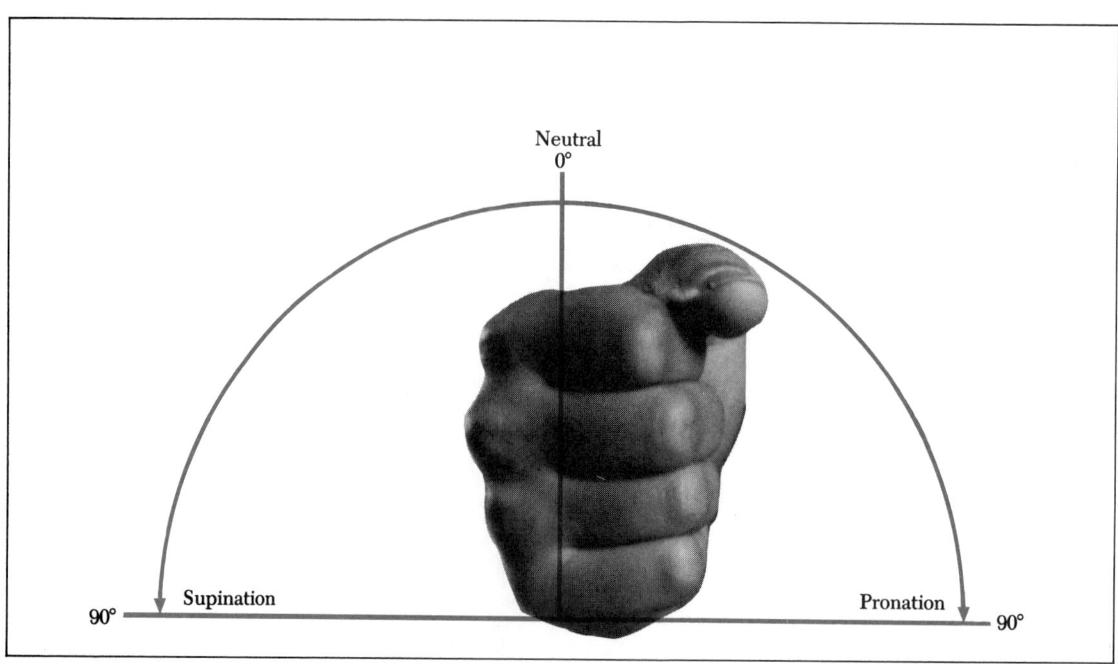

160° Flexion
0° Extended

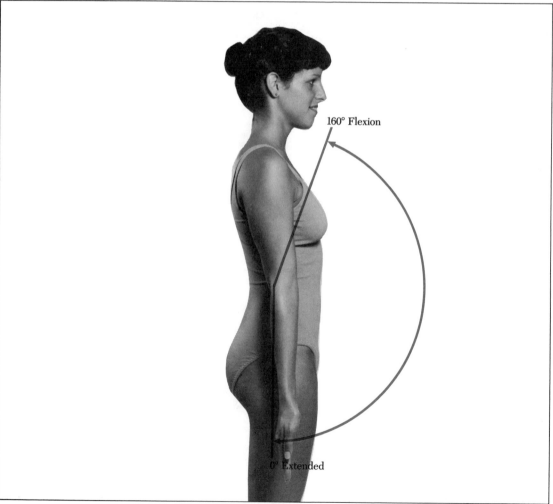

Figure 17-19 Range of motion of the elbow.

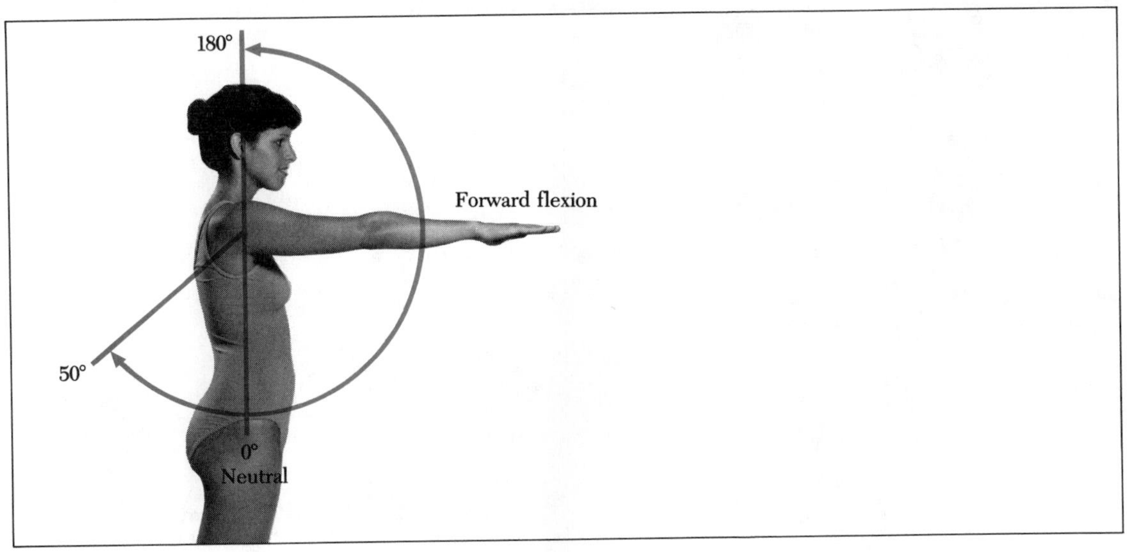

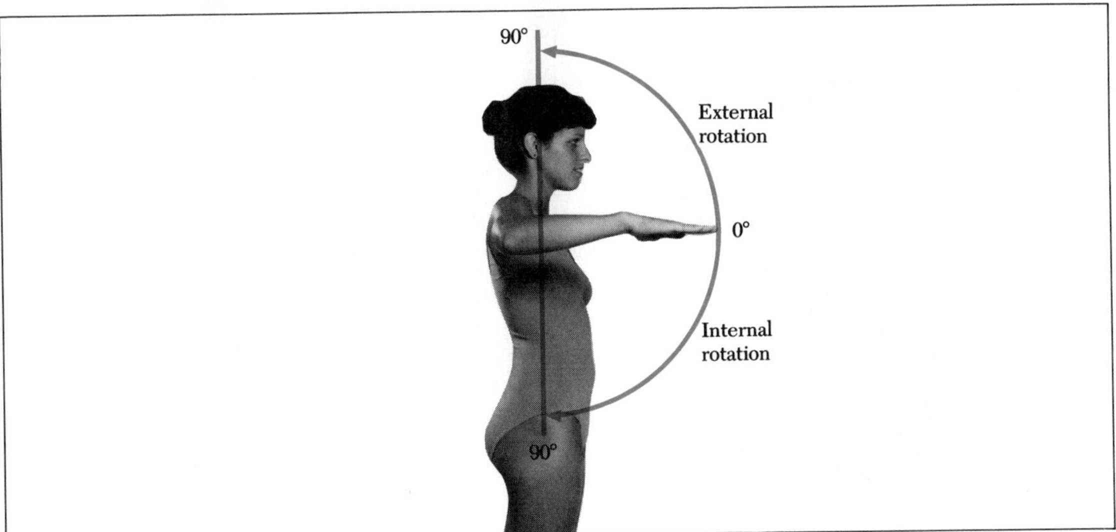

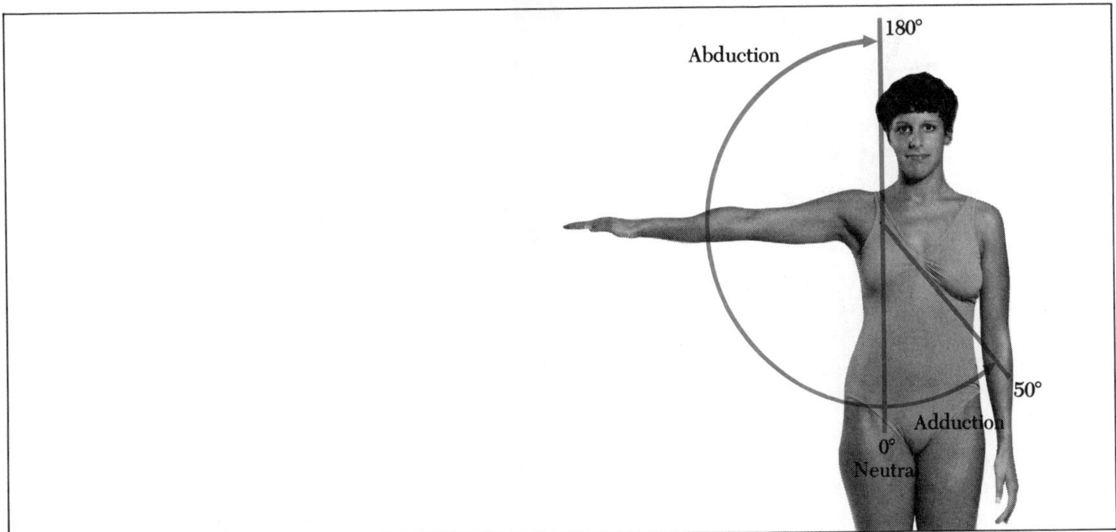

Figure 17-20 Range of motion of the shoulder.

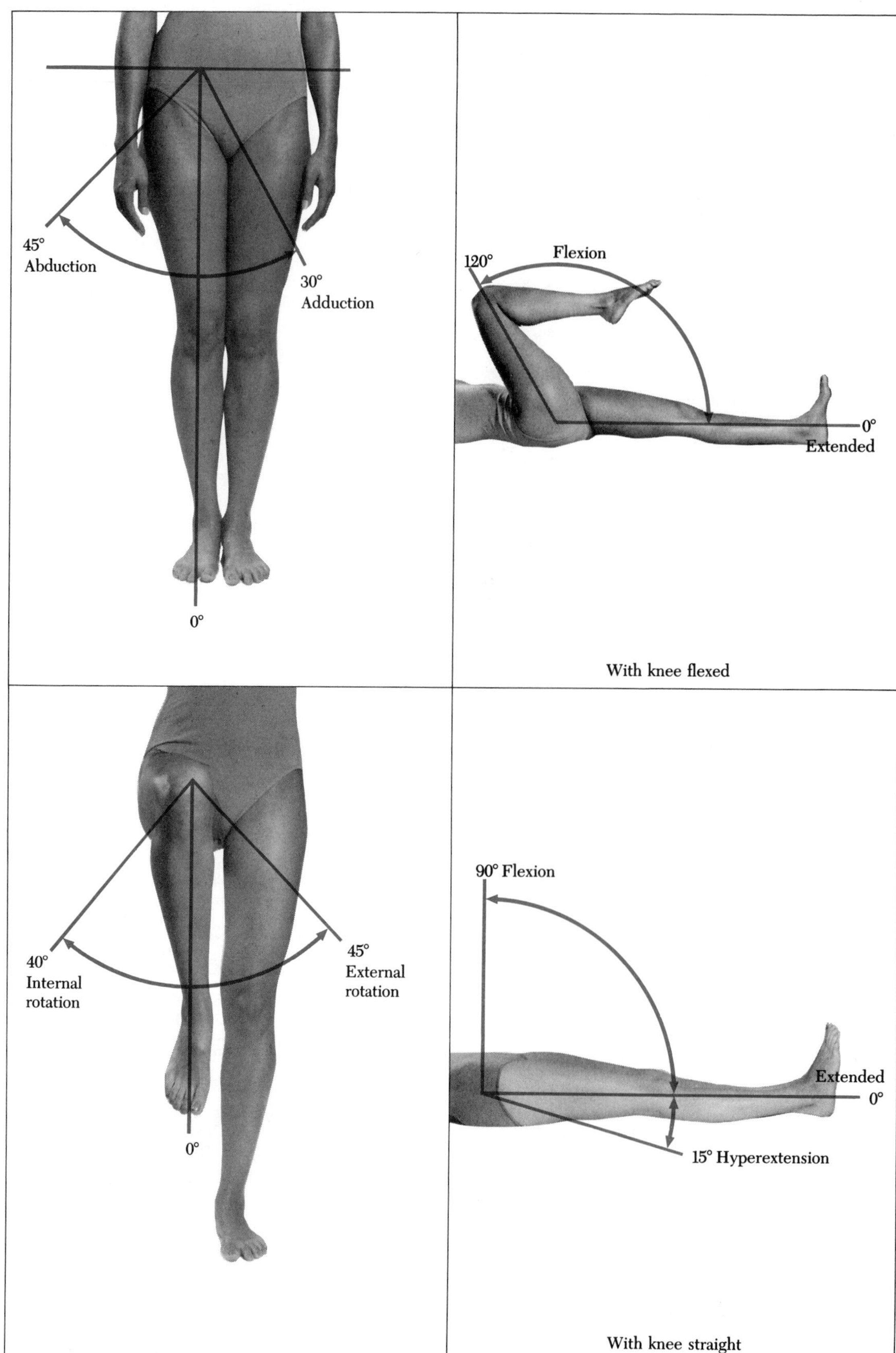

Figure 17-21 Range of motion of the hip.

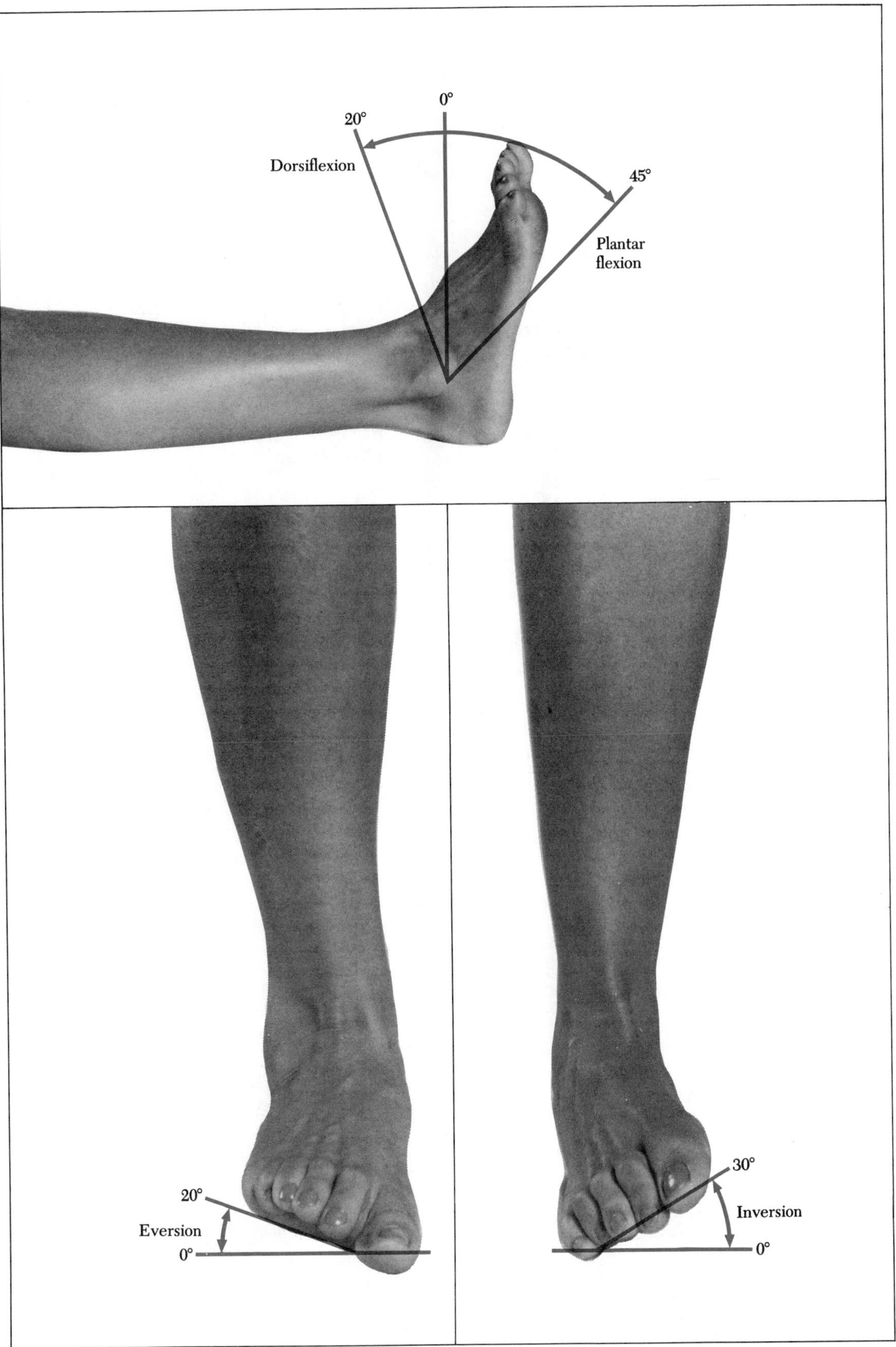

Figure 17-22 Range of motion of the ankle and foot.

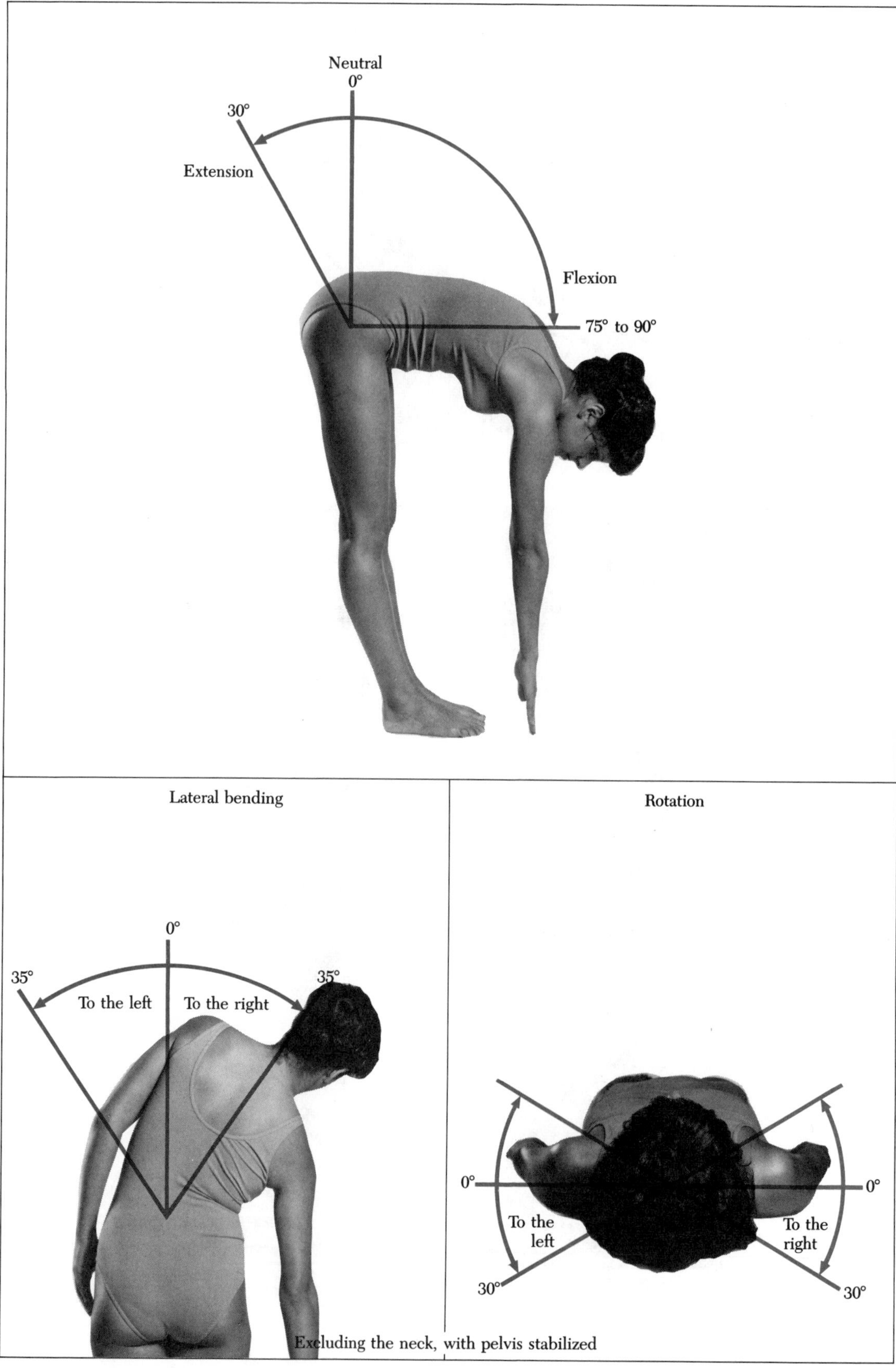

Figure 17-23 Range of motion of the spine.

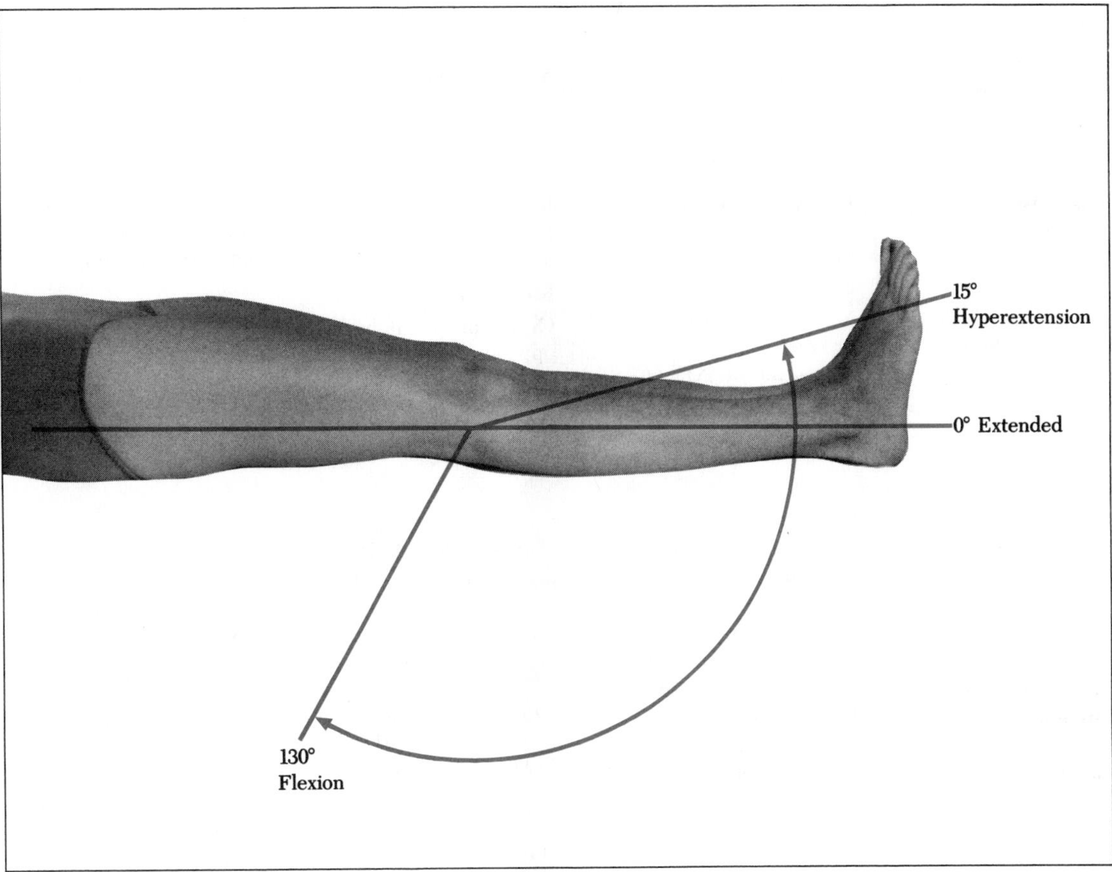

Figure 17-24 Range of motion of the knee.

There are several means of documenting joint motion. The easiest and best is to note the comparison between the corresponding joints of the client. You may also use your own range of movement as a gauge if you have no limitations. A standard method is based on the neutral position of a joint (when the extremity is extended) being zero degrees (0°). Tables that list degrees of range of joint motion are useful; however, you need to realize that there are differences between individuals and between age groups. Joint motion can also be measured with a goniometer, a device that incorporates a protractor.

Sports injuries and nursing management are delineated in Table 17-3. Common signs and symptoms resulting from musculoskeletal involvement are fasciculations, tremors, and acute and chronic bone pain. Characteristics and comments regarding these signs and symptoms, deformities, and disease states affecting the musculoskeletal system are listed in Table 17.4.

Technique for Inspection and Palpation of the Joints

1. Inspect and palpate:
   Temporomandibular joints
   Neck
   Interphalangeal, intermetacarpal, carpal bones and joints
   Elbows
   Shoulders
   Hips
   Patellar areas
   Ankles and feet
   Vertebral column and thoracic cage
2. Range of motion:
   Active
   Passive

Table 17-3. Sports Injuries

Injury	Etiology	Behavioral assessment	Medical therapy	Nursing management
Acute Injuries				
Knee				
Contusion	Blunt force to soft tissue; common in gymnastics, hockey	Ecchymosis, edema, tenderness *Mild*—full ROM 24 hr later *Moderate*—½ ROM 24 hr later *Severe*—⅓ ROM 24 hr later	Ice Compression wrap ankle to thigh Elevation Crutch or cane in hand opposite side of injury	Demonstrate correct application of compression wrap.
Sprain	Force is exerted that exceeds normal range of motion: *Mild*—few fibers of ligaments torn *Moderate*—ligament torn, some functional loss *Severe*—fibers completely torn	*Mild*—pain, swelling; joint stable with no locking *Moderate*—pain, swelling, limitation of movement; join stable but may lock *Severe*—pain, immediate swelling; joint unstable and may lock	*Mild*—ice for 24–28 hr, aspirin, activity limited as necessary *Moderate*—knee immobilizer splint 2–3 weeks; exercises: 10 straight leg lifts per hour while awake, quad sets, ROM; resume sports 6–8 weeks *Severe*—surgical repair of ligaments; cast 3–4 weeks; no weight bearing; may be 6–10 months before resuming sports	Assess neurovascular status of affected leg. Apply ice and elevate leg. Reinforce explanations regarding purpose of knee immobilizers, compression wraps, casts. Demonstrate correct application of immobilizers, compression wrap. Explain cast care. Demonstrate crutch walking, if needed. Demonstrate leg lifts, isometric exercises. Give specific explanations regarding limitations of movement.
Cruciate ligaments	Hyperextension or excessive external rotation on anterior ligament, especially with abrupt stops Fall on flexed knee injures posterior ligament	"Pop" as knee gives way		
Collateral ligaments	Valgus stress to knee injures medial collateral ligament Varus stress injuries lateral collateral ligament	Tearing, ripping sound		

Table 17-3. *Continued*

Injury	Etiology	Behavioral assessment	Medical therapy	Nursing management
Acute Injuries				
Meniscal tears	Vigorous rotation of femur on tibia Internal rotation injures medial meniscus External rotation injures lateral meniscus	Sudden and severe pain Click heard when rotating tibia on femur when knee is flexed Inability to extend joint fully Swelling Occasionally knee locks Buckling during walking	*Conservative*—evacuate joint of intraarticular fluid; ice 24–36 hr followed by heat; avoidance of weight bearing; quadriceps exercises *Surgical*—Removal of meniscus surgically; ice, compression dressing, elevation of affected leg; quadriceps setting exercises beginning on 2nd day postoperatively, done 10–15 min 3–4 times daily; progress to straight leg raising; return to sports within 10 weeks. Immobilization in extension for 4–6 weeks May require surgery to repair Quadriceps exercises	Demonstrate exercises. Teach crutch walking or use of cane. Postoperatively, apply ice; elevate extremity; assess neurovascular status.
Patellar dislocation	Lateral (valgus) rotation stress or direct blow to medial aspect of knee	Buckling Pain in medial aspect of knee Can feel knee "go out of place" but return to normal when leg is extended Excessive movement of patella is possible in lateral direction Crepitation between patella and femoral groove Reports having heard sound "like canvas ripping" at time of injury	Immobilization in extension for 4–6 weeks May require surgery to repair Quadriceps exercises	
Shoulder Dislocation	Force causing excessive abduction, extension, and external rotation Humerus is displaced anteriorly and inferiorly	Pain Humeral head palpable in anterior axilla	With child lying prone on examination table and arm suspended over side, sustained anterior traction (toward floor) is manually applied	Assess for injury of axillary nerve by testing for sensation where deltoid inserts on humerus and by asking child to attempt to abduct arm. Assess for ulnar nerve injury by asking child to abduct and adduct the four medial digits. Administer analgesic prior to reduction procedure.

(continued on page 366)

Table 17-3. *Continued*

Injury	Etiology	Behavioral assessment	Medical therapy	Nursing management
Acute Injuries				
Ankle Sprain	Violent force at high speed exceeding normal range of motion: *Mild*—ligament stretched but not torn *Moderate*—ligament partially torn *Severe*—ligament(s) completely torn	"Pop" or "snap" heard with injury Obvious deformity Swelling Pain when moved through range of motion Discoloration at joint	Ice or cold water applied during acute phase Compression bandages or tape strapping Crutches After 48 hr, contrast baths or whirlpool	Apply ice and elevate leg. Apply compression bandage. Demonstrate both non-weight-bearing and weight-bearing gaits on crutches. Demonstrate ROM exercises.
Leg Quadriceps contusion	Excessive force applied usually to anterior or anterolateral portion of muscle	Decreased ability to bend knee Occasionally, a palpable hematoma is present; discoloration after 48 hr	Ice Compression bandage Crutches or bedrest Rehabilitation exercises: quadriceps contractions, ROM exercises	Apply ice. Apply compression bandage. Demonstrate crutch walking. Demonstrate exercises.
Overuse Injuries				
Achilles tendinitis	Repeated forcible stretching of short Achilles tendon	Pain usually around tendon itself when exercising or when plantar flexing the foot	*For all overuse injuries:* Rest, decreased training activities, alternate exercise such as cycling instead of running, crutches or casting for 4–5 days	*For all overuse injuries:* Stress the need to change those activities that brought on the pain of the injury. Teach stretching exercises:
Stress fractures	Repeated stress, usually in tibia	Swelling in area of fracture Limp Pain may be sharp and persistent or dull and aching Tenderness over a specific point	Stretching exercises Restrengthening exercises Ice for 30–40 min over injury Whirlpool at 10°–20°C Alternate cold with heat Ultrasound	1. Stretch affected muscle for 15–20 sec almost to where pain occurs. 2. Relax 15–20 sec. 3. Repeat 5–6 times at least 3 times daily or as ordered. Teach restrengthening exercises:
Plantar fascitis	Repeated stretching of plantar fascia	Pain in arch or heel Limp Walks on lateral aspect of foot	Tape strapping, splints, braces High-intensity galvanic stimulation Aspirin 2–3 tablets 4 times daily	*Isometric* 1. Tighten involved muscle for 8–10 sec. 2. Relax briefly. 3. Repeat 8–10 times at least 3 times daily or as ordered.

Table 17-3. *Continued*

Injury	Etiology	Behavioral assessment	Medical therapy	Nursing management
Overuse Injuries				
Anterior leg pain ("shin splints")	Repeated traction on anterior or posterior tibialis muscles	Pain and tenderness along middle or distal portions of tibia		*Isotonic* 1. Lift prescribed weight with affected muscle through range of motion for 3 sec. 2. Relax briefly. 3. Repeat 10 times at least 3 times daily or as ordered. Apply ice. Teach patient to check condition of skin beneath splints, braces daily. Review purpose and side effects of aspirin.

From Servonsky/Opas: *Nursing Management of Children* © 1987 Boston: Jones and Bartlett Publishers.

Table 17-4. Common Abnormalities of the Musculoskeletal System

Terminology	Characteristics	Comments
Fasciculations	Slight twitching in a resting muscle.	Frequently occurs. Associated with strain, muscle weakness, and atrophy. May be due to denervation of muscle fibers.
Tremors		
Resting tremor	Accentuated by rest. Diminishes upon movement. More rhythmic.	Seen in Parkinson's disease. Usually indicates basal ganglia disease.
Intention tremor	Increases with voluntary movement. Irregular movement.	Seen in multiple sclerosis. Could suggest cerebellar disease.
Flapping tremor	Hand falls momentarily, only to raise again.	Transient loss of extensor tone at the wrist. Seen in hepatic failure, hypercapnia, uremia.
Bone pain		
Acute	Localized tenderness. Redness, swelling, increased warmth. Intensified by movement, abnormal mobility, loss of function, bony crepitus.	Associated with trauma.
Chronic	Bone pain only symptom—no other physical signs.	Especially occurs in vertebrae and pelvic bones. Incidence increases with age, due to disuse, inadequate nutrition, and excessive loss of minerals.
Pain of multiple myeloma	Pain localized or general. On x-ray punched-out areas in bone. Anemia and high globulin levels in blood.	Invasion and destruction of bone and bone marrow by malignant cells. Most common malignant bone tumor. More frequent in men and in the sixth decade.
Osteoporosis	Back pain, loss of stature, "dowager's hump" from vertebral compression. Increase of fractures, particularly of hip.	Common in women past menopause. Results from inadequate calcium intake, insufficient exercise, and unknown effects of reduced steroid levels.

(continued on page 368)

Table 17-4. *Continued*

Terminology	Characteristics	Comments
Abnormal spinal curvatures		
Arthritis		
Osteoarthritis	Stiffness after periods of rest. Exacerbation of symptoms with changes in barometric pressure. Signs include joint crepitation and pain, limitation of motion, changes in shape of affected joints. Signs of inflammation minimal.	Increases in prevalence with age.
Rheumatoid arthritis	Morning stiffness, pain and swelling of joints, subcutaneous nodules, positive rheumatoid factor, typical x-ray joint changes.	Adult form develops insidiously. Specific cause unknown but generally believed that joint changes are related to antibody reaction.
Abnormal spinal curvatures		
Kyphosis	Excessive rounding of the back due to an increase in the posterior curvature of the thoracic spinal column.	Frequently associated with osteoporosis; ankylosing spondylitis. Senile kyphosis of osteoporosis caused by collapse and anterior wedging of thoracic vertebrae. Adolescent round back or juvenile kyphosis caused by epiphysitis of lower thoracic vertebrae or Scheuermann's disease. Occupationally induced.
Lordosis	Abnormal anterior convexity of lumbar spinal column.	Increased lordosis found in clients with spondylolysis, those with tight hamstring muscle. Also seen in clients with hip disease, especially congenital dislocation of hips, and in persons with flexion contractions of the hips who hyperextend lumbar spine to stand erect.
Scoliosis	Lateral curvature of spine.	Usually consists of two curves, the original abnormal curve and a compensatory curve in the opposite direction; most commonly idiopathic and occurs most frequently in adolescent girls.
Vitamin D deficiency	Defective mineralization of bone resulting in sides of thorax flattening, sternum protruding. Knobs on end of ribs (rachitic rosary). May have lordosis, kyphosis, scoliosis, liver and spleen enlargement, curvature of long bone.	Rickets (children). Osteomalacia (adults). Renal insufficiency.
Paget's disease	Chronic inflammation of bones, resulting in thickening, softening, and bowing of long bones.	Also called osteitis deformans. Among most common of chronic skeletal diseases of elderly.
Legg-Calvé-Perthes disease	Protective limp, limited movement of hip joint. Atrophy of thigh muscle.	Occurs in children, onset between ages 3 and 12. Occurs more often in boys.
Ankylosing spondylitis (Marie-Strümpell disease)	Stiff back, gradual ankylosis with kyphosis, involvement of sacroiliac and spinal apophyseal joints. Decreased chest expansion.	Affects young men, familial. Measure chest expansion at nipple line (4ICS level). Normal expansion for young adults is at least 5 cm.

Table 17-4. *Continued*

Terminology	Characteristics	Comments
Osteogenesis imperfecta	Blue sclera, early deafness, multiple fractures—"loose" joints in some forms, backache.	Inherited disorder—autosomal dominant trait. Tendency to fracture decreases and often disappears later in life.
Gout	Podagra (of the foot or great toe) and weight-bearing joints affected; involves more joints as progresses. Tophi with joint destruction. Acute attacks, severe pain.	Occurs more frequently in males. Increased serum uric acid level.
Sickle cell disease	Acute crisis with bone and abdominal pain, fever, and shortness of breath. Edema of hands and feet. Tenderness of joints and limited range of motion.	Hereditary, chronic form of anemia. Frequency of gene that causes disease high in Mediterraneans and blacks. Physical and emotional stress can precipitate a crisis.
Acromegaly	Hypertrophy of articular cartilage and joint enlargement, particularly in fingers and knees. Elongation and enlargement of bones of extremities and certain head bones, especially frontal bones and jaws.	A chronic disease of middle age. First sign may be that client needs to buy a larger hat and gloves.

Summary

This chapter discussed the basic structure and function of the musculoskeletal system and described the characteristics and techniques used in the examination of the muscles, bones, and joints. Muscles must be examined for strength and joints examined for range of motion. The client should be checked for fasciculations, tremors, muscle tone, skeletal deformities, and bone tenderness.

Discussion Questions/Activities

1. What are the three specific structures of the musculoskeletal system that are examined during a routine physical assessment?
2. What areas of the body would you assess in regard to muscle strength? Perform this assessment, step by step.
3. What other aspects of the muscular system would you assess in addition to muscle strength?
4. Demonstrate the technique used to assess whether fluid is present in the knee joint.
5. Demonstrate how you would assess the nine joint areas of the body.
6. By what means can you assess and document range of joint motion?

Recording of Findings

Normal findings are recorded in the first box. Findings for a client diagnosed as having suffered a right cerebrovascular accident are recorded in the second box.

Normal	Right cerebrovascular accident
Muscles **INSPECTION** Symmetrical; no hypertropy or atrophy noted; no tremors; no fasciculations; no abnormal muscle movements. **PALPATION** No tenderness; proximal and distal strength equal. Good muscle tone upon palpation.	**Muscles** **INSPECTION** Atrophied fine muscles of left hand; left hemiplegia. **PALPATION** Strength good on right side with equal proximal and distal strength; muscle tone rigid on left side.
Bones **INSPECTION** Body and limb symmetry; no increase in normal spinal curvatures; no deformities. **PALPATION** No tenderness.	**Bones** **INSPECTION** Body and limb symmetry; no increase in normal spinal curvatures; no deformities. **PALPATION** No tenderness.
Joints **INSPECTION** Full range of movement—smooth without limitations; no swelling. **PALPATION** No tenderness; no crepitation.	**Joints** **INSPECTION** Full active range of movement on right side; full passive range of movement on left side; no swelling. **PALPATION** No tenderness; no crepitation.

CHAPTER 18

Assessment of the Neurologic System

LEARNING OBJECTIVES

1. State the primary functions of the frontal, parietal, occipital, and temporal lobes.
2. State the various sensory modalities and explain how to test for them.
3. Describe the difference between expressive and receptive aphasia.
4. Describe tests used to evaluate balance and coordination.
5. Name the 12 cranial nerves and explain how each is evaluated.
6. Name the site for percussion of each of the deep tendon reflexes (DTRs).
7. Interpret reflex findings and categorize into appropriate grading scale.
8. Name the superficial reflexes and the normal response for each.
9. Recognize common pathologic reflexes.
10. Compare the findings of upper motor neuron damage to those of lower motor neuron damage.

The extent of physical assessment of the neurologic system depends on the presence and type of signs and symptoms elicited during the health history. A health history that is negative for signs of dysfunction shortens the assessment procedure considerably, as you will understand better after reading about the assessment of the neurologic system. A detailed neurologic assessment may take from 2 to 3 hours. Such a long and tedious in-depth assessment may anger, frustrate, or fatigue the client. Therefore, you need to be aware of this fact and proceed in a tactful, kind, and understanding manner.

The areas assessed are the cerebrum, the cerebellum, the cranial nerves, and the neurologic reflexes. The assessment technique primarily employed in evaluating the neurologic system is inspection—observation of behavior and body movement. In other chapters structure and function are discussed first, followed by a section on characteristics and techniques of examination. In this chapter these aspects will be discussed simultaneously because, more so than with any other physiologic system, the techniques of examining the neurologic system are relatively simple. It is the complexity of the functioning of the neurologic system that is difficult to understand; therefore, it is necessary to provide a great deal of discussion of the structure and physiologic functioning of a part of the neurological system to enable an understanding of the scientific rationale for, in many cases, one simple observation.

Within the neurologic system the major areas of the cerebrum, cerebellum, brain stem, and spinal cord are assessed. The *cerebrum* is the major portion of the human brain; it is responsible for sensations, voluntary actions, thoughts, and personality. The *cerebellum* is located at the posterior aspect and inferior to the cerebrum. It controls coordination and equilibrium. Within the *brain stem* are the respiratory and vasomotor centers, which regulate respirations and heart rate and blood pressure respectively. These functions are generally evaluated during assessment of the respiratory and cardiovascular systems. The majority of the cranial nerve nuclei are housed in the brain stem; it is during neurologic assessment that these are tested and evaluated. The *spinal cord* is the communication line through which impulses and messages are transmitted to and from the brain. When assessing this area, you will become aware of the functioning of the sensory and motor tracts, the reflex arc, and the end areas in the cerebrum.

Assessment of the Cerebrum

The four distinct areas of the cerebrum are the frontal, parietal, occipital, and temporal lobes.

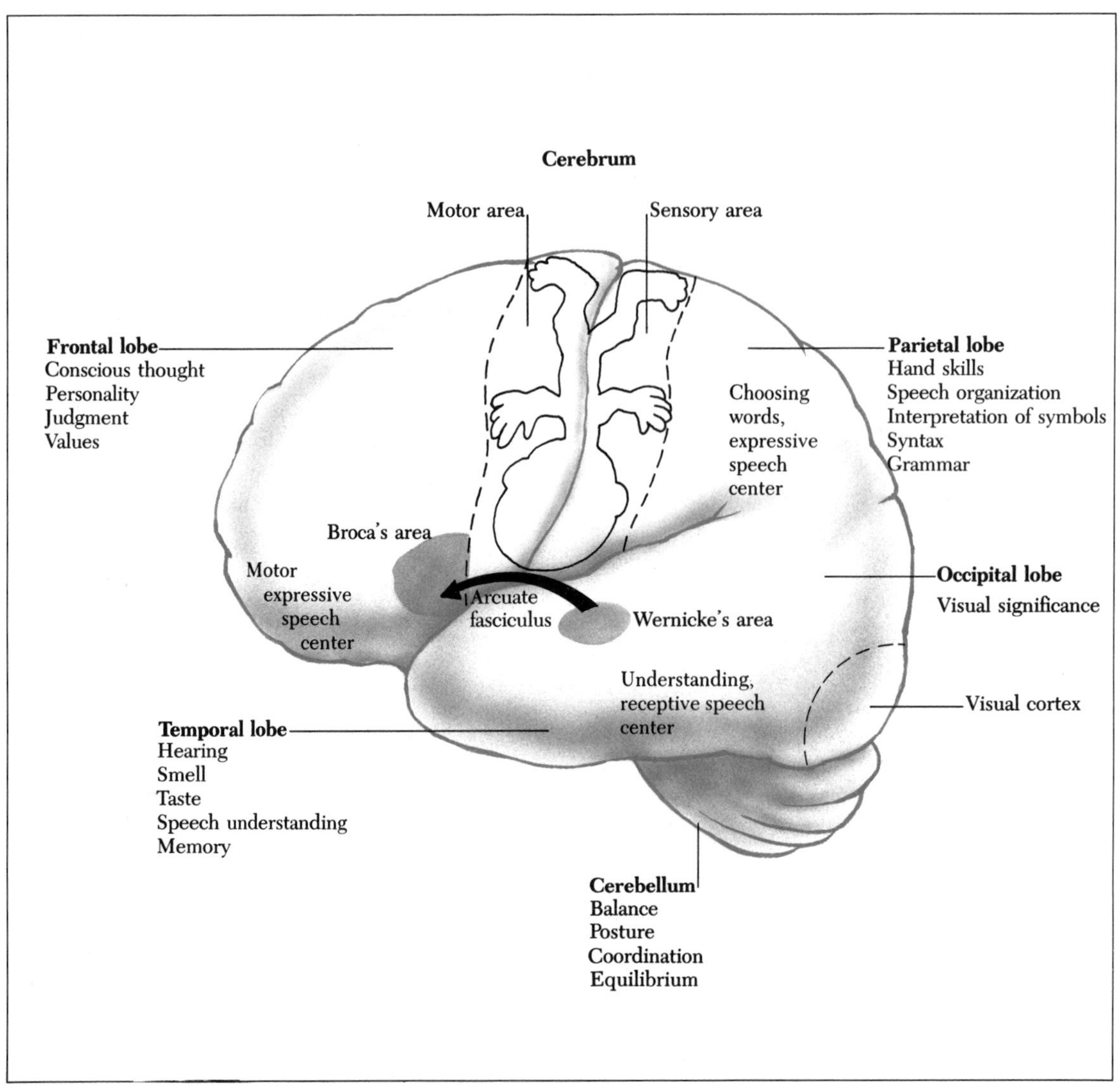

Figure 18-1 Functions of the cerebrum and cerebellum, including three major speech centers in the frontal, parietal, and temporal lobes.

Frontal Lobe Areas

As Figure 18-1 shows, the frontal lobes are responsible for higher thought functions and for regulating personality and behavior. The key function of the frontal lobe is to regulate cortical tone—in other words, the state of consciousness. Dysfunction of the anterior portion of the frontal lobes may produce alternating personality/mood/attitude changes or may result in difficulties in thought content, learning, decision making, and the ability to generalize or to perform mathematical computations. Thus, interpersonal relationships and the management of one's household or employment are commonly disrupted. A client with frontal lobe pathology may display behaviors that range from apathy to preoccupation with self to irritability, hostility, suspicion, or grandiose ideation. The individual may become quite rigid and may be difficult to deal with because of impaired reasoning. The individual also is not able to adequately assess the emotionality of others in a given situation. For instance, he cannot detect when another person is sad. This places him at a social disadvantage. Emotional stress (anxiety, depression, psychosis) or physical stress (tumor, infarction, abscess, penetrating head wound) may be an etiological factor underlying such altered behavior. If you suspect cerebral dysfunction, you should conduct a meticulous mental status assessment employing the tests of cerebral function discussed in Chapter 5, Mental Health Assessment. It is noteworthy to comment that generalized convulsions occur in 50% of the clinical cases involving frontal lobe lesions. Therefore, precaution should be taken not to examine a client under artificial lighting that may be going bad. Lighting that tends to flicker may trigger convulsive seizures.

A *motor tract area* is located in the posterior portion of the frontal lobe. Each part of the body is represented by large pyramidal cells (motor neurons) in this tract. Figure 18-1 shows that the arrangement of these representative cells resembles an "upside-down" person, with the head and face areas just superior to the temporal lobes and constituting more than half of the motor tract; the remainder of the body is represented in the superior portion of the tract. Figure 18-2 illustrates how nerve fibers from the motor cortex tracts converge and descend through the *internal capsule*. Some motor nerve fibers project down the *corticobulbar tract* directly without crossing and end in the various

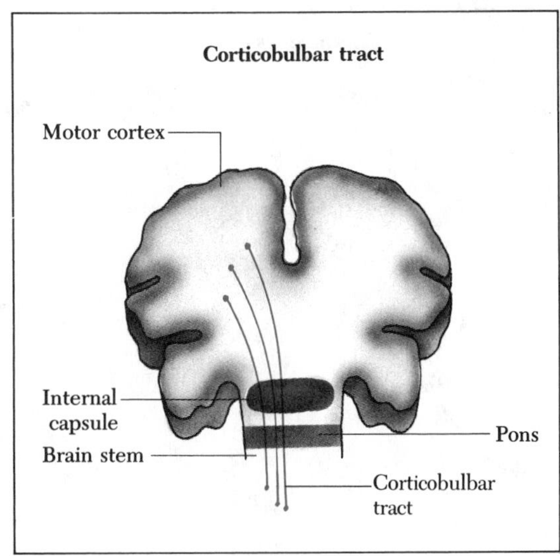

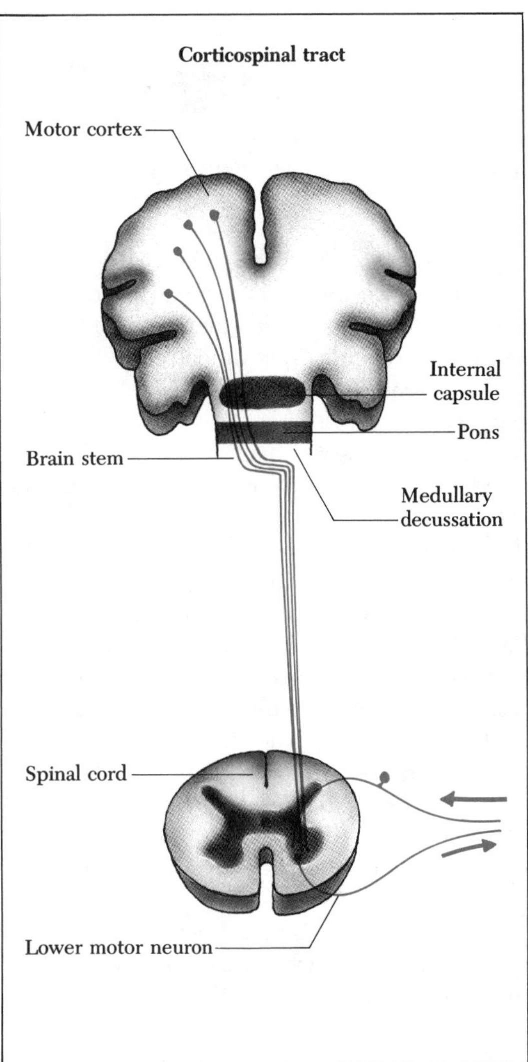

Figure 18-2 The corticobulbar tract and the corticospinal tract.

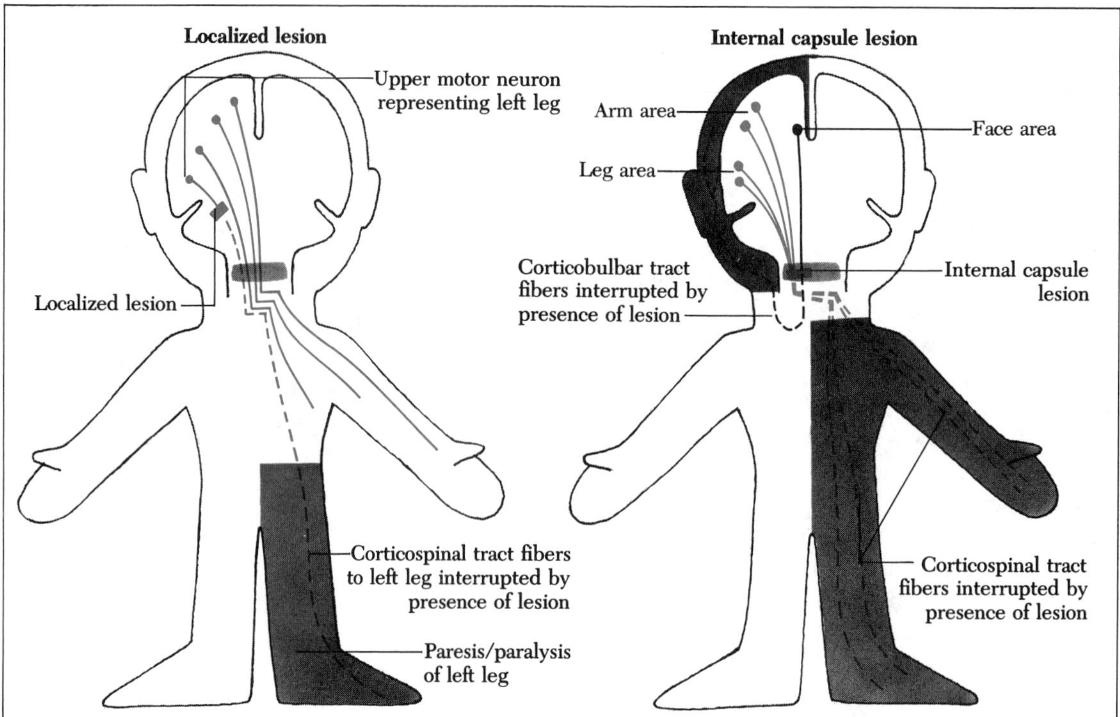

Figure 18-3 Localized and internal capsule lesion with corresponding paresis/paralysis areas of the body.

cranial nerve nuclei in the brain stem; others continue down the *corticospinal tract*, cross over in the lower medulla, and descend in the spinal cord, eventually terminating in the anterior gray motor horn of the spinal cord at all of the correlating levels from the cervical cord area through the sacral.

As Figure 18-3 illustrates, the extent and location of a lesion within the cerebral motor area determines the degree of paresis/paralysis experienced. A localized lesion of an isolated represented area of the cerebral motor tract confines the paresis/paralysis to that contralateral portion of the body, such as arm or leg weakness. A lesion involving the internal capsule disrupts all the neural fibers of the motor tract and results in ipsilateral paresis/paralysis of the face and contralateral hemiparesis. Thus you should make note of any weakness or lack of ability to move a body part as part of your assessment of frontal lobe function.

Irritation of the motor tract, such as by a slowgrowing meningioma, can initiate a jacksonian seizure beginning on the opposite side of the body. Observation of this type of seizure readily reveals the typical jacksonian march. Characteristically, clonic contractions start in one portion of the body, such as the face or fingers, and can march along to eventually include the entire half of the body and may even spread to the opposite side of the body, culminating in a grand mal seizure and unconsciousness. However, this is not always the case; the seizure motor march may stop at any point along the way.

The upper motor system includes the cerebral cortex, the cerebellum, and the brain stem. Cranial nerve nuclei I and II are contained in the cerebral cortex, while cranial nerves III–XII are contained in the brain stem.The lower motor neuron system is located within the ventral (anterior motor) horn of the spinal cord. In the evaluation of clinical signs and symptoms, a distinction can be made between upper motor neuron damage and lower motor neuron damage by the motor system findings and those of the deep tendon reflexes. These distinctions will be discussed later in this chapter in the section on reflexes.

A lesion in *Broca's area*, which is in the inferior frontal gyrus just anterior to the motor tract of the left frontal lobe, can cause expressive or nonfluent aphasia (see Figure 18-1). A lesion of the posterior frontal area will produce disturbances in expressive writing. Anosmia (loss of

Techniques for Assessing Frontal Lobe Areas

1. *Mental status:* Refer to Chapter 5.
2. *Motor status:* Refer to Chapter 16.
3. *Motor speech:* Note ability to speak and articulate words.
4. *Sense of smell:* Client closes eyes; press one naris closed with your index finger; ask client to identify common scent—e.g., soap, mint, tobacco; repeat with opposite naris.

smell) suggests the possibility of a lesion of the anterior-inferior portion of the frontal lobe, where the olfactory fiber tracts are situated.

Parietal Lobe Area

A tract similar to the motor tract of the frontal lobes lies in the anterior portion of the parietal lobes and deals with body sensation. In this *sensory tract*, as in the motor tract, each part of the body is represented by cortical cells. A lesion interfering with these sensory cells may result in numbness, tingling, or other unusual sensations. Such symptoms would most likely be mentioned during an investigation of a chief complaint or the review of systems while collecting the health history. Episodic bouts of numbness and tingling may occur, as well as a focal seizure followed by a sensory march similar to the motor march. Other sensory disturbances that may be experienced by clients with cortical lesions of the sensory tract are hyperesthesia (increased sensitivity to touch stimuli) and paresthesia (spontaneous sensations such as pins, needles, "crawling" sensations).

In evaluating sensory system status, test the perception of the following modalities: touch, pain, temperature, proprioception (position sense), and vibration. Obviously you cannot test the entire body surface, but you should be guided by the client's history and other neurologic findings in determining the areas to be more closely scrutinized. Testing is difficult to evaluate and depends on the cooperation of the client. The client's eyes should be closed during the testing. The sensitivity of each modality should be compared with the opposite side of the body or with corresponding extremities. The difference between sensitivity of proximal and distal parts of the extremity should also be noted.

Normally all sensations are perceived equally. Should sensory disturbances be detected, construct sketches to show the areas or pattern of involvement, such as on one side, dermatomal or peripherally confined. Figure 18-4 locates the body surface areas associated with the major nerves. Cortical sensory tract and discriminatory sensations are not routinely tested.

Within the spinal cord are pathways for transporting the various sensations to the thalamus for awareness and on to the cerebrum for location and intensity. In assessing the sensory system it is important to have a basic understanding of the spinal tracts and their routes. Of particular importance are (1) the posterior (dorsal) columns tract, (2) the lateral spinothalamic tract, and (3) the ventral spinothalamic tract. In Figure 18-5 you can see the location of these various tracts on the right; the functions of these ascending tracts are indicated on the left.

Sensory impulses are picked up by the receptors in the skin, mucous membranes, muscles, and body organs. Figure 18-6 illustrates how *afferent nerves* transmit these impulses from the receptors to the cell body in the *ganglion* on the posterior root of a *spinal nerve* and on the posterior or *dorsal horn* (gray matter of the cord). From the sensory or dorsal horn the impulses ascend, according to the type of sensation, up either the *dorsal column* (solid color), the *lateral spinothalamic tract* (broken color), or the *ventral spinothalamic tract* (solid black).

The dorsal column transmits the impulse sensations of vibration, proprioception, two-point discrimination, stereognosis, and graphesthesia up to the thalamus; from there the impulses proceed to the parietal cortex.

Vibration is tested by holding a vibrating fork on the bony prominences of the body (finger joints, wrists, elbows, shoulders, hips, knees, shins, ankles, and toes). Note the ability of the client to determine the presence of the vibrations and when they stop. You can grossly countercheck the client's responses by comparing them to your own sensations, providing you have no sensory deficit. In other words, when the client states that the vibration sensation has stopped, place the tuning fork on your own wrist to see if it has indeed ceased. Sensitivity to vibration should be compared between one side of

Anterior
I
II
III
Great auricular
Anterior cutaneous
Supraclavicular
Axillary (circumflex)
T2
3
4
5
6
7
8
9
10
11
12
Lower lateral cutaneous
Lateral cutaneous rami
Anterior cutaneous rami
Medial cutaneous
Medial cutaneous
Ilioinguinal
Lateral cutaneous
Iliohypogastric
Femoral branch of genitofemoral
Radial
Genital branch of genitofemoral
Ulnar
Median
Scrotal branch of perineal nerve
Dorsal nerve of penis
Lateral cutaneous
Obturator
Intermediate and medial cutaneous
Saphenous
Lateral cutaneous
Superficial peroneal
Deep peroneal
Sural
Medial and lateral plantar

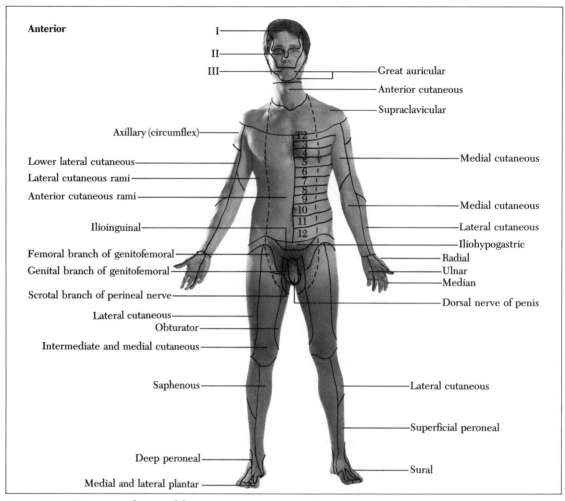

Figure 18-4A Dermatomal areas of the major nerves, anterior view.

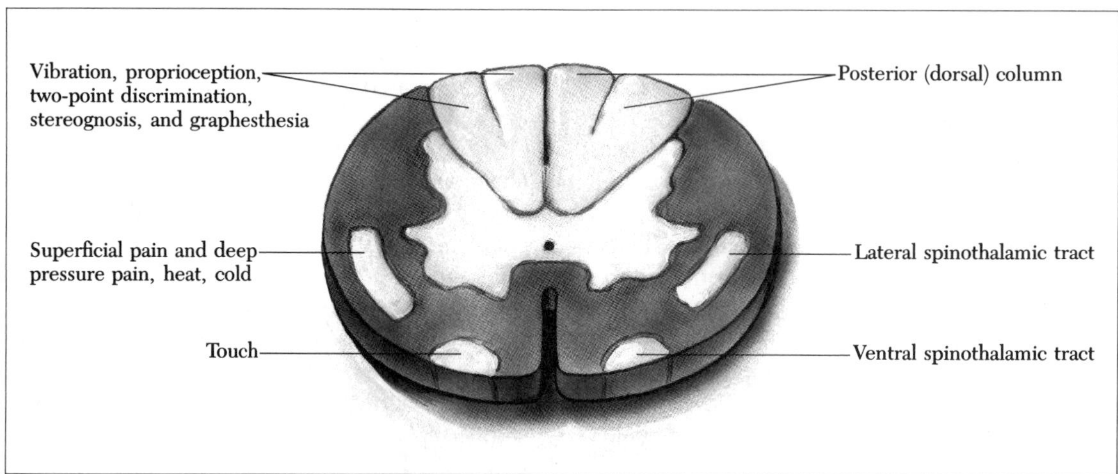

Figure 18-5 Cross-section of the spinal cord.

Posterior

Lesser occipital
Greater occipital
Great auricular
Anterior cutaneous
C5
C6
T1
T2
3
4
5
6
7
8
9
10
11
12
L1
S1
Supraclavicular
Axillary (circumflex)
Posterior cutaneous rami
Posterior cutaneous
Medial cutaneous and intercostobrachial
Lateral cutaneous rami
Lower lateral cutaneous
Medial cutaneous
Posterior cutaneous
Lateral cutaneous
Posterior rami of lumbar, sacral and coccygeal
Radial
Iliohypogastric
Ulnar
Median
Inferior medial clunial
Inferior lateral clunial
Lateral cutaneous
Posterior cutaneous
Obturator
Medial cutaneous
Lateral cutaneous
Saphenous
Superficial peroneal
Calcanean branches of sural and tibial nerves
Sural
Medial plantar
Lateral plantar
Calcanean branches of sural and tibial nerves
Saphenous
Sural
Superficial peroneal

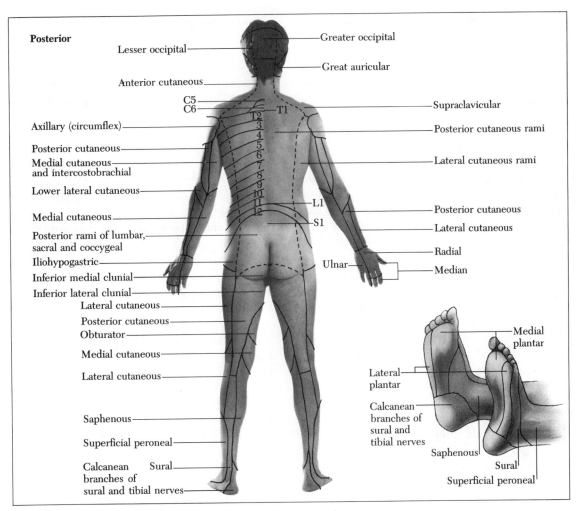

Figure 18-4B Dermatomal areas of the major nerves, posterior view.

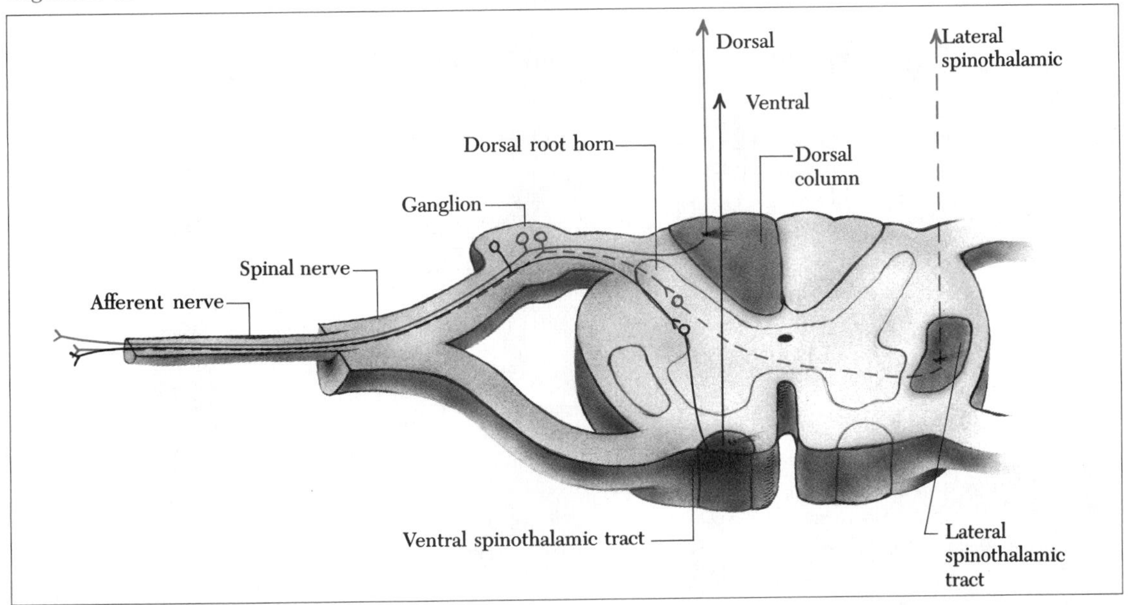

Figure 18-6 Sensory impulse transmission from receptor site to the appropriate tract according to type of sensation.

the body and the other and between the proximal and distal portions of the extremities.

Every extremity should be evaluated for *proprioception* (position and joint motion sense). As you move the client's fingers and toes passively, ask him to state whether the movement is upward or downward. When passively moving the digits, it is important that you hold the sides of the finger or toe being tested, since upward or downward pressure upon the client's skin may reveal the direction of the movement. It is not necessary to test position sense of proximal joints if the perception of the distal (finger and toe) joints is normal, as position sense is always lacking distally in organic lesions.

The sensory impulses of superficial and deep pain and of temperature (hot and cold) enter the dorsal horn of the spinal cord, ascend a segment or two, and then decussate to the lateral spinothalamic tract to continue to ascend to the thalamus and on to the sensory cortical tract of the anterior parietal lobe (see Figure 18-6). In assessing the lateral spinothalamic tract, test both superficial and deep pain perception, as only one may be deficient. For instance, in tabes dorsalis the client may perceive superficial pinpricks but lack all perception of deep pressure pain. To assess superficial pain, randomly alternate use of the blunt and sharp ends of a safety pin, asking the client, whose eyes should be closed, to identify whether the sensation is "sharp" or "dull." Evaluate the perception of deep pressure pain by squeezing the intrinsic muscles of the hands, the forearm muscles, the Achilles tendon, or the calf muscles.

Because temperature sensations travel over the same spinal tract as those of pain, temperature perception is not routinely tested if pain testing demonstrates the tract to be functioning. However, if you suspect a lesion of the lateral spinothalamic tract, if there are doubtful findings regarding pain perception, or if the client complains of a lack of perception of temperature, then evaluate temperature perception by placing test tubes containing hot and cold water against the client's skin for identification.

Both crossed and uncrossed peripheral fibers carry the sensation of touch. Some enter the dorsal ipsilateral (same) side of the spinal cord via the thalamus to the parietal lobe on the same side. Others travel the ventral spinothalamic tract, which ascends and decussates at the medullary level. Thus, the touch sensation is rarely absent except in cases of severe damage to the spinal cord or cerebrum.

Evaluate the perception of touch by having the client, with eyes closed, point to the areas of his body where he has been touched lightly with a wisp of cotton. Loss of touch perception is generally accompanied by absence of other sensations. This is a common finding in peripheral neuropathies. Ordinarily, the feet and legs

Techniques for Assessing Parietal Lobe Areas

Client's eyes should be closed for all testing of parietal lobe areas.

1. *Sensory status:* Stimuli applied in dermatomal areas of the body; ask client to identify whether sensation is "dull" or "sharp" and hot or cold, and to point to areas of body where touched by cotton wisp.
   a. Pain (pinprick)
   b. Temperature (test tubes of hot and cold water)
   c. Light touch (cotton wisp applied to body)
2. *Vibration:* Place vibrating tuning fork on major bony prominences—i.e., toes, ankles, knees, iliac crests, knuckles, wrists, elbows, shoulder; ask client to identify presence of vibration and when it stops; place your hand on upper end of tuning fork to stop vibration to detect if client senses cessation of vibration.
3. *Proprioception:* Hold digit with your index and thumb on either side; move in up and down direction; ask client to identify direction of movement; test each extremity.
4. *Stereognosis:* Place two objects in succession in each hand; ask client to identify the shape, and to compare the size and weight of the two objects; this tests both left and right parietal lobes.
5. *Decision making:* If neurologic problem is suspected, perform additional special techniques for assessing parietal lobe function.

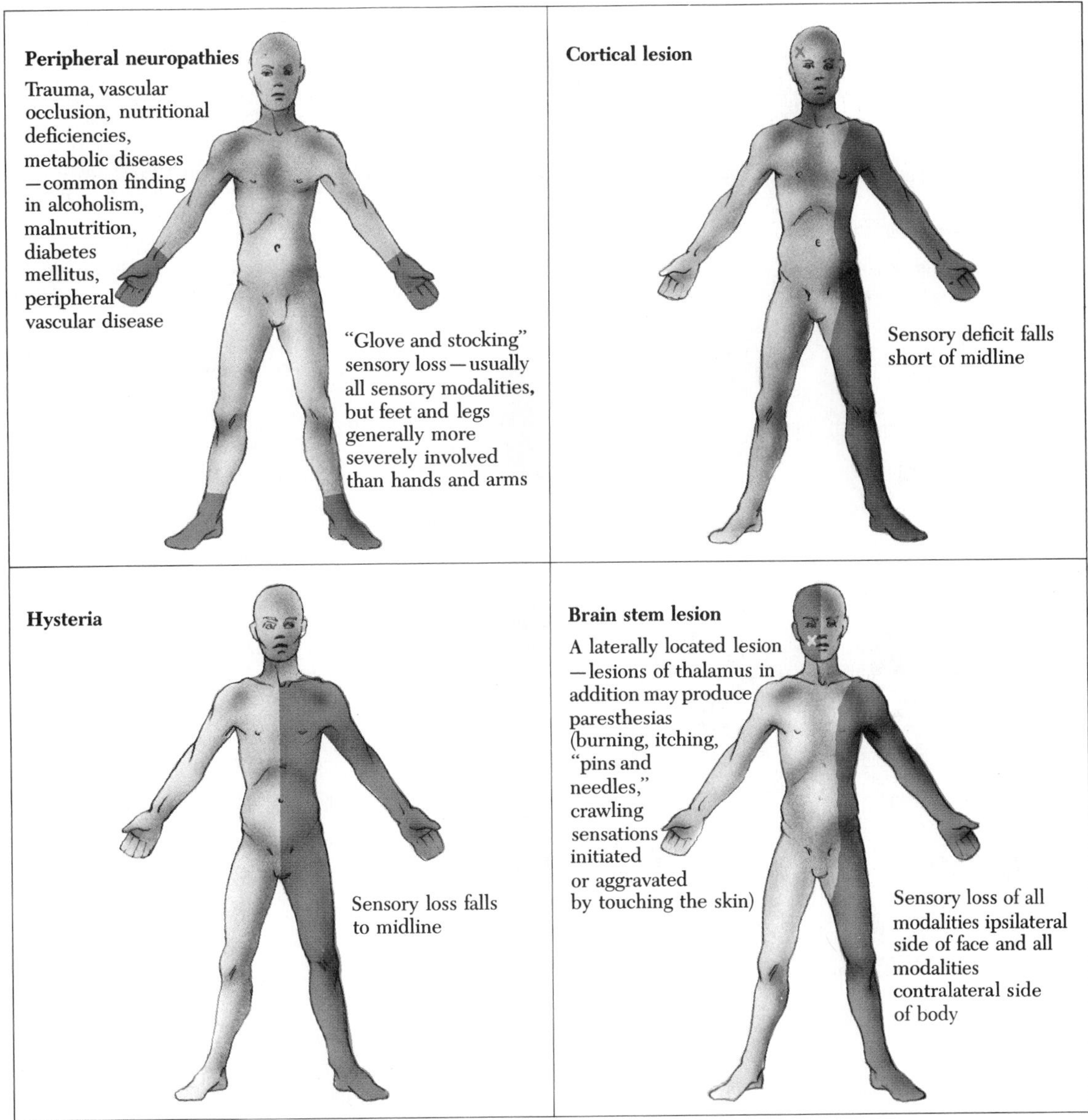
Peripheral neuropathies
Trauma, vascular occlusion, nutritional deficiencies, metabolic diseases —common finding in alcoholism, malnutrition, diabetes mellitus, peripheral vascular disease
"Glove and stocking" sensory loss—usually all sensory modalities, but feet and legs generally more severely involved than hands and arms
Cortical lesion
Sensory deficit falls short of midline
Hysteria
Sensory loss falls to midline
Brain stem lesion
A laterally located lesion —lesions of thalamus in addition may produce paresthesias (burning, itching, "pins and needles," crawling sensations initiated or aggravated by touching the skin)
Sensory loss of all modalities ipsilateral side of face and all modalities contralateral side of body

Figure 18-7 Common patterns of sensory loss.

are more severely involved than the upper extremities, and the loss may manifest as a "glove and stocking" pattern: a sensory loss in which all sensory modalities, including pain, temperature, touch, vibration, and proprioception, are diminished.

Peripheral nerve pathology is often associated with decreased perspiration as well as diminished sensation, since the peripheral nerves also carry sympathetic fibers to the corresponding sensory distribution of the nerve. The peripheral nerves most commonly affected are the medial, ulnar, radial, tibial, and common peroneal.

Peripheral nerves may be affected by such conditions as direct trauma, vascular insufficiency, nutritional deficiencies, and metabolic disease processes. The dorsal root ganglion may be attacked by such diseases as tumors, a herniated intervertebral disk, herpes zoster, or tabes dorsalis. A lesion of the dorsal root ganglion will cause sensation to be lost in the related dermatome distribution. Figure 18-7 illustrates common patterns of sensory loss. Figure 18-8 illustrates how the position of a lesion affects sensory loss.

An expressive aphasia may occur with a pari-

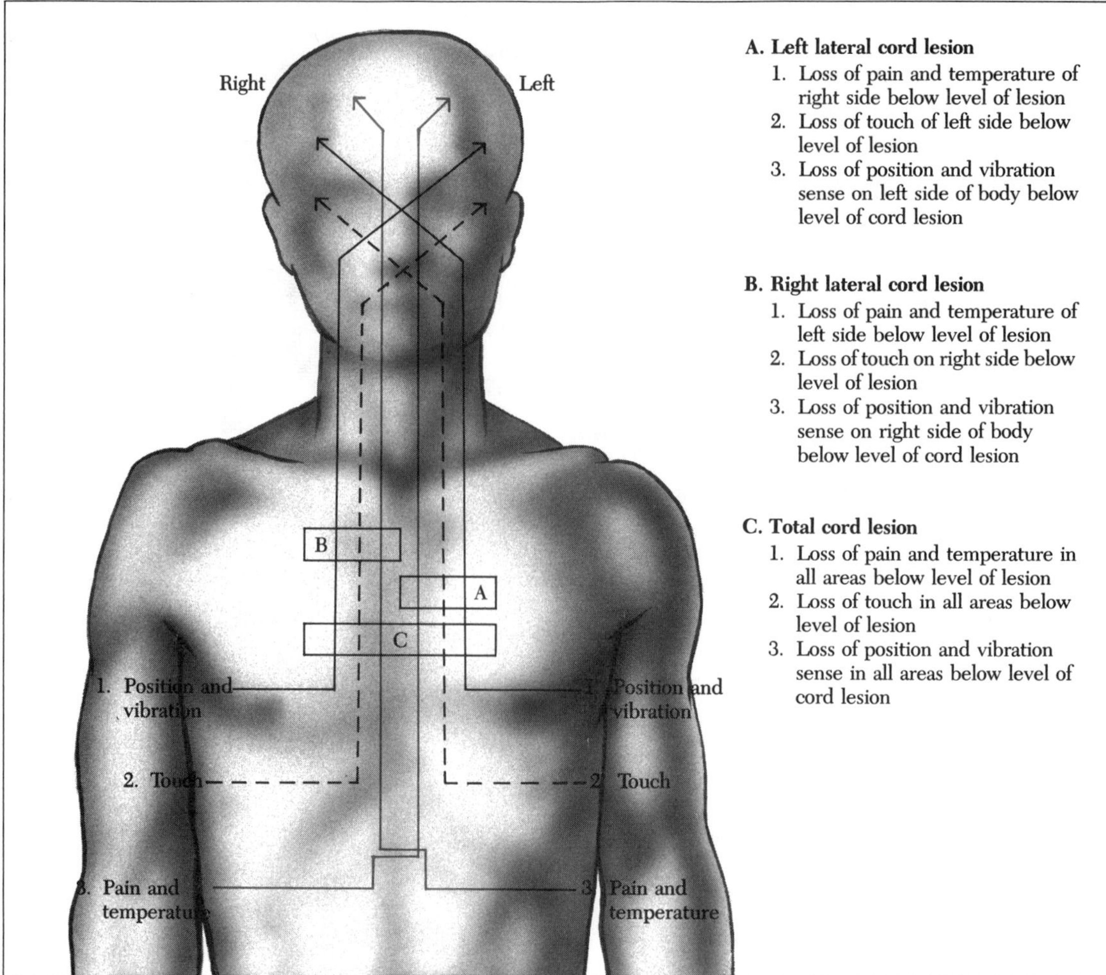

Figure 18-8 Cord lesions and sensory loss.

etal lesion if the speech center responsible for choosing the words for verbal communication is affected. If this speech center is destroyed, the client's speech is gibberish (see Figure 18-1).

The parietal lobes are also involved in specific sensory interpretations. They are the seat of *stereognosis*, the ability to recognize the shape, size, and relative weight of objects. A lesion involving this area of the parietal lobes would interfere with this discriminatory ability. To test intactness of this area, place two objects in succession in the client's hand while his eyes are closed. For instance, first place a golf ball in the client's left hand, and ask him to identify the form and approximate size of the object. Next place a coin in the *same* hand and ask about its size and shape. Then ask the client which object weighs more. You have then tested right parietal lobe functioning. Left parietal lobe functioning is tested by placing two different objects in succession in the client's right hand, such as a pencil, a matchbook, a drinking glass, and a paperweight. Inability to discriminate between objects is abnormal and is termed *a*stereognosis.

Other discriminatory tests performed in an extensive neurologic assessment are two-point discrimination, point localization, texture discrimination, the extinction phenomenon, and graphesthesia. These tests are *not* ordinarily performed during a routine screening of health assessment.

In testing *two-point discrimination,* touch various parts of the body with two closely approximated sharp points, while the client keeps his eyes closed. The normal individual is able to identify that he is being touched by two points. With cortical pathology the client cannot discriminate two sharp points placed close to-

Special Techniques

1. *Two-point discrimination*: Touch various areas with two closely approximated points. Ask client to identify if touched by one or two points.
2. *Point localization*: Touch various body areas. Ask client to name and point to the area where he is being touched.
3. *Texture discrimination*: Place such materials as sandpaper, silk, and velvet in client's hand to identify rough, smooth, and soft textures.
4. *Extinction phenomenon*: Simultaneously touch the same areas of the body on both left and right sides. Ask client to identify whether he feels the touch on one or both sides.
5. *Graphesthesia*: With your fingertip, write letters or numbers on the client's palm or other body part. Ask client to identify the letters or numbers.

gether. The distances that a client can detect two points varies on different parts of the body. However, a minimal distance of 2–3 mm can be found on the fingertips of the normal client. To test *point localization*, ask the client to keep his eyes closed and name and point to the area where he is being touched. To test *texture discrimination*, check whether the client is able to recognize the feel (rough, smooth, soft) of materials such as sandpaper, silk, velvet, and so on. In proceeding with the assessment, touch the same area on both sides of the body simultaneously to assess whether the *extinction phenomenon* is present. Ask the client whether he feels the touch on one side or on both sides. With a parietal cortical lesion the client will be inattentive to the diseased side; in addition to not noticing the touch on the affected side, the client will also have difficulty identifying left from right body parts.

To test the sense of *graphesthesia*, ask the client to name the letters or numbers you write with your fingers on his palms or on other parts of the body. The normal individual is able to discriminate point localization, texture, left from right body parts, and letters or numbers written on a portion of his body while his eyes remain closed. Inability to do this is called *a*graphesthesia.

The parietal lobe does not become fully functioning until 7–8 years of age. This is why young children can easily get lost because they are unable to find their spatial bearings. The parietal lobe also is necessary for understanding grammatically complex instructions. Therefore, an adult client with a parietal lesion, or a young child, will respond better when instructions are short and simple. For example, do not give them three instructions in one command. Give each command separately and pause for response before continuing to next command.

A summary of the assessment of tactile perception is seen in Table 18-1.

Occipital Lobe Area

The cortical functions of vision and visual interpretation lie in the occipital lobes. The visual center is assessed during testing of visual acuity and visual field. A lesion involving the whole of the visual center of both occipital lobes would result in total "cortical blindness" in spite of normal eyes and optic tract. Destruction of the visual center in only one lobe would result in contralateral homonymous hemianopia.

When neurologic difficulties exist, the functions of the occipital lobes should be carefully examined. To assess visual object recognition, ask the client to identify familiar objects, such as a glass or wristwatch. Evaluate visual-verbal comprehension by asking the client to read a sentence from a newspaper or magazine and explain its meaning. If the client is unable to follow this verbal command, print the instructions and evaluate whether the client can follow the writ-

Techniques for Assessing Occipital Lobe Areas

1. *Visual object recognition*: Ask client to identify familiar objects.
2. *Visual-verbal comprehension*: Ask client to read a sentence from newspaper or magazine and explain it.
3. *Visual acuity and visual fields*: Refer to Chapter 11.

Table 18-1. Summary Assessment of Tactile Perception

Sensation	Assessment technique	Behaviors: Normal	Behaviors: Abnormal
Primary Sensation			
Light touch	A wisp of cottom is touched to each of the designated areas bilaterally to elicit sensation.	Perceives and identifies the area lightly touched	Anesthesia, hyperesthesia
Pain/temperature			
Superficial	Superficial sharp and dull points tested using a hypodermic needle and the hub. Each area is tested bilaterally for sharp and dull.	Easily and bilaterally distinguishes sharp and dull	Hypoesthesia, hyperesthesia, paresthesia, anesthesia
Deep	Achilles tendon or biceps squeezed.	States pain is felt	
Temperature	Hot or cold temperature is tested bilaterally in all designated areas (if pain tests abnormal)	Easily and bilaterally differentiates heat and cold	
Vibration	Vibrating tuning fork is applied over bony prominences (ankle or wrist) to elicit sensation.	Easily indentifies when vibrations felt and when they stop	Hypoesthesia, anesthesia
Kinesthesia/Proprioception			
Position sense	With child's finger or toe in a neutral position, examiner gently elevates or depresses digit to elicit position sense.	Easily distinguishes whether digit is elevated or depressed	Inability to correctly indentify position
Romberg test	Child stands feet together, arms down, with eyes open. If normal, retest with eyes closed.	Slight swaying but maintains balance and upright posture	Loses balance
Alternating motion	Child rapidly alternates pronation and supination of both hands.	Rate and rhythm bilaterally equal	Lacks coordination
Finger-to-nose test	Child, the eyes closed, touches forefinger to nose.	Touches nose easily	Unable to directly locate nose
Secondary Sensation			
Graphesthesia	A blunt object is used to draw a number or letter on child's hand, arm, or back.	Easily identifies number or letter bilaterally	Unable to identify or indentifies incorrectly
Stereognosis	A familiar object is placed in child's hand, and after feeling it child is asked to identify the object (paper clip, button, coin).	Easily, correctly, and bilaterally identifies object	Unable to identify or identifies incorrectly
Two-point Discrimination	Using a compass or two sharp objects, examiner touches client simultaneously with both points and asks if one or two points are felt.	Two points can be discriminated at the following separations: fingertips 2.8 mm toes 3–8 mm chest and forearm 40 mm back 40–70 mm	

Source: Adapted from J. P. Bellack and P. Bamford, *Nursing assessment: A multidimensional approach* (Boston: Jones and Bartlett Publishers, 1987), pp. 333–334. Used with permission.

ten command. With occipital lobe tumors, visual disturbances and seizures, preceded by an aura of light and visual hallucinations, are common. Headache and papilledema may also exist.

Temporal Lobe Area

Much of the visual (optic) tract projects through the temporal lobes, so visual defects are also common with temporal lobe lesions. The most common defect is homonymous hemianopia contralateral to the side of the temporal lesion, but if the lesion is small a homonymous superior quadrant may result (see the discussion of the cranial nerves, particularly the optic nerve, later in this chapter).

Damage to a center for speech understanding in the temporal lobe results in receptive aphasia, in which the client is unable to interpret the meaning of words. The speech center, *Wernicke's area* (see Figure 18-1), is central in the left temporal lobe and is joined to Broca's area by a nerve bundle called the arcuate fasciculus. When this nerve bundle is disrupted, the client can comprehend words, but cannot repeat them. When Wernicke's area per se is damaged, speech is fluent but is wordy and has little substance to its content; comprehension is usually lost—that is, sentences do not make much sense (see Figure 18-1).

Because the posterior temporal lobes are in close proximity to the visual association areas, visual hallucinations may occur, consisting of familiar sights including people, animals, and places. Some clients with temporal lobe tumors may have distorted vision, such as micropsia (seeing things as smaller than they actually are), macropsia (seeing things as larger), or wavy-deformed vision, or they may experience colors in unusual ways.

Because portions of the auditory, olfactory, and gustatory systems are located in the temporal lobes, lesions of these areas may produce tinnitus, auditory hallucinations (such as voices, unusual noises, or music), and olfactory hallucinations, sometimes accompanied by smacking movements of the lips. Singing of a melody all day long may occur with a temporal lesion. So, too, auditory agnosia (difficulty in recognition of verbal words) may result. These attacks are similar to behaviors manifested in psychiatric disorders but differ in the fact that temporal lobe attacks are episodic and of brief duration.

Some "psychic" phenomena are related to temporal lobe structures—temporal lobe pathology may result in such experiences as déjà vu, dreamy states, and psychomotor seizures. *Déjà vu* is the dreamlike impression that one is in a situation that is an exact repetition of a previous experience. Occasionally, *jamais vu* occurs, in which a familiar situation suddenly becomes totally strange. In *psychomotor seizures* the client suddenly performs inappropriate or, at times, appropriate behavior ranging from nonsignificant movements to states of rage, after which he has no memory of his behavior. The client may "wake up" and find himself in a strange place or may suddenly find himself home with amnesia as to how or why he got there. The duration of psychomotor seizures is generally 20–30 minutes. Longer episodes must be differentiated from the fugue states of psychiatric origin.

Techniques for Assessing Temporal Lobe Areas

1. *Visual fields*: Refer to Chapter 11.
2. *Speech understanding*: Receptive aphasia. Check if client can follow command and if client can repeat command verbally.

Assessment of the Cerebellum

The cerebellum, or hindbrain, which consists of two hemispheres, is located posteriorly and inferiorly to the cerebrum. It is connected to the cerebrum, pons, and medulla oblongata by three fiber bundles: the superior peduncles, middle peduncles, and inferior peduncles, respectively. Thus, some of the nerve fibers from these anterior portions of the brain pass through the cerebellum. Of particular importance are the impulses received from the cortical motor tract, the semicircular canals of the inner ear, and the muscles, as these structures play a major role in body position and movement. The cerebellum receives, sorts, and synergizes these impulses, after which they are sent out to maintain posture, balance, muscle coordination, and the tone of the voluntary muscles.

Injury to the cerebellum, manifested in hypotonia (extremely poor muscle tone) and lack of coordination, may be so great that the individual is rendered helpless. The severity of the signs and symptoms of cerebellar dysfunction vary, depending on the location and extent of the cerebellar lesion. Cerebellar dysfunction may also be associated with cranial nerve palsies (frequently of nerves V, VI, and VII) because of pressure on the pons and the medulla. Tender neck muscles and occipital headaches may also be major complaints. Trauma, tumors, abscesses, diffuse infection, demyelinating diseases, and various drugs (including alcohol) and toxins frequently alter the functioning of the cerebellum.

Cerebellar assessment procedures focus on balance and coordination. As the client performs the various tests for balance and coordination, you should observe closely for any abnormalities in rhythm and smoothness.

Balance Assessment

Observe the client's gait. Pathology may cause *ataxia*, in which the client displays the tendency to fall toward the affected cerebellar hemisphere. When the vermis, the midline structure of the cerebellum, is affected, the gait is characteristically wide-based and the client staggers from side to side. The vermis also has reign over truncal movements. Thus, misdirected or jerky movements of the trunk and neck may be observed as the client attempts to maintain his balance. The character of an ataxic gait may change over time as a lesion extends from one cerebellar hemisphere into the vermis.

Gait is best assessed by having the client walk barefoot across the room away from you and back. Closely observe the movements of the extremities. The arms normally swing smoothly in opposition to the advancement of the foot. The client should be able to start and stop locomotion easily. Abnormalities in gait sometimes appear in relation to the position of the torso, the size and speed of steps, and the width of stance. These aspects should therefore be taken into consideration.

In Parkinson's disease the arms are held stiffly and do not move, the body lunges forward, and the steps are small and shuffling. In the client with hemiparesis the rhythmic arm swing on the affected side is diminished or absent; the leg is stiff and is swung in a wide arc, with the toe scraping the floor as the client ambulates. Neurosyphilis and cerebellar lesions cause the client to be unsteady and to walk with a staggering (ataxic) broad-based gait.

Romberg's sign, the inability to stand with feet together and eyes closed, may indicate cerebellar disease, among others. It is also observed in clients with vestibular damage. When requesting a client to perform this test of balance, you should stand nearby to catch the client if necessary. With cerebellar dysfunction the client will fall toward the affected side. A small amount of swaying during this test is normal.

If you discover difficulty, you may ask the client to perform several other tests to verify the suspected finding of loss of balance. One such test is tandem walking—the familiar heel to toe along a straight line—frequently associated with the testing of balance control when inebriation is suspected. Another test is to have the client hop on one leg or perform a deep knee bend, first on one leg and then on the other. Taking the client's age and general status into consideration, these maneuvers are normally accomplished with little difficulty.

Coordination Assessment

Test both upper and lower extremities, one limb at a time. To assess the upper extremities, use the finger-to-nose tests. Ask the client to touch his nose and then your finger; change the position of your finger and have the client follow the same procedure. Repeat this action with increasing rapidity. Test one hand at a time. Another test calls for the client to close his eyes and hold his arms straight out from his sides. Then, with each hand in succession, he touches his nose. With pathology, "past pointing" will occur on the

Techniques for Assessing Balance

1. *Observe gait:* Have client walk barefooted away from you and toward you. Characteristics: movement of extremities, position of torso, size and speed of steps, width of stance.
2. *Romberg's sign:* Stand close to the client. Ask the client to place feet together and close eyes.
3. *Tandem walking:* Have client walk in a straight line alternating the placement of the heel of one foot in front of the toe of the opposite foot.
4. *Have the client hop or do a shallow knee bend* on one leg and then on the other.

diseased side. Fine coordination does not develop until age 5 or 6; therefore, if a younger child can point to 2 inches away from his nose, this is within normal limits.

The lower extremities are assessed in a similar fashion. Ask the client to perform the heel-to-shin test by placing the heel of one foot on the knee of the opposite leg and moving it down the shin. This is normally performed without difficulty, both with the eyes open and then closed. Another maneuver used to assess the lower extremities is testing the client's ability to "write" a figure 8 in the air with each foot or to point to your hand with each big toe while lying down. Normally this feat is easily and smoothly accomplished.

Another feat of coordination that is normally easily performed is the rapid tapping of the fingers on a table and the toes on the floor. Other skills that reveal inability or clumsiness in the presence of cerebellar disease are the touching of each finger to the thumb in rapid succession and rapidly alternating pronation and supination of the forearms. Observe the equilibrial position of the eyes. Nystagmus may be present with inner ear difficulties, but it, too, may indicate cerebellar involvement. With cerebellar involvement the nystagmus is most marked when the client gazes toward the side with the lesion.

During the testing of coordination, note any tremors or impairment in rhythm and coordination in body movements and speech. A cerebellar lesion can be manifested in a characteristic staccato, explosive speech pattern. The most common findings in cerebellar disease are disturbances in walking and making alternating movements, and the presence of tremors. The characteristic tremor of cerebellar pathology is the *intention tremor*, a tremor that is associated with every voluntary movement of the body. However, clients with multiple sclerosis may also demonstrate an intention tremor with voluntary efforts.

Assessment of the Cranial Nerves

The routine assessment of each of the cranial nerves has been discussed throughout the text in the appropriate anatomic section. Generally, the first cranial nerve, the olfactory, is not routinely tested. However, when there is suspicion of neurologic disorder, each of the cranial nerves is meticulously assessed.

In Figure 18-9 the location of each of the cranial nerve nuclei from oculomotor (III) to hypoglossal (XII) is illustrated in relation to the ventricular system, the spinal cord, and other brain structures. The olfactory (I) and optic (II) nuclei are located in the cerebrum in the temporal lobe and occipital lobe, respectively. The midbrain houses the oculomotor (III) and trochlear (IV) nuclei, whereas the pons houses the next four cranial nerves: the trigeminal (V), the abducens (VI), the facial (VII), and the auditory or acoustic (VIII). The four remaining cranial nerve nuclei are located in the medulla: the glossopharyngeal (IX), the vagus (X), the spinal accessory (XI), and the hypoglossal (XII).

To ensure assessment of all twelve cranial nerves, the first hurdle is to memorize their sequence and names. This may be facilitated by the use of the following mnemonic device "On Old Olympus' Towering Tops A Finn and German Viewed Some Hops." Another mnemonic that helps to remember whether the cranial nerve is sensory, motor, or both sensory and motor is "Some Say Marry Money But My Brother Says Bad Business Marrying Money." Sensory is designated by words beginning with the letter "S," motor by "M," and both motor and sensory by "B" words (see accompanying box).

(I) Olfactory

The sense of smell is tested by closing each nostril separately and requesting the client to identify a familiar odor while his eyes are closed. Substances such as coffee, tobacco, lemon, peppermint, may be used, but avoid such volatile substances as ammonia. Most important is whether the client can make a distinction between odors, not whether he is able to identify precisely the given substances. It must be remembered that loss of smell can be affected by many factors, including a cold, aging, sinusitis, heavy cigarette smoking, and nasal obstruction. Pathology such as tumors at the base of the frontal lobes, involving the olfactory groove, or trauma of the olfactory bulbs or the ethmoid plate may result in anosmia—complete loss of smell. It is important to assess the function of smell in clients who have had trauma to the head, meningitis, or subarachnoid hemorrhage, in clients who complain of visual failure, and in clients who have demonstrated progressive intellectual deterioration. Olfactory hallucinations may also occur with brain lesions, particularly those of the temporal lobes.

BIOLOGICAL AND CULTURAL VARIATIONS

Tay-Sachs Disease in Ashkenazic Jews

The Jewish population is often divided into three major groups based on historical migrations and geographic location (Groen 1973). The Ashkenazic Jews are the descendants of Jews who migrated from Judea and Jerusalem to France and Germany in the first century, and who were later forced to migrate to northern, central, and eastern Europe. The United States Jewish population is largely Ashkenazim. The Sephardic Jews left Palestine and Galilee in the fifth century and settled in Spain and Portugal. After total expulsion in the late fifteenth century, they migrated to all parts of the Mediterranean. The Oriental Jews are the descendants of groups that left the Middle East and migrated to the Near and Far East.

A large number of simple inherited genetic disorders occur in relatively high frequencies in the Ashkenazim. These disorders include dystonia musculorum deformans, Riley-Day syndrome (familial autonomic dysfunction), Gaucher's disease (familial splenic anemia), Niemann-Pick disease (lipid histiocytosis), and Tay-Sachs disease (infantile amaurotic idiocy).

Tay-Sachs disease has one of the highest incidence rates of this group of genetic conditions. In the United States the disease occurs in approximately 1 out of 6,000 Jewish births, as opposed to 1 in approximately 500,000 non-Jewish births (Myrianthopoulos & Aronson 1973). It has been shown to be due to the inheritance of a recessive gene from both parents. Thus, symptoms of the disease only appear in recessive homozygotes (who have inherited two Tay-Sachs genes). From the incidence rate of Tay-Sachs disease, the frequency rate of the recessive gene in heterozygotes (those who have inherited one normal gene and one Tay-Sachs gene) can be computed. Thus, it has been estimated that 1 of 40 Jewish persons and one of 380 non-Jewish persons is a heterozygote for the Tay-Sachs gene.

Among Ashkenazic Jews, symptoms of the disease generally appear in infancy. Nerve cell degeneration and muscle weakness occur in the first few months after birth. These symptoms are due to the accumulation of lipid deposits in the cytoplasm of brain neurons. Cerebral function and mental development fail as the brain atrophies. Death usually occurs within the first or second year of life.

Various researchers have addressed the question of how such a gene, which is fatal to recessive homozygotes in infancy, could have risen to such a high frequency in a population. Homozygotes for the Tay-Sachs gene

(II) Optic

Loss of visual acuity, defects in peripheral vision, and changes in the optic nerve disk characterize optic nerve tract difficulties. Therefore, vision should be tested for accuracy by means of a Snellen chart, and the visual fields should be assessed with a perimeter and tangent screen. The ophthalmoscope examination of the retina and the optic nerve head is also a pertinent part of the assessment of the optic nerve. See Chapter 11 for a more detailed discussion of the procedures used to assess the eyes.

Figure 18-10 illustrates how the optic nerve receives visual images from the retina of the eye. At the optic chiasm, the temporal portion of each visual field crosses over, and both temporal and nasal impulses are transported to the occipital lobe of the cerebral cortex. Here the images are recognized and interpreted. If the visual cortex of the occipital lobe is damaged, "cortical blindness" results. Disturbances in vision are better understood and detected if you possess knowledge of the anatomy of this system. Figure 18-10 will help you to visualize the bases for the various hemianopias (the color portions represent areas of no vision). *Hemianopia* refers to visual defects that involve half of the visual field. The term is generally used to refer to bilateral defects resulting from a single lesion.

It can be seen with visual field defect 1 that the occurrence of a lesion anterior to the optic chiasm could cause a totally blind eye. A lateral lesion at the optic chiasm would cause a unilateral medial defect (2). Remember that the me-die well before reproductive age and do not pass the gene on to their offspring. In such cases of early mortality from a recessive homozygotic genetic condition, the recessive gene usually falls to a much lower frequency than the 1 heterozygote out of 40 found in Tay-Sachs disease.

The most plausible explanation is that heterozygotes for the Tay-Sachs gene have some advantage over dominant homozygotes (those individuals who have inherited two normal genes and do not carry the Tay-Sachs gene). This advantage might be that they have more children than the dominant homozygotes and that they live longer and thus tend to complete their reproductive years. Greater fertility for the heterozygotes would result in the Tay-Sachs gene remaining in the population from one generation to the next.

Some investigators think that the heterozygotic condition might offer an individual an increased resistance to certain infectious diseases. Such disease resistance would have been a great advantage in the past few centuries, for Ashkenazic Jews tended to live in the cities of northern, eastern, and central Europe, which had continuous epidemics of infectious diseases such as bubonic plague, cholera, smallpox, and diphtheria. If the Tay-Sachs gene offered a selective advantage in the face of these severe infectious diseases, we might expect heterozygous carriers to have greater survival and fertility rates than dominant homozygotes.

This hypothesis has received partial support from the findings of at least one study. Myrianthopoulos and Aronson (1973) compared the fertility of grandparents of a Tay-Sachs child, as measured by completed family size, with the fertility of a control group of grandparents with no Tay-Sachs grandchildren. It was assumed that at least one maternal and one paternal grandparent of an affected child was a heterozygote. Overall, they found that grandparents of Tay-Sachs children had produced 6% more offspring than grandparents who presumably did not carry the gene. The results were most marked for offspring not born in the United States. These findings suggest that there is a selective advantage associated with being a heterozygote for the Tay-Sachs gene. This heterozygote advantage might explain the rather high rate of this lethal homozygotic disease among United States and European Ashkenazic Jewish population groups.

Techniques for Assessing Coordination

1. Upper Extremities:
   a. *Finger-to-nose tests:* Have client touch index finger of each hand to nose. Have client touch nose and then your moving finger with his index finger.
   b. *Rapid alternating movements:* Have client rapidly move hands to and from supination to pronation positions. Tap fingers of each hand on a table surface; rapidly oppose each finger of each hand to the thumb.
2. Lower Extremities:
   a. *Heel to shin:* Have client place the heel of one foot at the knee of the opposite leg and run the heel down the shin to the ankle level. Perform with eyes both opened and closed.
   b. *Figure "8":* Have client write an imaginary "8" in the air with each foot.
   c. *Toe to finger:* Have the client point his great toe to your finger as you move it in different left/right/up/down directions.
   d. *Tapping toes:* Have client rapidly tap toes of both feet on the floor.

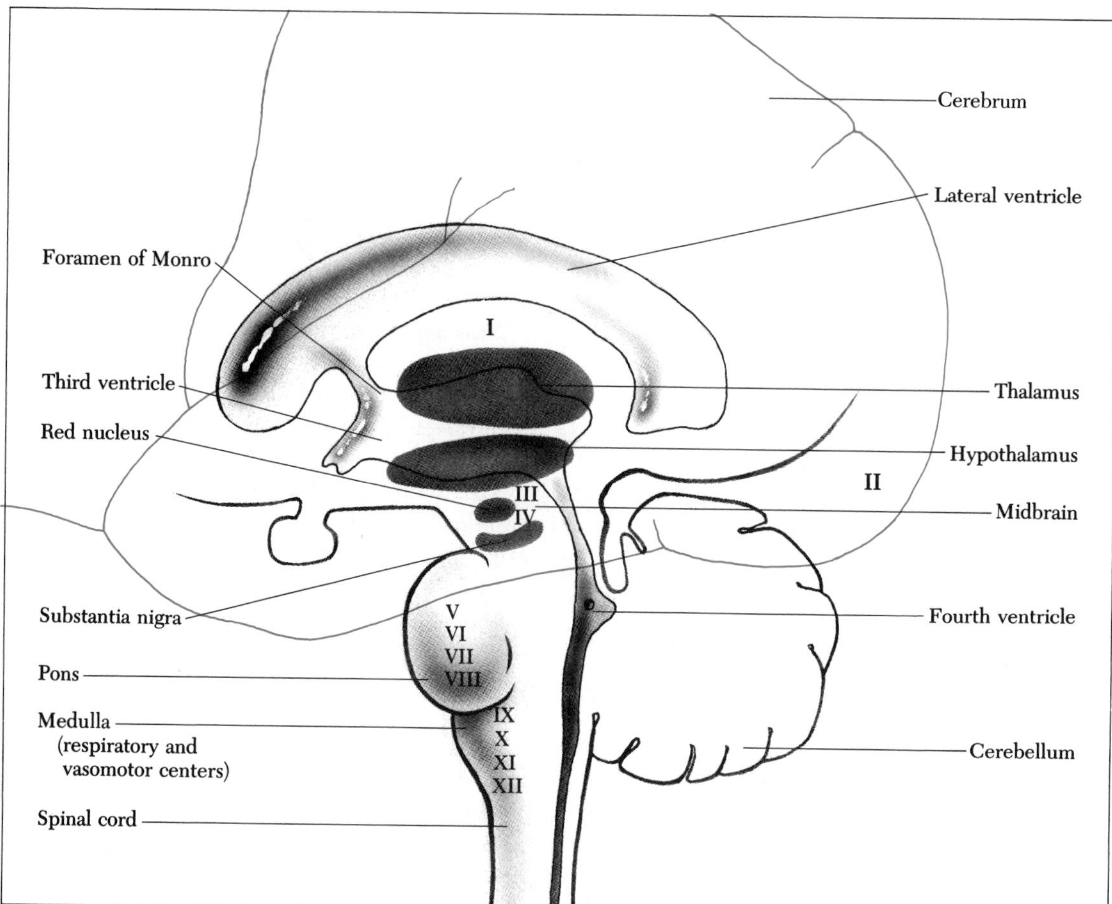

Figure 18-9 Location of cranial nerve nuclei.

Mnemonics for Remembering Cranial Nerves

On	I Olfactory	Some—Sensory
Old	II Optic	Say—Sensory
Olympus'	III Oculomotor	Marry—Motor
Towering	IV Trochlear	Money—Motor
Tops	V Trigeminal	But—Motor and Sensory
A	VI Abducens	My—Motor
Finn	VII Facial	Brother—Motor and Sensory
And	VIII Auditory or Acoustic	Says—Sensory
German	IX Glossopharyngeal	Bad—Motor and Sensory
Viewed	X Vagus	Business—Motor and Sensory
Some	XI Spinal accessory	Marrying—Motor
Hops	XII Hypoglossal	Money—Motor

dial aspect of each retina is served by optic nerve fibers that decussate at the optic chiasm before continuing to the contralateral occipital lobe. A lesion at this point may involve only those medial tracts and would therefore result in a bitemporal hemianopia because of the inversion of the field of vision upon the retinas (see defect 3). Bitemporal hemianopia commonly occurs in the

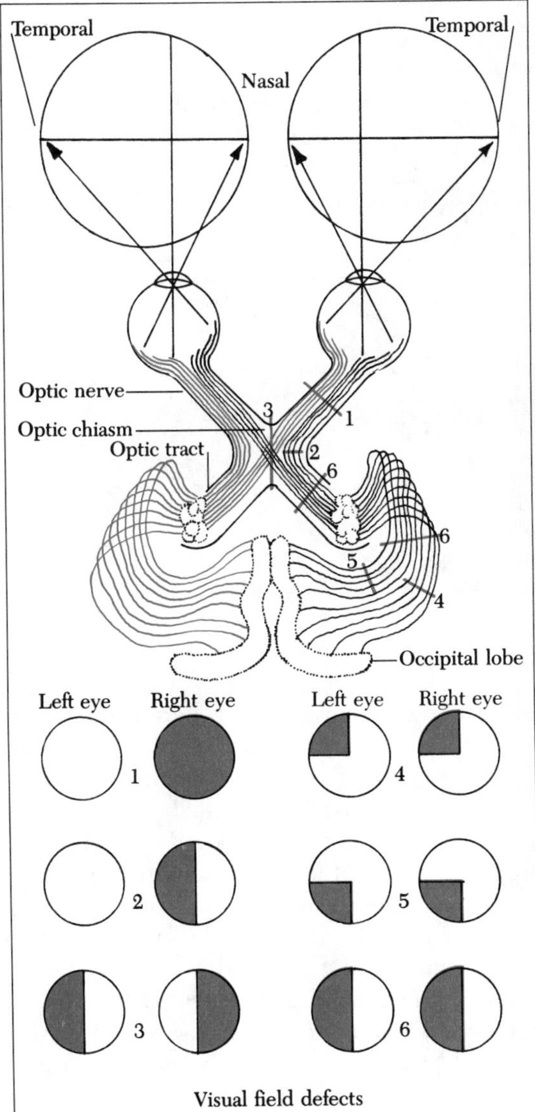

Figure 18-10 Lesions of the optic tract and resultant visual field defects.

presence of a pituitary tumor, as the pituitary gland is nestled anteriorly in the arms of the optic chiasm. When the optic tract between the chiasm and the geniculate body in the temporal and occipital lobes is interrupted, a homonymous (same) hemianopia occurs, wherein the field of vision is obliterated on the same side of both eyes (6). Generally, homonymous hemianopia is accompanied by pupillary abnormalities. A lesion of only a portion of the optic tract fibers may cause a homonymous quadrantic defect. In this situation the field of vision is lost in a similar quadrant of both eyes (4 and 5). Detection of visual defects is important not only for detection of client problems and for diagnostic purposes but is extremely pertinent for the planning of nursing care.

(III) Oculomotor, (IV) Trochlear, (VI) Abducens

The oculomotor, trochlear, and abducens nerves innervate the extraocular muscles of the eyes, and all three nerves pass in close proximity to the internal carotid artery; therefore, it is not uncommon for vascular aneurysms in this area to cause disturbances in visual gaze. Besides innervation of certain extraocular eye muscles, the oculomotor nerve serves to contract the iris muscles and to constrict the pupils, as well as elevate the eyelid. Thus, defects of this nerve may result in the eyeball turning downward and out, a dilated pupil, or ptosis of the eyelid.

In Adie's syndrome, the pupil is dilated and sluggish in reacting to light. However, on sustained accommodation the pupil may actually become smaller than the normal pupil. This syndrome usually occurs in young women and is an idiopathic, benign condition.

With trochlear paralysis the client is unable to rotate the eyeball nasally downward, and with abducens paralysis the client is unable to rotate the eyeball outward. However, weakness of the lateral rectus muscle is not always a focal sign but may result indirectly from increased intracranial pressure, which may stretch the abducens nerve as it traverses its long course from the pons within the brain stem to the lateral rectus muscles of the eyes.

Frequently, frontal lobe lesions will cause the eyes to deviate toward the location of the lesion—"the client looks at his lesion."

In Parinaud's syndrome the client is initially unable to gaze upward, and eventually the ability to look downward is also affected, designating increased pressure from an upper midbrain lesion. This phenomenon may be accompanied by dilated pupils.

Strabismus and diplopia can occur in conditions in which the extraocular muscles are rendered weak, such as muscular dystrophies, myasthenia gravis, and occasionally hyperthyroidism. Nystagmus may be observed in clients with multiple sclerosis, cerebellar lesions, or inner ear inflammation, as well as in clients who are taking barbiturates and tranquilizers (these

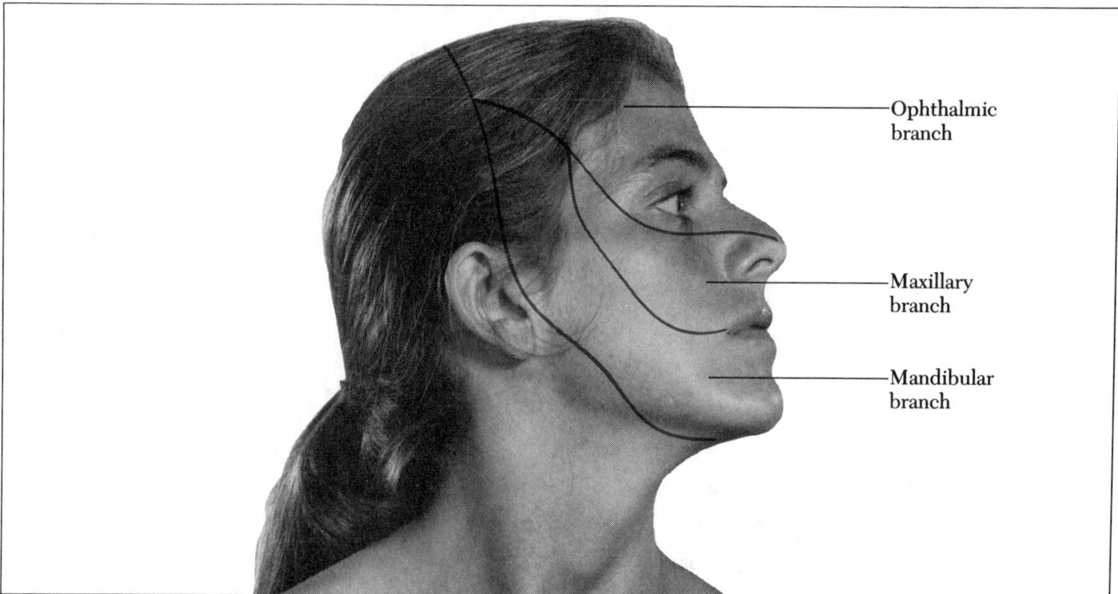

Figure 18-11 Sensory divisions of the trigeminal nerve.

medications interfere with the intricate pathways between the vestibular system and the nuclei of the third, fourth, and sixth cranial nerves).

Assessment of the oculomotor, trochlear, and abducens nerves requires that you observe the client following through the six cardinal gaze positions and that you note whether the eyes are symmetrical at rest.

(V) Trigeminal

The trigeminal nerve is a mixed nerve; that is, it contains both sensory and motor fibers. Its distribution evolves in three branches, as shown in Figure 18-11: (1) ophthalmic, (2) maxillary, (3) mandibular. These divisions consist of superficial sensory nerves of the cornea, the oral and nasal mucosa, and the skin of the face. These anatomical areas are normally sensitive to pain, temperature, and light touch. In addition, the motor fibers of the trigeminal nerve innervate the masseter and temporalis muscles.

To assess the ophthalmic tract, lightly touch the cornea with a wisp of cotton; be sure to touch the cornea and not just the sclera of the eye. This procedure normally results in a blink of the eye, known as the corneal reflex. Assess the pain and light touch sensation of all the branches by using a pinprick and by touching the three areas of the face lightly with a cotton ball. Temperature and pain perception travel essentially the same nerve tracts. Therefore, testing for the presence of temperature sensation is generally done only when there appears to be a loss or a questionable finding regarding pain perception. Should an area of sensory loss be identified, determine its outermost margins by proceeding outwardly from the center of loss until sensation is felt. A loss of sensation should be documented by a sketch of the area of sensory loss in the context of the anatomic part involved.

With trigeminal damage, all modalities (pain, touch, and temperature) may be affected, or you may find that there is only a loss of pain and temperature sensation on one side of the client's face but that the perception of touch is intact. These variations in findings are relevant to the level of the lesion in the brain stem. A high brain stem lesion will generally obliterate all modalities, whereas a lower brain stem lesion will not impair touch perception. A tumor involving the mandibular branch is rare, but it is helpful to remember that numbness of the chin is the first client complaint.

Two afflictions of the trigeminal nerve are herpes zoster and tic douloureux. Herpes zoster (shingles) is a very painful, acute virus infection that appears as a vesicular eruption along the area of distribution of a sensory nerve. Its symptoms of constant itching and pain render it an exhausting disease, particularly for the elderly client. Herpes zoster of the eye produces a severe conjunctivitis and presents the potential danger of corneal ulceration and scarring if untreated. Tic douloureux (trigeminal neuralgia) is characterized by sharp pain spasms of one side of the face, which may be triggered by brushing the teeth, drinking cold liquids, chewing, talking, blowing the nose, shaving, washing the face, or brushing the hair, or by cold drafts. Surgical treatment is resorted to if a medical regimen proves unsuccessful. When surgery is performed the client has a complete loss of facial sensation on the affected side. Thus, infection of the eye may develop as a result of the loss of the corneal reflex. The client should therefore be instructed to watch for signs of corneal infection and to examine the eye frequently for signs of any foreign particles.

The motor portion of the mandibular branch can be assessed by observing for any deviation of the lower jaw as the client opens his mouth and by having the client open his mouth while you use your hand to place resistance under his lower jaw. Normally the jaw is in mid-alignment and the client is able to open his mouth against resistance. Another means of evaluation is to palpate the muscles of mastication as the jaw is clenched. This will aid in the detection of any muscle atrophy, paresis, or paralysis. Weakness of the masseter and temporalis muscles is characteristic in clients with myasthenia gravis and amyotrophic lateral sclerosis (ALS).

(VII) Facial

The facial nerve is also a mixed nerve, with motor fibers to the facial muscles and sensory fibers mediating taste perception of sweet and salty on the anterior two-thirds of the tongue. Therefore, the normal client displays facial symmetry and the ability to identify sweet and salty tastes. (Other taste sensations are involved with the glossopharyngeal nerve and will be mentioned later.) The facial nerve also innervates the lacrimal glands and certain salivary glands. Damage to the motor component results in paralysis of the face muscles of expression. A change in taste sensation and an increase or decrease in salivation and tearing occurs with damage to the sensory component. Sometimes, when trauma has severed the facial nerve fibers, they regenerate and heal incorrectly. This has been evidenced by clients who will weep instead of salivate at the sight of food.

The anatomic tract of the facial nerve extends from the nucleus in the lower pons through the temporal bone and the internal auditory meatus to one side of the face. Its close proximity to the middle ear makes it susceptible to trauma by diseases or surgery in that area, such as otitis media, mastoiditis, fractured temporal bone, or parotid gland tumor.

In routine health assessment, the status of the facial muscles should be observed. Peripheral facial nerve and facial nuclei damage (Bell's palsy) are manifested by weakness or paralysis of all the facial musculature on one side of the face. Generalized weakness of the facial muscles is observed in myasthenia gravis and Guillain-Barré syndrome. You will be able to note that the usual wrinkles seen on the forehead are absent on the weak side.

Should the function of the forehead muscles remain intact but weakness or drooping of the mouth exist, a lesion along the tract from the cerebral cortex motor area of the opposite hemisphere to the nucleus of the facial nerve in the pons (brain stem lesion) should be suspected. This type of facial involvement is commonly observed in cerebrovascular accidents. This is because the lower facial musculature receives fibers only from the opposite cerebral cortex.

The taste sensation ability of the sensory component of the facial nerve is not assessed during a routine health screening. It is pursued only if the client complains of an abnormality regarding taste or if facial nerve damage or a brain stem lesion is suspected.

To test taste perception, dip an applicator stick in a preparation solution and place it on a portion of the client's tongue. Figure 18-12 identifies the various taste regions of the tongue. It is important that the client keep his tongue out until the taste is identified—the material will spread to all areas of the tongue if the client retracts it before identifying the taste. Test each side of the tongue separately and in succession with the various solutions for salty (salt solution), sweet (sugar water), bitter (quinine water), and sour (vinegar solution) tastes. After each application to the tongue and identification of the solution by the client, have him rinse his mouth well with water.

(VIII) Auditory or Acoustic

The auditory nerve has two divisions: the cochlear branch and the vestibular branch. The cochlear portion is concerned with hearing and is routinely assessed on health screening. The

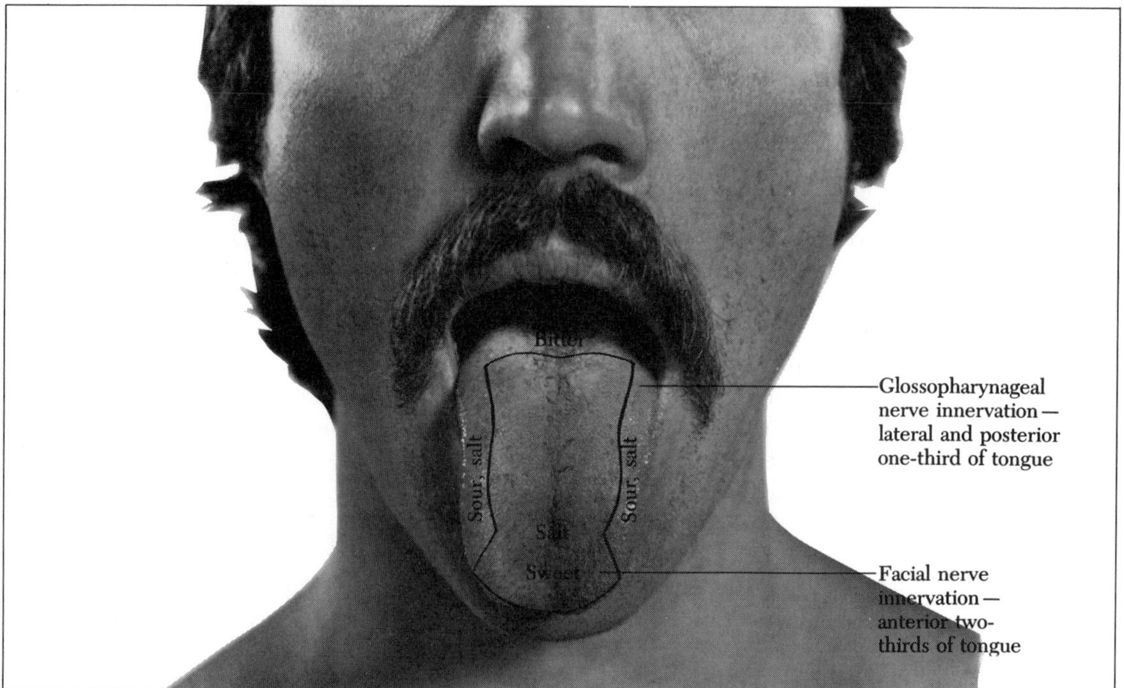

Figure 18-12 Taste regions of the tongue.

gross assessment procedures are described in Chapter 12. When difficulties arise with this portion of the auditory nerve, audiometry examination must be conducted for a more accurate evaluation.

The vestibular portion of the auditory nerve is concerned with equilibrium. Unless there is suspicion of disease of the vestibular system, evaluative tests of its function are not performed. However, symptoms of vertigo, ataxia, nausea, and vomiting warrant investigation of this system, and you should observe closely for signs of nystagmus (involuntary oscillation of the eyeball) and past pointing. Nystagmus or vertigo will present in neural disease when the client is made to perform sudden alterations in head position.

A specific test for evaluating vestibular function is the caloric test, in which the client is placed in supine position with his head elevated approximately 30 degrees. (This is done in order to place the horizontal semicircular canals in a vertical position). With a syringe and a soft-tipped rubber catheter, introduce 5 ml of ice water into the ear under gentle pressure. In the normal individual this will produce vertigo, nystagmus, nausea, and often vomiting, since the vestibular branch is functioning. These symptoms occur because the vestibular nuclei are connected to the cranial nerves governing the extraocular muscles and to the visceral organs of the abdomen and thorax. Test both ears. If there is no reaction to the caloric test, the vestibular branch on that side is affected.

(IX) Glossopharyngeal, (X) Vagus

The glossopharyngeal and vagus nerves are discussed under a single heading to emphasize their close anatomic and functional relationship. The glossopharyngeal nerve innervates the pharynx, palate, and posterior third of the tongue. Its motor function to the stylopharyngeus muscle is minimal; this muscle widens the pharynx during the process of swallowing, and its impairment is not usually recognized clinically.

To determine the presence of sensation and gag reflex, touch the sides of the pharynx lightly. The gag reflex is often brisk in heavy smokers and nervous individuals. The gag reflex is not routinely tested because it is an unpleasant experience. It is checked, however, when a neural disorder is suspected. With glossopharyngeal nerve damage the gag reflex may be dampened. Also, a rare disease called glossopharyngeal neuralgia may result from insult to the glossopharyngeal nerve. This affliction is characterized by severe paroxysms of pain in the throat initiated by swallowing.

In light of neurologic complaints or signs, the taste sensation of the posterior third of the tongue, which is for bitter and sour, should be tested to evaluate the glossopharyngeal nerve (see Figure 18-12). With a lesion, there is a loss of taste over the posterior third of the tongue and decreased sensation in the pharynx and palate. The normal individual has no difficulty with swallowing or with identifying bitter and sour tastes.

The vagus nerve has motor fibers supplying the larynx, pharynx, and palate (external laryngeal, recurrent laryngeal, and pharyngeal nerves, respectively); visceromotor fibers also innervate the heart, lungs, and alimentary tract. The sensory function of the vagus is widespread, as it receives impulses from the pharynx, larynx, epiglottis, trachea, esophagus, heart, lungs, stomach, and small intestine.

Basically, swallowing and phonation are the most important functions of the vagus nerve neurologically and are checked routinely. To evaluate these functions, have the client swallow water. Regurgitation of the water through the nose would indicate weakness of the soft palate and an inability to close off the nasopharynx; this inability is commonly found in hemiplegic clients, but it can occur with other conditions, such as multiple sclerosis, amyotrophic lateral sclerosis, meningitis, encephalitis, cerebral and aortic aneurysms, enlarged glands, and tumors in the neck and thorax, as well as trauma to the neck or thorax from injury or surgical procedures (particularly thyroid operations). It is also important to study the timbre of the client's voice. Dysphagia (weakness or paralysis of swallowing), aphonia (loss of voice), or hoarseness may indicate vagal damage, and direct mirror laryngoscopy is advisable. Hoarseness persisting over two weeks requires physician consultation. Ordinarily, in routine assessment the position of the uvula is checked at rest and during phonation to aid in evaluation of the vagus nerve. When the client says "aah," the uvula will normally rise symmetrically in midline. With vagus nerve damage, the uvula will deviate away from the affected side. If both sides are affected, movement will be absent.

(XI) Spinal Accessory

The function of the spinal accessory nerve is clear-cut. It innervates the trapezius and sternocleidomastoid muscles. Therefore, the normal client has strength in these muscles and displays symmetry of the shoulders, neck, and scapulae. This nerve is rarely affected alone but is seen in accompaniment with other cranial nerve palsies. Spinal accessory involvement may be observed in trauma to the neck. To specifically test the function of the spinal accessory nerve, apply resistance to the client's shoulders and ask him to shrug his shoulders. Next ask the client to turn his head from side to side against applied resistance. The sternocleidomastoid muscles can be evaluated by having the client flex his head against the resistance of your hand on his forehead. When nerve involvement is suspected, observe for drooping of the shoulder as well as difficulty or inability to raise the arm above the head. With involvement, the scapula is displaced downward and there may be a slight winging (outward displacement). Atrophy and flatness of the neck may be noted on the affected side, and weakness in neck flexion occurs with paralysis of both sternocleidomastoid muscles.

(XII) Hypoglossal

The hypoglossal is a motor nerve that innervates the tongue. The appearance, movement, and strength of the tongue should be evaluated by observation, both with the tongue inside the mouth and sticking out. You can have the client move his tongue against the inside of his cheek as you apply resistance to the outside of the cheek with a finger, or you can have the client move it against resistance supplied by a tongue blade. Atrophy and increased coating may be observed on a paralyzed side. In early involvement, atrophy is quite difficult to detect, but it will manifest as scalloping or indentation along the edge of the tongue. In corticobulbar tract damage, pseudobulbar palsy occurs, displaying severe tongue weakness. Severe tongue weakness also occurs in poliomyelitis and amyotrophic lateral sclerosis, diseases that affect the cranial nerve nuclei and, therefore, are of lower motor neuron damage. Differentiation of lesion origin is possible, since these diseases involving lower motor neuron damage will have accompanying signs of muscle atrophy and fasciculations. Unilateral hypoglossal nucleus damage, which

Table 18-2. Techniques for Cranial Nerve Assessment

Cranial Nerve	Technique	Common Problems
I. Olfactory	1. Have client close eyes. 2. Close off client's naris by placing pressure against the side with an index finger. 3. Hold substance—e.g., soap, lemon, coffee—near naris. 4. Ask client to identify substance. 5. Repeat procedure for the remaining naris.	Anosmia.
II. Optic	See techniques described in Chapter 11 "Assessment of the Eye," e.g., visual acuity, visual fields, eye grounds.	Decreased or loss of visual acuity, visual field defects, changes in optic nerve disk.
III. Oculomotor	1. Inspect eyelids 2. Inspect pupil sizes and reaction to light, accommodation, and convergence (see Chapter 11). 3. Check EOMS. 4. Note whether eyes are symmetrical at rest.	Ptosis of eyelid. Dilated pupil.
IV. Trochlear	1. Check EOMS. 2. Note whether eyes are symmetrical at rest.	Unable to gaze in nasally downward direction.
V. Trigeminal	1. Check corneal reflex (see Chapter 11) and three sensory divisions (ophthalmic, maxillary, and mandibular) with a cotton wisp, pinprick, and temperature (hot and cold water–filled test tubes). 2. Observe for jaw deviation. 3. Palpate masseter muscle while teeth are clenched and unclenched. 4. Have client open lower jaw against resistance (place your hand under lower jaw to provide resistance).	Brain stem lesion, herpes zoster, tic douloureux. Masseter and temporalis muscle weakness with myasthenia gravis and amyotrophic lateral sclerosis (ALS).
VI. Abducens	1. Check EOMS. 2. Note whether eyes are symmetrical at rest.	Unable to gaze in lateral direction.
VII. Facial	1. Observe for symmetry at rest and while client smiles, frowns, clenches teeth, blows out cheeks, purses lips.	Bell's palsy.

may result from a neck injury, would manifest unilateral weakness, atrophy, and fasciculations of the tongue. In this case, the strong, intact side of the tongue would push and cause the tongue to deviate toward the affected, weak side as it protrudes. Normally the tongue is symmetrical in shape, protrudes midline, and possesses motor strength.

In summary, if the client displays signs and symptoms, the cranial nerves should be meticulously tested. If time limits are imposed during routine health assessment, the most pertinent evaluations to be performed regarding the cranial nerves are assessment of the visual fields, extraocular muscle movements, pupillary reflexes, facial innervation, tongue movement, and swallowing. See Table 18-2.

Assessment of Neurologic Reflexes

A *reflex* is elicited by applying a sensory stimulus that initiates the transmission of a muscle-stretch

Table 18-2. *Continued*

Cranial Nerve	Technique	Common Problems
	2. Test for sweet and salty taste sensation on anterior two-thirds of tongue. 3. Dip applicator in salt-water solution. 4. Ask client to extend tongue and identify taste before retracting tongue into mouth. 5. Place applicator on anterior portion of tongue. 6. Rinse mouth with water. 7. Repeat procedure with sugar-water solution.	Change in taste sensation. Decrease in salivation and tearing.
VIII. Auditory or acoustic	1. Weber test (see Chapter 12). 2. Rinne test (see Chapter 12). 3. Special tests a. Audiometry examination. b. Caloric test (see page 359).	Decreased or loss of hearing. Acoustic neuroma.
IX. Glossopharyngeal	1. Observe for difficulty swallowing. 2. Check gag reflex. 3. Test for bitter and sour taste sensation on posterior one-third of tongue using quinine water and vinegar respectively.	Dysphasia, decreased gag reflex, glossopharyngeal neuralgia, and change in taste sensation.
X. Vagus	1. Observe for difficulty swallowing as client drinks water. 2. Check uvular reflex.	Hoarseness or aphonia, regurgitation of water through the nose.
XI. Spinal accessory	1. Have client shrug shoulders against resistance (place your hands on client's shoulders). 2. Observe scapula. 3. Place hand on side of client's forehead. 4. Ask client to flex his head against your hand. 5. Repeat on opposite side of face.	Drooping of shoulder, unable to raise arm above head. Scapula displaced downward and maybe slight winging.
XII. Hypoglossal	1. Have client stick out tongue. 2. Have client move tongue against resistance (tongue blades or examiner's finger on outside of cheek). 3. Observe for scalloping or indentation along edge of tongue.	Tongue deviation, weakness, atrophy.

impulse or a cutaneous stimulation through the reflex arc in the spinal cord. Figure 18-13 shows that the reflex arc involves the union of a sensory and a motor nerve fiber. The sensory stimulus creates a sensory impulse that is carried by a sensory nerve fiber within a peripheral nerve to the posterior root horn. It synapses with a motor neuron in the anterior root horn, and the motor nerve fiber carries the impulse back to the muscle, which contracts. Should any of the fibers of the reflex arc be interrupted, the reflex is absent (lower motor nerve damage). The briskness of the intact reflex arc is regulated by the upper motor neurons of the cerebral cortex. Therefore, cortical motor tract damage, characteristically present in the majority of cerebrovascular accidents, manifests exaggerated reflexes or hyperreflexia because the cord reflex arc is still intact but there is loss of the cerebral "dampening" ability.

It is extremely important for the client's muscles to be *relaxed* in order to elicit and accurately evaluate the neurologic reflexes. The stimulus should be applied evenly to corresponding sides

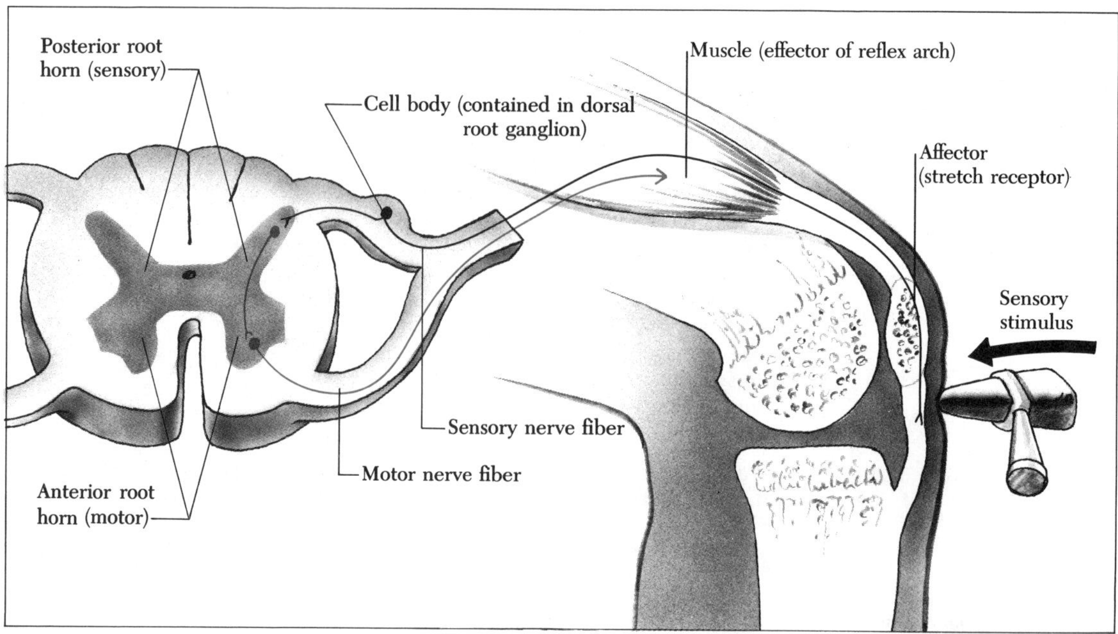

Figure 18-13 The reflex arc.

of the client's body and the results then compared.

For assessment purposes the reflexes are considered in three basic categories: (1) deep tendon reflexes (DTRs), (2) superficial (cutaneous) reflexes, and (3) pathologic reflexes.

Deep Tendon Reflexes

DTRs are unstable in the newborn, so testing results are of little significance at this age. DTRs may be absent during neural shock, which generally lasts from 4 to 7 days following a severe injury. They are also absent in increased intracranial pressure of a high degree, as well as in lower motor neuron damage, such as in poliomyelitis, tumor, or injury to the anterior motor horn of the spinal cord. Peripheral nerve diseases and herniated intervertebral disks can also cause absent DTRs. Diseases of the muscles (muscular dystrophy) may result in decreased or absent DTRs, not because of neural/reflex arc damage but because of the muscle fiber involvement. Gradually diminishing DTRs are observed in myasthenia gravis with successive testing; that is, when the percussion site is struck 3 or 4 times in a row, each response decreases in quality. With myxedema a slowed relaxation phase may be noted. However, some individuals are normally areflexic and may not have any demonstrable DTRs.

With an absence of DTRs or with diminished responses, you should instruct the client to perform isometric muscular contractions elsewhere in the body before drawing your final conclusions regarding his reflex status. Ask him to lock his fingers together and pull when you test his reflexes in the lower extremities and to squeeze his thigh as you test the reflexes in his upper extremities. At the moment of muscle tenseness during these maneuvers, strike the tendon with the percussion hammer. These reinforcement techniques usually facilitate neural conduction in the reflex arc if the arc is intact.

The most common DTR tests are presented in Table 18-3. The grading system for tendon reflexes shown in Table 18-4 is an arbitrary method of categorizing deep tendon reflexes. Figure 18-14 gives examples of how the grading system is implemented for a client with normal tendon reflexes and for a client diagnosed with a right cerebrovascular accident.

Superficial (Cutaneous) Reflexes

The commonly tested superficial reflexes, illustrated in Table 18-5, are the abdominal, cremasteric, plantar, and anal. These reflexes are present by approximately 6 months of age. The upper and lower abdominal reflex is difficult to elicit if the abdominal muscles are not relaxed. To perform this test, briskly stroke the skin of

Table 18-3. Deep Tendon Reflexes

Reflex	Percussion Site	Response	CNS dermatomes
Biceps	Biceps tendon 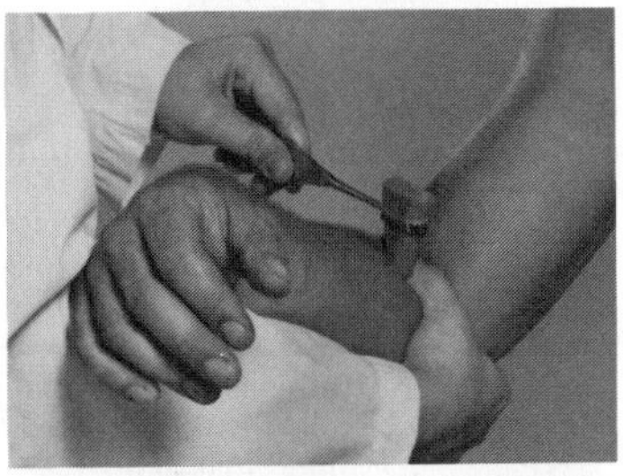	Biceps contraction (Place your thumb on tendon cord in midantecubital space with client's elbow flexed. Strike your thumbnail with percussion hammer.)	Cervical 5 and 6
Triceps	Triceps tendon 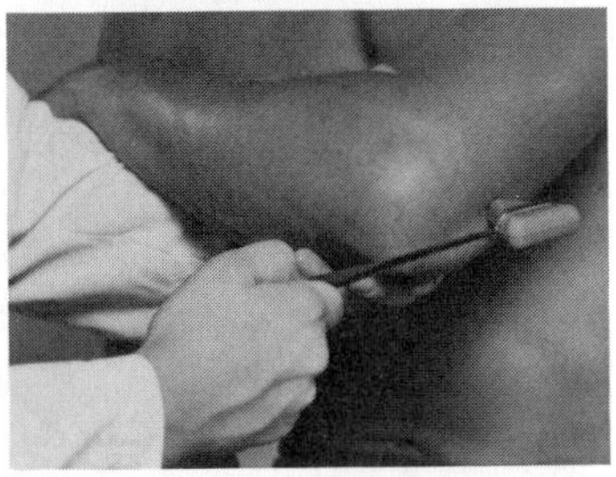	Elbow extension; triceps contraction (Strike tendon with percussion hammer about 1.5 inches above the olecranon process.)	Cervical 6–8
Brachioradialis	Styloid process of radius 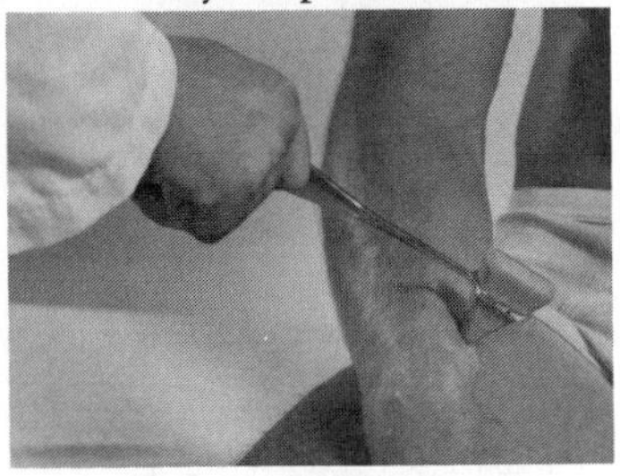	Pronation of forearm and hand (Strike tendon about 2 inches above the wrist on the radial [thumb] side of the arm.)	Cervical 5 and 6
Patellar	Patellar tendon 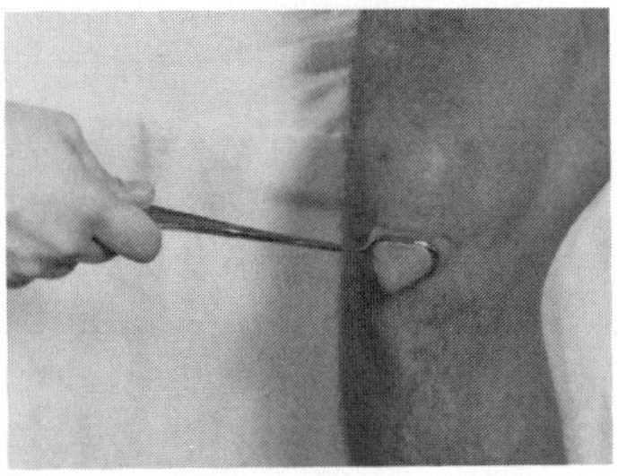	Knee extension (Strike tendon immediately below the patella [knee cap].)	Lumbar 2–4
Achilles	Achilles tendon 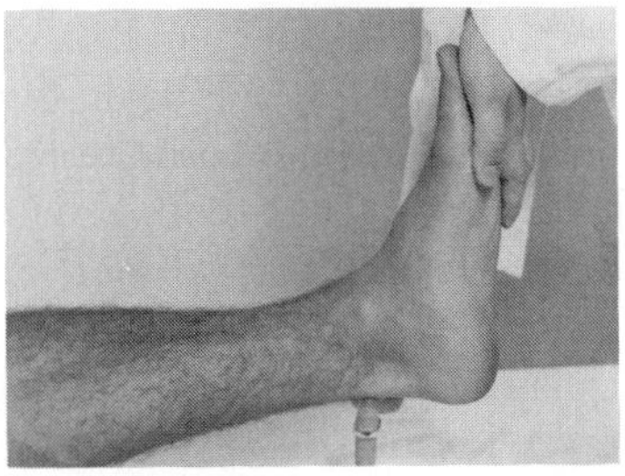	Plantar flexion of foot (Strike heelcord as you gently apply pressure to bottom of foot.)	Sacral 1 and 2

Table 18-4. Grading System for Tendon Reflexes

Grade	Symbols	Interpretation
0	0	Absent (indicate whether reinforcement used)
1	+	Diminished but present
2	+ +	Normal; average
3	+ + +	Normal; brisker than average—may or may not indicate pathology
4	+ + + +	Hyperactive; very brisk—most often pathologic
5	+ + + + +	Hyperactive with clonus

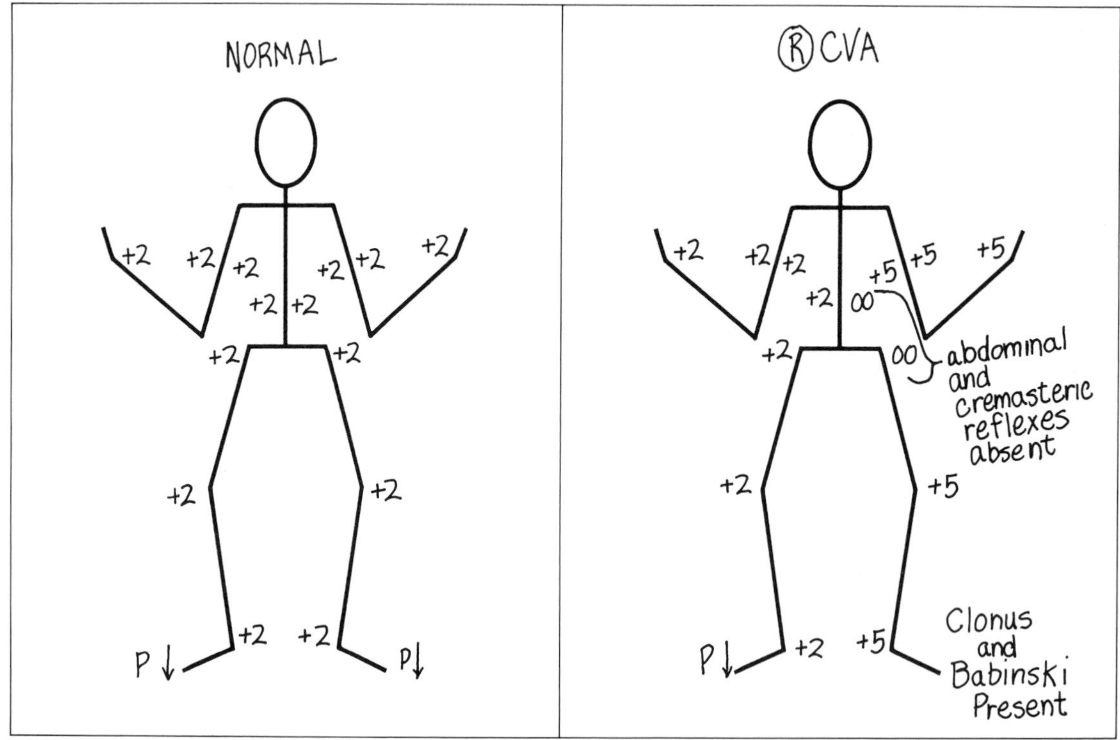

Figure 18-14 Grading of tendon reflexes.

the upper abdomen in the four quadrants from periphery to umbilicus with a sharp object (key, tongue blade, end of applicator). Normally the umbilicus will move toward the area stimulated. The lower abdominal reflex is similarly tested, resulting in a downward movement of the umbilicus. The abdominal reflex is generally elicited quite easily in the young. However, it may be absent in the elderly, in the obese, or in persons having a history of multiple abdominal surgeries or several pregnancies. In the obese client you may be able to palpate the presence of muscular contraction if you first retract and hold the umbilicus away from the direction being stimulated.

The cremasteric reflex is tested in the male client by stroking the inner aspect of each thigh with a sharp object. The normal response is elevation of the scrotum on the side stroked.

Absence of these cutaneous reflexes will be contralateral to damage of the corticospinal tract above the level of the medulla (cortex damage), whereas the absence will be on the same side of a lesion involving the corticospinal tract below medullary level. Thus, both abdominal and cremasteric reflexes may be absent with both upper and lower motor tract damage.

Stroking the bottom of the foot elicits the plantar reflex, in which the toes curl under. This normal response is recorded as "plantar."

Table 18-5. Superficial Reflexes

Reflex	Stimulus site	Response	CNS dermatomes
Abdominal		Umbilicus moves toward area stroked	Upper thoracic 7–9
Cremasteric		Scrotum elevates	Thoracic 12 and lumbar 1
Plantar		Toes flex	Sacral 1 and 2
Anal	Rectal stimulation by gloved finger	Contraction of anal sphincter	Sacral

To evaluate the intactness of the sacral neural dermatome, insert a gloved finger into the rectum. The normal response is contraction of the anal sphincter muscle.

Pathologic Reflexes

Pathologic reflexes (see Table 18-6) are documented as being absent or present. In the healthy individual they should be absent. However, these reflexes may normally be present at birth and remain up until 2 years of age because of the immaturity of the infant nervous system. Their appearance in the individuals over age 2 is a sign of pathology and requires medical consultation and evaluation.

The Babinski reflex is tested for during a routine physical assessment, since it is elicited, if present, by the same stimulus used for testing the plantar reflex. Ankle clonus is tested for if the DTRs or superficial reflexes are hyperactive. The pathologic reflexes—Babinski, Chaddock, Oppenheim, Gordon, Hoffmann, and ankle clonus—are significant signs of upper motor neuron (cortex) damage.

When meningeal irritation (meningitis, encephalitis, head trauma, blood in the cerebrospinal fluid) is suspected, the presence of Kernig's and Brudzinski's signs should be determined.

Table 18-7 attempts to summarize the findings of upper motor neuron (UMN) damage typically observed in such conditions as cerebrovascular accidents, brain tumors, and cerebral aneurysms, as compared to those findings characteristic of lower motor neuron (LMN) damage, as in clients with paraplegia and quadriplegia.

Summary

Learning the assessment techniques and normal functioning of the neurologic system is facilitated by understanding this system's structure and

Table 18-6. Pathologic Reflexes

Reflex	How elicited	Response if present
Babinski	Stroke lateral aspect of sole of foot	Extension of great toe and fanning of the toes
Chaddock	Stroke lateral aspect of foot beneath the lateral malleolus	Same response as above
Oppenheim	Stroke anteromedial tibial surface	Same as above
Gordon	Squeeze calf muscles firmly	Same as above
Hoffmann	Flick terminal phalanx of middle finger downward	Flexion of thumb and/or fingers (clawing)
Ankle clonus	Sudden, brisk dorsiflexion of foot with knee flexed and applying sustained and moderate pressure	Exaggerated rhythmic up-and-down movements of foot (a rapidly exhaustible clonus may be normal)
Kernig's sign (meningeal irritation)	Straight leg raising or below knee extension with thigh flexed on abdomen	Limitation with pain down posterior thigh
Brudzinski's sign (meningeal irritation)	Flexing chin on chest	Limitation with pain

Table 18-7. Comparison of Findings: Damage to Upper Motor Neurons and Lower Motor Neurons

Signs	UMN damage	LMN damage
Muscle tone	Increased/spastic—greater in flexors in arms and extensors in legs	Flaccid, hypotonus, loss of tone, wasting of muscles (atrophy)
Reflexes	Hyperreflexia; Babinski present; ankle/knee clonus	Areflexic; Babinski absent; clonus absent
Fasciculations	Absent	Present
Paralysis or weakness	Paralysis or weakness in limb(s) according to degree of pressure damage to the pyramidal distribution of lesion; weakness usually in hand grip, arm extensors, and leg flexors	Paralysis or weakness in appropriate muscles, depending on which spinal segment, root, or peripheral nerve is damaged

physiologic functioning. The main areas to be assessed are the cerebrum, cerebellum, cranial nerves, and reflexes.

Assessment of this system begins with initial contact with the client. Data on mental status are recorded during the history-taking, and mental status continues to be noted throughout the nursing assessment process. Cerebral assessment includes observation of frontal, parietal, occipital, and temporal lobe functions. Cerebellar assessment includes balance and coordination examination techniques. The functions of the cranial nerves are assessed in sequence. Reflexes to be examined include the deep tendon reflexes, superficial or cutaneous reflexes, and pathologic reflexes.

Discussion Questions/Activities

1. Draw a diagram of the cerebrum and label the various lobes, indicating the major functions of each.
2. What manifestations would be present with damage to Broca's area? to Wernicke's area? Where are these areas located in the cerebrum?
3. What are some of the signs and symptoms characteristic of a client with a temporal lobe tumor? What would be a differentiating factor between a temporal lobe attack and a psychiatric disorder?
4. What cranial nerve palsies frequently accompany cerebellar dysfunction?

5. Discuss the factors considered when assessing gait.
6. What are the two categories of cerebellar assessment? Demonstrate the techniques used to test them.
7. Name the cranial nerves; discuss how you would assess each one; state the normal findings for each cranial nerve.
8. Where along the optic tract would you find a lesion causing each of the following conditions: (a) cortical blindness? (b) bitemporal hemianopia? (c) homonymous hemianopia?
9. What two cranial nerves are concerned with taste? In what circumstances and how would you assess the sensation of taste?
10. State the signs and symptoms that would alert you to the need for investigation of the vestibular branch of the auditory system.
11. If you have only a short period of time to test the cranial nerves, what are the seven most pertinent evaluations that you would perform?
12. Name the DTRs that are routinely assessed and the normal response of each.
13. Discuss how the commonly assessed superficial reflexes are each tested, and state the normal response of each.
14. State the physical responses that you would observe if the following pathological reflexes were present: Babinski, ankle clonus, Hoffmann, Kernig's sign, and Brudzinski's sign. What techniques would you use to attempt to elicit each of these responses?

Recording of Findings

The first box contains normal findings; the second box contains recordings of abnormal findings.

Cerebrum

INSPECTION

Oriented to person, time, and place; recent and remote memory intact; appropriate behavior and speech; alert and cooperative; stereognosis, two-point discrimination, and graphesthesia intact.

Cerebellum

INSPECTION

Normal gait; Romberg's sign absent; tandem walking, finger to nose, heel to shin smoothly intact; rapid alternating hand movements and fingers intact; thumb opposition without difficulty; no tremors.

Cranial Nerves

INSPECTION

Grossly intact. I: able to discriminate between soap, tobacco; II: OU 20/20 with corrective lenses; peripheral vision intact; III, IV, VI: PERRLA; no ptosis; EOMs intact without nystagmus; no strabismus; V: corneal reflex present; light touch and pain sensation intact; can open mandible against resistance; VII: facial symmetry; no weakness; sweet and salty taste discrimination; VIII: hearing intact; IX, X: gag reflex present; bitter and sour taste intact; no dysphagia; uvular reflex intact; XI: neck-head movement and shoulder shrug intact; no weakness; scapulae in horizontal plane; XII: tongue protrudes midline; no weakness; no atrophy; no fasciculations.

Reflexes

INSPECTION

Plantar reflex; no Babinski; no clonus; normal abdominal reflexes.

	B	T	BR	P	A	PR
R	+ +	+ +	+ +	+ +	+ +	↓
L	+ +	+ +	+ +	+ +	+ +	↓

Cerebrum

(Client with cerebral arteriosclerosis)

INSPECTION

Oriented to person; disoriented to time and place; poor immediate recall and recent memory; remote memory fair at times; slow to respond; short attention span.

Cerebellum

(Client with Parkinson's disease)

INSPECTION

Forward lunging gait; short shuffling steps; difficulty stopping; arms held stiffly at sides; resting tremors.

Cranial Nerves

(Client with amyotrophic lateral sclerosis)

INSPECTION

I, II, III, IV, VI, VIII: intact; V: light touch and pain intact; corneal blink; weak masseter muscles; unable to hold eyes closed tightly; IX, X: slurred speech; mild dysphagia with occasional nasal regurgitation of liquids; diminished gag and uvular reflex; XI: decreased shoulder shrug and movement of head from side to side against resistance; XII: decreased strength of tongue, atrophy and fasciculations present.

Reflexes

(Client with right cerebrovascular accident)

INSPECTION

Right plantar reflex; left clonus; left Babinski present; cremasteric and abdominal reflexes absent on left side.

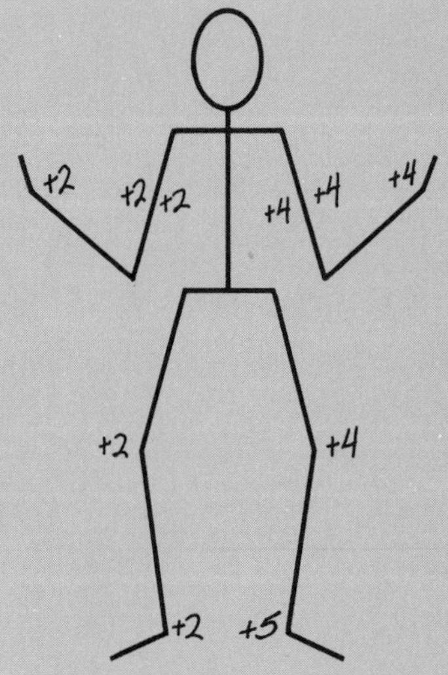

CHAPTER 19

Assessment of the Genitals and Rectum

LEARNING OBJECTIVES

1. Review structure and function of the genitals.
2. List the characteristics of the genitals that are considered during inspection.
3. Describe the techniques for palpation of the testes and scrotum.
4. Describe the procedure for insertion of a vaginal speculum.
5. State the areas from which smears are obtained for a Pap test.
6. Describe the bimanual pelvic examination and the reason for doing this procedure.
7. Describe the rectovaginal-abdominal examination and the reason for doing this procedure.
8. Recognize the importance for putting on a new glove when proceeding from the genital exam to the rectovaginal-abdominal exam.
9. State the characteristics noted in inspection and palpation of the anus and rectum.
10. Describe the technique used in performing a rectal exam.

It is not uncommon to discover in the client's record that the genital and rectal examination has been deferred. In most cases such deferment is due to cultural and sexual attitudes or problems on the part of both clients and health workers, including nurses. Because pathology can occur in the genitals and rectum as well as in any other anatomic region of the body, it is important to have a positive attitude toward assessment of this region, geared toward promotion of health and detection of disease. Infection is a reality, so you should wear gloves while performing assessment of these two areas of the body. Assure the client that the gloves are used to avoid cross-contamination and for the client's welfare.

Because this particular portion of the physical assessment may be embarrassing and uncomfortable, proper client preparation and support during the assessment is essential. Assemble the equipment to be used beforehand, and arrange the environment to provide comfort and privacy for the client. As you progress through the assessment, explain each step to the client prior to performing it. Before beginning the examination of the genitals and rectum, tell the client that it may be uncomfortable at moments but that you will proceed as gently as possible. Ask the client to tell you immediately if he experiences any

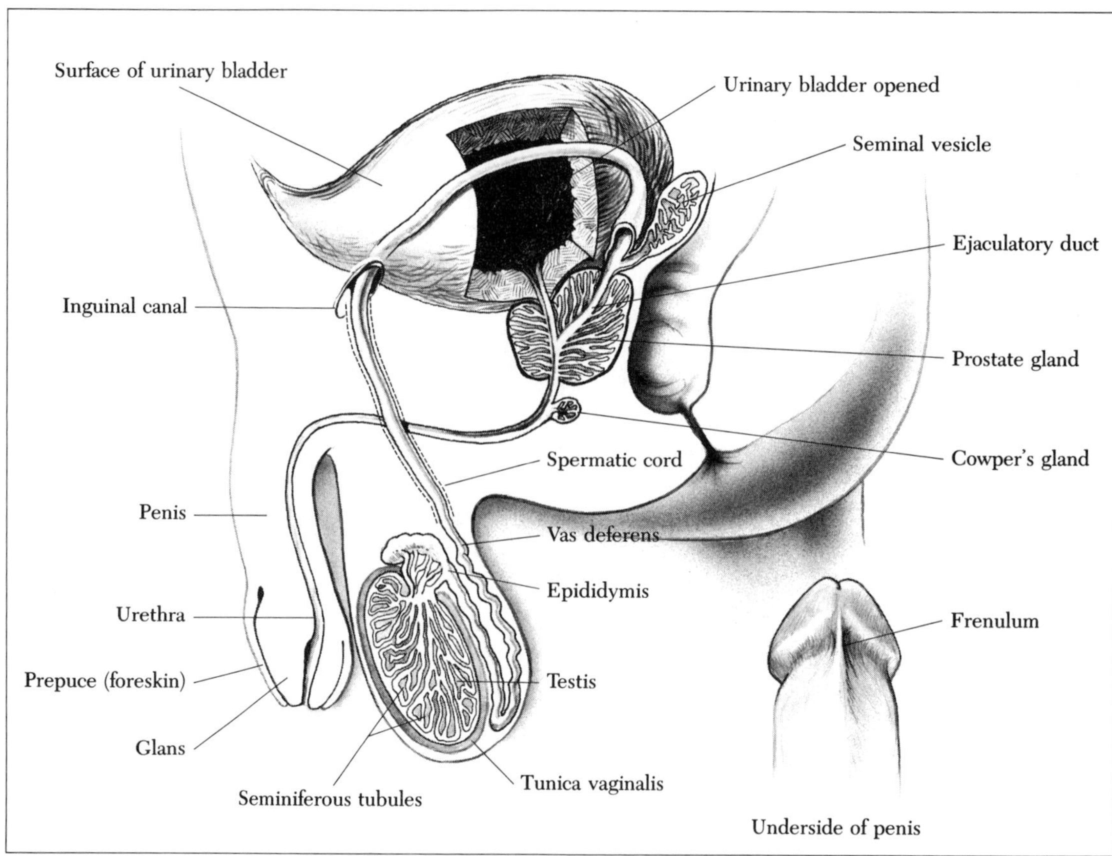

Figure 19-1 The male genitals.

pain. Assure the client that if pain should develop the examination will be stopped.

Structure and Function of the Male Genitals

Figure 19-1 identifies the major structures of the male reproductive system. The function of the *testes* is the production of spermatozoa (by the *seminiferous tubules*) and the production of testosterone (by the Leydig's cells). The *epididymis* is located posterolateral to the testis. The distal portion of the epididymis, called the *vas deferens,* is part of the *spermatic cord.* Encased within the spermatic fascia and constituting the spermatic cord are the vas deferens, arteries, veins, nerves, and lymphatic vessels. The spermatic cord passes through the *inguinal canal* and enters the abdominal cavity. It continues upward to join the *seminal vesicle* behind the *bladder.* The seminal vesicle secretes a nutritious protective fluid for the sperm. Another protective (alkaline) fluid is produced for the sperm by *Cowper's gland.* This latter fluid also serves as a lubricant.

Characteristics and Techniques of Examination

On inspection of the male genitals, first note the pubic hair distribution. This may vary somewhat from person to person; only the absence or extreme sparseness of pubic hair in the adult male need be reported. Usually the diamond-shape pattern is observed.

Penis

Figure 19-2 shows the normal male penis. Gross inspection will reveal the size of the penis, which also varies from person to person. Only wide deviations in size are likely to be of significance. Usually the left testis will be lower than the right. Inspect the skin covering the penis and scrotum to detect the presence of any abnormal-

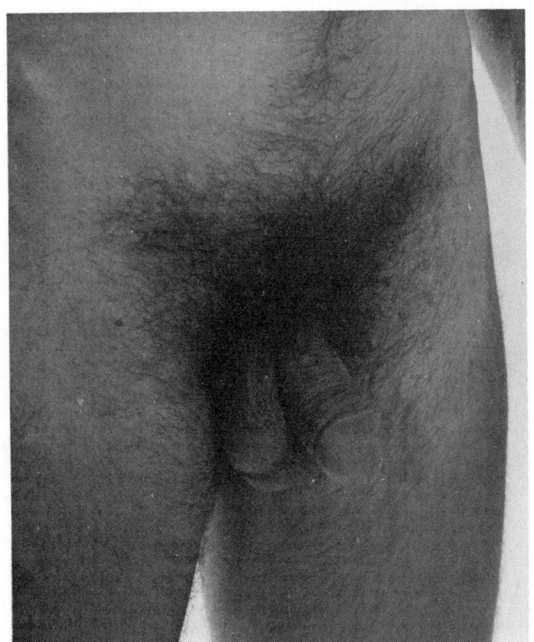

Figure 19-2 Normal male genitals.

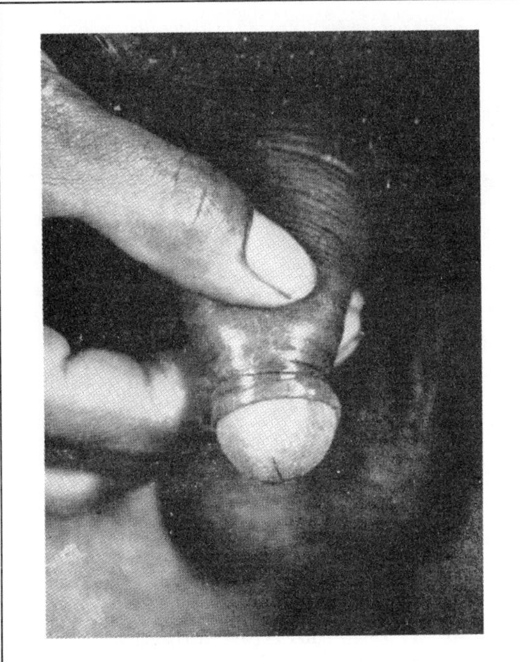

Figure 19-3 Phimosis of moderate degree. Note constriction of the glans as foreskin is retracted.

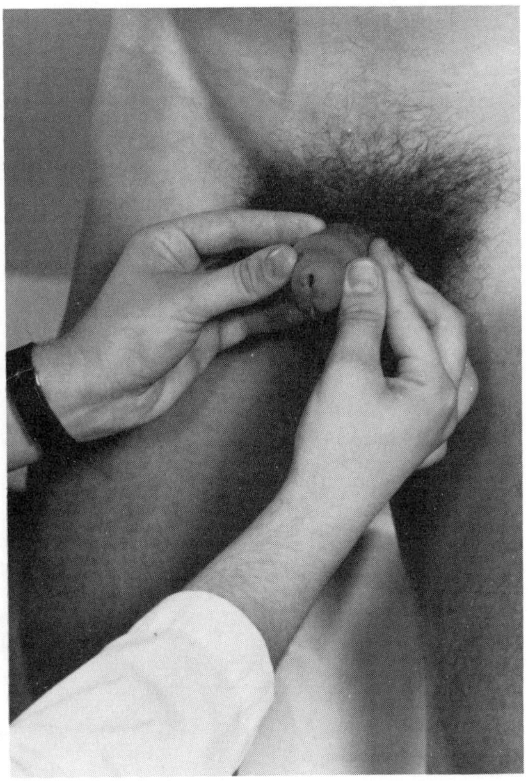

Figure 19-4 Inspection of the urethra.

ities. Inspection of the skin for lesions or scars can be accomplished simultaneously with palpation. Note whether the client is circumcised or uncircumcised.

The *foreskin* of the penis (see Figure 19-1) should be easily retracted back over the *glans*. This is not possible in phimosis, a condition in which the foreskin adheres to the glans (see Figure 19-3). A small amount of thick white secretion may be observed between the foreskin and the glans; this is a normal secretion called smegma. Next palpate the penile shaft for any signs of tenderness or induration. Normally the *urethral meatus* is present at the distal end of the *frenulum*. Variations are hypospadias, in which the meatus is located on the underside of the penile shaft, and epispadias, in which it is on the top surface of the penis. Such abnormalities are generally corrected by plastic surgery at a young age. To inspect the *urethra*, use your thumbs to separate the meatus, as shown in Figure 19-4. A culture should be taken if a thick, purulent discharge is noted, as this suggests gonorrhea. Gonorrhea may also manifest associated urinary symptoms. If untreated, the disease process could lead to sterility, arthritis, and endocarditis. A thin, mucoid discharge may indicate urethritis.

If, during the health history, the client has complained of dysuria or a change in urination stream, try to observe the client's voiding, if possible. A deviated or poor stream suggests such

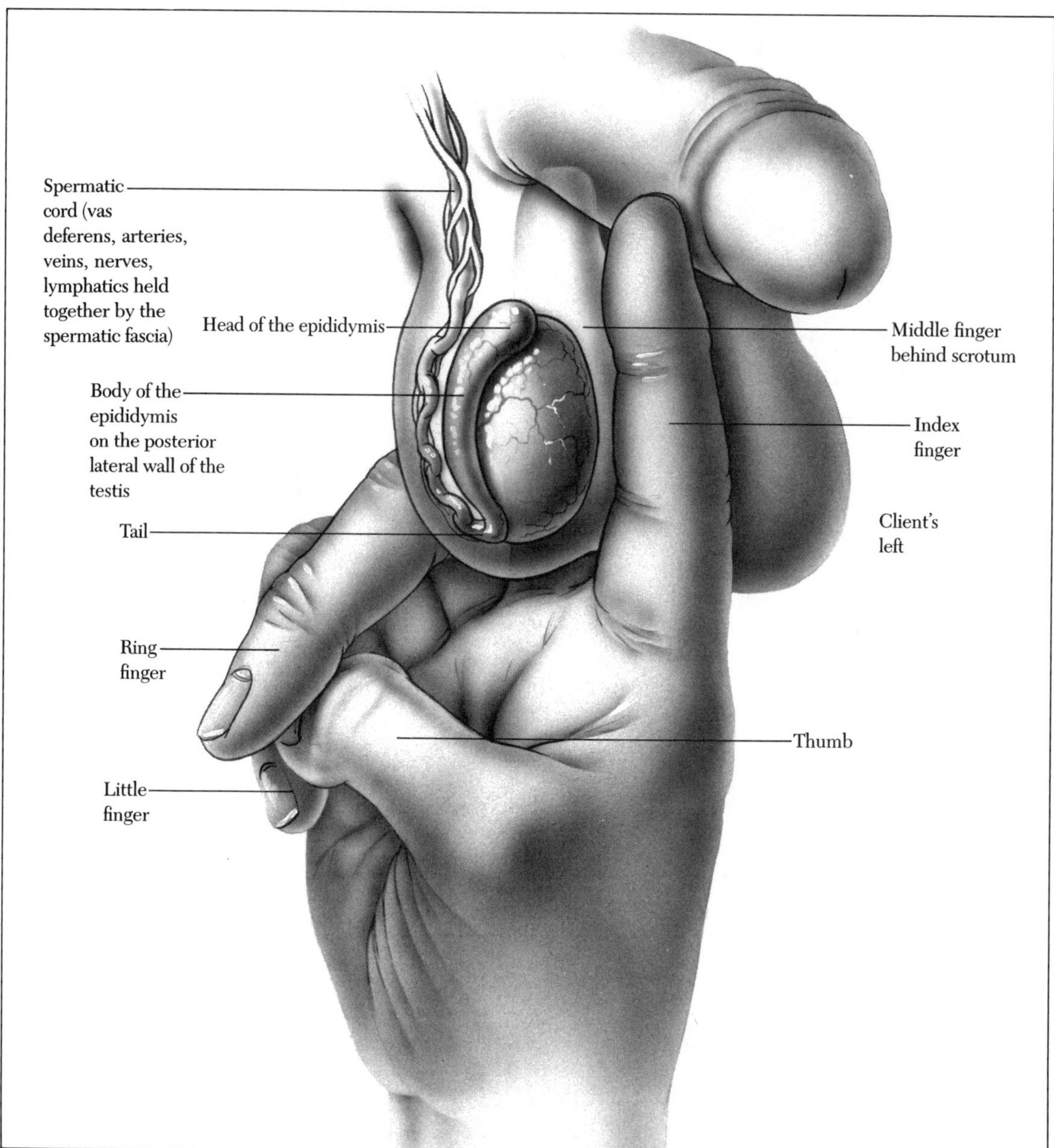

Figure 19-5 Palpation of the scrotum.

conditions as urethral stricture, urethral polyp, or urethral obstruction from prostatic hyperplasia.

Scrotum

To best examine and palpate the scrotum, the client should be standing and you should sit in front of him. To assess the scrotum, use your index and middle fingers like a pair of scissors, to separate the testes and divide the scrotum in half. Figure 19-5 illustrates this technique. The right testis and epididymis should be examined with the left hand, and vice versa. Gentle palpation is warranted; normally the testes are tender. The testes are 2 × 4 cm in size and are rubbery (neither hard nor soft) in consistency. They become softer and decrease in size during middle age. Both the epididymis and the spermatic cord should be palpable. The cord is of a harder consistency than the epididymis and is best palpated high in the lateral portion of the

Techniques for Inspection and Palpation of Penis

1. Arrange for client comfort and privacy.
2. Have adequate lighting.
3. Sit on chair facing standing client.
4. Put on gloves.
5. Explain each step prior to doing it.
6. Characteristics of inspection:
   Hair distribution
   Size and contour
   Skin surfaces
   Position of urethral meatus
   Abnormalities
7. Palpate penile shaft between thumb and first couple fingers.
8. Retract foreskin.
9. Separate meatus with thumbs.
10. Decision making: If client complains of dysuria or change in urination stream, observe client voiding.
11. Decision making: If thick, purulent urethral discharge, take culture of discharge.

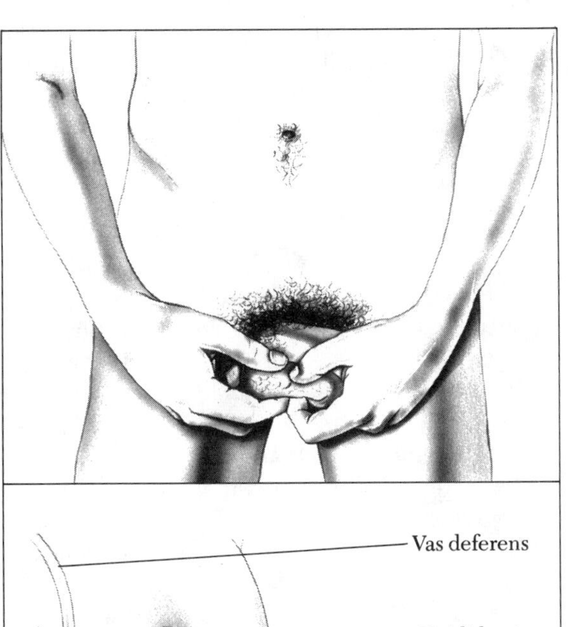

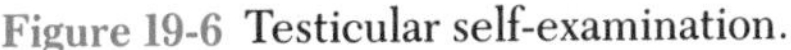

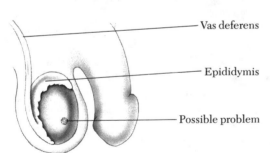

Figure 19-6 Testicular self-examination.

scrotum as it ascends toward the inguinal canal. For palpation use your thumb on the anterior surface of the scrotum and your index finger behind the scrotum. This same technique of using the thumbs on the anterior surface is explained to the male clients when teaching them how to perform the testicular self-examination (STE) (see Figure 19-6). Any nodule found within the testis must be held suspicious and warrants medical referral. With epididymitis there is extreme tenderness, and you should be unable to distinguish the epididymis from the testis. If there is any evidence of swelling in the scrotal area, use the technique of transillumination. Scrotal edema causes the skin to stretch, and there is less wrinkling of the scrotum. It is usually associated with generalized edema as in cardiac and renal disease (see Figure 19-7). A hernia or fluid should be suspected with enlargement. The normal testis, a tumor, or a hernia that has

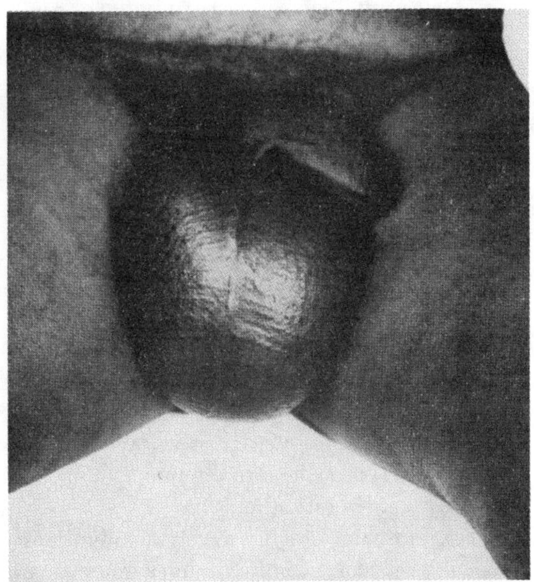

Figure 19-7 Edema of the scrotum and penis in congestive cardiac failure.

BIOLOGICAL AND CULTURAL VARIATIONS

Cancer and Circumcision

Mortality rates for different types of cancer vary by region, degree of urbanization, population group, and religious affiliation. Two interesting associations are those of cancer of the uterine cervix and cancer of the penis in different religious groups. Because cancer of the cervix is extremely rare among Jewish women, it has been hypothesized that this may be linked to the fact that Jewish women often have as sexual partners Jewish men, who are uniformly circumcised after birth. Jewish men also have extremely low rates of cancer of the penis, which is also hypothesized to be associated with circumcision. Moslem men, who are circumcised at puberty, have intermediate cancer rates. Hindus, who are uncircumcised, have rather high rates (Damon 1977).

Technique for Inspection and Palpation of Scrotum

1. Sit in chair facing standing client.
2. Characteristics of inspection:
   Size and contour
   Skin surfaces
   Abnormalities
3. Decision making: If swelling, use technique of transillumination.
4. Separate scrotal sac into two sides with index and middle finger of right hand.
5. Palpate right testis and epididymis with left thumb and index finger.
6. Continue to palpate upward on lateral aspect for right spermatic cord between right testis and inguinal canal.
7. Separate scrotal sac with left hand and palpate left testis, epididymis, and spermatic cord with right hand.

descended into the scrotal sac will not transilluminate, whereas fluid (hydrocele) will transilluminate. Also the indirect inguinal hernia will be palpated as a continuous structure to the external inguinal canal, whereas the hydrocele will present as a mass above which you will be able to palpate. Hydroceles are commonly found in toddlers and are nontender.

A common abnormality that is readily identified is a varicocele, a soft irregular mass within the scrotum resulting from varicosities. It has been appropriately termed a "bag of worms" because it truly feels like one. These varicose veins of the scrotum will collapse gradually as the scrotum is elevated while the client is lying down.

Structure and Function of the Female Genitals

The *mons pubis* (see Figure 19-8) is an eminent fatty pad that lies over the symphysis pubis and is covered by pubic hair. Lip-shaped structures, the *labia majora* and *labia minora*, straddle the more delicate structures of the external genitals and provide protection. The labia majora are composed of adipose tissue, while the labia minora are constructed of thin, pink-appearing stratified squamous epithelium. The elongated oval area between the labia minora is termed the *vestibule*. The *clitoris*, located at the anterior angle of the vestibule, is the site of concentrated sensory nerve endings and is homologous to the glans penis in the male. Posterior to the clitoris is the *urethral meatus*, which displays the openings of the *paraurethral* or *Skene's glands* on either side. In the posterior portion of the vestibule is the *vaginal introitus*. Nearby (sometimes on the inferior surface of the vaginal introitus) are the ducts of the *Bartholin's glands*. These ducts are not generally visible. The *fourchette* is the posterior boundary of the vestibule.

The internal genitals include the *vagina*, a flexible channel that leads to the uterus; the *cervix*, which connects the vagina and uterus; the *uterus*, which is the site for development and nourishment of a growing fetus; the *ovaries*, which produce ova and hormones; and the *fal-*

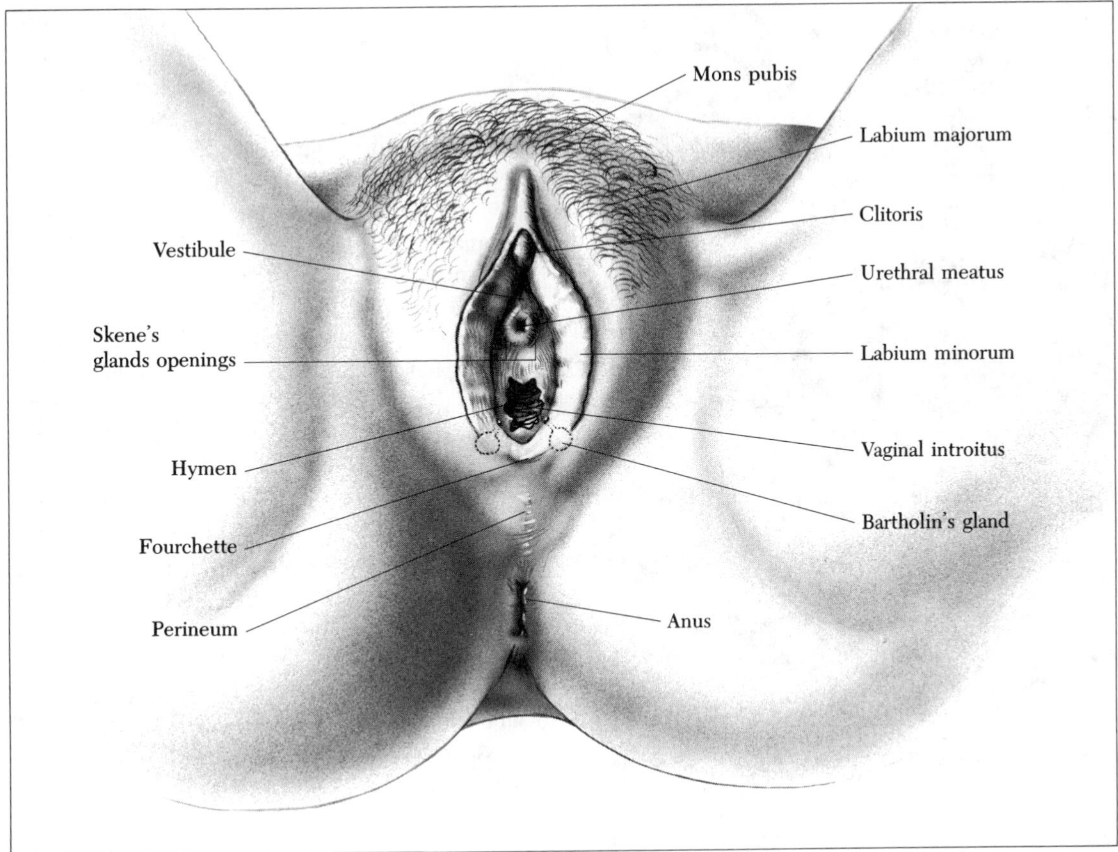

Figure 19-8 The female external genitals.

lopian tubes, through which ova travel from the ovaries to the uterus.

Characteristics and Techniques of Examination

The female client should be instructed *not* to douche 24 hours prior to a pelvic examination, as douching may interfere with smears, cultures, and cytology. Immediately before the examination takes place, have the client empty her bladder. The urine specimen should be collected, as in most cases a routine urinalysis is performed. Your approach, in addition to nurse-client rapport, is important for promoting cooperation. Relaxation of the client is necessary to ensure a good exam and to avoid unnecessary discomfort. Good lighting is needed. Adequate draping should be used so the client will not be overexposed. A mirror may be used for the client to view her own genital area; this technique facilitates health teaching and client learning.

Position the client on the examining table with her buttocks down to the very edge of the bottom of the table. Adjust the foot stirrups for comfortable flexion of the knees. The legs should be relaxed, with the knees apart. The client's head should be elevated sufficiently to use the viewing mirror.

Inspection and Palpation

The mons pubis should be inspected for amount and distribution of pubic hair. The pubic hair pattern of the female presents as an inverted triangle. Absence of pubic hair by age 16 is abnormal. The labia majora and the perineum should be inspected for lesions, fissures, excoriations, erythema, edema, and leukoplakia (white, thick precancerous patches).

As you explain what you are going to do, touch the inner aspect of the client's thigh to

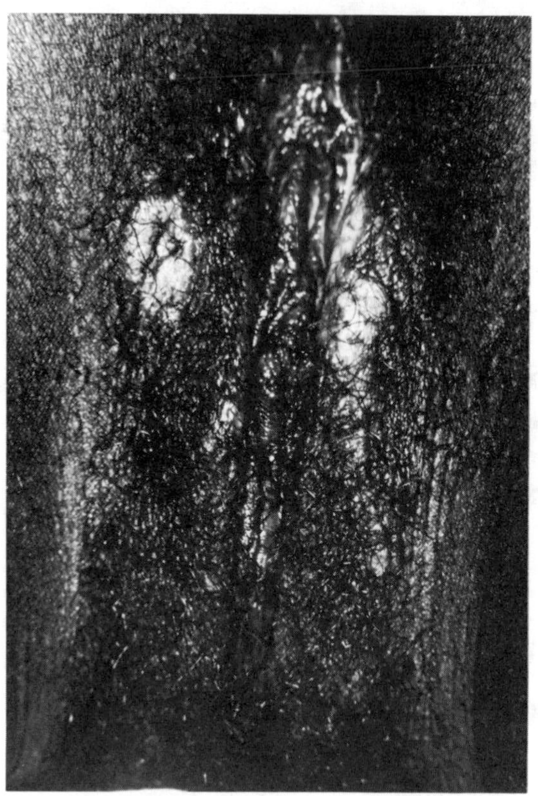

Figure 19-9 Syphilitic chancres of the left and right labia. Note scooped out appearance and red-raw floor. This condition heals without leaving a scar.

the labia. This aids in the prevention of tenseness. With the labia separated, inspect the interior of the labia majora and the surfaces of the labia minora. The genitals are next inspected in an anteroposterior direction. The clitoris should be examined first. It should be 0.5 cm or less in diameter. Carefully inspect the vestibule for erythema and ulcerations, as this is the most common site of venereal lesions and malignant changes. Primary syphilitic chancres are shown in Figure 19-9. Inspect the urethral meatus and the vaginal introitus. The Skene's glands, or paraurethral glands, on either side of the urethral meatus should be barely distinguishable unless infected. Observe the fourchette, where the labial folds join together posteriorly, for the strength of the walls as the client "strains" and for the presence of an anterior or posterior bulging of the vaginal wall, suggesting a cystocele or a rectocele, respectively (see Figures 19-10 and 19-11). The Bartholin's glands, which open into either side of the vagina just outside the hymen, cannot be visualized. However, this area should be carefully checked for inflammation, erythema, tenderness, and swelling. With the presence of any of these signs and if the client has a history of labial swelling, palpate this area on each side by using the index finger on the inside

Technique for Inspection and Palpation of Female External Genitals

1. Have client empty bladder.
2. Provide comfort, privacy, and adequate draping and lighting.
3. Ask client to lie on examining table with buttocks at bottom edge of table.
4. Place client's feet in stirrups.
5. Adjust foot stirrups for comfortable flexion of knees.
6. Use mirror for client to view genitalia (aids health teaching).
7. Explain each step prior to doing it.
8. Put on a pair of gloves.
9. Characteristics of inspection:
   Pubic hair distribution
   Symmetry
   Skin
   Abnormalities
10. Touch inner aspect of thigh and inform client that you are going to separate the labia for further inspection.
11. Inspect surfaces of labia majora and labia minora.
12. Inspect size of clitoris.
13. Inspect vestibule, urethral meatus, Skene's glands, and vaginal introitus.
14. Instruct client to "bear down" and examine fourchette.
15. Inspect Bartholin gland areas on either side of the vaginal introitus.
16. Insert lubricated gloved index finger into vagina with palmar side up.
17. Milk urethra by pressing gently upward and withdrawing your finger from the vagina.
18. Decision making: If a greenish yellow discharge is present or if a discharge is elicited upon milking the urethra, take a culture of the discharge.

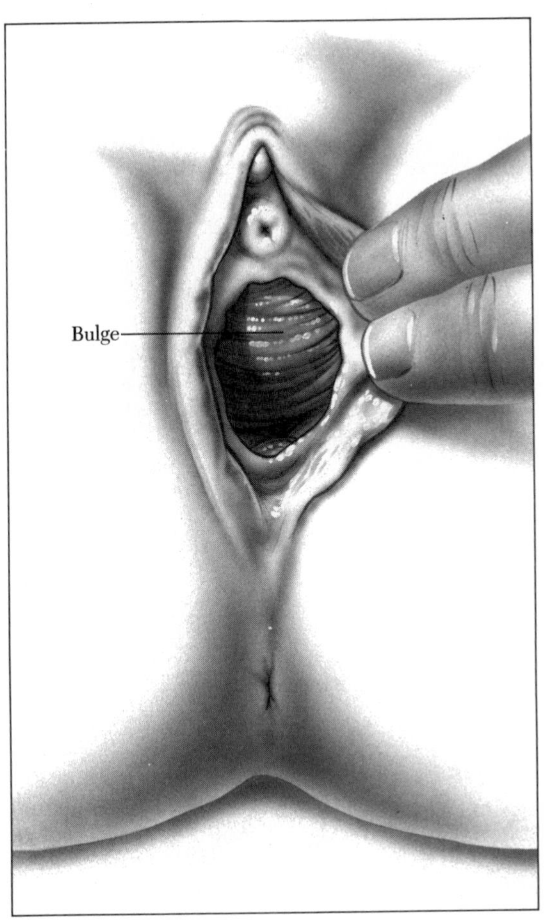

Figure 19-10 Cystocele: a bladder hernia that protrudes into the anterior wall of the vagina. Inspect for bulging of the anterior vaginal wall as the client strains down. Occasionally the bulging may extend out of the introitus.

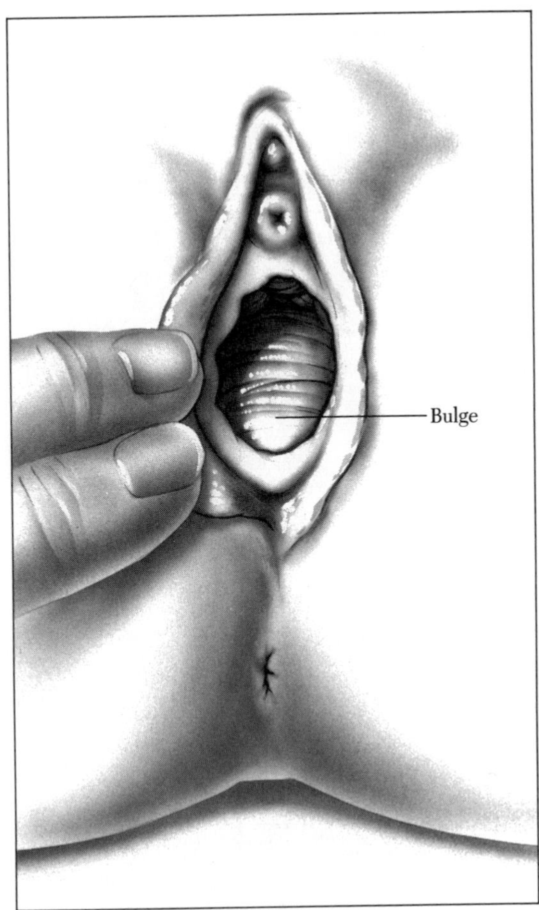

Figure 19-11 Rectocele: herniation of the posterior vaginal wall and the anterior rectal wall into the vagina. Inspect vaginal wall as client strains down.

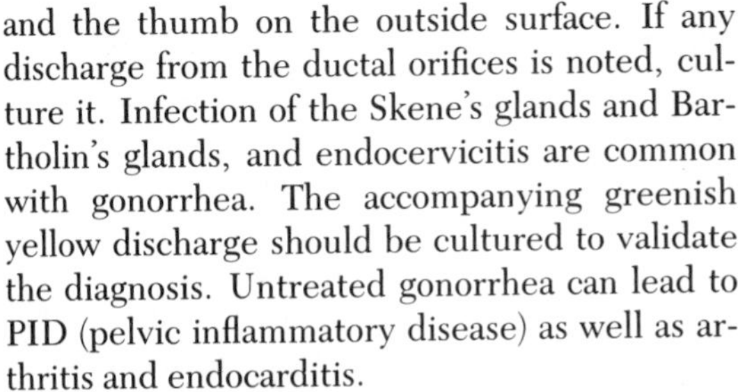

and the thumb on the outside surface. If any discharge from the ductal orifices is noted, culture it. Infection of the Skene's glands and Bartholin's glands, and endocervicitis are common with gonorrhea. The accompanying greenish yellow discharge should be cultured to validate the diagnosis. Untreated gonorrhea can lead to PID (pelvic inflammatory disease) as well as arthritis and endocarditis.

Next, gently insert a gloved index finger into the vagina with the palmar surface up. The urethra should be "milked" by withdrawing the finger while exerting gentle pressure on the anterior wall of the vagina. Figure 19-12 illustrates the technique for "milking." Normally there is no discharge from the urethra or pain during this maneuver. If a discharge is elicited, a culture should be done to identify the causative organism and to establish a diagnosis.

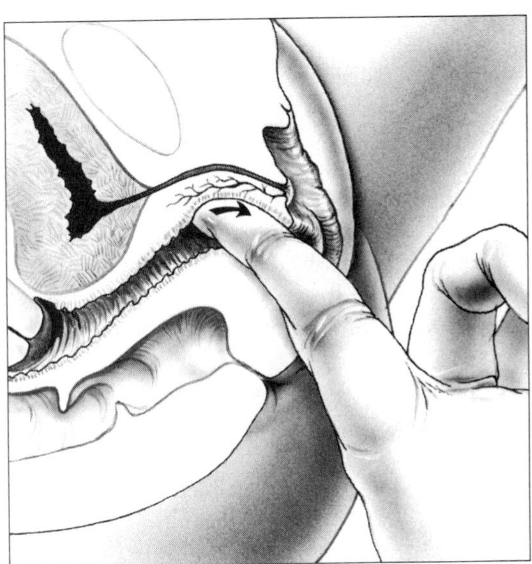

Figure 19-12 "Milking" the urethra.

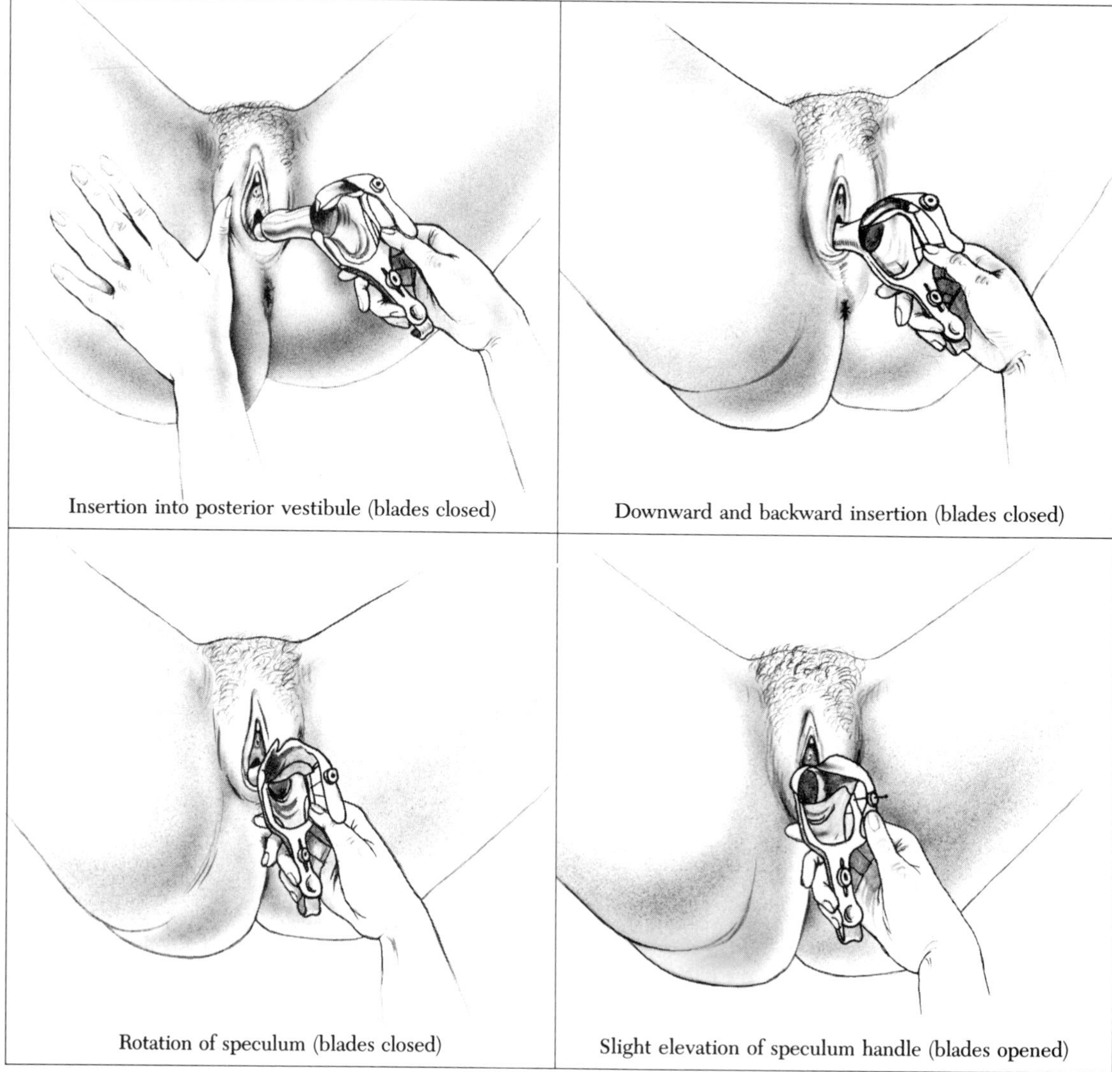

Insertion into posterior vestibule (blades closed)
Downward and backward insertion (blades closed)
Rotation of speculum (blades closed)
Slight elevation of speculum handle (blades opened)

Figure 19-13 Speculum insertion.

Speculum Exam

To examine the internal genitals use a speculum, as shown in Figure 19-13. The vaginal speculum should be lubricated with warm water, as jelly lubricant interferes with cytologic studies. After all smears and cultures have been collected, a jelly lubricant may be used to facilitate further examination.

When first inserted into the introitus, the blades of the speculum should be in a vertical position. Once they are within the vagina, the blades should be rotated to a horizontal position. During the insertion of the speculum, or later of the examining fingers, the labia should be widely separated and the pubic hair should be cupped away from the vaginal area to avoid pulling the pubic hair with the speculum or examining fingers. As the speculum insertion is continued, a downward 45 degree angle should be maintained in order to avoid trauma to the sensitive anterior tissue over the urethral area. When the cervix is located, the blades of the speculum should be locked open. You may not be able to visualize the cervix if the speculum blades are too short or if the blades have been inadvertently opened anteriorly or posteriorly to the cervix. Observance of rugae suggests that the blades have been opened anterior to the cervix, whereas a smooth surface suggests the position to be posterior to the cervix. If this occurs,

Technique for Speculum Examination

1. Decision making: If client is a virgin or elderly woman with vaginal atrophy, use small vaginal speculum or nasal speculum as warranted.
2. Lubricate vaginal speculum with warm water.
3. Spread labia apart with thumb and index finger cupping the pubic hair back from the vaginal area.
4. Insert the vaginal speculum gently downward at a 45° angle with the blades in a vertical position.
5. When blades are within the vagina, rotate them horizontally.
6. Locate the cervix and lock the speculum blades in open position.
7. Characteristics of cervical inspection:
   Color
   Surface
   Os
   Abnormalities

withdraw the speculum a short distance and attempt to better position the distal ends of the blades.

The normal cervix is pink, about 2–3 cm in diameter, and free from lacerations, erosions, and growths. The normal cervical os of a nulliparous female, shown in Figure 19-14, is small and either round or oval; the os of the normal parous female, shown in Figure 19-15, has a slitlike appearance.

Transverse or stellate lacerations (see Figure 19-16) of the cervix may occur with difficult deliveries. Also, the normal color of the cervix changes from a pink to a purplish color during pregnancy.

Generally, a beefy red color will present with ulcerations and erosions. Early carcinomas can appear beefy red also, but with progression they may appear as a hard granulated or cauliflower growth. Both erosions and carcinomas bleed easily when sponged with an applicator or spongestick.

If the cervix appears abnormal, perform the Schiller test. In this test normal areas of the cervix and upper vagina stain brown when painted with Lugol's solution (iodine in potassium iodide). Abnormal areas remain colorless due to the lack of glycogen; these areas warrant biopsy, which can be performed in the office with a biopsy punch. The bleeding that occurs with biopsy can easily be controlled by a tampon, silver nitrate stick, or electrocauterization. Biopsy specimens should be placed immediately in 10% formalin. Cervical cancer usually has its beginnings at or near the cervical os and may be present in a cervix that appears normal. Thus it is important for all women over 20 years of age to have annual routine Papanicolaou smears (cytology studies) to increase early detection of cervical cancer.

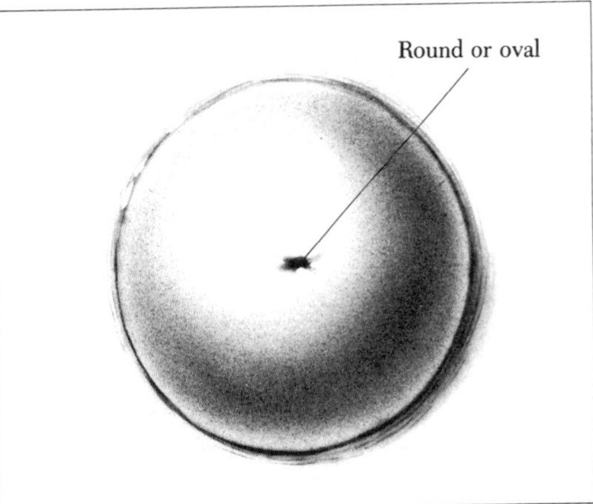

Figure 19-14 Normal nulliparous cervical os.

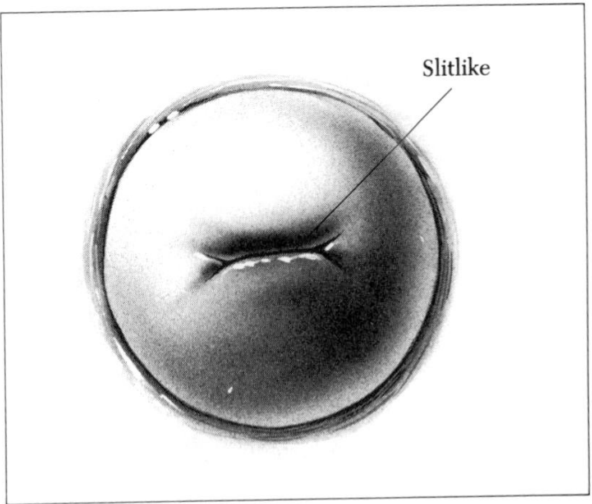

Figure 19-15 Normal parous cervical os.

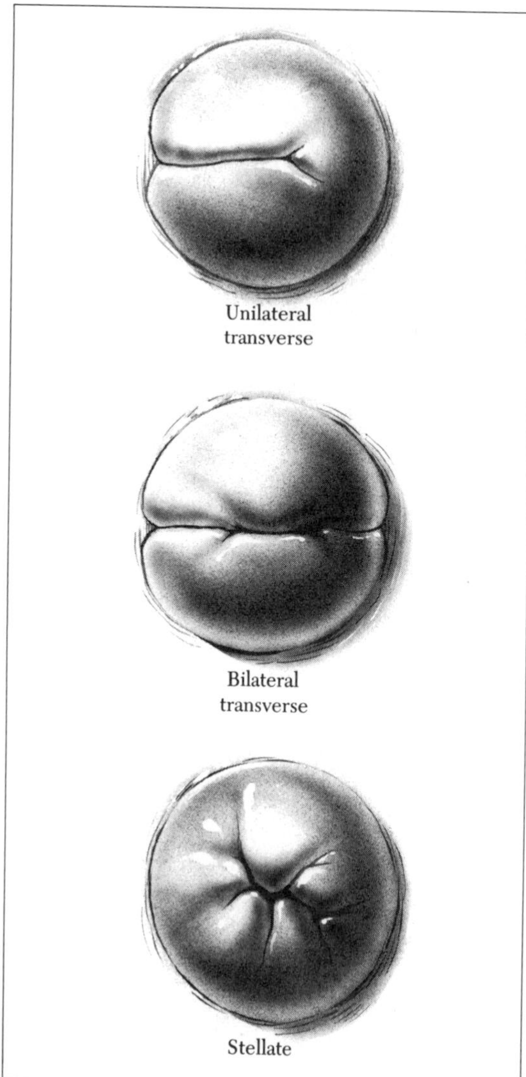

Figure 19-16 Cervical lacerations.

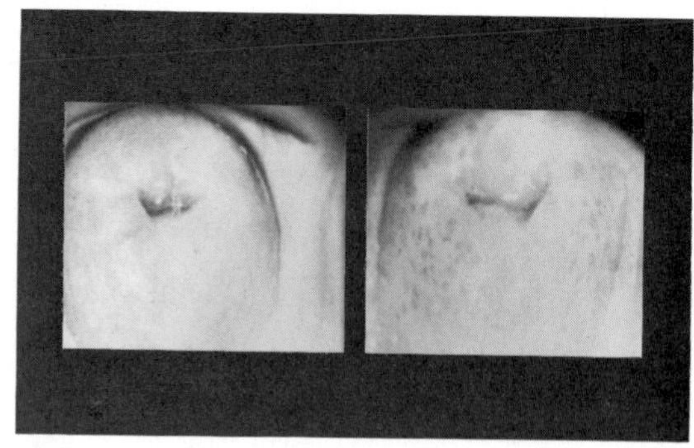

Figure 19-17 Trichomonas vaginitis. (See also endsheet plate 28.)

Other abnormalities that may be observed are cervical polyps, the "strawberry spots" associated with trichomonas vaginitis (see Figure 19-17); translucent nabothian cysts, which accompany chronic cervicitis; eversion; and erosion (see Figure 19-18).

When performing a Pap test it is best to secure three specimens for cytology as shown in Figure 19-19; one from the cervical os (the *endocervical smear*), one from the cervical surface (the *cervical scrape*), and another from the vaginal pool (the *vaginal smear*). The endocervical smear is secured by inserting a cotton applicator that has been moistened with normal saline into the os. The applicator is rotated both clockwise and counter-clockwise before removal; it is then rolled upon a glass slide numbered 1 and is either fixed with fixative spray or placed in a bottle of fixative solution. Should the latter technique of fixation be used, paper clips should be placed on the slides to prevent the surfaces from

Technique for Papanicolaou Smears

1. Moisten cotton applicator in saline.
2. Insert applicator into cervical os.
3. Rotate applicator clockwise and then counterclockwise and remove.
4. Roll applicator upon a glass slide.
5. Spray glass slide with fixative or place it in a container of fixative.
6. Label slide "E" (endocervical specimen).
7. Place the longer side of the tip of an Ayre spatula into the cervical os.
8. Rotate the spatula in a full circle, scraping the surface of the cervix.
9. Place scrapings on glass slide; fix and label "C" (cervix specimen).
10. Roll applicator wet with saline in cul-de-sac area between inferior aspect of cervix and posterior vaginal wall or aspirate specimen from this area with soft aspiration syringe.
11. Place smear on glass slide; fix and label "V" (vaginal specimen).
12. Release lock on speculum blades.
13. Hold blades in comfortable open position and withdraw slowly, inspecting the vaginal mucosa.

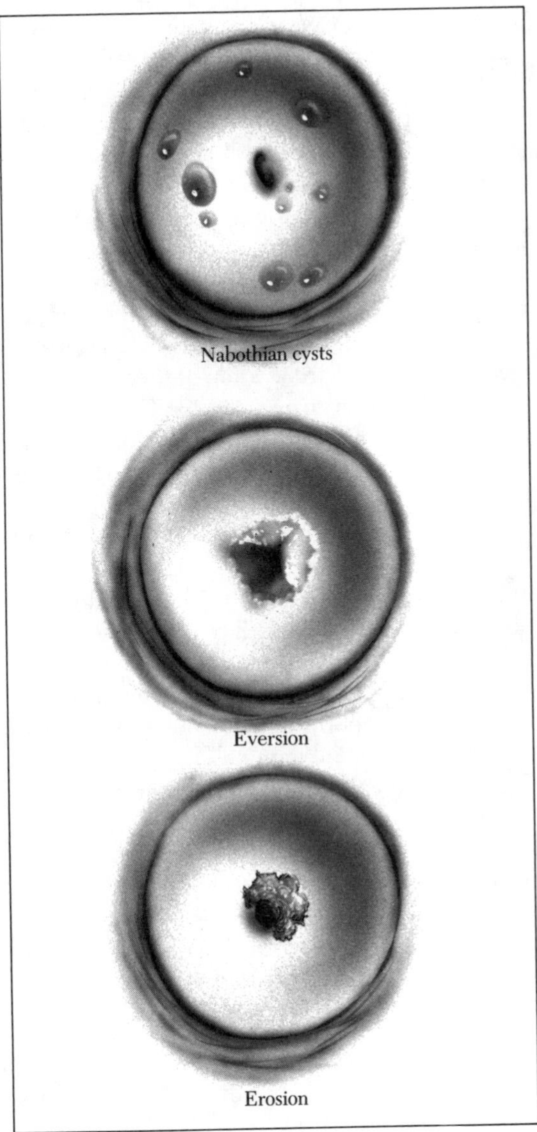

Figure 19-18 Surface irregularities of the cervix.

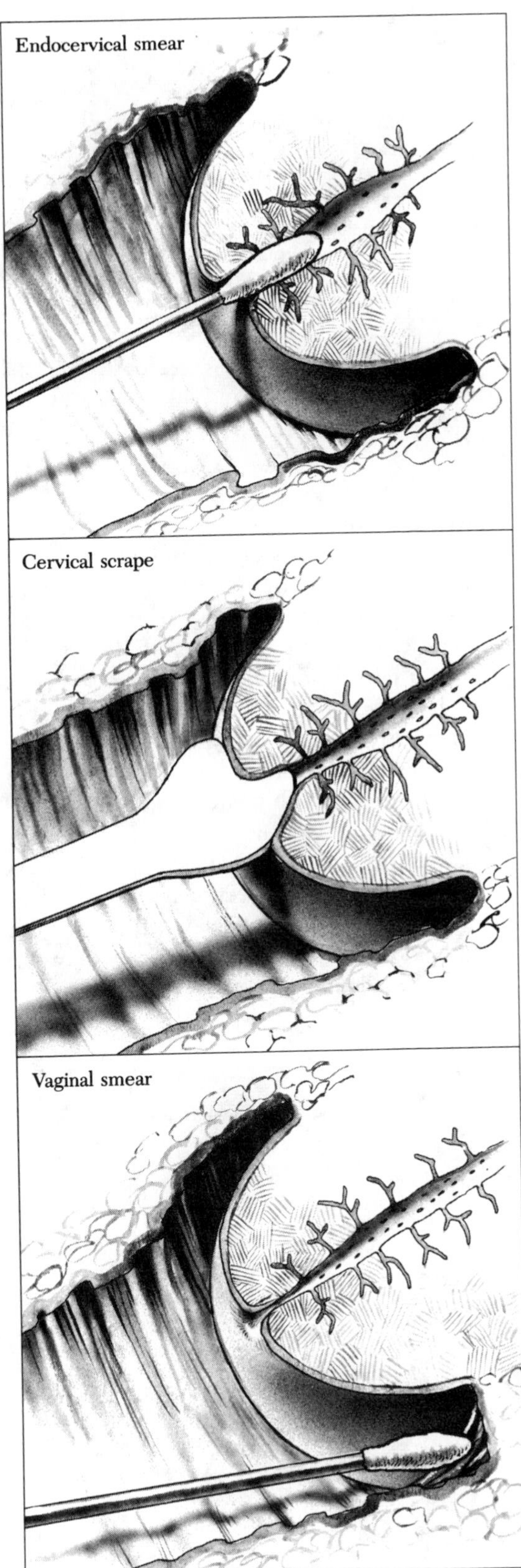

Figure 19-19 Sites and techniques for Pap test.

rubbing together. The cervical scrape is obtained by using an Ayre spatula. The longer arm of the spatula is placed in the cervical os and is then rotated in a full circle. The scraping is placed on the number 2 slide and is fixed. The specimen from the vaginal pool is collected by rolling a wet applicator over the vaginal wall beneath the cervix or by using an aspiration technique; the specimen is then placed on the number 3 slide.

After the cervix and cervical os have been inspected and the Pap smear specimens have been collected, slowly remove the vaginal speculum as you inspect the vaginal mucosa.

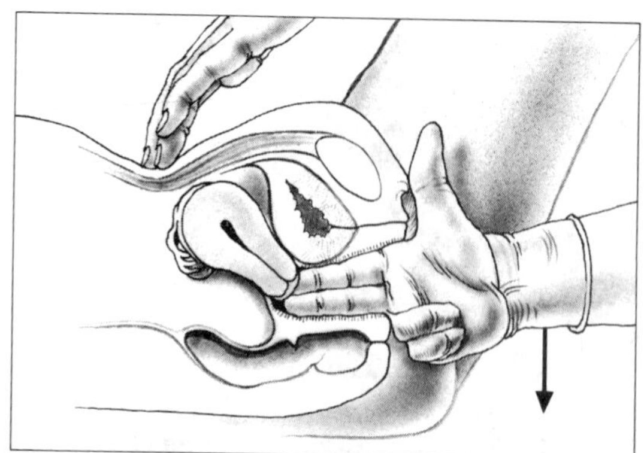

Figure 19-20 Bimanual palpation technique.

Bimanual Exam

Next, the bimanual pelvic examination should be performed to attempt palpation of the uterus and ovaries. The examining finger should be well lubricated before insertion into the vagina. Once you have inserted the finger, place your other hand between the umbilicus and pubic symphysis to steady the body of the uterus as the vaginal finger palpates the entire surface of the cervix. Figure 19-20 illustrates the bimanual palpation technique. Normally the cervix is smooth and of a firm consistency; it should be freely movable 2–3 cm in all directions, and the movement should be painless. Pain will occur with inflammation, and the cervix may be immovable with pelvic inflammatory disease or with malignant infiltration. Cervical polyps are palpable as soft, spongy masses.

With the palm upward, position a finger of the vaginal hand on either side of the cervix to stabilize the uterus in midline position. Simultaneously, press the abdominal hand downward between the umbilicus and pubic symphysis in order to judge the size, consistency, position, and contour of the uterus. Figure 19-21 illustrates retroversion, the backward tilting of the entire uterus (both body and cervix), and retroflexion, the backward angling of the body of the uterus in relation to the cervix. The fundus of the retroverted uterus is palpable through the rectum; the fundus of the retroflexed uterus may be palpable rectally.

Palpation of the *adnexa* (fallopian tubes and ovaries), illustrated in Figure 19-22, is the most difficult maneuver of the pelvic examination, especially for the beginner. Even the expert is occasionally foiled when the client is obese, is tense, has a full bladder, or has abdominal-pelvic tenderness. To perform assessment of the right ovary, press the abdominal hand gently but deeply into the right lower quadrant while placing the vaginal finger firmly in the right lateral fornix. Try to palpate the adnexa between the finger inserted into the vagina and the hand, which is flat upon the abdomen. The vaginal finger should be moved to the left lateral fornix and the abdominal hand pressed in the left lower quadrant for assessment of the left adnexa. The

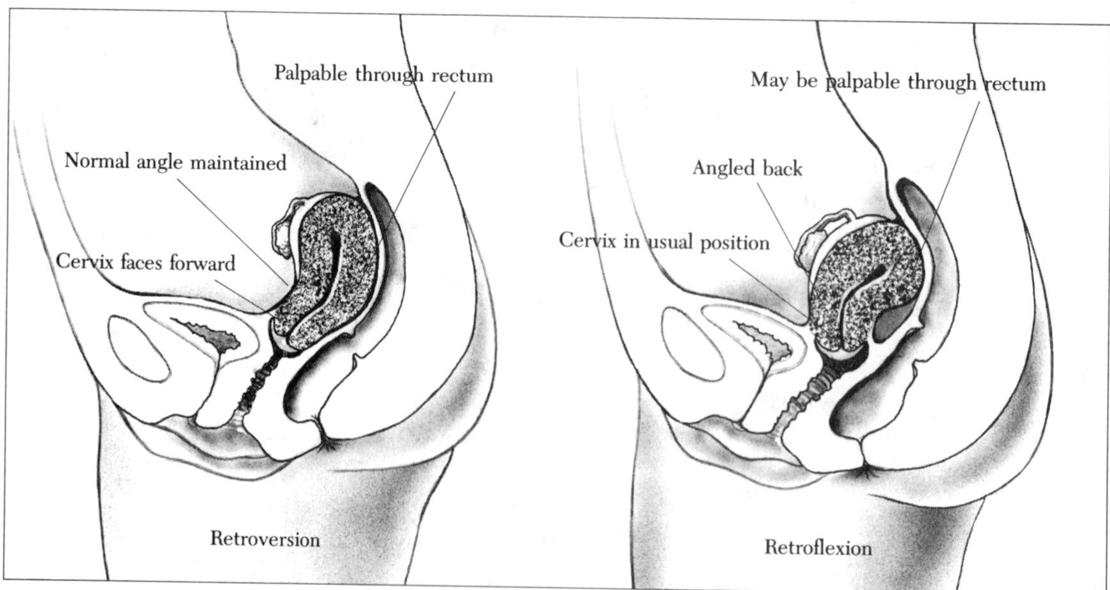

Figure 19-21 Retroversion and retroflexion of the uterus.

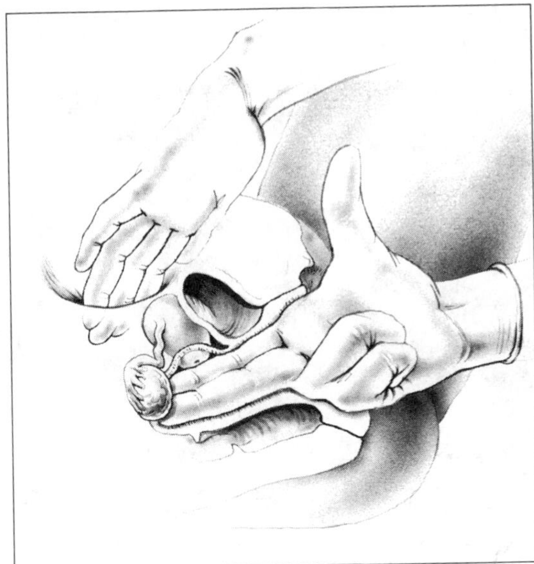

Figure 19-22 Bimanual palpation of the adnexa.

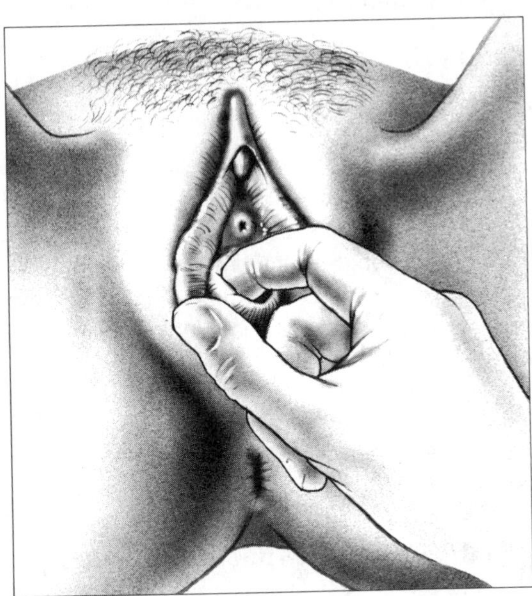

Figure 19-23 Palpation of the Bartholin's glands.

normal fallopian tube is usually nonpalpable, and rarely is the normal ovary palpable.

As you withdraw the vaginal finger, at the completion of the adnexal assessment, palpate the area of the Bartholin's glands, as shown in Figure 19-23. Hold the area firmly between the index finger, which should be slightly inside the margin of the vaginal introitus, and the thumb, which should be positioned on the outside perineal skin. Normally the Bartholin's glands are not palpable unless they are infected (see Figure 19-24).

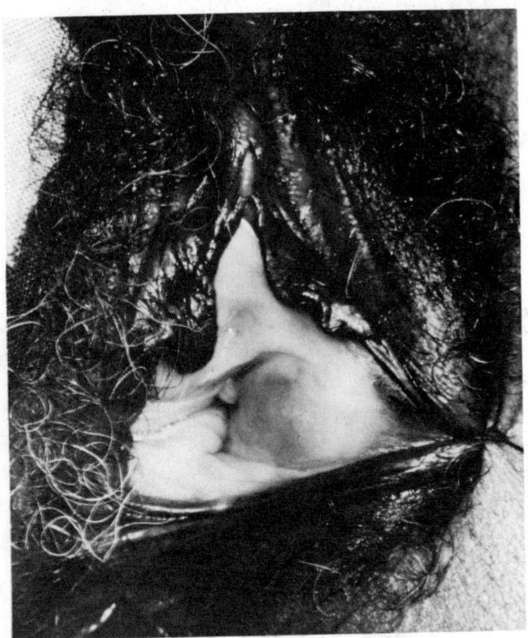

Figure 19-24 Bartholin abscess in a Black female. Note swelling of the left labia.

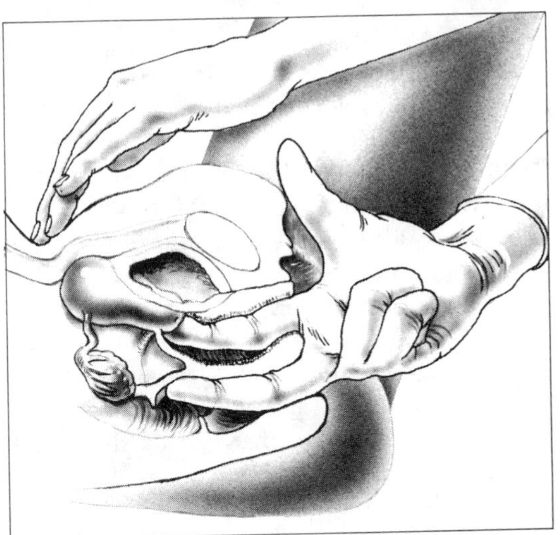

Figure 19-25 Rectovaginal-abdominal palpation technique.

Rectovaginal-Abdominal Exam

The last portion of the pelvic examination is rectovaginal-abdominal palpation illustrated in Figure 19-25. You should put on a new examining glove for this procedure to prevent possible cross-contamination between the genitals and the rectum. The index finger should be inserted into the vagina and the middle finger into the rectum. Inform the client that this procedure may cause her to feel as if her bowels must move.

Assess the strength of the rectovaginal wall.

Technique for Bimanual Examination

1. Lubricate gloved examining finger.
2. Insert finger into vagina.
3. Characteristics of cervical palpation:
   Surface
   Consistency
   Movability
   Abnormalities
4. Place other hand on abdomen between umbilicus and pubic symphysis.
5. Place index finger on one side of the cervix and middle finger on the other side to steady cervix.
6. Press abdominal hand downward to palpate uterus.
7. Characteristics of uterine palpation:
   Size and contour
   Consistency
   Position
   Abnormalities
8. Place vaginal examining finger(s) in right lateral fornix.
9. Place abdominal hand in right lower quadrant.
10. Bring abdominal hand downward and vaginal fingers upward to attempt palpation of right adnexa.
11. Transfer abdominal hand to left lower quadrant and vaginal finger(s) into left fornix.
12. Press abdominal hand downward to meet vaginal finger(s) in attempt to palpate the left adnexa.
13. Withdraw finger(s) to vaginal opening.
14. Place tip of index finger slightly inside lateral aspect of vaginal introitus.
15. Place thumb in opposition on the outside.
16. Palpate Bartholin's gland area on either side of the vaginal opening.

With this technique it is possible to detect herniation of the small bowel dissecting between the rectal and vaginal walls. Direct careful attention to the area beneath the cervix. Apply pressure with the abdominal hand to move the uterus backward so that its posterior surface may be palpated with the rectal finger. Ordinarily the pelvic tissues, particularly the broad ligaments, are inaccessible to manual assessment. The rectovaginal-abdominal technique allows palpation of inflamed areas and indurated areas of malignant tumor invasion that can be done *only* from the rectum.

In conducting a pelvic assessment of virgins or elderly women in whom the introitus has become atrophied and small, use a single examining finger, a small vaginal speculum or a nasal speculum, or the bimanual examination with one finger in the rectum and a hand on the abdomen, whichever technique is most appropriate for comfort of examination.

Structure and Function of the Anus and Rectum

The anus is the most distal portion of the gastrointestinal tract. The anus is demarcated from the rectum by a line at which skin changes to the mucous membrane lining of the rectum. The anus has an abundance of somatic nerves, which renders it highly susceptible to discomfort caused by a rough examination technique. The rectum, located between the anus and the sigmoid colon, is about 12 cm long. It is in the rectum that the urge to defecate is stimulated as a result of stretching of the nerve fibers by the bulk of descending feces.

Technique for Rectovaginal-Abdominal Exam

1. If you have gloves on and have completed prior examination of the female genitals, put on new examining gloves.
2. Tell client that this may make her feel as if her bowels must move.
3. Insert lubricated index finger into the vagina.
4. Insert lubricated middle finger simultaneously into the rectum.
5. Assess strength of rectovaginal wall.
6. Next place other hand on abdomen over uterus.
7. Push uterus backward, palpating posterior surface with rectal finger.

Characteristics and Techniques of Examination

The rectum is very accessible to physical examination, and the procedure takes but a few minutes. Rectal examination is an essential part of any routine assessment and is a quick and easy means for early detection of carcinoma of the prostate gland in the male as well as of carcinoma of the rectum. Early prostatic carcinoma produces no symptoms to prompt the client to seek medical attention. Therefore, the rectal examination should be routinely performed on an annual basis, especially for every male over the age of 40.

Out of fear that stimulating the vagus nerve will result in a decreased heart rate, physicians and nurses have been reluctant to perform rectal exams on clients with acute myocardial infarction. When Earnest and Fletcher (1969) conducted a closely monitored study involving eighty-six clients admitted to a coronary care unit, none of whom displayed any symptoms of shock or life-threatening arrhythmias, they found no adverse effects from a gentle digital rectal exam. The clients were monitored before, during, and for 3 minutes following the exam. No negative effects were noted either clinically or electrocardiographically, and there were no incidents of angina pectoris. The researchers concluded that there were no adverse effects and, furthermore, that immediate value may be forthcoming from a brief gentle rectal exam of clients diagnosed with acute myocardial infarction, assuming the absence of shock or life-threatening arrhythmia. Information obtained from the rectal examinations of the study clients included thirty-eight potential fecal impactions, nine with 3+ to 4+ benzidine tests (occult blood), twenty out of fifty-six with prostatism, and eight with symptomatic prostatism.

Inspection

First inspect the superior cleft area of the buttocks for presence of a pilonidal cyst. With both male and female clients, the buttocks should be spread in order to visualize the anus. This may be very painful for the client with an anal fissure. Inspect the anus and perineum for any lesions, fistulas, fissures, or skin tabs; note the presence of hemorrhoids. Instruct the client to "bear down"; this normally causes the anal sphincter to contract and indicates intact innervation. However prolapse of the rectum may be observed.

Technique for Inspection of the Anus

1. Position in Sim's or have client stand and lean over bed or examining table.
2. Spread buttocks gently with a hand positioned on each buttock.
3. Examine crevice of buttocks from sacrum to anterior genitals.
4. Characteristics of inspection:
   Anus
   Perineal skin surface
   Abnormalities
5. Instruct client to "bear down" while examining the anus.

Palpation

If the genitals have been examined prior to the rectal examination, and particularly if gonorrhea is suspected, you should put on a new pair of examining gloves. Gonorrhea can infect the rectum as well as the genitals.

Use a well-lubricated finger to gently press against the anus; as relaxation occurs, slowly insert the finger into the rectum. By using a rotating motion, you can palpate all sides of the rectal wall with the palmar aspect of the examining finger. Note any tenderness, nodules, or masses.

In the male the prostate gland can be palpated through the anterior wall of the rectum. Figure 19-26 illustrates the technique for palpation of the prostate gland. The best position for palpation is to have the client stand and lean over the bed or table. Identify the well-marked median sulcus, which divides the two lobes of the gland. The prostate is normally firm and rubbery and is approximately 4 cm in diameter; the borders are discrete, and there is normally no fixation of the gland. During palpation of the prostate, the client may experience the urge to urinate, but there should be no tenderness. Tenderness of the prostate is commonly experienced during the examination of clients with benign prostatic hyperplasia and urinary abnormalities. The cause of prostatic hypertrophy is not known, although it is definitely linked with aging and is a common occurrence in men over 50 years of age.

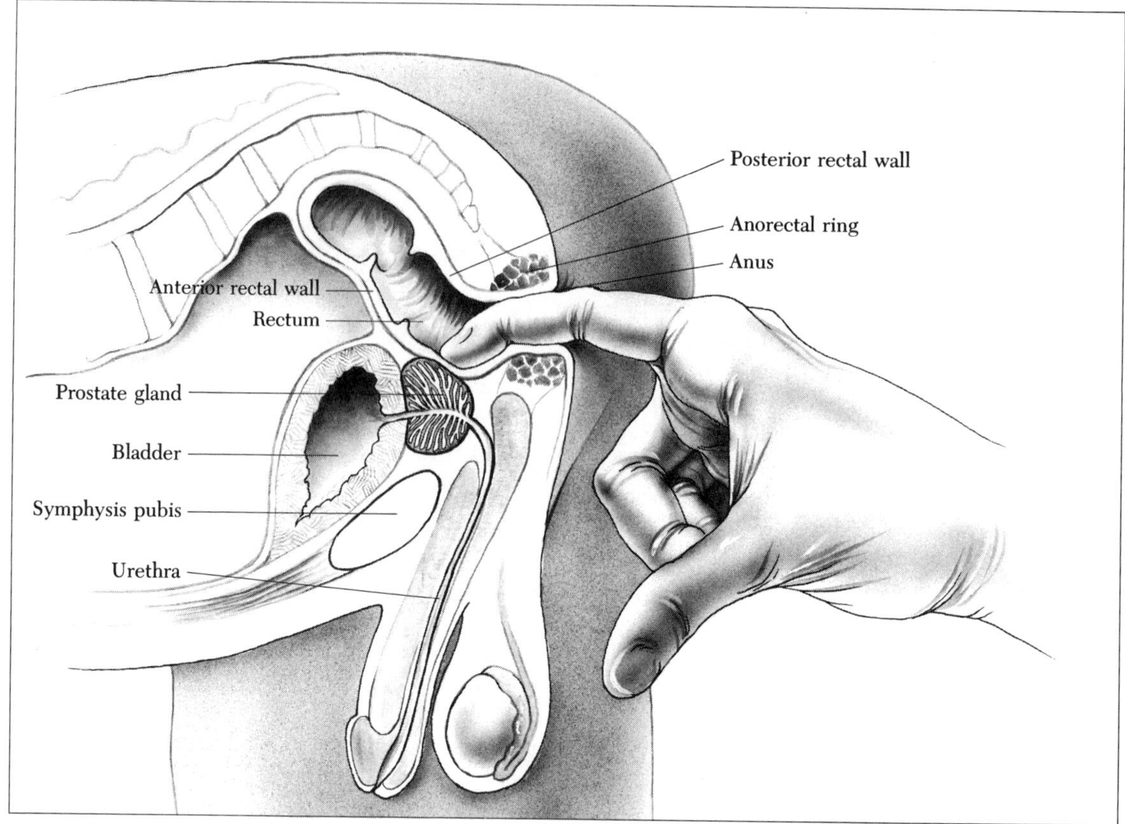

Figure 19-26 Technique for palpation of the prostate gland.

Technique for Palpation of the Anus

1. Have client remain in same position as for inspection of the anus.
2. If you have on examining gloves from prior examination of the genitals, put on a new pair.
3. Place your well-lubricated index finger gently against the anus.
4. As client relaxes, slowly insert index finger into rectum.
5. Note sphincter muscle action.
6. With the palmar aspect of your examining finger, palpate the posterior rectal wall.
7. Rotate your examining finger and palpate the left rectal wall.
8. Rotate finger to palpate the right rectal wall.
9. Rotate finger to palpate the anterior rectal wall.
10. Withdraw examining finger slowly.
11. Observe finger for presence of feces.
12. Note characteristics of feces.
13. If feces present, test for occult blood.
14. Wipe anus with tissue.

When the examining finger is withdrawn from the rectum, it should be observed for the presence of feces. Feces should be tested for occult blood, and the color of the feces should be recorded, as well as any presence of mucus or visible blood. See Table 19-1 for common abnormalities of the genitals.

Technique for Palpation of the Prostate Gland

1. Performed at completion of palpation of the rectum in men prior to withdrawing examining finger.
2. Tell the client to inform you if the area is tender.
3. Tell the client that he may experience the urge to urinate during the procedure and that this is common.
4. Through the anterior rectal wall identify the median sulcus.
5. Palpate the surface of the left and right prostatic lobes.
6. Characteristics of palpation:
   Size
   Consistency
   Borders
   Movability
   Abnormalities
7. Wipe lubricant and feces from anus with tissue.

Table 19-1. Common Abnormalities of the Genitals

Condition	Characteristics	Comments
Phimosis	Narrow preputial orifice, resulting in inability to retract foreskin back over the glans penis.	Health teaching regarding peri-care. Acute stage treated with saline soaks. Medical referral for evaluation of need for circumcision.
Hypospadias	Congenital opening of urethra on underside of penis; congenital opening of urethra into vagina.	Medical referral for evaluation regarding reconstructive surgery.
Epispadias	Congenital opening of urethra on superior surface of the penis.	Medical referral for evaluation regarding reconstructive surgery.
Epididymitis	Swollen, tender epididymis; fever, chills, inguinal pain.	Investigate past medical history—may be complication of prostatic and urinary infections, mumps, TB, sexually transmitted disease, or prolonged use of foley catheter. Medical referral. Rx consists of bedrest, scrotal support, antibiotics.
Prostatitis	Fever; chills; tender, swollen prostate, which frequently is slightly asymmetrical.	Check for history of low back or perineal pains and urinary, erection, and ejaculation difficulties. Urine culture. Medical referral warranted. Prostatic massage may decrease congestion.
Hydrocele	Enlarged scrotal sac; transilluminates.	Medical referral warranted.
Varicocele	Varicose veins of the spermatic cord; occasionally purplish appearance, palpable full vessels or side(s) of scrotum.	Investigate whether dull ache and/or dragging sensation in area of cord. Rx: suspensory. Medical referral warranted with persistent symptoms.
Syphilis	*Primary stage:* ulcerated papule or erosion (chancre); painless hard ulcer with shiny red, raw, scooped-out appearance; purulent secretion; generalized lymphadenopathy. *Secondary stage:* skin rash, condylomata lata (syphilis warts) occurring 6–8 weeks after chancre. *Latent stage:* usually asymptomatic.	Highly contagious primary syphilitic ulcer during chancre stage—wear gloves; examine rectum, mouth, genital area, woman's breast, and eyelids and conjunctiva; heals without leaving scar. Take culture and order serology. Medical referral warranted for antibiotic therapy.
Gonorrhea	Men—thick opaque or purulent urethral discharge; red, swollen urethral meatus.	Check for history of sore throat; urinary urgency; take throat (oral sex), urethral, and rectal culture.

(continued on page 426)

Table 19-1. *Continued*

Condition	Characteristics	Comments
Gonorrhea	Women—may be asymptomatic carrier; purulent urethral discharge; cervical discharge; red, swollen Skene's or Bartholin's glands and/or edema of vulva is usual.	"Milk" urethra; check for history of sore throat, dysuria, and abnormal uterine bleeding; cervical, vaginal, rectal and throat secretions cultured. Increased incidence in 15- to 30-year-olds.
Genital herpes	Painful blisters or sores, which eventually form scabs and heal; occasionally headache, fatigue, fever, dysuria, and enlarged and tender inguinal lymph nodes, fever.	Most common STD in upper-income and college-educated people. Cervical pap smear in women every 6 months (linked with cervical carcinoma). Check for history of headaches, anorexia, general malaise, premature deliveries, and spontaneous miscarriages. Medical referral warranted for pharmacologic control of disease.
Trichomoniasis	Women—vulvar irritation and pruritis, foul greenish-yellow foamy vaginal discharge. Men—may be asymptomatic; urethritis; prostatitis.	Obtain saline slides, Pap smear, and urinalysis.
Moniliasis (Candida)	Vulvar irritation and pruritis, thick cottage cheese-like vaginal discharge.	Obtain culture of discharge, wet smear, Pap smear, and urine culture.
Crabs (public lice)	Pruritus—especially nocturnal. Presence of parasite (gray colored but rusty red after feeding on human blood 4–5 times per day) in pubic hair, eyebrows, eyelashes, and/or beard; occasionally mild fever and cervical lymphadenopathy.	Health teaching: spreads via close contact, clothing, bedding, toilet seats. Rx for patient and all sexual partners: Kwell cream or shampoo, and washing of clothing and bedding (Rand C Spray).
AIDS (acquired immune deficiency syndrome)	General malaise, fever, 10–20 lb weight loss over few months; ecchymosis; painful and enlarged lymph nodes (over 10 days' duration); persistent herpes sores (over 5 weeks' duration); sensory or motor loss.	Etiology unknown. Higher incidence in homosexual men. Believed to be sexually transmitted and via contaminated blood or blood products. Check for respiratory signs and skin lesions. Check for history of syphilis, nitrate inhalants ("poppers"), and sexual practices—i.e., oral-anal, penile-anal, and manual-anal contacts.
Cystitis	Fever, pyuria.	Check for history of burning upon urination, urgency, low back or abdominal pain. Obtain clean-catch (midstream) urine for urinalysis. Health teaching: hot tub bath t.i.d., force fluids, avoid bladder irritants (alcohol, coffee, tea, and spices). Medical referral warranted.
Endocervicitis	White or yellow mucoid vaginal discharge, cervical erosion on inspection.	Medical referral for electrocauterization of cervix.
Ovarian carcinoma	Distended abdomen and/or ascites (shifting dullness), signs of hyperthyroidism, feminization or virilization; anemia and cachexia in advanced cases.	Check for vague lower abdominal discomfort/pain and mild digestive complaints. Medical referral warranted.
Cervical carcinoma	Friable cervical mass or ulcer upon inspection.	Obtain Pap smears. Medical referral warranted.

Table 19-1. *Continued*

Condition	Characteristics	Comments
Vaginal carcinoma	Tumor of vaginal wall upon inspection (commonly posterior upper one-third of vaginal wall), watery discharge, urinary frequency.	Check for history of bleeding after coitus, dyspareunia, involvement of bladder or rectum may result in urgency and/or painful defecation. Obtain Pap smear, perform Schiller's test. Medical referral is warranted.
Uterine carcinoma	Recurrent metrorrhagia in menstruating woman, postmenopausal bleeding, mucosanguineous vaginal discharge with vaginal metastasis.	Peak incidence 50–60 years of age. Check for stormy menstrual history, infertility, and suspicious predispositional factors (obesity, hypertension, diabetes mellitus, familial history). Obtain Pap smear and make medical referral.
Prostatic carcinoma	Change in urinary stream, hematuria, pyuria, palpable stony hard induration and/or nodule(s).	Check for history of bone pain (pelvis and/or lumbar spine metastasis). Medical referral warranted. Do annual rectal exam for all men 40 years of age and older.
Testicular carcinoma	Firm or cystic scrotal mass, occasionally painful.	Health teaching: self-testicular exam (STE), check for history of cryptorchid testis, trauma in young men 17–35 years old (increased incidence). Immediate medical referral when signs present.

Summary

This chapter described the structure and function of the male and female reproductive organs. The main techniques used to examine the male genitals are inspection and palpation of the penis and scrotum. The external female genitals are inspected for lesions and infections. The internal female genitals are examined using the speculum and bimanual palpation. The anus and rectum should be inspected and palpated routinely as a preventive measure for carcinomas of the rectum and prostate gland.

Discussion Questions/Activities

1. What feelings have you had personally when having a genital and/or rectal examination? What approaches by the attending health personnel facilitated your comfort? What factors added to your discomfort?
2. Do you believe that the genital examination is imperative for all age groups? Substantiate your answer.
3. What can you do to raise the consciousness of health workers regarding the importance of performing a rectal and genital examination on all routine health assessments and assessments conducted for the purpose of diagnosing illness?
4. What position best facilitates examination of the prostate gland in the adult male?
5. What is the reason for "milking" the urethra in the female client? How is this procedure performed?
6. Describe the procedure for obtaining a Pap smear from the three recommended female genital sites.
7. State the rationale for changing gloves between the vaginal and rectal examinations.
8. Role-play health teaching a young man the procedure for testicular self-examination.
9. Incorporate assessment of the genitals in your clinical practice of nursing.
10. Document the findings of clients for whom you have assessed the genitals and rectum.

Recording of Findings

Normal findings are presented in the first box. Abnormal findings are presented in the second box.

Male Genitals

INSPECTION
Diamond-shaped pubic hair distribution; urethral meatus at penile tip; uncircumcised; no lesions, scars, edema, discharge, or erythema.

PALPATION
No nodules; foreskin freely movable; testicles descended; no tenderness.

Female External Genitals

INSPECTION
Inverted pyramid-shaped pubic hair pattern; labia majora/minora and perineum intact; no lesions, scars, fissures, excoriations, swelling, or erythema; normal clitoris; vestibule clear; meatus clear; fourchette intact.

PALPATION
No urethral discharge with "milking"; Skene's and Bartholin's glands nontender and without inflammation.

Female Internal Genitals

INSPECTION
Vaginal walls intact—negative for cystocele and rectocele; mucosa pink; no discharge; cervix positioned posteriorly; cervix pink with no lacerations, erosions, or masses.

PALPATION
Pap smears (3) done; bimanual exam: cervix firm, smooth, freely movable, uterus normal size and shape, smooth, firm, mobile, positioned anteriorly; adnexa nonpalpable; rectal wall normal consistency; cul-de-sac free of bulging and lesions; posterior uterine aspect smooth.

Anus and Rectum

INSPECTION
Anal sphincter intact; no lesions, fissures, skin tabs, or external hemorrhoids; stool brown with no visible blood or mucus; negative for occult blood.

PALPATION
No tenderness, masses, or internal hemorrhoids; (male) prostate firm, discrete borders, mobile, normal size, no tenderness or nodules.

Male Genitals

INSPECTION
Severe bilateral scrotal edema; transillumination present.

PALPATION
Unable to palpate epididymis or spermatic cord; nontender.

Female Internal Genitals

(Client has inflammation of a Bartholin's gland secondary to gonococcal infection)

INSPECTION
Left lower labial edema with tenderness; erythematous; copious purulent vaginal discharge; urethral orifice edematous and red.

PALPATION
Tenderness and greenish yellow urethral discharge upon "milking" urethra; dysuria; endocervical and urethral cultures done.

Anus and Rectum

(Client diagnosed as having prostatic carcinoma)

INSPECTION
Anal sphincter intact; no lesions, fissures, skin tabs, or external hemorrhoids; stool brown with no visible blood or mucus; negative for occult blood.

PALPATION
No tenderness, masses, or internal hemorrhoids; enlarged prostate 6–7 cm with multiple stony-hard nodules, no tenderness, fixated.

CHAPTER 20

Assessment of the Newborn

LEARNING OBJECTIVES

1. Describe the role of the nurse in newborn assessment.
2. List specific areas and questions that guide the collection of a complete newborn history.
3. Evaluate infant development using both birth weight and gestational age as criteria.
4. Develop a flexible approach to systematic newborn assessment.
5. Explain the techniques of inspection, palpation, percussion, and auscultation used to gather data constituting a complete newborn assessment.
6. Describe normal variations in findings of the newborn assessment.
7. Identify abnormal conditions of the newborn that require further evaluation and treatment.

This chapter was written by Mary Lou Rusin, R.N., Ed.D., Daemen College.

Newborn assessment is a critical component of the nursing process, since it provides the nurse with baseline assessment data that can be used as a parameter for future growth and development of the infant. The assessment findings are the foundation of nursing planning, intervention, and evaluation and yield important information for the nurse to share with the parents in order to initiate rapport, begin teaching activities, and commence anticipatory guidance with the parents to achieve holistic client care.

Because newborn infants are anatomically and physiologically unique, many techniques of physical assessment have to be modified to meet the infant's specific needs. Also, findings associated with newborn appraisal must be evaluated in the context of the newborn's specific individual characteristics. This chapter is designed to present a total approach to newborn assessment; it describes in detail common findings and their significance.

Health History

The newborn's health history is essentially the pregnancy history of the mother. This information can be gathered by examining previous records and interviewing the mother.

A complete prenatal history includes information regarding the mother's general state of health during her pregnancy. The determination of the length of her prenatal care, when it was begun, where it was obtained, and whether the mother kept regular appointments is essential. Ask the mother about the milestones of pregnancy, and evaluate them in terms of timing and sequence. Note any infections and the month of their occurrence. Discuss any illnesses and accidents, the month of occurrence, and the method of treatment. Determine the infant's blood type, along with the blood types of both mother and father. Also important is such information as prenatal diet history of the mother and a total family history. Finally, include the emotional reactions of the parents to the pregnancy.

Examine the mother's labor and delivery room record to determine the length and type of labor, time the membranes ruptured, type of delivery, anesthesia, analgesia, and any problems during delivery of the child and the placenta. Analyze the infant's delivery room record for information, including presentation, position, weight (which should be plotted on a gestational age chart), Apgar score, eye prophylaxis, first voiding and first stool, and the infant's response to feeding. If fetal monitoring was done, include information regarding the infant's vital signs during labor and delivery.

Evaluate the infant according to birth weight, gestational age, or a combination of these two. Classification by birth weight alone defines premature infants as those weighing less than 2500 g at birth and labels as full term those infants with a birth weight over 2500 g. When gestational age alone is used as an evaluation criterion, the gestational weeks are calculated from the first day of the last menstrual period (LMP). Premature or preterm infants are defined as being born before the end of the 37th week. Infants born between the beginning of the 38th week and the end of the 41st week are classified as term infants. Postmature or postterm infants are those born at the beginning of the 42nd week or later. Intrauterine growth curves were devised by plotting a chart using both birth weight and gestational age as coordinates (see Figure 20-1). This method of evaluation determines the appropriateness of the infant's growth.

Specific criteria regarding the neuromuscular and physical maturity of the newborn can be

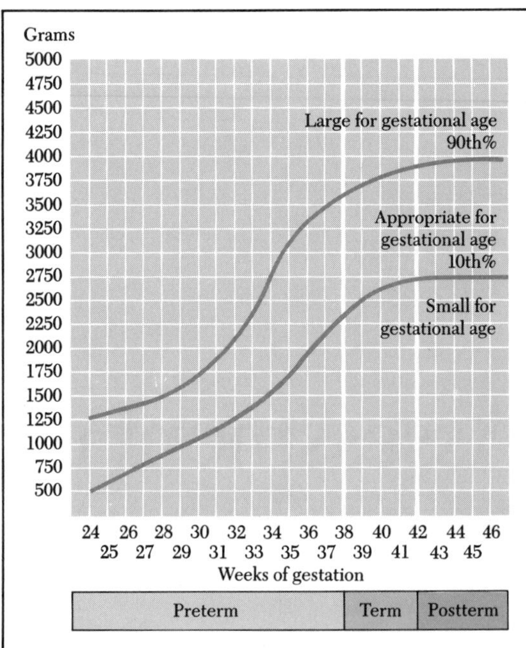

Figure 20-1 University of Colorado Medical Center classification of newborns by birth weight and gestational age.

measured and rated postnatally using a classification system (see Figure 20-2). This method yields extremely accurate information regarding exact gestational age.

The Apgar score measures the infant's immediate reaction to extrauterine life on the basis of five criteria, which are evaluated immediately at birth and at one minute and five minutes following birth. These criteria include heart rate, respiratory effort, muscle tone, reflex irritability, and color (see Table 20-1).

Physical Assessment

Physical assessment of the newborn begins with inspection of the infant in a cephalocaudal direction. The sequence of the examination should be flexible to allow the examiner to take advantage of a sleeping infant to auscultate the heart and lungs, or to take advantage of a crying infant to assess the mouth, throat and palate, gums, and facial movement. This chapter is organized following the sequence of systems discussed throughout the textbook; however, the examiner should be able to organize the assessment to ad-

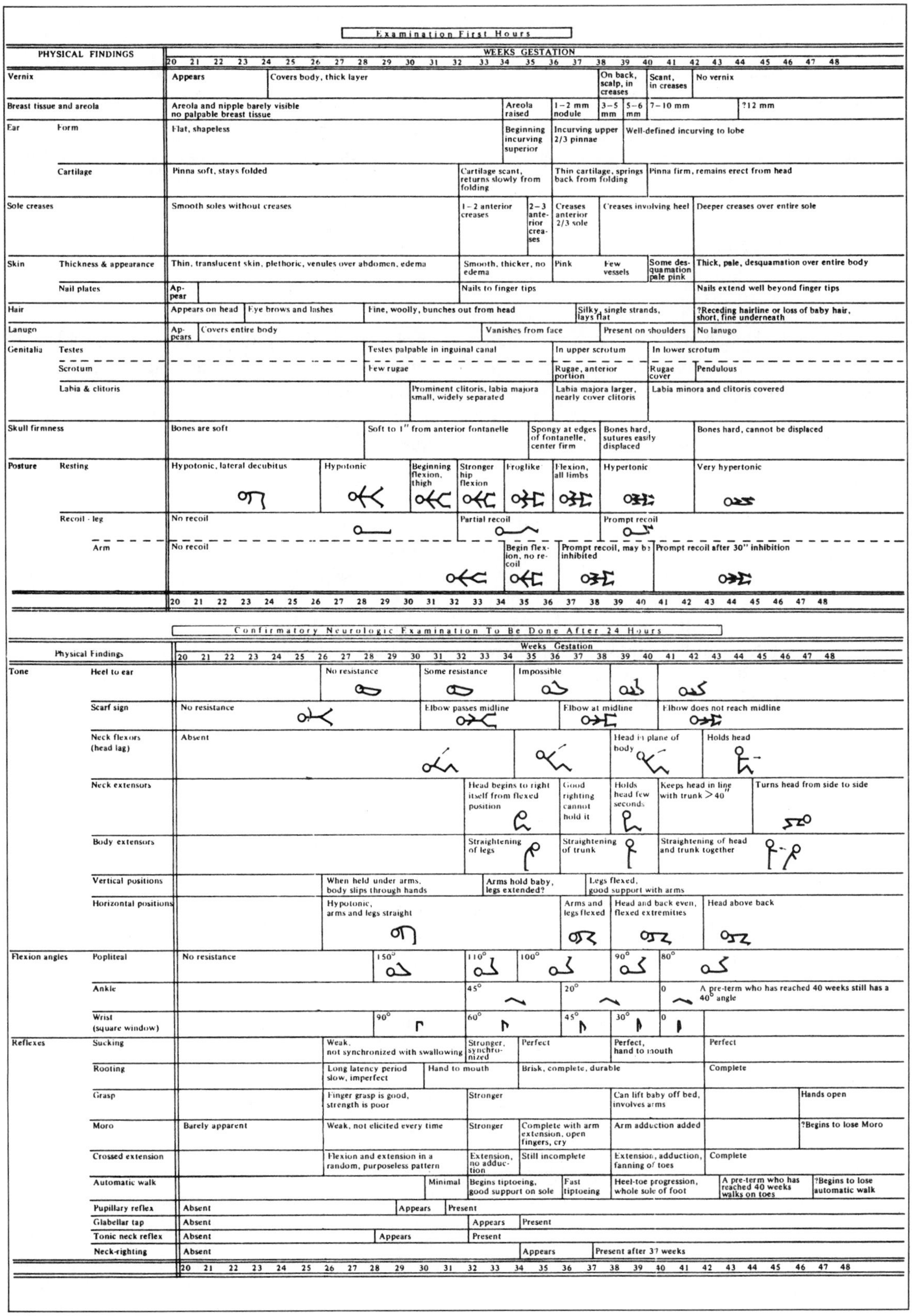

Examination First Hours

WEEKS GESTATION: 20 21 22 23 24 25 26 27 28 29 30 31 32 33 34 35 36 37 38 39 40 41 42 43 44 45 46 47 48

PHYSICAL FINDINGS									
Vernix		Appears	Covers body, thick layer	On back, scalp, in creases	Scant, in creases	No vernix			
Breast tissue and areola		Areola and nipple barely visible no palpable breast tissue	Areola raised	1–2 mm nodule	3–5 mm	5–6 mm	7–10 mm	?12 mm	
Ear	Form	Flat, shapeless	Beginning incurving superior	Incurving upper 2/3 pinnae	Well-defined incurving to lobe				
	Cartilage	Pinna soft, stays folded	Cartilage scant, returns slowly from folding	Thin cartilage, springs back from folding	Pinna firm, remains erect from head				
Sole creases		Smooth soles without creases	1–2 anterior creases	2–3 anterior creases	Creases anterior 2/3 sole	Creases involving heel	Deeper creases over entire sole		
Skin	Thickness & appearance	Thin, translucent skin, plethoric, venules over abdomen, edema	Smooth, thicker, no edema	Pink	Few vessels	Some desquamation pale pink	Thick, pale, desquamation over entire body		
	Nail plates	Appear		Nails to finger tips	Nails extend well beyond finger tips				
Hair		Appears on head	Eye brows and lashes	Fine, woolly, bunches out from head	Silky, single strands, lays flat	?Receding hairline or loss of baby hair, short, fine underneath			
Lanugo		Appears	Covers entire body	Vanishes from face	Present on shoulders	No lanugo			
Genitalia	Testes		Testes palpable in inguinal canal	In upper scrotum	In lower scrotum				
	Scrotum		Few rugae	Rugae, anterior portion	Rugae cover	Pendulous			
	Labia & clitoris		Prominent clitoris, labia majora small, widely separated	Labia majora larger, nearly cover clitoris	Labia minora and clitoris covered				
Skull firmness		Bones are soft	Soft to 1" from anterior fontanelle	Spongy at edges of fontanelle, center firm	Bones hard, sutures easily displaced	Bones hard, cannot be displaced			
Posture	Resting	Hypotonic, lateral decubitus	Hypotonic	Beginning flexion, thigh	Stronger hip flexion	Froglike	Flexion, all limbs	Hypertonic	Very hypertonic
	Recoil - leg	No recoil	Partial recoil	Prompt recoil					
	Arm	No recoil	Begin flexion, no recoil	Prompt recoil, may be inhibited	Prompt recoil after 30" inhibition				

Confirmatory Neurologic Examination To Be Done After 24 Hours

Weeks Gestation: 20 21 22 23 24 25 26 27 28 29 30 31 32 33 34 35 36 37 38 39 40 41 42 43 44 45 46 47 48

Physical Findings								
Tone	Heel to ear	No resistance	Some resistance	Impossible				
	Scarf sign	No resistance	Elbow passes midline	Elbow at midline	Elbow does not reach midline			
	Neck flexors (head lag)	Absent	Head in plane of body	Holds head				
	Neck extensors	Head begins to right itself from flexed position	Good righting cannot hold it	Holds head few seconds	Keeps head in line with trunk > 40°	Turns head from side to side		
	Body extensors	Straightening of legs	Straightening of trunk	Straightening of head and trunk together				
	Vertical positions	When held under arms, body slips through hands	Arms hold baby, legs extended?	Legs flexed, good support with arms				
	Horizontal positions	Hypotonic, arms and legs straight	Arms and legs flexed	Head and back even, flexed extremities	Head above back			
Flexion angles	Popliteal	No resistance	150°	110°	100°	90°	80°	
	Ankle	45°	20°	0	A pre-term who has reached 40 weeks still has a 40° angle			
	Wrist (square window)	90°	60°	45°	30°	0		
Reflexes	Sucking	Weak, not synchronized with swallowing	Stronger, synchronized	Perfect	Perfect, hand to mouth	Perfect		
	Rooting	Long latency period slow, imperfect	Hand to mouth	Brisk, complete, durable	Complete			
	Grasp	Finger grasp is good, strength is poor	Stronger	Can lift baby off bed, involves arms	Hands open			
	Moro	Barely apparent	Weak, not elicited every time	Stronger	Complete with arm extension, open fingers, cry	Arm adduction added	?Begins to lose Moro	
	Crossed extension	Flexion and extension in a random, purposeless pattern	Extension, no adduction	Still incomplete	Extension, adduction, fanning of toes	Complete		
	Automatic walk	Minimal	Begins tiptoeing, good support on sole	Fast tiptoeing	Heel-toe progression, whole sole of foot	A pre-term who has reached 40 weeks walks on toes	?Begins to lose automatic walk	
	Pupillary reflex	Absent	Appears	Present				
	Glabellar tap	Absent	Appears	Present				
	Tonic neck reflex	Absent	Appears	Present				
	Neck-righting	Absent	Appears	Present after 37 weeks				

Figure 20-2 The Dubowitz scoring system for clinical estimation of gestational age.

Table 20-1. Infant Evaluation at Birth (Apgar score).

Points	0	1	2
1. Heart rate	Absent	Slow (<100)	> 100
2. Respiratory effort	Absent	Slow, irregular	Good, crying
3. Muscle tone	Limp	Some flexion of extremities	Active motion
4. Response to catheter in nostril (tested after oropharynx is clear)	No response	Grimace	Cough or sneeze
5. Color	Blue or pale	Body pink; extremities blue	Completely pink

Reproduced with permission from V. Apgar, *JAMA* 168:1985, 1958.

just to the individual infant's activity level. Table 20-2 lists the identifying characteristics of the most common abnormalities found in newborns.

The examiner should observe the infant lying undisturbed on the examining table or crib. This inspection should be made with the infant completely undressed; thus, a warm examination room is essential. Body proportions should be assessed. Head circumference is normally greater than chest circumference in the newborn, and the arms and legs of the infant commonly appear short in proportion to the trunk. The position of the infant should be noted. Newborns commonly lie in a somewhat symmetrical position with the arms and legs semiflexed and hips partially abducted. The head is slightly flexed and in midline or turned to one side. The lying position of the infant should correspond with the delivery presentation and also with the established gestational age. When placed in a prone position, the infant displaying normal muscle tone will pull the knees under the abdomen, thus raising the midsection off of the examining table or crib. Sucking motions of the mouth should also be observed in the resting infant along with easy respiratory exchange. Some sporadic retractions may be noted in the normal infant, but any consistent respiratory retractions may be indicative of respiratory distress. The infant's color should also be evaluated during the general inspection.

Table 20-2. Common Abnormalities of the Newborn

Terminology	Characteristics	Comments
Skin		
Acrocyanosis	Cyanosis of the hands and/or feet during the early hours of life.	Related to limited development of the peripheral capillary circulation in the skin. May also occur in older infants, especially during periods of exposure or chilling.
Harlequin sign	In a side-lying position, the dependent half of the body remains pink; the superior half of the body becomes very pale. A sharp line of demarcation appears at midline.	A vasomotor phenomenon related to functional immaturity of the higher centers controlling peripheral vascular tone. No pathologic significance.
Physiologic jaundice (icterus neonatorum)	Yellowish discoloration most readily seen on face and brow, which can be checked by applying direct pressure with index finger over forehead.	One-third to one-half of all newborns develop jaundice during the first week of life. Usually appears at 48–72 hours after birth and disappears by 2 weeks of age. Related to increased destruction of red blood cells no longer needed after birth and functional immaturity of newborn liver, which is unable to secrete resulting elevated serum bilirubin.

Table 20-2. *Continued*

Terminology	Characteristics	Comments
Café au lait spots	Hyperpigmented, macular areas, which are variable in size, light tan to brown in color, and have regular borders.	Six or more are a cardinal sign of neurofibromatosis. Solitary café au lait spots are usually insignificant.
Mongolian spot	Bluish gray, bruiselike macular areas of discoloration located over the buttocks, sacrum, and back.	Common finding in darker-complexioned infants of all races. Caused by collections of dopa-positive melanocytes in the dermis. Frequently seen in Black, East Indian, and Oriental infants.
Storkbite (stork's beak mark)	Pale pink to mauve spots seen most frequently on the eyelids, glabella, and occipital areas.	Common finding in light-complexioned newborns. Tend to blanch on pressure and fade promptly and disappear before the end of the first year.
Port wine stain	Pink to reddish purple in color; variable in size, shape, and location. Most commonly found at center of forehead and nape of neck.	Composed of plexus of newly formed capillaries in papillary layer of corium. Does not blanch with pressure or disappear spontaneously. Use of a covering cosmetic is most acceptable treatment.
Strawberry mark (nevus vasculosus)	Elevated, lobulated, bright red or red-purple, soft lesion. Usually located in head region.	Consists of dilated, newly formed capillaries occupying entire dermal and subdermal layers with associated connective tissue hypertrophy. Tend to grow rapidly in size until about 8 months and will completely disappear in most cases by 7 years.
Cavernous hemangioma	Poorly circumscribed, deep-seated, soft, compressible swelling, which may elevate and impart a bluish hue to the overlying skin.	Composed of mature blood vessels and located in subcutaneous tissue. Rapid growth or episodic bleeding may necessitate surgical removal, although conservative treatment is method of choice.
Nevus spilus	Pale yellow to brown or black, flat, hairless nevus.	Color is dependent on amount of melanin within nevus cells. Rarely requires removal except when location causes irritation or when rapid change in size or color is noted.
Nevus pilosus	Pigmented nevus covered with short fine or coarse hair.	Spina bifida is often associated with nevi located around the base of the spine. Tends to be rare in newborns.
Milia	Small whitish papules found on midline of palate (Epstein's pearls), forehead, cheeks, nose and/or chin. In approximately 50% of all infants.	Tiny sebaceous retention cysts. Usually disappear spontaneously during first weeks.
Erythema toxicum neonatorum	Diffuse rash consisting of 3–4 mm erythemic areas with a small, raised, yellowish white wheal in the center.	Typically appears during first 24 hours on trunk and diaper area. May persist for up to 7–10 days. No other related symptomatology is usually evident and treatment is rarely necessary.
Forceps marks	Consist of depression or edema with erythema, ecchymosis, and sometimes abrasions, usually located on cheek and jaw areas.	Signify a traumatic delivery and may rarely be associated with cranial nerve injuries or fractures. Usually disappear within one to two days.

(continued on page 436)

Table 20-2. *Continued*

Terminology	Characteristics	Comments
Head		
Molding	Asymmetrical head shape found in vaginally delivered infants.	Due to intrauterine position and passage through birth canal. Normal head shape is usually regained by end of first week.
Caput succedaneum	Diffuse, edematous swelling of soft tissues of the scalp that involves the presenting part during labor and delivery. May also be associated with petechiae, purpura, or ecchymoses.	Swelling may extend across suture lines and is not well defined. Disappears within first days of life.
Cephalhematoma	Unilateral edema located over parietal bones that does not extend across suture lines.	Due to periostial hemorrhage. No discoloration of overlying scalp and visible swelling; is usually not noticed until several hours after birth. Swelling typically disappears in an average of 6 weeks.
Eyes		
Subconjunctival hemorrhage	Bright red crescent-shaped band located around iris.	Due to rupture of a small conjunctival capillary as a result of pressures exerted during delivery. Blood is reabsorbed within 7–10 days.
Chemical conjunctivitis	Edematous eyelids, and erythematous palpebral and bulbar conjunctivae.	Related to irritation of the eyes induced by instillation of silver nitrate drops used in prophylaxis of gonorrheal ophthalmia. May be differentiated from bacterial conjunctivitis by prompt onset of inflammation. Spontaneously subsides within 2–5 days.
Pseudostrabismus	Illusion of crossed eyes.	This illusion is due to the combination of epicanthal folds and wide, flat bridge of the newborn's nose. May be differentiated from true strabismus by performing Hirschberg's test/corneal light reflex test.
Mouth		
Epstein's pearls/Bohn's nodules	Small, superficial, firm, white cysts found along gum margins or in palate.	Occur in approximately 85% of newborns. Usually asymptomatic and spontaneously disappear within a few weeks.
Abdomen		
Umbilical hernia	Midline defect, which measures 0.5 to 2 cm in diameter at site of umbilical cord.	A common finding; usually closes by 2–3 years of age.
Diastasis recti abdominis	Palpable cleft found midline on abdomen.	Due to wide separation between the two rectus muscles of the abdomen. Tends to disappear spontaneously by school age.
Genitals		
Epispadias	External urinary meatus lies on dorsal aspect of penis.	Requires surgical intervention.

Table 20-2. *Continued*

Terminology	Characteristics	Comments
Hypospadias	External urinary meatus lies on ventral aspect of penis proximal to the normal site.	Requires surgical intervention.
Phimosis	Very narrow preputial orifice.	Requires surgical intervention.
Cryptorchidism	Unilateral or bilateral absence of testicles.	It is extremely important to differentiate between retractile testes and undescended testes. The testes may descend by the second month; over 80% of all undescended testes are within the scrotum at age 1. However, close supervision is mandatory.
Extremities		
Polydactyly	Supernumerary digit on either hands or feet.	Frequently these digits are no more than simple skin tags, which can be ligated and allowed to slough. In more complicated cases, more complex surgical intervention is indicated.
Syndactyly	Abnormal fusion of digits, either partial or complete. Webbing of skin and/or the bony structure may be involved. May be present in either upper or lower extremities.	Requires surgical intervention.
Hip dysplasia/dislocation	The femoral head can be dislocated from the acetabular cavity when the femur is extended and adducted (Ortolani's maneuver). Accompanying signs and symptoms may include asymmetry of skinfolds and creases on dorsal thigh, along with apparent shortening or lengthening of affected leg.	Due to abnormal development of hip joint and related ligaments and soft tissues.
Talipes equinovarus (clubfoot)	Foot is turned downward and inward so that plantar surface is turned medially. May be unilateral or bilateral.	May be a consequence of unusual in utero position. Treatment mode is determined by mobility of foot.
Metatarsus varus/adductus	Medial deviation of forepart of foot. Heel maintains a normal position. May be unilateral or bilateral.	In most cases, condition will correct itself spontaneously. However, early detection is important since a series of manipulative exercises serve to improve correction.

Integumentary Assessment

Integumentary assessment of the newborn is accomplished primarily through the techniques of inspection and palpation. The general inspection may reveal vernix caseosa, a cheesy white material covering the entire body. Postmature infants might present with a noted desquamation after one day of life.

Skin Color

The color of the newborn infant is extremely labile and prone to individual differences due to genetic characteristics but tends to be reddish

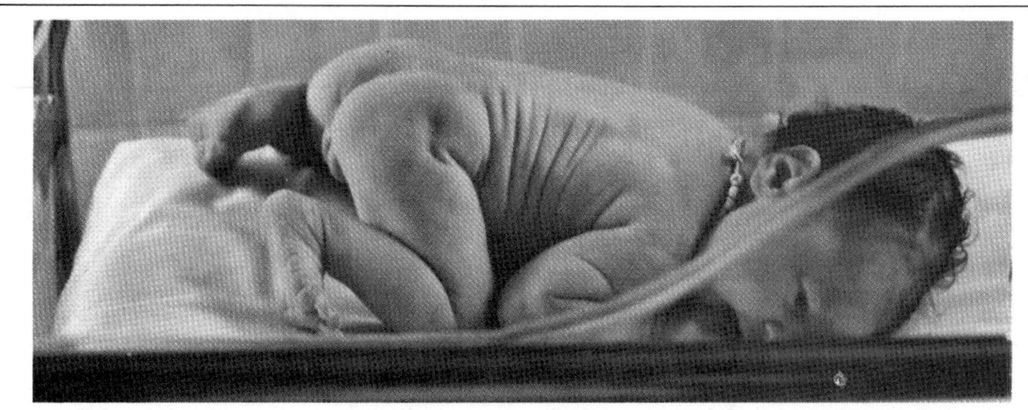

Figure 20-3 Acrocyanosis.

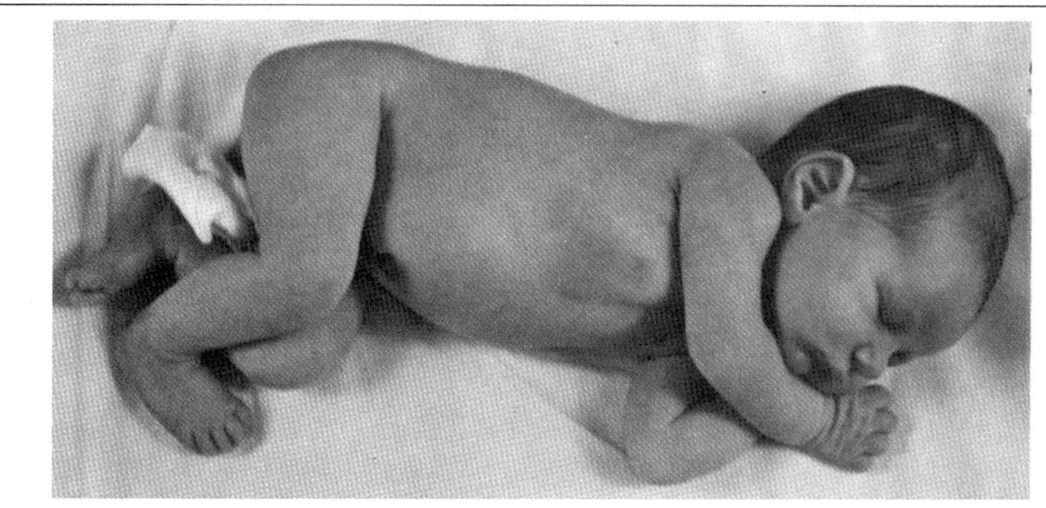

Figure 20-4 Icterus neonatorum (physiological jaundice).

for the first 8 to 24 hours after birth. Also, skin color in a given infant may vary from one moment to the next depending on the activity level of the infant and room temperature. A usual guideline is that the newborn's color should be pink at rest and change to a deep red color with crying. Acrocyanosis presents as cyanosis of the hands and feet during the first hours after delivery and tends to be increased by exposure and chilling (see Figure 20-3). Any cyanosis of the hands, of the feet, or around the mouth should disappear by about 4 hours after birth. The newborn may exhibit a generalized mottled appearance, especially when undressed or exposed to the environment; this usually disappears with warming.

Any alterations in the surface of the skin, such as scratches, petechiae, and ecchymotic areas, should be noted. Bruised areas over the cranium may be associated with the birth process. Lab values should be checked in a newborn who exhibits generalized pallor; such pallor may be caused by anemia or may be indicative of shock or circulatory failure. A beefy red color may be associated with hypoglycemia. Some newborns may exhibit a color discrepancy from one side of the body to the other and appear to be half-reddened and half-pale. This phenomenon is referred to as the harlequin sign and is usually transitory and not pathologic.

Physiologic jaundice (icterus neonatorum) may appear after 24 hours and is best detected by inspection of the sclerae, mucous membranes, and skin (see Figure 20-4). The examiner should ascertain the presence of jaundice by applying direct pressure to the forehead with the index fingertip, which blanches the blood from the head area and leaves a yellowish cast. The

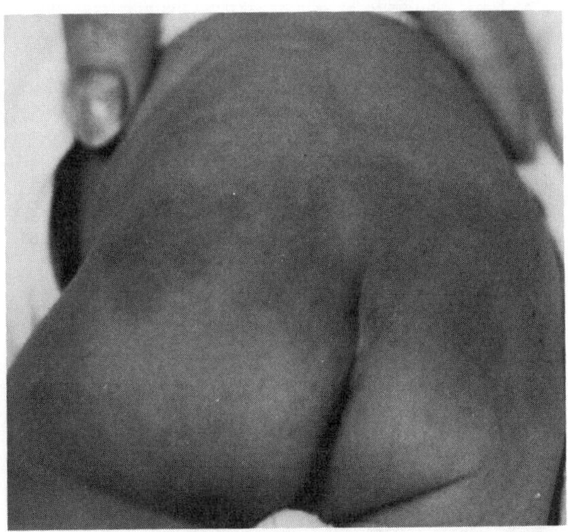

Figure 20-5 Mongolian spots.

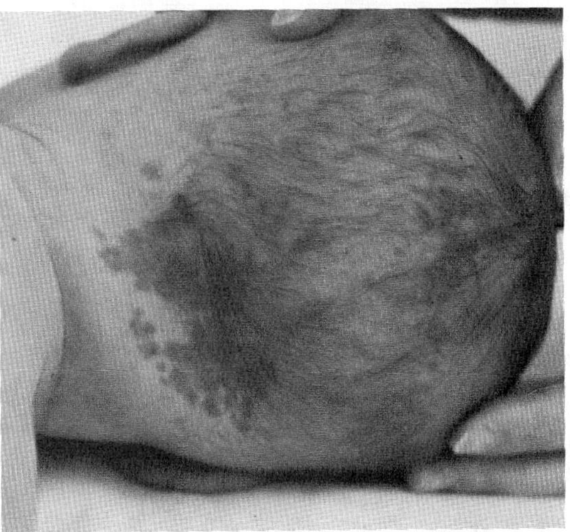

Figure 20-6 Stork's beak mark.

presence of jaundice may also be secondary to some abnormal conditions such as erythroblastosis fetalis, ABO incompatibility, sepsis, viral hepatitis, or bile duct obstruction.

Birthmarks

Minor pigmentation changes are a common finding in newborns, but since they tend to be quite apparent, they are the cause of much anxiety for the parents. A multitude of myths and old wives' tales add to the anxiety and guilt of the parents regarding causative factors behind the existence of such marks. Therefore, the nurse should stress the physiologic etiology of the pigmentation changes and the high incidence of their occurrence; the nurse should also offer support and factual evidence regarding the lack of association between prenatal influences and the occurrence of such blemishes.

The first group of birthmarks present as flat areas of skin discoloration. Café au lait spots are small, light-brown patches that should be assessed in terms of size, location, and number. If more than six are found, the examiner should suspect neurofibromas or fibromas. Mongolian spots are irregularly shaped, bruiselike, dark blue or purple flat areas over the buttocks and sacral area, which may even extend into the lumbar area and dorsal aspects of the extremities (see Figure 20-5). They are more commonly found in dark-skinned and Black clients. The examiner should note size and location of any mongolian spots. These marks tend to spontaneously disappear by age 4.

Another group of birthmarks are classified as hemangiomas or vascular nevi. A storkbite (or stork's beak mark) is a flat capillary hemangioma that presents as a pale pink or reddish spot seen most frequently on the eyelids, the upper lip, and the posterior aspect of the neck (see Figure 20-6). These marks tend to blanch on direct pressure, and the majority fade and disappear during the first year. Port wine stains, or nevi flammeus, are red to purplish blue flat marks that are variable in size, shape, and location, although they are most frequently found on the face along the distribution of the facial nerve (see Figure 20-7). Port wine stains do not blanch on pressure and will not resolve spontaneously; however, radical treatments such as surgical removal and radiation have proved to be of limited value, and more conservative treatment such as the use of masking cosmetics has been more successful. Infants who have port wine–type birthmarks should be referred for nervous system screening.

One type of raised capillary hemangioma is the strawberry mark (nevus vasculosus), which is sharply defined, rough surfaced, and pink to red in color (see Figure 20-8). Strawberry marks are more commonly found singly, but often multiple birthmarks are apparent. The vast majority of these strawberry marks appear on the head and face, which causes great concern for parents. However, increase in growth usually stops by 8 months and the birthmark will normally then recede in size and disappear by age 7, leaving little evidence of its presence. Therefore, the nurse examiner must be supportive of the parents' concern while at the same time engaging in

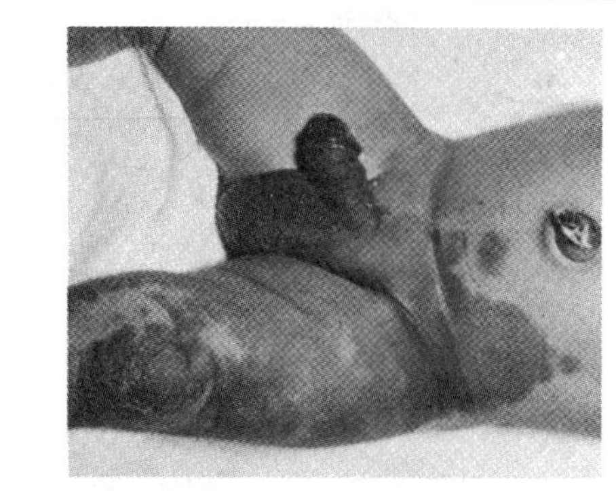

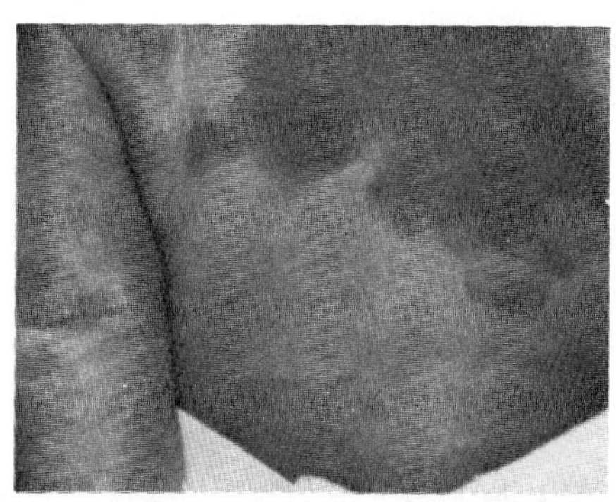

Figure 20-7 Port wine stain.

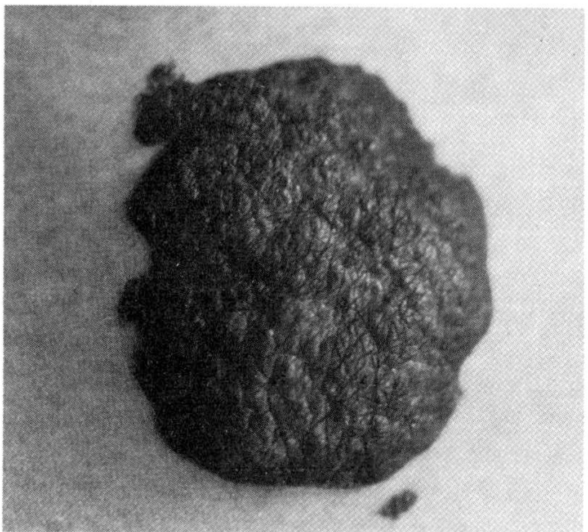

Figure 20-8 Strawberry mark.

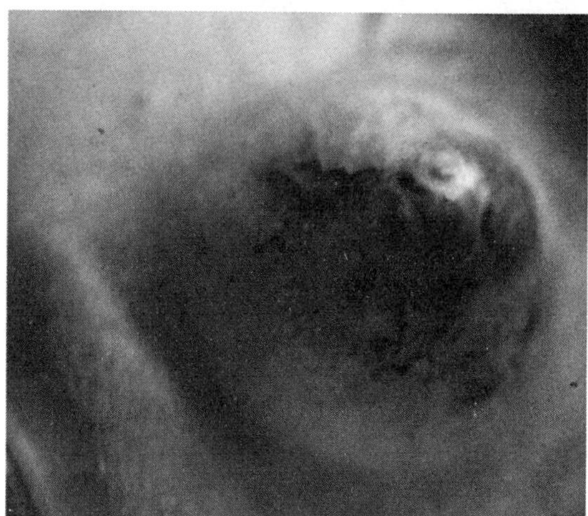

Figure 20-9 Cavernous hemangioma.

health teaching and counseling regarding the normal progression of the strawberry mark.

Cavernous hemangiomas are another type of vascular nevus. Cavernous hemangiomas are poorly delineated, soft, deep, compressible swellings that are elevated and impart a bluish coloration to the overlying skin (see Figure 20-9). The size and location of these marks should be noted, and frequent evaluation of the infant is necessary since problems with rapid growth or bleeding may occur that would necessitate surgical removal. Treatment is, however, usually conservative. There may be a period of variable growth before the cavernous hemangioma regresses.

The final group of birthmarks are pigmented nevi or moles, which are usually brown in color but have a wide variation in size, location, and pigmentation. A nevus spilus is a flat, hairless nevus varying in color from pale yellow to brown or black (see Figure 20-10). In contrast, short, fine or coarse hair covers the nevus pilosus (see Figure 20-11). These nevi should be assessed for size, number, and location. Nevi located in areas of the body prone to friction irritation should be reevaluated periodically for any changes.

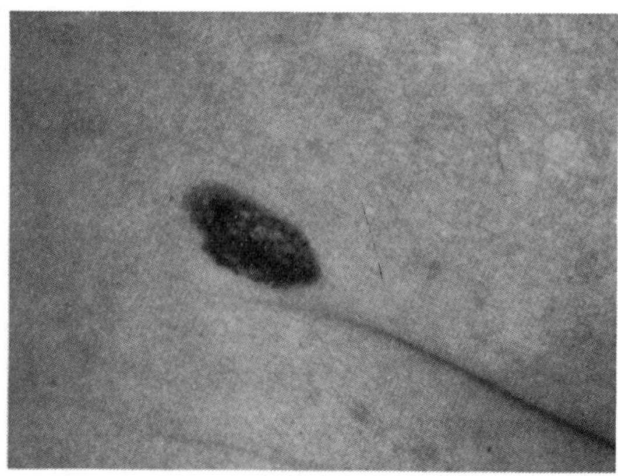

Figure 20-10 Nevus spilus.

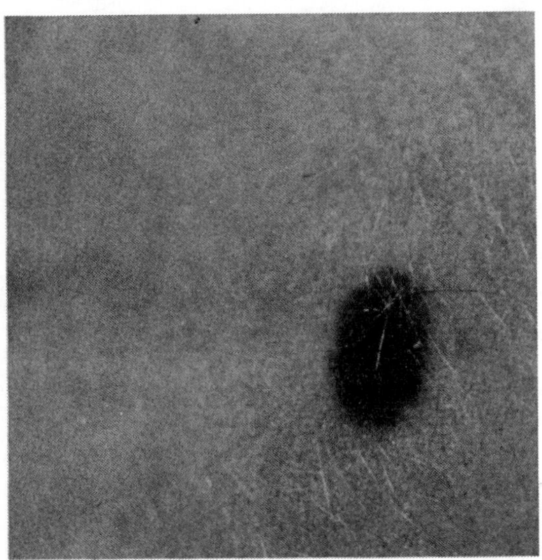

Figure 20-11 Nevus pilosus.

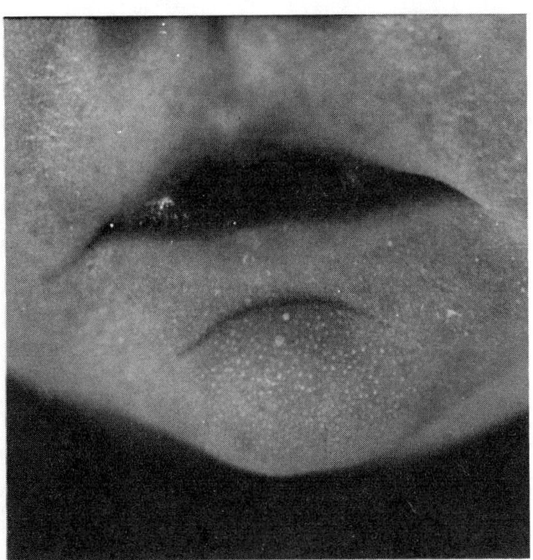

Figure 20-12 Milia.

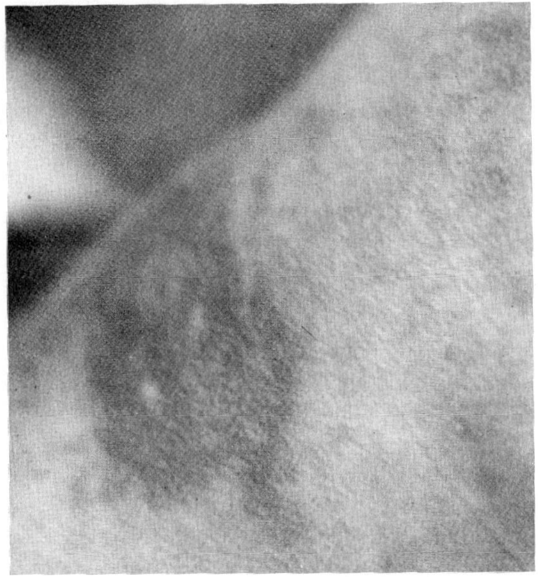

Figure 20-13 Erythema toxicum (urticaria neonatorum).

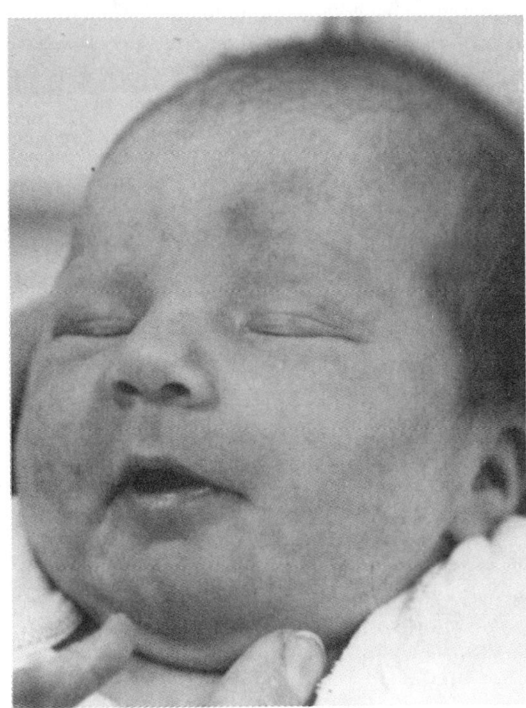

Figure 20-14 Forceps marks.

Other Common Skin Findings

Milia are small opalescent plaques that appear on the nose, cheeks, and chin of the newborn and are caused by sebaceous retention cysts (see Figure 20-12). These usually disappear within a few weeks.

Erythema toxicum neonatorum (urticaria neonatorum) presents as small, discrete areas of redness on the cheeks or trunk that usually appear within the first day (see Figure 20-13). This condition is usually transient and rarely requires treatment.

Forceps marks on the face along the jaw line and cheek area are common findings in infants delivered with the use of instruments (see Figure 20-14). Since these bruiselike marks are very apparent, they may alarm the parents; however, forceps marks usually disappear within one to two days. Table 20-3 lists some normal variations in the integumentary system.

Table 20-3. Normal Variations in the Integumentary System of Newborns

Variation	Description
Vernix caseosa	Cheesy, white substance covering the body at birth; absorbed or rubbed off within 24 to 48 hours
Desquamation	Peeling 2 or 3 days after birth
Milia	Tiny (pinpoint) white spots on the nose, chin, and forehead. Disappear in 2 to 4 weeks
Lanugo	Fine, soft hair covering the body in various amounts which sheds within the neonatal period
Birthmarks	Single, brown or reddish colorations; flat or slightly elevated. Remain throughout life
Café au lait	Flat, irregular, light brown colorations. Appear as dark brown colorations in dark-toned children. Remain throughout life. Five or more areas greater than 1.5 cm each are considered abnormal
Stork bites	Flat, pink-purple areas usually found above the nose, on the upper lip and eyelids, and above the hairline on the back of the neck
Port wine stain	Nonelevated, irregular, red-purple area found on one side of the body. Remains throughout life
Strawberry mark	Slightly raised capillary 2 to 3 cm in diameter; contracts with increasing age
Cavernous hemangioma	Round red-blue mass of blood vessels; may increase in size
Mongolian spots	Flat, blue colorations on the buttocks, back, and/or outer surfaces of the hands and feet of dark-toned children. Fade with increasing age
Cutis marmorata	Mottling of skin caused by exposure to a cool environment. Disappears with warming
Erythema toxicum (newborn rash)	Pinpoint, red areas found on the cheeks or trunk. Appears during the first 3 days of life and disappears within 8 hours

From Servonsky/Opas: *Nursing Management of Children*, © 1987 Boston: Jones and Bartlett Publishers.

Nails

The newborn's nails should be assessed for size, shape, color, and configuration. The nails are normally longer than they are wide, nail color should be pink, and the nails are commonly soft in infants. Deviations in nail size and shape may be associated with congenital disorders including Down's syndrome. Postmature infants may have yellowish nail beds. Vernix caseosa may be found under the newborn's nails.

Hair

Newborns may have *lanugo*, a fine downy hair over the shoulders, back, or sacral areas that will disappear by the third month. Tufts of hair over the spine and sacral area may be indicative of spina bifida, and a newborn with such tufts should be referred. The amount and texture of scalp hair varies greatly from newborn to newborn, but the color should be consistent throughout the entire strand of hair. Darker hair usually replaces the newborn's hair by three months of age.

Skin Turgor

Skin turgor may be assessed by pinching a fold of skin over the infant's lower abdomen or thigh. When the skin is released, it should return to its original position immediately.

Assessment of the Head, Face, and Neck

Central nervous system growth and development of the infant is directly related to cranial assessment. Evaluation of the head provides the examiner with information related to a number of congenital disorders and systemic diseases.

Head

The newborn's head should be inspected and palpated for symmetry, noting the typical frontal, parietal, and occipital prominences (see Figure 20-15). Bossing, or excessive frontal prominence, may be associated with rickets or syphilis, and a newborn with bossing should be referred. The examiner should be sure to assess the head from all aspects, including a superior position. Head shape may also be indicative of the ethnic background of the infant; for example, children of Nordic descent commonly have long-shaped heads while Oriental children tend to exhibit a somewhat wide appearance of the head.

There are a number of common deviations of head shape related to the birth process that may result in asymmetry of the cranium (see Figure 20-16). In vaginal deliveries, molding of the newborn's head is a typical finding during the first week. This asymmetrical appearance of the cranium is caused by the movement of the flexible suture lines to accommodate the infant within the birth canal (see Figure 20-17). Therefore, molding of the head is not present in breech or Caesarean section births. Caput succedaneum presents as a diffuse, edematous swelling that involves the soft tissues of the head and scalp (see Figure 20-18). As with molding, the presenting part during labor and delivery is directly affected. Bruiselike discoloration of the scalp frequently accompanies caput succedaneum, and the generalized swelling may extend across the

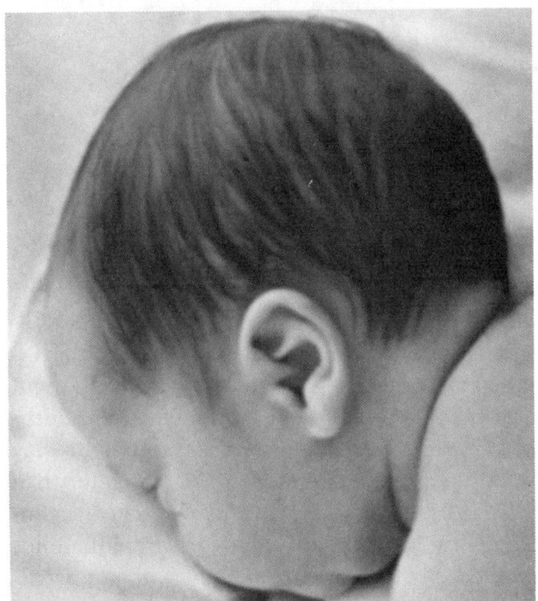

Figure 20-15 Normal head shape.

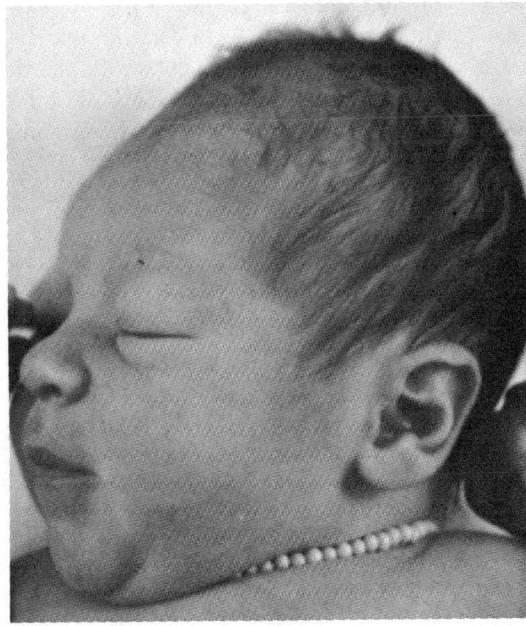

Figure 20-16 Molding.

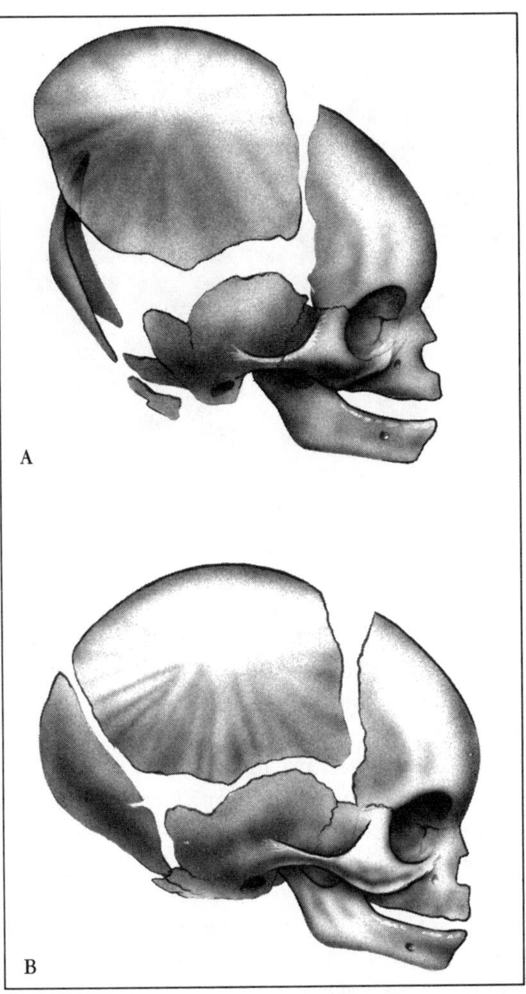

Figure 20-17 The newborn skull. (A) Typical configuration of the skull on the first day of life due to the normal compression from passage through the birth canal. (B) Resolution to normal cranial configuration on the third day of life.

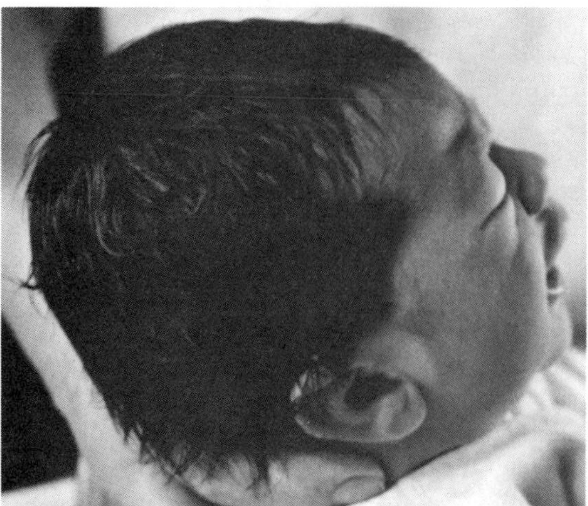

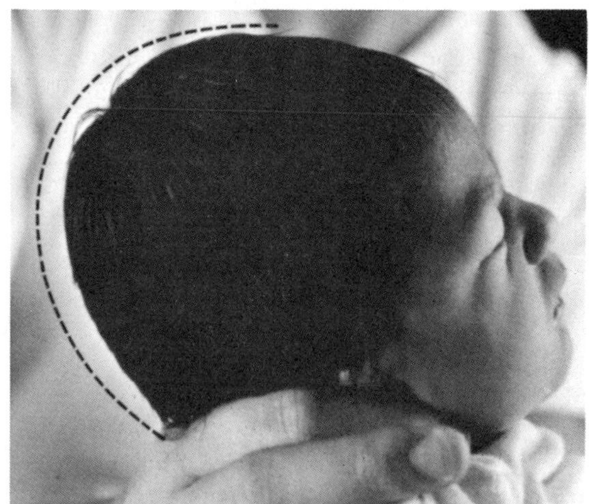

Figure 20-18 (A) Caput succedaneum. (B) Resolution of edematous swelling typical of caput succedaneum. Dotted line indicates original swelling.

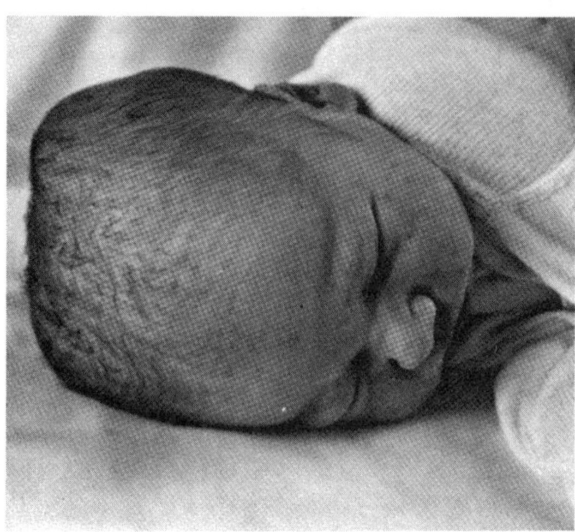

Figure 20-19 Cephalhematoma.

cranial suture lines. A cephalhematoma may be differentiated from caput succedaneum since the bleeding is below the periosteum of the cranium; therefore, the associated swelling does not extend across the suture lines (see Figure 20-19). Unilateral swelling is apparent. Cephalhematomas may not be noticeable until several hours after birth, and they tend to remain until approximately 6 weeks of age.

The anterior and posterior fontanelles and cranial suture lines should be palpated by the examiner. The suture lines are palpated immediately following birth as small ridges and then as slight depressions within the first 24 hours. The suture lines may be felt until about 6 months of age. Any overriding of the cranial bones resulting in pronounced palpable ridges should be referred.

The anterior fontanelle may be small or absent at birth, but it normally grows to about 2.5 × 2.5 cm before closing between 9 months and 2 years of age. The posterior fontanelle may be difficult to palpate at birth. It is smaller than the anterior fontanelle and usually closes completely by 1 to 2 months of age. Both fontanelles should be palpated with the infant in an upright position and also while lying supine. No bulging should be apparent with the infant placed upright; however, when the child is lying supine or crying, the fontanelles may have a full appearance. Slight depression of the fontanelles may be noted with an infant in an upright position. An extreme depression or sunken appearance of the fontanelles is indicative of dehydration in an infant.

Head circumference should be measured by the examiner. An accurate measurement of cranial size is essential as a baseline indicator. To ensure exactness of this measurement, a paper or metal tape measure should be placed around the infant's head at the point of greatest circumference, making sure that the tape is placed at midforehead and over the bilateral occipital protuberances. At birth, normal head circumference is approximately 32–38 cm with an average measurement of 34 cm. The normal head circumference is also about 2 cm larger than chest circumference. Head circumference of the newborn should be plotted on a graph in relation to gestational age to determine appropriateness.

An infant whose head circumference falls within the normal range is said to be normocephalic. Infants whose head circumference is small for age and body size are termed microcephalic, while those with larger than normal head size for body size and age are referred to as macrocephalic. A larger than normal head circumference accompanied by excessive fluid in the cranial cavity denotes hydrocephalus.

Face

The newborn's face should be assessed for symmetry, the position of the facial features, and full and equal range of movement. Motion can best be assessed when the infant is crying, yawning, or grimacing. The eyes should be set at the same level on the face. In hypotelorism, the infant exhibits close-set or narrowly set eyes; hypertelorism is present in infants with widely spaced eyes. The nose should be placed centrally on the face and the nostrils should be of equal size and position. The lips and mouth should be positioned equidistant from midline. The ears should be inspected for placement. The examiner should note any major deviations in ear placement bilaterally. The nasolabial folds should also be symmetrically placed. Occasionally, position of the infant in utero will result in a transitory asymmetry of the face and neck that is apparent at birth. If the infant's head was in a definite laterally flexed position in utero, an asymmetry of the mandible and noted depression in the neck may be apparent (see Figure 20-20). This condition will usually diminish completely during the first few weeks or months depending on its severity.

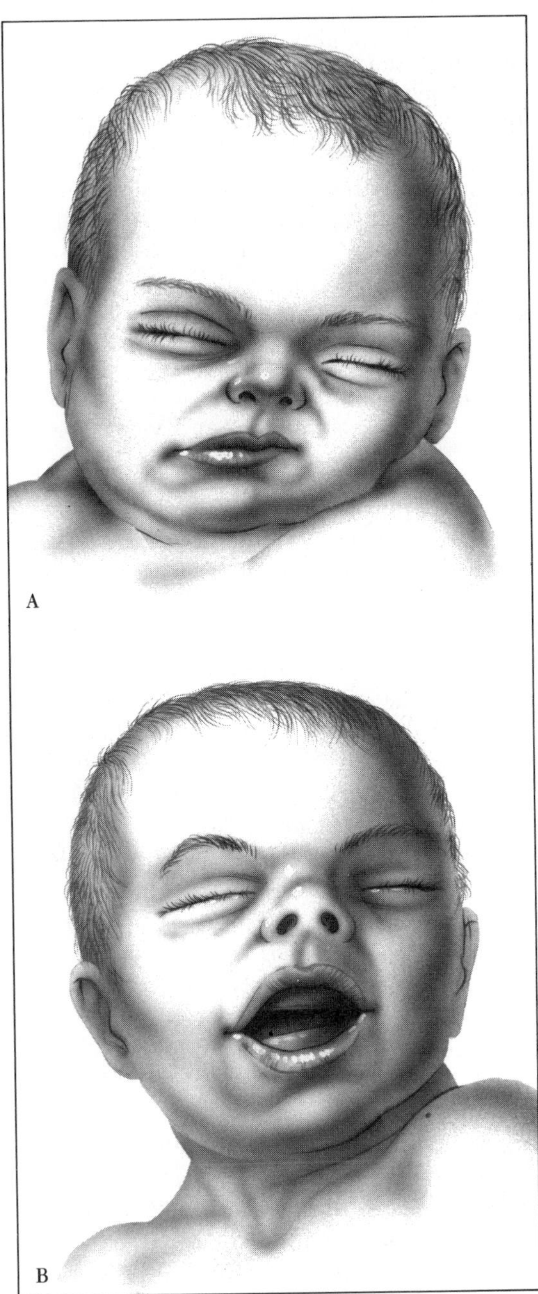

Figure 20-20 Facial asymmetry. (A) In utero position. (B) Resultant newborn appearance.

Neck

The neck should be observed from all angles for symmetry. The head should be centered on the neck, and the neck musculature (trapezius and sternocleidomastoid) should appear equal in size and placement. Any extra folds of skin or webbing of the neck may be associated with a number of congenital syndromes and should be referred for additional investigation. The examiner can evaluate the movement and control of the infant's neck by passively moving the head in all directions with one hand while simultaneously palpating the opposite aspect of the neck musculature for symmetry of tension and size with the other hand. An additional maneuver to assess neck control consists of the examiner slowly pulling the supine newborn to a sitting position by holding the infant's hands. Some head lag is usually evident until about three months of age, although a "rag doll" lack of control should be referred.

The resting position of the head should be assessed to rule out torticollis, a constant deviation of the head and neck to one side. Any pulsations of the neck should be inspected and palpated. Constant bounding pulsations of the neck may indicate cardiac abnormality. The trachea should be palpated as a series of concentric cartilage rings in the midline of the neck. Since newborns have extremely short necks, this assessment may be facilitated by supporting the infant's shoulders and allowing the head and neck to fall backward to more fully expose the neck area. The thyroid gland is rarely palpable in a newborn.

Assessment of the Eyes

The examiner should begin by inspecting the eyes and eyebrows for alignment and symmetrical placement and movement. The eyes should be observed for their relationship to each other as well as their position in relationship to ear placement. The outer canthus of the eye should be in line with the external ear. Movement should be smooth and controlled. Some edema of the eyelid may be noted in newborns who have received silver nitrate drops at birth. This edema can be differentiated from periorbital edema, which is characterized by a bulging of the eye globe. The eyelids should completely close and cover the cornea and conjunctivae at rest. There should be no evidence of any lid retraction. Lagophthalmos, a condition resulting from facial nerve paralysis, may cause incomplete closure of the lids.

Since most newborns exhibit moderate photophobia, the eyes are usually closed. In order to evaluate the structures of the eye occluded by the lids, the examiner may lift the infant's head, causing the eyes to open. The slant of the palpebral fissures can be noted by drawing an imaginary line through both medial canthi. No slant should be noted in non-Oriental children. Down's syndrome may be present in a non-Oriental newborn who exhibits a slanting appearance of the eyes. A phenomenon termed the setting sun expression may be elicited by quickly changing the infant from a sitting to a lying position (see Figure 20-21). This maneuver tends to expose the sclera above the iris and may be a normal finding in many premature and some full-term infants. Oriental infants and approximately 20% of Caucasian infants have epicanthal folds, which are vertical folds of skin occluding the medial canthus of the eye (see Figure 20-22). These are normal in persons of Oriental heredity and tend to diminish by 10 years of age in the Caucasian population. Epicanthal folds tend to be an associated finding in infants with Down's syndrome. The lacrimal apparatus should be inspected and palpated. Normally there is no tear production during the first month; a moderate discharge may be present secondary to the installation of silver nitrate.

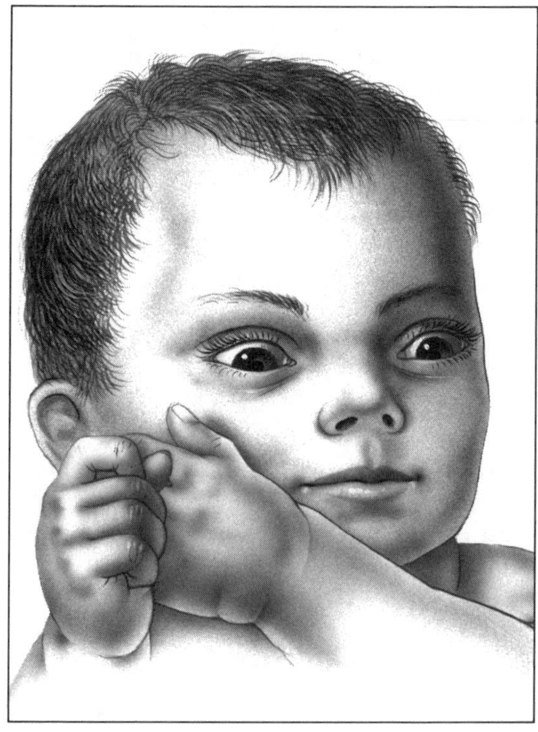

Figure 20-21 The setting sun expression.

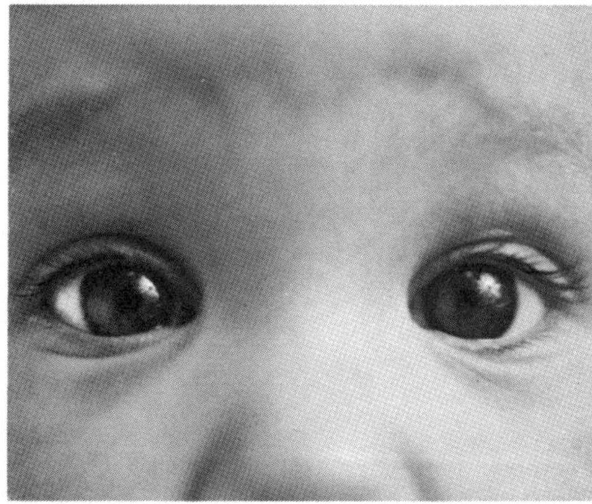

Figure 20-22 Epicanthal folds and resultant pseudostrabismus.

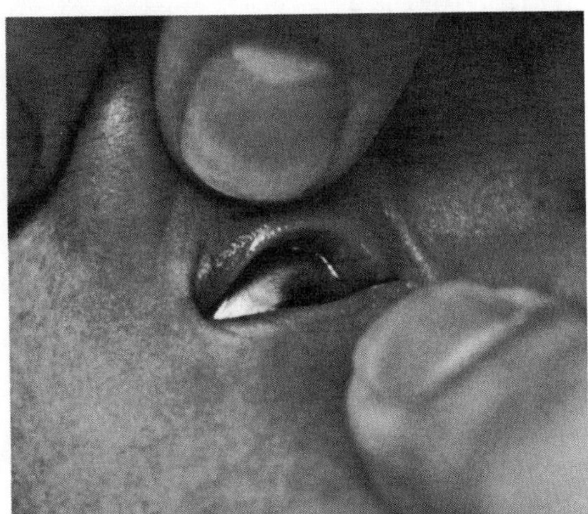

Figure 20-23 Subconjunctival hemorrhages.

The bulbar conjunctivae and sclerae should be observed for color and integrity. The sclerae may present as white or as having a bluish tint; however, there should be no erythema as associated with hemorrhage or yellowish color due to jaundice. Subconjunctival hemorrhages are a common occurrence in newborns due to the rupture of small conjunctival capillaries (see Figure 20-23). Normally, this finding resolves spontaneously within seven to ten days. Chemical conjunctivitis due to silver nitrate installation causes a generalized erythema of the conjunctivae and has a rapid onset. Bacterial conjunctivitis also results in conjunctival erythema but has a much slower, more progressive onset of symptomatology.

The cornea should be assessed by using oblique lighting to rule out any surface irregularities or opacities. Normally, the cornea is shiny, smooth, and transparent. The corneal reflex should be present in the newborn. To elicit this reflex, the examiner should touch the cornea with a wisp of cotton; the infant should blink in response. The iris of the newborn is concentrically round and usually slate blue or very dark in color until about 6 months. The pupils should be assessed for equality, shape, and direct and consensual reaction to light. The infant should have an intact blink response when a light stimulus is presented. Some involuntary movement and blinking of the eyes is common.

Generally, infants are able to fix their gaze on large objects and follow them to midline. Any absence of response or blink reflex must be referred. Anteroposterior alignment of the eyes or the position of the globes within the sockets should be evaluated to determine the function of the eye muscles. Infants with pronounced epicanthal folds may exhibit pseudostrabismus. To differentiate this phenomenon from true strabismus, the examiner should elicit the corneal light reflex (Hirschberg's test) by shining a light source on the face and noting the clock position of the light reflection on the infant's pupils. Symmetrical points of reflected light are noted in infants with normal eye alignment. However, this finding may be of questionable value since some transitory strabismus is frequent in infants. Nystagmus, an involuntary rapid, jerking movement of the eye, may also be normally present in the newborn and may be stimulated by rotating the infant in a lateral direction. Nystagmus should not persist when the infant lies down; any persistent incoordinate movement should be referred for further evaluation.

A complete ophthalmoscopic exam is impossible to conduct on an infant without the use of dilating drops and retractors. However, it is essential that the examiner use the ophthalmoscope to elicit the red reflex in each eye. The presence of the bilateral red reflex is a gross indicator that the retina is intact and that no opacity of the lens exists.

Assessment of the Ears

The external ear should be inspected and palpated for symmetry of alignment, size, and configuration. The examiner should visually imagine a line drawn from the outer canthus of the eye to the occipital prominence. This line should intersect the pinna of the ear (see Figure 20-24). Also, the ear position should be within about 10 degrees of true vertical. There are numerous normal variations of ears in terms of their size, shape, and attachment. It is sometimes helpful to trace such individual differences back through family history; however, usually such findings have little, if any, medical significance. In utero position sometimes results in folded or creased ears. This will usually resolve soon after birth. The amount of cartilage in the external ear varies with the gestational age and maturity of the newborn.

The skin of the external ear canal should be pink and have a uniform appearance. Vernix caseosa and amniotic fluid commonly occlude the

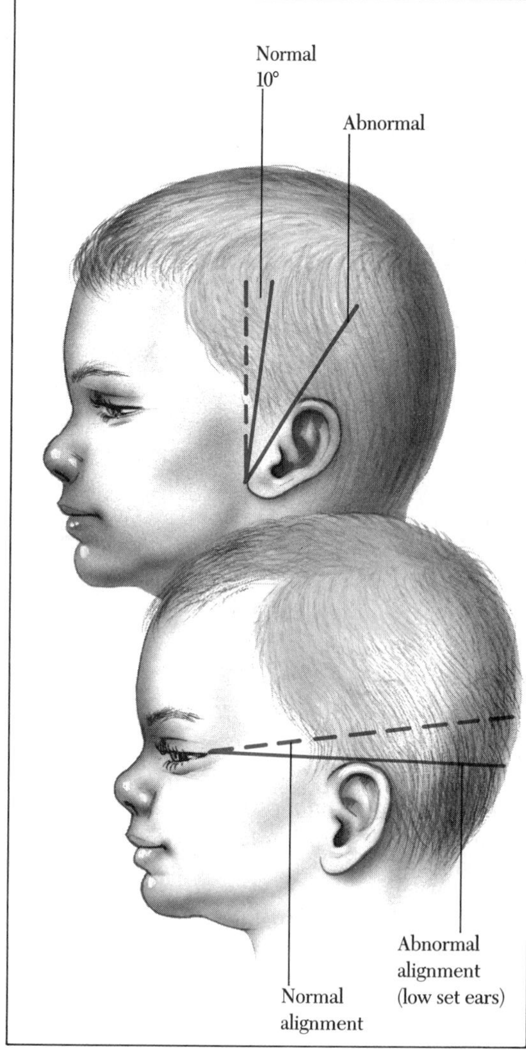

Figure 20-24 Normal and abnormal ear alignment.

tympanic membranes from direct observation using an otoscope.

Auditory acuity should be determined by assessing the infant's startle or blink reflex in response to a fingersnap or bell. The examiner should be sure that the sound stimulus is out of the line of vision of the infant and that the stimulus does not initiate a tactile response in the infant.

Assessment of the Nose

The newborn's nose should appear smooth and exhibit the same coloration as the face. The nose should be positioned in the midline and the external alignment should be symmetrical, although many newborns present with a somewhat flattened appearance of the nose.

Because newborns are obligatory nasal breathers, the examiner must verify the patency of the nares. This can be accomplished by occluding one naris at a time and determining that the infant can breathe easily through the unobliterated naris. Choanal atresia is a condition in which one or both of the nares are not patent. The presence of mucus may interfere somewhat with breathing; however, the infant should not show any indication of nasal flaring, which would signal respiratory distress.

Assessment of the Mouth and Throat

The nurse should inspect the lips for color, placement, and symmetry. The lips of the newborn should be pink, although transient circumoral pallor is common. The lips should be observed both at rest and during movement to ascertain both vertical and lateral symmetry of position and motion. Sucking and rooting reflexes should be intact. Using a tongue blade and light source, the nurse should inspect the inner lips and buccal mucosa of the infant. The color should be pink. The gums should also be pink, although the posterior gum area may appear whitish. There may normally be a rather jagged or uneven appearance of the gums. Epstein's pearls or Bohn's nodules are small, pearly white cysts seen along the gums of infants (see Figure 20-25). They usually disappear by age 2–3 months. Normally, no salivation is present in the newborn.

The tongue should be inspected for color and position. The tongue should be pink and located within the mouth. An infant with macroglossia

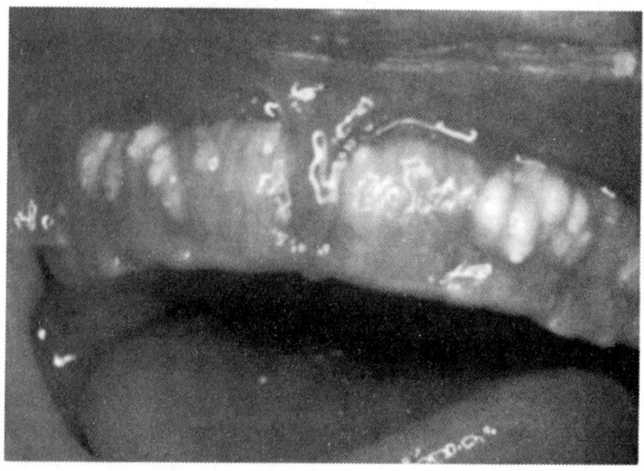

Figure 20-25 Epstein's pearls, or Bohn's nodules.

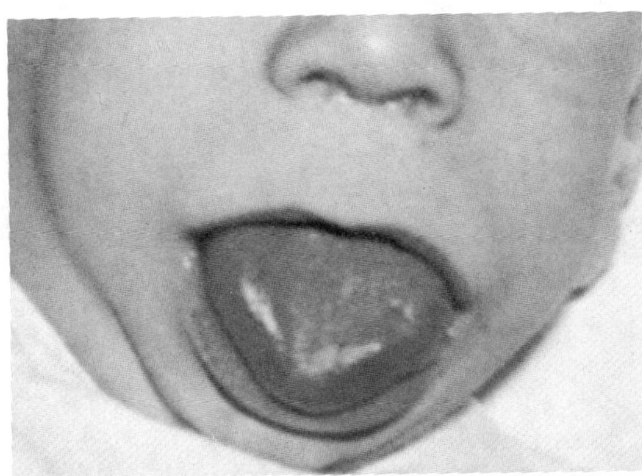

Figure 20-26 Macroglossia.

has a protruding tongue that appears to be too large for the mouth. Macroglossia may be a sign of a congenital defect such as Down's syndrome (see Figure 20-26). The attachment of the tongue should also be assessed. In glossoptosis the tongue attachment is more anterior than usual. Frequently, glossoptosis is accompanied by a small mandible, which may lead to feeding problems as well as respiratory distress, hypoxia, and cyanosis. This combination of findings is also commonly associated with cleft palate.

The hard and soft palates of the newborn should be both inspected and palpated. The palates should be pink and completely formed. No cleft should be evident as the examiner palpates the palate using the index finger. The nurse should refer any infant who exhibits an extremely high or narrow palatal arch.

The gag reflex can be elicited by pressing on the posterior tongue with a tongue blade. A light source should also be used. The extrusion reflex should also be elicited.

Assessment of the Chest

The nurse should inspect the newborn's chest to determine that the skin color is pink and that the anteroposterior diameter is approximately equal to the lateral diameter. Thus, the chest should appear almost circular; the normal chest wall configuration is somewhat rounded. No gross abnormalities, such as areas of bulging or depression, should be apparent. The sternum should be straight, not raised or sunken in relationship to the chest wall. Using a tape measure, the nurse can measure the chest circumference and plot the measurement on a graph depicting normal distributions of chest circumference as related to gestational age (see Figure 20-27). Normal chest circumference ranges between 30 and 37.5 cm in the newborn.

The entire chest should be palpated by the examiner. The clavicles should be smooth and straight and present no evidence of fracture or dislocation, which is a common birth-related trauma. Any crepitus felt in the clavicular area may be associated with fracture. Bony prominence of the clavicles may also signify early callous formation related to fracture. The ribs and all costochondral junctions of the newborn should feel smooth and have no sharp, angular bumps. Such bumps are termed rachitic rosary and are usually due to rickets. A mild flaring of the rib cage just below the level of the diaphragm in conjunction with a horizontal groove (Harrison's groove) at diaphragmatic level is sometimes present normally in the newborn.

The breast tissue should be inspected and palpated. Normally some breast tissue is present in both sexes; the amount varies with gestational age of the newborn (see Figure 20-2). The nipples should be positioned symmetrically. Supernumerary nipples are sometimes found along the milk line, which extends on a diagonal from the anterior axillary line through the true nipples and inferiorly to the medial pubic bone. The nipples should evidence no signs of infection, although a milky discharge may be present accompanied by palpable engorgement of the breast tissue.

Infants typically display abdominal and nasal breathing patterns. The respiratory rate is normally 30–60 breaths per minute. Some infants may demonstrate Cheyne-Stokes type breathing; this will usually disappear by 4 weeks of age. The supraclavicular and intercostal areas should be inspected to rule out any retractions associated with respiratory distress. The nurse should auscultate both the anterior and posterior chest to determine the quality and intensity of breath sounds using the diaphragm of a pediatric stethoscope. Bronchovesicular and vesicular breath sounds should prevail over the entire chest. No rales, rhonchi, wheezes, or other adventitious sounds should be heard.

The anterior chest should be inspected and palpated to assess the point of maximum intensity (PMI). No cardiac thrills should be palpated. The nurse should then auscultate the anterior chest to determine the rate, rhythm, and quality of the heart sounds and to assess any cardiac murmurs. All five auscultatory sites should be

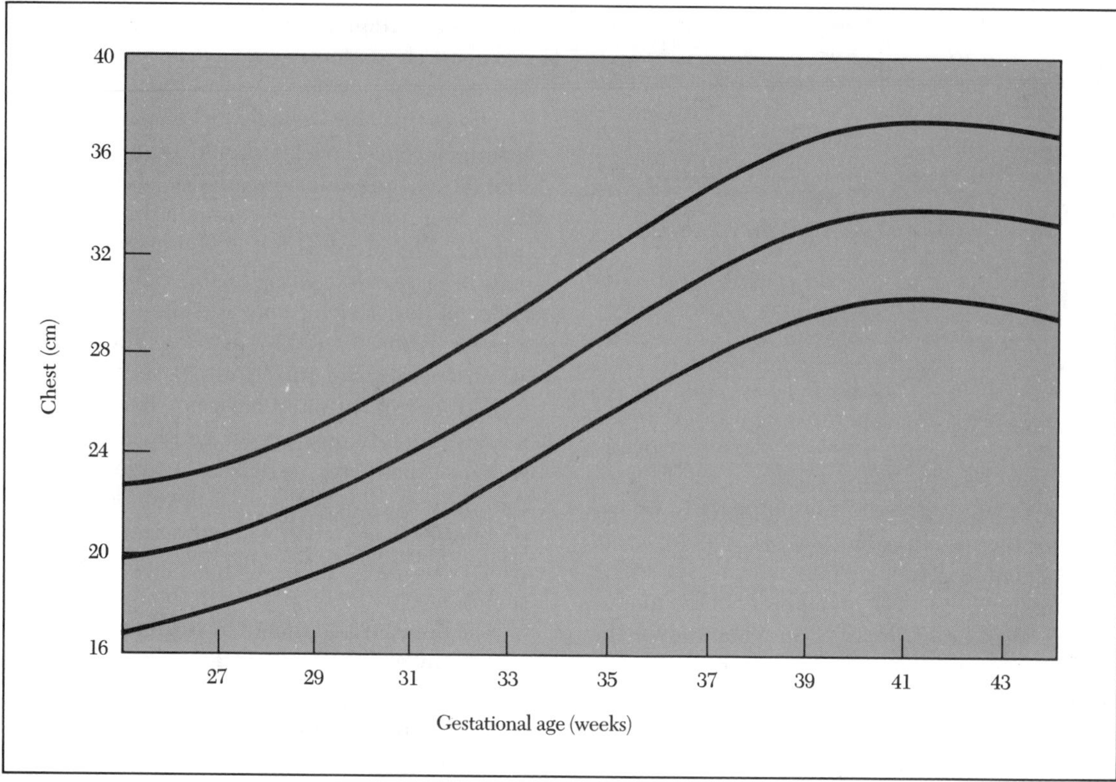

Figure 20-27 Chest circumference related to gestational age.

used to evaluate heart sounds along with auscultating at the posterior chest to evaluate any radiating heart sounds. Normal heart rate varies from 120 to 150 beats per minute. The heart sound rhythm is usually regular, although a short period of irregularity may be apparent following either physical or emotional stimuli. Sound one (S_1) and sound two (S_2) should be sharp, distinct sounds. There should be no extra sounds or murmurs heard during systole or diastole. However, because cardiac composition of the newborn is often incomplete during the first 24 hours, there may be some transitory Grade I or Grade II systolic murmurs during this time. Such murmurs should be followed, though generally they have no clinical significance. The blood pressure of the newborn is commonly measured at the thigh and is normally between 96/62 and 64/30. Major tetratogenic factors and common syndromes with cardiovascular involvement are listed in Table 20-4. Findings and medical management of cyanotic and acyanotic congenital heart defects are shown in Tables 20-5 and 20-6.

Assessment of the Abdomen

On inspection, the newborn's abdomen should appear smooth and soft. A faint venous network may be visible. The contour of the abdomen is commonly cylindrical. Since the abdomen of the newborn is typically quite prominent, the infant might exhibit a "pot belly" appearance in both the upright and supine positions; however, there should be no generalized distention or scaphoid contour of the abdomen. Peristalsis is normally not visible on the abdomen. Visible peristaltic waves moving from left to right across the abdomen are classic symptoms of pyloric stenosis and should be referred immediately.

The umbilicus should be centrally located on the abdomen and, on an infant who is only a few hours old, the two arteries and one vein that compose the cord might be evident. The cord stump is normally bluish white and dry within several hours after birth. There should not be any odor, discharge, or periumbilical redness, induration, or skin warmth, which would signify

Table 20-4. Major Teratogenic Factors and Common Syndromes with Cardiovascular Involvement

Category	Factors	Associated defects
Teratogens	*Viruses*	
	Congenital rubella	Patent ductus arteriosus
	Maternal cytomegalovirus (CMV)	Pulmonary stenosis
	Coxsackie B	
	Herpes virus hominus B	
	Drugs	
	Thalidomide	
	Folic acid antagonists	
	Maternal therapy with anticonvulsants such as diphenylhydantoin and trimethadione	
	Dextroamphetamine, lithium chloride, alcohol, progesterone, estrogen, warfarin	Ventricular septal defect
	Deficiency or excess of vitamins	
	Other Environmental Factors	
	Radiation	
	High altitude	Patent ductus arteriosus
	Diabetic mothers	Transposition of the great vessels, ventricular septal defects
	Maternal lupus erythematosus	Heart block
	Toxoplasmosis	
	Congenital syphilis	
Chromosomal abnormalities	Trisomy 21 (Down's syndrome)	Endocardial cushion defect, atrial or ventricular septal defect, tetralogy of Fallot
	Turner's syndrome	Coarctation of the aorta
Heritable and possibly heritable	Noonan's syndrome	Pulmonic valve dysplasia
	Muscular dystrophy	Cardiomyopathy
	Cystic fibrosis	Cor pulmonale
	Sickle cell anemia	Cardiomyopathy, mitral regurgitation
	Familial deafness	Arrhythmia, sudden death
	Familial dwarfism and nevi	Cardiomyopathy
	Neurofibromatosis	Pulmonary stenosis, coarctation
Connective tissue disorders	Marfan's syndrome	Aortic dilation, aortic and mitral incompetence
	Osteogenesis imperfecta	Aortic incompetence

From Servonsky/Opas: *Nursing Management of Children*, © 1987 Boston: Jones and Bartlett Publishers.

Table 20-5. Findings and Medical Management of Acyanotic Congenital Heart Defects

Defect	Pathophysiology
Patent ductus arteriosus (PDA)	Results from persistence of opening between descending aorta and pulmonary artery. Blood is shunted from aorta to pulmonary artery. Usually asymptomatic. Accounts for 12% of all heart defects. Spontaneous closure may occur within first year of life. Associated with history of first-trimester rubella, birth at high altitude, coxsackie virus, prematurity. Twice as common in females. Coarctation of aorta and ventricular septal defect are frequently associated. May be life-saving when other defects are present. May lead to complications, such as pulmonary congestion, especially in premature infants.

(continued on page 452)

Table 20-5. *Continued*

Defect	Pathophysiology
Atrial septal defect (ASD) 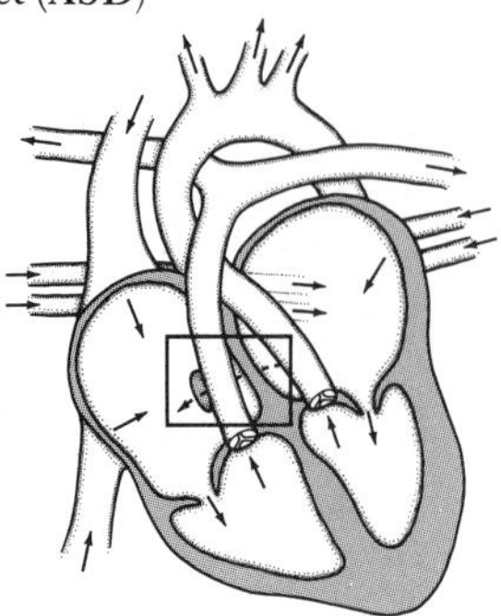	One or more openings located between the left and right atria, permitting left-to-right shunting of blood between the atria. Ostium secundum type located in an intermediate position of atrial wall. Ostium primum type is low in position and is a form of endocardial cushion defect. May be asymptomatic. If presenting behaviors occur, they usually do so by the third decade of life. Ostium secundum type most common, twice as common in females. Left atrial pressure is higher than right. Left-to-right shunt may cause pulmonary artery hypertension. If associated with cyanotic defects such as transposition, this defect may be life-saving.
Ventricular septal defect (VSD) 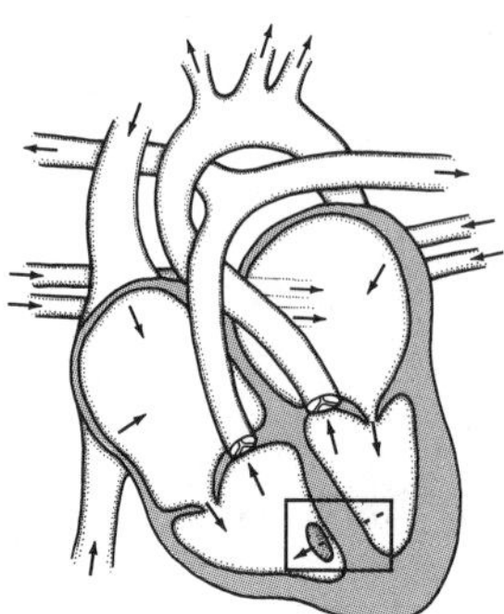	Abnormal opening in ventricular septum (usually membranous area), allowing shunting of blood between left and right ventricles. Blood usually shunts left to right due to less resistance in the pulmonary vascular bed than systemic arteries. The shunt causes an increased pulmonary blood flow. Simple ventricular septal defect most common. More than 50% of small defects may close spontaneously. Closure usually occurs in the first 6 months of life. May be life-saving when associated with other defects. Mortality from a large VSD is highest during the first year of life due to cardiac failure.

Behavioral assessment	Diagnostic criteria	Medical therapy
Clinical findings and clinical course are dependent on degree of pulmonary hypertension and size of shunt. Characteristic machinery murmur maximal at second intercostal space and left sternal border and below left clavicle. Bounding pulses. Pulse pressure is widened. Normal first heart sound. Second sound is narrowly split.	X-ray findings negative with small shunts. Left atrial and left ventricular enlargement with large shunts. ECG may be normal or may indicate left ventricular hypertrophy with large shunt. Evidence of increased oxygen saturation at the level of the pulmonary artery on cardiac catheterization.	Surgical correction is recommended except in patients with pulmonary vascular obstruction. Patients with pulmonary hypertension and large left-to-right shunts should have surgery early (before one year of age). Simple patent ductus should be corrected after the child reaches one year of age. Indomethicin has proven successful in closing patent ductus in low-birth-weight infants.
If symptomatic, easy fatigability with severe murmurs. Congestive heart failure uncommon. Pulmonary systemic ejection murmur heard best at the second left intercostal space, wide split second heart sound. Middiastolic murmur may be present. Arterial pulses are normal and equal. Atrial arrhythmias may result from right atrial overload.	Chest x-ray usually demonstrates slight cardiac enlargement. ECG may be normal or may indicate right ventricular hypertrophy. Echocardiography reveals two features: abnormal motion of right ventricular wall and ilation of the right ventricle. Cardiac catheterization reveals increased oxygen saturation at the atrial level.	Generally, defects do not require surgery early. Large defects are usually repaired before the child enters school. Surgical correction is direct closure of the defect with a dacron patch.

Table 20-5. *Continued*

Behavioral assessment	Diagnostic criteria	Medical therapy
Small left-to-right shunt usually asymptomatic. Child may have frequent respiratory infections in infancy and childhood. Large left-to-right shunts usually cause behaviors of dyspnea, poor weight gain, exercise intolerance, frequent respiratory infections. Congestive failure may develop in the first six months of life. Typical murmur is harsh and pansystolic, best heard at left sternal border in third and fourth intercostal space.	X-ray and electrocardiogram findings normal with small defects. X-ray findings with large defects demonstrate cardiac enlargement and increased pulmonary vasculature. ECG findings with large defects indicate combined ventricular hypertrophy.	Treatment by pulmonary artery banding may be performed to decrease pulmonary blood flow and relieve behaviors of congestive heart failure. Surgical repair is achieved through dacron-patch closure at defect. Age for elective surgery is becoming progressively earlier (usual range is two to five years). Pulmonary artery banding is generally being replaced by early total correction.

Defect	Pathophysiology
Pulmonary stenosis 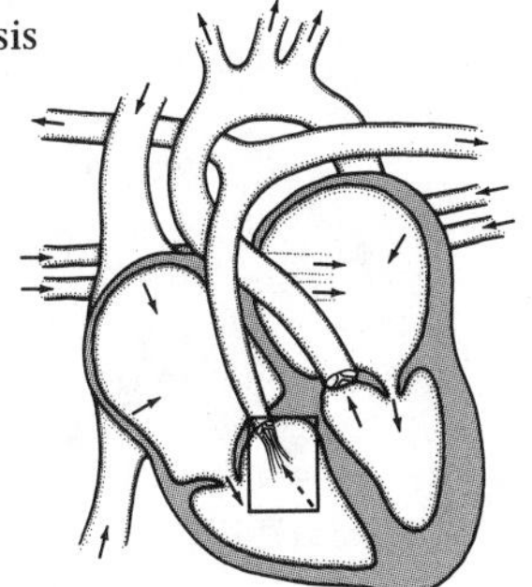	Cusps of pulmonary valve are fused to form a membrane with an opening in the center. Obstruction of blood flow across the pulmonary valve results in increased pressure developed by the right ventricle to maintain adequate output. Asymptomatic and acyanotic unless defect is severe. Associated with maternal rubella. Right ventricular pressure increases to overcome obstruction. Right atrial pressure increases, and finally systemic pressure rises. Right ventricular failure may result. In severe cases, a patent foramen ovale may persist.
Endocardial cushion defect	Results from incomplete fusion of membranous portion of ventricular septum, atrial septum, and leaflets of the tricuspid and mitral valves. Defect may be complete or incomplete. Complete form consists of a high ventricular defect and a low atrial defect continuous with the ventricular defect. A cleft is also present in both the septal leaflet of the tricuspid valve and the anterior leaflet of the mitral valve. The incomplete form involves as small atrial septal defect. Incomplete defect may present few problems. With severe defects, may develop congestive heart failure. Large defect allows blood flow between chambers of heart. First-degree heart blocks present in 50% of cases. High incidence of defect associated with Down's syndrome.
Aortic valvular stenosis 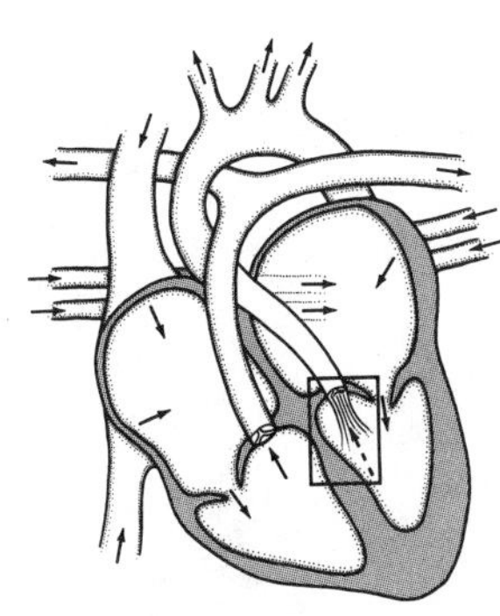	At valvular level may be caused by fusion of the valve cusps. The valve is frequently bicuspid rather than tricuspid and has thickened leaflets. Subaortic and supravalvular stenosis may also occur. Subvalvular obstruction may be due to fibrous ring or muscular obstruction below the aortic valve. Usually asymptomatic and acyanotic in infants and children. Severe obstruction causes increased left ventricular pressure to maintain aortic pressure. Left ventricular hypertrophy may result. Pulse pressure in the aorta is narrowed. More common in males.

(continued on page 454)

Table 20-5. *Continued*

Behavioral assessment	Diagnostic criteria	Medical therapy
Progressive cyanosis. Easy fatigability. Dyspnea on exertion. Systolic ejection murmur associated with a thrill heard best at left sternal border.	X-ray findings in mild forms indicate normal heart. In moderate to severe cases, cardiac enlargement and decreased perfusion to the pulmonary vasculature may occur. ECG indicates varying degrees of right ventricular hypertrophy.	Surgical correction is recommended immediately for all children who have right ventricular pressure equal to or greater than systemic pressure or who have cyanosis. Valvotomy is performed for a valvular obstruction. Elective surgery is usually performed by two to three years of age.
In severe cases, chronic congestive heart failure, growth failure, and persistent respiratory infections may occur. A systolic thrill may be palpated. A loud, hard holosystolic murmur is heard best at the lower left sternal border. Diastolic flow murmur heard at the apex and lower left sternal border. Cyanosis may be present in severe cases and with predominant right-to-left shunts.	X-ray may reveal enlarged heart with increased pulmonary vascular markings. ECG shows left axis deviation and ventricular hypertrophy.	Corrective surgery involves patch closure of septal defect, and mitral and tricuspid valve repair. Surgery for incomplete forms has significantly higher mortality. Complete correction is advised in first year of life before irreversible behaviors occur. Primary repair is performed on children who have intractable heart failure or severe pulmonary hypertension.
If symptomatic, mild exercise intolerance. Easy fatigability. A prominent aortic ejection click. Systolic ejection murmur with a thrill felt at the second right intercostal space.	Chest x-ray frequently shows a normal heart. Dilation of ascending aorta may be seen with subvalvular aortic stenosis. ECG may be normal, even with severe obstruction. Left ventricular hypertrophy may be present. Cardiac catheterization demonstrates pressure differential between left ventricle and aorta.	Major criterion for considering surgery is a large resting pressure gradient of (60–80 mm Hg). Surgery frequently unsuccessful. Aortic insufficiency may result from repair. Surgical outcome is better for discrete subvalvular disease. Close follow-up and limitation of exertion are necessary for nonsurgical management.

Defect	Pathophysiology
Coarctation of the aorta 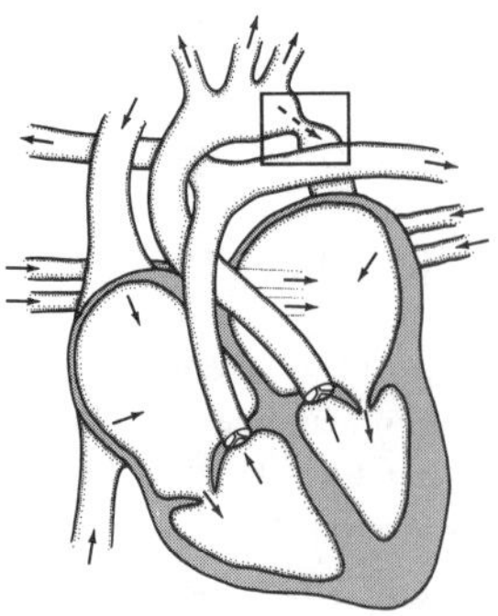	Constriction of aorta, occurring most frequently in thoracic portion of descending aorta. Commonly classified as pre- or postductal. May, however, be juxtaductal. Usually associated with other anomalies, such as patent ductus arteriosus, ventricular septal defect, and bicuspid aortic valve.

Table 20–5. *Continued*

Behavorial assessment	Diagnostic criteria	Medical therapy
Hypertension. Bounding pulses proximal to defect. Weak or absent pulses distal to defect (femoral pulses). Stenotic murmur across the back. Systolic ejection murmur heard best at aortic area and lower left sternal border. Dizziness, fainting, headache, decreased exercise tolerance, easy fatigability. Increased pallor and cool lower extremity on manual compression. Behaviors of this defect usually occur in either early infancy or adulthood.	X-ray findings indicate left ventricular enlargement. Ascending aorta is usually normal in size. ECG may show evidence of slight left ventricular hypertrophy. Infants with marked congestive failure indicate marked cardiac enlargement with right ventricular hypertrophy. Cardiac catheterization demonstrates severity, degree, and location of coarctation.	Infants with severe coarctation require measures to correct congestive heart failure. Surgical resection and end-to-end anastomosis of uncomplicated juxtaductal coarctation can be accomplished with excellent results. Asymptomatic children may have surgery delayed until four to six years of age.

Table 20-6. Findings and Medical Management of Cynoatic Congenital Heart Defects

Defect	Pathophysiology
Tetralogy of Fallot 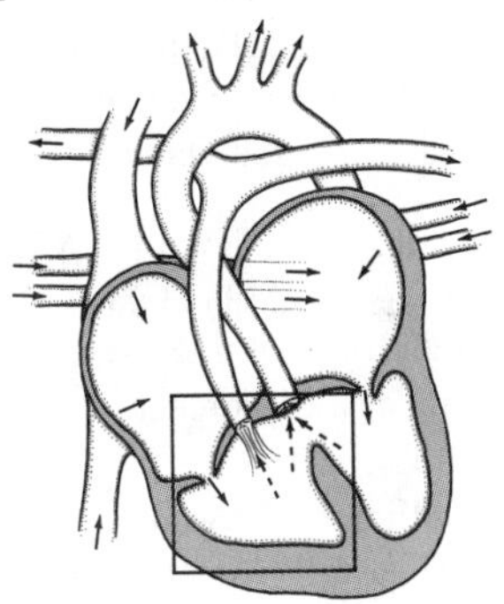	Consists of four anatomic abnormalities: ventricular septal defect, overriding aorta, pulmonary stenosis (right ventricular outflow obstruction), and right ventricular hypertrophy. Right-to-left shunting of blood results from severe right ventricle outflow obstruction and large ventricular septal defect. Unoxygenated blood shunted through ventricular septal defect. Partially oxygenated blood is pumped to systemic circulation. Most common cyanotic defect.

Behavioral assessment	Diagnostic criteria	Medical therapy
Cyanosis (determined by size of defect and amount of outflow obstruction). Clubbing of nailbeds in older infants and children. Dyspnea and easy fatigability. Delayed growth and development. Feeding problems. Hypoxic spells. Knee-chest position or squatting to relieve respiratory distress. Rough, ejection type systolic murmur, best heard at left sternal border, third intercostal space. Murmur radiates over anterior and posterior lung fields.	Chest x-ray usually reveals boot-shaped heart; aorta often on right; right ventricle may be hypertrophied. Pulmonary vascular markings are usually decreased. ECG indicates right ventricular hypertrophy. Cardiac catheterization demonstrates a right-to-left shunt at ventricular level.	Immediate palliative surgery is required for the cyanotic infant. Surgery may be postponed for infants who have minimal behaviors of distress. Most common palliative surgery is joining of right pulmonary artery to right subclavian artery (Blalock-Taussig). Waterston anastomosis is less frequently used. Procedure is an anastomosis between right pulmonary artery and ascending aorta. A third procedure involves an anastomosis between ascending aorta and main pulmonary artery.

(continued on page 456)

Table 20-6. *Continued*

Behavioral assessment	Diagnostic criteria	Medical therapy
		Palliative procedures are performed to reduce hypoxemia and reduced pulmonary blood flow. Total correction is recommended for nearly all patients. Total correction is achieved by relieving the pulmonary stenosis and patching the septal defect. Cardiopulmonary bypass under deep hypothermia is used for infants; heart/lung bypass in older children. Early repair, even in infancy, is advocated in most cardiovascular centers.

Defect	Pathophysiology
Tricuspid atresia 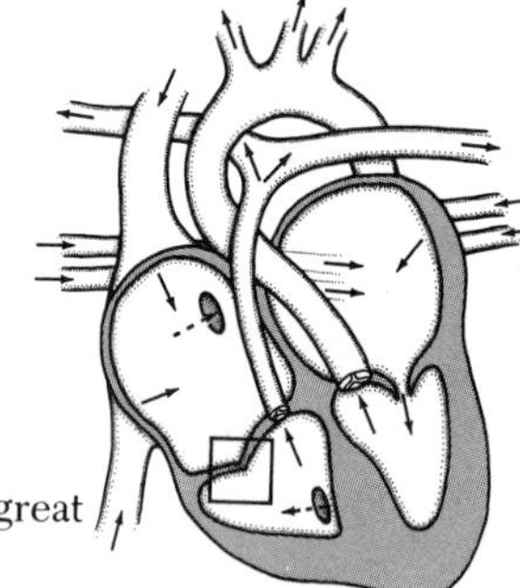	Tricuspid valve fails to form. No direct communication exists between right atrium and right ventricle. The two types are those with normally related great arteries and those with transposition of the great vessels. Right-to-left shunting occurs through a stretched foramen ovale into the left heart. Pulmonary blood flows through a left-to-right shunt at ventricular level. Relatively rare; often associated with other cardiovascular defects, such as ventricular septal defect.
Transposition of the great vessels 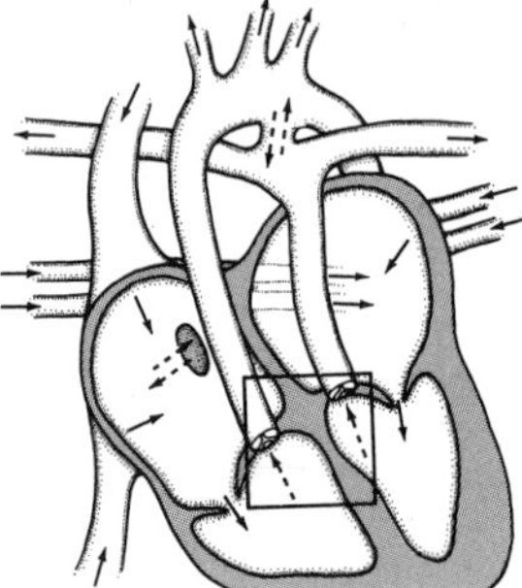	Pulmonary artery leaves the left ventricle, and aorta leaves the right ventricle. Oxygenated blood flows through left heart and is recirculated through lungs. Unoxygenated blood flows through right heart into aorta and through the systemic circulation. Second most common cyanotic defect. Male/female ratio: 3:1. May be associated with life-savings defects, ventricular septal defect, patent ductus, and artial septal defect. Newborns are often large-for-gestational-age. May have family history of diabetes.
Truncus arteriosus 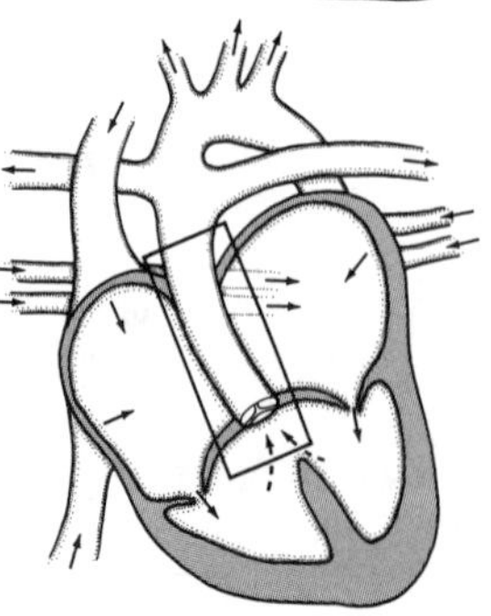	A great vessel arises from the heart supplying both pulmonary and systemic circulations. A high ventricular septal defect is always present. Valve leaflets usually number from 2 to 6. Clinical picture depends on the degree of pulmonary blood flow. Pulmonary vascular obstruction does not usually become restrictive until one to two years of age. Early development of pulmonary vascular obstructive disease is responsible for a poor prognosis in truncus arteriosus.

Table 20-6. *Continued*

Behavioral assessment	Diagnostic criteria	Medical therapy
Severe cyanosis from diminished pulmonary flow. Congestive heart failure may occur if ventricular septal defect is large. Delayed growth and development. Easy fatigability on feeding. Tachypnea, dyspnea, and hypoxic spells. Clubbing may be present in older children. Harsh, blowing murmur best heard at left sternal border.	X-ray findings indicate diminished pulmonary vascular markings and a right atrium varying in size from huge to moderately enlarged. ECG findings of left axis deviation, right atrial enlargement, and left ventricular hypertrophy suggest tricuspid atresia in a cyanotic infant.	A palliative shunting procedure may be done in the neonatal period—Blalock-Hanlon septectomy or anastomosis of the superior vena cava to right pulmonary artery. Functional correction has been accomplished by insertion of a prosthetic conduit with a valve between right atrium and pulmonary artery. Closure of the interatrial communication (Fontan procedure). With appropriate palliative surgery in early life, approximately half of patients survive to first decade. Candidates for corrective surgery must have normal pulmonary vascular pressure and a mean pulmonary artery pressure less than 20 mm Hg, adequate left ventricular function, and pulmonary arteries of near normal size.
Cyanosis (minimal with large PDA and VSD). Retarded growth and development after neonatal period. Congestive heart failure, dyspnea, and hypoxia are the major complications. Murmur usually not a significant finding unless large ventricular defect is present.	Chest x-ray demonstrates cardiac enlargement with increased pulmonary vasculature. ECG findings include right atrial enlargement and right ventricular hypertrophy.	Palliative procedures are usually performed to create interatrial mixing of blood. Common procedures are: Blalock-Hanlon (surgical creation of an atrial septal defect); balloon septostomy (passing a balloon catheter through the foramen ovale, inflating the balloon, and withdrawing it to rupture the atrial septum); pulmonary artery banding, and creation of a ductus arteriosus if pulmonic stenosis is present. Complete repair is done by performing a Mustard procedure. This physiologically corrects the defect by rerouting systemic and pulmonary venous return to heart with a pericardial intra-atrial baffle.
Congestive heart failure and poor physical development occur early in infancy. Mild cyanosis becoming progressively more severe with age. Harsh systolic murmur and low-pitched, rumbling middiastolic murmur and bounding pulses are usually present.	X-ray findings indicate gross cardiomegaly, with left or combined ventricular enlargement. Main pulmonary artery segment may be small or absent. Left ventricular hypertrophy, alone or in combination with right ventricular hypertrophy, is usually present on ECG.	A palliative procedure of surgical banding of one or both pulmonary arteries is usually performed to reduce blood flow to lungs. A corrective procedure is usually performed before one or two years of age. The procedure consists of closing the ventricular septal defect using a valve-containing prosthetic conduit to establish communication between right ventricle and pulmonary arteries.

(continued on page 458)

Table 20-6. *Continued*

Defect	Pathophysiology
Total anomalous pulmonary venous return 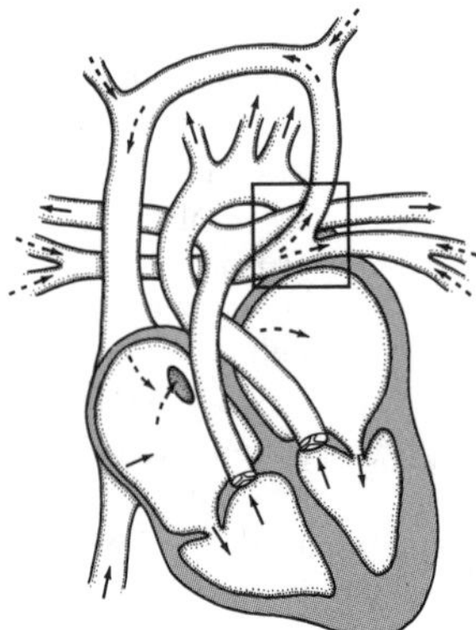	Total venous drainage empties into right atrium via a systemic venous connection. Malformation is classified by site of entry of pulmonary veins into right atrium: *Type 1* Left superior vena cava is point of entry (43%) or right superior vena cava is the point of entry (12%). *Type 2* Right atrium or coronary sinus is point of entry. *Type 3* Portal vein is usually point of entry. *Type 4* Multiple entry points. Oxygen saturation is determined by ratio of systemic blood flow to pulmonary blood flow. If pulmonary vascular resistance is normal, pulmonary artery blood flow is greater than blood entering left side of the heart. Pulmonary return is increased with high O_2 saturation within the right atrium. If pulmonary vascular resistance is increased, ratio of pulmonary to systemic blood flow is lower. When equal amounts of blood flow in both directions, marked O_2 desaturation of blood occurs and child is extremely cyanotic. Defect is rare, accounting for 2% of all malformations. Right-to-left shunt is always present at the atrial level. Half of the infants with increased vascular resistance die by six months of age. High mortality due to congestive heart failure. Children who survive beyond 2 years of age do not have pulmonary arterial hypertension.
Hypoplastic left heart	Underdevelopment of the left heart. Anomalies include underdeveloped left atrium and ventricle, stenosis or atresia of aortic or mitral orifices, and hypoplasia of ascending aorta. Following birth there is marked impairment of circulation due to small left ventricle and obstructive lesions. Congestive heart failure usually occurs by first week of life.

Behavioral assessment	Diagnostic criteria	Medical therapy
Normal pulmonary vascular resistance: Majority of patients have an increased pulmonary blood flow. Mild cyanosis in early life. Respiratory infections occur frequently. Growth failure may occur. Right ventricular heaving pulse may be present. Third and fourth heart sound may be heard. A systolic murmur is heard in the pulmonary area. A middiastolic flow murmur may be heard at the lower left sternal border. *Increased vascular resistance:* Cyanosis usually present at birth—pronounced by one week of age. Tachypneas is as early presenting behavior.	*Normal vascular resistance:* Chest x-ray reveals cardiac enlargement. Pulmonary vascular markings are increased. ECG reveals right axis deviation with hypertrophy of right and left ventricle. *Increased vascular resistance:* Chest x-ray reveals marked pulmonary venous congestion with a small heart. ECG shows right atrial and right ventricle hypertrophy. Cardiac catheterization is diagnostic and confirms the presence of the defect along with associated features.	Atrial balloon septostomy should be performed at initial diagnostic cardiac catheterization, if immediate surgical correction is not contemplated. Surgical treatment during cardiopulmonary bypass involves anastomosing common pulmonary trunk to left atrium. The atrial septal defect is usually closed, and the systemic venous circuit eliminated. Surgical results have improved even with symptomatic infants. The prognosis appears to be excellent if postoperative hemodynamics are normal.

Table 20-6. *Continued*

Behavioral assessment	Diagnostic criteria	Medical therapy
Congestive heart failure may develop later in life. A very noticeable right ventricular point of maximum impulse is present. A systolic murmur grade I–IV/V is heard over the pulmonary area. Diastolic murmurs are uncommon.		
Clinical picture depends on type of obstructive lesions. Dyspnea and hepatomegaly are usually present. Peripheral pulses are weak. A right ventricular lift is present due to cardiac enlargement. Murmurs, if present, are short and midsystolic. Cyanosis is usually present and visible early in life.	Chest x-ray may be normal at birth with rapid and progressive cardiac enlargement associated with pulmonary venous congestion. ECG frequently indicates right axis deviation and right ventricular hypertrophy with absence of left ventricular forces.	Therapy is symptomatic. Most patients die in first few weeks of life. Surgical procedures have been attempted to decompress left atrium by septectomy, creation of a systemic-pulmonary shunt, and banding of both pulmonary arteries. Heart transplant is becoming an increasingly viable option. The mortality associated with these procedures is high, and long-term prognosis is not known.

From Servonsky/Opas: *Nursing Management of Children*, © 1987 Boston: Jones and Bartlett Publishers.

possible infection. Infection of the cord stump is extremely dangerous, since the invading bacteria can rapidly travel up the open arteries into the peritoneum, which may result in fatal sepsis. Umbilical hernias are a common finding, especially in black infants. These hernias vary in size from a few millimeters to 3 cms; however, any hernia that grows in size after one month should be referred and further evaluated.

The nurse should auscultate the abdomen with a stethoscope before palpating and percussing to prevent distorting the bowel sounds. During auscultation the presence of bowel sounds should be verified. The nurse should also listen for vascular sounds in the abdomen. Venous hums may be found in cases of congenital abnormalities of the umbilical vein, vascular problems in the portal system, or hemangiomas of the liver.

Palpation of the newborn's abdomen begins by assessing the skin for turgor. All four quadrants of the abdomen should be palpated lightly, then more deeply, progressing to deep palpation for the purpose of specific organ identification. The liver edge is normally palpable 1–2 cm below the right costal margin; the border of the spleen is usually felt 1–2 cm below the left costal margin. During deep palpation, the nurse should not feel any areas of weakness or muscle herniation; also, no tenderness should be apparent. The kidneys are able to be felt using deep palpation techniques. The lower pole of the right kidney can usually be felt. Since the left kidney is obliterated by the intestine and is also normally positioned higher in the abdomen, it is not as commonly palpable. Kidney size should be noted. The umbilical ring should be palpated. Generally, rings greater than 2 cm in diameter will not close spontaneously. Diastasis recti abdominis is palpated as a wide separation between the two rectus muscles and is a common finding in the Black population.

Finally, the abdomen should be percussed to determine tympany and to confirm the presence and location of the liver, spleen, and the superior margin of the bladder.

Assessment of the Genitals and Rectum

The newborn's genitals typically appear large in relationship to the rest of the body. Some edema of the genitals may be present in breech birth infants. Genital development is a criterion used to determine gestational age (see Figure 20-2).

Male Genitals

The size of the genitals in newborn male infants varies. Commonly, the penis is between 2 and 3 cm and the testes are between 1 and 2 cm. The foreskin should be retracted to visualize the urinary meatus and its placement on the glans. If the prepuce adheres to the glans, the end of the prepuce should be peeled back to ascertain the position of the urinary meatus. The meatus should appear as a slit centrally located on the glans. In epispadias, the urinary meatus is located on the dorsal side of the penis, and in hypospadias, the opening is found ventrally at the junction of the glans and the penile shaft (see Figure 20-28). Both conditions should be referred since surgical intervention is usually necessary. Phimosis, or a pinpoint opening of the urinary meatus, should also be referred. There should be no discharge from the urinary meatus.

Normally the scrotum is slightly asymmetrical, with the left side appearing slightly larger than the right. The nurse should note the development of rugae on the scrotal sack and palpate both testes to confirm that they are descended. It is helpful to palpate using one hand to block the inguinal canal, which prevents the testes from slipping upward as the other hand palpates. Cryptorchidism is a term used to describe undescended testicles. This condition should be referred immediately. Hydrocele, whether unilateral or bilateral, usually disappears spontaneously and is insignificant.

Female Genitals

The nurse should inspect the female genitals for the presence of the gross structures. The labia majora and labia minora are often enlarged. In fact, the labia minora may be so prominent that they protrude over the labia majora. Many times the urethral and vaginal openings are obliterated

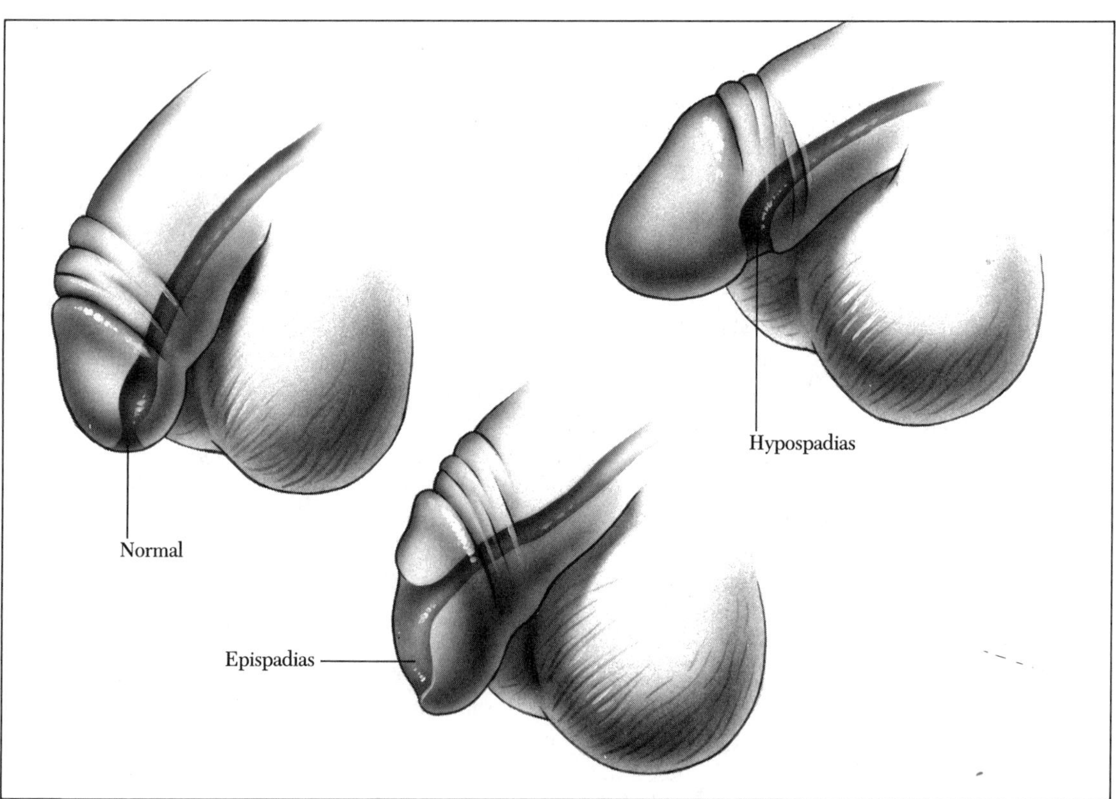

Figure 20-28 Three types of meatal openings: normal, hypospadias, and epispadias.

by edema of the labia. Smegma and vaginal secretions are routinely present and are often blood tinged in response to the withdrawal of maternal hormone. A mucoid vaginal discharge is often commonly present for about 7–10 days.

Anus

The nurse's finger-cotted little finger may be inserted into the anus to verify patency. Patency can also be determined by the presence of meconium or stool on a rectal thermometer. There should be no evidence of anal fissures, bleeding, or imperforate anus.

Assessment of the Extremities

The nurse should inspect the infant, confirming that no gross abnormalities exist and verifying that all body parts are present, intact, and symmetrically aligned. The infant generally assumes a flexed resting position, and the nurse can conduct full passive range of motion to determine the mobility of the extremities. Any paralysis or limitation of range of motion of an upper extremity may be due to a fractured clavicle, brachial or cervical plexus injury, or fracture of one of the long bones of the arm. Polydactyly is the presence of a supernumerary digit on the hand or foot. This is a common finding and the digit is usually rudimentary. Syndactyly is an absence of a digit on the hand or foot.

Spine

The spinal curve is convex in the newborn, and as head control is gained a cervical curve gradually develops.

Upper Extremities

The nurse may test muscle tone by unflexing the newborn's arm for about five seconds. When the arm is released, it should return to the flexed position immediately. This finding would suggest normal muscle tone. The length of the arms can be evaluated by holding the infant's arm down parallel with the thigh. If the arms appear to be unusually short, the existence of achondroplastic dwarfism may be indicated.

The hands should be inspected. Infants who have webbing between the fingers, an unusual curve and shortness of the little finger, and a simian crease may be suspected as having Down's syndrome. The range of motion of the wrist should be assessed. The radial pulses should be palpated and compared. The entire extremity should be palpated to rule out any fractures of the bones. The scarf sign may also be conducted as a test for gestational age (see Figure 20-2). Shoulder muscle strength is assessed by lifting the infant under the arms. The infant should be able to maintain this position and not slip through the nurse's hands.

Lower Extremities

On inspection of the lower extremities, a mild degree of bowing or medial rotation is common. After a frank breech presentation, the lower extremities tend to be abducted and externally rotated; therefore, only gross abnormalities of the lower extremities are able to be confirmed immediately after birth.

The hip joint should be evaluated to determine whether it is intact. The nurse should inspect the anterior and posterior thighs for symmetry of medial skinfolds. The gluteal folds should also be even and bilaterally symmetrical. The nurse should perform the Ortolani maneuver by placing the index and middle fingers under the hip joints and laterally abducting and flexing the hips (see Figure 20-29). Normal range of motion is approximately 160–170 degrees in flexion and extension. When flexed at the hip, the thighs should abduct to an angle of 160 degrees between the thighs. There should be no click or feeling of the hip joint slipping due to the head of the femur striking the acetabulum ridge. If such a click is noted, it should be referred and reported immediately and the Ortolani maneuver should not be repeated, since subsequent motion will serve to further weaken and damage the hip joint.

The knee joint should be flexed and extended to verify range of motion. The legs should be aligned and inspected for an increased degree of bowing, which is referred to as tibial torsion.

Foot position should be evaluated. The intrauterine position of the infant may have caused the feet to turn in (varus). If the foot can be turned passively in the opposite direction without forceful manual stretching, this finding is usually transient and insignificant. Putting the ankle through range of motion determines the flexibility of the heel cords. Normally 120 degrees of motion between flexion and extension is

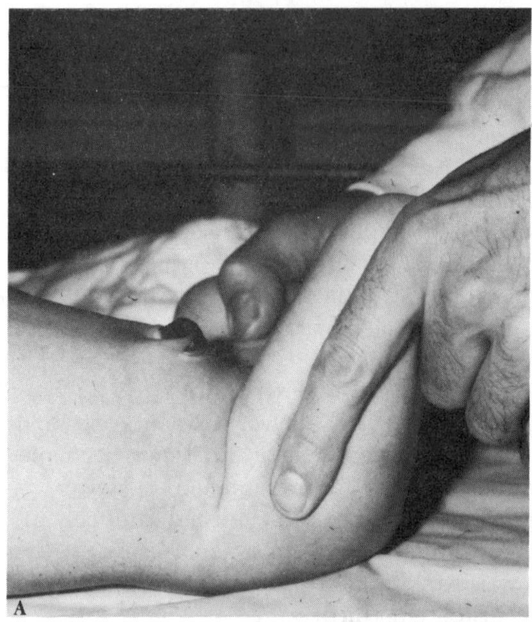

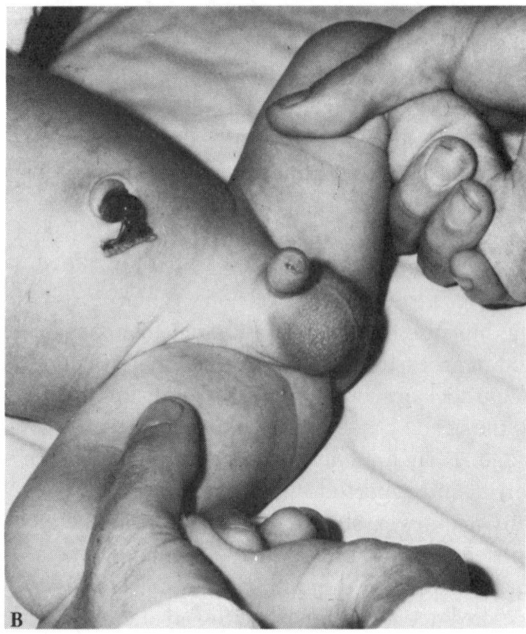

Figure 20-29 Method of inducing Ortolani's sign. (A) With the infant's knees bent, hips flexed to 90 degrees, the examiner's fingers are placed over the femoral head, exerting pressure downward. (B) The thighs are then fully abducted to induce the characteristic "click."

apparent. Any evidence of clubfoot (talipes equinovarus) should be referred promptly. Clubfoot is a relatively common deformity, which usually involves plantar flexion, inversion, and adduction. Ankle clonus may be tested by sharply dorsiflexing the foot. One or two clonic beats are normal; however, any evidence of clonic movement should be referred.

Assessment of the Neurologic System

Neurologic assessment of the newborn aims to determine the general integrity of the central nervous system. The central nervous system develops more rapidly than any other body system during the first year (see Figure 20-30). Many of the reflexive behaviors tested will be present only during the first weeks of life. Persistence beyond the normal time may be a signal of central nervous system disease and should be referred, although many reflexes are variable and their significance is uncertain. The nurse should observe the infant's reflex pattern and development, motor skill development, and socialization development. Table 20-7 lists normal newborn reflexive patterns along with typical ages of onset and disappearance.

Mental Assessment

The newborn should appear quiet and content. A fretful or tense appearance would not be typical.

Speech

The infant's basic verbal communication with the environment is the cry. The cry may normally be loud and even sound rather angry; however, a high-pitched, shrill cry should be noted and referred.

Cranial Nerves

Some cranial nerves can be tested indirectly by observation of the newborn's functioning. Cranial nerves III, IV, and VI can be assessed by observing the infant's ability to visually follow an object a short distance. Any total nonrecognition or absence of the blink reflex should be referred.

Cranial nerve V function can be demonstrated by observing the rooting reflex. This reflex is elicited by stroking the infant's upper or lower lips or the side of the cheek. The normal response is that the infant will turn his face toward the stimulus and open his mouth. This reflex is present at 32 gestational weeks and is fully developed by 34 weeks of gestation. The rooting reflex tends to disappear by 3 to 4 months when the baby is awake, and by 7 to 8 months when the infant is asleep. It is important to note that

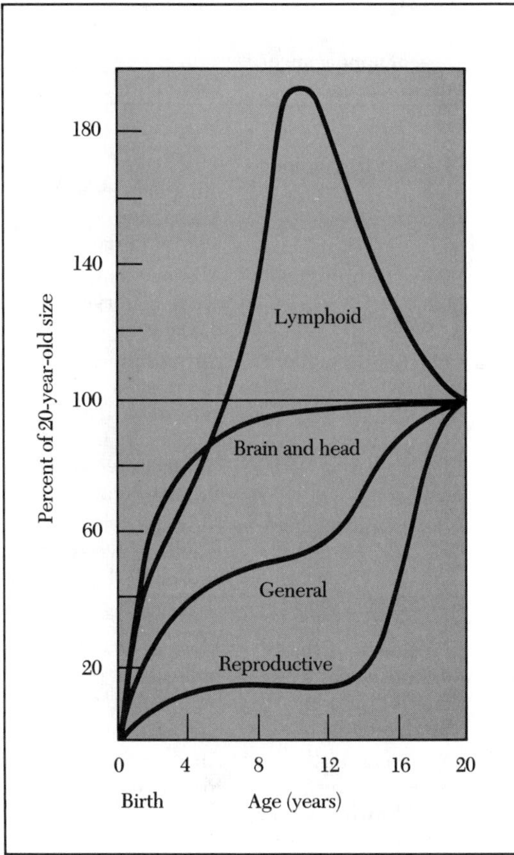

Figure 20-30 Growth patterns of various systems.

this reflex may be depressed, especially after feeding. The rooting reflex also is somewhat less vigorous during the first two days of life.

The sucking reflex also indicates the integrity of cranial nerve V function. This reflex is vital to life, although it tends to be less intense during the first 3 to 4 days. The nurse can elicit the sucking reflex by stroking the lips, which should produce a sucking motion. Complete evaluation of the suck can be made by placing the index finger in the infant's mouth and noting the action of the tongue, which should push the nurse's finger up and back. The rate, pressure, strength, and pattern of grouping of the suck should also be noted. The sucking reflex is normally strong at 32 weeks and is completely developed at 34 weeks of gestation. It tends to diminish by 3 to 4 months and gradually disappears by 12 months. It also is difficult to elicit in a recently fed baby. Absence of the sucking reflex is a strong indicator of possible brain damage.

Cranial nerve VIII function can be demonstrated by eliciting the startle or Moro reflex using an auditory stimulus. The nurse may use a bell or hand clap. A complete Moro reflex would include extension of the trunk and extension and abduction of the limbs. Extension of the fingers with a "C" formed by the thumb and index finger followed by flexion and adduction of the limbs would also be present to constitute a complete reflex response (see Figure 20-31). The Moro or startle reflex may also be elicited by any loss of equilibrium of the infant as with sudden movement. However, when the establishment of disequilibrium is used as a stimulus, cranial nerve VIII function is not tested. The Moro reflex is typically present at 32 gestational weeks and tends to diminish and disappear at between 1 and 4 months. A consistent absence before this time is a sign of possible brain damage. Unilateral absence of the startle reflex may be due to brain damage, a fractured clavicle, or injury to the brachial plexus.

Cranial nerves IX and X can be tested by placing an object on the back of the tongue to assess the infant's swallowing reflex. This reflex is present at 34–36 gestational weeks and persists throughout life. The gag reflex is another indicator of cranial nerve IX and X function.

Cerebellar Function

Cerebellar function including proprioception can be tested by observing the infant's spontaneous activity and noting symmetrical, smooth movements. The infant should also swallow easily. Sensory function is not normally tested in the

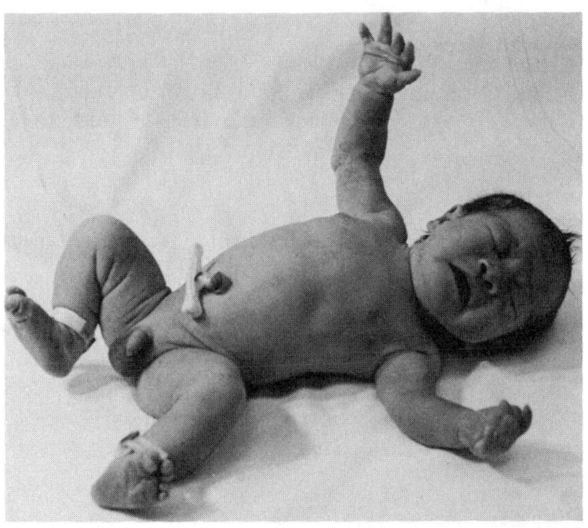

Figure 20-31 An infant demonstrating a Moro reflex.

Table 20-7. Newborn Reflexes

Reflex	Stimulus	Normal response	Age of appearance/ disappearance	Comments
Eyes				
Optical blink reflex	Shine penlight into infant's eyes	Bilateral eyelid closure	Persists throughout life	Absence or unilateral blink may indicate cranial nerve III, IV, and/or VI damage.
Acoustic blink reflex	Clap hands next to infant's ear	Bilateral eyelid closure	Persists throughout life	Absence may indicate acoustic nerve damage.
Pupillary reflex	Shine penlight into infant's eyes	Pupillary constriction	Persists throughout life	Any asymmetrical response or evidence of fixed or dilated pupils may indicate cranial nerve II, III, IV, or VI damage.
Glabella reflex	Tap index finger on bridge of infant's nose	Symmetrical eyelid closure	Persists throughout life	Absence may indicate cranial nerve III, IV, and/or VI damage.
Mouth and throat				
Sucking reflex	Stroke infant's lips; place clean finger in infant's mouth	Strong sucking movement; tongue pushes finger up and back	Present at birth; diminishes by 3–4 months; disappears by 12 months	Absence is a strong indicator of possible brain damage.
Rooting reflex	Stroke infant's upper or lower lip or lateral aspect of lips	Face turns toward the stimulus and mouth opens	Present at birth; disappears by 3–4 months when awake; disappears by 7–8 months when asleep	Absence may be due to cranial nerve V damage.
Extrusion reflex	Touch infant's tongue	Tongue thrusts outward	Present at birth; disappears at 2–4 months	A continuous tongue protrusion may indicate Down's syndrome or macroglossia.
Gag reflex	Stimulate posterior pharynx with tongue blade	Gag	Persists throughout life	Absence may indicate cranial nerve IX or X damage.
Swallowing reflex	Place an object on posterior tongue	Swallow	Persists throughout life	Absence may indicate cranial nerve IX or X damage.
Extremities				
Palmar grasp reflex	Place index finger in infant's palm from ulnar side.	Infant grasps finger and forcefully holds	Present from birth until about 3–4 months; replaced by voluntary grasping	Any asymmetry of response may indicate a neurological problem.
Plantar grasp reflex	Touch sole of infant's foot	Plantar flexion of toes	Present from birth until 8–10 months	Absence may indicate defect of lower spinal column.
Babinski reflex	Stroke lateral surface of infant's sole beginning at heel and moving in a curve to great toe	Fanning of toes; dorsiflexion of great toe	Present from birth until about 18 months	Absent response may indicate lower spinal cord defect; unilateral absence may be due to peripheral nerve damage on affected side.

Table 20-7. *Continued*

Reflex	Stimulus	Normal response	Age of appearance/ disappearance	Comments
Moro reflex (startle response)	May be elicited by jarring the infant's bed, using an auditory stimulus (loud hand clap, bell) or suddenly dropping infant's head (loss of equilibrium)	Extension of trunk and extension and abduction of limbs; also, extension of fingers followed by flexion and adduction of the limbs	Present from birth until about 1–4 months	Asymmetry of response may indicate fracture of clavicle or injury to brachial plexus. Consistent absence before 1–4 months may be due to brain damage.
Parachute	Lower infant in prone position quickly downward	Infant will extend arms, hands, and fingers out as if trying to break the fall	Begins 7–9 months; persists	Absence is significant of CNS defect.
Tonic neck reflex	Rotate infant's head to one side in prone or supine position	Arm and leg on same side as head is turned will extend; opposite arm and leg will flex; classic "fencer" position	Appears at birth to 2 months and disappears at 4–6 months	Asymmetry may indicate cerebral lesion. Many normal infants never exhibit this response.
Trunk incurvation reflex (Galant's reflex)	Stroke dorsal skin along vertebral column from shoulders to buttocks using a sharp object (infant should be lying in a symmetrical, prone position)	Trunk curves toward side stimulated	Easily elicited at 3–6 days of age; disappears at 2 months	Absence may indicate spinal cord damage (T2 to S1).
Placing reflex	Hold infant upright with dorsum of one foot gently touching underside of a surface (table, shelf)	Knees and hips flex; stimulated foot should rise and be placed on surface	Present from birth until about 6 weeks	May be difficult to elicit during first 4 days.
Step-in-place/ stepping reflex	Hold infant upright with feet flat on table.	Infant will demonstrate alternating stepping movements	Easily elicited at 3–4 days; diminishes at 2–3 months; disappears at 7–8 months	Asymmetry may indicate neurological abnormality. Some breech infants will not exhibit this reflex.
Landau	Hold infant in prone position and flex head downward	Legs will flex	Elicited at 3–12 months; disappears at 2 years	Absence is significant of CNS defect.

newborn. Muscular tone and function can be assessed by inspecting the infant's resting position and using the pull-to-sit maneuver. Muscle tone should also be evaluated by holding the infant in a ventral position supporting the chest. A full-term infant should hold the head at a 45-degree angle or less, exhibit a straight or slightly flexed back, flex the arms at the elbows, and partially extend at the shoulders and moderately flex the legs. Range of motion will also provide information as to motor function and muscle tone.

Other Reflexes

Deep tendon reflex testing is not usually done in the infant. Rather, a series of infant reflexes should be evaluated by the nurse. These include the optical and acoustic blink reflexes, which both result normally in eyelid closure but use different stimuli. In the optical blink reflex a light source is used, whereas the acoustic blink reflex is elicited by using a loud clap or other sound stimulus. These reflexes might be difficult to elicit during the first days of life; however, if the infant is unable to demonstrate them after 2–3 days, the absence may indicate visual or auditory problems.

The glabella reflex is elicited by tapping on the bridge of the infant's nose. The normal response would be a symmetrical closing of the eyes.

The tonic neck reflex is an important reflex for the nurse to assess. The typical posture associated with this reflex consists of turning the face to one side with the jaw over one shoulder. The arm and leg on the jaw side will extend and the opposite arm and leg flex, placing the infant in the classic "fencer" position (see Figure 20-32). The tonic neck or fencing reflex can be elicited by turning the infant's head. It usually appears from birth to 6 weeks and disappears at 4 to 6 months. Some normal infants never exhibit this response.

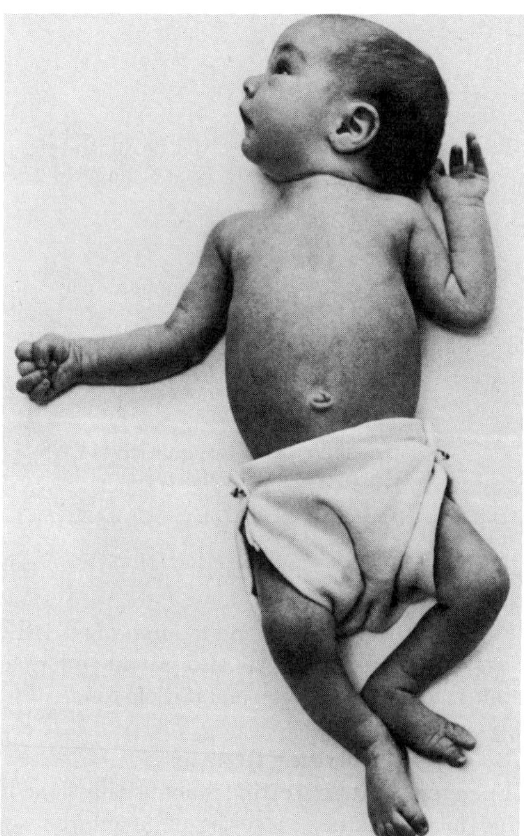

Figure 20-32 An infant displaying the tonic neck reflex.

The palmar grasp reflex is tested by placing the nurse's finger in the palm of the infant's hand from the ulnar side. Typically, the infant will grasp the finger with his hand, and the grasp should be of sufficient strength so that the nurse can lift the infant into a sitting position (see Figure 20-33). This reflex is present from birth until about 3–4 months of age and is then replaced by voluntary grasping.

The plantar grasp is elicited by touching an object to the sole of the infant's foot, resulting in flexion of the toes downward (see Figure 20-34). This reflex is normally present from birth to about 8–10 months.

The Babinski reflex is stimulated by stroking the lateral surface of the infant's sole beginning at the heel and moving in a curve to the great toe. The normal infant response of fanning of the toes and dorsiflexion of the great toe is present from birth to 18 months (see Figure 20-35). This is described as a positive response.

Galant's reflex or the trunk incurvation reflex is demonstrated by lightly scratching a pin or other sharp object from the shoulders to the buttocks parallel to the spinal cord and about 3 cm from midline. The trunk should curve toward the side stimulated. This reflex is easily elicited at about 5–6 days of age.

The placing reflex is elicited by holding the infant upright with the dorsum of one foot gently touching the table edge. The infant's knees and hips should flex and the stimulated foot should

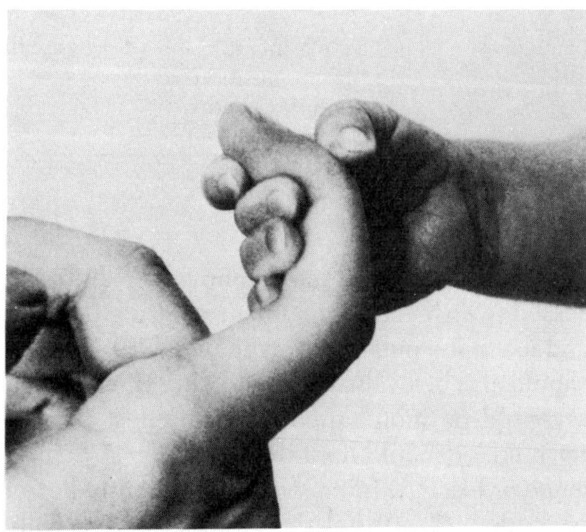

Figure 20-33 Palmar grasp reflex.

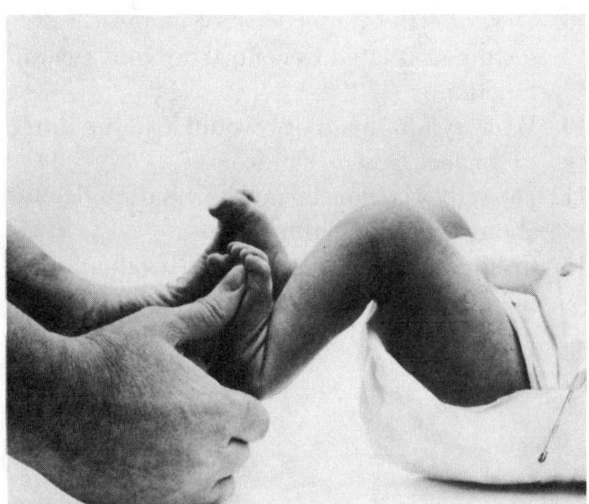

Figure 20-34 Plantar grasp reflex.

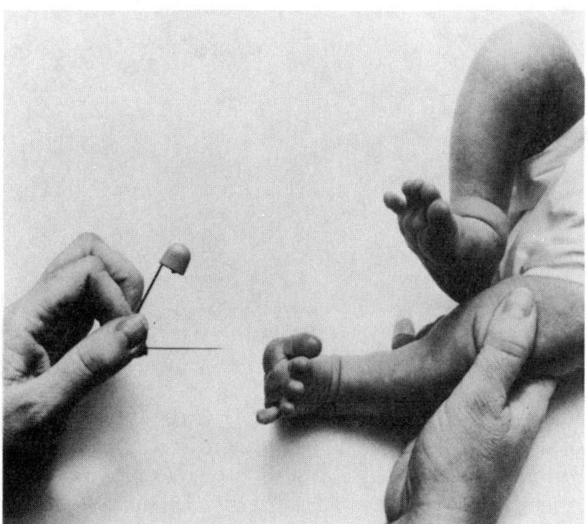

Figure 20-35 The Babinski reflex.

rise and be placed on the table. This reflex may be difficult to elicit during the first four days. The step-in-place or stepping reflex is similar, but the baby is placed with feet flat on the table (see Figure 20-36). Normally, the infant will respond by demonstrating alternating stepping movements. This reflex is more difficult to elicit in the first 2–3 days and tends to fade at about 2–3 months. Some breech infants will not exhibit the stepping reflex.

Summary

This chapter discussed the health assessment of the newborn infant, including the history. A complete newborn assessment comprises all aspects of physical assessment and provides the nurse with important baseline data about the infant's status. Many typical variations and conditions of the newborn were presented. The newborn assessment is a prime opportunity for the nurse to initiate rapport with the parents as well as to reassure and counsel the parents regarding any obvious deviations. The general techniques of physical assessment must be modified in many areas to apply to the newborn.

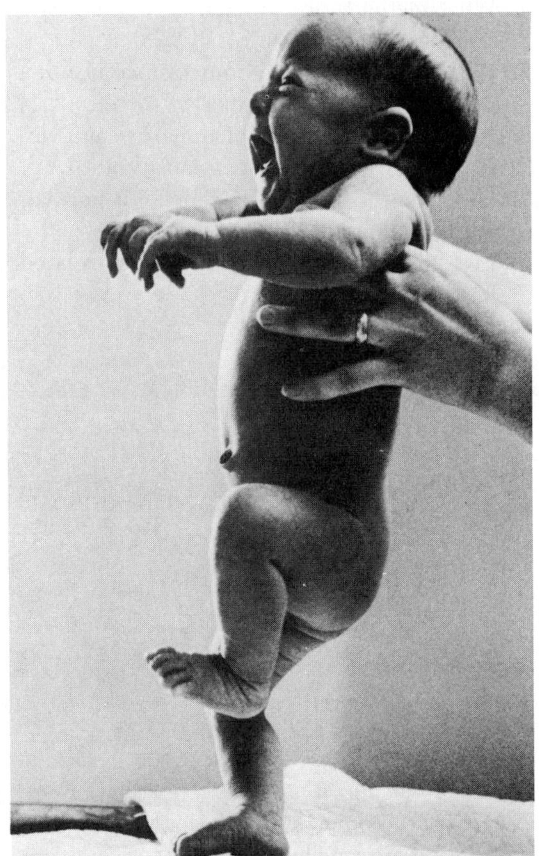

Figure 20-36 The step-in-place, or stepping, reflex.

Discussion Questions/Activities

1. Discuss the value of the newborn assessment in establishing rapport with the family.
2. Give the rationale behind having a flexible sequence of examination when doing a newborn assessment.
3. Collect a complete history on a newborn. What specific questions need to be answered?

4. What methods are utilized to assess gestational age?
5. What is the role of the nurse in counseling parents regarding birthmarks?
6. Name three types of birthmarks, and describe their characteristics and resolution.
7. Describe the resting position of a normal, full-term infant.
8. List three common birth-trauma–related head-shape deviations.
9. Describe the importance of infantile refle testing as related to central nervous syster function.
10. What symptomatology would lead the nurs to suspect Down's syndrome?
11. Describe the normal newborn's umbilicus at about four hours after birth.
12. Conduct an examination and evaluation of the health status of a newborn.

EXAMPLE OF A NEWBORN HISTORY AND PHYSICAL EXAMINATION

HEALTH HISTORY

Name: Megan M.
Address: 16 Clark Road, Amherst, New York
Sex: Female
Age: 2 days
Birthdate: 1/10/86
Race: Caucasian
Ethnic origin: Irish
Informant: Mother; reliable historian
History of present illness: Normal newborn assessment

Past History

Prenatal—Megan is the first child of Mr. and Mrs. M. Mother was in good general health throughout the pregnancy. Prenatal care was provided beginning in the first month through the ninth month by a private physician. Prenatal vitamin and iron supplement was taken as prescribed by the physician. No illnesses, infections, accidents, x-rays, or medications reported. Mother's blood type O+; father's blood type O+. A sonogram was done at 16 weeks to determine the EDC more exactly. Mother consumed a balanced diet; weight gain of 30 pounds. No alcohol, cigarette, or drug use. No previous abortions or miscarriages. Both parents were excited about this planned pregnancy.

Natal—Spontaneous rupture of amniotic membranes followed by a labor of 6½ hours. No anesthesia or medication. Father was present and coached throughout. Baby born at Sister's Hospital, Buffalo, New York. Gestational age 40 weeks. Vertex delivery. Length: 21"; weight: 7 lb 5 oz. Infant cried spontaneously. Apgar 8 and 10. No jaundice, cyanosis, or respiratory problems.

Postnatal—Infant placed in regular nursery. Breast-feeding successfully. Both parents very happy about and comfortable with baby.

Family History

Family members: Mother—29 years, good health; father—29 years, with seasonal allergies.

Family diseases—Denies history of diabetes, arthritis, TB, alcoholism, bleeding disorders, mental illness, stomach problems, liver disorders, hypertension, heart disease, kidney disease, birth defects, and infant deaths.

Family history significant for cancer and allergies. Geographic exposure: not significant.

Review of Systems

Eyes, ears, nose, throat: No discharge, swelling, swallowing difficulties.
Cardiorespiratory: No labored breathing, cyanosis.
Gastrointestinal: No vomiting, diarrhea, constipation.
Genitourinary: No irritation, rashes, discharge.
Neurological: No convulsions.
Musculoskeletal: No dislocations, congenital malformations.

Physical Assessment

General impression: Megan M. is a 2-day-old female, well developed, well nourished, and in no acute distress. No gross abnormalities.
Length—21″
Weight—7 lb 2 oz.
TPR—98.4F/136/38.

Integument: Color pink to reddish, somewhat mottled. No excoriations, fissures or lesions. No birthmarks evident. Numerous white papules over chin, nose, and forehead. Pale pink area over medial aspect of left eyelid that blanches with pressure. Finger and toe nails intact, pink in color. Fine, downy hair over the shoulders and back. Scalp hair fine, soft, and dark. Normal skin turgor.

Head, face and neck: Normocephalic, head circumference 35 cm. No molding apparent. Anterior fontanelle 2 cm × 2 cm. Unable to palpate posterior fontanelle. No bulging of fontanelles noted. Normal facial symmetry with full range of motion. Eyes, ears, and nose, symmetrically placed. Neck is symmetrical; no webbing. Full range of motion present. No apparent neck pulsations. Trachea at midline, thyroid not palpable.

Eyes: Normal alignment and position of eyes and eyebrows. Noted edema of eyelids. Palpebral fissures normal, no slanting noted. Sclerae white; corneas clear, shiny smooth, transparent. Lacrimal apparatus patent bilaterally. Corneal reflex intact. PERRL. Iris color slate gray. Blink response present. Hirschberg's test normal. No nystagmus. Bilateral red reflex present.

Ears: Symmetrically placed. Normal placement in relation to eyes. External ear canals pink. Startle reflex intact in response to sound stimulus.

Nose: Smooth, centrally placed. Nares patent bilaterally. No nasal flaring.

Mouth and throat: Lips are deep pink, symmetrically positioned. Inner lips and buccal mucosa pink. Tongue pink and centrally located within the mouth. Hard and soft palates intact on palpation. Palatal arch normal. Sucking, rooting, gag, and extrusion reflexes intact.

Chest: Skin color pink. AP diameter = lateral diameter. Chest circumference 33 cm. No bulging or depression. Sternum straight, smooth. Clavicles smooth and straight, no fracture or dislocation. Nipples positioned symmetrically. No retractions. Vesicular breath sounds auscultated throughout. PMI palpated, normal heart sounds auscultated.

Abdomen: Cylindrical contour, no visible peristaltic waves. Umbilicus centrally located. Cord stump dry. No odor, discharge, or redness at stump site. Normal bowel sounds present. Liver edge palpable. Spleen not palpable. Lower pole of right kidney felt on deep palpation. General abdominal tympany.

Genitals and rectum: Labia majora and labia minora present, slightly enlarged. Urinary meatus patent. Vaginal meatus present.

Anus: Patent. No anal fissures or bleeding.

Extremities: Infant resting in a flexed position. All extremities present, intact, in appropriate alignment. No polydactyly or syndactyly. Complete range of motion of all extremities. Convex spinal configuration. Normal muscle tone in upper extremities. Lower extremities slightly bowed. Hip joints intact bilaterally. Foot position slightly inverted; able to passively straighten without force. No ankle clonus present.

Neurologic:
Speech—Cry loud and strong. No high-pitched or shrill sound.
Cranial Nerves—III, IV, V, VIII, IX, and X intact. Rooting, sucking, startle, swallowing, and gag reflexes intact.
Cerebellar function—Movement is generally symmetrical and smooth. Normal muscle tone.
Other reflexive behaviors—Optical and acoustic blink, glabella, tonic neck, palmar and plantar grasp, Babinski, and placing reflexes present.

CHAPTER 21

Assessment of the Child and Adolescent

LEARNING OBJECTIVES

1. Identify the developmental milestones of the child and adolescent.
2. Recognize that cultural assessment is a pertinent part of health assessment in the child and adolescent.
3. State principles of communication specific to the child and adolescent during the interview process.
4. Discuss the specific areas of the health history of the child and adolescent that differ from those of the adult.
5. Differentiate the body measurements recorded in the general appearance section for that of a young child from those of an adult.
6. Recognize the need to differ the approach and the sequence of the physical assessment process for various aged children and for the adolescent.
7. Identify physical assessment techniques and norms specific to various aged children and the adolescent.

When assessing the health status of the child and adolescent, the nurse applies many of the same basic principles of interpersonal relationships and communication, and uses many of the same cultural, mental, and physical assessment techniques, used in collecting data from and about the adult client. With children and adolescents, however, the analysis of the findings is acutely attuned to the parameters of growth and development, which change rapidly during the early years of life. Knowledge of growth and development milestones is the basis of health assessment of the child at various ages. It provides criteria by which to detect normal range and progression of physical growth and development in skill and capacity of functioning and by which to recognize abnormalities. Those growth and development changes occurring during adolescence are particularly challenging to the adolescent, parents, relatives, teachers, and neighbors alike. The child and adolescent both need and deserve special attention. They should not be talked down to, around, or about; when being interviewed and examined, they are the primary focus. This principle does not ignore the fact that contact with the parents does lend data for evaluation of the child's or youth's health status. (We use the word *parent* in this chapter to indicate the responsible adult. Keep in mind, however, that there are many family patterns, at least one of which does not have parents in the home.) Attention must be given evenly to what the client says in relation to what is said by the parents. However, contact with the parents provides the opportunity for important health teaching, facilitating the client's compliance with a nursing or medical regimen. In the interchange the nurse can also learn the parents' attitudes and practices of child-rearing.

Cultural Assessment

Children are strongly influenced by cultural patterns. The parents have each brought with them certain beliefs and practices into the marriage and family pattern. Moreover, the merging of these beliefs and practices produces a redefined perspective of the culture(s). According to social and ethnic customs, the mother, father, and child generally assume their assigned positions and roles within the family. Furthermore, the character of interactions among family members and the child-rearing practices, including punishment for wrongdoing, stems from these roots. Likewise religious beliefs and practices are cultural ingredients that influence and mold those of the child as well as becoming a factor in personality development.

The health care that the child receives is usually dependent on many cultural factors. An ethnic medicine man may be sought out, or religious beliefs may dictate a "laying on of hands," faith healing, or the denial of blood transfusions or surgical procedures. At such times traditional medicine is caught up in ethical dilemmas. Often it has been fruitful to combine such cultural approaches, in mutual respect, with traditional medicine. In many family patterns the day-to-day care of the child is conducted by someone other than the parents; this other person could be a "nanny," siblings, grandparents, or teachers in a day-care center. Whoever this person may be, he or she provides the locus of a social and cultural heritage. The child's health care is also dependent on the parent's knowledge level and decision-making skills. The parent may not know when and where to go to obtain needed health care and how to create and maintain a healthy physical and healthy mental environment. The parent may have only a limited knowledge of sanitation principles, nutritional needs, and adequate food, shelter, and clothing necessary to ward off disease. These material things may also be lacking due to inadequate income. You should not assume that the lack of these things implies a lack of love. Love may be very real and recognized and felt by both child and parents.

Interviewing the Child and Adolescent

With very small children you must obtain the historical information from the parents. The principles of communication and interviewing discussed in Chapter 3 would apply here. However, in this situation, periodic interaction with the child is very important; this interaction could take the form of play, calling the child's attention to something pleasant, or just a friendly word or so to acknowledge the child's presence. With children who are older, you involve them as much as possible and to the extent that they are capable in contributing directly to the interview. Much patience and tact are necessary with an overprotective or dominating parent. You may need to keep eye contact with the child and address the child by name as you interview.

A loud voice or sudden, loud, strange sounds may frighten the child. If you speak softly, you will find that you are better able to hold the child's attention. A pleasant environment and privacy are just as important for the child and adolescent client as for the adult client. You need to remember that the young child thinks concretely rather than abstractly. Thus, your communication content must be simple, clear, and concrete. As well, your directives to the child should be very specific and in as few words as possible. Accompanying hand movements and gestures (nonverbal communication patterns) should be used. A friendly reassuring voice is the key. However, when you give the child directions, your voice must reflect confidence and gentle firmness. You would not ask the child, "Will you please roll over onto your belly?" This style is inviting to a "no" and noncompliance. Instead, say "Please roll over onto your belly." Make the content of your statements positive and a gentle command. Avoid using the word *don't.* For instance, instead of "Don't write on the walls with that crayon!" reach out for the crayon and say, "Please, I need walls without crayon marks."

When interviewing children, you must assume an active, verbal role. Children are turned off by the nondirective head-nodding nurse; they respond better to concrete examples rather than abstract concepts. In assessing the child you must have a working knowledge of developmental theory. Children's problems, more than those of individuals in any other age group, have more significance when viewed within a developmental framework. Such techniques as storytelling and doll play can be helpful in getting children to express their feelings and adjust to impending losses. The parents should not be forgotten, as they can be an asset to your assessment; they should therefore have sufficient understanding of the situation and should be incorporated in the planning and implementation of care.

Another point to take into consideration with the young child is his short attention span. This demands frequent change in activities during the interview. You should assess as much as possible the mental and physical functioning of the child while you are gathering the history. Take note of the child's general development, physical abilities, gait, posture, and behaviors that reflect his level of mental functioning and personality characteristics as he moves about the room. At the same time you can observe the child-parent interactions as well as obtain information about the parents' outlook and child-rearing practices. Attempt to involve the child in the process to the greatest degree possible, appropriate to his age and intellect. Generally the adolescent is able to assume a greater role in the interview process, having reached by midadolescence (14–15 years old) the period of reasoning and abstract thinking that Piaget termed the period of "formal operations."

The adolescent is more complex and does not readily reveal inner feelings. More frequent contacts and observation periods are often necessary to gather sufficient sampling of behavior for analysis. You will do well to interact "straight from the shoulder" and to avoid a condescending attitude when working with the adolescent. Adolescents rarely, if ever, appreciate an older nurse's obvious attempts at teenage slang. They readily recognize such a phony facade, which only hampers the establishment of mutual respect.

Particularly with the adolescent, you must determine whether the parents' presence facilitates or inhibits the assessment process. Facilitation occurs when the parents are supportive and accepting of the child. Inhibition occurs when the parents dominate the interview and do not allow the child to participate. Furthermore, sensitive topics such as sexual activity and drugs are often more freely discussed in the parents' absence.

The adolescent appreciates honesty from interactions with adults. Also, as you work with the adolescent, the assurance of confidentiality is of utmost importance. However, the adolescent, like the adult, must *fully* understand prior to self-disclosure that you have both legal and ethical obligations to share with the appropriate person(s) any information that is seemingly of potential harm to self or a danger to another. This developmental stage, dependence versus independence (refer to Appendix B), is one of turmoil for both youth and parents. The generation gap seems to become widened as the youth struggles to establish a sense of identity. The adolescent may adopt a new slang-type language, teenage music and idols, or a particular type of clothing or hairstyle as the ticket into his or her peer group.

The young nurse may find it difficult working with the adolescent client who is so near in age, since the nurse himself or herself may well be striving for autonomy, too. In such situations guidance and support should be sought from an older professional. The establishment of an identity permits the tasks of late adolescence (engaging in love relationships, defining career goals, and finding one's own lifestyle) to be pursued. If you are an older nurse, clarification becomes a much needed communication technique when interacting with the adolescent and his slang language with which you may be unfamiliar. Clarification of what the adolescent is saying is a form of expressing your interest and concern. A nonjudgmental approach and good listening skills are necessary for both the young and older nurse when interacting with the adolescent.

Parents, for most part, react out of love and their own needs, experience, and background.

Some are overly protective and others quite permissive. As in all situations, the midway of these two extremes is most likely the ideal. In reality the adolescent needs love, support, assistance, and limitations in the not-so-easy transition from childhood to adulthood. Most adolescents have their physiological and safety needs generally met; they are developing the means to meet the needs stated in Maslow's next hierarchical level—those for loving and belonging. The conflicts between youth and parent usually derive from a superficial day-to-day disagreement regarding curfew and car keys, not regarding basic moral and cultural values.

If youth and parents are basically in agreement, then working with both poses no problem. The difficulty arises when major disagreements between youth and parents exist. However, in this case, you must also work tactfully with each person because of the legality of the parents' responsibility for the care and behavior of their children.

For the purpose of interview and data collection regarding the youth's health status, it may be more to your advantage to talk with the parent(s) and the youth separately before bringing them together for a family group session. The purpose of this approach is to permit the youth the freedom from being controlled by the parent(s). Adolescents tend not to say anything or tend to say what they think people want them to say. They also tend to become very defensive, particularly if they feel they are being publicly humiliated or threatened. By interviewing each person separately, the nurse can avoid such conflict situations and may glean information that may not otherwise have been obtained. For example, you could approach the family and, after appropriate introductions, invite the youth to accompany you to an area providing privacy in the following manner: "My practice is to first speak separately with the client and then separately with the parent(s). I then follow these separate interviews with a family session. So Jason, I would like you to come with me, please."

In the separate sessions you explain confidentiality and its limits and evaluate the client's understanding. You assure the parties that what they say will not be disclosed to the other parties without their prior consent. In other words, you tell the adolescent that the information that he shares with you will not be given to his parent(s) without his permission. If the youth does disclose information to you that demands sharing with other health care professionals, it is appropriate to tell the youth what information needs to be shared, why, and with whom. You may need to determine within the guidelines of the state in which you are practicing whether or not the parent(s) need to know this information along with the appropriate medical personnel.

After you have determined the client's understanding of confidentiality, you explain the interview process (see "Interview Structure" in Chapter 4). With the adolescent, it is important to point out that some of the questions will involve personal habits of which his parent(s) may or may not be aware, such as use of alcohol, tobacco, or other drugs and sexual activity. Tell him that it is for this reason that you requested that you and he meet alone; however, give him the option of inviting his parent(s) to be present during the interview. If he desires that the parent(s) be with him, this is the appropriate time to include them. In summing up each session, ask whether any specific information was disclosed that the participant does not wish to have revealed in the family session. This request must be honored. The same privileges and procedure are accorded the parent(s).

The History

The historical data base for the child and adolescent is quite similar to that of the adult in regard to the major categories investigated. The focus of the inquiries is adapted to the specific age group. However, in contrast to the history of an adult, a pertinent part of the infant's and toddler's total health history includes the child's fetal, delivery, and newborn evaluations. Also, data regarding the mother's prenatal and labor-delivery events are significant for assessment of the infant's and toddler's health status (see Chapter 20).

Biographic Information

The biographic information includes the name, age, sex, birthdate, father's name, mother's name, marital status and age of each parent, home address, religion, race, and ethnic origin.

Chief Concern/Complaint

The chief concern for the child's health visit, for most part, in the early years of life is for preventive measures and anticipatory guidance, and for the promotion and maintenance of wellness. However, if a health problem is found to exist, it is recorded using the child's or parent's own words. Then the history of present illness is documented in a chronological fashion using the seven variables of investigation (see "Current Health Status or History of Present Illness" in Chapter 4) and exploring related areas of possible influence or involvement.

Past History

The past history contains the previously mentioned information regarding mother and child during prenatal, labor-delivery, and postnatal periods. It also includes a developmental history of the child's language and motor abilities compared to the achievement landmarks of siblings and the norm ranges for the child's specific age group (see Tables 21-1 and 21-2). The Denver Developmental Screening Test forms and evaluation may be filed at this point (see Figures 21-1 and 21-2).

Personal History and Patterns of Living

The investigation of the personal history and patterns of living yields a large amount of information, as it also does for the adult. In contrast to

Table 21-1. Milestones in Language Development: Infancy Through Preschool Years

Age	Developmental milestone
Birth–1 month	Has full, strong cry; makes throaty sounds
1–3 months	Coos
4–6 months	Babbles; laughs
7–9 months	Repeats self-produced sounds
10–12 months	Imitates sounds, understands about 10 words (e.g., *bye-bye, hot*); uses jargon
13–15 months	Uses jargon; uses at least 3 words other than *mama* and *dada*
15–18 months	Identifies three body parts, such as mouth, eyes, belly; uses jargon and syncretic speech; has vocabulary of 20 words; names familiar objects, such as dog, cat, toy
18 months–2½years	Uses telegraphic speech; uses pronouns such as *I* and *me*; uses adverbs; has vocabulary of 200–300 words; speech becomes more intelligible
3 years	Has vocabulary of 900 words; uses 3- to 4-word sentences; uses more pronouns, adjectives, and adverbs; speech is intelligible
4 years	Has vocabulary of 1,500 words; uses 5- to 6-word sentences; recites poems or sings from memory; speech is intelligible
5 years	Has vocabulary of 2,200 words; uses average of 6 words in a sentence; speech is intelligible

From Servonsky/Opas: *Nursing Management of Children*, © 1987. Boston: Jones and Bartlett Publishers.

Table 21-2. Milestones in Motor Development: Infancy Through Preschool Years

Age	Gross motor skills	Fine motor skills
1 month	When prone, may lift head occasionally, but unsteadily. Will turn head from side to side. Will make crawling movements when prone. Is able to push feet against a bare surface to propel self forward. When head is turned to one side, extends arm on the same side and flexes the opposite arm to the shoulder (tonic neck reflex). "Dancing" or "stepping" reflex when held upright. Symmetrical Moro reflex.	Hands are predominantly in fists. Demonstrates a tight hand grasp. Head and eyes move together. Rooting reflex. Sucking reflex. Shows flaring of toes when sole of the foot is stroked gently (positive Babinski reflex).
2 months	Holds head erect in midposition. Can turn from side to back. When prone, can raise head and chest slightly up and off surface lying on. Tonic neck reflex beginning to fade.	May hold toy placed in hand for brief time. Good palmar grasp. Follows movements of objects or people easily with eyes and head turn. Smiles.

(continued on page 476)

Table 21-2. *Continued*

Age	Gross motor skills	Fine motor skills
3 months	Holds head erect and steady. When prone, holds head at 45- to 90-degree angle, keeping legs outstretched. Stepping and crawling reflexes absent. When supported, sits with rounded back and flexed knees. May turn from front to back.	Plays with fingers and hands. Will reach for bright objects, but will obtain them only by chance. Is able to carry an object in hand to mouth. Grasping, rooting, and sucking reflexes beginning to fade.
4 months	Uses arms to support self at 90-degree angle when on abdomen. Can turn from back to side. Can sustain part of own weight when held upright. Will sit upright if adequately supported and safely propped. Tonic neck reflex disappearing.	Spreads fingers to grasp. Hands held predominantly open. Will hold on to and shake small objects. Will bring hands to midline and watch them for prolonged periods of time.
5 months	Will hold back straight when pulled to sitting position with no head lag. Reaches for objects. Moro reflex disappearing. Tonic neck reflex absent. Can turn from back to front.	Beginning to use thumb in partial apposition to fingers. Grasps with whole hand ("mitten grasp"), reaches for objects handed to child with two hands. Can transfer small object from hand to hand.
6 months	Can pull self up to a sitting position. Sits briefly without support if in a comfortable leaning position. Can turn completely over in either direction. Voluntary crawling may appear. May "hitch" (propel self in a sitting position using arms and legs to move body). Moro reflex absent.	Bangs object held in hand. Can release object. Reaches for and grasps object, usually carrying it to mouth. Uses all four fingers in apposition to base of the thumb for grasping.
7 months	Will sit briefly, using arms thrust forward for support. Enjoys bouncing when sitting or held in a standing position.	Can approach toy and grasp with one hand. Uses tips of all fingers against thumb. Will bring feet to midline and watch them for prolonged period of time. May grasp feet and suck on toes.
8 months	Sits well alone. Will attempt to flee from an unpleasant event.	Uses index and middle fingers to form crude pincer grasp with thumb.
9 months	Although children exhibit unique styles, just about all are crawling (infant is prone with abdomen touching floor; body is pulled by arm movement with legs dragging). May "creep" (trunk is above and parallel to floor, with both hands and knees used in locomotion).	Complete thumb apposition. Uses pincer grasp (thumb and forefinger) for small objects. Manipulates objects by pushing, pulling, sliding, squeezing. Holds bottle and places nipple in mouth when wants it.
10 months	Pulls self to feel, holding on to something for support. Can walk sideways holding on to something ("cruising"). May cry when unable to sit down by self.	Uses index finger to "poke" at objects. Feeds self finger foods (crackers etc.). Can bring hands together and play "peek-a-boo." Enjoys throwing objects.
11 months	Can stand erect while holding on to some form of support with one hand. Will walk holding on to adult hands.	Picks up tiny objects with very precise pincer grasp.
12 months	Stands alone momentarily. Walks alone (some before this; some after). Climbs onto sofas, chairs. May sit down from standing by self.	Positive Babinski reflex beginning to fade. Can stroke with a crayon. Can drink holding cup, but needs assistance.
13 months	Climbs stairs well on hands and knees.	Holds adult's hand when being spoon-fed. Will position body to assist with dressing.
14 months	Steps off one step well. May walk backwards.	Pats pictures in books. Holds spoon to feed, but needs assistance.
15 months	Creeps up stairs. Falls frequently; falling often used as a way of sitting down.	Builds tower of two to three blocks. Opens most boxes. Pokes fingers into holes.

Table 21-2. *Continued*

Age	Gross motor skills	Fine motor skills
18 months	Runs with less falling; climbs; pulls toys and large objects, followed soon by pushing them; throws small balls, with minimal directionality; walks up or down stairs with adult holding hand; rolls large ball on floor.	Puts blocks in large holes, rings on peg, or beads into bottle; scribbles and may attempt straight lines; can drink from cup without much spilling; still has frequent spills in getting spoon contents properly inserted into mouth; turns several pages of a book together; unzips large zipper; unties bow by pulling string; builds tower of four to five blocks.
2 years	Tries to jump; can walk up and down stairs, without adult help, holding on to handrail or using wall for support; sits self in small chair; puts on coat with assistance; throws large ball with both hands.	Can line up blocks horizontally to make train; can turn doorknobs within reach; can imitate vertical stroke while scribbling; can drink from small cup, using only one hand; still spills liquids (e.g., soup, milk) from spoon when eating; turns pages of book one at a time; unbuttons large buttons; builds tower of six to seven blocks.
2½ years	Rides various forms of "kiddie" cars; can stand on one foot alone for at least 1 second; can throw large ball about 5 feet; can walk on tiptoe; may run fast and be unable to slow down to round corner; jumps in place; can pick up objects from floor without losing balance; gets down from adult chair without assistance; catches soft object with both arms and body.	Is able to make tower of nine large blocks; likes to fill containers with objects; will disassemble objects; can take off socks and other easy-to-manipulate clothing; zips larger zipper with help; snaps large snaps; buttons large buttons; moves fingers and thumb separately in imitation games; twists caps off bottles; places simple shapes in correct holes.
3 years	Pedals tricycle; jumps from low step; can go to toilet by self; can undress self in most situations; can go up and down stairs using alternating feet without holding on; throws large ball with one hand; can put on own coat without assistance; catches soft object with both arms.	Begins to use blunt scissors; strings large beads on shoelace; can copy circle; can help with simple household tasks (dusting, picking up); can wash and dry hands, with some wetting of clothes; can brush teeth, but not adequately; can imitate making bridge with three blocks; can pull pants up and down for toileting without assistance.
3½ years	Skips on one foot; hops forward on both feet; runs well without falling; kicks large ball; twists upper body while holding feet in one place; uses hands to get up from floor; catches soft object with hands; catches large ball with arms.	Can cut straight lines with scissors without tearing paper; manipulates pieces into position for simple puzzles; can weave yarn randomly through card; places small pegs in pegboard; unbuttons small buttons; can eat from spoon without spilling
4 years	Jumps well; hops forward on one foot; may catch large bounced ball with hands; walks backward; catches soft object with one hand; catches small ball with arms.	Cuts around pictures with scissors; can copy square; can button side buttons; may bathe self, with assistance; folds napkin into triangle or rectangle; outlines picture with yarn; buttons small buttons.
5 years	Can jump rope; runs lightly on toes; alternates feet to skip; gets up without using hands; catches small ball with two hands.	May be able to print own name; copies triangle; dresses without assistance; may be able to lace shoes; can put toys away neatly; bathes self; threads small beads on a string; eats with fork.

Source: From *The process of human development: a holistic approach*, by C. Schuster and S. Ashburn, pp. 141, 142, and 231.

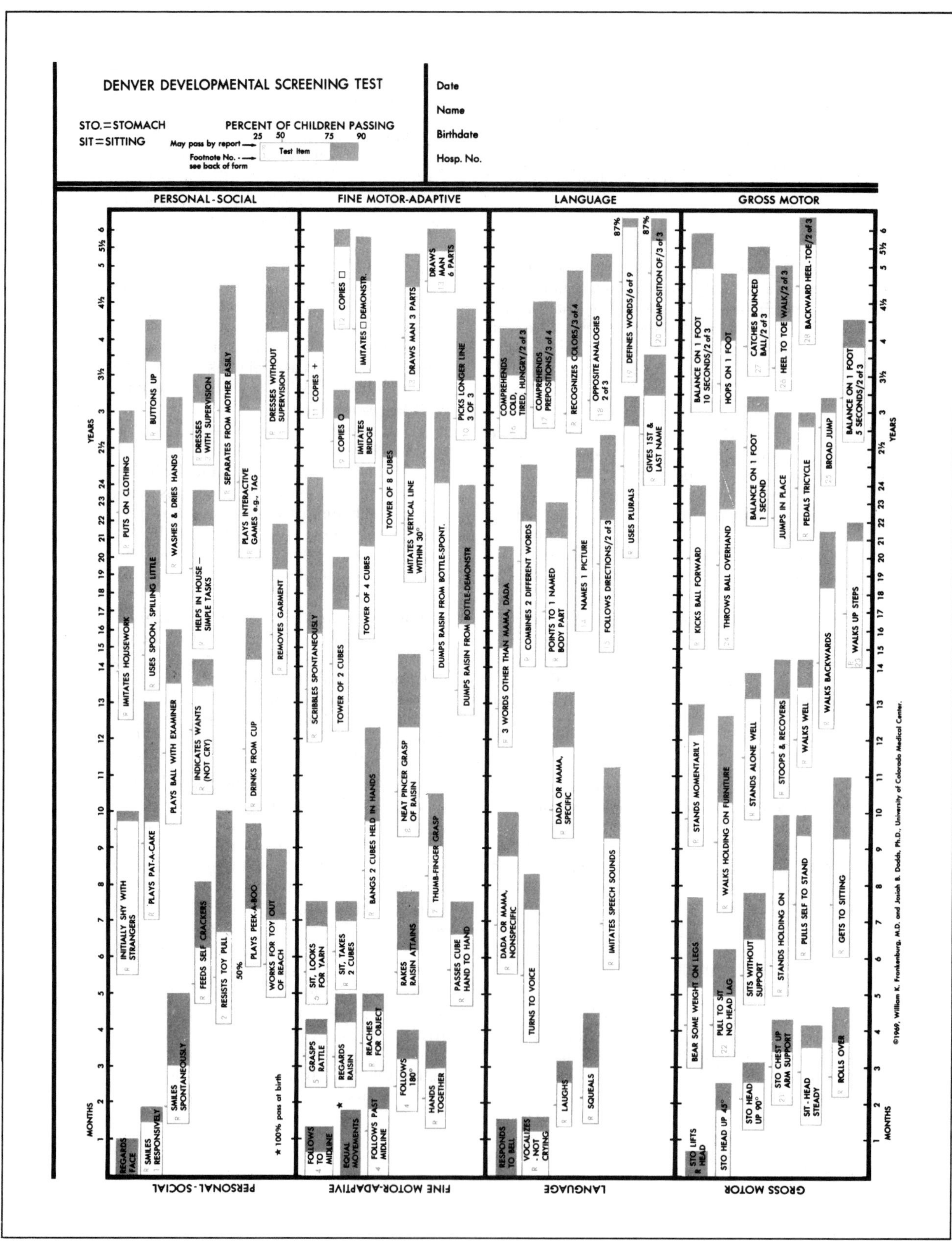

Figure 21-1 Denver Developmental Screening Test.

1. Try to get child to smile by smiling, talking or waving to him. Do not touch him.
2. When child is playing with toy, pull it away from him. Pass if he resists.
3. Child does not have to be able to tie shoes or button in the back.
4. Move yarn slowly in an arc from one side to the other, about 6" above child's face. Pass if eyes follow 90° to midline. (Past midline; 180°)
5. Pass if child grasps rattle when it is touched to the backs or tips of fingers.
6. Pass if child continues to look where yarn disappeared or tries to see where it went. Yarn should be dropped quickly from sight from tester's hand without arm movement.
7. Pass if child picks up raisin with any part of thumb and a finger.
8. Pass if child picks up raisin with the ends of thumb and index finger using an over hand approach.

9. Pass any enclosed form. Fail continuous round motions.
10. Which line is longer? (Not bigger.) Turn paper upside down and repeat. (3/3 or 5/6)
11. Pass any crossing lines.
12. Have child copy first. If failed, demonstrate

When giving items 9, 11 and 12, do not name the forms. Do not demonstrate 9 and 11.

13. When scoring, each pair (2 arms, 2 legs, etc.) counts as one part.
14. Point to picture and have child name it. (No credit is given for sounds only.)

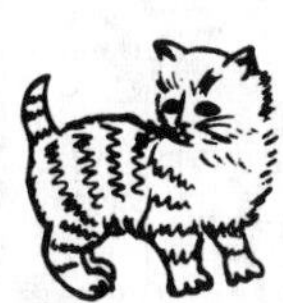  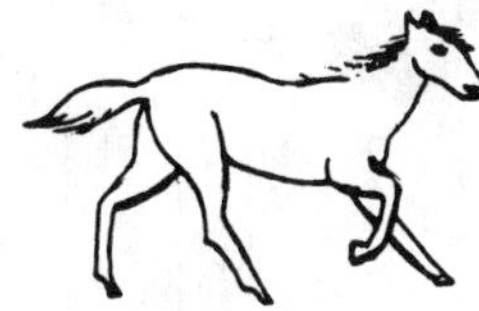 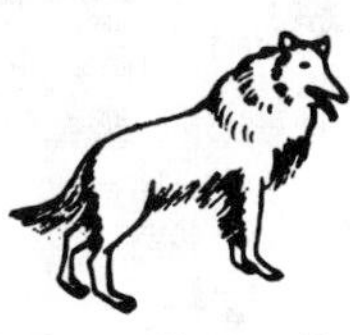 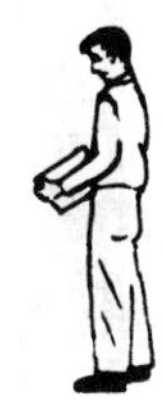

15. Tell child to: Give block to Mommie; put block on table; put block on floor. Pass 2 of 3. (Do not help child by pointing, moving head or eyes.)
16. Ask child: What do you do when you are cold? ..hungry? ..tired? Pass 2 of 3.
17. Tell child to: Put block <u>on</u> table; <u>under</u> table; <u>in front</u> of chair, <u>behind</u> chair. Pass 3 of 4. (Do not help child by pointing, moving head or eyes.)
18. Ask child: If fire is hot, ice is ?; Mother is a woman, Dad is a ?; a horse is big, a mouse is ?. Pass 2 of 3.
19. Ask child: What is a ball? ..lake? ..desk? ..house? ..banana? ..curtain? ..ceiling? ..hedge? ..pavement? Pass if defined in terms of use, shape, what it is made of or general category (such as banana is fruit, not just yellow). Pass 6 of 9.
20. Ask child: What is a spoon made of? ..a shoe made of? ..a door made of? (No other objects may be substituted.) Pass 3 of 3.
21. When placed on stomach, child lifts chest off table with support of forearms and/or hands.
22. When child is on back, grasp his hands and pull him to sitting. Pass if head does not hang back.
23. Child may use wall or rail only, not person. May not crawl.
24. Child must throw ball overhand 3 feet to within arm's reach of tester.
25. Child must perform standing broad jump over width of test sheet. (8-1/2 inches)
26. Tell child to walk forward, → heel within 1 inch of toe. Tester may demonstrate. Child must walk 4 consecutive steps, 2 out of 3 trials.
27. Bounce ball to child who should stand 3 feet away from tester. Child must catch ball with hands, not arms, 2 out of 3 trials.
28. Tell child to walk backward, ← toe within 1 inch of heel. Tester may demonstrate. Child must walk 4 consecutive steps, 2 out of 3 trials.

<u>DATE AND BEHAVIORAL OBSERVATIONS</u> (how child feels at time of test, relation to tester, attention span, verbal behavior, self-confidence, etc,):

Figure 21-1 *Continued*

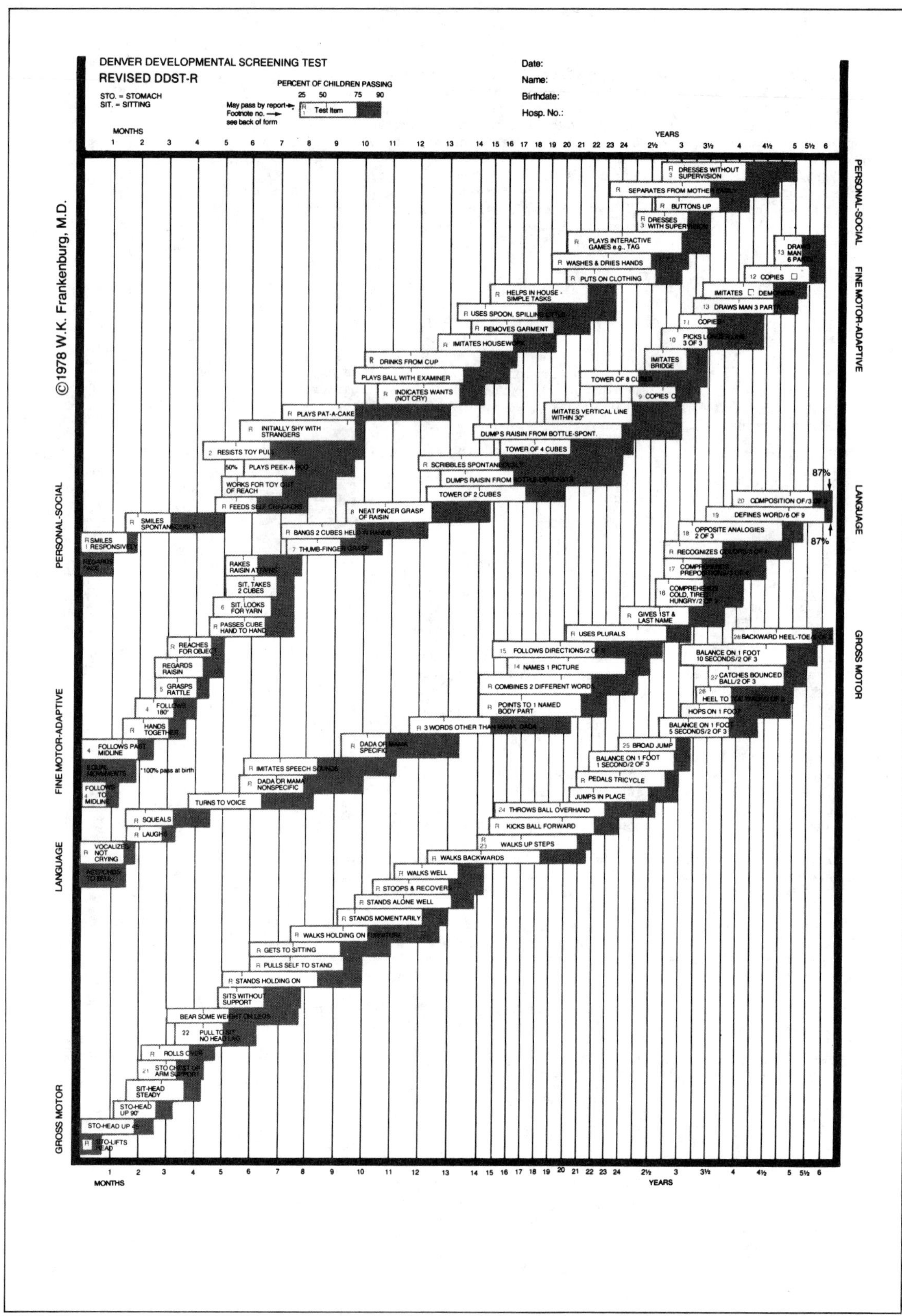

Figure 21-2 Revised Denver test.

assessing the late adolescent's and adult's occupational history, the nurse assesses the play and school activity in the child and early-mid adolescent, since this generally constitutes "work" for them. However, information is also sought regarding whether the child does have a job, what his home responsibilities are, and whether he receives an allowance. The nurse looks at the play patterns—whether the child mostly plays alone, parallel plays, plays with same-sex groups or opposite-sex groups or mixed-sex groups—and the amount of play and daily physical exercise. In this area, too, the nurse inquires about the school grades, study habits, school progress, and standing, in addition to whether or not the child has any problems at school or with the law. Is school worthwhile? Does the adolescent have a career choice? Does the child get along well with his peers, teachers, other adults, and authority figures? Have the parents met the teacher(s)? Are absences from school excessive (more than 3 days/month), and, if so, what are the causes for the absenteeism? Does the child attend a house of worship? Is this a family activity?

Family Health History

The history of each family member's health status, his or her age, and illnesses and anomalies is recorded in the same manner as would be for the adult (see "Family History of Illness" in Chapter 4). Geographic exposure may be quite relevant to the health status of the child and adolescent. Travel may be closely related to the occupation of the family breadwinner (for example, international business executive, ambassador to a foreign country, missionary, or military personnel).

Diet

Considered within the lifestyle pattern is diet. The same guideline questions used in assessing the dietary habits of the adult can be used in assessing those of the child and adolescent (see "Diet" in Chapter 4).

Feeding protocols in the first year of life are very defined. Therefore, you need to collect specific data about the infant's diet (see Table 21-3).

If the new infant is being breast-fed, you need to investigate adequacy of breast milk and the mother's diet and drug use, including prescriptive and social drugs and birth control pills. Table 21-4 lists substances that are secreted in breast milk. Table 21-5 identifies adverse effects that may arise in the child when particular medications are taken by the mother during pregnancy.

Other factors important to investigate are: Who prepares the food? What are the patterns for acquisition, storage, and cooking of the food? What equipment, such as freezer, refrigerator, food processor, and stove, is available?

For all ages, an important part of the nutritional evaluation is assessment of ability to feed oneself, regularity, amount and content of meals, as well as vitamin or other diet supplements,

Table 21-3. Assessment of Diet for Infants

Formula:
brand ______
type ______
ounces per feeding ______
number of feedings ______

Food texture:
liquids
soft baby foods
mashed table foods
cut fine table foods

Food additions:
juices: ______ diluted ______ undiluted ______
type ______
amount ______
enriched baby cereal ______
strained fruits ______
strained vegetables ______
strained meats ______
egg yolk or baby egg yolk ______
teething biscuit ______
whole milk ______
fortified cereal ______
fruit, canned ______
or fresh ______
vegetables ______
meat, poultry, fish ______
bread ______
butter ______
starch, potato ______
rice ______
pasta ______
dessert, custard ______
pudding ______

Table 21-4. Examples of Medications in Breast Milk

Drug	Explanation of effects on infant
Analgesics	
Codeine	Insignificant with therapeutic doses (60 mg PO,SC,IM)
Heroin	Sufficient concentration in habituated mothers to prevent withdrawals in habituated infant
Meperidine	Insignificant in therapeutic doses (100 mg IM)
Morphine	Sufficient concentration in habituated mothers to prevent withdrawals in habituated infants; insignificant levels with therapeutic dose (10 mg SC,IM)
Propoxyphene	Insignificant with therapeutic dose (65–130 mg PO); probably significant effect when used IV, but not studied
Sodium salicylate	1–3 mg/ml serum level with 4 g dose (equivalent to 4 g ASA), which is insignificant; may be a problem with rheumatics with continual high dose
Antacids	Rarely absorbed to an appreciable extent; no problem unless mother develops an electrolyte imbalance
Antiemetics	
Antihistamines	Cause decreased lactation with large doses even though they may not be appreciably excreted
Antimicrobials	The use of these may lead to microbial resistance
Ampicillin	Excreted; safe to use, but may cause diarrhea and allergic sensitization
Chloramphenicol	Excreted to 50% of serum levels and possible but remote chance of "gray syndrome" with neonate
Erythromycin	Excreted but safe to use
INH	Excreted but safe to use
Oxacillin	Excreted but safe to use
Penicillin	Excreted but safe to use; possible allergic sensitization
Streptomycin	Excreted but safe to use
Sulfonamides	Excreted, with possible occurrences of kernicterus in neonates
Tetracyclines	Excreted to 20–90% of serum levels and may cause decreased bone growth and tooth staining
Depressants	
Barbiturates	
Long-acting	Barbital: insignificant effects with hypnotic doses (650 mg); phenobarbital: sedative effects with hypnotic doses (100 mg), no effect with sedative doses (30 mg t.i.d.); phenobarbital and diphenylhydantoin (390 and 300 mg): methemoglobinemia reported in one infant, no effect on infant with 300-600 mg diphenylhydantoin alone
Short-acting	Secobarbital and pentobarbital: no effect with sedative doses; possible effect with hypnotic doses
Others	
Alcohol	Small amounts have no effect; large doses (750 ml wine over 24 hours or equivalent) cause sedation
Bromides	Rashes and sedation with hypnotic doses
Chloral hydrate	1.33 g rectally (approximately 2 g orally) has caused sedation
Diazepam	Large oral doses cause sedation (10 mg q.i.d.)
Reserpine	Nasal stuffiness with doses greater than 0.5 mg
Diuretics	
Hydrochlorothiazide, chlorothiazide	Excreted with remote possibility of causing problems
Hormonal compounds	
Iodides	Therapeutic doses will cause goiters
Oral contraceptives	Decreased lactation in a minority of women, but most can take low dose preparations from the first day postpartum without decreasing lactation; possibility of causing idiopathic jaundice

From R. Levin, in E. T. Herfindal and J. Hirschman, eds., *Clinical Pharmacy and Therapeutics* (Baltimore: Williams & Wilkins, 1975);

Table 21-4. *(Continued)*

Drug	Explanation of effects on infant
Pregnane beta-diol	Abnormal progesterone metabolite produced and excreted in some mothers and leads to jaundice
Propythiouracil	Excreted and will cause thyroid suppression
Thyroid	Excreted and will also cause increased milk production
Laxatives and fecal softeners	Bulk formers, castor oil, Dulcolax, mineral oil, DOSS, saline, phenopthalein, and other nonabsorbed types cause no problems and are safe to use
Anthraquinone derivatives	
Cascara	Increased bowel activity with usual doses
Danthron	Increased bowel activity with usual doses
Social drugs (legal)	
Alcohol	See under *Depressants*
Caffeine	1% of ingested dose of coffee or tea secreted; no effect on infant with moderate intake
Tobacco	More than 20 cigarettes per day have caused nicotine effects in infant—i.e., restlessness, diarrhea, vomiting, and rapid pulse
Social drugs (illegal)	
Abuse drugs	Stimulants, depressants, narcotics, psychedelics, and others used in high doses have not been studied or reported and probably are excreted in high concentrations and should not be used
Miscellaneous	
Anticoagulants, oral	Not adequately studied and should be avoided
DDT	Excreted in milk at four times the level of cow's milk but less than maximum permissible amount; death has occurred in infant whose mother inhaled a large amount
Ergotrate maleate	Excreted and causes ergotism—i.e., decreased circulation, vomiting, diarrhea, tremors
Fluorides	Levels of 1.13 ppm in drinking water achieve milk concentrations of 0.25 ppm
Foods	White navy beans, corn, egg white, chocolate, unripe fruit, pickles, peanuts, cottonseed, and wheat are all reported to cause allergic reactions—i.e., colic and rash; should be used sparingly or avoided

Table 21-5. Examples of Teratogenic Medications

Drug	Adverse effect	Stage of pregnancy	Significance
Analeptics			
Dextroamphetamine sulfate	Transposition of great vessels, biliary atresia	First trimester	More evidence needed
Serotonin	Multiple anomalies of skeleton and organs	4th–12th week	More evidence needed
Analgesics			
Heroin	Respiratory depression, withdrawal symptoms	Near term	Fairly well documented
Methadone	Prolonged withdrawal	Term	Fairly well documented
Morphine	Neonatal death	Near term	More evidence needed
Salicylates	Neonatal bleeding, thrombocytopenia	Near term	More evidence needed
Anesthetics (inhaled)			
Cyclopropane, ether, halothane	Neonatal depression	Near term	Established

Continued on page 440

From R. Levin, in E. T. Herfindal and J. Hirschman, eds., *Clinical Pharmacy and Therapeutics* (Baltimore: Williams & Wilkins, 1975); © 1975 The Williams & Wilkins Co., Baltimore.

Table 21-5. *Continued*

Drug	Adverse effect	Stage of pregnancy	Significance
Anesthetics (local)			
Lidocaine	Neonatal depression	Near term	More evidence needed
Mepivicaine	Fetal bradycardia	Near term	Not established
Anticoagulants			
Sodium warfarin	Fetal death, hemorrhage	Throughout pregnancy	More evidence needed
Antidiabetics			
Chlorpropamide	Prolonged neonatal hypoglycemia, anomalies	Throughout pregnancy	More evidence needed before implication
Tolbutamide	Congenital anomalies, hypoglycemia	Throughout pregnancy	More evidence needed
Antiepileptics			
Diphenylhydantoin	Cleft gum, lip, or palate; syndactyly, polydactyly; microcephaly, anencephaly	1st and 2nd trimesters	Fairly well documented
	Neonatal bleeding	Near term	Fairly well documented
Mysoline	Neonatal bleeding	Near term	Fairly well documented
Antihistamines			
Diphenhydramine	Thrombocytopenia	Near term	More evidence needed
Promethazine	Thrombocytopenia	Near term	More evidence needed
Anti-inflammatory agents			
Cortisone	Cleft palate	Very early in gestation	More evidence needed
Antimicrobials			
Chloramphenicol	"Gray syndrome" and death	Near term	Fairly well documented
Isonicotinic acid hydrazide (INH)	Retarded psychomotor activity		More evidence needed
Streptomycin	8th-nerve damage, micromelia, hearing loss, multiple skeletal anomalies	Throughout pregnancy	Debatable; more evidence needed
Sulfonamides (long-acting)	Hyperbilirubinemia and kernicterus	Near term	Fairly well documented
Tetracyclines	Inhibition of bone growth, discoloration of teeth, micromelia, syndactyly	2nd and 3rd trimesters	Fairly well documented
Antineoplastics			
Amethopterin	Abortefacient, retarded growth, cleft palate, cranial anomalies, encephaloceles	1st trimester	Fairly well documented
Aminopterin	Abortefacient, retarded growth, cleft palate, cranial anomalies, encephaloceles	1st trimester	Known teratogen
Antithyroid agents			
Potassium iodide	Goiter and mental retardation	From 14th week on	Fairly well documented
Propylthiouracil	Goiter and mental retardation	From 14th week on	Fairly well documented
Depressants			
Alcohol	Vacuolization of bone-marrow cells, neonatal depression, decreased birth weight	Throughout and near delivery	More evidence needed
Barbiturates and other hypnotics	Respiratory depression, hemorrhage	Near delivery	Fairly well documented
	Malformations	1st and 2nd trimesters	More evidence needed

Table 21-5. *Continued*

Drug	Adverse effect	Stage of pregnancy	Significance
Thalidomide	Phocomelia, hearing defect	28th–42nd days	Known teratogen
Diuretics			
Thiazides (hydrochlorothiazide, chlorothiazide)	Thrombocytopenia, neonatal death	Later part of pregnancy	One report only; more evidence needed
Hormonal steroids			
Androgens	Masculinization, labial fusion, and clitoris enlargement	Throughout pregnancy	Well documented
Estrogens (stilbestrol)	Adenocarcinoma	Throughout pregnancy	More evidence needed
Oral progestogens	Masculinization, labial fusion, and clitoris enlargement	Throughout pregnancy	Fairly well documented
Immunizations (live)			
Measles vaccine	Infected fetus	Throughout pregnancy	More evidence needed
Mumps vaccine	Infected fetus	Throughout pregnancy	More evidence needed
Rubella vaccine	Congenital rubella, anomalies	Throughout pregnancy	Fairly well documented
Smallpox vaccine	Fetal vaccinia	Throughout pregnancy	Fairly well documented
Social drugs (legal)			
Nicotine and smoking	Small babies, early birth, irritable	Throughout pregnancy	Probably significant
Social drugs (illegal)			
Lysergic acid diethyl-amide (LSD)	Chromosomal damage, stunted offspring, other malformations	1st trimester	Could be significant; more evidence needed
Tranquilizers			
Chlordiazepoxide	Thrombocytopenia	Near term	More evidence needed
Diazepam	Thrombocytopenia	Near term	More evidence needed
Imipramine	Thrombocytopenia	Near term	More evidence needed
Phenothiazines (in general)	Retinopathy, urinary retention, extra-pyramidal reactions, hyperbilirubinemia	Close to delivery	More evidence needed
Chlorpromazine	Chromosome changes, possible goiter	Throughout pregnancy	More evidence needed
	Thrombocytopenia	Near term	
Prochlorperazine	Thrombocytopenia	Near term	More evidence needed
Reserpine	Nasal blockage	Near term	More evidence needed
Vitamins			
Vitamin A	Retarded growth, intracranial hypertension	Throughout pregnancy	In large doses only
Vitamin C	Scurvy develops after birth	Near term	More evidence needed
Vitamin D	Excessive blood calcium, mental retardation	Throughout pregnancy	In large doses only
Vitamin K analogues	Hyperbilirubinemia, kernicterus	Near term	In large doses only
Pyridoxine	Withdrawal seizures	Near term	More evidence needed (in large doses only)
Miscellaneous			
Acetophenetidin	Methemoglobinemia	Near term	More evidence needed
Glyceryl guaiacolate	Thrombocytopenia	Near term	More evidence needed

food preferences, dislikes, intolerances, food allergies (allergy to cow's milk is a common problem), and gastrointestinal problems. With teenagers the major health problems related to diet are inadequate nutrition and being overweight. Physical and mental behaviors need to be analyzed in association with nutrition. Table 21-7 shows a comparison of findings for Marasmus and Kwashiorkor in children.

Sexuality

In addressing the area of sexuality, history-taking for the preschool and school age child, the parents are questioned since they exert much influence on this area of the child's development. Examples of inquiries regarding sexual health are contained in Table 21-8. Adolescents are questioned in the same manner as adults (see Chapters 4 and 24).

Habits

Frequently in the school-age child, you may find excessive use of tobacco, alcohol, and other social drugs. Presently there seems to be a shift from smoking cigarettes to that of using chewing tobacco by young males. Documented cases of oral carcinoma have been associated with "chew." Young girls are smoking cigarettes more; this has the potential for increased incidence of lung carcinoma in women. Alcohol has been the legal depressant for adults. The role model phenomenon may be the impetus for the increase in the use of alcohol in teenagers as they struggle to "be adults." Grown-ups use alcohol, why not us? Do drugs make you feel good? Do you take drugs when you are alone? What drugs do you take? Caffeine seems to be the most commonly abused substance in the high school and college student. Cup after cup or glass after glass of coffee, tea, or cola is downed to stimulate alertness for an all-nighter session of study for examinations and term paper completions (see Table 21-6).

Table 21-6. Caffeine Content of Beverages and Some Nonprescription Drugs

Item	Caffeine Content (mg)
Beverages	
Coffee	
Decaffeinated	2–70/cup
Ground	85–200/cup
Instant	30–80/cup
Cola	40–60/glass
Tea	20–150/cup
Nonprescription drugs	
Aspirin-containing preparations	30–35/tablet
Excedrin	60/tablet
Stimulants, nonprescription	80–150/tablet

From Y. H. Hui, *Human Nutrition and Diet Therapy* (Boston: Jones & Bartlett, 1983).

Sleep

From the time an individual is born, changes are occurring in his sleep patterns. A newborn will spend about 16 hours per 24 hours asleep. The newborn child spends most of his sleeping time in the third and fourth stages of sleep, the deepest stages of sleep. During these stages the growth hormone peaks and produces the products to be used in REM sleep. According to Oswald (1972), perhaps this is why 50% of the newborn's sleeping time is spent in REM sleep. This stage of sleep has also been associated with the learning process. Hales (1981) believes that failure of a newborn to receive an adequate amount of REM sleep may result in a lower level of development.

The amount of time a child spends sleeping at any one length is about half as long as that of an adult's cycle. Children are unable to consolidate their sleeping time, so they nap frequently. As the child grows older, he develops the ability to consolidate his sleeping, and naps are no longer needed and eventually are eliminated.

Parasomnia, a sleeping disorder that affects mostly children, is composed of three individual behaviors: night terrors, sleepwalking, and bedwetting. They may all occur together or individually. Some unique aspects of each behavior warrant attenion. In night terrors, also termed pavor nocturnus, there appears to be an immature development of the central nervous system. However, by adolescence this disorder usually disappears. Evidence has indicated that sleepwalking, or somnambulism, has a familial history. Finally, bedwetting (enuresis) is a completely involuntary act; this fact must be kept in mind and parents must be made aware in order that the child is not punished for something over which he has no control. Parasomnias are common sleep disorders that occur in children.

Another common sleep disorder that occurs in children between the ages of 1 and 12 months is sudden infant death syndrome (SIDS). This disease claims the lives of approximately 10,000

Table 21-7. Comparison of Marasmus and Kwashiorkor in Children

Characteristic	Marasmus	Kwashiorkor
Etiology	Inadequate calorie intake due to diet insufficiency and disturbed parent-child relations Obstructive disease of the upper gastrointestinal tract, malabsorption syndromes	Severe deficiency of protein, although adequate calories may be ingested
Age of onset	Any age, but commonly seen in infants under age one	Classically, at time of weaning from breast milk
General appearance	Emaciated and wrinkled	Pallor and generalized edema, with multiple skin lesions
Weight	Extreme loss with depletion of fat and muscles	Some loss despite edema
Face	Loss of fat from cheeks (buccal fat pad)	Moon face from retention of buccal fat pad and edema
Hair	Growth retarded, with atrophied hair follicles	Hair is either lost or easily pulled out; depigmentation of hair in bands
Skin	No lesions	Dermatitis is common; darkening of areas of irritation but not those exposed to sunlight; desquamation may occur
Abdomen	Shrunken with visible peristalsis; may be distended with gas	Potbelly
Behavioral assessment	Fretful at first, then listless	Neurological changes; irritability and apathy to stupor and coma Marked psychomotor impairment
Physical assessment	No hepatomegaly Behaviors of severe vitamin deficiencies	Hepatomegaly with or without fatty infiltration Usually other vitamin and mineral deficiencies present as well
Laboratory findings	Reduced basal metabolic rate	Prolonged prothrombin time Total body potassium depletion Immune system deficits Increased total body sodium, but decreased serum levels
Prognosis	Neurologic status vulnerable in early, severe marasmus Mortality rate is high	Mortality of treated severe, acute kwashiorkor is 30 percent or greater

Source: Developed by Gayle Giboney Page, R.N., M.N., Children's Hospital of Los Angeles.

infants each year in the United States. The etiology is unknown. The phenomenon seems to be that a healthy child is placed in bed and is found dead the next morning. One theory is that this disorder may be brought about by an immature nervous system. When the infant is placed in the bed and the room is darkened, little stimulation is provided. This lack of stimulation upon the reticular formation may cause the infant to stop breathing. The reticular formation plays a key part in respiratory functioning and requires additional stimulation when REM sleep normally begins to decrease after the first two months of life.

Home and Neighborhood

The home and neighborhood environment are important and can be assessed by investigating the same areas as you would with the adult (see "Home and Neighborhood" in Chapter 4). Additional kinds of information are the mother-child relationship and interpersonal relationships between the child and adolescent and siblings and other family members. Some guidelines for assessing mother-infant relationship and for assistance in identifying common inhibiting factors to adequate mothering are presented in the accompanying box, "Criteria for Assessing Adequate Motherhood."

Table 21-8. Sexual Health History for the Parents of the Preadolescent Child

1. How have you answered your child's questions about sex?
2. Whom else does your child ask about sex?
3. How old was your child when you first talked about reproduction (intercourse, how babies are made)? Does your child know about menstruation? Erection? Wet dreams?
4. Describe your child's sexual activity:
   a. When he or she was younger.
   b. Now.
   c. What changes do you expect in the next year?
5. Is there anything you would change about your child's sexual activity?
6. Do you have any concerns about your child's relationship with friends or with family members?
7. Is there anything you think your child needs to or wants to know that you are unable to discuss with him or her?
8. Would you like help from someone in discussing that difficult area?
9. Do you have any questions about your own sexuality, sexual activity, or sexual health?

Source: F. H. Mims and M. Swenson, *Sexuality: A nursing perspective.* Copyright © 1980 by McGraw-Hill Book Company. Reprinted by permission.

How does the client get along with brothers, sisters, parents, grandparents, neighbors? Does the client make friends easily? Have a lot of friends? Are siblings favored over the client? Could things be better in the home? Who disciplines the child? What types of disciplinary methods are used? Do parents understand him? Are they fair? Do they care about him? Are the parents too strict or too old fashioned in his estimation? Is his family life basically happy? Violent? Do his parents get along well with each other? Are there any concerns about specific problems such as obedience, temper tantrums, toilet training, phobias, enuresis, stuttering, masturbation, thumb sucking, and nail biting? If problems exist, how are they being managed? The life event stressors can be analyzed by use of a stress scale for children (see Table 21-9).

Recreation and Hobbies

Recreation and hobbies are a very real part of the child's and adolescent's lifestyle. In what types of activities is the child interested? What activities does the child participate in and enjoy? Is the child active in sports? To what extent? Are there any activities that he does not like but in which, in his opinion, he is coerced to participate? Does the youth date? Double date? Go out in groups? What types of activities are engaged in on dates? What do the youth and his friends do in their leisure time and for entertainment? Does the youth have friends? Who are his close friends? Do his parents know his friends and his friends' families? What plans does the youth have for himself? What are the parents' and family members' expectations of the youth?

Occupation/Socioeconomic Level

What is the socioeconomic level of the family? What are the occupations of the parent(s) and significant others? Are there adequate finances available to support good health practices? Are the family members literate? What is the educational background of the various family members? What is the prevailing atmosphere and physical environment of the neighborhood?

Previous Experiences with Illness/ Immunizations

The collection of data regarding previous experiences with illness is the same as that when interviewing the adult. The nurse inquires about the types of common illness suffered, major diseases experienced, surgery that had been done, and any accidents and injuries that had occurred. Also investigated is how the client reacts to illness, stress, hospitalization, and separation, if the latter two situations have been experienced to date. Particularly with this age group it is important to assess the youth's immunization schedule. See Chapter 4 for a schedule for first vaccinations based on the recommendations of the American Medical Association and the American Academy of Pediatrics. Injections, however, are not administered when the child has an upper respiratory infection or other illness. Because of immunizations against childhood diseases, the mortality rate from such illnesses has declined significantly. However, danger does exist for those children who do not receive a comprehensive immunization program as a result of ignorance, religious tenets, inadequate finances, or inadequate health care.

The most common illnesses in the younger child are respiratory afflictions, including the common cold. High causes of mortality in teenagers are accidents, suicide, and homicide. Does the client use seatbelts when driving or riding in a car? Does he know how to swim? Are there firearms and ammunition in the home? In

Criteria for Assessing Adequate Motherhood in the Early Weeks of Infant Life

Mother-infant unity can be said to be satisfactory when a mother can:

1. Find pleasure in her infant and in tasks for and with him.
2. Understand his affective states and can comfort him by relieving his states of unbearable tension.
3. Read his cues for new experience; sense his fatigue level.

Examples: *Can receive his eye contact with pleasure. Promotes his new learnings with use of her face, hands, and objects. Does not overstimulate for her own pleasure.*

Signs mothers give when not adapting to their infants:

1. See their infants as ugly or unattractive.
2. Perceive the odor of their infants as revolting.
3. Disgusted by drooling of infants.
4. Disgusted by sucking sounds of infants.
5. Upset by vomiting, but seem fascinated by it.
6. Revolted by any of infant's body fluids which touch them, or which they touch.
7. Annoyed at having to clean up infant's stools.
8. Preoccupied by odor, consistency, and number of stools.
9. Let infant's head dangle, without support or concern.
10. Hold infants away from their own bodies.
11. Pick up infant without warning him by a touch or by speech.
12. Juggle and play with infant, roughly, after feeding him even though he often vomits at this behavior.
13. Think infant's natural motor activity is unnatural.
14. Worry about infant's relaxation following feeding.
15. Avoid eye contact with infants, or stare fixedly into their eyes.
16. Do not coo or talk with their infant.
17. Think that their infants do not love them.
18. Consider that their infants expose them as unlovable, unloving parents.
19. Think of their infants as judging them and their efforts as an adult would.
20. Perceive their infant's natural dependent needs as dangerous.
21. Fears of infant's death appear at mild diarrhea or minor cold.
22. Convinced that their infant has some defect, in spite of repeated physical examinations which prove negative.
23. This feared defect tends to migrate from body system to disease, and back again.
24. Conceal the defect site, or disease feared. If asked what they fear they disclaim knowing. They will reply to the reverse question of, "What do you hope it is *not?*"
25. Major maternal fears are often connected with diseases perceived as "eating" diseases (leukemia, or one of the other malignancies; diabetes; cystic fibrosis).
26. Constantly demand reassurance that no defect or disease exists, cannot believe relieving facts when they are given.
27. Demand that feared defect be found and relieved.
28. Cannot find in their infants any physical or psychological attribute which they value in themselves. (Probably the most diagnostic of these signs and readily elicited)
29. Cannot discriminate between infant signs signaling hunger or fatigue, need for soothing or stimulating speech, comforting body contact, or for eye contact.

(continued on page 490)

From M. G. Morris, "Maternal Claiming-Identification Processes: Their Meaning for Mother-Infant Mental Health," in *Parent-Child Relationships: The Role of the Nurse,* papers presented at Continuing Education Program for Nurses, workshops held in May and June 1968, ed. by Ann Clark and others. New Brunswick, N.J., Nursing Programs, University Extension Division, Rutgers University, The State University of New Jersey, 1968, pp. 34–35.

Criteria for Assessing Adequate Motherhood (*Continued*)

30. Develop inappropriate responses to infant needs:
    a. Over or under-feed.
    b. Over or under-hold.
    c. Tickle or bounce the baby when he is fatigued.
    d. Talk too much, too little, and at the wrong time.
    e. Force eye contact, or refuse it.
    f. Leave infant in room alone.
    g. Leave infant in noisy room and ignore him.
31. Develop paradoxical attitudes and behaviors.
    Example: *Bitterly insist that infant cannot be pleased, no matter what is done, but continue to demand more and better methods for pleasing him.*

Deterrents to adequate mothering

1. General personal immaturity.
2. Current stress in mother's life situation.
    a. Loss or threatened loss of love object or objects (including her infant).
    b. Disappointments of severe nature.
    c. Excessive fear of significant family member (own or in-laws).
    d. Father's criticism of mother *or* her infant.
    e. Rejection by her own mother, her in-laws of her *or* her infant.
    f. Financial worries.
    g. Husband's loss of job. This often provokes excessive fear of starvation on deep level, for self and infant.
    h. Father punishing mother (openly or subtly) for own dependent needs.
    i. Serious illness of original parents or in-laws. The illness replaces the real infant as the "first child," especially when a mother is directly involved in care of her original parents or parents of her infant's father.
3. Current depersonalized and unrelated parturition and neonatal hospital practices.
4. Early discharge (from the second to fifth day) without sufficient help at home for maternal-infant adaptive tasks.
5. Failure in mother-doctor-family support system.

friends' homes? Health teaching about principles of safety, measures to strengthen self-esteem, and values clarification are paramount with the adolescent client and his parents.

Review of Systems

The review of systems (ROS) is essentially the same as that for the adult. Special tact is necessary, however, when discussing menarche and seminal emissions and problems or concerns regarding sexuality and sexual functioning. You could ask the client whether he is aware of how a woman becomes pregnant, whether he would like to learn about the prevention of pregnancy, and, since some young people engage in sexual activity before marriage, how his actions fit with his beliefs. Also, this portion of history-taking is an excellent time for health teaching and answering questions the client may have. When interviewing the 16- to 21-year-old (late adolescent) female, inquire whether a Pap smear has ever been performed and, if so, when.

The adolescent is able to provide a great majority of the data base. It is usually with regard to his immunization schedule, family history of illnesses, and own past illnesses that he may fall short. In such cases you need to tap other sources of information such as parents, school, private physician, and other medical records that may be available. On some occasions, too, you may want and need to validate the information given to you by the client.

Mental Status

Consideration of specific developmental tasks is helpful in evaluating mental status and growth (see Table 21-11). However, the basic indices for assessing mental status and mental functioning

Table 21-9. Stress Scale for Children*

Life event	Preschool age	Elementary school age	Junior high school age
Beginning nursery school, first grade, or high school	42	46	45
Change to a different school	33	46	52
Birth or adoption of a brother or sister	50	50	50
Brother or sister leaving home	39	36	33
Hospitalization of a brother or sister	37	41	44
Death of a brother or sister	59	68	71
Change of father's occupation requiring increased absence from home	36	45	42
Loss of job by parent	23	38	48
Marital separation of parents	74	78	77
Divorce of parents	78	84	84
Hospitalization of a parent (serious illness)	51	56	54
Death of a parent	89	91	94
Death of a grandparent	30	38	35
Marriage of a parent to a stepparent	62	65	63
Jail sentence of a parent of 30 days or less	34	44	50
Jail sentence of a parent of 1 year or more	67	67	76
Addition of third adult to family (ie, grandparent)	39	41	34
Change in parents' financial status	21	29	40
Mother beginning to work	47	44	36
Decrease in number of arguments between parents	21	25	29
Increase in number of arguments between parents	44	51	48
Decrease in number of arguments with parents	22	27	29
Increase in number of arguments with parents	39	47	46
Discovery of being an adopted child	33	52	70
Acquiring a visible deformity	52	69	83
Having a visible congenital deformity	39	60	70
Hospitalization of self (child)	59	62	59
Change in acceptance by peers	38	51	68
Outstanding personal achievement	23	53	65
Death of a close friend (child's friend)	38	53	65
Failure of a grade in school	—	57	62
Suspension from school	—	46	54
Pregnancy in unwed adolescent sister	—	36	60
Becoming involved with drugs or alcohol	—	61	70
Becoming a full-fledged member of a church or synagogue	—	25	28
Not being accepted into an extracurricular activity the child wanted to be involved in (ie, team, band)	—	—	49
Breaking up with a boyfriend or girlfriend	—	—	47
Beginning to date	—	—	55
Fathering an unwed pregnancy	—	—	76
Unwed pregnancy	—	—	95

*Different life events produce varying amounts of stress for children—the more points, the greater the stress. The chart is arranged in order of how frequently the events occur.

Source: Heisel JS et al: The significance of life events as contributing factors in the diseases of children. *J Pediatr* 1973; 83(1):119.

Table 21-10. Revised Infant Temperament Questionnaire

Mother's general impressions of infant's temperament

A. How would you describe your baby's temperament in your own words?

B. In comparison with what you know of other babies of the same age, how would you rate your baby as to the following criteria? (Circle one)

I. *Activity level*—the amount of physical activity during sleep, feeding, play, dressing, etc.
(1) high (2) medium (3) low

II. *Regularity*—of bodily functioning in sleep, hunger, bowel movements, etc.
(1) fairly regular (2) variable
(3) fairly irregular

III. *Adaptability to change in routine*—the ease or difficulty with which initial response can be modified in socially desirable way.
(1) generally acceptable (2) variable (3) generally slow at adaptation

IV. *Response to new situations*—initial reaction to new stimuli, to food, people, places, toys, or procedures:
(1) approach (2) variable
(3) withdrawal

V. *Level of sensory threshold*—the amount of external stimulation, such as sounds or changes in food or people, necessary to produce a response in the baby.
(1) high threshold (much stimulation needed)
(2) medium
(3) low threshold (little stimulation)

VI. *Intensity of response*—the energy content of responses regardless of their quality.
(1) generally intense (2) variable
(3) generally mild

VII. *Positive or negative mood*—amount of pleasant or unpleasant behavior throughout day.
(1) generally positive (2) variable
(3) generally negative

VIII. *Distractibility*—the effectiveness of external stimuli (sounds, toys, people, etc.) in interfering with ongoing behavior.
(1) easily distractible (2) variable
(3) non-distractible

IX. *Persistence and attention span*—duration of maintaining specific activities with or without external obstacles.
(1) persistent (2) variable
(3) non-persistent

C. How has the baby's temperament been a problem for you?

D. In general, temperament of baby is:
(a) about average
(b) more difficult than average
(c) easier than average

Sample items by category from the Revised Infant Temperament Questionnaire

The mother rates each of the following items as follows:

Almost Never 1	2	3	4	5	Almost Always 6

Category	Description
1. Activity	The infant moves about much (kicks, grabs, squirms) during diapering and dressing. The infant plays actively with parents—much movement of arms, legs, body.
2. Rhythmicity	The infant wants and takes milk feedings at about the same times (within one hour) from day to day. The infant's bowel movements come at different times day to day (over one hour's difference).
3. Approach	The infant accepts right away any change in place or position of feeding or person giving it. For the first few minutes in a new place or situation (new store or home), the infant is fretful.
4. Adaptability	The infant objects to being bathed in a different place or by a different person, even after two or three tries. The infant accepts regular procedures (hair brushing, face washing, etc.) any time without protest.
5. Intensity	The infant reacts strongly to foods, whether positively (smacks lips, laughs, squeals) or negatively (cries). The infant reacts mildly to meeting familiar people (quiet smiles or no response).

Table 21-10. *Continued*

Category	Description
6. Mood	The infant is pleasant (smiles, laughs) when first arriving in unfamiliar places (friend's house, store). The infant cries when left to play alone.
7. Persistence	The infant amuses self for half an hour or more in crib or playpen (looking at mobile, playing with toy). The infant watches other children playing for under a minute and then looks elsewhere.
8. Distractibility	The infant stops play and watches when someone walks by. The infant continues to cry in spite of several minutes of soothing.
9. Threshold	The infant reacts even to a gentle touch (startle, wriggle, laugh, cry). The infant reacts to a disliked food even if it is mixed with a preferred one.

From "Revision of the Infant Temperament Questionnaire," by W. B. Carey and S. C. McDevitt, *Pediatrics*, 1978, 61:735–739.

are those of affect, orientation, memory, knowledge, calculations, generalizations, judgment, and abstract thinking.

Affect

The normal infant's affect will be identifiable at approximately 3 months of age when smiles and laughs appear as a response to stimuli. Gradually additional emotional responses will appropriately be added to the child's repertoire. The toddler or preschool child presents affect that matches with his verbal and nonverbal communication. The school-age or adolescent youth demonstrates congruency between thought, interaction content, and verbalizations.

Orientation

Orientation to person, place, and time—as we think of it when testing the adult—begins to emerge in the toddler stage when the child is generally able to state his first name. The preschooler is able to state his first and last name and those of others. The school-age child, and many times the preschooler, is able to identify place and time or season of the year. The school-age child and older is able to state the date (day, month, and year).

Memory

Memory for the 6-month-old infant manifests itself as signs of recognition of familiar faces and persons and signs of differentiation of strangers from known persons. At 9 months of age the infant can repeat remembered activities such as wave bye-bye or play pat-a-cake. As the child ages, he is readily able to remember and imitate behaviors by the age of 1–2 years. The 2- to 4-year-old child has recent memory recall when tested similar to the adult. The school-age child and older normally has no difficulty with either recent or remote memory.

Knowledge and Its Application

When you are assessing knowledge level, calculations, judgment, generalization, and abstract thinking of the child, Piaget's stages of cognitive development are helpful. Table 21-12 presents the major abilities within each stage. Generally the preschool child understands such concepts as hungry, thirsty, tired, and parts of the body; he recognizes colors and is able to count numbers in correct sequence. The school-age child's cognitive capabilities are able to be tested in the same manner as an adult's (see Chapter 5).

Table 21-13 gives helpful guidelines to identify mental health dysfunction in the child and to differentiate characteristics common to the abnormal mental functioning of a child who is autistic, mentally retarded, or suffering from brain dysfunction.

Table 21-11. Developmental Tasks in Ten Categories of Behavior from Birth to Late Adolescence

	Infancy (birth to 1 or 2)	Early childhood (2–3 to 5–6–7)	Late childhood (5–6–7 to pubescence)	Early adolescence (pubescence to puberty)	Late adolescence (puberty to early maturity)
I. Achieving an appropriate dependence-independence pattern	1. Establishing oneself as a very dependent being 2. Beginning establishment of self-awareness	1. Adjusting to less private attention; becoming independent physically (while remaining strongly dependent emotionally)	1. Freeing oneself from primary identification with adults	1. Establishing one's independence from adults in all areas of behavior	1. Establishing oneself as an independent individual in an adult manner
II. Achieving an appropriate giving-receiving pattern of affection	1. Developing a feeling for affection	1. Developing ability to give affection 2. Learning to share affection	1. Learning to give as much love as one receives; forming friendships with peers	1. Accepting oneself as a worthwhile person really worthy of love	1. Building a strong mutual affectional bond with a (possible) marriage partner
III. Relating to changing social groups	1. Becoming aware of alive as against inanimate, and familiar as against unfamiliar 2. Developing rudimentary social interaction	1. Beginning to develop ability to interact with age-mates 2. Adjusting in family to expectations it has for the child as a member of social unit	1. Clarifying adult world as over against child's world 2. Establishing peer groupness and learning to belong	1. Behaving according to a shifting peer code	1. Adopting an adult-patterned set of social values by learning a new peer code
IV. Developing a conscience	1. Beginning to adjust to expectations of others	1. Developing ability to take directions and to be obedient in presence of authority 2. Developing ability to be obedient in absence of authority where conscience substitutes for authority	1. Learning more rules and developing true morality		1. Learning to verbalize contradictions in moral codes, as well as discrepancies between principle and practice, and resolving these problems in a responsible manner

From Lida F. Thompson, Michael H. Miller, and Helen F. Bigler, *Sociology—Nurses and Their Patients in a Modern Society,* 9th ed. (St. Louis: C. V. Mosby, 1975).

Table 21-11. *Continued*

	Infancy (birth to 1 or 2)	Early childhood (2–3 to 5–6–7)	Late childhood (5–6–7 to pubescence)	Early adolescence (pubescence to puberty)	Late adolescence (puberty to early maturity)
V. Learning one's psychosocio-biological sex role		1. Learning to identify with male adult and female adult roles	1. Beginning to identify with one's social contemporaries of same sex	1. Strong identification with one's own sex mates 2. Learning one's role in heterosexual relationships	1. Exploring possibilities for a future mate and acquiring "desirability" 2. Choosing an occupation 3. Preparing to accept one's future role in manhood or womanhood as a responsible citizen of larger community
VI. Accepting and adjusting to a changing body	1. Adjusting to adult feeding demands 2. Adjusting to adult cleanliness demands 3. Adjusting to adult attitudes toward genital manipulation	1. Adjusting to expectations resulting from one's improving muscular abilities 2. Developing sex modesty		1. Reorganizing one's thoughts and feelings about oneself in face of significant bodily changes and their concomitants 2. Accepting reality of one's appearance	1. Learning appropriate outlets for sexual drives
VII. Managing a changing body and learning new motor patterns	1. Developing physiological equilibrium 2. Developing eye-hand coordination 3. Establishing satisfactory rhythms of rest and activity	1. Developing large muscle control 2. Learning to coordinate large muscles and small muscles	1. Refining and elaborating skill in use of small muscles	1. Controlling and using a "new" body	

(*continued on page 496*)

Table 21-11. *Continued*

	Infancy (birth to 1 or 2)	Early childhood (2–3 to 5–6–7)	Late childhood (5–6–7 to pubescence)	Early adolescence (pubescence to puberty)	Late adolescence (puberty to early maturity)
VIII. Learning to understand and control the physical world	1. Exploring physical world	1. Meeting adult expectations for restrictive exploration and manipulation of an expanding environment	1. Learning more realistic ways of studying and controlling physical world		
IX. Developing an appropriate symbol system and conceptual abilities	1. Developing preverbal communication 2. Developing verbal communication 3. Rudimentary concept formation	1. Improving one's use of symbol system 2. Enormous elaboration of concept pattern	1. Learning to use language actually to exchange ideas or to influence one's hearers 2. Beginning understanding of real causal relations 3. Making finer conceptual distinctions and thinking reflectively	1. Using language to express and to clarify more complex concepts 2. Moving from the concrete to the abstract and applying general principles to the particular	1. Achieving level of reasoning of which one is capable
X. Relating oneself to the cosmos		1. Developing a genuine, though uncritical, notion about one's place in the cosmos	1. Developing a scientific approach		1. Formulating a workable belief and value system

Table 21-12. Piaget's Stages of Cognitive Development

Stages	Major abilities
Sensorimotor (birth–2 years)	The child progresses from instinctive, reflexive behavior to that of organizing his experiences and moving toward intentional behaviors. He develops the ability to differentiate himself from his environment and to anticipate consequences as a result of his behavior (cause and effect).
Preoperational (2½–7 years)	The child's memory and anticipation abilities expand. Preconceptual thinking emerges, wherein each object and event is dealt with separately; usually one dimension is focused upon, and others are ignored. This applies to the self also—the child is egocentric and is unable to empathize with another person.
Concrete operational (7–11 years)	Ability to perform intellectual operations is present. The child can consider several dimensions of an object or event; he can retrace steps and make conclusions and correct himself. He is able to understand the other person's point of view. He is able to conceptualize numbers, sequencing, mass, and categories.
Formal operational (12 years and older)	The adolescent is able to think abstractly, hypothesize, and test hypotheses through logic; symbolic logic becomes the primary pattern of problem solving.

Table 21-13. How to Differentiate Organic from Genetic Difficulties

Measure	Autism	Mental retardation	Brain dysfunction
Intellectual function	Usually functions below age level in all areas, but performance levels are inconsistent; may show potential in good memory	Deficit levels are uniform and consistent—level depends on degree of retardation	Wide range, but generally normal potential
Tests that help decide	Hard to test	IQ test	EEG, psychology, Ritalin
Speech	Lack of speech, echolalia; wooden, flat speech; pause in phrases and sentences	Delayed development, degree depending on degree of retardation	Normal for age—there may be articulation difficulties
Motor coordination	Usually good	Poor in both gross and fine motor, related to degree of retardation	Poor in both gross and fine motor
Physical appearance	Healthy, often intelligent looking	Physically underdeveloped, delayed milestones, such as walking	Usually normal
Perception	Often use only one sense for recognizing objects	Impaired in the severely retarded	Higher sensory CNS functions, such as auditory discrimination, are affected
Behavior	Withdrawn, ritualistic	Normal to sluggish, depending on degree of retardation; possibly aggressive outbursts	Hyperactive, aggressive, low attention span; responds well to medication, especially to amphetamines
Ego functions	Severely impaired; lack of reality testing; preoccupied	Fairly normal, but low frustration tolerance	Low frustration tolerance

From V. Whillam, "The Autistic Child," *Canadian Nurse*, 66 (November 1970), 44–47.

General Impression

The general impression for the child and adolescent includes the essential components as previously discussed in Chapter 8. The major differences from that of the adult are the ranges of norm according to age for the vital signs and height and weight. Also, chest and abdominal circumferences are routinely measured until approximately age 2–2½ years.

Height and Weight

The height of toddlers and younger children is measured with the child lying down (see Figure 21-3). The preschool and older child are measured as they stand with their shoulders and heels against a calibrated measure on a wall (see Figure 21-4). For measuring the child's weight, a beam balance scale is preferably used.

Height and weight are generally recorded in centimeters and kilograms, respectively. Table 21-14 provides an English (feet, inches, and pounds) measurement reference for metric equivalents. Figures 21-5 to 21-8 show the average growth for males and females from birth to 36 months and from 2 to 18 years. Some children will consistently fall within a certain percentile, suggesting a lag in growth, below the 5th percentile, or excessive growth rate, above the 95th percentile. This may or may not constitute a growth problem; family genetic background must be investigated. It may be that parents and ancestors have all been small or very tall. Further assessment is needed when you note a

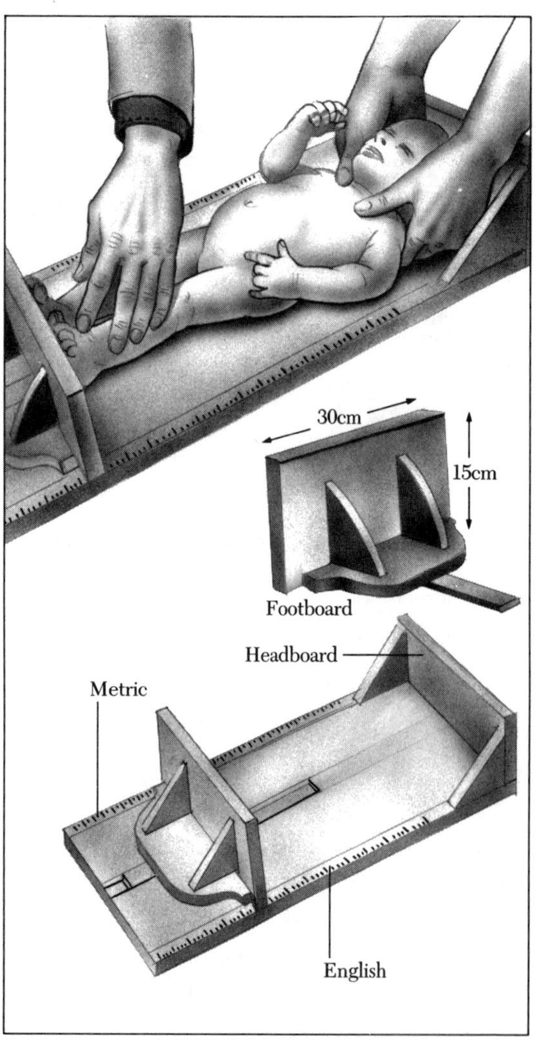

Figure 21-3 The proper way to measure the length of a child under 3 years old.

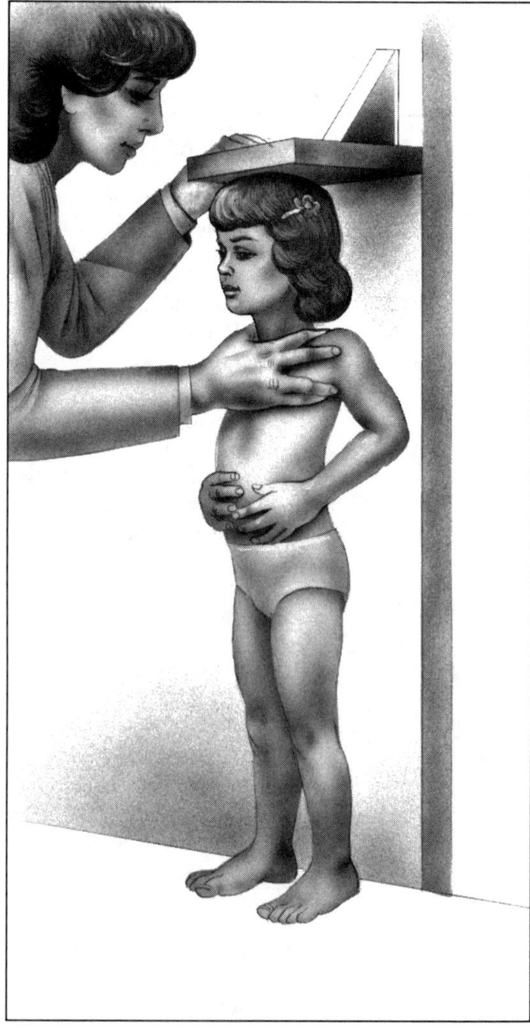

Figure 21-4 The proper way to measure the height of a child older than 3 years.

Table 21-14. Conversions of Metric Measures for Weight and Height

Pounds to kilograms (for weight reference)

Pounds	Kilograms	Pounds	Kilograms	Pounds	Kilograms	Pounds	Kilograms	Pounds	Kilograms
5	2.3	50	22.7	95	43.1	140	63.5	185	83.9
10	4.5	55	25.0	100	45.4	145	65.8	190	86.2
15	6.8	60	27.2	105	47.6	150	68.0	195	88.5
20	9.1	65	29.5	110	49.9	155	70.3	200	90.7
25	11.3	70	31.7	115	52.2	160	72.6	205	93.0
30	13.6	75	34.0	120	54.4	165	74.8	210	95.3
35	15.9	80	36.3	125	56.7	170	77.1	215	97.5
40	18.1	85	38.6	130	58.9	175	79.4	220	99.8
45	20.4	90	40.8	135	61.2	180	81.6		

Feet and inches to centimeters (for height reference)

Feet and inches	Centimeters	Feet and inches	Centimeters	Feet and inches	Centimeters	Feet and inches	Centimeters	Feet and inches	Centimeters
0 6	15.2	2 4	71.1	3 4	101.6	4 4	132.0	5 4	162.6
1 0	30.5	2 5	73.6	3 5	104.1	4 5	134.6	5 5	165.1
1 6	45.7	2 6	76.1	3 6	106.6	4 6	137.1	5 6	167.6
1 7	48.3	2 7	78.7	3 7	109.2	4 7	139.6	5 7	170.2
1 8	50.8	2 8	81.2	3 8	111.7	4 8	142.2	5 8	172.7
1 9	53.3	2 9	83.8	3 9	114.2	4 9	144.7	5 9	175.3
1 10	55.9	2 10	86.3	3 10	116.8	4 10	147.3	5 10	177.8
1 11	58.4	2 11	88.8	3 11	119.3	4 11	149.8	5 11	180.3
2 0	61.0	3 0	91.4	4 0	121.9	5 0	152.4	6 0	182.9
2 1	63.5	3 1	93.9	4 1	124.4	5 1	154.9	6 1	185.4
2 2	66.0	3 2	96.4	4 2	127.0	5 2	157.5	6 2	188.0
2 3	68.6	3 3	99.0	4 3	129.5	5 3	160.0	6 3	190.5

child's measurement pattern is reflecting a gradual consistent decline or progression from his usual percentile level.

Routinely the child's head is measured on each visit and is recorded on standardized head growth charts, which facilitate assessment of whether growth is proceeding at a normal pace or whether there is inadequate growth (microcephaly) or excessive growth (macrocephaly).

The proper technique for measuring the head is to use a metal or paper tape, as a cloth tape tends to become stretched with use (see Chapter 20, "Assessment of the Head, Face, and Neck"). This measurement is called the occipitofrontal circumference (OFC). The measurement of the head circumference is generally performed on each assessment until the child is 2 years old. Two other body circumferences to be measured are the chest and the abdomen. The chest span is measured at the nipple level, and the abdomen is measured at the level of the umbilicus. Table 21-15 lists the mean head, chest, and abdominal circumferences in the various age groups.

Temperature

The usual method of measuring the body temperature in the infant and very young child is by axillary or rectal thermometer. With a rectal temperature measurement, the thermometer is

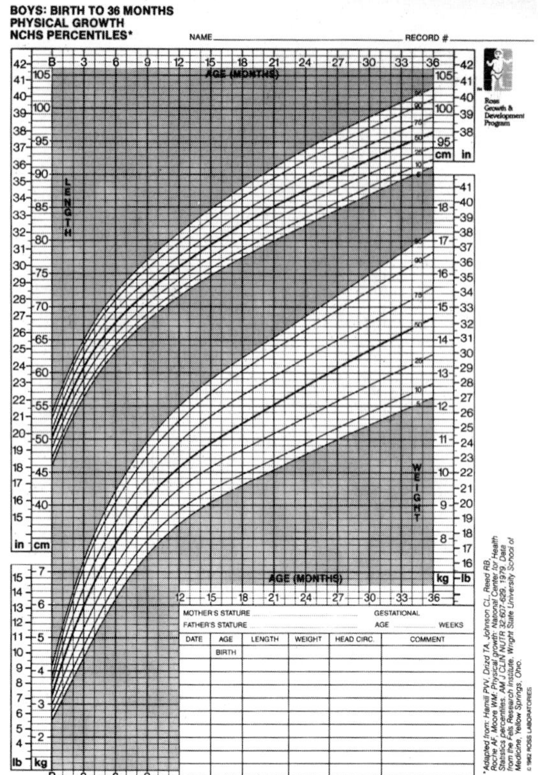

Figure 21-5 Physical growth chart for boys, birth to 36 months.

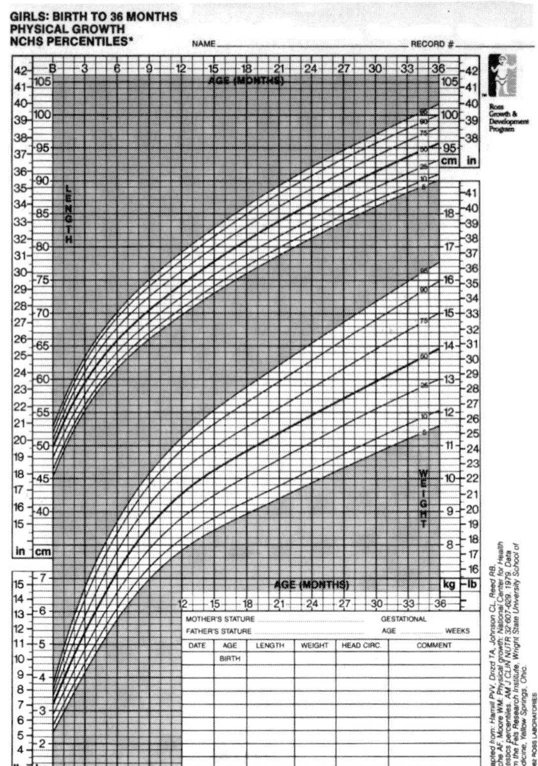

Figure 21-6 Physical growth chart for girls, birth to 36 months.

inserted just immediately inside the anus. Keep in mind that the infant's rectum is very short, and the danger of perforating the rectum is a reality. When the child reaches age 4–5 years, an oral temperature reading can be obtained safely and accurately. The child's normal temperature is usually higher than that of the adult; thus, a temperature as high as 100°F (37.8°C) is considered high normal range in a child. As you take the child's temperature, you can also teach

Table 21-15. Average Head, Chest, and Abdominal Circumference in Centimeters by Age

	Boys			Girls		
Age	**Head**	**Chest**	**Abdomen**	**Head**	**Chest**	**Abdomen**
Newborn	35.3	33.2	—	34.7	32.9	—
3 months	40.9	40.6	38.5	40.0	39.8	38.4
6 months	43.9	43.7	41.4	42.8	43.0	41.4
9 months	46.0	46.0	43.4	44.6	45.4	43.4
12 months	47.3	47.6	44.6	45.8	47.0	44.5
15 months	48.0	48.6	45.1	46.5	47.9	45.0
18 months	48.7	49.5	45.5	47.1	48.8	45.5
2 years	49.7	50.8	46.2	48.1	50.1	46.3
2½ years	50.2	51.7	46.7	48.8	51.2	47.0
3 years	50.4	52.4	47.2	49.3	51.9	47.7

From Victor C. Vaughan and R. James McKay, *Nelson Textbook of Pediatrics*, 10th ed. © 1975 by the W. B. Saunders Co., Philadelphia, pp. 46, 47.

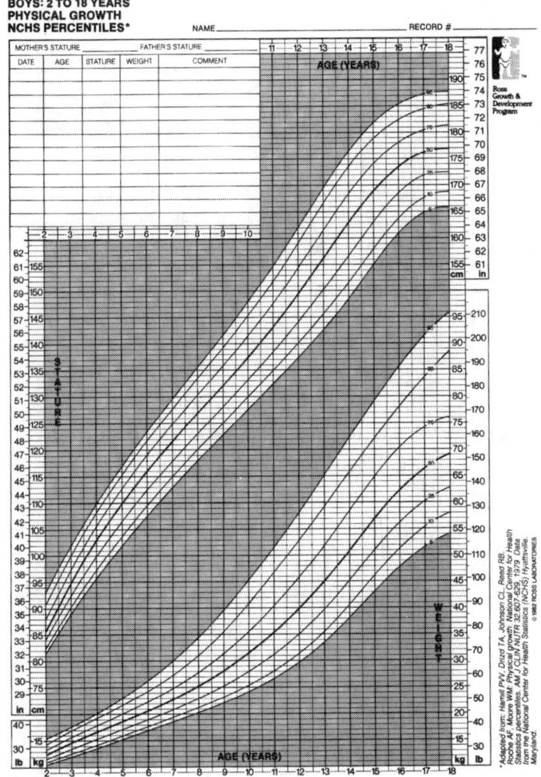

Figure 21-7 Physical growth chart for boys, 2 to 18 years.

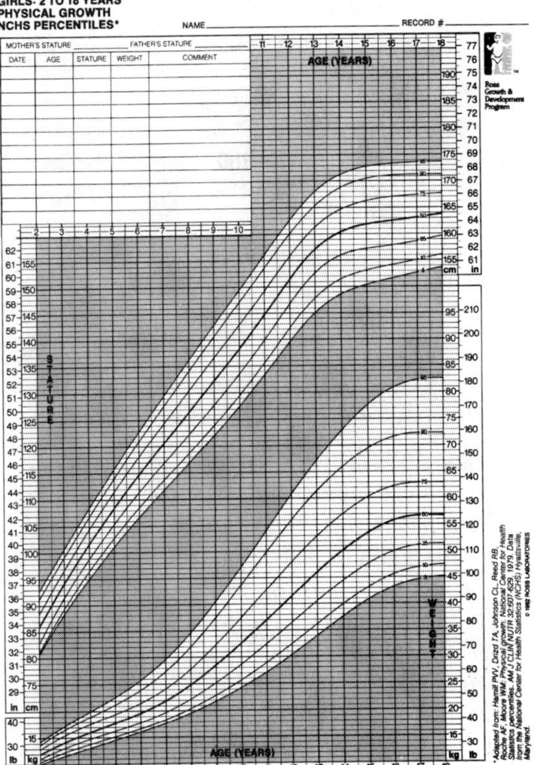

Figure 21-8 Physical growth chart for girls, 2 to 18 years.

the parents how to perform this procedure and read the thermometer, if they do not already know how.

To convert Celsius degrees to Fahrenheit, multiply by 9/5 and add 32:

$$37.8°C = (37.8 \times 9/5 + 32)F$$
$$= (68 + 32)F = 100.05°F$$

To convert Fahrenheit degrees to Celsius, subtract 32 and multiply by 5/9:

$$100° F = (100 - 32) \times 5/9\ C$$
$$= 68 \times 5/9\ C = 37.75°C$$

Pulse and Respirations

The average rates of pulse and respirations differ with each age level. The normal ranges for the various ages are delineated in Table 21-16. If these two parameters are assessed while the child is crying, fearful, excited, or upset in any way, neither will reflect the norm status. The pulse is generally taken radially in the older child and adolescent; however, an apical pulse is more accurate for the infant and young child, because children at these ages normally have a rapid heart rate. An apical measurement is also much more accurate if arrhythmias are present. The apex of the heart in the young child and infant is best heard with the bell of the stethoscope or a small diaphragm head placed in the third intercostal space near the left sternal border.

Blood Pressure

Take the child's blood pressure at the earliest age possible. It is routinely done on all preschool children and older. The child's arm is much smaller than the adult's; therefore, cuff size is important to ensure a correct reading. The cuff must cover two-thirds of the length of the upper arm and should encircle the arm without a copious amount of overlapping and bulk. The flush method for blood pressure measurement for newborns or infants is described in Chapter 8. The values of blood pressure norms differ according to age. They are presented in Table 21-16.

Table 21-16. Norms for Vital Signs in Children

Vital signs	0–1 year	1–2 years	2–3 years	3–4 years
Blood pressure	90 ± 25 systolic 61 ± 19 diastolic	96 ± 27 systolic 65 ± 27 diastolic	95 ± 24 systolic 61 ± 24 diastolic	99 ± 23 systolic 65 ± 19 diastolic
Pulse	70–180	80–140	80–140	80–120
Temperature	99.6F rectal 98.6F oral 97.4F axillary	99.6F rectal 98.6F oral 97.4F axillary	99.6F rectal 98.6F oral 97.4F axillary	99.6F rectal 98.6F oral 97.4F axillary
Respirations	30–40	28–32	28–32	24–28

Approach to the Physical Examination

The approach to the physical examination of the child and adolescent differs with the client's level of cognitive development. The examination of the infant over 6 months of age and the young child is usually performed with the parent present, and most of the examination can take place with the child in the parent's arms or on the parent's lap. While the infant is asleep or contented in the parent's arms, the nurse can note skin color and respirations, because touching the infant generally startles him. When palpation is begun, the infant may begin to cry. With crying the skin color takes on a red-purplish haze, which under ordinary circumstances would be an abnormal finding, and the normal rate and depth of the respirations would then be impossible to assess. It is best to auscultate the heart and lungs of the infant during the initial period also because it is very difficult, if not almost impossible, to do so once the infant is crying (see Figure 21-9).

Provision of comfort for the young child may involve allowing him to keep a security object during the examination; this is particularly comforting for the 1- to 3-year-old. The child of this age group generally will move freely about the room with the attitude of exploration, making it quite easy to assess general appearance and psychomotor skills before touching the child.

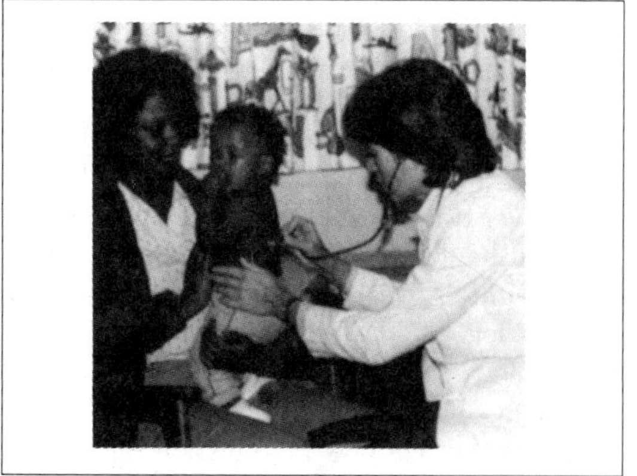

Figure 21-9 Initially auscultate the heart and lungs.

It is best to begin the examination without the use of instruments and to examine the nonvulnerable areas such as the extremities and the abdomen. The more invasive areas of the head—ears, nose, and mouth—are assessed last in the toddler and preschooler (3–6 years). Table 21-17 presents a schema of approaches to the physical assessment of the child at the various age levels. If at any time the child starts to cry during the examination, this may be the most opportune time to inspect the oropharynx.

Have the preschooler sit on the side of the examining table, chair, or bed during the examination. In this position he can see his parent at all times. This decreases the fear of abandonment and the continuous wiggling to keep an eye on the parent, which many times happens when you have the child lying down on the table. Also from the lying-down position the perspective of you is that of a towering, looming giant.

Constant attentiveness is a must when working with infants and children. Do not turn your back to an infant or child and assume that he is too small, weak, or ill to turn over and fall off the table. Also infants and young children are curious and have quick little arms and hands; therefore, needles, pins, scissors, medications, solutions, hot objects, and the like need to be kept out of their reach.

When examining the child, gradually introduce instruments in a playful manner. Demonstrating the procedures on yourself and blowing out the examining light are effective approaches. You can use the stethoscope like a telephone and allow the child to handle it, thus reinforcing a

Table 21-17. Approaches to Physical Examination of Child by Developmental Level

Newborn	Infant	Toddler	Preschool child	School-age child	Adolescent
Perform most of exam while baby is held by parent.	Perform most of exam while baby is held by parent.	Begin with nonthreatening interactions first, such as DDST.	Begin with nonthreatening interactions, such as DDST.	Show equipment and explain its use.	Show equipment and explain its use.
Avoid abrupt, sudden movements that may startle baby.	Avoid abrupt, sudden movements that may startle baby.	Examine child while child is standing near parent or on parent's lap.	Allow child opportunity to play with some equipment, such as stethoscope.	Allow child opportunity to ask questions and discuss feelings about examination.	Discuss adolescent's questions and feelings about examination.
Avoid prolonged exposure of baby to cool environment.	Use toys, pacifier, or bottle to distract baby. Parent can assist with distraction.	Use toys or simple games to distract child. Parent can assist with distraction.	Allow child opportunity to ask questions and state feelings.	Give concrete answers to questions.	Describe how body functions during examination.
Perform intrusive tasks, such as taking rectal temperature or examining ears, after less intrusive ones, such as assessing heart and breath sounds.	Perform intrusive tasks, such as taking rectal temperature or examining ears, after less intrusive ones, such as assessing heart and breath sounds.	Perform intrusive tasks, such as taking rectal temperature or examining ears, after less intrusive ones, such as assessing heart and breath sounds.	Give simple, honest answers to questions. Indicate how and when child may help during examination.	Determine if child will be more comfortable with parent present or absent during examination.	Perform examination while parent is not in the room.
Examine skin color, respirations, and heart rate while baby is quiet or asleep.	Examine skin color, respirations, and heart rate while baby is quiet or asleep.	Use words that will decrease fantasies (*measure* blood pressure instead of *take*).	Use words that will decrease fantasies (*measure* blood pressure instead of *take*).	Indicate how and when child may help during examination.	Indicate how and when adolescent may help during examination.
Talk to baby in soothing voice.	Talk to baby in soothing voice.	Offer limited choices when appropriate. Provide an opportunity for child to play with or handle some equipment, such as stethoscope. Remove one article of clothing at a time. Have parent assist child. Give simple directions. Demonstrate techniques on a doll, parent, or older sibling. Measure rectal temperature and examine genital area last.	Give simple explanations and feedback during examination. Provide privacy while child undresses. Allow child to leave underwear on until it is necessary to examine covered areas. Demonstrate techniques on a doll, parent, or older sibling. Measure rectal temperature and examine genital area last.	Describe how body functions during examination. Provide privacy while child undresses. Allow child to leave underwear on until it is necessary to examine covered areas. Examine genital area last.	Provide privacy while adolescent undresses. Examine genital area last.

Sources: Fernholt, J. D., 1980; Hansen, B., and Evans, M., 1981; Yoos, L., 1981.

trusting relationship by showing the harmlessness of the instrument.

The early adolescent (12–14 years) is easily embarrassed and is experiencing ambivalent feelings regarding the rapid changes taking place in his body appearance. Providing privacy indicates that you have respect and are thoughtful concerning the adolescent's difficulty with accepting his newly developing body. The male client should be permitted to keep his undershorts on through most of the examination, and the female client should be allowed to keep on the undershirt or bra and underpants and remove them only for the amount of time it takes to examine the breast and the genital-rectal areas. At the time of examination of these areas the client must be carefully and adequately draped. Important health teaching can occur at this time. Privacy also decreases the potential for humiliation in front of others if a procedure or treatment causes discomfort and crying. All clients, regardless of age, appreciate honesty regarding uncomfortableness of procedures, because the client can anticipate and bolster himself to better withstand the discomfort.

The sequence of physical assessment of the school-age child and adolescent proceeds systematically and follows that used for the adult; you begin with the examination of the head and end with the genitourinary system and rectal examination.

Skin

When assessing the skin of the child and adolescent, follow the same indices as for assessing the skin in the adult. Skin turgor is best assessed on the infant's abdomen. In the child the common findings of play injuries are cuts and abrasions. Also frequently observed are the lesions characteristic of the common childhood diseases, such as vesicles of measles. The high production of the pituitary hormones influences the changes evidenced in the skin of the adolescent. There is generally some increase in pigmentation, a change in fat distribution, and the appearance of body hair growth reflective of secondary sexual characteristics. The most common integumentary problem of the teenager is acne.

Head

Inspect the fontanelles. They should not be bulging or sunken or show marked pulsation. The anterior fontanelle is open in the infant and ranges from 4 to 6 cm in diameter. The anterior fontanelle is normally closed by the age of 18 months. The posterior fontanelle is open and ranges in diameter from 0.5 to 2 cm. It generally closes by 2 months of age.

Ears

Note placement of the ears. The external ear is inspected and palpated. In the infant and toddler hearing acuity is assessed by observing the child as you talk and watching to see the response. For instance, does the child look toward you? With the very young infant you may wish to use a rattle to see whether the sound attracts the infant's attention. However, the reliability of testing hearing by observing response to sound is poor before 9 months of age.

If you can gain the cooperation of the child, a 3-year-old usually can identify what is being heard in response to the Weber and Rinne Tests (see "Characteristics and Techniques of Examination [of the Ear]" in Chapter 12).

The examination of the auditory canal and tympanic membrane in the newborn and young child must be done carefully. The least bit of movement may result in the speculum injuring the walls of the canal or the tympanic membrane itself. Therefore, positioning of the child is very important. With a very small child who is clinging to the parent, the best position may be for the parent to hold the child upright with the child's head turned sideways and held against the parent's chest or shoulder (see Figure 21-10). Another helpful position for maintaining limited motion of the child's head is the prone position with the head turned to the side to facilitate examination. The child can be placed prone on the parent's lap, on a bed, or on an examining table (see Figure 21-11). If the parent is useful in calming the child, he or she can stand near the head of the bed or table within the child's view and close enough to offer a stroking, soothing touch if needed.

Because of the angle of the child's auditory canal, the pinna must be pulled downward and slightly back to straighten the canal for easy insertion of the speculum and visualization of the tympanic membrane. The handle of the otoscope is held in the upward position, and the ulnar surface of the hand holding the otoscope is placed firmly against the side of the child's head just above the ear (see Figure 21-12).

The light reflex of the tympanic membrane in

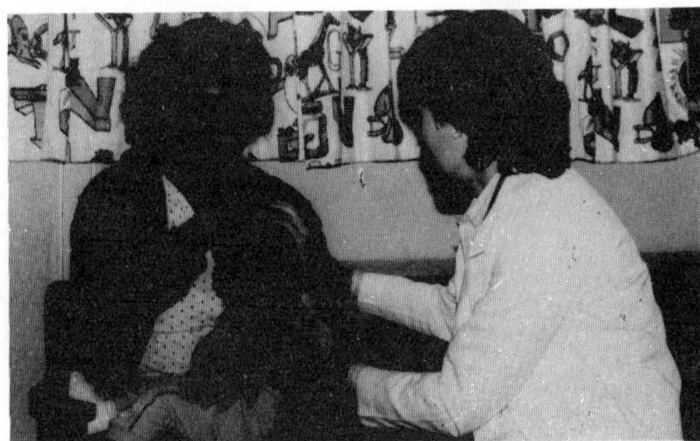

Figure 21-10 Position for holding child to facilitate ear exam.

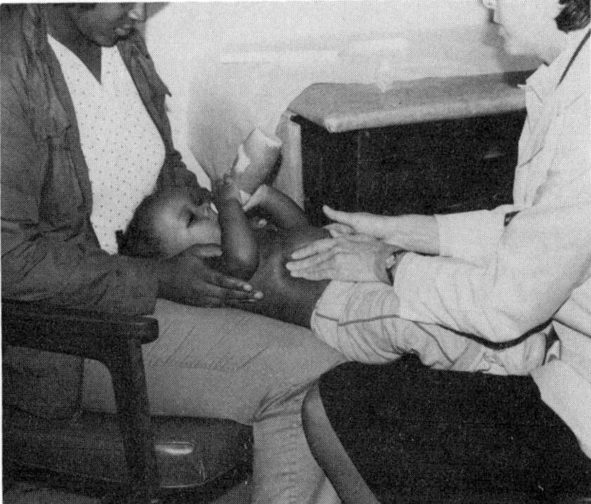

Figure 21-11 Security for the child during an exam is found on the mother's lap.

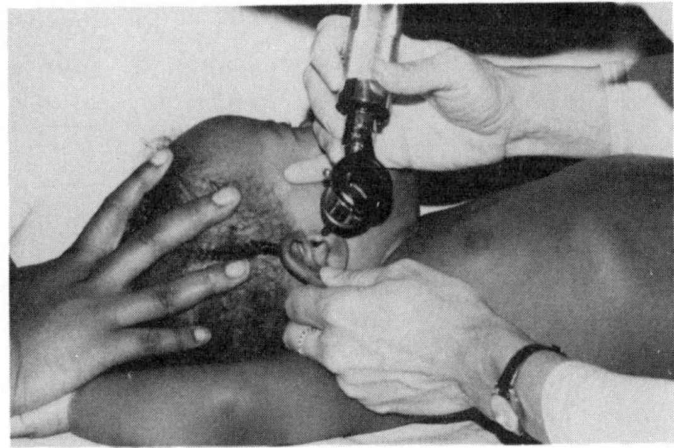

Figure 21-12 Safety position that allows otoscope to move with any turning of the child's head.

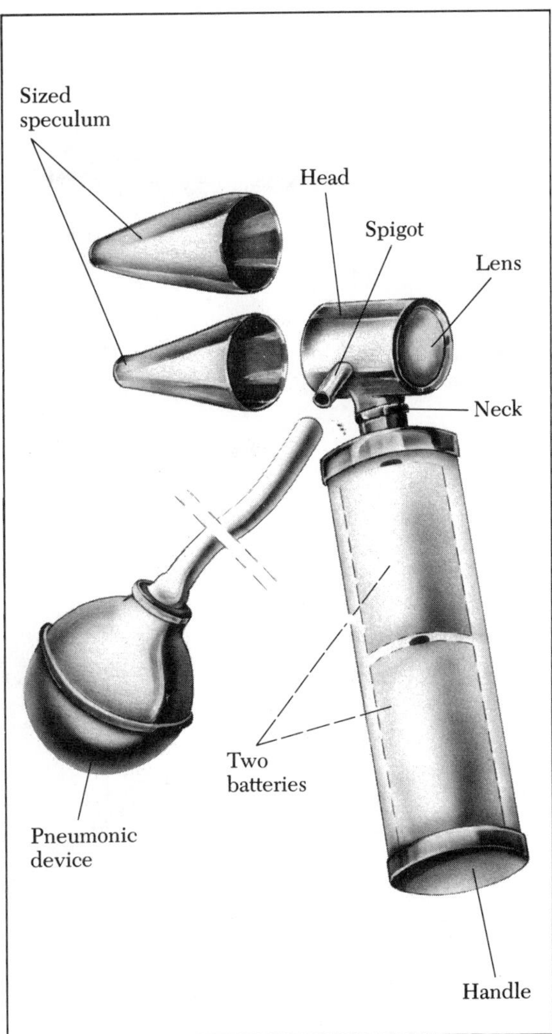

Figure 21-13 Pneumatic otoscope.

the child is more diffuse than that of an adult because of the shortened, "straight-shot" characteristics of the auditory canal compared to the longer and more angulated canal of the adult. Should you have some doubts as to whether the physical findings of the otoscope examination of the child are within the norm, the movability of the drum warrants evaluation. This is accomplished by the use of a pneumatic otoscope—an otoscope with a bulb attached, which enables you to direct a gentle air current toward the drum (see Figure 21-13). The tympanic membrane normally will vibrate. The absence of movability can indicate dysfunction, and the child should be referred for further medical evaluation.

Eyes

In children it is important to observe the angle of eye placement. An upward slanting of the eyes may be indicative of a chromosomal abnormality, but it can also be a racial or genetic characteristic.

The sclerae are normally white, and the clarity of the corneas are checked by use of tangen-

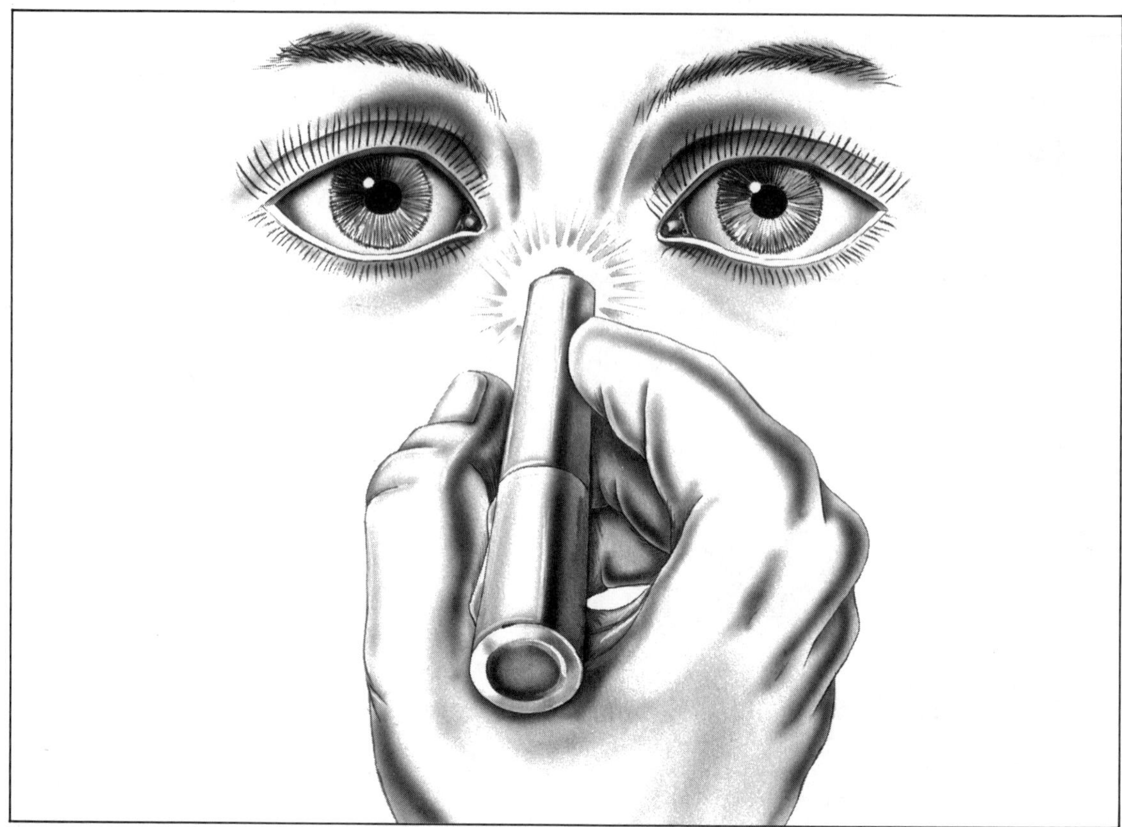

Figure 21-14 The Hirschberg test involves shining light into eyes from 1–2 feet away.

tial lighting of a penlight. The pupils of the child compared to those of the adult are larger. With aging the size of the pupils normally decreases and is miotic in the older adult. The pupils normally react to direct light and display consensual reaction. The pupils are also round and of equal size.

You would not expect to see the infant's eyes converge on an object as it is brought toward the nose until the child is about 3 months old. Also, when testing tracking or the extraocular muscle movements (EOMs), you would not observe conjugate movement of the eyes until the infant is approximately 6 months old. Then the paired or joined movement of the eyes will be only with slow-moving objects.

Hirschberg's test is helpful to assess the position of the eyes. While the child looks straight ahead, a light is shone into the eyes from a distance of 1–2 feet (see Figure 21-14). This is best done in a dimly lit room. The light reflected from the eyes normally is in the same position on each eye. If there is a positional deviation of one eye, the light reflex will be asymmetrical. Note the displaced light reflex in Figure 21-15.

The cover test is another method of assessing eye position. This method can be used with children over 6 months old. An object is held approximately 1 foot away from the child, and the child is allowed time to focus upon it. Then a cover is held in front of one eye for several seconds; care is taken not to touch the child or the eyelashes. The cover is then quickly removed, and the eye that was covered is observed for any jerky movements, deviation, and movements to refocus on the object. These latter movements are suggestive of strabismus. The presence of strabismus warrants prompt referral to an ophthalmologist. The cover test is generally successfully used with the toddler and preschool child.

Visual acuity is difficult to assess in the infant. An infant 2 months old will look at objects, but if an object is moved out of the central field of vision, the infant will not move his head to follow it. The 3-month-old infant will follow objects with his eyes and the turning of his head.

To screen the vision of the infant and toddler (6 months to 3 years old), use the fixation test. Cover one of the child's eyes and hold a penlight

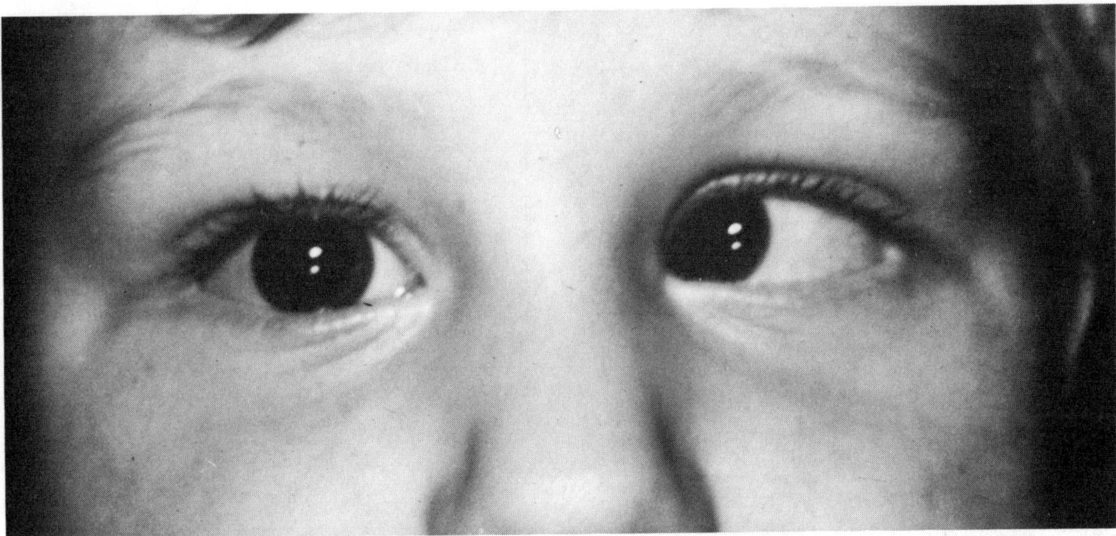

Figure 21-15 Convergent squint of left eye. Note asymmetry of light reflection.

at a distance of 1½ feet; move the light from a midline position to the right and then to the left. Then cover the other eye and repeat the process. The child will normally track the light. If the child loses interest in the light, use a spinning toy to attract attention. If the child does not track with either eye, the test is failed.

For children 2½ to 3 years old, use the picture vision card test included in the Denver Developmental Screening Test kit. First, ascertain that the child knows the name of each picture. Then give the child a 15-foot string and ask him to walk that distance away from you. Test one eye at a time. Tell the child to place the plastic eye cover over one eye. Then present five pictures; the child normally should be able to identify at least three with each eye.

For children under 7 years old and illiterate persons who are unable to read letters as on the Snellen letter eye chart, you can use a Snellen symbol eye chart for distant vision screening. *E*'s in various sizes and positions are on the chart. Ask the client to point in the same direction the "fingers" or the "legs" of the table are pointing. Test each eye separately. A child stands 15 feet from the chart, while an adult would stand 20 feet away. The scoring is the same as for the conventional Snellen chart (see Figure 21-16).

A 20/30 vision is normal for children between the ages of 4 and 8. Children age 9 and older test out normally at approximately 20/20. If visual acuity is questionable, referral for further evaluation and ophthalmoscopic examination of the eyegrounds by an expert is warranted.

Visual fields of the preschool child and older are tested in the same manner as for the adult (see "Visual Fields" in Chapter 11). The same indices of fundoscopic examination are assessed in the child as in the adult (see "Ophthalmoscopic Examinations" in Chapter 11), except the retinal background of the child will present highlights (shiny light reflections) as the light of the ophthalmoscope falls upon it.

Nose

The patency of the nares is assessed in the child by occluding one naris at a time and instructing the child to blow through his nose. A partially occluded naris will produce a higher pitch with forced nasal expiration compared to a nonoccluded naris; you may encounter this finding frequently, as toddlers and preschool children have a tendency to stick small objects in their body orifices.

Testing of the olfactory nerve (cranial nerve I) is not very reliable in the preschooler and younger ages.

Nose shape and symmetry should be noted. Palpation is performed to detect any deviation and tenderness. The nasal mucosa is normally free of lesions and red in color.

Sinuses

The sinuses are not usually assessed until the child is of school age. The frontal and maxillary sinuses are assessed by inspection, palpation or direct percussion, and transillumination in the same manner as for an adult (see Chapter 12).

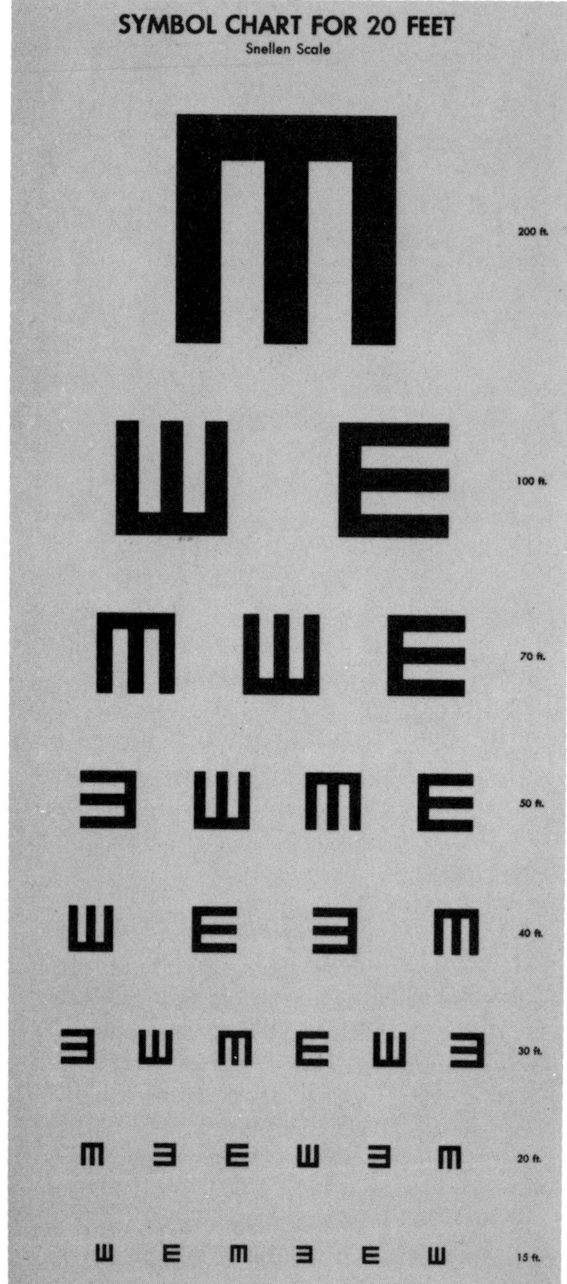

Figure 21-16 Snellen chart.

The difference, however, is in the anatomical location throughout the growth from infancy to adulthood. In the infant the sinuses are small and cylindrically shaped and lie near the bridge of the nose; in the child the maxillary sinuses enlarge somewhat in a horizontal fashion toward the cheekbones. Prepubescence brings a widening and elongation of both frontal and maxillary sinuses; in the adolescent the sinuses assume more of a blocklike pattern with the frontal

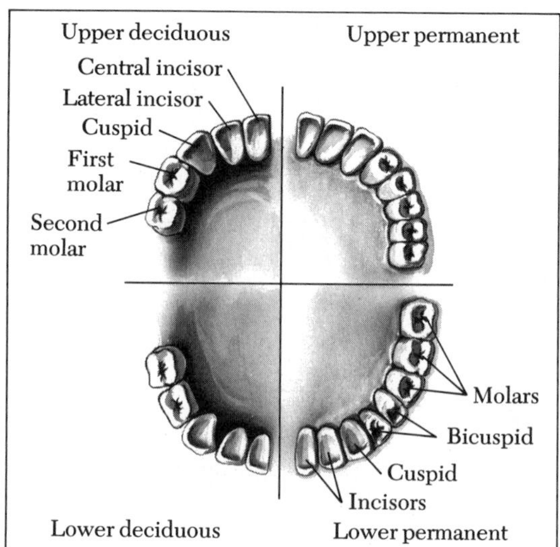

Figure 21-17 Maxillary and mandibular positions of both deciduous and permanent teeth at full eruption.

sinuses positioned above the level of the brows. In the adult the sinuses are larger, and the maxillary sinuses are distributed over a wider area of the cheeks.

Mouth

At about 6 months of age the deciduous teeth begin to erupt and the complete 20 teeth are present by the age of 3. There are 4 incisors, 2 canine, and 4 bicuspids on the upper jaw and the same number and type on the lower jaw. For the ages that each of these teeth normally erupt, see Table 12-2. The child begins losing these teeth about the age of 6 or 7, and they become replaced by 32 permanent teeth (see Figure 21-17).

The uvular reflex can be assessed as the child cries or phonates, and the gag reflex is tested as you would in the adult (cranial nerves IX and X, see "Oropharynx" in Chapter 12). Also you need to use a special approach in the infant to test whether or not the hypoglossal nerve is intact (cranial nerve XII, see "Tongue" in Chapter 12). The infant is unable to follow your instructions to "stick out his tongue and say aaah." Therefore, you gently pinch the infant's nares closed. In response he will open his mouth to breathe; with this the tongue will normally extend out in the midline and up. Lateral deviation of the tongue would suggest pathology, just as in the adult.

The lymph system in the child displays palpable lymph nodes, which normally are nontender. If they are tender, you need to assess whether there are additional signs of infection such as fever, erythema, or tenderness. Likewise, the tonsils are proportionately larger in the child than in the adult because they are a part of the lymphatic system. Further enlargement of the tonsils may interfere in eating and swallowing. Hypertrophied adenoids frequently accompany serous otitis media. Excessive mouth breathing and a voice of nasal quality may indicate enlarged adenoids. Mumps, a childhood disease affecting one or both of the parotid glands, manifests as swelling anterior to the lower part of the ear, which may extend behind the ear above the angle of the jaw to the mastoid process. The area is generally tender to palpation.

Respiratory System

The respiratory rate varies according to age (see Table 21-16). You will note that the child up to approximately age 7 breathes abdominally rather than costally. Also, about age 7, the thorax of the child assumes a more elliptical shape like that of the adult rather than the round, barrel-shape characteristic of the newborn or preschooler. A round thorax in the school-age child would cause you to suspect respiratory dysfunction, such as asthma.

The intercostal spaces are carefully observed in the infant/child for retraction or bulging, which would indicate respiratory dysfunction. Inspection reveals as much as palpation in the infant because of the smallness of the chest.

Generally the suprasternal notch is palpated to detect any abnormal cardiac pulsations in this area and to determine whether the trachea is midline. Increased fremitus may be indicative of consolidation in the lung tissue; however, in the infant and child, fremitus is normally of great intensity upon palpation due to the thinness of the chest wall and paucity of adipose and muscle tissue in the area. For this reason it is not usually necessary to palpate for fremitus in the child under 7 years of age.

In the infant and small child the percussion note will be much more resonant than in the adult. It is best, therefore, to use a light, direct percussion technique. Direct percussion of the small chest is lightly performed by using the pad of the index finger, and striking it directly, but gently, over the lung fields. Any area of decreased resonance is significant, as it would be in an adult, and warrants medical validation. The auscultatory sites in the young child are fewer and somewhat different than those of the adult. It is best to use the bell of your stethoscope so that you will be better able to localize the source of sounds. It is preferable to use a bell that has soft rubber margins, because it makes a more complete contact on the small curved thorax of the infant and small child.

The normal breath sounds that you will hear in the child are harsher than those heard in the adult. Even at the periphery of the child's lung fields, the breath sounds are bronchovesicular because of the thinness of the chest wall, which allows for greater transmission of sounds to the outside. Therefore, auscultation is of little diagnostic benefit in the young child. A technique to detect rhonchi in the infant is to hold your stethoscope in front of the mouth. This technique, however, does not reveal the presence of rales. Adventitious sounds within the lungs are able to be detected in the older child; thus, auscultation of the lungs is of greater diagnostic benefit in the school-age child. In prepubescence the normal, auscultated lung sounds become similar to those of the adult.

Cardiovascular System

Epigastric pulsations may be normally detected upon inspection of the anterior thorax of the young child; they may also be detected in very thin adults. These pulsations are normal if they correspond to the timing of the arterial pulse. Abnormal epigastric pulsations in the infant may indicate an enlarged heart.

The PMI, in contrast to being in the left fifth to sixth intercostal space slightly right of the midclavicular line in the school-age child and adult, is located in the fourth left intercostal space to the left of the midclavicular line until the age of 7.

Auscultation of the heart will reveal sinus arrhythmia. Over 50% of children have innocent systolic heart murmurs of Grade III or less. Generally they are heard loudest along the left sternal border at the level of the second or third intercostal space. There are no other associated cardiovascular symptoms. Murmurs heard in the child may or may not be pathologic, but they warrant medical referral for evaluation and follow-up.

Breast

Breast tissue growth begins in the preadolescent period. In the female the growth may begin in only one breast, and the breast may be tender.

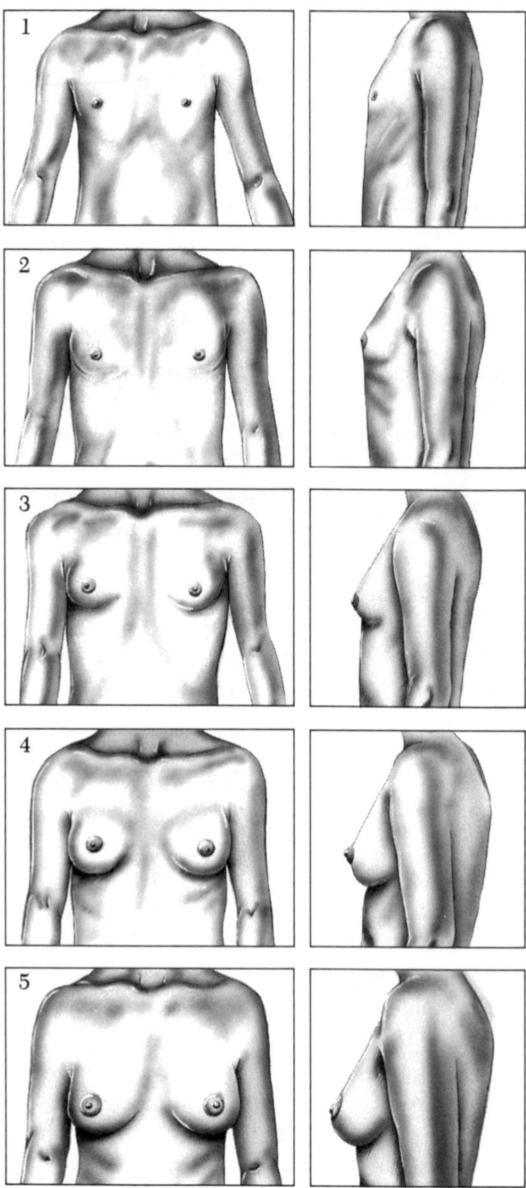

Figure 21-18 Stages of breast development in adolescent girls. (1) Prepubertal flat appearance like that of a child. (2) Small, raised breast bud. (3) General enlargement and raising of breast and areola. (4) Areola and papilla (nipple) form contour separate from that of breast. (5) Adult breast—areola is in same contour as breast. (Based on Tanner, J. M. *Growth in Adolescence*, 2nd ed. Oxford: Blackwell, 1962. Used by permission of the author.)

It is not uncommon for males during adolescence to have some breast engorgement and tenderness. This may persist for several years. In this situation there will be no local or systemic signs of infection. Injury to the area must be ruled out at the onset. Stages of breast development have been identified by Tanner (see Figure 21-18).

Abdomen

Infants and toddlers have a round, slightly protruding abdomen, and it is not uncommon to see slight umbilical protrusions in the toddler. Referral for further evaluation is needed if a child in this age range presents with a scaphoid abdomen. On inspection of the child's abdomen, the superficial veins are readily observed, but they should not be prominent.

In the toddler and preschool child bowel sounds are normally heard every 10–30 seconds and are of greater frequency shortly after eating or when the stomach has been empty for several hours. The bowel sounds of the school-age child, as well as those of the adult, occur 5–6 times per minute. They will also increase in frequency with an empty stomach and after a recent meal.

Palpation of the liver in the infant is performed lightly, using only the fingertips to 1–2 cm deep. The liver edge may be felt 2 cm below the right costal margin in contrast to that of the adult, which is palpated immediately above or at the costal margin.

Percussion for liver size in the young child reveals a normal size liver of 4–6 cm approximately in the right MCL (midclavicular line). Normal liver size in the older child and adolescent ranges from 6 to 10 cm.

The kidneys are usually palpable in the infant and thin child; the procedure is performed in the same manner as for the adult (see Chapter 16).

Palpation of a distended bladder above the pubic symphysis in the infant requires the retention of 90 ml, whereas 180 ml of urine is required to extend the adult bladder above this level.

Genitals

Developmental changes in pubic hair pattern and genitals in the male are heralded between the ages of 12 and 16. Before this age there is no pubic hair. Then sparse, soft, straight hairs begin to grow at the base of the penis, and the scrotal skin reddens and becomes more thick. Gradually the pubic hair gets darker, coarser, and more curled and eventually covers the total pubic region. At the completion of puberty the hair distribution is diamond shaped with the far ends at the level of the umbilicus and anus, and the genitals are of adult size and shape (see Figure 21-19). Pubic hair growth and enlarged genitals in the male prior to age 10 may indicate endocrine pathology. The penis is inspected and palpated with care to note any abnormalities (see Chapter 19). The prepuce up to 6 months of age

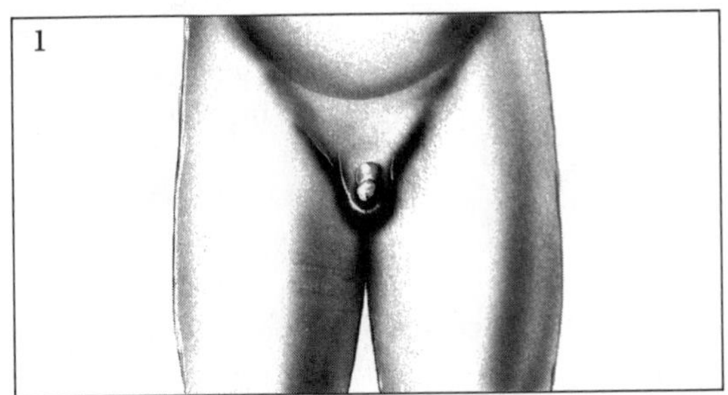

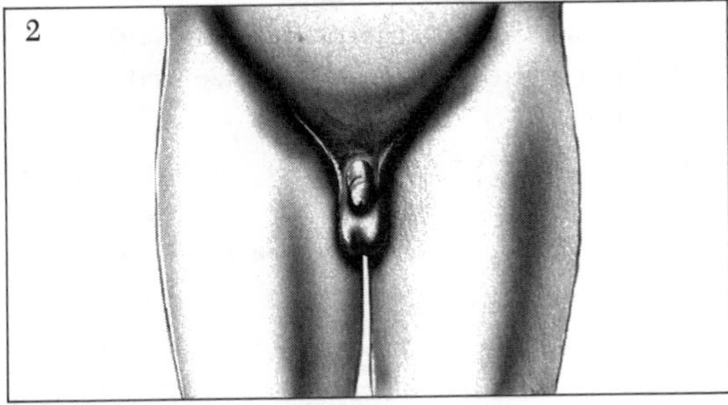

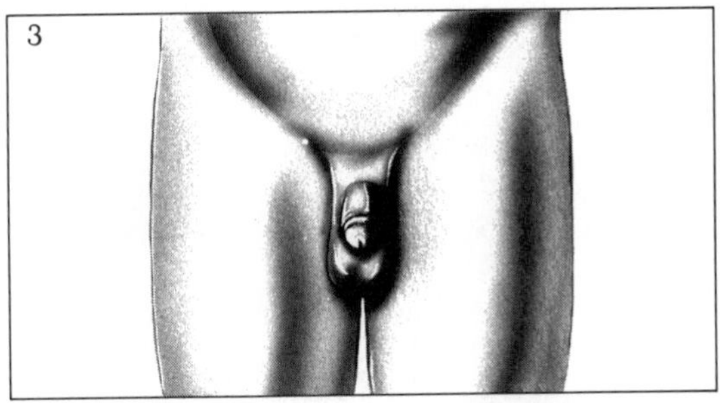

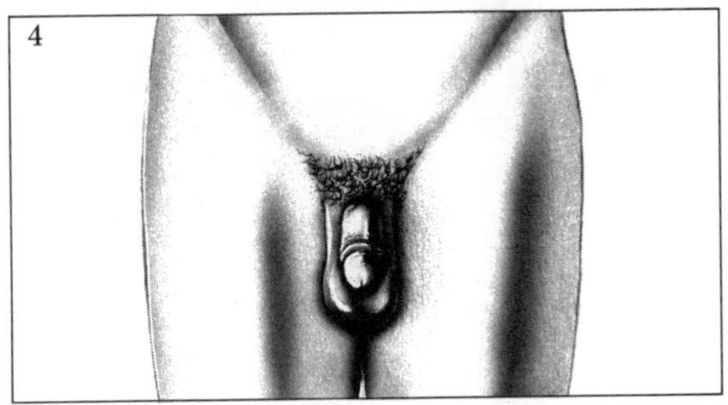

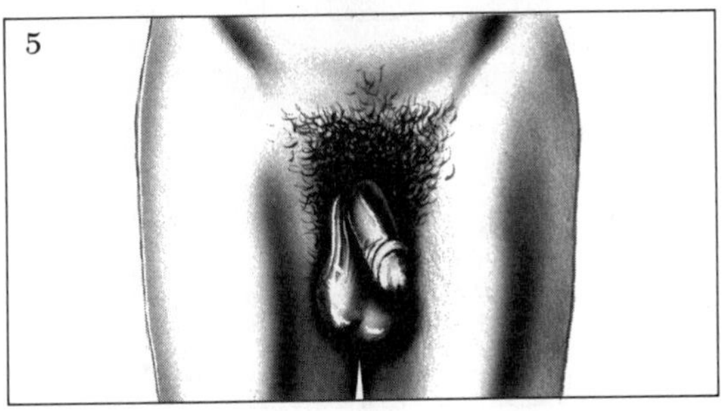

Figure 21-19 Stages of male genital development. (1) Prepubertal in which the size of the testes and penis is similar to that in early childhood. (2) Testes become larger and scrotal skin reddens and coarsens. (3) Continuation of stage 2, with lengthening of penis. (4) Penis enlarges in general size, and scrotal skin becomes pigmented. (5) Adult genitals.

may remain adherent to the glans. After this age, however, it should easily retract.

The scrotum and its contents, testes and epididymises, are palpated in the same manner as that of the adult (see Chapter 19). The epididymis may be difficult to distinguish before school age. However, the epididymis and the inguinal ring on both sides of the scrotum are assessed in the school-age child. The little finger, rather than the index finger, is used to palpate the inguinal ring.

The best position in which to place the child for assessment of the anus and rectum is the supine position with the legs flexed at the knees and laterally rotated at the hips (frog legged). The prostate gland is not assessed until the child is in the adolescence period.

Generally the pubic hair pattern of the female is established between the ages of 11 and 13 (see Figure 21-20). It is shaped like an inverted triangle. Assessment of the female genitals in children employs only the techniques of inspection and external palpation. Internal vaginal inspection and palpation of the Bartholin's glands, vaginal walls, uterus, and adnexa are not performed. The position assumed by the female child for inspection of the genitals is the same as that for assessment of the anus and rectum (supine and frog legged).

Adhesion of the labia minora may be present in infants and toddlers; these children will be more prone to urinary infections due to urine collected in a sac formed by the labial adhesion.

When performing a pelvic examination of the adolescent female, use a small or medium vaginal speculum. A summary of pubertal development is seen in Table 21-18.

Musculoskeletal System

The center of gravity in the child before the age of 4 is higher than that of the adult. The latter is about the level of the iliac crest. As a result the child has a wide gait and stance. As well, until the age of 4, the child normally has an increase in the lumbar curvature, giving a slightly swayback appearance. All children are examined for the presence of scoliosis, a lateral spinal curvature deviation. To inhibit further deviation of structure, the nurse must refer any sign of sco-

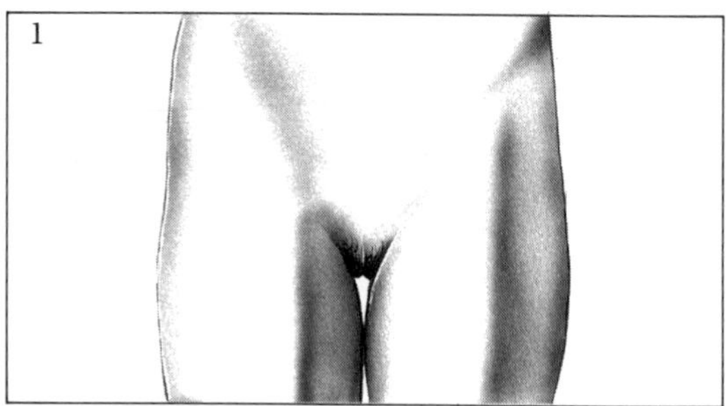

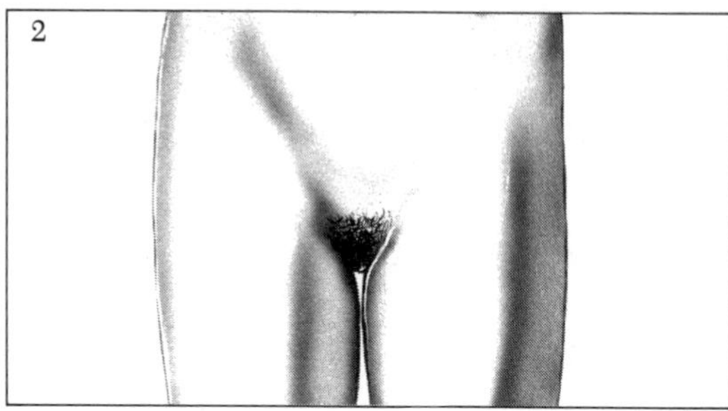

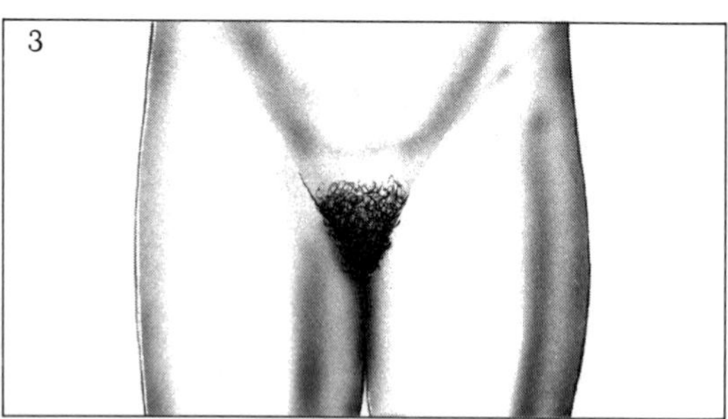

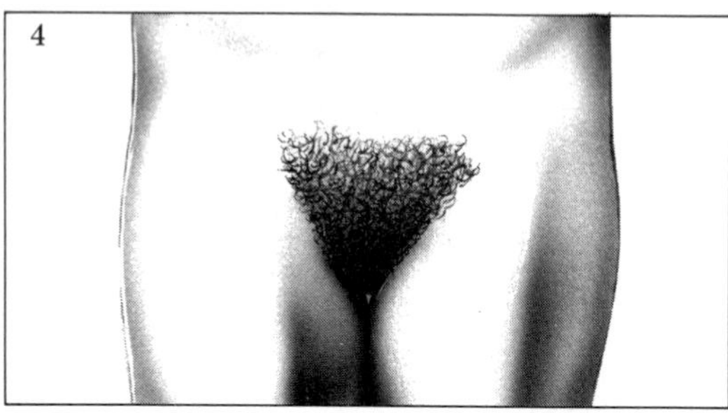

Figure 21-20 Stages of pubic hair development in adolescent girls. (1) Sparse growth of downy hair mainly at sides of labia. (2) Pigmentation, coarsening, and curling, with an increase in the amount of hair. (3) Adult hair, but limited in area. (4) Adult hair with horizontal upper border.

liosis, no matter how mild. The best method for inspection is to view the child from the back as he bends over at the waist and leans forward dangling his hands toward his toes. With scoliosis, the scapulae no longer are on a horizontal plane; instead the scapula on the deviated side is displaced laterally and superiorly (see Figure 21-21). In the young child the Denver Developmental Screening Test is used to assess muscle strength. The school-age and older child's muscle strength is assessed in the same way as the adult. As muscle strength and intellect develop, so does the child's abilities.

Neurologic System

The Denver Developmental Screening Test is used initially at the age of 3 months and repeated about every 6 months up to about age 6. Children 5 to 6 years old can be tested like an adult for balance, using the Romberg test, and for coordination ability of upper and lower extremities (see Figures 21-22 and 21-23).

Children six years of age and older can be tested for sensory function as an adult would. Infants will respond to a pinprick (pain sensation) by crying and/or withdrawal. Hot and cold sensation and sharp and dull sensation can be tested in the 3-year-old. Vibration and position sense is not tested in the infant or toddler because of the difficulty in gaining cooperation. These sensations, as well as stereognosis and graphesthesia, can be readily assessed in the 6-year-old and up (see Chapter 18).

At approximately 6 months of age the superficial reflexes are present. When testing for the plantar reflex, you may normally observe a Babinski response up until the age of 2. The appearance of any pathologic reflexes after the age of 2 is abnormal and warrants referral (see Chapter 18). Any child, regardless of age, who displays a high-pitched cry, irritability, extended posturing, or is unresponsive, must be seen by a physician.

Summary

The health assessment of the child and adolescent uses developmental parameters for each age level as a base for evaluation. These activities and functions were incorporated throughout the chapter. How cultural history is pertinent to the health assessment of the child was discussed. Also presented were specific communication and interview principles that need to be used with the child and the adolescent. The components of the health history were reviewed in light of the areas of inquiry, and sample questions were given relevant to the child and adolescent. The specific techniques of measurement (head, chest, and abdomen circumferences) included in the general appearance section for the very young child were explained. Rationales and

Table 21-18. Sequence of Pubertal Development

Male		
Average age onset	**Physiologic changes**	**Average age completion**
11.5 years	*Genital development* (see Figure 21-19) —Testicular volume increases —Penile enlargement and lengthening	2–5 years after onset
12.5	*Adrenarche* (growth of body hair) —Pubic hair development (see Figure 10-1) —Axillary and facial hair development	Late teens
About 2 years after onset of pubic hair growth		
13.5	*Growth spurt* —Pattern: hands and feet, calves and forearms, hips, chest, shoulders, trunk —Height: increases about 7–12 cm/year at peak —Weight: almost doubles between 12 and 16 years —Larynx growth and voice deepening occur at end of penile growth	Late teens
About 3 years after onset of genital development	*Ejaculation* via masturbation or nocturnal emissions —Mature sperm are produced between 14.5 and 17.5 years of age	14.5 to 17.5 years
	Breast development —Areola darkens and enlarges —Transient gynecomastia may occur between 10 and 16 years of age	

Female		
Average age onset	**Physiologic changes**	**Average age completion**
9.0 to 11.0 years	*Breast development* (see Figure 21-18) —Breast bud appears followed by general enlargement and raising of the breast and areola —Areola and nipple are raised from breast —Adult breast contour	14.0 to 17.0 years
About 1 year after breast buds appear	*Adrenarche* —Pubic hair development (see Figure 21-20)	Late teens
About 1 year after onset of pubic hair growth	—Axillary hair development	
10.5 years	*Growth spurt*—same sequence as male —Height: increases 6–11 cm/year at peak	16 years
12.5 to 13.5 years	*Menarche* (onset of menstruation) —Initial cycles are usually anovulatory and irregular —Ovulatory cycles usually occur within two years of menarche —Dysmenorrhea more often associated with ovulatory cycles	

From Bellack/Bamford: *Nursing Assessment: A Multidimensional Approach*, © 1987 Boston: Jones and Bartlett Publishers.

examples for approaching the physical assessment of the child and of the adolescent in a particular way were given. Specific techniques used with the child for each body system as well as the normal findings were included. If an assessment technique is used for the child and adolescent in the same manner as used for the adult, the reader was referred to the chapter or section in the text for the purpose of learning or reviewing the specific principles and steps of the technique.

Discussion Questions/Activities

1. Role-play a history-taking session with an adolescent and parents who do not allow the

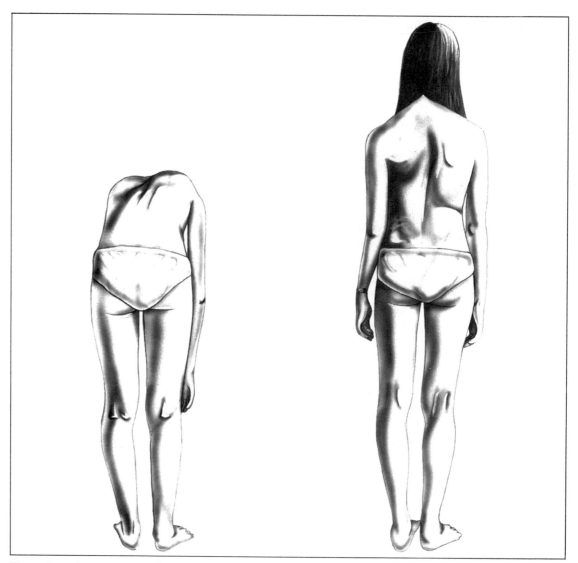

Figure 21-21 Screening procedure for scoliosis.

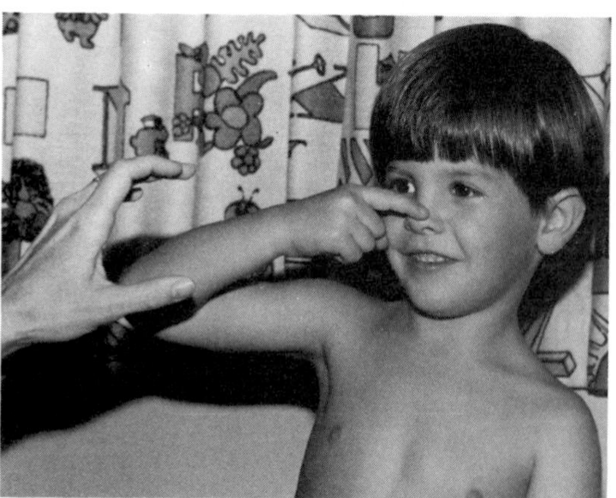

Figure 21-22 Finger-to-nose test for cerebellar functioning.

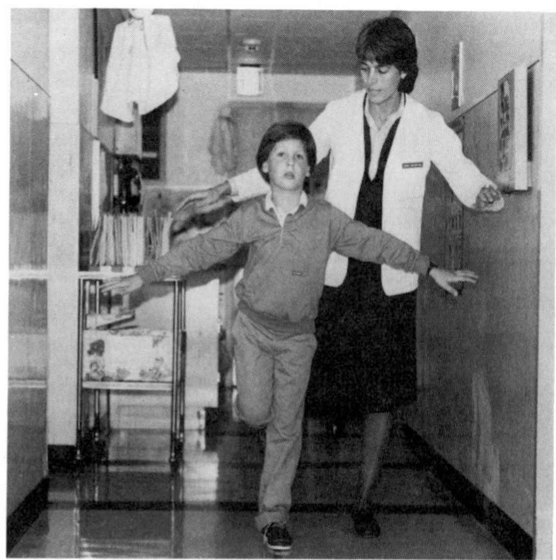

Figure 21-23 Assessing balance for cerebellar functioning.

client to answer questions or talk very much to you.

2. Perform a health assessment on a toddler, preschool child, school-age child, prepubescent child, and a mid- to late-adolescent child.
3. Describe some ways that you might approach children and adolescents that would decrease anxiety and facilitate communication and examination.
4. List areas of history-taking that would likely be sensitive for the adolescent and how you would plan to approach these areas.
5. Discuss how cultural history is pertinent to the health assessment of the child.
6. Describe how aspects of your cultural history influence your health status and behavior.
7. Develop projects that will enhance wellness and health maintenance in children and adolescents.

EXAMPLE OF A HEALTH ASSESSMENT OF A CHILD

HEALTH HISTORY

Name: Kevin Cain Jones, Jr.
Address: 82 Brushlee St., Carlsburg, N.M.
Sex: Male
Age: 5 years
Birthdate: 5/9/82
Mother: Ann Marie *Age:* 30 *Address:* Same as client *Education:* High school graduate
Religion: Catholic *Race:* Caucasian *Ethnic origin:* Italian
Father: Kevin Cain Jones *Age:* 28 *Address:* same as client *Education:* B.S. in business
Religion: Protestant *Race:* Caucasian *Ethnic Origin:* English
Informant: Parents; reliable source
Chief Concern/Complaint: "Sore throat"

History of Present Illness (HPI)
Client has been "cranky" for past 3 days. Nonproductive cough and runny nose. Asking for more fluids. Appetite poor. Temperature 102°F since midnight. History of 1–2 strep throat infections/yr for past 2 yrs. No earaches, stomachaches, diarrhea, or changes in bowel habits.

Personal History and Patterns of Living
Prenatal—Healthy pregnancy. Kevin was 1st child. No x-rays, special diet, or hospitalization during pregnancy. Followed from 4th–9th month at Saver's Prenatal Clinic. On vitamins and iron for duration of pregnancy. No abortions or miscarriages. Mother, father, and client have RH+ blood types.
Natal—Uneventful 10 hr labor. Father present most of labor and present at delivery. Vaginal delivery. Vertex presentation, caudal anesthesia at Carlsburg General Hospital. Apgar 9; birth weight: 7 lb 2 oz; length: 20 inches. Color was good—spontaneous cry; no O_2 needed.
Postnatal—Uneventful, mother and Kevin discharged on 2nd day postdelivery. Client had slight bilateral breast hypertrophy that lasted about 2 wks without tenderness or erythema. No jaundice or cyanosis. Cord and circumcision healed without complications. Breast-fed. Lost 5 oz 1st wk at home.
Present—Kevin attends kindergarten, which he enjoys; has formed friendships with peers. He gets along with most people. Protective and sharing with 3½ yr old sister, Cindy. Talks constantly; appropriate interaction content; asks relevant questions; egocentrism, normal for his age, displayed; talks about grandparents, aunts and uncles; knows his name, age, address, telephone number, and where his daddy works and mommy goes to school; knows basic colors, days of week; able to print name and few other short words and write numbers 1–20. Cindy spends time on weekdays at Happy Child Day Care Center. Mother attends Catholic church school most Sundays with both children. Father attends infrequently. No outstanding financial debts. Maternal grandparents are helping with cost for mother to attend baccalaureate nursing program at Carlsburg University. She is ending her 4th semester.

Family Health History
Denies family history of TB, alcoholism, mental illness, bleeding disorders, stomach problems, liver and kidney disorders, cancer, heart disease. Family history significant for hypertension, arthritis, and diabetes.

Geographic Exposure: Disneyland at age 4. Family has traveled and vacationed mainly in state and Texas.

Lifestyle
Sexuality—Mimics father. Plays with building blocks, tricycle. Has favorite teddy bear for naps and bedtime. Girls are mommies, boys are daddys.

(continued on page 516)

Personal habits: Brushes teeth after breakfast and before bedtime. Likes soda and popsicles—allowed 2–3 times/wk. Has been on penicillin when strep throat past couple years. Tylenol liquid for fever.
Diet: Generally has good appetite. Meat, vegetables, fruit, cereal, and milk daily. Pasta 2–3 times/wk. Loves fruit. Weekdays has brown bag lunch—sandwich, cookies, raw carrots or celery, apple, carton of milk. No eating difficulties except when past strep throat and present "sore throat." Does not like raw tomatoes or cooked peas. Takes Flintstone daily vitamin.
Sleep and rest patterns: 8 P.M. bedtime. Wakes 7–8 A.M. Short nap in afternoons (½ hr). No bedwetting. "Bad" dreams—ghosts, witches 4–5 times/month. Sleepwalks 2–3 times/month.
Activities of daily living: Feeds, washes, and dresses self. Needs help with tying shoelaces and combing hair. Brushes teeth. Toilet trained at 3½ yrs. Picks up toys—usually after reminded to do so.
Home and neighborhood: Family rents small bungalow in young family residential area. No basement, small backyard. 3 BR (each child has own bedroom).
Interpersonal relationships: Contact with grandparents, aunts, and uncles. Closest to maternal grandparents. Father and mother share chores, child care, and responsibilities. Stressful at times—father works in bank; mother is college student. Discipline seems consistent, with father and mother consciously working at it. Removal of privileges seems most effective discipline with client—occasional spanking 2–3 times/yr.
Recreation: Likes to go for walks, to the local playground. Watches Saturday A.M. cartoons. Enjoys building with blocks, Leggos, Tinkertoys.

Previous experiences with illnesses

Mumps at 3 yrs of age. No history of measles, chickenpox, scarlet fever, or rheumatic fever.
Immunizations: DPT and TOPV 2 mos old, 4 mos old, 6 mos old, 18 mos old. Tine Test 1 yr old. Measles, rubella, mumps vaccine 1½ yrs old. DPT and TOPV booster 4½ yrs old.
Allergies: Animal fur—breaks out in rash.
Past illness, injuries, surgery: Strep throat past 2 years. Rx with penicillin by Dr. Rouse. Mumps at 3 yrs of age. Fell 2 mos ago at kindergarten and lacerated base of left palm—needed 3 sutures. No surgeries or hospitalizations.

Review of Systems

General health: Very strong and active except for strep throat. No history of polydipsia, ecchymosis, bleeding tendencies, easily fatigued.
Integument: Papular rash when around furry pets. No jaundice, diaphoresis, hives, pruritus, skin lesions. 3 cm diameter port wine birthmark on lower, lateral quadrant of left buttock. Lately, past couple of months, has begun biting nails. No changes in daily routine.
Head: Never complained of headache or held head when crying. No head injuries known.
Eyes: No history of infections or pain. No excessive lacrimation, crossed-eyes, or photophobia. No history of walking into walls or doors. Can see blackboard from seat.
Ears: Earache last winter with last episode of strep throat. No vertigo noted.
Nose, nasopharynx, and paranasal sinuses: No epistaxis, strep throat 1–2 times/yr for past 2 yrs with tenacious white-yellow nasal drainage.
Mouth and throat: No toothaches, sores of mouth or tongue. Dysphagia when strep throat episodes. Annual dental visits.
Neck: Complains of pain (see HPI).
Breasts: No scaling, edema, or discharge.
Cardiorespiratory system: Nonproductive cough past couple days (see HPI). No history of pneumonia or asthma. No dyspnea or wheezing. Dr. Rouse, pediatrician, told family that client had slight murmur but that it appeared to be "innocent." Annual pediatrician exam done.
Gastrointestinal system: Client goes to toilet by self; no known recent diarrhea or constipation. No bloody stools, pain, or vomiting. No food intolerances.
Genitourinary system: Straight, strong urinary stream. No dribbling, nocturia, hematuria, or polyuria noted.
Musculoskeletal system: No broken bones, sprains, pain, or swelling in joints, lameness, weakness, dislocations, or congenital defects.
Neurologic system: No history of convulsions, twitching, tremors, vertigo, "blackouts," fainting, or difficulty with motor activities. No stuttering or other speech difficulties.

PHYSICAL ASSESSMENT

General impression: Kevin Cain Jones, 5-year-old white male presents with "sore throat" and dysphagia. Appears within cognitive and physical developmental norms. Raspy cough and visible swollen glands in neck; nasal congestion. No gross deformities.
Ht.—45".
Wt.—43 lbs.
TPR—102.6°F./88/26.
BP—98/66 left arm lying.
Chest circumference—54.5 cm.

Integument: Moist, flushed, and warm to touch; skin turgor—fair; port wine birthmark noted lower, lateral quadrant of left buttock; curly, short blond hair; moderate degree of nail-biting observed; no clubbing of digits; no nailbed cyanosis; good capillary refill.

Head and neck: Normocephalic; atraumatic; clean clear scalp; tonsillar and anterior cervical lymph nodes enlarged and tender to touch bilaterally; trachea midline.

Respiratory: Rate 26; abdominal respirations; no ICS or sternal retractions noted; round thoracic cage; symmetrical breathing; no cyanosis; resonance; bronchovesicular breath sounds; no crackles, wheezes, or rubs.

Cardiovascular: Slight epigastric pulsations concomitant with arterial pulse; no heaves or thrills; PMI at left 4ICS slightly left of MCL; rate 88; sinus arrhythmia; summation gallop; physiological splitting of S_2; $A_2 = P_2$. Grade I systolic murmur at left 2ICS; no radiation into neck or axilla.

Abdomen: Flat; B.S. every 10–30 seconds; tympany; liver dullness = 5 cm; splenic dullness = 4 cm; no pain or masses with light and deep palpation.

Musculoskeletal: Full ROM; no joint tenderness or edema noted; good bilateral, proximal, and distal strength; normal gait; tires easily from present fever; no spinal deviations noted.

Neurologic: Scapulae on horizontal plane. Slow mental processes 2° to pyrexia. Sensitive to hot and cold, light touch, and vibration. Able to button and unbutton shirt. Can tap toes. Romberg sign absent. Able to touch nose with finger. Babinski sign absent. Abdominal, anal, and cremasteric reflexes present.

Eyes: No edema; sclerae white; corneas clear; no lid lag; EOMs intact; PERRLA/consensual reaction; convergence; Hirschberg test—symmetrical reflection; cover test—no jerking movements, no deviation. Snellen Chart results—O.U. 20/30 does not wear glasses; field vision WNL by gross confrontation.

Ears: Appropriate placement; no lesions or drainage noted. No mastoid tenderness. TMs—pearly gray, landmarks visible, membranes moveable; Weber without lateralization; Rinne—AC>BC. Watch ticking 12" bilaterally.

Nose: Congested; thick, whitish yellow exudate; no deviation; pale bluish mucosa.

Mouth/pharynx: Free of lesions; all deciduous teeth (#20); tongue midline; uvular reflex; pink, firm gums; posterior pharynx erythemic; purulent, exudative, enlarged tonsils bilaterally; culture taken (to be referred to pediatrician, Dr. Rouse for medical Rx).

Genitourinary: No public hair; descended testicles; urethral opening and penile size appropriate; prepuce retracts easily; circumsized; no drainage, masses, or hernias noted.

DTR's		T	B	BR	P	A	PR
	L	2+	2+	2+	2+	2+	↓
	R	2+	2+	2+	2+	2+	↓

CHAPTER 22

Assessment of the Older Adult

LEARNING OBJECTIVES

1. Appreciate the ways in which culture dictates the behavior of the older adult.
2. Recognize that chronological age is a poor index of mental functioning and physiologic performance.
3. Acquire a general understanding of the older adult.
4. Identify changes in lifestyle patterns of the older adult.
5. Analyze physical assessment findings in light of criteria that includes physiological changes of aging.

The United States grows grayer every year, despite the obsession with youth. In the past decade, according to the U.S. Census Bureau, the number of people over age 65 has increased 37%, which is more than double the growth of the general population. According to the Bureau's projections, the country will continue to age, and by 2010 people 55 and older will number about 74 million, or one quarter of the total population. This fact alone warrants that this group of people needs to be understood in regard to the influence of the aging process on health status. The "elderly image" has been one of frailness, confusion, and doddering; however, research is shattering the myths of aging. The elderly are not a homogeneous group with identical developmental changes and behaviors that can be categorized. Indeed, they are unique individuals with the commonality merely of having lived a longer time than other people. The perceptions of old age are based on obsolete information and have been associated with the term *elderly;* therefore, in an attempt to move away from such an undeserved image, we have chosen to discuss health assessment of the *older adult*.

The quality of health assessment is dependent on not stereotyping or making assumptions. Moreover, it is dependent on the awareness, understanding, and attitudes of each nurse regarding each age group, including the older adult.

It has been said that aging is a process to become old. But what does this mean? Does this mean that the individual is decrepit and cannot or should not be salvaged? Chronologic age is a poor index of mental functioning and physiologic performance. Aging is highly individualized. Therefore, a careful health assessment must be performed. More research is needed in the area of health and health status regarding the older adult to better meet the needs of this large population group. Contained in this chapter is a discussion of specifics regarding the health assessment of the older adult with indices inherent in cultural, mental health, and physical assessment aspects—the knowledge divisions of health assessment used throughout this text.

Cultural Assessment of the Older Adult

Investigation of a client's cultural background brings out the beauty and uniqueness of the individual. For the most part the older adults within our society are the ones who uphold and transmit culture and ultimately are the preservers of culture. The many life experiences—some difficult learning experiences and others emotionally, intellectually, and physically pleasurable—have profited the value system formation of the older adult. If the adage "practice makes perfect" is true, the older adult has much to teach each of us if we will only listen. Moreover, by being aware of the values, beliefs, attitudes, and practices of older individuals, which may differ greatly from our own, we can conscientiously afford them respect as individuals and come to understand the rationale behind some of their behavior.

Health Practices

The majority of older adults today continue to view the use of health care systems as a source of help only in times of severe illness or injury. They are often reluctant to leave their home and forfeit their independence.

Religion

As one ages, the concern of mortality becomes more paramount, and the spiritual sphere enlarges. Faith is a tenet of everyday living, though it is not often verbalized. If the older adult had interrupted formal religious practices earlier in life, it is not uncommon for him to return to active participation in the later years of his life. Most likely the return is due to a combination of religious reawakening and a means for socializing.

Social Aspects

In the many years of lifework the person has developed networks for socialization and support systems to help cope with stressful life events. Most central to an individual's social support network is the family. Research by D. Preston and J. Grimes (1987) found that married persons rely a good deal on their spouses as confidants for help. The married male relies significantly more on his spouse, whereas the married female tends to rely on family and friends as well as her spouse. Therefore, if the wife should die first, the social support system of most widowers is devastated. The nurse can help the married male, preferably with the aid of his wife, to broaden his network. To identify the social support system with the older adult becomes a mutual task within the cultural assessment component of the total health assessment. A good social support system is highly correlated with well-being. Along with knowledge of support systems, the nurse needs to consider the available resources, the client's assets, and his effective coping skills.

The occupational history aids in the identification of predisposing factors to particular disease entities and infirmities and may be of significance in determining a diagnosis. When assessing the older adult, you would be greatly amiss if you ceased investigation of occupational experiences at the mention of "I am retired." A person may have worked as a clerk in a hardware store for a few years prior to retirement; however, as you continue investigation, you may find that he spent 10 years as a coal miner and another 30 years shoveling coal into blast furnaces in a steel mill. This would call your attention to the possibility of existing or potential respiratory problems. Inadvertently you may learn about interests and support networks as you have the client talk about his lifework. For instance, you may hear a client say, "I've worked with Joe for the past 30 years; he will always be my friend. We go fishing together almost every weekend, and we help each other in planting our gardens."

Lifestyle

The eating habits of the older adult sometimes fail to change, although exercise and other physical activities are generally modified. Given the sustained daily caloric intake, the client tends to put on weight. With a lowered basal metabolic rate (BMR), the need for high caloric intake no longer exists. Or the client may have lost weight and is thin or actually malnourished; this may have an etiology of just not cooking for oneself for a variety of reasons or of not having financial means, or it may be due to a disease state.

The sleep pattern changes with age. Around the age of 50 the fourth stage of sleep is decreased by 20% of what it was during the second decade of life. The void is replaced by an increase in stages two and three and is accompanied by an increase in the frequency and duration of spontaneous awakening.

Most nurses probably do not pursue an assessment of sexuality in the older adult. Once again, though, recent research has debunked the myth that sexuality and sexual activity are dead past age 50. However, the older woman may find that suitable partners are lacking. Because women tend to live longer than men, the ratio of women to men becomes greater with age. Many times social customs must be breached in order for the older woman to satisfy this social-physical need. She may engage in an alternative lifestyle, find a younger partner, have a married partner, or cohabit with a widower. The practice of marriage may not be exercised by the older adult at times because of the attitudes of children or other relatives. Thus the older adult makes a sacrifice of moral values in the name of love for his family. Perhaps family members do not have difficulty accepting the sexuality of parents, but they are fearful of losing part or all of an inheritance if marriage occurs. Premarital contracts regarding already accrued property and assets may be a solution. (See Figure 22-1.)

Those older adults in nursing homes find themselves deprived of human intimacy. Nurses can be advocates by ensuring privacy and coupling activities that promote the expression of sexuality by the residents. Despite long-term institutionalization, illness, and disease, sexual needs continue. Because of cultural attitudes and myths, the older adult may experience feel-

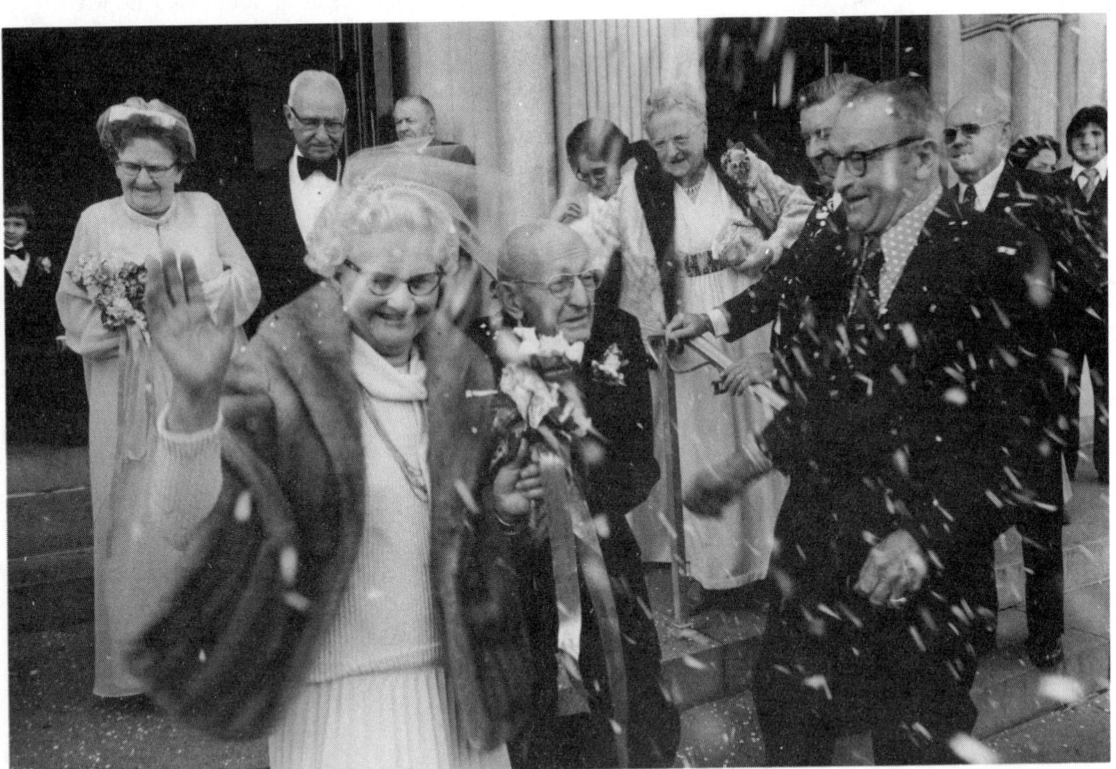

Figure 22-1 Marital bliss can be a reality for the older adult.

ings of guilt and embarrassment. Sexual activity may even be avoided in order to conform to these cultural "norms." However, some older adults may have never had much interest and enthusiasm in sexual matters. Some may have a decreased self-image and lack the self-esteem necessary for a healthy expression of sexuality. Ebersole and Hess (1981) point out that impaired physical health may interfere directly or indirectly with sexual activities. Effects of chronic illness, such as fatigue, shortness of breath, and alterations in blood or nerve supply, may impair sexual functioning. Also medications used by the older adult can alter sexual behavior. The phenothiazines increase libido in older women; L-dopa increases libido in older men. This effect may be very distressing for the client. Medications commonly used by older adults that depress sexual behavior are listed in Table 22-1.

If the older adult is aware of the effects of medications and is knowledgeable of the changes in sexual response that commonly occur as a normal part of the aging process, he will understand the effects rather than fear that sexual powers are being lost (see Table 22-2).

The use of alcohol by the older adult should be investigated. Because of the diminished basal metabolic rate in the older adult, alcohol tends to remain in the body longer. Thus, even though the older adult drinks less, he may not necessarily be less intoxicated. The same alcohol intake criteria for other ages cannot be used, because the older adult has changes in fat and water composition and in body weight. The older adult who lives alone is at greater risk; the identifica-

Table 22-1. Drugs That May Suppress the Libido in the Older Adult

Antianxiety agents (in large doses causing CNS depression)
Clorazepate dipotassium
Chlordiazepoxide
Diazepam
Meprobamate
Oxazepam
Antidepressants
Monoamine oxidase (MAO) inhibitors
Tricyclics
Antihypertensives
Chlorothiazide
Guanethidine
Hydralazine
Methyldopa
Pargyline
Rauwolfia alkaloids
Antispasmodics/Anticholinergics
Atropine
Diphenhydramine
Propantheline bromide
Trihexyphenidyl
Narcotics
Codeine
Heroin
Meperidine
Oxycodone
Sedatives
Alcohol
Antiasthmatics
Barbiturates
Flurazepam
Stimulants
Amphetamines
Anorexic agents
Caffeine (small amounts)
Ephedrine
Epinephrine
Methylphenidate
Tranquilizers
Butyrophenones
Dihydroindolones
Haloperidol
Phenothiazines
Thioxanthenes

Source: B. H. Glover. Sex Counseling of the Elderly. *Hospital Practice*, 12:101–113, June 1977.

Table 22-2. Age-Related Changes in Sexual Response

Phase of response cycle	Age-related changes
Excitement phase	Female—may require from 1–5 minutes of sexual play for vaginal lubrication. Male—less intense and slower erection.
Plateau phase	Female—less change in labia color; clitoral hood and fatty tissue of mons decrease. Male—decreased or absence of Cowper's lubrication.
Orgasmic phase	Female—fewer orgasmic contractions. Male—fewer penile and rectal sphincter contractions; decreased force of ejaculation; decreased semen.
Resolution phase	Female—vasoconstriction of clitoris and orgasmic platform quickly subsides. Male—refractory period lengthens (time required for another erection ranges from several to 24 hours or longer).

tion of alcohol abuse is more difficult. Many times well-caring families are not aware that such a problem exists. The family members may live far away; they may lack knowledge to identify the signs and symptoms; they literally may not care, or they may be preoccupied with their own life. In addition, the older adult may tend to withdraw and isolate himself from the family so as not to be a burden or interfere. He may attempt "to drown in the bottle" feelings of unworthiness, guilt, loneliness, and the like. A stigma remains attached to seeking help, and fear of being institutionalized is common.

Signs of alcohol abuse in the older adult are similar to many other problems frequently observed in this age group. For example, memory loss can be due to decreased cardiac output; alcohol will exacerbate this memory loss problem. This could have a ripple effect, wherein the older adult becomes less and less capable of handling his household and everyday affairs. The effects of alcohol may become altered because of the pattern of polydrug use by this age group. Older adults constitute about 25% of the users of prescription tranquilizers such as Valium and Librium. They are generally heavy OTC (over-the-counter) drug users. The use of a combination of drugs and alcohol is practiced by over half of the older adult population. This is a deadly combination; unintentional overdose can be a result. The interaction of drugs and nutrition needs to be analyzed (see Table 22-3).

The stereotypic image of exercise in the older adult is knitting in a rocking chair and playing checkers. This image is rapidly fading as we see our mothers, fathers, grandmothers, grandfathers, and even great-grandparents, aunts, and uncles running in the marathons. The older adult can sometimes have more stamina than the most active of the young. Also research is showing that walking, gardening, and similar activities contribute to health maintenance almost as much, if not as much, as aerobic dancing, jogging, and swimming. The older adult need not exercise to the point of severe sweating for 20-minute periods three times a week to maintain health as was previously thought. In fact, this type of regimen may be detrimental. Particularly when initiating an exercise regimen that is vigorous and a great change from normal exercise activity, the older adult needs to begin gradually and consult with his physician. (See Figure 22-2.)

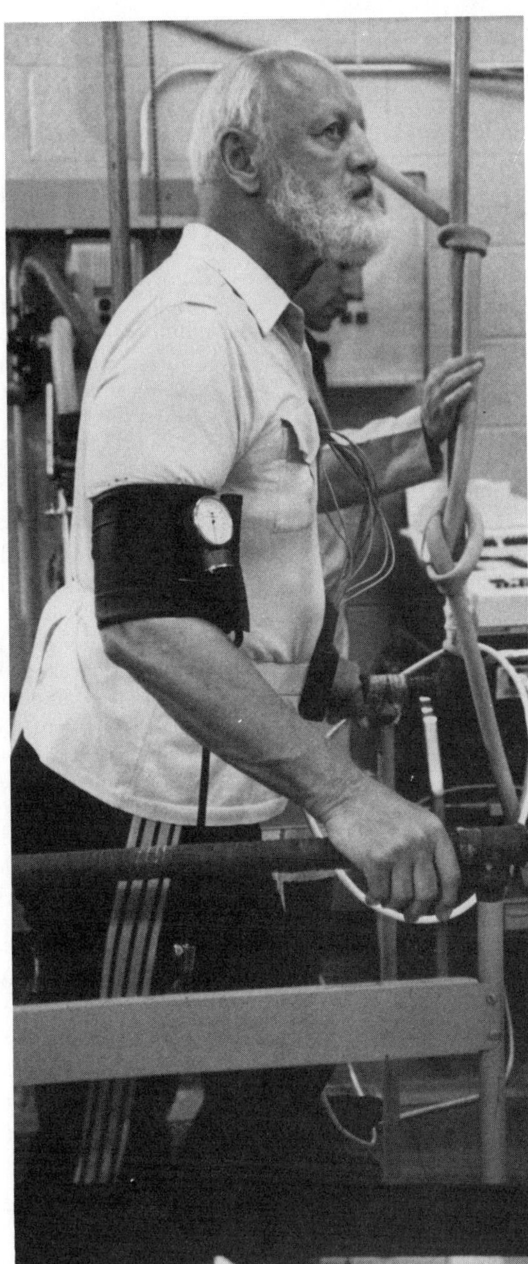

Figure 22-2 Older adults should not begin an exercise program without first getting a physical exam and physician input.

The nurse can explore thoughts and plans about retirement with older adults. What changes do they anticipate? What are their goals in regard to retirement? Do they belong to groups and engage in activities with persons other than co-workers? Do they enjoy activities with their spouse? Do they foresee financial problems? If already retired, how are they en-

Table 22-3. Nutrient/Drug Interactions to Be Aware of in Elderly Persons

Drug	Nutritional effects
Alcohol	Can lead to deficiencies in all nutrients, especially B vitamins Can replace eating
Aminopterin Methotrexate (used to treat leukemia)	Inhibits folate utilizations. However, if folate is supplemented, drug may not be as effective.
Antacids	Magnesium salts can cause diarrhea, limiting absorption of all nutrients. Protein absorption may be adversely affected when stomach acidity is reduced. Aluminum hydroxide binds phosphates.
Antibiotics	1. Tetracycline can bind iron, magnesium and calcium salts. 2. Many antibiotics are antagonistic to folic acid and can result in deficiencies of other nutrients. 3. Can lead to malabsorption. 4. Neomycin binds bile acids and affects fat-soluble vitamin absorption. 5. Neomycin causes intestinal structural changes that result in malabsorption of N, Na, K, Ca, Iactose.
Anticoagulants	Can cause vitamin K deficiency
Anticonvulsants	Primadone, phenobarbitol induce folate deficiency and vitamin D deficiency.
Antidepressants	Some cause accelerated breakdown of vitamin D. If the monamine oxidase (MAO) inhibitor-type is used, patients become intolerant to foods containing tyramine, such as aged cheese, red wine, beer, dry salami and chocolate. These foods can precipitate hypertensive crisis when MAO inhibitors are being used.
Aspirin and other anti-inflammatory drugs	1. Many cause gastrointestinal bleeding; arthritic patients who ingest large quantities may develop iron-deficiency anemia secondary to blood loss. 2. Aspirin usage can affect folic-acid status. 3. Aspirin and indomethacin can increase need for vitamin C by impairing its effectiveness.
Barbiturates	1. Some cause breakdown of vitamin D 2. Excessive sedation of nursing home patients for behavior control can result in missed meals. 3. Folic acid is malabsorbed.
Cathartics	Reduce intestinal transit time necessary for proper absorption of some nutrients
Cholesterol-lowering drugs such as chlofibrate	Any drug-altering blood lipids can affect absorption of fat-soluble vitamins. Vitamin K deficiencies can be produced.
Colchicine, used in gout	Causes malabsorption of fat, carotene, sodium, potassium, vitamin B12, folic acid and lactose
Diuretics	Most diuretics cause potassium to be lost in urine. Blood levels of potassium must be monitored, since mental confusion can result from low levels of potassium. Dietary sources of potassium should be consumed. (Magnesium may be deficient in long-term diuretics.)
Glucocorticoids, used in allergy and collagen disease	Impair calcium transport across mucosa
Hormones	1. ACTH and cortisone therapy increases excretion of sodium, potassium and calcium, and may contribute to the development of diabetes, hypertension, obesity and water retention. Calcium and potassium supplements may be needed, as well as special diet prescriptions if hypertension and diabetes develop. 2. Calcitonin treatment: Decreases serum calcium levels as calcium is deposited into bone. Tetany may develop without oral calcium supplements. 3. Estrogen therapy: Over an extended period, may result in deficiencies of folic acid and vitamin B6. Patient should not receive folic acid supplements until vitamin B12 status is confirmed to be satisfactory. 4. Hormone therapy can cause peptic ulcers, which require dietary management. 5. Prednisone causes malabsorption of calcium.

Isoniazid (INH) (a drug used to treat tuberculosis)	Causes B6 deficiency in some persons because it is an antagonist to the vitamin
Laxatives	Harsh laxatives may cause diarrhealike effects: Food passes through the GI tract too fast to be absorbed. Mineral oil absorbs vitamins A and D, preventing them from being absorbed.
Licorice candy	Limits potassium absorption
Metformin and Phenformin Hypoglycemic agents used in diabetics	Competitively inhibit vitamin B12 absorption
Para-amino salicylic acid, used to treat tuberculosis	Can cause malabsorption of fat and folic acid; blocks absorption of vitamin B12
Potassium chloride, used to replenish potassium lost due to diuretic use	Depresses absorption of vitamin B12

From Kart/Metress/Metress: *Aging, Health and Society*, © 1988 Boston: Jones and Bartlett Publishers.

joying it? How and why does it seem to be miserable for them? Are they goal-setting and identifying realistic ways to meet their goals? What are the stumbling blocks and problems? Have their living arrangements changed?

Economic Status

The stereotype is that the older adult is in the lower income bracket. About 15–20% of older persons fit this picture, and of this percentage, 40% are minority groups, with the black female being at the lowest level. Conversely, the majority of older adults are in a higher income bracket; they usually own their home and have relatively low expenses.

Stress

It has been said that aging is the ability to survive stress and, laughingly, that gray hair is hereditary—you get it from your kids! However, changes attributed to aging are most apparent when the individual is under stress. Such is the source for comments like "That took 10 years off my life!" and "He looks 40 years older!" The nurse must assess the degree of stressful life events that the older adult has experienced. The more common ones are dealing with death, disease, accidents, and retirement. The major health problems of older adults fall into the category of chronic disease. Commonly occurring conditions are accidental injuries, mental health problems, nutritional problems, colon/breast/cervical cancer, hearing and visual defects, anemia, diabetes, renal disease, poorly fitting dentures, dental caries, and periodontal disease. The leading causes of death in people over age 65 are congestive heart failure, stroke, cancer, and accidents.

Assessment of Mental Health Status in the Older Adult

In the not too distant past it was thought that chronic and acute organic brain syndromes were consequences of aging. Any signs of disorientation, delirium, confusion, decreased cognitive ability, excitement, or poor judgment were attributed to the aging process. Yet young and middle-aged clients who are afflicted by such conditions as hypoglycemia, hypokalemia, anemia, dehydration, cardiac failure, and stroke will manifest many of these same mental changes. The old stereotype of intellectual decline in the older adult has become a self-fulfilling prophecy in many cases. Most people assume that intellectual decrement in the later years of life is a universal and unavoidable phenomenon. In a 7-year longitudinal study of older adults (Schaie, 1985), it was found that on the average, intellectual functioning did decline in the sixth decade of life; however, even by age 81 about 50% of the subjects maintained their intellectual functioning level over the 7 years. Other than genetic factors, those individuals who maintained function were free of cardiovascular disease, were of at least middle-class socioeconomic status, and had a stimulating and engaged lifestyle. They also described themselves as having flexible attitudes and behaviors during the middle-aged years. In light of these findings, professionals and the media need to educate the public and focus attention on those 95% of the elderly who are not institutionalized, who are living in the community, and who possess full cognitive competence.

The older adult must be approached with respect and value of equal worth and importance. Nurses can play a significant role in teaching and encouraging the older adult to seek compensation for sensory changes and to remain active in lifestream activity. More effort needs to be placed on developing flexible retirement plans and on preretirement counseling. Chronological age, in the form of mandatory retirement, has become nothing more than a constraining time frame.

The usual parameters of mental health and techniques used for assessing intellectual functioning are the same as described in Chapter 5. Depression and suicide have a high incidence in the older age group and are due to the same kind of problems experienced by persons of a younger age group who also manifest depression and attempt or commit suicide. A decrease in self-esteem may be a basis. Disengagement from society may contribute to a lowered self-image. Sensory deprivation brought about by living alone and ignored by society may give rise to depression. Sensory stimulation, or "future shock" due to increased technological changes, may also be the cause of mental stress and dysfunction. Research has shown that the degree of participation in family and community is positively correlated with an individual's mental state and functioning. Assessment therefore needs to include an investigation of family life and participation in such aspects of community life as volunteer work, senior citizen groups, and pastoral visits. (See Figure 22-3.)

Physical Assessment of the Older Adult

The following information addresses the physical assessment of the older adult in ways that differ from the process of assessment found in the major portion of the textbook. For example, the normal physiologic changes attributed to the aging process will be reflected in criteria of norms for this age group. However, at the present there is much doubt regarding whether the changes commonly observed in the older adult are due to aging, since wide variations are observed. In other words, in regard to physical changes that are thought to be due to aging, a 70-year-old may actually be in better physical shape than a 30-year-old. This is dependent on many things, such as lifestyle, genetics, life stresses, and environment. Logically, though, one would expect that such changes would be present after many years of wear and tear on all of the body parts and systems. Therefore, in assessment of the older adult, you must be careful not to stereotype; you must approach the process with an objective attitude.

Assessment of the Integument

Assessment techniques or procedures learned in earlier chapters will not be repeated.

Inspection

Over the years the skin begins to lose its elasticity and becomes thinner, particularly over the dorsum of the hands. Skin turgor is poor to fair, and because of the thinning phenomenon, the superficial blood vessels are more visible. The skin appears wrinkled and sagging is prominent. The skin color is generally paler than in the middle-aged adult, even in the absence of anemia. However, anemia is a common problem; it may be due in part to decreased iron absorption in the stomach. Hydrochloric acid is needed for this iron absorption, and the production of hydrochloric acid by the gastric mucosal cells diminishes with age. Becauses of the iron deficiency state, vascular skin lesions such as petechiae and ecchymosis may be frequently observed. Another reason for the presence of vascular lesions may be medications such as anticoagulants and aspirin. Types of nonpathologic lesions commonly seen are cherry angiomas (small ruby-red round papular lesions) and hyperkeratosis (raised flat brown-black lesions). Because of the increased incidence of diabetes in the older adult, xanthomas are common. In the presence of diabetes, the older adult, like the younger client with diabetes, will be prone to yeast, fungal, and bacterial infections.

The hair of the older adult may be thinner on all parts of the body as well as on the head. Older women may develop upper lip and chin whiskers. Older men do not usually need to shave as often because facial hair growth is retarded. The

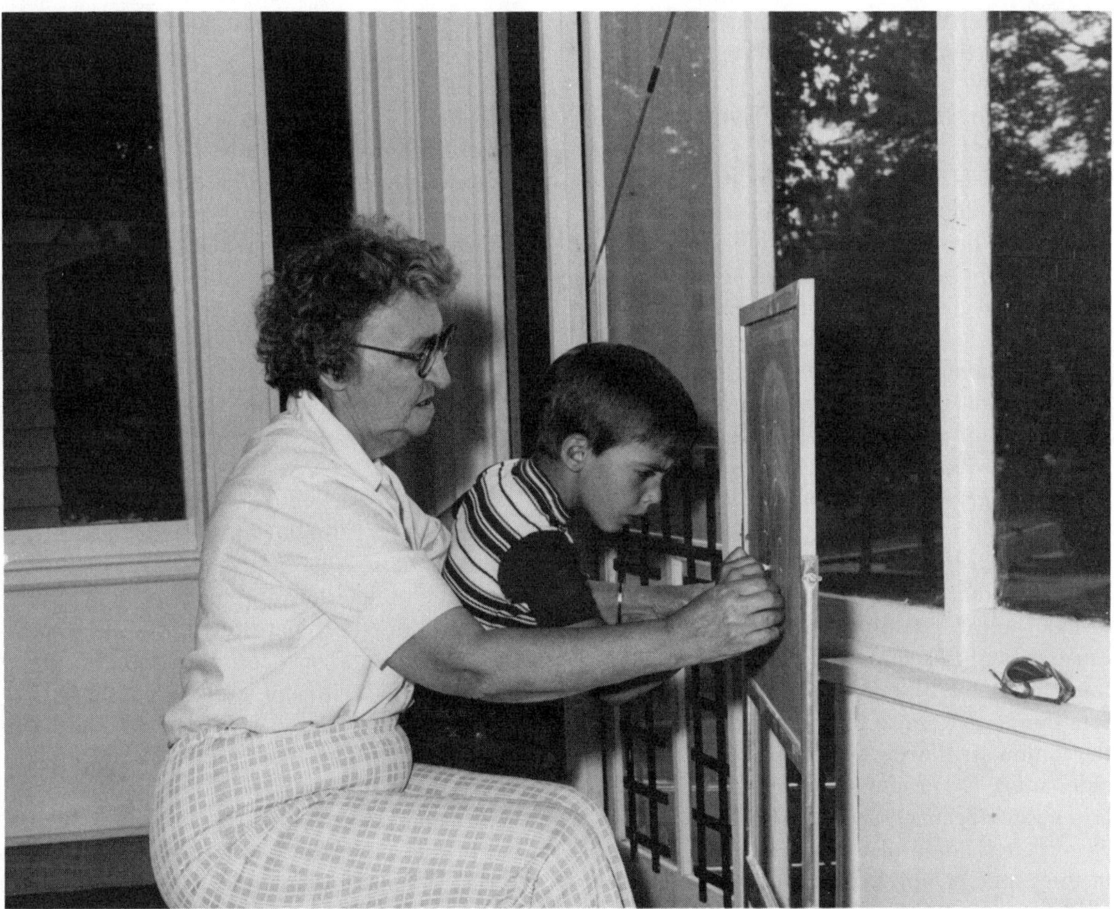

Figure 22-3 Involvement has been highly correlated with an individual's mental state and functioning.

color of the hair may vary from the natural coloring of the middle years to a dull gray, silver, white, or yellow.

The nail growth slows and the thickness increases.

Palpation
The skin of the older adult is dry to the touch because of diminished functioning of the sebaceous and sweat glands. Additional factors promoting dryness are exposure to wind and sun, hot climates, increased use of soap with inadequate rinsing, frequent bathing, and central heating systems. Frequently, pruritus becomes a problem with dry skin.

Assessment of the Neck

Inspection
Difficulty in swallowing (dysphagia) may be noted due to diminished salivary gland function. Jugular venous distention (JVD) may be noted with regard to the common incidence of impending or existing heart failure (see discussion in Chapter 14).

Palpation
Palpation of the carotid pulses must be performed with caution so as not to massage the carotid bodies, thereby causing bradycardia to occur. Moreover, both carotid arteries should not be palpated at the same time; this could result in vertigo (dizziness) or syncope (fainting) should the vertebral arteries, which extend up the posterior portion of the neck, have a high degree of atherosclerosis.

Auscultation
Because of the potential of a higher degree of atherosclerosis, which begins early in childhood

(about age 9), the carotids should be auscultated for the detection of bruits (see Chapter 14).

Assessment of the Eye

Inspection

Loss of the lateral third of the eyebrows is a common sign accompanying hypothyroid state, especially in the older woman. There may be increased signs and symptoms of irritation and infection because of diminished tearing and the subsequent loss of protection afforded by this process. Increased vulnerability to irritation and infection can be caused by the commonly occurring condition of extropion (eyelids turn outward), in which the palpebral conjunctiva is readily observed, giving the eyes a sagging or "sad sack" appearance. With entropion (eyelids turn inward) the inward turning of the lashes onto the bulbar conjunctiva and cornea gives rise to mechanical irritation. These conditions may cause enough discomfort to require correction; this is a relatively simple surgical procedure. It is not unusual to see a thinning and yellowing of the conjunctiva. Arcus senilis, particularly in the older adult, is considered a normal variation and is of no significance (see Chapter 11). Because of changes in the neurologic system some decrease in the range of upward gaze may be observed when checking the extraocular muscle movements (EOMs). In addition, the eyes may be unable to converge. Also, decrease in the peripheral fields of vision is commonly noted. The older adult requires corrective lens because of the atrophied/fibrosed condition of the ciliary bodies and resultant loss of accommodation and loss of elasticity in the lens per se. Cataract phenomenon is common, and the nurse should carefully check for this via oblique lighting (see "Ophthalmoscopic Examination" in Chapter 11).

Ophthalmic examination of the eyegrounds typically reveals tortuosity and silverwire retinal vessel changes despite the blood pressure of the older adult. Be aware though that the presence of A-V nicking signifies arteriosclerosis of the retinal arteries. The incidence of diabetes in the older adult is higher than in any other age group. It is therefore common to observe the fundoscopic changes characteristic of diabetics, such as hard exudates, cotton wool patches, flame-shaped hemorrhages, microaneurysm, and narrowed arteries (see "Ophthalmoscopic Examination" in Chapter 11).

Palpation

Palpation for extraocular pressure may reveal an increase. Because glaucoma commonly occurs in the older adult, a more accurate assessment of intraocular pressure should be performed every 2 years in persons over 40 years of age using a tonometer (see "Intraocular Pressure" in Chapter 11).

Assessment of the Nose, Mouth, Pharynx, and Ear

Inspection

With aging, especially in older men, there is an increase in hair growth in the nares. Additionally, it is not unusual for the sense of smell to be diminished bilaterally and for taste acuity to be decreased due to the atrophy of the taste buds. The latter change may account for the practice, often observed with aging, of increasing the use of seasoning on food. Conditions attributing to inadequate intake of vitamins, whether decreased finances, loss of teeth, or inability to exercise social desire for eating due to being alone, may manifest as cheilosis, crusted or tender lips, and an edematous tongue. The mouth should also be carefully inspected for abrasions and sores caused by ill-fitting dentures. It is not unusual to find a decreased response to the gag reflex. The cilia in the ear become coarser and stiff with aging and present interference with the sound waves reaching the tympanic membrane. In addition there appears to be an accumulation of cerumen, which is influential in the decreased hearing commonly observed in the older adult. Otosclerosis and neurosensory changes further compound the problem. The chief difficulty begins with the perception of high-frequency tones; communication may be impaired, resulting in inadequate history taking. This inability to communicate adequately due to hearing loss tends to give the older adult the appearance of being confused or unsociable. This problem could be an impetus for withdrawal from interacting with others because of embarrassment and frustration and for the state of depression frequently observed in the older adult. The older adult should be screened for hearing defects and should undergo dental examination every 2 years.

Assessment of the Lungs

Inspection

An increased anteroposterior diameter may be observed due to senile emphysema, secondary to loss of lung tissue elasticity and resulting from degenerative changes in the ribs and vertebrae and increase in rigidity of the rib cage. The first sign of these changes is a shortness of breath. Adding to this is the atrophy and decreased strength of the respiratory muscles and the decreased efficiency of neurologic innervation of the respiratory muscles. There is debate as to whether a Tine test should be done once in this age group (60–80 years old). However, the older adult is at risk for tuberculosis, even though the incidence of tuberculosis is rare today. The theory underlying this belief is that the older adult lived through a time when tuberculosis had a high incidence and treatment was inadequate and that the disease can surface years after the primary infection dissipates.

Percussion

When percussing the lung fields, pay careful attention to the apices of the lungs, which extend above the level of the clavicles, because that is the most common site for tuberculosis. Also, the diaphragmatic excursion is generally decreased in the older adult due to the changes that occur in the respiratory system.

Auscultation

Auscultation is not as diagnostic in the older adult as in the younger client because there is less movement of air, particularly in the bases of the lungs, compared to the apices. This is because of the gradual decrease in lung tissue elasticity and limitation of chest movement and expansion due to calcification of the costal cartilages.

Assessment of the Cardiovascular System

Inspection

The face and extremities may be pale or mottled. At 80 years of age the person has approximately one-half the cardiac output (amount of blood forced out of the heart with ventricular contraction) of the younger years. With the decrease in stroke volume, there is a decrease in circulation to all of the organs, including the heart.

Palpation

The extremities, especially the feet, are generally cold to the touch. Wearing socks or "footies" to bed is recommended. Overall the arteries are more easily palpated because of the loss of connective tissue and thinning of the overlying skin. However, due to generalized and localized arteriosclerosis, weak and absent pulses in the lower extremities may be found without additional local signs of decreased circulation.

Auscultation

Heart rate does not change with age at normal rest. Progressive arteriosclerosis, however, leads to peripheral resistance. A significant rise in the systolic blood pressure occurs, and there is a slight rise in the diastolic pressure. This results in an increase in pulse pressure (the difference between the systolic and the diastolic pressure; see "Heart Sounds" in Chapter 14).

Systolic murmurs are present in 60% of the older population. Diastolic murmurs and ventricular gallops are significant of pathology and deserve referral to the physician and follow-up (see "Heart Murmurs" in Chapter 14). Any complaint of chest pain, even mild chest pain, should be thoroughly investigated because the older adult does not experience pain to the degree that the younger person does. A slight feeling of tightness in the chest may be a manifestation of cardiac angina. The typical pattern of precordial site and radiation down one or both arms will be seen. In the older adult the primary symptom of myocardial infarction may be fatigue. Because the pain is of less intensity than in the younger person, it may be ignored in light of the more apparent signs of dyspnea and confusion. Thus, the clinical picture may not appear as serious as it realistically is. Attention must be given to chest pain, no matter how mild, in the older adult.

Assessment of the Breast

The procedure for examining the breasts of the older adult is the same as for any age group (see Chapter 15). However, the incidence of breast carcinoma increases with age. Therefore, breast examination screening should be done annually by a professional, and the examiner can review the procedure for self-breast examination with the client at that time. A regular time each month, perhaps the first day of each month, should be earmarked by the postmenopausal woman for performing the self-breast examination.

Inspection

The breasts may have a sagging appearance, and the nipple line, which is usually at the level of the fourth rib, may fall lower. Gynecomastia may be seen in the older man. This may be due to the decrease in testosterone, leaving a greater effect on the body by adrenal-produced estrogen; it has also been seen in clients who are taking digoxin. In the woman, diminished breast tissue is noted.

Palpation

The consistency of the breast tissue in the older woman may be stringy and more nodular in character. You might detect small, nontender, firm, mobile axillary lymph nodes due to minor trauma and infection that occurred in the hands.

Assessment of the Abdomen

A large number of gastrointestinal problems are commonly found in the older adult. The etiology of most is secondary to decreased circulation. For example, the following sequence of events can follow decreased circulation to the stomach: (1) degeneration of the gastric mucosa results in decreased hydrochloric acid production; (2) achlorhydria or decreased gastric acidity leads to bone disease and iron deficiency anemia, since an acid medium is necessary for the absorption of calcium and iron. Also periumbilical pain may be due to ischemia of the colon.

The weakening of musculature also results in gastrointestinal problems. Diverticulosis is common as well as the incidence of hiatal hernia. Approximately 80–90% of persons age 70 and older have a hiatal hernia. In the older adult who has an acute abdomen, the characteristic sign of abdominal muscle rigidity may be missing. Medications frequently taken by the older adult, such as aspirin and cortisone for arthritis and muscular aches and pains, may cause gastric ulcers. Antacids, such as calcium carbonate, have a constipating effect, and they slow gastrointestinal motility. However, constipation can also be caused by emotional stress via the stress response of sympathetic stimulation, which inhibits intestinal peristalsis. Sedatives, opiates, and tranquilizers all tend to diminish gastric motility. Prolonged use of laxatives tends to weaken the intestinal musculature and contribute to decreased motility and constipation. Laxatives also tend to deplete the body of potassium, further compounding the situation since potassium is essential for neural transmission in muscular contraction.

Inspection

Lipid distribution tends to be concentrated in the trunk of the older adult, and the extremities tend to be thin with little fat deposit. Increased visualization of the vascularity of the abdomen may be noted due to thinning of the skin and abdominal distention secondary to muscular weakness of the abdominal rectus muscles and flatus accumulation secondary to decreased intestinal motility.

Palpation

The liver may be palpable below the right costal margin, but it will be smooth and nontender. Percussion for size will reveal a normal-size liver. The downward displacement of the liver in absence of disease is due to senile emphysema, wherein the overinflation of the lungs maintains the diaphragm at a lower position. Refer to Chapter 16 for the palpation and percussion techniques used in assessing the abdomen. Palpation of the lymph nodes in the groin may reveal nontender, small, mobile nodes secondary to multiple minor injuries and infections in the feet and legs.

Auscultation

Abdominal aortic aneurysms resulting from weakening of the vessel wall may give rise to a bruit heard mid-abdomen above the umbilicus. The bruits of stenotic renal arteries will be heard above the umbilicus on either side of the midline area (see Chapter 16). Decrease in the frequency of bowel sounds may be observed.

Assessment of the Musculoskeletal System

Osteoporosis is common in the older adult; postmenopausal Caucasian women are at highest risk. Other factors predisposing the client to osteoporosis are inadequate calcium intake and lack of vitamin D, although the latter does not occur as often if the person is exposed to sunshine. Good sources of vitamin D are milk, eggs, liver, and fish. Osteoporosis presents the hazard of fractures occurring. Osteoarthritis can be seen due to the wear and tear of joint motion over the years.

Inspection

Height may decrease 1 to 4 inches from lifetime maximum height. Changes in the joints and tendons influence the overall appearance of the older adult. The appearance may be one of some kyphosis and slight flexion of the elbows, knees, and hips. There is generally a decrease in muscle mass, and with this, the bony prominences are usually more visible. Because of fibrotic changes in the muscles, tendons, and joints, range of motion is limited and the arms swing less when the client is walking. The use of Brudzinski's sign to diagnose meningitis is futile when the older adult has difficulty bending his head forward because of cervical spondylosis.

Palpation

Atrophy of the musculature can most often be detected by palpation.

Assessment of the Neurologic System

Inspection

With diminished neurologic functioning, primarily affected by vascular changes and decreased oxygen, it is not uncommon to observe senile tremors in the older adult. These are benign involuntary movements involving the head, face, and hands. They appear slightly as a jerking vertical or horizontal movement of the head and continuous facial and tongue movements.

Percussion

The voluntary and automatic reflexes are more sluggish. This is seen in the pupillary response to light and also at times with the deep tendon reflexes. Although the deep tendon reflexes remain present in the healthy aged, the lack of elasticity of the tendons and arthritic involvement of the joints may result in a diminished or absent deep tendon reflex, particularly of the knees and the Achilles tendon reflex. The sense of light touch, pain, and vibration is depressed in the feet, but if this occurs above mid-shin level, pathology such as peripheral neuropathies or spinal cord tumor may be present.

Assessment of the Genitals and Rectum

Inspection

Decreased cardiac output from reduced cardiac muscle efficiency and arteriosclerosis results in less blood flow to the kidneys and thus decreased filtration rate. The degenerative changes in the kidneys per se lead to a decrease in the number of nephrons. The tubular walls become less permeable, and toxic levels of drugs accumulate as a result of decreased tubular excretion. On the other hand, dehydration occurs because of diminished tubular reabsorption. You must therefore be attuned to observing for drug overdose signs and symptoms and hallmarks of dehydration. Decreased urine output could be a sign of dehydration, but it should be thoroughly investigated because there are many additional problems that would cause this sign as well. With polyuria a urinalysis should be done, since there is an increased incidence of diabetes in this age group. Furthermore, a routine urinalysis should be done every 4–5 years for the purpose of screening for diabetes. An annual urinalysis is recommended for the older woman because urinary tract infections are common and many times asymptomatic.

A prolapsed uterus is a commonly observed problem in the older woman due to muscle weakness. When inspecting the perineum, pay special attention to the vestibule (the area beneath the clitoris and urethra), since this is a common site for carcinoma of the genitals in the woman. During a pelvic exam the nurse may find that the vaginal walls appear thinner and drier; it is not uncommon for vaginal pruritus to result. Additionally, narrowing and shortening of the vaginal canal may be noted. In the older man the size of the testes is decreased.

Palpation

Rectal examination may reveal constipation or fecal impaction and commonly occurring problems like a cystocele in women and benign prostatic hyperplasia in men. The incidence of colonic cancer increases with age and should, therefore, be an object of screening in annual health history-taking. Also the occurrence of prostatic carcinoma rises for older men. Men over 40 years old should have an annual rectal examination.

Summary

The older population is steadily growing faster than any other age group; therefore, it is important that the older adult be understood in order to promote well-being and meet health needs. Stereotyping has placed limitations on how the older adult is viewed by the general society and on how older adults live in order that their behavior conforms to society's expectations. Sexual behaviors, living arrangements, need for privacy, capability to make decisions, and control of personal finances are a few of the areas in which the American society questions and restricts this group by stereotyping. Fears of institutionalization and an invasion of privacy deter the older adult from seeking health care. Fear of losing independence and self-sufficiency keep them from enlarging their social support networks. Fear of the stigma of being considered a "charity" case results in avoiding welfare and free services. Older adults have, to a great extent, become the victims of society. Ironically, they are the primary transmitters of culture.

The many signs and symptoms attributed to the aging process must be regarded cautiously. Myths surrounding mental abilities have been shattered with research revealing that intellectual functioning, learning, and decision making do continue to grow even in 81-year-old adults. Also, physiologically, some older adults are in "better shape" than persons of much younger years.

The older adult is fitting into a self-fulfilled prophecy of what society dictates. However, the myths and stereotypes are gradually dissipating as older adults are becoming more assertive and active in such spheres as academia, politics, and sports. The lifestyles of older adults are changing accordingly. In this chapter each phase of physical assessment was discussed in light of norms of the older adult and health risks of the older adult age group.

Discussion Questions/Activities

1. Give some examples to illustrate how culture dictates the behavior of an older adult.
2. Choose a seemingly healthy older adult and take his health history.
3. Compare the similarities between the health histories of several older adults.
4. Compare the health history and physical and mental status of two older adults—one with a broad social support system and one without such a support system.
5. Analyze physical findings from several physical assessments of older adults and identify physiologic changes that are attributed to the aging process.
6. Role-play the part of an older adult with normal mental functioning who is institutionalized and is being cared for by a nurse's aide who holds stereotypic beliefs regarding the older adult.

EXAMPLE OF A HEALTH ASSESSMENT OF AN OLDER ADULT

HEALTH HISTORY

Name: James Guisweite
Address: RD#3, Easton, Maryland
Sex: Male
Age: 70
Birthdate: 12/3/18
Marital status: Widower since 10/86
Occupation: Retired dairy farmer since 2/84, worked 5 years in sawmill as a young man 21-26 yrs of age.
Religion: Methodist (attends church regularly)
Race: Caucasian
Ethnic origin: German
Education: High school graduate
Informant: Client, a reliable historian

History of Present Illness
Comes to clinic every third week for blood pressure check. Stiffness and discomfort in hands due to arthritis has increased over the past three months. Grief acceptance (see next topic).

Personal History and Patterns of Living
Was "always self-sufficient." Very close relationship with wife—"We worked, played, laughed and cried together." Acceptance of wife's death as "God's will." Was very depressed and antisocial first year following her death. Youngest daughter strongest support. Quite active recently in farmers market and livestock auction—selling vegetables and regular socializing. Sold all of farm buildings, equipment, and land at the time of his retirement. Retained home, 1 acre orchard and 1 acre garden area (total 3.5 acres). Traveled to Europe and across the United States with wife before her death. These trips and photos taken provide pleasant reminiscing. He states no financial difficulties. Has health insurance—Mutual Benefit Corporation, and Medicare.

Family Health History
Denies family history of cancer, diabetes, heart disease, alcoholism, bleeding disorders, mental illness, stomach problems, liver disorders, kidney diseases. Family history significant for arthritis, hypertension, and TB.

Geographic Exposure
Within-state travel until retirement, then trip to Europe and across U.S. and to sons in Vermont and Pennsylvania and eldest daughter in Delaware.

Lifestyle
Sexuality: Very polite and traditional gentleman behavior, i.e., opening doors, standing when woman enters room, jokes tastefully with both young and older women. Traditional values of monogamy. Discomfort/conflict with separation of eldest daughter from her husband. Recently spending time with a "lady friend." His children encourage and support the latter relationship. "Too soon to think about marriage—I'll cross that bridge when I come to it!"
Personal Habits: Drinks a beer or wine cooler 1–2/wk. No coffee or tobacco. Takes over-the-counter pain pills for arthritis (Advil, Excedrin extra-strength) 2–4 tabs/day in the past 3–4 months.
Diet: Cooks for self. Eats 3–4 evenings at youngest daughter's home. Has cut down on his salt intake. Reads labels and buys low-salt food products and no-caffeine products. Breakfast—fruit, cereal, milk, toast. Lunch—soup and sandwich. Dinner—meat or fish (trying to eat more chicken and turkey than red meats), baked or broiled potatoes, vegetable, milk. Snacks on saltless pretzels before dinner and/or before bedtime. Has taken daily multivitamin capsules for last 5–6 years. Appetite is "not as good as it used to be."
Sleep and rest patterns: Slept 10–12 hrs/24 hr day after wife died. Lately is sleeping 6–7 hrs—feels rested. Up usually one time during night to urinate around 3–4 A.M.
Activities of daily living: No difficulties caring for self. Daughter does laundry and "helps keep the house clean."
Home and neighborhood: Close neighbor across the road and several good friends within 2–3 miles. Sleeps and lives mostly on first floor of home.
Interpersonal relationships: Doesn't see sons and eldest daughter as much as he would like, but youngest daughter "has been a blessing—I don't know what I would have done without her and the grandchildren."

(continued on page 534)

Recreation: Loves to walk in the woods. Works about his home, garden and orchard almost every day. Helps youngest daughter and her husband frequently with projects for home improvement. They live 8 miles from the client. Enjoys socializing every Tuesday and Thursday nights at the livestock auction barn. Going square and round dancing "some" on Saturday nights with lady friend. Doesn't watch much TV. Reads the local daily newspaper.

Previous Experience with Illness

Had measles and mumps as a young child. Smallpox vaccination when 6 years old and before traveling to Europe (3 years ago). Flu shot—5 years and 3 years ago. Denies any known allergies. Hospitalized for fractured left leg at 56 years of age (kicked by a bull). Appendectomy at age 23.

Review of Systems

General health: No significant loss or gain in weight; denies fatigue, weakness, night sweats, cold or heat intolerance, easily bruised, excessive thirst or perspiration.

Integument: No history of skin diseases; some brown "liver" spots on face and arms. Nails—"seem thicker than younger years." Denies jaundice, eczema, psoriasis, hives, rashes, boils, ecchymoses, nevi that have changed in color or size, open sores that are slow to heal. Hair—"is thinning." Some pruritus and dry skin experienced. Mild seborrhea of scalp.

Head: Denies unusually frequent or severe headaches.

Eyes: Wears bifocals. Last eye exam two years ago. No history of infections or pain. Denies blurring, diplopia, photophobia, excessive lacrimation. No spots or halo-rainbows experienced.

Ears: "Hearing is somewhat diminished." No history of infections. Denies pain, discharge, tinnitus, auditory hallucinations and vertigo.

Nose, nasopharynx, and paranasal sinuses: No discharge. Denies epistaxis, allergies, postnasal drip, pain, and tenderness. Very seldom had colds except the past two years had winter-spring seasonal change cold. Smell lost when colds present.

Mouth and throat: New dentures in May of this year (old dentures were loose and rubbed). Denies bleeding gums; soreness of mouth, tongue, and throat; dysphagia, hoarseness. Edentulous.

Neck: Denies pain, edema, swollen glands, limitation of movement. Some stiffness in early morning experienced past 6 months.

Breasts: Denies drainage, soreness, masses, hypertrophy, skin changes. Did not realize men should examine breasts monthly.

Cardiorespiratory system: Chest x-ray when had severe cold 2 years ago (Dr. Madison). Denies cough, sputum, dyspnea, orthopnea, and PND. No chest pain, history of anemia, heart disease, palpitations, and varicosities. Takes hydrodiuril tablet 2 times/day when edema occurs (Rx Dr. Madison).

Gastrointestinal system: Denies nausea, vomiting, anorexia, dyspepsia, pyrosis, bright blood in stools, tarry stools, flatulence, pain, rectal pain. Hemorrhoidal discomfort when straining with "hard" stool. Switches to Bran Buds and more fruit in diet when this occurs. Does not drink much water (1–2 glasses/day), likes milk 3–4 glasses/day.

Genitourinary system: Denies frequency, burning upon urination, dribbling, hematuria, difficulty in starting stream, pain, polyuria, and discharge. Has not been sexually active with a partner since death of wife.

Musculoskeletal system: (see neck) Stiffness and some "turning of my fingers and knuckle-swelling." Occasional ankle swelling every 3–4 months for past year (hydrodiuril). Denies muscular pain, weakness, leg cramps, sprains, deformities, limp. Fracture of left femur (see previous experience with illness). Some hip and knee pain when cold, damp weather. No joint swelling except "knuckles."

Neurologic system: No history of unconsciousness, seizures. Denies vertigo, syncope, difficulty walking, pain in arms or legs, decreased strength in arms and legs, weakness in one part of his body. Has not experienced tingling, numbness, burning, or crawling sensations anywhere in body. Was "very down in the dumps after my wife died." Has had more energy recently and enjoys friends, family, and activities more. His memory "isn't what it used to be."

Client profile

Mr. James Guisweite, 70-year-old white male, appeared jovial and cooperative. Essentially healthy appearance. Logical thought processes. Mild discomfort presently with arthritis of hands. Able to care for self.

PHYSICAL ASSESSMENT

General impression: Mr. James Guisweite, a 70-year-old white male in NAD. WD/WN. Ruddy complexion, stocky frame, "laughing eyes," friendly but quiet manner. No gross abnormalities noted. 5′10″, 180 lb (weight stable for past 10 years ± 5 lb).

TPR—98.2°F, 76, 22.

BP—148/86 left arm sitting; 140/86 right arm sitting; left leg BP 160/82 (see clinic BP flow sheet for record of BP readings).

Integument: Thinning of skin over hands; good skin turgor; ruddy complexion; small brown macular lesions (½—1½ cm) on face, forearms, and hands; hyperkeratosis—mild, generalized over body (papular, flat black lesions, approx. ¼–½ cm). Silver, thin hair slightly receding. Nails—no clubbing and good capillary refill. No cyanosis noted; no ecchymosis; a few cherry angiomas on shoulders and anterior chest; skin warm, rough-dry texture.

Head: Normocephalic; atraumatic; scalp clear; no tenderness. Face—symmetrical. No sinus tenderness.

Neck: Limited flexion, extension, and lateral flexion: 10–15 degrees short of normal range of motion. No JVD noted. Carotids equal bilaterally. No bruits noted. No thyroid enlargement; no masses; trachea midline; no lymphadenopathy.

Eyes: Arcus senilis noted; eyebrows full; no edema. Sclera white; small opacities noted left cornea; EOMs intact; PERRLA. Consensual reaction; sluggish on accommodation; unable to converge smoothly or sustain convergence. Corneal reflex. Peripheral fields slightly decreased 10–20 degrees by gross confrontation technique. Fundoscopy—red reflex; well-demarcated disk; slight arterial narrowing; no A-V nicking, exudates, or hemorrhages noted. Referral for visual acuity and tonometry check. No increase in ocular tension noted on palpation.

Nose, mouth, pharynx: No nasal obstruction; nasal mucosa red; lips, tongue, buccal mucosa, pharynx free of lesions on inspection and palpation; sluggish gag reflex; uvular reflex symmetrical; tongue midline.

Ears: No lesions; no discharge; no mastoid tenderness; large amount cerumen bilaterally—Rx with cerumenex. T.M.'s pearly gray; landmarks present; Weber s̄ lateralization; Rinne—AC > BC; can hear whispered voice; clock ticking 10″ from right ear and 8″ from left ear.

Respiratory: Mild increase in AP diameter; respirations 22–24; pink skin color; symmetrical respirations. No use of respiratory accessory muscles; fremitus present; resonant percussion notes; bilateral diaphragmatic excursion, 3–4 cm.; vesicular breath sounds.

Cardiovascular: NSR; 76 apical; feet warm, good color. Peripheral pulses:

	T	C	B	R	F	P	PT	DP
L	1+	2+	2+	2+	2+	2+	2+	1+
R	2+	2+	2+	2+	2+	2+	0	1+

No abnormal pulsations; no thrills; PMI at left 5ICS/MCL; MSL → LCBD = 10 cm at 5ICS; Grade I systolic murmur at apex—does not radiate; heart sounds distant; normal S_1 and S_2; $A_2 = P_2$; no abnormal splitting, ventricular gallops, or rub noted.

Breast: No tissue enlargement; everted nipples; no dimpling or retraction; no discharge; slight sagging; no masses noted; no lymphadenopathy—axillary, supra, and infraclavicular.

Abdomen: Flat and symmetrical; no hernias noted; B.S. present. No renal/aortic/femoral bruits noted; tympany in all four quadrants; spleenic dullness—7 cm at left MAL; liver dullness at right MCL = 10 cm; palpable liver 2 cm below RCM—smooth and nontender. Kidneys nonpalpable; palpable lymph nodes in left inguinal area—small, nontender, mobile.

Musculoskeletal: Mild kyphosis; body and limb symmetry; tenderness in PIPS, MIPS, and DIPs of all fingers. Slight enlargement of MIPS: Full ROM except for neck, fingers, and hips—latter 10–20 degrees less than norm; no crepitation. Muscles—symmetrical and good strength; proximal—distal muscle strength equal; muscle atrophy noted in biceps and fine muscles of the hands; no muscle tenderness; no edema or masses noted.

Neurologic: Slight horizontal tremors of head; no difficulty with gait; Romberg sign absent; smooth coordination of upper and lower extremities; CN I—not tested; CN II—referred for eye exam and tonometry; CN III–XII grossly intact (taste not tested); sensitive to pain, light touch, and vibration; position sense intact. DTRs:

	B	T	BR	P	A	PR
L	2+	2+	2+	1+	1+	↓
R	2+	2+	2+	2+	1+	↓

(continued on page 536)

Abdominal reflex intact; no clonus, Babinski absent. Mental status—Logical thought processes; alert; no speech difficulties; has calendar for notes to remind him of events; recent and remote memory intact; affect and mood congruent; "Christian—law abiding man"; intellectual functioning intact; cultivating new affectional and satisfying roles with family, friends, and initiating social activities appropriate to health, energy, and interests.

Genitals/rectum: Urinalysis WNL; circumcised; normal male pubic hair distribution; body and pubic hair thinning; no lesions or discharge noted; urethral meatus at end of penis; foreskin easily retracted; no abnormalities noted; no testicular masses; no indirect inguinal or femoral hernia noted; no rectal masses; several small anal tabs noted; sphincter and cremasteric reflex intact; stool negative for occult blood; prostate slightly enlarged, nontender and firm consistency.

CHAPTER 23

Assessment of Women's Health

LEARNING OBJECTIVES

1. Discuss the morbidity and mortality rate for women, and describe the differences in these rates between men and women.
2. Review and describe the physiology of menstruation.
3. Describe the components of a health history pertinent to distinguishing between primary and secondary dysmenorrhea and amenorrhea.
4. Describe the characteristics and symptoms of metrorrhagia and dysfunctional uterine bleeding.
5. Describe premenstrual syndrome.
6. Identify common physical changes of menopause.
7. Discuss anorexia nervosa and bulimia, and describe specific changes noted during assessment.
8. Describe those components of the health history specifically related to pregnancy.
9. Identify physiologic changes occurring throughout pregnancy.

Female mortality has always been less than that for males; however, the morbidity rate for women is higher than that of men. Women of all ages make more visits to the physician than men. Several theories have been advanced to explain this phenomenon. For example, women report more illness than men presumably because it is more culturally acceptable for them to do so. Women's social role carries with it more stresses and anxiety, especially in confronting the more nurturant and circumscribed roles defined by society. Also, women are urged to seek more help in relation to contraception, prepartum and postpartum care, and relief of menopausal symptoms.

In the 1960s the women's movement drew attention to the special health needs of women resulting from their anatomy and physiology and the demands placed on them as they gave birth, raised families, and entered the workforce in increasing numbers. Greater numbers of women expressed dissatisfaction with the health care options available to them. Parameters of health or the absence of health were described by men who appeared to know little about normal functioning of women because most of the parameters of pathology had been gathered using male subjects as guides. Women became aware that functions such as menstruation, menopause, childbearing, and lactation are normal, healthy functions and in fact do not mean that women are less than or weaker than men. Women became critical of treatment that directly impinges on their lives as women, such as gynecologic examinations, birth control, sexuality, childbirth, and psychotherapy.

This chapter provides guidelines for assessing specific events that affect women's lives and health. Assessment data are presented for normal events and for several deviations from normal.

Menstruation

One of the most constant reminders women have of their uniqueness is the occurrence of menstruation every month. This important event prepares women for other unique functions such as pregnancy, lactation, and menopause. Menstruation has been misunderstood by many, and in fact many women have been socialized to feel that it is shameful, dirty, and to be considered an illness. Increased understanding of the event and education are helping women to view menstruation as a healthy and essential biologic and emotional experience.

Problems that occur with menstruation should never be dismissed lightly. The menstrual history must include information regarding onset of menarche, pattern of menstruation, method of contraception, reproductive history, sexual activity, feelings about menstruation, understanding of the event, and the effect of menstruation on lifestyle.

Abnormal vaginal bleeding or lack of bleeding can cause great anxiety for clients. Both are common symptoms, and emotional support must be provided while the cause is determined and treatment prescribed. Women may seek care for absence of bleeding (amenorrhea), painful menstruation (dysmenorrhea), or changes in the menstrual cycle.

Menstruation starts generally at age 11 or 12, although some girls have begun menstruation as early as 9 or as late as 18. Very few have an absolutely regular cycle. The length of the cycle ranges from 20 to 36 days, with the average cycle at 28 days. The menstrual flow lasts 2 to 8 days, with the average flow from 4 to 6 days.

It is important that adolescents and adult women understand menstruation and be aware that it is normal. Old wives' tales warning against activity, bathing, and sexual activity should be ignored. These fears have been passed from one generation to the next, creating fear, anxiety, and embarrassment that continues through life.

The menstrual fluid contains cervical and vaginal mucus as well as degenerated endometrial particles and blood. Sometimes clots appear in the fluid. About 2 to 3 ounces of fluid are lost with the menses, but the amount of flow is highly individual. The fluid does not smell until it makes contact with bacteria in the air and begins to decompose. Sanitary napkins and tampons are common methods of absorbing the flow. Caution is advised when using tampons, however, since toxic shock syndrome appears to be linked to the heavy use of them.

The nurse should also be aware of several other methods to absorb the flow. For instance, some women use a natural sponge. Before insertion a piece of dental floss is tied around the sponge and the sponge is dampened. When the sponge is full, it is removed, washed in cool water and soap, and squeezed to remove excess water before being reinserted. A diaphragm with a little K-Y jelly or contraceptive cream on the edge to hold it in place can be used to collect the flow. In another method, called menstrual extraction, a small tube attached to a suction device is inserted in the uterus when the flow starts and the menstrual fluid is sucked out in 5 minutes. Advocates of this method note that there is no research to indicate the long-range effects of regular menstrual fluid extraction.

Problems Related to Menstruation

Dysmenorrhea

Dysmenorrhea, painful menstruation, is one of the most common gynecologic problems of women. More than half the women in this country experience some discomfort; about 10% are so incapacitated they miss work or school. One study found that 35% of older adolescent girls, 25% of college students, and 60% to 70% of single women in their 30s and 40s experience discomfort severe enough to interfere with normal activities for 1 or 2 days (Green 1977). The degree of pain or discomfort varies with the individual and may be manifested as lower abdominal cramping pain, backache, or aching thighs. Two types of dysmenorrhea are *primary dysmenorrhea*, in which pelvic organs are normal, and *secondary dysmenorrhea,* in which a diagnosed pelvic disease or condition is present.

Primary dysmenorrhea usually develops 1 to 2 years after the onset of menstruation. It appears to be self-limiting and primarily a problem of teenagers and young adults. It disappears or is markedly better by age 25 or following pregnancy. The pain is either sharp or a steady dull ache accompanied by bearing down sensations with referred pain to the legs and suprapubic area. Many women also experience abdominal distention, breast tenderness, nausea and vomiting, dizziness, headache, palpitations, and flushing.

Secondary dysmenorrhea may occur due to such conditions as large uterine or cervical polyps, submucous fibroids, endometriosis, pelvic infection, a fixed malpositioned uterus, the presence of an intrauterine device, or cervical stenosis following recent gynecologic surgery or procedures. Secondary dysmenorrhea generally occurs after a pattern of problem-free periods had been present for some time. The pain is generally more constant in nature and continues throughout the period. A careful history must be obtained to distinguish between primary and secondary dysmenorrhea.

Information must be elicited as to when the client's periods began, since this is an important factor in determining whether primary dysmenorrhea is occurring. Although this problem is now thought to be related to the presence of prostaglandins, some experts still feel the problem is partly or wholly due to psychogenic factors. For this reason the nurse should explore with the client the type of preparation she received prior to onset of menarche and attitude of the client and siblings or female relatives to menstruation.

Information on frequency and duration of menstruation is important so that the nurse can note where the client falls within the range of normal responses. Changes in the character and amount of flow should be noted. The nurse must also determine the time when cramps begin, their duration, and their severity. The relationship between pain and bleeding is significant. Any clotting should also be noted.

The client should be asked about the use of contraceptives since they may affect cramping. The IUD is often associated with more severe cramping, while oral contraceptives suppress ovulation and thereby alleviate dysmenorrhea associated with ovulation. Reproductive history is important because traumatic labor and delivery, cervical lacerations, infections, and gynecologic procedures predispose to secondary dysmenorrhea.

The client's pain threshold and response to pain should be determined. As mentioned previously, the nurse should explore the client's and family's attitudes toward menstruation to help determine whether there is a psychological component to the problem.

Amenorrhea

Amenorrhea, the absence of menstruation, is classified as primary or secondary. It is termed primary if the client has never menstruated and secondary if she has had normal periods. Primary amenorrhea exists if the client has had no menstrual period by age 14 and there is absence of growth and development of secondary sexual characteristics or if there is no menstrual period by age 16 regardless of the presence of secondary sexual characteristics. It may be caused by a variety of factors, including hormonal imbalance, chromosomal disorders, infection, congenital absence of the uterus (müllerian abnormalities), disorders of the anterior pituitary, and disorders in the central nervous system or hypothalamus.

Secondary amenorrhea exists when a client has been menstruating and stops for a period of at least 3 months. The existence of pregnancy should be determined; however, pregnancy is just one of many causes of secondary amenorrhea.

A careful history to determine whether the mother and grandmother had a late menarche can be significant to the diagnosis of primary amenorrhea, since girls tend to menstruate at the same time as their mothers and grandmothers. A history of systemic disease such as diabetes mellitus, tuberculosis, hyperthyroidism, or mitral stenosis may give a clue to the cause of secondary amenorrhea. It is also significant if the client is taking oral contraceptives or tranquilizers, especially chlorpromazine or phenothiazine. Some women experience "post-Pill" amenorrhea in which menstruation is not reestablished up to 12 months following discontinuation of the Pill. A history of stress, anxiety, and fatigue may also be significant. Women athletes frequently stop menstruating when they train very hard. This probably occurs because they have a low ratio of body fat to body muscle, resulting in an excessive secretion of prolactin, which in turn decreases release of gonadotropin releasing factor, causing a decrease in FSH, follicular development, and estrogen levels. Anorexia nervosa may cause stress-related anovulation due to the same increase in prolactin seen in athletes. In the obese client it may be the result of increased conversion of androstenedione to estrone by adipose tissue.

Menorrhagia and Metrorrhagia

Menorrhagia is an abnormally excessive menstrual flow. It can occur as the result of anovulatory cycles just prior to puberty and in women nearing menopause. As you assess the client, you must determine what the client considers a heavy flow. For example, women who have discontinued the Pill often describe heavy flow when it may be normal. A woman who saturates a pad every hour for more than 2 hours has an excessive flow, as does a woman who saturates a tampon or pad every 2 hours for 7 to 9 days. Women using IUDs often experience a very heavy flow. Heavy flow may be indicative of anemia, endometriosis, a blood dyscrasia, or the presence of a tumor. A single episode of excessive bleeding may be due to a spontaneous abortion or an ectopic pregnancy. Women at menopause are at great risk for uterine cancer, which often has as a symptom increased bleeding.

Metrorrhagia describes bleeding between periods. Vaginal bleeding is a symptom of ovarian cysts and uterine cancer. When such bleeding occurs for more than 1 month and the client is not taking oral contraceptives, there is cause for concern. There are instances when this is normal. For example, some women have spotting at the time they ovulate. Women who take oral contraceptives may have "breakthrough" bleeding for the first 3 to 4 months. Vaginal infection may also be responsible. Any bleeding in the postmenopausal woman is considered to be abnormal. Bleeding that is continuously occurring in women around the time of menopause is referred to as dysfunctional uterine bleeding (DUB). This specific type of metrorrhagia is usually caused by prolonged estrogen stimulation of the endometrium after long periods of no ovulation secondary to faulty neuroendocrine or ovarian function. These factors cause the continuous proliferation of the endometrium.

A list of causes of menstrual alterations is in Table 23-1.

Premenstrual Syndrome

In recent years a cluster of symptoms appearing just before menstruation and disappearing with the menstrual flow have been referred to as *premenstrual syndrome* (PMS). The awareness that the menstrual period is about to start is experienced by almost all women. For some the symptoms are more dramatic and incapacitating. Examples of symptoms range from mild abdominal fullness, breast tenderness, and mild irritability to severe nervousness, fatigue, crying spells, decreased concentration, and depression.

Katharina Dalton, a pioneer in work on PMS, defines the syndrome as recurrent premenstrual difficulties followed by at least one week entirely free of symptoms. If a woman is experiencing difficulties in her life, these difficulties may not go away completely during the week that is free of premenstrual symptoms but will certainly become more severe premenstrually. For example, a woman whose symptom premenstrually is depression will have at least one week free of depression; on the other hand, a woman who is generally depressed will not have a week where she is not depressed, but her depression will be more severe premenstrually.

Many theories have been offered to explain PMS symptoms. Explanations have included progesterone deficiency, estrogen excess, or a relatively high estrogen-progesterone ratio, vitamin deficiency, hypoglycemia, hormone allergy, fluid retention, prolactin excess, stress, endorphins, and psychosomatic causes. Several studies have been carried out in an attempt to correlate a wide variety of symptoms and behaviors with the premenstrual phase of the menstrual cycle. Most of these have been inconclusive and in fact have been criticized for their methodology. Much research needs to be done, not only related to the premenstrual phase but about all the phases of the cycle.

As nurses we must be aware of the problems experienced by women related to menstruation and assess the health and symptoms that are occurring with a goal of helping her take steps to alleviate those symptoms. When taking the history of the client, keep in mind several characteristics that are suggestive of premenstrual syndrome:

1. Painless periods are more common than painful ones.
2. The onset is often seen at puberty, after stop-

Table 23-1. Causes of Menstrual Alterations

Alteration	Causes	Alteration	Causes
Amenorrhea		Amenorrhea	
Primary	Anatomical alterations	Secondary	Pregnancy
	Imperforate hymen		Psychological alterations
	Blind end to vagina		Crash dieting (anorexia nervosa)
	Cervical stenosis		Drugs: cytotoxic agents, phenothiazines, contraceptives, narcotics
	Agenesis of cervix		Pituitary or ovarian tumors
	Agenesis of uterus		Chronic disease (as per primary amenorrhea)
	Gonadal alterations	Dysmenorrhea	Anatomical alteration
	Turner's syndrome		Intrauterine device
	Androgen-secreting ovarian tumor		Prostaglandin overproduction
	Pituitary alterations		Infection
	Hypopituitarism		Endometriosis
	Hypothalamic tumors		Idiopathic
	Adrenal alterations	Menometorrhagia	Anovulatory cycles (dysfunctional uterine bleeding)
	Adrenogenital syndrome		Hematological disorders
	Androgen-secreting tumor		Hemophilia
	Chronic disease		von Willebrand's disease
	Renal failure		Thrombocytopenia
	Inflammatory bowel disease		Spontaneous abortion
	Collagen-vascular disease		Ectopic pregnancy
	Hypothyroidism		Birth control pills
	Cushing's syndrome		Trauma
	Addison's disease		Tumor
	Cardiopulmonary disease		

From Servonsky/Opas: *Nursing Management of Children*, © 1987 Boston: Jones and Bartlett Publishers.

ping birth control pills, after pregnancy, or after a period of amenorrhea.

3. The severity also seems to increase after stopping birth control pills, pregnancy, amenorrhea, tubal ligation, or hysterectomy.
4. Pregnancies may be complicated by miscarriage, toxemia, or postpartum depression.
5. There may be an onset of acute symptoms such as migraine headaches, panic attacks, epilepsy, or severe depression after long food gaps (5 hours in the day or 13 hours overnight).
6. The woman may experience food cravings, binges, or increased sensitivity to alcohol premenstrually.
7. Client may notice significant weight gain, water and salt retention, abdominal bloating, and mastalgia.

Women who have symptoms should be encouraged to use a calendar to chart which symptoms are occurring and when they occur. Those who are ovulating can correlate their temperature change with symptoms. At ovulation the body temperature rises 0.5 to 1.0 degree and stays elevated until the next menstrual period.

Many women can be helped to alleviate or minimize their symptoms by changing their lifestyle (improved diet and exercise). Some may have to be medicated with progesterone. All women with symptoms need to have support and encouragement to manage their lives and avoid the stereotype of women as unreliable or out of control once a month because of menstruation.

Menopause

Menopause is the end of a cycle that began at puberty with the menarche. The most common age for the onset of the menarche is 12, while menstruation stops from 45 to 53. Unfortunately, menopause has been felt by many, including health professionals, to be a negative experience and is often described by the symptoms of dysfunction, rather than a healthy and normal part of life's experience. *The Merck Manual* lists menopause not under "Gynecology" as a natural physiological function, but under "Ovarian Dysfunction." In her very informative book about menopause, Rosetta Reitz objected to this approach because the attitude promotes the idea that a woman's life is normal for the 30 years she ovulates and abnormal before and after (Reitz 1977). The nurse can help to convey the normality of the period of menopause. Changes take place in the woman's body during menopause, and some of these can cause discomfort just as with the menarche. Discomfort can be minimized through education of the client about the changes, a healthy mental and physical lifestyle, and occasionally the use of hormone therapy.

When taking the health history of the premenopausal client, ask the age at which menopause occurred for the client's mother. As with menarche, mothers and daughters appear to begin and end their menstrual periods about the same time. Menopause that occurs through the normal process of age tends to happen gradually. Many authorities feel it takes about 5 years to complete the cycle. The events of the climacteric can be divided into three phases:

1. *Premenopausal*—a time in which menstruation is still occurring but may become irregular. At this stage estrogen decline begins and the fertility index declines.
2. *Menopausal*—at this stage the ovaries are unable to respond to gonadotropins, resulting in the cessation of the menses and infertility.
3. *Postmenopausal*—all traces of ovarian activity are gone and signs of estrogen decline may occur.

During the history taking the nurse must determine how the client views this experience. Often there is a fear of aging, and some women will still anticipate this time in their lives as one in which they will not feel well. Some women may view the menses as having been bothersome and are happy that it is ending. However, as many or more women equate the menses with femininity and may react with depression at the loss of this function. Some women find the period of menopause to be one of renewed interest and satisfaction in themselves. With a sense of how the client views this time, the nurse can help the client achieve a positive state of wellness.

Several physical changes occur with menopause. Vasomotor instability, referred to as "hot flashes," is the sensation of overwhelming heat spreading from the chest upward over the neck, face, and arms. The skin on the affected areas may become flushed, and excessive perspiration may occur. The episodes last from several seconds to a minute and occur most frequently at night, disturbing sleep. The precise mechanism for the vasomotor instability is unknown. One factor relates to the increased production of FSH (follicle-stimulating hormone) in response to the decreased production of estrogen and progesterone. The large amount of FSH upsets the delicate balance in the relationship between the ovaries, hypothalamus, and pituitary gland. The overactive pituitary is responsible for the increased production of FSH. Another cause given is the decreasing production of estrogen. Hot flashes are harmless, but they can cause great distress for some women. For those experiencing great discomfort, estrogen replacement may be prescribed. Other suggested means of controlling the symptoms of this instability are the use of the herb ginseng, vitamin B complex, and vitamin E.

Changes due to estrogen decrease can occur in the vulva, vagina, and uterus. The epidermis of the *vulva* thins, causing the labia and introitus to shrink. The vagina loses elasticity and becomes shorter and narrower. There is increased susceptibility to irritation and vaginal infection. This may result in atrophic vaginitis. Regular sexual activity makes these changes hardly noticeable and helps to prevent this condition. The use of vaginal creams has also helped some women. Dyspareunia occurs as a result of thinning of the vulva, but it can be helped by using K-Y jelly.

The *uterus* decreases in size and weight after menopause, and the cervix shrinks and becomes pale. The usual position of the uterus is anteroflexed. During the menopause the uterosacral ligaments may relax and the position of the uterus will change.

Changes in the structure and function of the *ovaries* relate to decrease in fertility and the decrease in size of the organs. Normally they are nonpalpable.

Estrogen decline at menopause causes a negative nitrogen balance and subsequently causes the *skin* to thin and the subcutaneous fat to atrophy and lose elasticity. Clients should be advised that these changes can be minimized by a good skin care regimen, including the use of skin oils, avoidance of drying soaps and detergents, and adherence to a healthy diet. About this time some women also develop freckles and brown spots, particularly on the face and hands. These skin changes appear to be due to the buildup of melanin that occurs as a process of aging. Occasionally these spots will develop into wartlike growths referred to as seborrheic keratoses. None of these changes is harmful unless the warts change in size or shape or begin to bleed. Many clients are upset about these brown spots, especially if they are on the face. Some women have suggested that the spots can be lightened by using diluted lemon or cranberry juice on the spots before going to bed or dabbing yogurt or buttermilk on the spots during the day.

On assessment no changes can usually be detected in the cardiovascular system. Women appear to be more susceptible to coronary artery disease after menopause, but it should be noted that the death rate for both sexes increases with age. Smoking, hypertension, and obesity are all risk factors that women should be counseled to control.

Musculoskeletal disorders, osteoporosis, and joint and muscle pain occur often in postmenopausal women. Both men and women lose bone after about age 35. The rate of bone loss appears to be greater in women. The many theoretical explanations given for the development of osteoporosis include inadequate intake of dietary calcium, fluoride, and vitamin D; alteration in the calcium-phosphorus ratio, probably precipitated by the lowered levels of estrogen and the subsequent increased removal of bone by parathyroid hormone; and lack of physical activity. An individual's lifestyle, diet, and cultural group may determine the increased likelihood of developing the condition. For example, people who are from vegetarian societies seem to have lower incidence than those from meat-eating societies like our own. (Seaman & Seaman 1977). Black women are less likely to suffer from the muscular and joint complaints and fractures (Seaman & Seaman 1977). At greatest risk seem to be Caucasian women who smoke and have a family history of osteoporosis. Estrogen therapy seems to have some positive effects on preventing or retarding this condition but only for the short term. Long-term therapy may contribute to decrease in bone formation.

To reduce the process of osteoporosis, women should be encouraged to select a diet with foods high in calcium and low in phosphorus, and some authorities recommend calcium supplements. Regular exercise should also become a part of the woman's lifestyle, since exercise not only helps to retard osteoporosis but helps to control weight and improve circulation.

Eating Disorders

Our society's emphasis on slimness has contributed to an increase in the incidence of serious eating disorders such as anorexia nervosa and bulimia. Anorexia nervosa, or self-induced starvation, affects about 1 of every 200 American girls between the ages of 12 and 18. Bulimia, a cycle of food binges followed by purging (induced by vomiting or by laxative or diuretic abuse), appears to be more prevalent, affecting an estimated 5% of adolescent and young adult females. Although both disorders occur less often among males, males are also victims of these ailments. A common feature of both disorders is the overwhelming desire to become and remain thin. Although a specific cause is unknown, a combination of interacting factors including psychological, familial, sociocultural, and biological determinants contributes to these complex disorders.

Psychoanalytic theory suggests that anorexia nervosa is an attempt to delay or prevent puberty. Psychodynamic theory attributes the problem to the individual's problems with self-image and adequacy, social interactions, and overcompliance. The pursuit of thinness is viewed as the struggle to exert control and self-direction. Family dynamics, including disturbed patterns of interactions, have also been thought to contribute.

Our society's emphasis on extreme thinness remains pervasive. Two cultural factors, idealization of the thin female form and pressures on women to be independent and successful, are believed to have contributed to the recent increase in the numbers of women with eating disorders.

Anorexia Nervosa

The typical client with anorexia nervosa is a white adolescent female from a middle- to upper-middle-class family. She is often described by her parents as the "perfect child." The anorectic tends to be a perfectionist, obedient, overcompliant, highly motivated, successful academically, well liked by peers, and a good athlete. Frequently, the anorectic's family is one that emphasizes high achievement, perfection, and physical appearance. Such families have been described as being overinvolved with one another, having a low tolerance for conflict, and being highly controlling.

Reason for Seeking Health Evaluation

Parents, alarmed by the girl's obvious weight loss, bizarre eating habits, purging, and often a loss of interest in school, may force their daughter to seek help. Other notable behavioral characteristics are extreme irritability, excessively overcontrolled behavior, an obsession with exercise, and changes in sleep patterns. In some cases, amenorrhea initially brings the client into contact with the health care system.

Current Health Status or History of Present Illness

In appearance these girls are emaciated, resembling walking skeletons. They do not see themselves as particularly thin, and often they underestimate their own body size and the size of others. Hunger is usually denied, and in fact appetite is described as too good.

Physical Assessment

On physical assessment the nurse will usually find weight loss of 20%–25% or more of total body weight or a reduced weight 20%–25% below average for the age-appropriate height. Reduced body fat and wasting of muscle can be noted along with other symptoms of decreased metabolic rate such as bradycardia, hypotension, and hypothermia. The anorectic client may also have abdominal tenderness, decreased motility, constipation, increased sensitivity to cold, dry inelastic skin with a yellowish caritonemic hue, brittle hair and nails, lanugo, and peripheral edema. Either during the history-taking or during the physical assessment the nurse should determine whether the client vomits to control her weight and uses laxatives. Typical laboratory values show leukopenia, anemia, hypoglycemia, hypercholesterolemia, and reduced gonadotropins.

Mental Status Assessment

Impaired mental performance may be found. In addition, anorectics have a disturbed body image, insisting that their body size is normal. Awareness of the usual senses of hunger and appetite is missing. Another misinterpretation of stimuli is their inability to acknowledge fatigue associated with their constant hyperactivity. They also display a tremendous sense of ineffectiveness, a feeling that they are helpless to change their lives. This is usually expressed as extreme negativism and stubborn defiance.

Most anorectic girls have difficulty accepting their sexual identity and fear pregnancy, which is described as getting fat. Anorectics are often very hostile. The hostility is usually toward their mother, who is frequently overprotective and overcontrolling. These clients try to solve their problems by changing their body through starvation and hyperactivity.

Bulimia

Bulimia is defined as recurrent episodes of rapid uncontrollable ingestion of large amounts of food in a short period of time, usually followed by purging, either by forced vomiting or by abuse of laxatives or diuretics. The purging techniques are used to prevent weight gain, relieve fullness, and restore the individual's sense of control. Like anorectics, bulimics have an exaggerated fear of fatness and are intent on pursuing slimness as a means of bringing control and a sense of effectiveness into their lives.

The typical bulimic is a white, single, college-educated female of normal weight-for-height in her early to middle twenties who has been involved in bulimic behavior for four to six years before seeking treatment. Bulimics tend to be slightly older and of more varied socioeconomic status than anorectics. While most are female, about 10%–13% are male.

Reasons for Seeking Health Evaluation

The reasons for seeking help vary. Using open-ended questions, which allow the client to express feelings, is the best approach and will probably elicit several reasons for finally entering the health care system.

Mental Status Assessment

Studies to date reveal that normal-weight bulimics have problems with impulse control (evidenced by stealing, abuse of alcohol or drugs), are chronically depressed or even suicidal, are intolerant of frustration, and have an exaggerated sense of guilt and recurrent anxiety. They feel alienated and self-conscious, are overly dependent on approval of others, and have low self-esteem and difficulties expressing feelings, especially anger.

Physical Assessment

Chronic self-induced vomiting can lead to enlarged parotid glands, esophageal inflammation, and many dental problems, such as caries and erosion of the enamel. Vomiting can also result in fluid and electrolyte disturbances, the most serious being hypokalemia. The client may also have urinary infections, renal failure, and cardiac arrhythmias. Laxative abuse may result in colon damage, disturbances of intestinal motility, and metabolic acidosis. Abuse of diuretics can lead to dehydration and hypokalemia and metabolic alkalosis. Bulimics complain of chronic indigestion, sore throats, facial puffiness, menstrual disturbances, muscle weakness, constipation, and lethargy.

Assessment of Pregnancy

Pregnancy is a normal physiological process that affects every organ system. The genital tract reflects the earliest changes; the others are more subtle and frequently develop later. During the prenatal period, complex emotional adjustments affect the women herself and also her family and significant others. Health care must include the assessment of the client's physiologic and emotional status as well as provide health education during pregnancy and assistance in preparing for labor, delivery, and the postpartum period.

Health History

Although the components of the history are similar to those described in Chapter 4, some areas should be given special emphasis. The information obtained in the initial interview assists the nurse in identifying the many factors that will affect the client during pregnancy. These factors include information about the client's past physical history as well as her emotional response to the pregnancy. Each woman is different, and the nurse must allow her to express her feelings and concerns about the pregnancy in an open, nonjudgmental fashion.

Age

Extremes of age put the woman in a high-risk category. Adolescents are considered at risk because they are still developing physically and psychologically. In addition, the very young mother might find the routine and responsibility of child care time consuming and an interference to a developing social life. Women who are older may resent additional responsibility and fear that they do not have the physical strength to raise a child. Genetic defects in the fetus are more often seen in older women. Other more common complications in this age group include hydatidiform mole, placenta previa, twinning, and low birth weight. Early identification and referral of high-risk clients enables the nurse to achieve maximal benefit for both client and fetus.

Marital Status

Obtain information about the length of the marriage and about the husband's name, age, and occupation. The father's effect on the pregnancy relates to his ability to give emotional and financial support. Some evidence suggests that the father's occupation as reflected in the family's socioeconomic status is related to the incidence of prematurity and infant mortality. Unmarried women face additional stress in our society. Mortality and morbidity rates are higher; prenatal care and advice are often not sought. When care is sought, the professional's advice is less likely to be followed. It may be that this is a denial of the pregnancy or that there is no significant other to give emotional support.

Current Occupation

The client's job is important in relation to the occupation's stress level and the degree to which heavy physical labor is required. Although women are encouraged to maintain an active lifestyle during pregnancy, certain physical activities may have to be altered as the pregnancy progresses. Of increasing importance is the exposure to possible toxic contamination at the place of employment. For example, women exposed to radiation are at definite risk. There is some question as to the health risks to the fetus for the mother who works with computers daily. Some are being advised to wear aprons with a lead shield during pregnancy. There is hard evidence that smoking causes low birth weights and a direct increase in infant mortality. A relationship between passive inhalation of environmental smoke and low birth weight has also been found in preliminary studies.

Ethnic Background and Religion

Ethnic origin may affect pregnancy outcome, as some diseases are more prevalent in certain races—for example, Tay-Sachs disease in Jews, thalassemia in Mediterranean and Asian populations, and sickle-cell anemia in blacks. Beliefs and practices specific to pregnancy, childbirth, and child rearing are common to every cultural group. Cultural beliefs about diet, role of the father, activity, labor, and delivery should be incorporated into prenatal care. Examples of cultural variables affecting health care can be seen in many groups. Spanish-speaking women view pregnancy as natural and are often reluctant to seek health care (Gibbs, Martin, & Gutierrez 1974). Some Chinese women are afraid that iron will harden their bones and make delivery difficult; as a result they don't want to take iron supplements (Mead 1956). Also, some Asian and Mexican American women, because of lactose intolerance, may not follow the nurse's advice to use dairy products (Rosenberg 1977). Food restrictions are noted almost universally. For example, Polynesian, Vietnamese, and Filipino pregnant women are forbidden to eat fruits that do not grow singly. They believe that fruits like bananas may cause twins (Brown 1976).

In many cultural groups excessive modesty and submissiveness to males are cultural patterns that may influence a woman's use of the health care system. To ensure the pregnancy's successful outcome, the nurse must understand and accept certain rituals prescribed by the woman's cultural group and use this awareness in carrying out the health assessment.

Because of religious beliefs, some women might object to using any contraceptive method. More research must be done on religion's influence on pregnant women's beliefs about contraception. The accuracy of information in this area is questionable because of the hesitancy of members of some cultural groups to share their beliefs on this sensitive subject (Orque, 1981).

Reason for Seeking Health Evaluation or Chief Complaint

Generally the client has experienced one or more of the signs and symptoms of pregnancy, which include amenorrhea, breast changes, nausea, and perhaps a positive pregnancy test. Since self-pregnancy tests are now available, the client may have confirmed her belief with one of these. The client may indicate at this time that this is an unwanted pregnancy, which is an extremely stressful experience for the woman. The nurse must have the skill to assist the woman in arriving at a decision and cousel her about preventing future unwanted pregnancies.

Current Health Status

The client's physiologic and emotional health has a bearing on whether she will experience a normal or high-risk pregnancy. Health habits such as cigarette smoking and alcohol or drug use can affect the growth of the fetus. The client's age may have a bearing on the pregnancy's progression. Clients who are suffering from diseases such as hypertension, diabetes, heart disease, or endocrine disorders certainly are at greater risk (see Table 23-2). Acute factors such as viral or bacterial infections can adversely affect the developing fetus.

Menstrual history should include such data as date of menarche and characteristics of the menstrual cycle, including length and amount of flow and date of last menstruation. This date is helpful in estimating the expected date of delivery. Frequently clients will have difficulty remembering when the last menstrual period was, particularly if the pregnancy was not planned. The skilled interviewer can use events that occur seasonally such as Christmas or Valentine's Day or special events in the client's life to help her remember.

The EDC (estimated delivery calculation) can be computed using Nagele's rule. Three months are subtracted and 7 days added to the first day of the last menstrual period. In simple terms, add 7 days to the LMP (last menstrual period) and count forward 9 months. The majority of women will deliver during the period extending 7 days before and 7 days after the EDC. This is only one determination of delivery date. If a woman does not know the date of her LMP or is very irregular, other methods are used to determine due date. In fact ultrasonic measurement is being used more frequently to assess progress and determine the EDC.

Table 23-2. Pregnancy Risk Factors

Physical	Psychologic	Environmental and social
Age: younger than 18 or older than 35	Family disorganization	Poverty
Height: less than 5 feet	Conflict about pregnancy	Poor nutrition
Obesity	Drug abuse	Poor access to health care
Poor weight gain	Reluctance to accept pregnancy	Contaminants in home
Pelvic inadequacy	Low self-esteem	Lack of education
Uterine incompetency	History of mental illness	Poor housing
Nutritional deficiency	Mental retardation	Highly mobile lifestyle
Bleeding after 20 weeks' gestation		Occupation involving dangerous or contaminated substances
Exposure to carcinogens		Lack of significant support person
Postmaturity		
Multiple gestation		
Presence of major illness (diabetes, hypertension, renal disease, heart disease, pulmonary disease, endocrine disorder, sickle-cell disease, anemia, pelvic inflammatory disease)		
Poor gynecologic or obstetric history		
History of child with congenital abnormalities		

At this time ask the client to indicate whether fetal movement has been felt and, if so, when it was first felt. This is also a good time to gather information about past obstetric history. Previous childbearing experiences can influence the course of the present pregnancy and can also be helpful to the nurse in predicting possible complications. Areas to explore include:

1. *Number and dates of previous pregnancies.*
2. *Duration of pregnancies:* If full-term deliveries, note date of delivery and birth weight of infant. If not full-term deliveries, note cause (if known) and gestational age of infant. *Gravida* and *para* are terms frequently used to describe pregnancy and the outcomes of pregnancy. A pregnant woman is described as gravida, and para is the number of pregnancies ending in the delivery of a baby or in the delivery of one weighing 500 g or of more than 20 weeks' gestation, either alive or stillborn. For example, a woman who has had three pregnancies, delivered two at term, and has had one miscarriage at 12 weeks would be described as gravida 3, para 2, or 3/2. A system referred to as G/TPAL is a five-digit means of expressing the woman's obstetric history more accurately.

   G = *gravida*
   T = number of babies born at *term* alive or stillborn
   P = number of babies born *prior* to term, alive or stillborn
   A = number of pregnancies ending in *abortion*
   L = number of children currently *living*

   In this example the recording would be 3/2102.
3. *Labor and delivery experience:* Onset—specifically, was labor spontaneous or induced? If induced, what was the reason for induction and the method? Also, what was the length of labor, complications, anesthesia, type of delivery (vaginal or Cesarean), and presentation of infant (vertex or breech).
4. *Abortions:* Spontaneous or induced.
5. *Problems experienced:* Types of complications and treatment.
6. *Postpartum experience:* Infections, hemor-

rhage, emotional difficulties, and course of recovery.

7. *Problems of the infant:* Jaundice, respiratory distress, infection, or stillbirth.
8. *Living children:* Course of growth and development and current health.

Personal History and Patterns of Living

Of particular concern is a family history of multiple pregnancy, cardiovascular disease, diabetes, renal disease, congenital abnormalities, genetic disorders, blood dyscrasias, and emotional problems. There is a familial and hereditary nature for many health problems. For example, if the client's mother suffered from hypertension, she is more likely to develop hypertension with pregnancy.

Since diet and lifestyle are implicated in maintaining wellness in the general population, they are certainly important in the pregnant woman. Increasing evidence links the mother's diet and habits to the infant's welfare. Note the wide dissemination of material related to smoking and drinking and infant wellness. Typically at risk are unmarried women, poorly nourished, often with a history of alcohol, drug, or tobacco abuse, chronic physical illness, or previous obstetric complications. Poor support systems and emotional disturbances may further complicate the problem. Poverty underlies many of these problems (Fogel & Woods 1981).

Previous Experience with Illness

Knowledge of past illness, including hospitalizations and surgery, helps the nurse determine whether any past problems may cause difficulties during the current pregnancy. Of particular importance are any past surgeries or injuries to the pelvis, urinary tract, bowel, or abdomen. Weakness or abnormalities in these areas could impede the progress of the pregnancy. Some previous conditions, such as hypertension, rheumatic fever, asthma, venereal disease, and allergies may be exacerbated by the pregnancy.

Physical Assessment

A complete assessment should be carried out when the client is first seen. She is then examined once a month until 32 weeks' gestation, every two weeks from 32 to 36 weeks, and weekly from that time until delivery. During these examinations special attention is paid to the breasts, abdomen, and pelvis. Changes can be noted in practically every body system during pregnancy. Most become more pronounced as the pregnancy progresses.

Developing a General Impression

During the general inspection you must focus on the client's state of consciousness, age, race, and development. As previously mentioned, age and concomitant physical and emotional development are important considerations. Nutrition may be one of the most important factors affecting the outcome of the pregnancy. Nutritional deficiency can have many consequences, such as retardation of fetal growth, increased incidence of spontaneous abortion, increased incidence of congenital malformation, and retarded motor and intellectual development. Observation of nutritional state should be made during the first visit, and the nurse might also carry out a complete nutritional assessment, as described in Chapter 7. In addition, a note should be made about the client's general state of health at the time of initial assessment.

Height and Weight The client's weight is often an indicator of nutritional status. Optimal weight gain is approximately 24–27 pounds during pregnancy (see Figures 23-1 and 23-2). The pattern should be no less than 3 pounds during the first trimester and 0.8 pounds each week after that unless the client is overweight at the beginning of pregnancy. There should be no more than 0.5 pound each week during the first 20 weeks of pregnancy and 1 pound each week after that period unless the client is underweight at the beginning of pregnancy. An overweight status is much more common even among the poor in this country. Clients with high weights prior to pregnancy face an increased risk of developing preeclampsia, and those who are underweight have low-birth-weight babies more frequently.

Blood Pressure The client's blood pressure in the first trimester should remain unchanged if she is healthy. A slight drop may be noted in the healthy client during the second trimester. This is the result of a decrease in peripheral resistance. Blood pressure should be measured in both arms on initial visit. If the pressure is elevated, measure again after a rest period with the client in the left lateral position because the

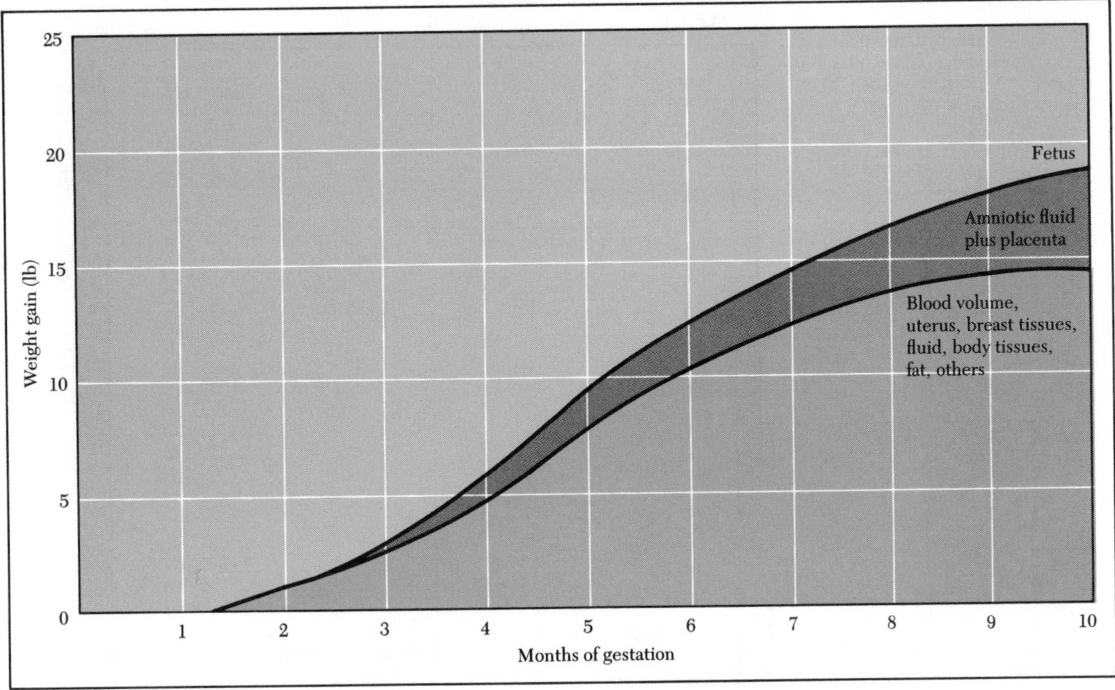

Figure 23-1 Components of weight gain in pregnancy.

pressure is lowest in this position in the pregnant woman. The rollover test should be carried out on all nulliparous women between 28 and 32 weeks' gestation. If positive, this screening test indicates the woman is more likely to develop preeclampsia. To conduct the test, take one blood pressure reading with the client in the left lateral position. Then have her roll on her back, let her rest for 5 minutes, and retake the pressure in the supine position. If the diastolic pressure is 20 mm Hg greater in the supine position than in the lateral position, the test is positive.

Assessment of the Integument

The hormonal changes that occur in pregnancy can be observed in some clients beginning about the 16th week. Pigmentation of the nipple and areola may be seen, particularly in dark-haired women. This increased deposition of melanin may also occur in the eyelids, vulva, and perianal area. Hyperpigmentation down the middle of the abdomen is called linea nigra. Mottling of the cheeks and forehead is called chloasma, or the "mask of pregnancy" (see Figure 23-3). Clients may express concern about these changes, especially those on the face. Dark pigmentation fades but does not completely go away after delivery. Other changes to note in the integument are localized areas of erythema over the fingers, fingertips, and palms. Striae may develop on the abdomen, breast, or buttocks. Fiery-red spider angiomas and bluish venous stars, the latter usually near varicose veins may be observed.

Assessment of the Head, Face, and Neck

An increase in facial and body hair may occur in pregnancy. It usually begins about the third month and appears as fine lanugo on the face and chest. This disappears two to three months after delivery. Hair on the head tends to straighten and hair loss occurs, usually beginning about two to four months after delivery. Regrowth occurs without treatment.

On palpation the thyroid will often be found to be enlarged. This is due to hyperplasia of the glandular tissue and increased vascularity. Pregnant women have a marked increase in their metabolic rates, most pronounced close to the delivery. This occurs because more oxygen is needed to maintain the metabolic activity of the mother and fetus.

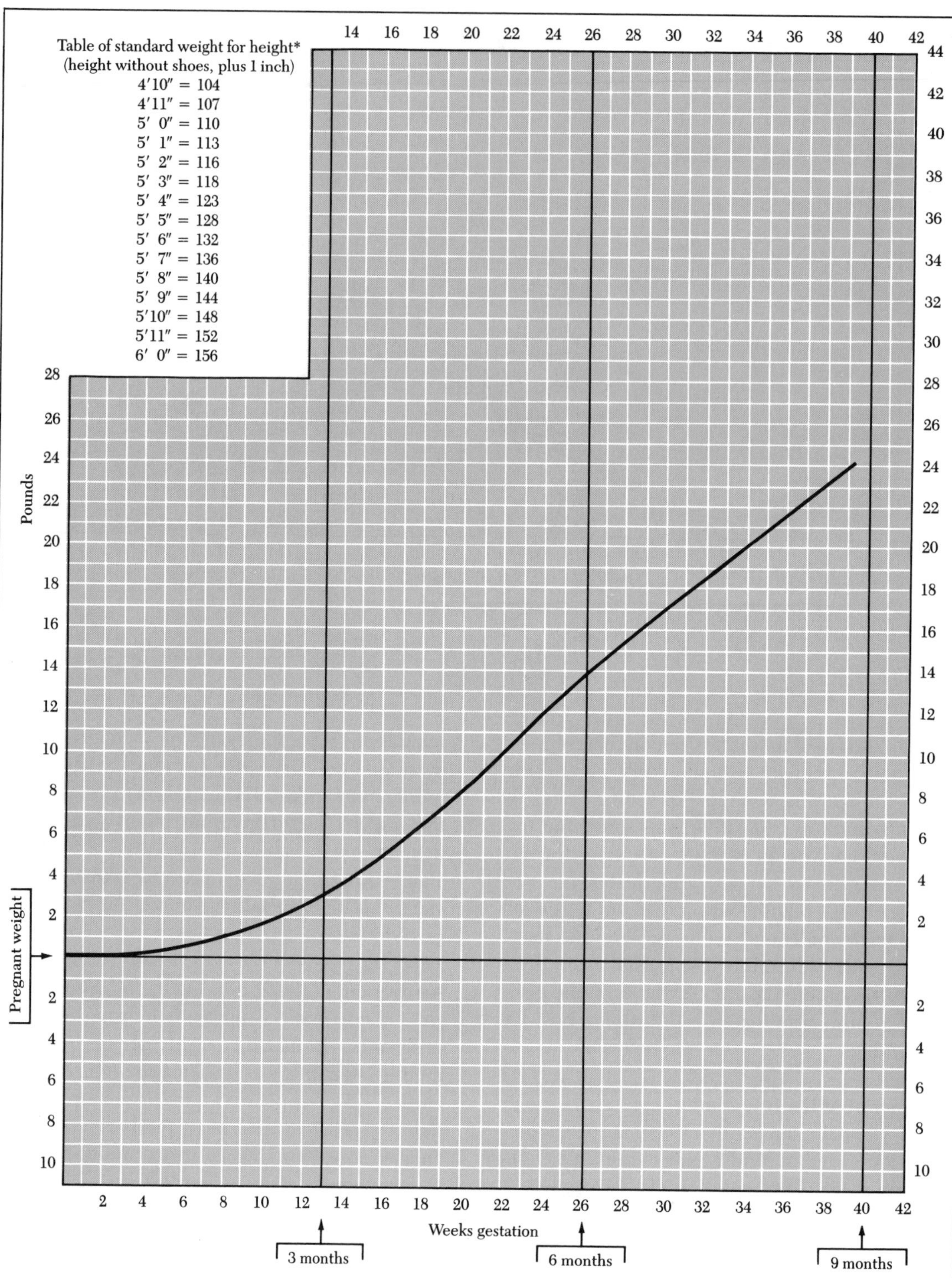

*The above weights were taken from Metropolitan Life Insurance Company Actuarial Tables, 1959 and adjusted to comply with instructions appearing on the Prenatal Weight Gain Grid, namely height in inches without shoes plus 1 inch to establish a standard for heels. Patients should be weighed with shoes as normally worn. The table above is for medium body build and, except for extreme body build deviations, these figures should be used. For example, a patient whose height, measured without shoes, is 5 feet 4 inches would have one inch added, therefore, her standard weight for height would be 128 pounds. Ranges are not acceptable in estimating standard weight since this is an objective observation and represents the mid-point. This mid-point must be used for recording purposes. For patients under age 25 one pound should be deducted for each year.

Figure 23-2 Prenatal weight gain grid.

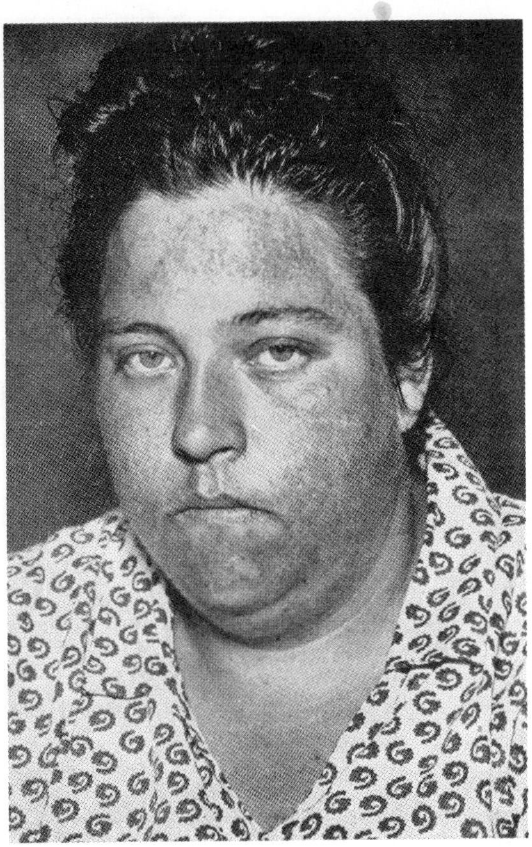

Figure 23-3 Mottling of cheeks and forehead, called chloasma of pregnancy.

Assessment of the Ear, Nose, Mouth, and Pharynx

No changes are usually noted in the ear, although some women complain of mild hearing loss due to Eustachian tube blockage. Nosebleeds are not uncommon during pregnancy and are the result of hormonal changes. Tissues of the mouth and gums may become hyperemic and swollen. Even brushing the teeth may cause bleeding. Hypertrophy of the gums causing epulides, which are small benign vascular lesions, may develop. These disappear after pregnancy.

Assessment of the Breasts

The breasts become progressively larger, and areolar hypertrophy causes them to have a nodular consistency. Areolar pigmentation deepens and widens; the veins in the breast become increasingly prominent (see Figure 23-4). About the 10th week, a secretion called colostrum may be expressed with gentle massage. The nurse should provide information regarding preparation for breastfeeding and should advise the client to wear a good, well-fitting bra for support.

Assessment of the Thorax and Lungs

There is an increase in respiratory rate as oxygen consumption increases. Breathing changes from abdominal to thoracic about the 24th week, and shortness of breath may occur late in pregnancy. Shortening and widening occurs at the base of the thoracic cage, and there is upward displacement of the diaphragm to allow for the expansion of the uterus.

Assessment of the Heart

As the uterus enlarges, it causes the diaphragm to elevate, which displaces the heart slightly upward and to the left, while at the same time causing a counterclockwise rotation (see Figure 23-5). The transverse diameter of the heart increases. The PMI is displaced laterally about 1 to 1.5 cm. Percussion and palpation of the heart will detect these changes. On auscultation systolic murmurs may be heard. They are generally soft and blowing and are usually heard best in the pulmonic area and at the apex.

The resting pulse is about 10 to 15 beats per minute faster during pregnancy. There is a slight fall in the blood pressure in the second trimester and then a rise as the pregnancy progresses. Any dramatic changes in the blood pressure are suspect and should be noted. A sustained systolic increase of 30mm Hg or diastolic increase of 15mm Hg after 20 weeks' gestation may be indicative of pathology.

There is an increase in plasma volume, which may cause a pseudoanemia. Hematocrits should be done periodically, and an iron supplement is usually necessary to keep the hemoglobin levels normal.

Assessment of the Abdomen

A complete abdominal examination, including palpation of the kidneys, liver, and spleen, should be done at the first prenatal visit because as the uterus enlarges it becomes more difficult to palpate these organs. In subsequent visits the abdominal examination is an objective measurement of fetal growth, as the fundal height changes at various gestational ages (see Figure 23-6).

Ask the client to empty her bladder before beginning the examination. Have her positioned with head slightly elevated and knees gently flexed. This position will relax the abdominal muscles. The liver and spleen should be palpated, although functions of both are normally

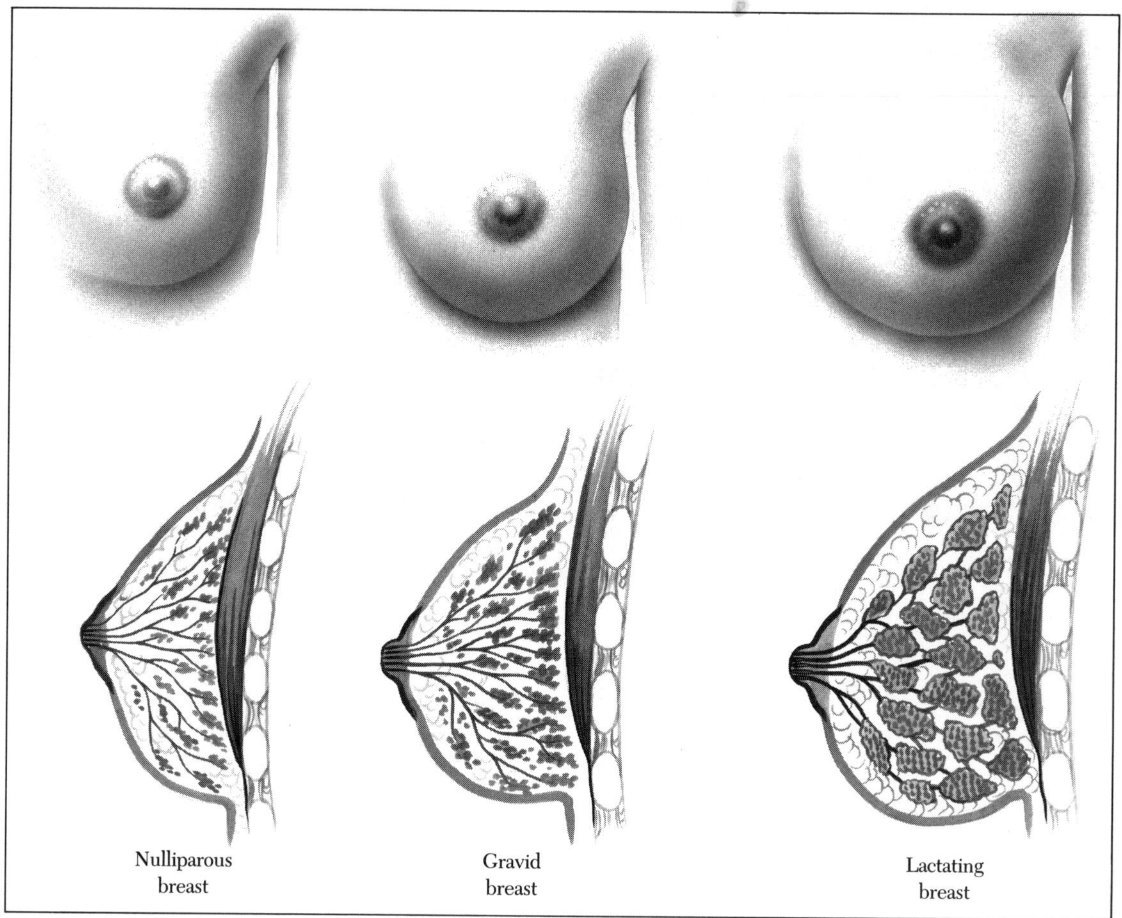

Figure 23-4 Changes in the breast during pregnancy and lactation.

unchanged during pregnancy. The kidneys should be palpated. Remember that renal blood flow increases by 25% during the first and second trimester. Percuss the abdomen, noting tympany. The bladder is more sensitive at this time and the enlarging uterus puts more pressure on it, resulting in frequency of urination during the first and third trimesters.

Inspection The nurse should note the presence or absence of scars and striations. These will vary for each client depending on past physical occurrences. Contour should be observed. Skin changes such as the linea nigra are not usually seen until the 16th week.

Palpation From the 12th week of pregnancy on, the abdomen should be palpated to note fundal height and fetal presentation and position. In Figure 23-6 you can see that at the 12th week the fundus is just above the symphysis pubis and at the 36th week it almost reaches the xiphoid.

To palpate the uterus, stand at the right side of the client in the supine position. Select a point about 3 to 4 cm above where the fundus is expected to be at that point of gestation. Using the ulnar surface of the hand or the fingertips, palpate downward until the soft abdomen becomes the firm, round, fundal edge. When you have located the fundus, measure its distance from the symphysis. There are several methods of doing this and the method used should be documented each time. It is also recommended that the same person measure the fundus throughout the pregnancy. The first method, using fingerbreadth measurements, is the most inaccurate. For example, you would record the fundus as being a certain number of fingerbreadths from the symphysis, umbilicus, or xiphoid (see Figure 23-7). The use of a measuring tape is more accu-

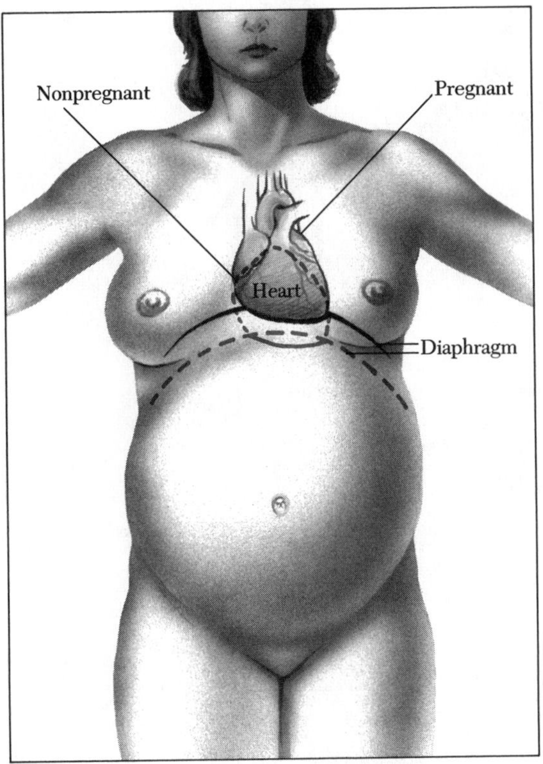

Figure 23-5 Changes in the heart and diaphragm during pregnancy.

rate. Place the tape at the superior border of the symphysis pubis and draw it up to the midline of the abdomen to the top edge of the fundus. After 22 to 24 weeks the number in centimeters should equal gestation (see Figure 23-8).

Following the measurement of fundal height the nurse should palpate the abdomen for lie, presentation, and position of the fetus. The relationship of the long axis of the mother to the long axis of the fetus is the lie. The lie can be longitudinal, oblique, or transverse (see Figure 23-9, page 557). Presentation denotes the part of the fetus that overlies the maternal pelvic inlet. The presentation can be vertex, brow, face, shoulder, or breech (see Figure 23-10, page 558). Position is the relationship of a designated point of the fetus (denominator) to a designated point in the maternal pelvis. For example, the occiput is the denominator in a vertex presentation. If the fetus has its occiput in the left inguinal area of the mother, the position would be described as LOA (left occipital anterior). The denominator in a breech presentation is the sacrum, and in a face presentation it is the chin.

One method of determining lie, presentation, and position is called Leopold's maneuvers (see Figure 23-11). For these to be most effective, the fetus should be large enough so that different parts can be felt through the uterine and abdominal walls, about 26 to 28 weeks' gestation. For the first step of these maneuvers, stand facing the client and place both hands on the abdomen. With fingertips nearly touching, cup your hands around the part of the fetus in the fundus. Usually the buttocks is in the fundus and it is rounded and somewhat soft. When moved, it causes the whole fetus to move. If the head is in the fundus, it is round and hard and moves independently of the rest of the fetus.

In step two, continue to face the client and place your hands on either side of the abdomen. Hold one hand steady and apply pressure to the fetus with your other hand. If the hand you are applying pressure with feels a long, smooth part, you are probably feeling the fetus's back. If the part is bumpy and has indentations and angles, you are probably feeling the arms, legs, and knees. You will most likely feel movement on this side as the fetus gets older. On each side palpate the flank to the midline, taking special note of the fetal back as a landmark in determining fetal position. If you feel the back more easily on the anterior abdomen, and the legs, knees, and so on more on the flank, the fetus is in an anterior position. If you feel the back more in the flank and the arms, legs, and so on more on the anterior abdomen, the fetus is probably in the posterior position.

To perform step three, face the client and take the thumb and middle finger of your right hand and place them at the symphysis pubis with your fingers on the left side and thumb on the right side. Grasp the presenting fetal part. If the presenting part is hard and rounded and can be moved independently of the part in the fundus, it is the head. If it is soft and rounded and causes the whole fetus to move when grasped, it is the bottom or breech.

The fourth step will help you to determine how far into the pelvis the presenting part has descended. Remain on the right side but face the patient's feet. Place both hands on either side of the lower abdomen just above the sym-

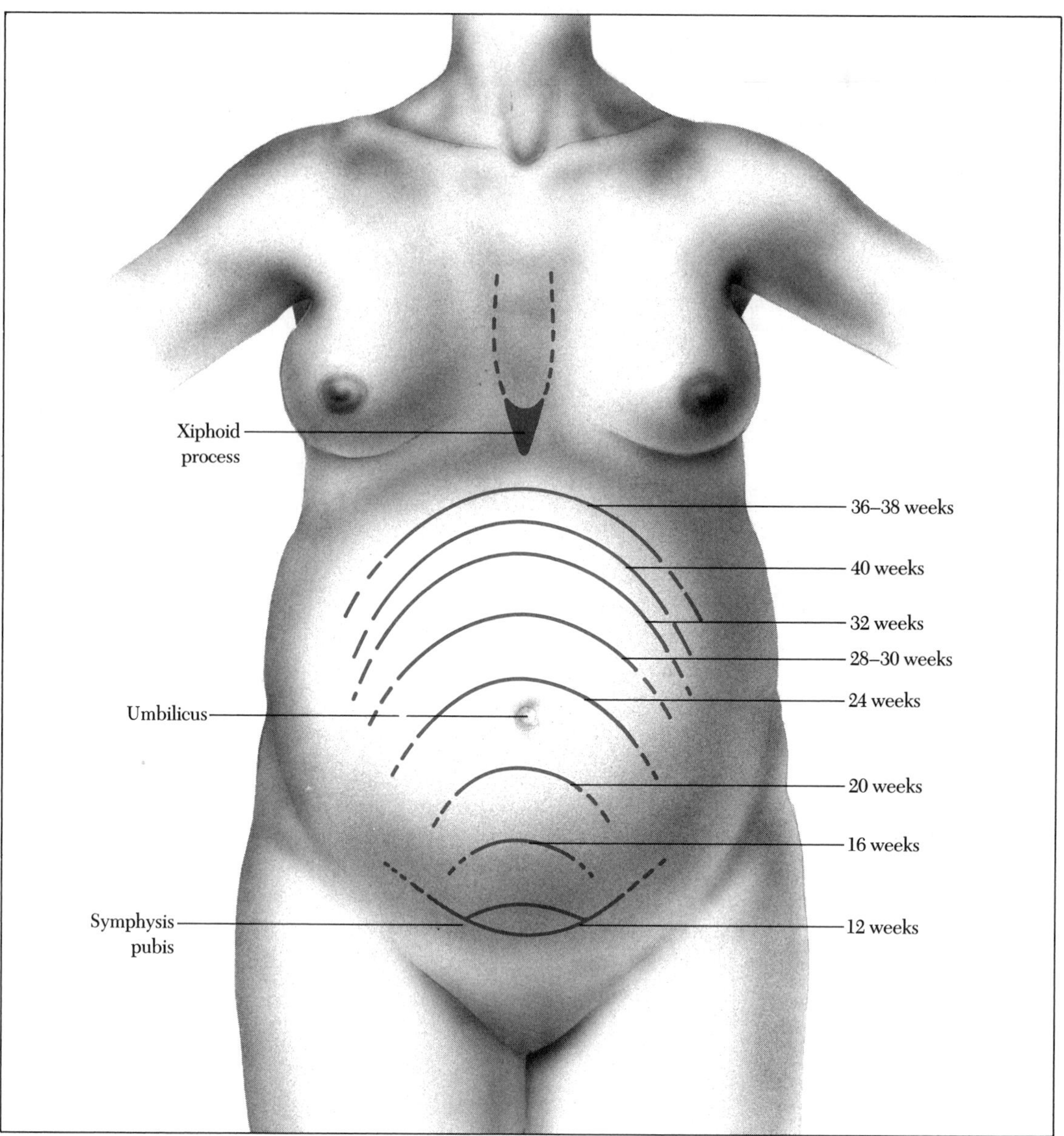

Figure 23-6 Fundal heights at various stages of pregnancy.

physis pubis. Ask the client to take a deep breath and dip your fingers deep into the pelvis to determine which side the cephalic prominence is on. The brow should be felt on the same side as the arms, legs, and elbows. If the bony prominence is felt on the same side as the back, it indicates that the head is extended, which may result in problems during labor.

Auscultation Monitoring the fetal heartbeat is an important part of each prenatal visit. Electronic equipment can be used to hear the heartbeat at about 10 weeks' gestation. The standard fetoscope is used from 20 weeks (see Figure 23-12). The normal heart rate is 120–160, but it varies according to length of gestation. Usually the heartbeat slows as the fetus grows and is closer to term. You can make some determinations about fetal presentation and position by locating the point of greatest intensity of fetal heart tones. Fetal heart sounds are heard best over a bony prominence. Therefore, if the fetal attitude is flexion, sounds will be best heard through the fetal scapula and shoulder. If the fetal attitude is extension, sounds will be best heard through the fetal anterior chest. When the fetus is in the

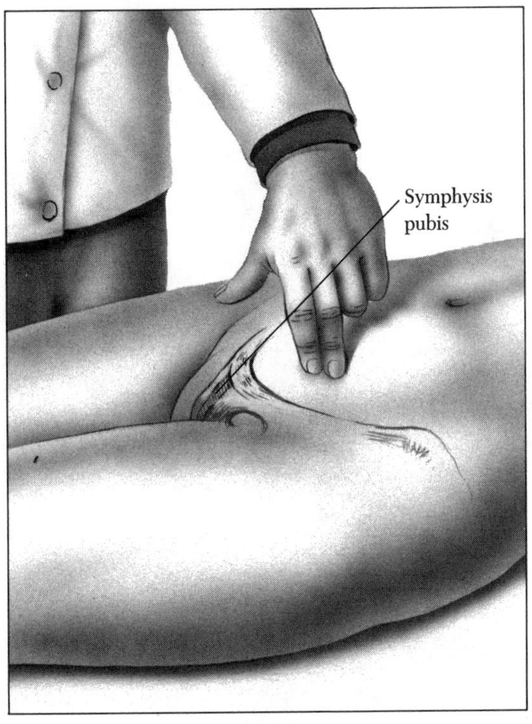

Figure 23-7 Measuring fundus using fingerbreadths.

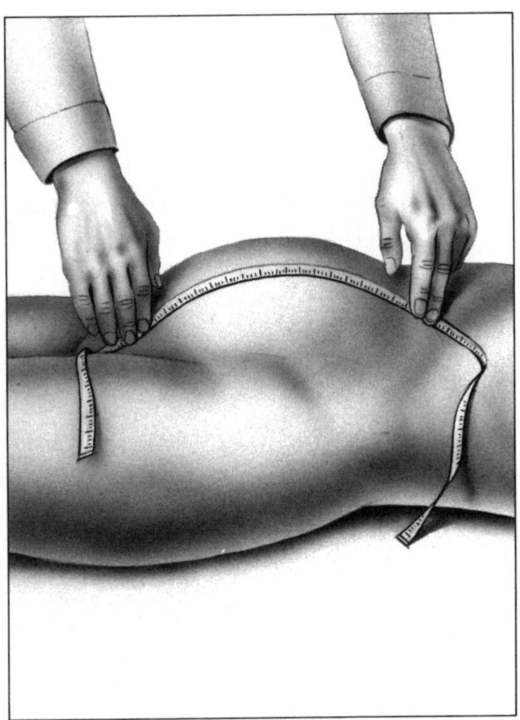

Figure 23-8 Measuring fundus with tape measure.

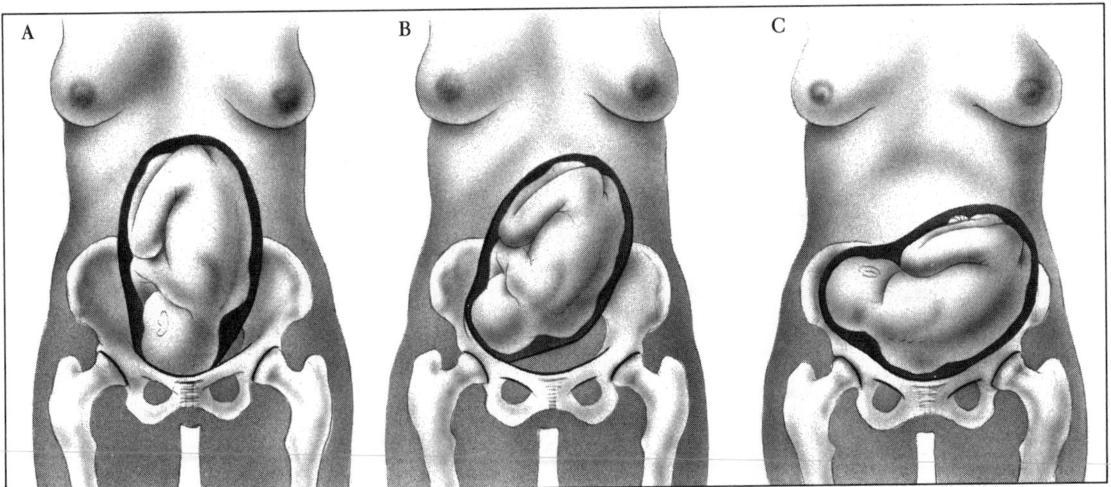

Figure 23-9 Examples of fetal lie. (A) Longitudinal lie. (B) Oblique lie. (C) Transverse lie.

anterior cephalic position LOA or ROA, you should place the stethoscope below the umbilicus to the right or left, depending on which side the back was felt. If the position is posterior, cephalic sounds are best heard by placing the stethoscope at the mother's flanks, again on whichever side the fetal back was felt. If the sounds are heard best above the mother's umbilicus, the fetus is probably in the breech position.

The fetal heart is rapid and sound. It is not synchronous with the mother's rate, so you can differentiate it by palpating the mother's pulse while auscultating the abdomen. Another sound that can be heard is called the uterine souffle, a

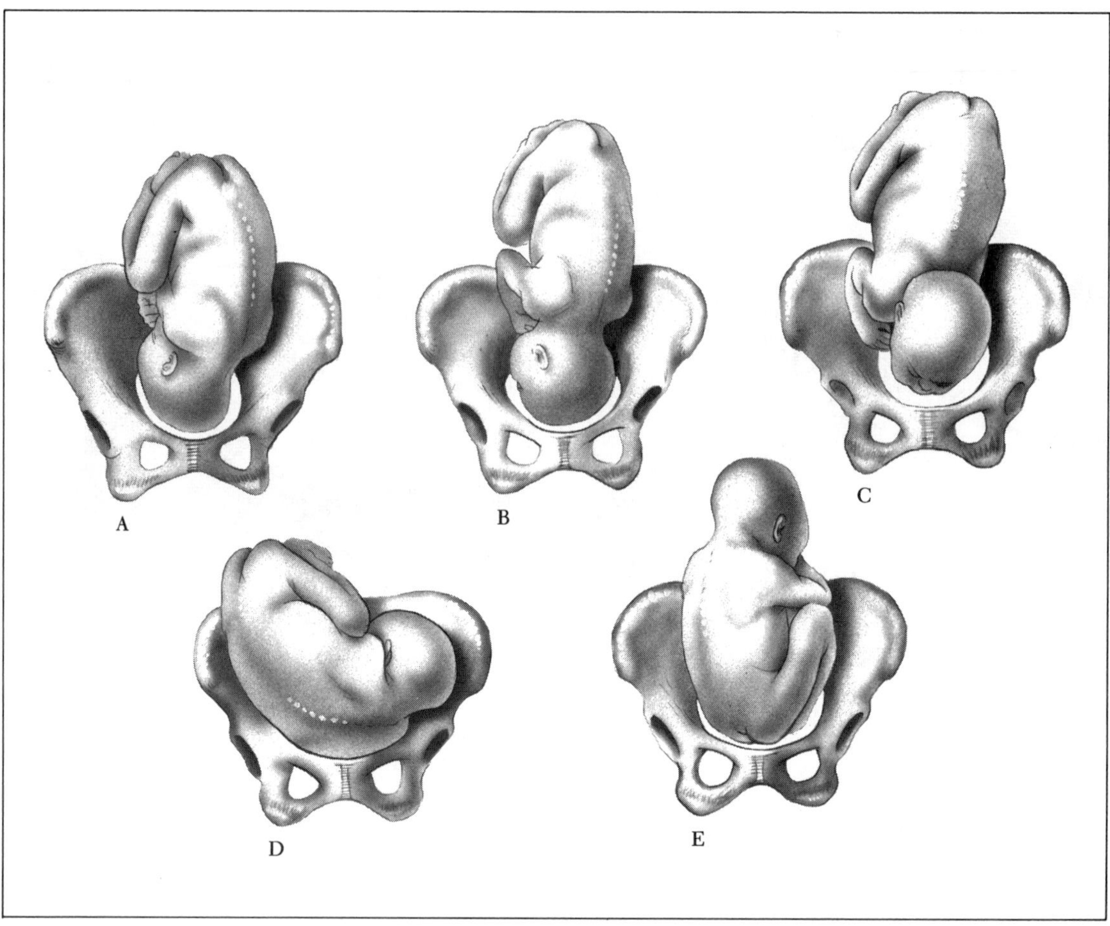

Figure 23-10 Examples of fetal presentation. (A) Vertex. (B) Brow. (C) Face. (D) Shoulder. (E) Breech.

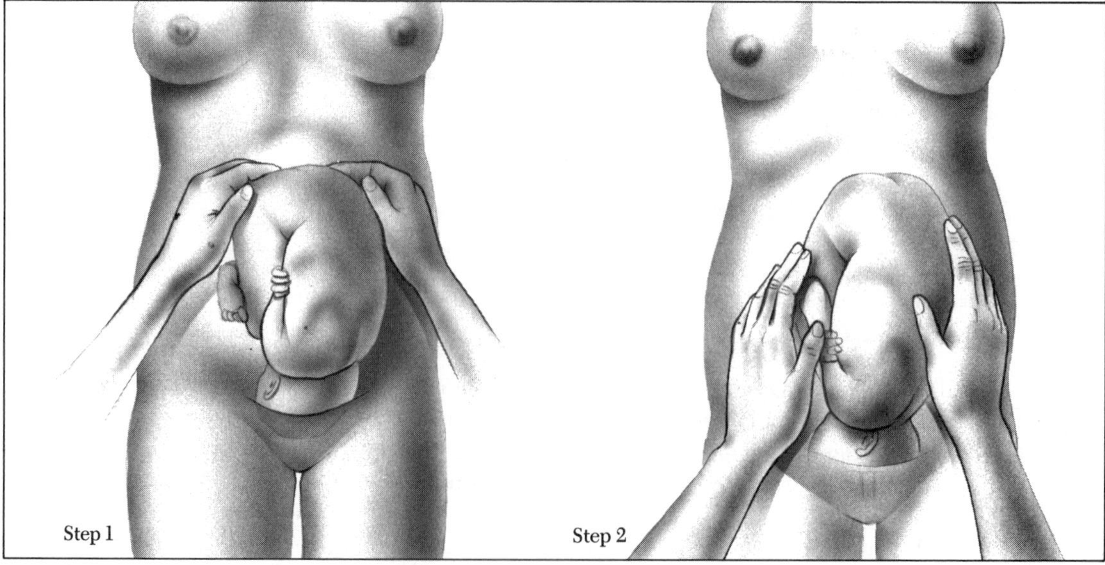

Figure 23-11 Leopold's maneuvers. *(Continued on next page)*

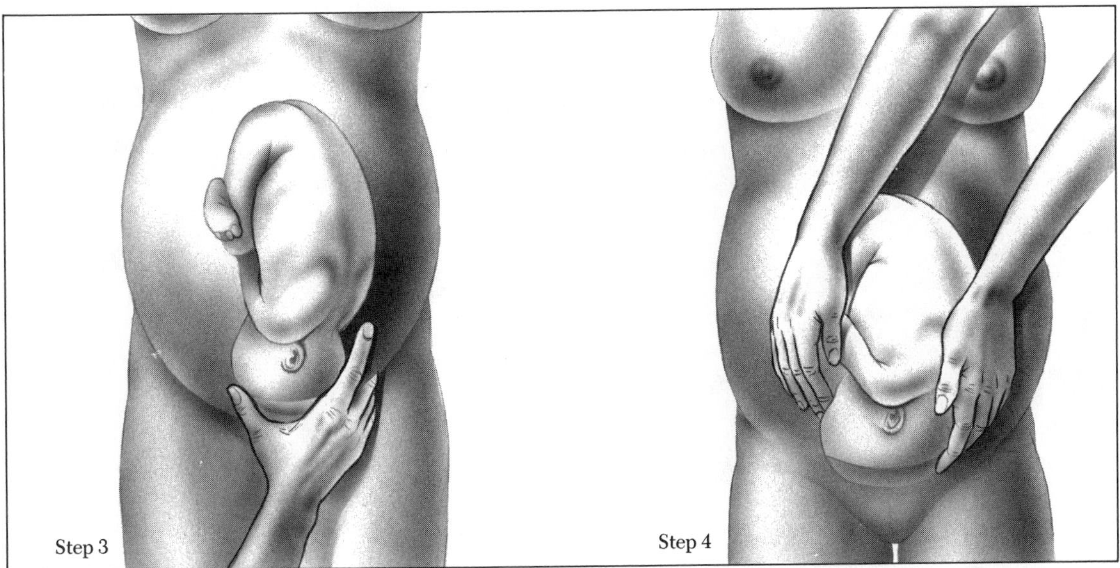

Figure 23-11 Leopold's maneuvers. (*Continued*)

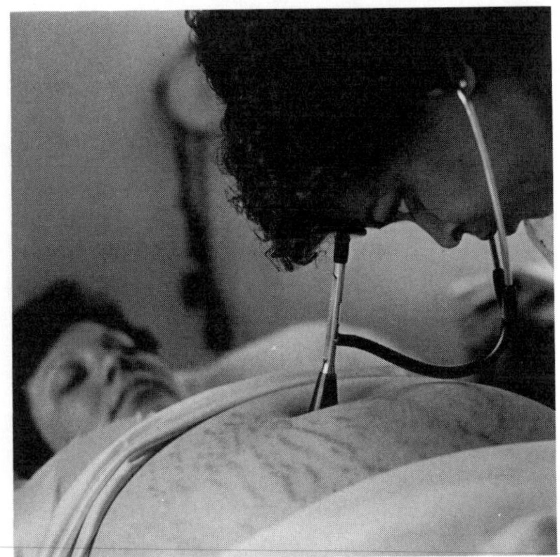

Figure 23-12 Using a fetoscope.

blowing noise synchronous with the mother's pulse and heard best in the lower portion of the uterus. This sound, which is normal in the pregnant woman, is the result of the increased blood supply to the uterus.

Assessment of the Pelvis

The technique for pelvic exam is described in Chapter 19. Some changes in pregnancy can be noted early in pregnancy. The first of these is *Goodell's sign*, in which softening of the cervix can be detected at about 5 to 6 weeks. *Hegar's sign* is noted at about 6 to 7 weeks. Place two fingers of one hand behind the cervix in the posterior vaginal fornix. Then compress the lower part of the corpus anteriorly by retropubic pressure with the other hand (see Figure 23-13). On palpation the dramatically enlarged globular uterus feels almost detached from the still not completely softened cervix. This occurs because the isthmus of the uterus is the first part to soften. At about the same time the examiner can easily flex the uterine body and the cervix against one another on bimanual examination. This is called *McDonald's sign* (see Figure 23-14). Frequently the uterus can be palpated asymmetrically, softening at the cornua when the ovum has implanted there. This is referred to as *Piskacek's sign* (see Figure 23-15). *Chadwick's sign* results from increased vascularity and is evidenced by the bluish violet of the vulva, vagina, and cervix.

Pelvic measurements should be obtained to evaluate whether the pelvic cavity is big enough to accommodate the fetus at delivery. The pelvis is composed of four bones: the two innominate bones, the sacrum, and the coccyx (see Figure 23-16). The innominates join in front at the symphysis and at the sacrum by sacroiliac synchondroses. That portion above the linea terminalis is referred to as the false pelvis, which supports the enlarged uterus (see Figure 23-17). The true pelvis, below the linea terminalis, is the bony birth canal through which the baby must pass at

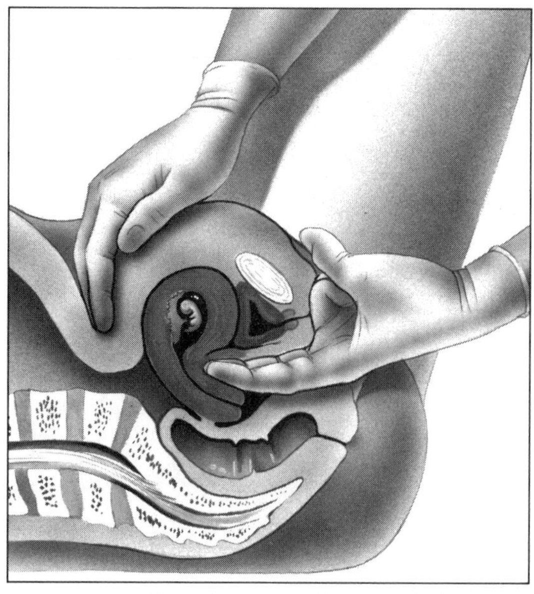

Figure 23-13 Hegar's sign: softening of the lower uterine segment.

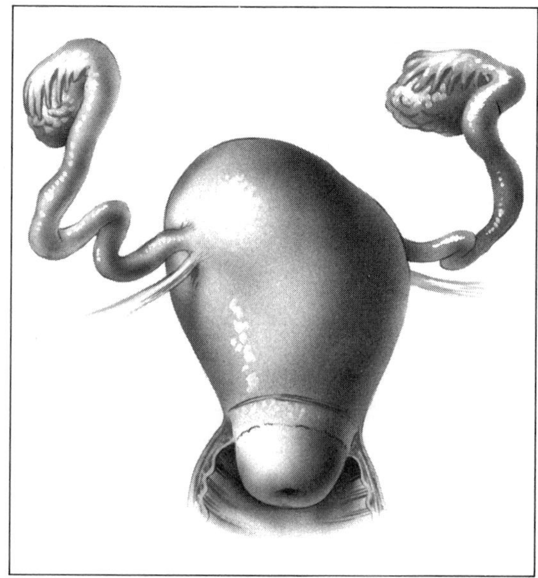

Figure 23-15 Piskacek's sign: asymmetrical enlargement of the uterine fundus.

delivery. If any of the planes or conjugates of this area are shortened or distorted, vaginal delivery may be difficult or impossible. The joints of the pelvis soften slightly during pregnancy in preparation for labor; the sacrococcygeal joint actually allows the coccyx to bend backward as the head is delivered.

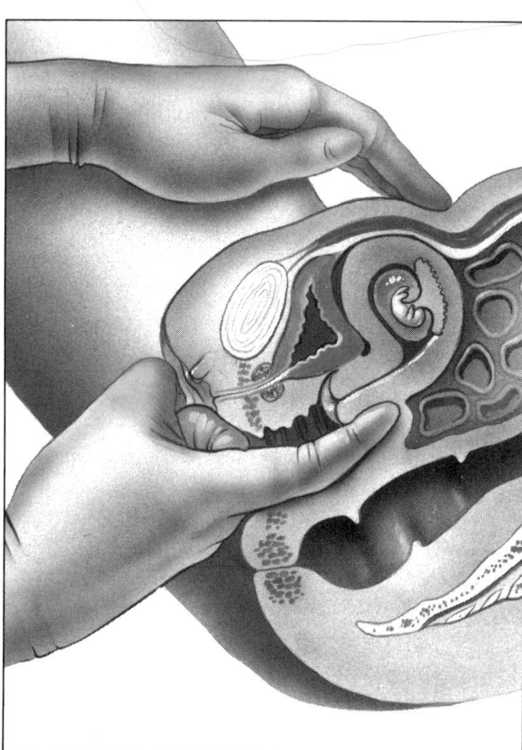

Figure 23-14 McDonald's sign: uterine body and cervix can be flexed against one another.

Race, sex, and age are responsible for the greatest variation in pelvic shape and size. Four types of pelvises have been identified (see Figure 23-18). Most often the pelvis is a mixture of types. The types are:

1. *Gynecoid*—The classic female type. The inlet is wide and the pubic arch is wide. This pelvis is found in about 40% of women and is fairly easy for the fetus to move through.
2. *Anthropoid*—Resembling the pelvis of anthropoid apes. This is a long, narrow pelvis. The inlet is oval shaped, ischial spines are prominent, and the pubic arch is narrow. This shape is found in approximately 25%–35% of women.
3. *Android*—Resembling the male pelvis. This pelvis is long and narrow. The pubic arch is narrow and the ischial spines are sharp and prominent. This pelvis is found in 15%–20% of women and is a difficult passage for the fetus.
4. *Platypelloid*—The flat pelvis. The inlet is wide with a narrow anterior-posterior diameter. The ischial spines are wide apart, the sacrum is short, and the pubic arch is wide, creating a shallow pelvis. This type is found in 3%–5% of women.

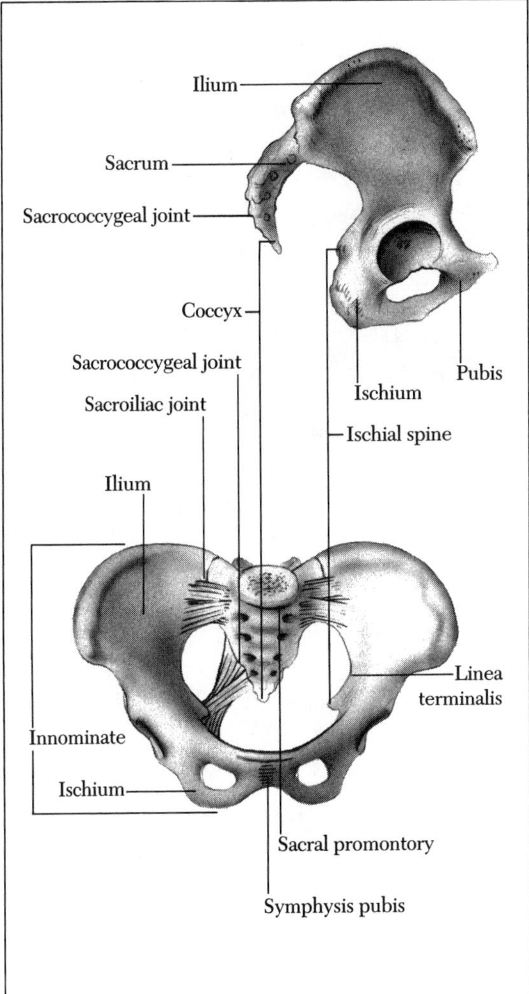

Figure 23-16 Bones and joints of pelvis.

The pelvis can be measured on the initial prenatal visit and repeated at 32–36 weeks if there is an indication of a problem or if client's tenseness and resulting muscular contraction make the exam too difficult. Since the joints and ligaments relax more in the third trimester, the examination may be more accurate at that time.

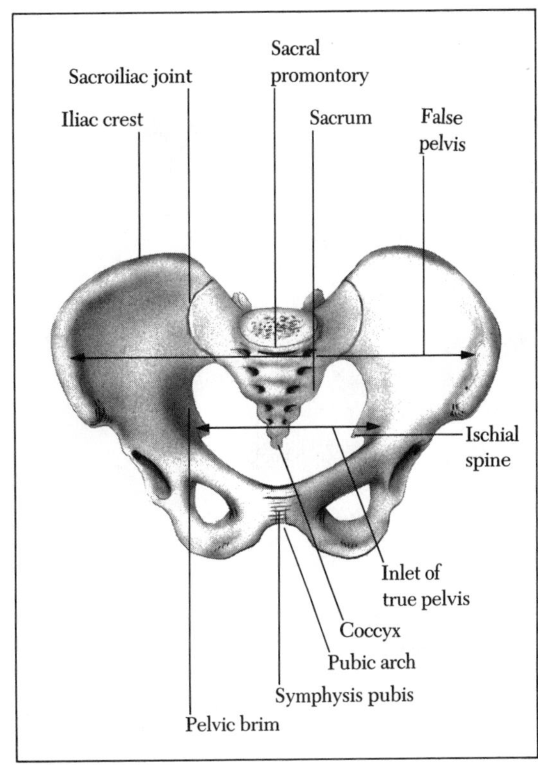

Figure 23-17 The pelvic cavity.

Another assessment can be made at the time of labor to compare pelvic measurements with data obtained on the presentation, position, and size of the fetus.

The first area to be assessed is the subpubic arch. To do this, press your right hand against the client's left ischiopubic ramus and the left hand against the right ischiopubic ramus so that the thumbs meet in the midline of the symphysis pubis (see Figure 23-19). Palpate the subpubic arch downward under the pubic bone until your right thumb rests on the left ischial tuberosity and the left thumb on the right ischial tuberosity. Mark each tuberosity with a small dot or *x* and then measure. Normally the line from the mid-

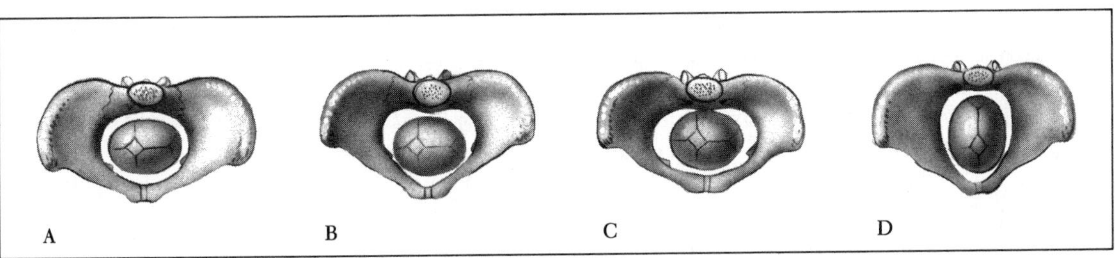

Figure 23-18 Four major pelvic types: (A) gynecoid, (B) android, (C) platypelloid (flat), and (D) anthropoid.

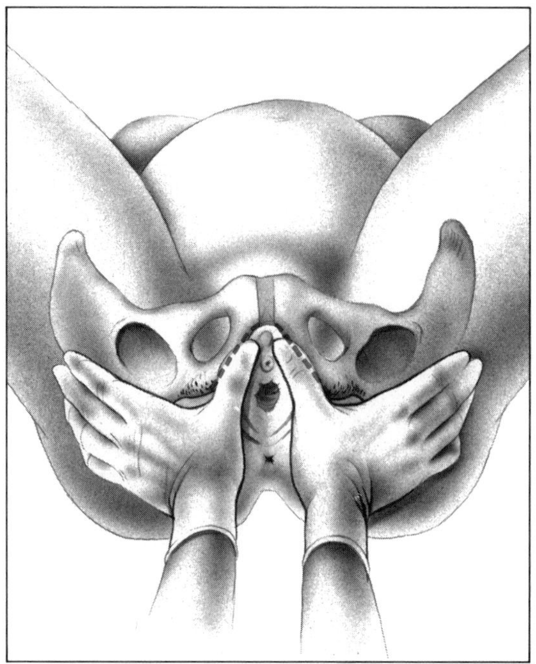

Figure 23-19 Method of estimating the angle of the subpubic arch.

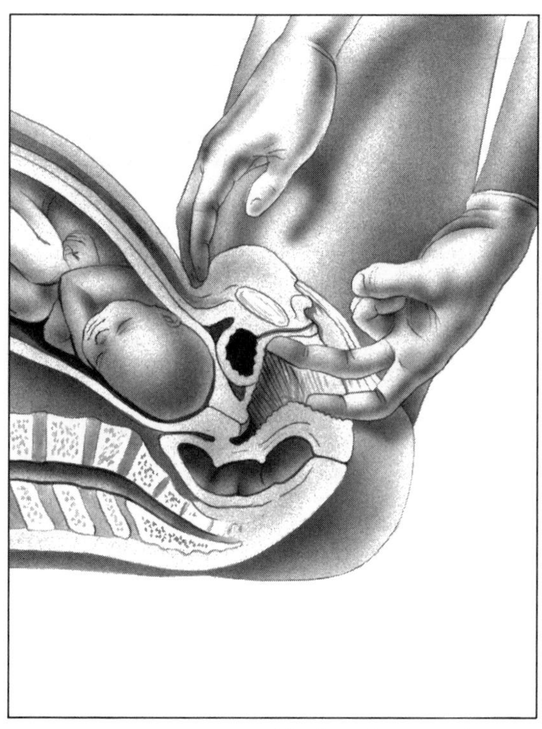

Figure 23-20 Estimation of the length and inclination of the symphysis pubis.

line of the symphysis to the ischial tuberosity should form an angle measuring slightly more than 90 degrees, which is a right angle.

To assess the thickness and inclination of the symphysis pubis, palpate the internal surface with the middle finger of your left hand and the external surface with your index and middle fingers of the right hand. The inclination can be estimated by sweeping the examining fingers under the symphysis. Judgments to be made at this time are related to screening for unusually long or steeply inclined symphysis and for an angular rather than a rounded forepelvis (see Figure 23-20).

Next assess the curvature of the right and left anterior segments of the pelvic inlet and the ischial side walls to gain an idea of overall pelvic symmetry. With your right hand, follow the client's right pubic bone from the symphysis to the right side of the pelvic inlet. Then sweep downward over the right ischial side wall to the right ischial tuberosity. Repeat the procedure on the left anterior segment using your left hand.

Examine the ischial spine and the sacrospinous ligament. Assess the spine as being blunt, prominent, or encroaching. If possible, the sacrosciatic notch is outlined with palpating fingers and the width determined in fingerbreadths or centimeters (see Figure 23-21). To do this, place the index and middle fingers of your right hand in the client's vagina. Palpate the right spine and then pass fingers across to the left ischial spine by pronating the right examining hand and following the conformation of the pelvic soft parts. This maneuver can be repeated several times. Ischial spines may be difficult to identify if they are not prominent. If that is the case, follow the sacrosciatic ligaments to their origins and reassess the spines during the rectal examination.

Measuring the transverse diameter of the midpelvis, also called interspinous or bispinous diameter, can be accomplished by using an examining finger or a pelvimeter. Insert the examining fingers into the vagina and move them in a straight line from one spine to the other. You may have to pronate your hand to do this estimation. The estimate is measured in centimeters and the average measure is 11 cm (see Figure 23-22).

The next important assessment is of the anterior-posterior diameter of the pelvic inlet (see Figure 23-23). There are three measurements of this diameter:

1. *True conjugate*—Distance from the top of

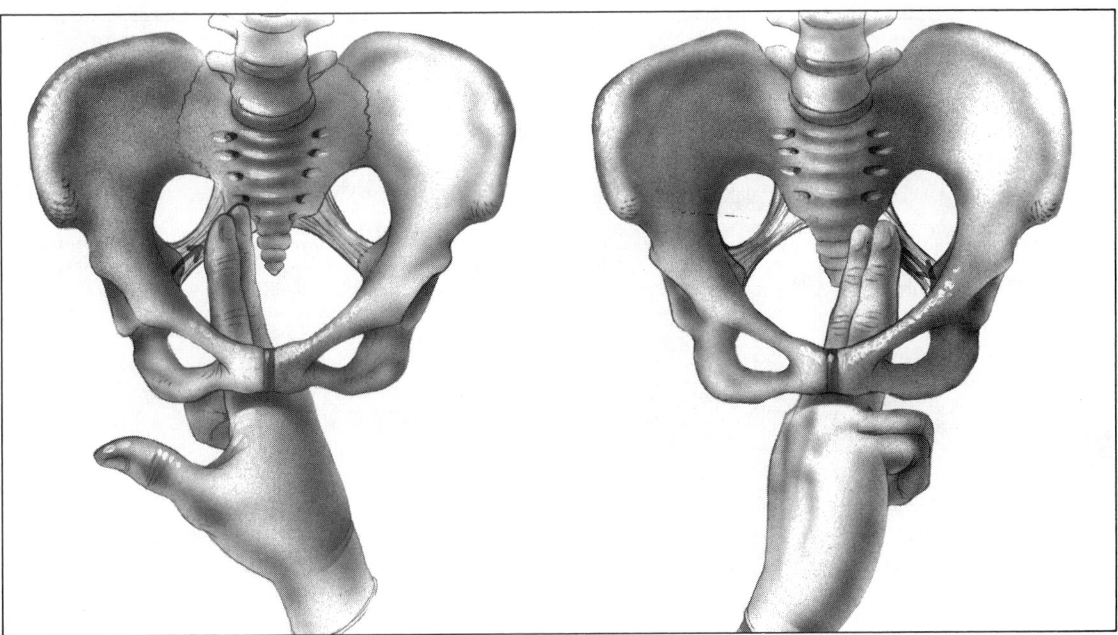

Figure 23-21 Measurement of the width of the sacrosciatic notch.

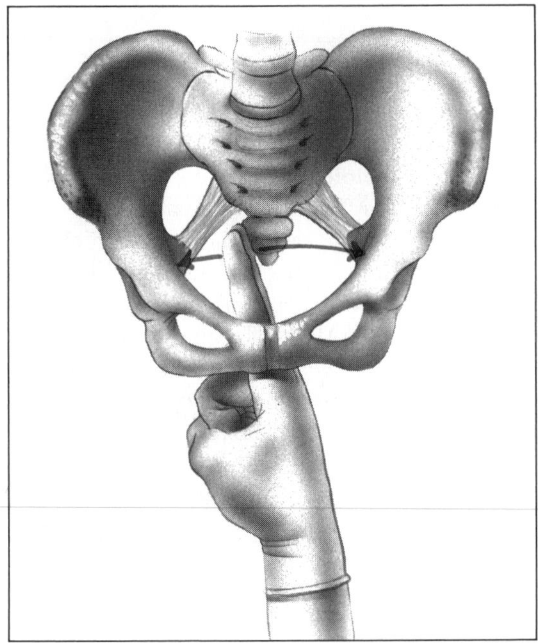

Figure 23-22 Measurement of the transverse, or interspinous, diameter.

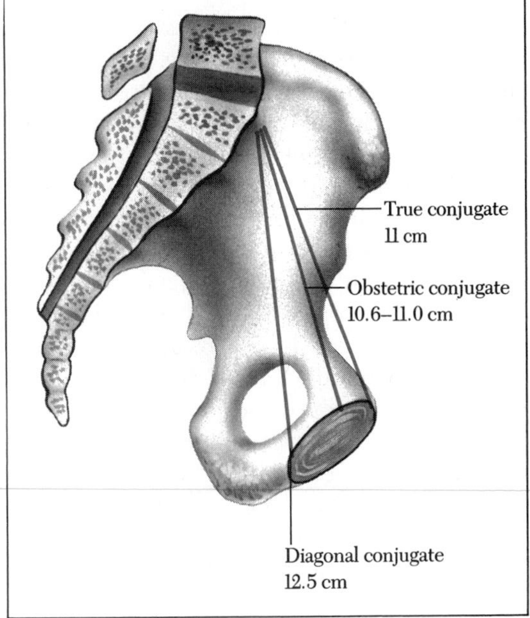

Figure 23-23 Assessing the anterior-posterior diameter of the pelvic inlet.

the symphysis pubis to the middle promontory of the sacrum.

2. *Obstetric conjugate*—Distance between the posterior surface of the symphysis and sacral promontory.
3. *Diagonal conjugate*—Distance from the inferior border of the symphysis to the sacral promontory.

The diagonal conjugate is the only diameter that can be measured without the use of x-ray. This examination may be uncomfortable, so you

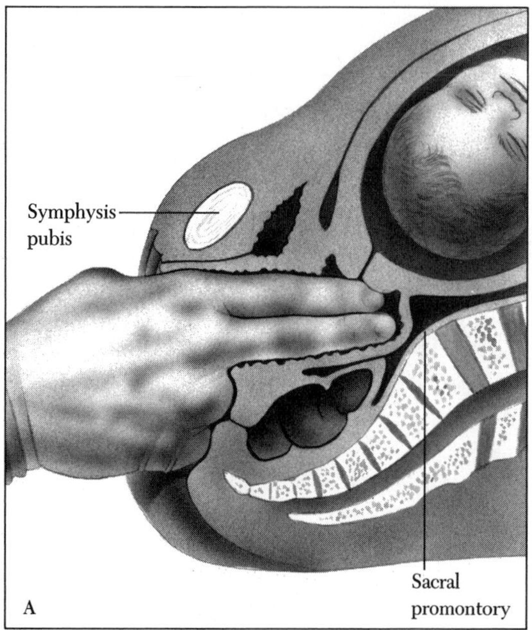

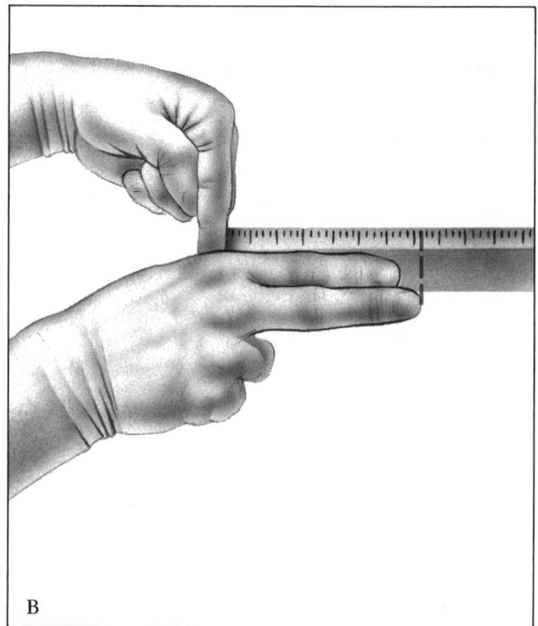

Figure 23-24 Measurement of the diagonal conjugate.

should instruct the client to relax and focus her attention on breathing slowly. A moderate amount of pressure is needed to depress the perineum. Position your own right foot on a small stool so that your right knee is bent and right thigh elevated. For this examination your fingers and wrist should be in a straight line with the forearm. Locate the sacrum with your examining fingers, and with the middle finger walk up the sacrum until the promontory is reached or until your finger can no longer reach the sacrum. Keeping your middle finger in place, raise your right wrist until your hand touches the inferior border of the symphysis pubis. Withdraw your hand and measure from the tip of the middle finger to the point on the examining hand that has touched the symphysis (see Figure 23-24). Normally the diagonal conjugate is greater than 12.5 cm. Estimation of the true conjugate can be made by subtracting 1.5 cm from the diagonal conjugate. An estimate of the obstetric conjugate can be arrived at by subtracting 2 cm from the diagonal conjugate.

The transverse diameter of the pelvic outlet is measured by the distance between the ischial tuberosities. The measurement can be made with a Thom's pelvimeter or can be estimated by placing a closed fist between the protrusions of the ischial tuberosities (see Figure 23-25). The usual distance is 10.5 cm.

Summary

This chapter has presented assessment in selected areas of women's health. The areas do not constitute a complete picture of women's health needs, however. Menstruation and menopause were presented because they are events all women experience. Specific health problems related to these events such as amenorrhea, dysmenorrhea, and PMS are frequent occurrences. Eating disorders were discussed, and there is evidence of increased incidence of these disorders occurring particularly among younger women.

The women's movement has had a profound influence on the care of women during pregnancy. The need to understand both physiologic and psychologic aspects of pregnancy is essential to the practice of nursing. Throughout the chapter normal findings, as well as selected deviations from normal, were described.

Discussion Questions/Activities

1. Describe the social factors that affect the health status of adolescent girls. Plan a health education program to counteract the negative responses that occur.

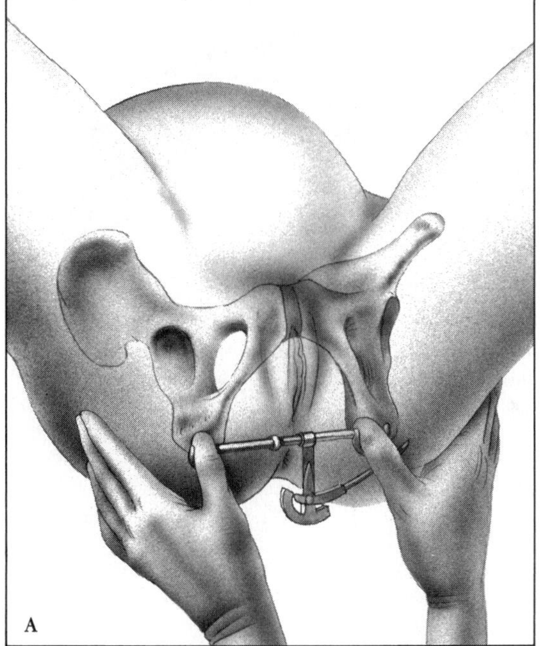

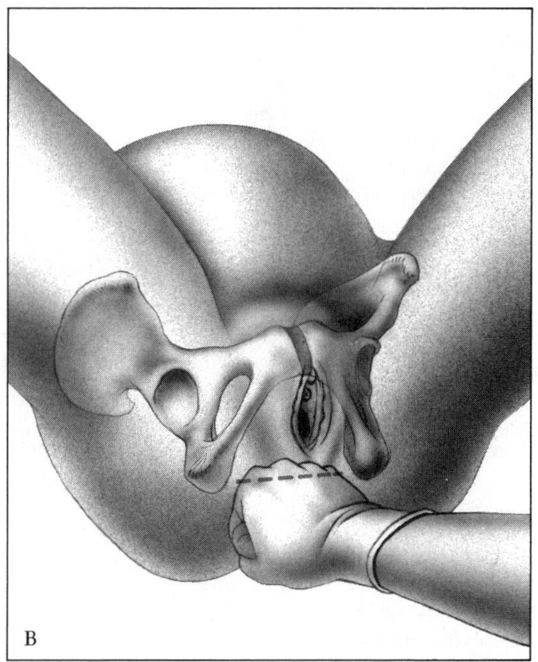

Figure 23-25 (A) Use of the Thom's pelvimeter to measure the intertuberous diameter. (B) Use of a fist to estimate the intertuberous diameter.

2. Research and discuss the historical development of women's health care as a specialty.
3. Plan a health education program related to menstruation and menopause.
4. Describe the assessment of the pregnant client on her initial health visit, at 16 weeks, and just prior to delivery.

EXAMPLE OF A HEALTH ASSESSMENT OF A PREGNANT WOMAN

HEALTH HISTORY

Name: Marianne Phillips
Address: 27 Lincoln Place
Sex: Female
Age: 34
Birthdate: 7/17/52
Marital status: Married since 1976
Occupation: Teacher
Religion: Protestant (attends church infrequently)
Race: Caucasian
Ethnic origin: English and Scotch
Education: College and graduate school
Informant: Client, a reliable historian

Reason for Seeking Health Care

Client has missed two menstrual periods and has been slightly nauseated upon arising for the past 10 days. Has also noted more frequent urination for several weeks. Client feels she is probably pregnant. She expresses hope that she is and states that she and her husband have been hoping to have a third child.

(continued on page 566)

Personal History and Patterns of Living
Client states she is happily married, has been teaching in a local college for two months, and in addition cares for two young children (both boys). She is able to handle all of these because her husband is very supportive, and she describes herself as being very ambitious. Her salary is $24,000 per year and her husband's is $50,000 per year. She describes financial status as very adequate for family needs; family has Blue Cross and Blue Shield health care coverage.

Family Health History
States family has a history of diabetes. Denies history of arthritis, alcoholism, bleeding disorders, kidney disease, hypertension, heart disease, endocrine disease, or mental illness.

Lifestyle
Client is currently attending diet classes but describes the plan as well balanced and one that with modifications for age and sex she can use for planning meals for her family. Wants to lose about 10 lb and, most important, to change the eating habits of herself and family to ensure good health. Client does not smoke and drinks only socially and then just wine. Describes family as very close and also close to grandparents, cousins, etc. Family is very active, swimming 3 times per week, cross-country skiing, and hiking.

Previous Experience with Illness/Hospitalization
Childhood illness: Mumps, age 8, chickenpox same year; measles (not sure of year); immunizations DPT.
Allergies: Allergic to grass and roses. Had series of allergy shots in early 1970s, which she describes as only moderately helpful. Uses over-the-counter medication (antihistamines) during June and August. She is aware that pregnancy will require change in that.
Past illness, injuries, surgery: Appendectomy age 11, hospitalized 6 days. Hospitalized for C-section in 1979 and 1981. Length of stay 2 weeks. Says she had to have sections due to high blood pressure and swelling.

Review of Systems
General health: In good health but has felt more fatigued in last few weeks with feeling of nausea and occasional vomiting in the morning. States she had same experience with previous pregnancies. Problem disappeared in several months. Never took medication to control symptoms in the past.
Integument: No history of skin disease but developed hyperpigmented areas on forehead and cheeks during last pregnancy. No itchy skin or scalp, denies rashes, hives, nevi, open sores, hair loss, or problems with nails. Has acne, which has become worse in last month.
Head: Denies frequent or severe headaches, dizziness.
Eyes: Denies infection or pain; does not wear glasses; last eye exam in 1983; denies diplopia, excessive lacrimation, blurring of vision, photophobia, or halo-rainbows around lights.
Ears: Has slight hearing loss in left ear since frequent infections as a child. Denies pain, discharge, tinnitus, auditory hallucinations, and vertigo.
Nose, nasopharynx, and paranasal sinuses: No discharge at present, infrequent colds, has allergies to roses and grass with seasonal copious discharge, itching, and sneezing. Notices decrease in sense of smell during middle and last part of pregnancy.
Mouth and throat: Denies bleeding gums at present but during last pregnancy noticed that gums were sensitive and bled easily when teeth brushed. Visits dentist yearly and was informed that gums often bleed more easily during pregnancy. Was advised by dentist to use softer bristles when brushing and to call if there was any increase in bleeding or increased soreness of gums. This did not occur.
Neck: Denies pain, edema, limitation of movement, swollen glands.
Cardiorespiratory system: Reports significant elevation in BP during both pregnancies especially during last trimester. States that following delivery BP returned to normal. Denies cough, sputum, othopnea, dyspnea, and PND. No history of pneumonia, TB, pain, wheezing, hemoptysis, anemia. Has some leg varicosities. Wears support hose.
Gastrointestinal system: Has had nausea and vomiting for last 10 days; denies blood in stools, melena, flatulence, pain. Has hemorrhoids since last pregnancy, occasional pain associated with constipation (infrequent). Usually has soft, formed stool daily after breakfast.
Genitourinary system: Has had frequency in last few weeks; denies pain, itching, blood. Describes sex life as very satisfying.
Gynecologic and obstetric: Menarche age 13, LMP 1/2/86. Has irregular cycle 28–35 days, flow moderate, uses tampons and pad interchangeably due to fear of toxic shock. Denies metrorrhagia, menorrhagia, dyspareunia. Has noted slight spotty bleeding following intercourse recently. Para 2 gravida 2—Had 2 C-sections following rapid increase in BP and significant swelling of feet and hands. No abortions. When practicing birth control, uses diaphragm.
Musculoskeletal system: Denies muscular pain, edema (currently). Had significant hand and pedal edema during last trimester of previous pregnancy.

Neurologic system: Has noticed some "lightheadedness" during last several weeks. Denies difficulty walking, convulsions, pain in arms or legs, numbness, paralysis, tingling or burning anywhere in body. Denies nightmares, sleepwalking, changes in feelings or speech patterns.

Client profile
Mrs. Marianne Phillips, 34-year-old female, feels she is pregnant, hoping she is, and anxious to confirm. In good health but expressed some concern about having to have another Caesarean delivery. She is also somewhat anxious because she and family have just moved to this area and she will be relating to a new nurse and physician.

PHYSICAL ASSESSMENT

General impression: Mrs. Phillips, 34-year-old female, WD/WN in NAD. Alert, well groomed.
Height: 5′4″
Weight: 160 lb
TPR—98.8F/a85/16
BP—left and right: 142/82 sitting and supine

Integument: Acne on face and anterior chest. Lesions are pustules, less than 1 cm in diameter and red. Remainder of skin is clear, pink with no fissures or lesions with no edema. Normal hair distribution, nails without deformities, clubbing, or cyanosis; good capillary refill; skin turgor good, warm to touch.

Head and face: Normocephalic; scalp healthy, no facial weakness or involuntary movements; eyebrows present and full; no facial edema; skin color WNL; no sinus tenderness.

Neck: Size, symmetry, and position WNL; normal ROM; thyroid palpable, firm without nodules. No thyroid bruit. No lymphadenopathy; no venous distention; carotids equal bilaterally and of good quality; no carotid bruits; trachea midline.

Eyes: Lashes and brows present; no orbital edema; palpebral fissures WNL; no lid lag, ptosis, nystagmus, or strabismus; conjunctiva pink and clear; sclerae white; cornea clear; PERRLA/consensual reaction; normal convergence; EOMs intact visual fields normal by gross confrontation: visual acuity—OD 20/20, OS 20/20 without glasses. Fundoscopy: red reflex clear, disk well demarcated and pinkish yellow in color; A/V 2:3 no AV nicking, OD two small flame-shaped hemorrhages 2DD at 2 o'clock. None in OS and no exudates. Occular tension on palpation WNL.

Nose, mouth, pharynx: No tenderness or deformity of nose; patent; pale gray mucosa; no edema; no discharge; no septal deviation or perforations; lips normal—no cracks, lesions; buccal mucosa pink; gums slightly hyperemic; soft and hard palate WNL; no ulcers, sores, or lacerations; tongue protrudes in midline; uvular reflex normal; tonsils absent; gag reflex present; teeth—several fillings, teeth well cared for.

Ears: Normal positioning; no deformities or lesions; no discharge; no cerumen; canals clear without redness or edema; eardrum pearly gray without perforation; light reflex present; watch ticking not heard in left ear; Weber test—lateralized to left ear; AC > BC in right ear, AC < BC in left.

Breasts: Breasts symmetrical, nipples everted; areola dark and Montgomery's glands enlarged; on palpation, slightly tender and client reports tingling sensation present; no dimpling, retraction; client has noted slight discharge with no itching or odor; no lymphadenopathy; slight bilateral venous engorgement; examines breasts regularly.

Thorax and Lungs: Thorax normal size and shape; symmetrical expansion; respirations—16/min; no abnormal pulsations; no tenderness; fremitus present; lung fields resonant; diaphragmmatic excursions 3.5 cm bilaterally; vesicular breath sounds in bases; no crackles, wheezes, or rubs.

Cardiovascular: Apical pulse at left fifth ICS at MCL; no heaves, thrills, rate 85 regular; $A_2 > P_2$; physiological splitting of S_2; no gallops, rubs, or murmurs. Peripheral pulses patent and good volume bilaterally.

Musculoskeletal: Full range of joint motion; no crepitation or deformities; body and limb symmetry; no pain, tenderness; muscle size, tone, and movements WNL; no atrophy, tremors, weakness, or fasciculations; proximal and distal strength WNL.

Neurologic: Oriented to person, place, and time; recent and remote memory intact; alert and cooperative; normal gait, good coordination; cranial nerves intact; DTRs present bilaterally.

Abdomen: Round with appendectomy scar LRQ; classical midline C-section scar at 8 cm; multiple abdominal striae; symmetrical without venous engorgement or flank edema; no bruits; bowel sound present; liver nonpalpable; spleen nonpalpable; no masses, tenderness; no CVA tenderness; kidneys nonpalpable; good muscle tone.

(continued on page 568)

Reproductive: Normal pubic hair pattern; external genitals normal in appearance; labia and vaginal walls show increased vascularity (positive Chadwick's sign); Skene's and Bartholin's glands not inflamed; normal vaginal discharge, no odor or itching. Cervix oval, external os appears as transverse slit. Cervix soft (Goodell's sign) at 12 weeks' gestation. Adnexa—nothing significant.

Uterus: Bimanual exam reveals uterus slightly antiflexed, larger and soft (Hegar's sign present). Pap smear to lab. Fundal height: 1.2 cm above symphysis pubis. Client notes periodic tightening across abdomen (Braxton-Hicks contractions). No cyctocele, rectocele, or prolapse.

Rectum: One small internal hemorrhoid; sphincter tone good; test for occult blood.

Bony Pelvis Examination
Subpubic arch—above 90 degrees
Side walls—parallel
Ischial spines—average
Sacrospinous notch—8.5 cm
Sacrospinous ligament—4 cm
Interspinous diameter—10.5 cm
Sacrum—straight
Coccyx—projects posteriorly
Diagonal conjugate—12.5 cm
Intertuberous diameter using Thom's pelvimeter—10.5 cm

Based on Mrs. Phillips's last menstrual period the expected date of delivery is: October 9, 1986.

CHAPTER 24

Assessment of Men's Health

LEARNING OBJECTIVES

1. Identify the impact of culture on men's health.
2. Analyze the value-belief pattern relative to male identity and its effect on client-health professional interactions.
3. Discuss the implications of male identity and health practices and status.
4. Identify the risk factors for cardiovascular disease.
5. List mental status alterations that may suggest cardiovascular difficulties.
6. Identify the physical findings that are reflective of cardiovascular disease.
7. State risk factors for lung cancer.
8. List signs and symptoms of lung cancer and potential metastatic sites and related symptomatology.
9. Discuss the ethnic epidemiologic findings associated with prostatic cancer.
10. Identify signs and symptoms of benign prostatic hyperplasia and prostatic cancer.
11. Discuss nursing implications relative to the incidence of testicular cancer.
12. State the signs and symptoms of testicular cancer.
13. Identify the primary causes of sexual dysfunctions.
14. Discuss the approach and components of history-taking with the client experiencing sexual dysfunction.
15. Cite diseases, surgeries, and drugs that are commonly associated with male sexual dysfunctions.

> Gender is perhaps the single characteristic which most fundamentally determines perceptions, behaviour and position in most societies. No other characteristic of individuals may be subject to the same degree of cultural and social learning (Dean 1989, p. 138).

The medico-nursing system readily attends to the pathophysiology, diagnosis and treatment of injuries and illnesses of prevalence in men (e.g., suicide, fractures, head and spinal injuries, cancers, hernias, peptic ulcers, cardiorespiratory diseases, and sex-related illnesses such as benign prostatic hyperplasia). Basic assessment skills and techniques of psychological and physical examination relative to these health problems that plague men are included in earlier chapters and will not be repeated here. This chapter will initially focus on the value-belief pattern pertinent to gender identity that is learned within the sociocultural context of men's lives. This will assist the nurse to generate a more holistic view of the male client when assessing his health. Then data associated with selected health problems encountered by men will be addressed.

Male Identity

Most cultures have child-rearing practices that instill a gender identity for the male as one who is in control of his emotionality; therefore, a boy is taught to be inexpressive—to hide his emotions. Feelings of hurt, pain, anxiety, and depression are not to be freely shared or overtly manifested. To do so would constitute a sign of weakness and inferiority. Whether each of us is male or female, we generally have a similar cultural view of how men and women are to behave. Our society teaches us that a man is competitive; he is a warrior. To live up to society's expectations, compensatory masculine role behaviors may take the form of risk-taking, aggression, and violence. Traditionally the male is thought of as being self-sufficient and strong. It follows then that these stereotypic characteristics of male identity will impact on health behaviors and health practices of clients and on practices and care rendered by health professionals.

Commonly, men feign good health to keep within society's expectations of the male identity as healthy and strong in spite of the fact that they might be ill. If not overtly, subconsciously the view that only the weak, dependent, and inferior become ill prevails in our society. It is not surprising that this ingrained belief leads men to psychologically deny health needs and find it difficult to seek preventive as well as curative care, and to accept assistance from others. This is a sad state in light of present health knowledge, and it likely contributes to the health statistics for men.

Chronic illnesses related to the leading causes of death such as chronic ischemic heart disease and chronic obstructive pulmonary disease are of a higher prevalence in men than in women. Men also have a higher risk of all the leading causes of death in the nation and a higher rate of injury at all ages compared to women. The higher rate of injuries may be related to occupational hazards in jobs done primarily by men and could be attributable somewhat to the more risk-taking behavior of men (Dean 1989). Issues of masculinity surround the high morbidity and mortality rates of motor vehicle accidents, homicides, and suicides involving men. Men tend to use seat belts less than women. Men have a greater use of alcohol and street drugs than women (Waldron 1982). The greater use of alcohol also is a contributing factor to men's higher morbidity and mortality from cirrhosis, laryngeal and bladder cancer as well as from heart disease. Men are more likely to use alcohol and tobacco as coping behaviors. Alcohol and cigarette smoking act synergistically, increasing the risk of development of cancer of the lungs and of the esophagus (Doll and Peto 1981).

Traditionally, more men have smoked than women, and men have a greater mortality rate from lung cancer. Men ingest smokeless tobacco far more than women and suffer a higher incidence of oral cancer as a result. The sex difference in cigarette smoking has lessened. In light of evidence and media focus on the dangers of tobacco, and legislation for "smoke-free areas" and individuals trying to "break the habit," it will be interesting to follow the morbidity and mortality rates for ischemic heart disease, lung cancer, emphysema, bronchitis, and other smoking-related diseases. Another interesting data find is that men have longer hospital stays than women (Dean 1989). Yet, in view of these statistics, men do not seek medical and nursing attention as frequently as women (Forrester 1986).

Women are more active in preventive spheres and adhere to regular check-ups that include cancer screening (pap smears, stool examinations for occult blood, breast examinations, pelvic examinations, mammograms) and routine monitoring of blood pressure, weight, and blood chemistry. At present, the majority of men are not attentive to preventive screening and to practices that safeguard their health, social beliefs being one influential factor; and neither men nor women health professionals are attentive to men's preventive health needs. This lack of preventive health measures by and for men was a major tenet of men's health that prompted Bozett and Forrester (1989) to propose the educational preparation of a nurse practitioner in men's health.

A male movement is growing out of the recognition of high morbidity and mortality rates for men and because of social emphasis on preventive practices and the reach for greater longevity in general. This holds implications for nursing practice and research. "One positive potential for the men's health movement would be to identify linkages between the way men die and the way they live as *men*" (Allen & Whatley 1986, p. 8).

Men and Health Professionals

Sex stereotyping occurs in health professionals as well as in other individuals. Most professionals hold traditional values and beliefs about masculinity and find it difficult to address and accept emotionality in men. Most male professionals find it difficult to deal with feelings and emotionality in either men or women clients. Men as professionals and as clients generally do not share health concerns on an emotional level but interact in a more factual, business-like exchange. Even more difficult is sharing health problems associated with sexuality. It is generally believed that "men do not discuss such things with each other" and that women "cannot possibly understand the unique male experience" (Forrester 1986, p. 17). The stereotypic beliefs that men must "bite the bullet," that men are strong and self-sufficient, that men don't cry, and that men are stoic and do not show their feelings shape the male client's responses not only to health practices but to illness and health personnel. So too, the practices of health professionals are influenced.

Quite some time ago, Jourard (1971) challenged health professionals to become aware of their cultural beliefs about men and to begin to help change the stereotypic image of men held by society in an effort to improve men's health and longevity. He emphatically addressed the need to encourage men to express their feelings of sorrow, pain, fear, tenderness, and love. He pointed out that, in turn, health professionals must be accepting of overtly manifested emotionality that does not fit the social stereotype. This is difficult for most individuals to do because of our deeply ingrained cultural values.

Some changes in values and attitudes surrounding masculinity are slowly evolving in parallel with the women's movement. Men are no longer viewed as the sole family breadwinner. When we find ourselves thinking this way, further investigation brings home to us the reality that today the breadwinner role is shared or reversed in some cases from the traditional role responsibility. Conversely, it is more acceptable for the male to engage in housekeeping chores and caring physically for the children without the shame that accompanied such behaviors in the past. It would seem that adaptation of a more androgynous model for social behaviors by health professionals, authors, media producers, teachers, parents, and society as a whole would decrease health risk behaviors in men. Health educators, nurses, and physicians need to convey the health hazards inherent in the traditional concept of masculinity. Health care professionals and those in the media and media production can incorporate guidance and reinforcement of positive health practices in their work so that more positive health behaviors may be fostered in men. All persons need to be conscientious role models. Storylines of books, films, and television programs could greatly help in this cause by incorporating positive health practices in the lifestyles of major male characters. In addition to the family, the public entertainment sphere is strongly influential in helping to form social values and beliefs.

Selected Health Problems of Men

Cardiovascular Disease

Health problems related to the heart and the cardiovascular system are heavily focused upon in nursing and medical education and are commented on in most discussions of men's health. This is because heart disease is the major cause of death and the major cause of differences in mortality rates between the sexes. Incident rates for coronary occlusions and myocardial infarctions are substantially higher for men than for women. Being male is in and of itself a documented risk factor for heart disease. Credence has been given to the presence of estrogen for the lower risk of heart disease in women. With menopause and the decrease of estrogen, the risk for heart disease in women increases. The woman's risk for heart disease also increases with high blood pressure, diabetes mellitus, hyperlipidemia, and when menopause is premature. White males between the ages of 35 and 55 are five times likelier to die of ischemic heart disease than white women in the United States. A bald man, reflective of higher testosterone levels, has an even greater risk than other men for cardiovascular disease. Such research findings have lead to the androgen hypothesis. However, not all research findings support this hypothesis.

Foreman (1986) pointed out the logic that if this androgen hypothesis were valid then men of all cultures and races would demonstrate similar rates of incidence of cardiovascular diseases. The incidence of cardiovascular heart disease is greatest in white American males and lowest in black African males. Furthermore, Foreman cited literature that attributed atherosclerosis to emotional inexpressiveness (a stereotypic characteristic of male identity). In addition he stated that a relationship was found between socially held beliefs of competitive and aggressive men and the characteristics of the Type A personality. Type A personality with underlying anger has been associated with an increased risk for heart disease. Another risk for cardiovascular heart disease is age—as one grows older, the risk of heart disease increases.

Reason for Seeking Health Evaluation

Signs of cardiovascular disease in men may be detected in a routine employment history and physical. Clinical symptoms may include weakness, extreme fatigue, palpitations, peripheral edema, extremity pain, tingling, and/or numbness in the arms or legs, dyspnea on exercise, hypotension, syncope, cyanosis, and chest discomfort. Severe chest pain that persists is a symptom that most likely motivates the male client to voluntarily seek medical attention with expediency.

Sociocultural Aspects, Lifestyle and Habits

Stress is a relevant factor in the development and progression of cardiovascular heart disease. Lifestyle, including leisure activities, habits of sleep-rest, recreation, exercise, drug use, eating patterns and diet, as well as values, beliefs, job satisfaction, family relationships, stressful life events, health practices, coping behaviors, and support systems requires investigation and evaluation. Specifically, we will comment on smoking, drug use (alcohol consumption, caffeine intake), diet, and exercise habits.

A history of smoking is important to ascertain because of a strong association between tobacco and cardiovascular disease. The responses of the cardiovascular system to the nicotine component of tobacco include a rise in both systolic and diastolic blood pressure, heart rate, myocardial oxygen uptake, force of cardiac contraction, myocardial excitability, and peripheral vasoconstriction. Free fatty acids, cortisol (an antidiuretic hormone), glucose and platelet aggregation also have been found to increase with nicotine use. Epidemiological studies of industry reveal that more disability due to chronic illness and more workdays lost are found among cigarette smokers than nonsmokers. Male smokers have a 60 to 70% greater risk for cardiovascular heart disease than nonsmokers. Respiratory problems that may cause cor pulmonale (enlargement of the right ventricle secondary to respiratory diseases) include the following disorders: pulmonary vascular disease, airway obstruction from tracheal stenosis, obstructive sleep apnea syndromes (which occur more in men than women), respiratory symptomatology of medullary dysfunction (hypoventilation and central sleep apnea syndromes), physical limitation of lung expansion and function by spinal-thoracic deformities (kyphoscoliosis, funnel breast, and pigeon breast), and obesity. Chronic obstructive lung disease, which is of higher prevalence in men, is viewed as an occupational hazard secondary to greater air pollutant exposure, including cigarette smoke. Cessation of smoking is associated with a dramatic decline in risk for both respiratory and cardiovascular heart disease.

Smokers drink more alcohol, coffee and tea (Braunwald et al 1987). If caffeinated coffee and tea are used, the amount consumed on a daily basis should be assessed. The use of street drugs or recreational drugs needs investigation. Cocaine use is especially a risk for cardiovascular heart disease. Endocarditis frequently occurs from "mainlining" habits (intravascular use of drugs). The use of tobacco, alcohol, and other psychoactive drugs by men is more culturally acceptable or tolerated. The use of such substances by women, particularly by pregnant women, is frowned upon because of the known influences of the fetus.

Alcohol can induce tachyarrhythmias (holiday heart syndrome); they frequently occur after a drinking binge. Alcoholic cardiomyopathy manifests a low cardiac output and peripheral and cardiac vasoconstriction. Progression of this cardiomyopathy may be halted by alcohol abstinence. If alcohol consumption continues, severe heart failure and death ensues generally within 1 to 3 years. The caffeine content in coffee and tea stimulates the heart and also may be a cause of arrhythmias. Chocolate may produce a similar effect; therefore diet investigation should question whether foods such as chocolate candybars, cocoa, and brownies are frequently eaten.

Other aspects of diet need assessment in relation to cardiovascular disease risks. It is believed that a diet consisting of fried foods, high salt, and high animal fats promotes the progression of atherosclerosis. Diet habits such as times for eating, amount of calories eaten, and types of foods consumed may be a cause of obesity. Obesity is considered to be another risk factor for cardiovascular disease. Obese men, especially over the age of 50, are more prone to cardiovascular heart disease. Lack of exercise may also be a proponent of obesity.

Exercise is viewed within the lifestyle; assess whether or not a regular exercise regimen is followed, and the amount of activity inherent in the type of occupation held, that is, the sedentary state versus degrees of physical activity. Exercise is postulated to clear the blood vessels of cholesterol and to raise the concentration of the high density lipoproteins (HDL).

Last, the family health history and the client's personal health history are scrutinized for any incidences of such diseases as hypertension, hypo or hyperthyroidism, obesity, diabetes mellitus, peripheral vascular disease, thrombophlebitis, pulmonary embolism, pulmonary infection, anemia, rheumatic heart fever, heart attack, and congestive heart disease.

Mental Health Assessment

Since Type A personality with underlying anger is strongly associated with the development of cardiovascular problems, it is important to assess if the characteristics representative of Type A personality, as well as undertones of anger, are manifested (see Chapter 5, Mental Status Assessment). Memory and other cognitive functions require evaluation, as alterations characterized by forgetfulness, difficulty in concentration, headaches, anxiety, insomnia, and confusion are reflective of cerebral arteriosclerosis, diminished cerebral blood flow and arterial hypoxemia as observed in severe congestive heart failure. Depression is a common finding in chronic, long-standing heart failure.

Physical Assessment

Abnormal blood pressure, and pulse and respiratory changes, may be found when checking the vital signs. The client may appear underweight and even cachectic as a result from congestion of the intestinal veins causing poor GI absorption of nutrients. The increased oxygen needs of an enlarged heart, and extra work demands met by the respiratory muscles, further deplete calories. Also the decreased intake of food may occur in conjunction with congestive hepatomegaly with associated anorexia and nausea. Weight loss, anorexia, and nausea also may be signs of digoxin toxicity.

For integumentary assessment, check for pallor of poor cardiac output and slow capillary refill of the nails. Note for the presence of intense rubor of the feet observed in Buerger's Disease (thromboangiitis obliterans). Buerger's Disease typically occurs in young men in the age range of 20 to 40. Observe for signs of cyanosis, particularly in the lips and nailbeds, and on the earlobes, tip of the nose, and under the tongue. Look for jaundice that appears late in congestive heart failure. The skin needs to be inspected for lesions such as skin ulcers, stasis dermatitis, petechae, and venous stars. Check for clubbing of the nails and increased thickness in the nails, especially the nails of the toes. Examine the fingertips for signs of nicotine stains from cigarette smoking. Look at the palms of the hands and the soles of the feet for Osler's nodes. The nodes are purple in appearance and are painful and tender; they are seen in infectious endocarditis. Observe the skin for diaphoresis and palpate for the presence of generalized or localized coldness. Increased tactile warmness and flushing may indicate fever that accompanies cardiovascular inflammation in such conditions as rheumatic heart fever and thrombophlebitis. Check for edema, especially in the pretibial area, about the ankles, and the flank and sacral region of clients who are bedfast. With cardiovascular disease the hair may be sparse and brittle, and may lack luster.

In assessment of the eyes, the appearance of the eyes may be dull in severe congestive heart failure. Check the lids and perinasal areas for any sign of xanthelasma. Note any pallor of the palpebral conjunctiva. Examine the eyegrounds for retinal changes such as papilledema, A-V nicking, hemorrhages, and exudates.

When assessing the throat and neck, check for sore throat as it may be a sign of rheumatic heart fever. Observe for the presence of jugular venous distention that is found in heart failure. Also look for abnormal pulsations in the neck region. Hemoptysis may signal pulmonary venous hypertension. Weak or absent carotid pulse(s) may be detected in heart failure and advanced arteriosclerosis. A carotid bruit may be auscultated in conjunction with a stenosed carotid artery or disorder accompanied by a dynamic blood flow.

For thorax and breast assessment, observe for thoracic deformities that may hamper adequate heart and lung function. Observe for the presence of gynecomastia that may be a sign of digoxin intoxication.

Within the cardiovascular assessment, check for paroxysmal nocturnal dyspnea, orthopnea, and dyspnea on exertion. Note whether there are any abnormal thoracic and epigastric pulsations or the presence of a cardiac heave (lift, thrust). Note the presence of the PMI at a location other than the apex of the heart. Palpate the thorax and the epigastric area for sign of a cardiac thrill. A thrill is associated with a Grade IV, V, or VI heart murmur. Check the chest x-ray for mention of cardiomegaly and/or percuss the LCBD to grossly assess heart size. Auscultate the cardiac region for abnormal heart sounds (e.g., murmur, gallop rhythm, wide-, fixed-, or paradoxical splitting, A2 < P2 ratio in the adult, opening snap, ejection click, and pericardial friction rub). Observe for varicose veins. Check for Homan's sign with any presence of vascular inflammation. Palpate the peripheral arteries for detecting weak, thready, and absent pulses. Review the ECG for any abnormalities.

During respiratory assessment, observe for abnormal breathing patterns and use of respiratory accessory muscles and sternal retraction. Note any retraction or bulging of intercostal spaces. Percuss for the dullness of pleural effusion or atelectasis. Auscultate for rales that accompany congestive heart failure.

When assessing the abdomen, note abnormal contour and abdominal asymmetry that may accompany congestive hepatomegaly. Check if the liver is palpable. Also percuss to assess whether the liver dullness span in the adult is greater than 12 centimeters. Abdominal pain and fullness generally is associated with hepatic congestion. Serum SGOT and SGPT enzymes are frequently elevated. Tricuspid valvular disease and constrictive pericarditis manifest marked ascites. Ascites is typically observed in clients with congestive heart disease. Percuss to detect the dullness of ascites and check for a fluid shift and fluid wave. Auscultate for bruits over the abdominal aorta, renal arteries, and femoral arteries that may denote such disorders as stenotic arteries and vascular aneurysms.

Renal changes within cardiovascular disease may include oliguria that results from a decrease in blood flow to the kidneys. Check urine for proteinuria and a high specific gravity. Investigate any signs of impotence that could result from diminished penile blood circulation.

Lung Cancer

Carcinoma of the lung is increasing throughout the world and is the leading cause of death in the United States. The great majority of incidence is linked with cigarette smoking. The younger the age when one starts to smoke, the more years one smokes, and heavy daily smoking (one pack per day) all increase the risk for lung cancer. The high risk profile is the male over 45 years of age who smokes two or more packs of cigarettes a day.

Reason for Seeking Health Evaluation

Lung cancer and other pulmonary conditions may manifest similar symptoms, and therefore the client may seek care for what may seem to him to be insignificant or nonserious respiratory symptoms. Such symptoms may be chronic cough, fatigue, wheezing, and a feeling of chest tightness. Some clients may put off seeking assessment until the symptoms become more frightening and include such events as hemoptysis, extreme weight loss, and the type of problems that arise with metastasis. Regional metastasis can cause tracheal obstruction and dyspnea, esophageal compression and dysphagia, and hoarseness. Neurologic defects would suggest brain metastasis. Bone pain, pathologic fractures, spinal cord compression syndromes, and cytopenias may herald skeletal and bone marrow involvement. Liver metastasis could result in anorexia, jaundice, and abdominal pain. Vascular occlusion can occur from metastasis and result in signs of cardiac failure and arrhythmias.

Sociocultural Aspects, Lifestyle and Habits

The incidence of lung cancer is highest in men, more in blacks than whites, and is steadily increasing in women. Variables that need investigation in association with lung cancer are the exposure to carcinogens in the workplace and home. Foremost is to assess smoking habits and exposure to the cigarette smoke of others. Were there smokers in the home when the client was growing up? Do other family members smoke in the home? Are there nonsmoking areas at work and in places that are frequented by the client? It is important to question exposure to asbestos. Asbestos has been used in insulation, pipes, filters, floor tiles, and highways. It has been detected in drinking water and acid rain. Nonsmokers with asbestos exposure have a five times greater risk of developing cancer of the lung than nonsmokers who have not experienced exposure to asbestos. Another toxic substance is nickel; it is found in asbestos as well as in coal and crude oil. Nickel is used in the stainless steel industry and is used as a fuel additive. Possible exposure to carcinogens is scrutinized through a careful occupational history. Increased risk also has been linked with exposure to uranium, chloromethyl ethers, synthetic rubber, pitchblends, radioactive ores, soaps, detergents, paints, industrial gas, and pharmaceutical preparations. Occupations that have an element of chronic irritation to lung tissue increase the risk (e.g., farmers, bakers, hairdressers, painters, gas station attendants, coal miners, truckers, auto body repairmen, stockcar and horse racers, cattlemen, and sawmill and grain mill workers, to name only a few). The home location may contribute to risk as well, depending on the degree of air pollution. The risk for lung cancer is twice as great in urban dwellers than in those living in rural areas. Lastly, the existence of a family history of cancer is important. The type of cancer that has occurred in a relative, and at what age, in addition to the age of death, if applicable, is helpful assessment information.

Mental Health Assessment

A diagnosis of cancer may result in feelings of anxiety, fear, and depression. Maladaptive coping may be present. Brain metastasis could display a difficulty with cognitive functioning and other neurologic dysfunctions, depending on the areas involved.

Physical Assessment

An overall appearance may or may not be cachexia. Integumentary assessment may reveal cyanosis, jaundice, and clubbing of the fingers. In assessing the respiratory system, observe particularly for an increased AP diameter, the use of respiratory accessory muscles, abnormal fremitus findings, dullness in percussion (detected over tumor and areas of pleural effusion), unequal diaphragmatic excursions with elevation of hemidiaphragm secondary to phrenic nerve involvement, and any adventitious lung sounds such as crackles, wheezes, and pleural friction rubs. Signs and symptoms of heart failure and arrhythmias should be noted when assessing the cardiovascular system. Abdominal assessment may reveal a liver mass or tenderness, and musculoskeletal examination may reveal localized bony pain and aching joints (hypertrophic pulmonary osteoarthropathy). With brain and nervous system metastasis, neurologic signs within a broad range could emerge, depending upon the specific site(s) of metastasis [e.g., cerebellum (ataxia, tremors) and cerebrum (personality changes, cognitive functioning difficulties)]. Tumors of the lung apicies that involve the bracheal plexus will produce symptoms of paresthesias and shoulder and arm pain, especially shoulder pain that tends to radiate down the ulnar distribution area of the arm.

Benign Prostatic Hyperplasia (BPH) and Prostatic Carcinoma

Prostatic hyperplasia is a common condition that occurs in 80% of men in the fifth to seventh decades of life and increases to over 95% thereafter. With the increase in longevity of men, there is an associated increase in the incidence of BPH. An increase in the number of prostatic cells thought to be caused by hormonal changes increases the overall size of the gland. Because of the location of the prostate gland, surrounding the prostatic urethra, the signs of BPH are urinary problems. Symptoms may include frequency, decreased size and force of the urinary stream, dribbling, hematuria, and urinary retention.

Similar symptomatology may occur in carcinoma of the prostate. However, metastasis may result in additional symptoms of back pain, hip pain, pathologic fractures, or pain from bony metastasis to the skull, ribs, thoracic vertebrae, and the long bones. Lymphedema can be secondary to cancer invasion of the pelvic lymph nodes, and ejaculation may be painful. Due to the close proximity of the prostate gland to the rectum, tumor growth may interfere with defecation. The client may experience changes in his stool and have pain upon defecation.

Sociocultural Aspects, Lifestyle and Habits

The frequency of prostate cancer varies throughout the world. Japanese men experience a lower incidence than caucasians. However, American-born Japanese men and Japanese immigrants to the United States show an increased incidence. Diet etiology has been proposed as an explanation for this epidemiological finding. Black men in the United States are at greater risk than white men. The risk for prostatic carcinoma increases with age and rarely occurs before the age of 50. Exposure to occupational carcinogens may be a factor in cancer of the prostate; therefore, an occupational history is important. Gonorrhea and exposure to a virus also is associated with an increased incidence of prostatic cancer.

Physical Assessment

As with any form of cancer, the potential for metastasis is there. With prostatic carcinoma, the most frequent site of metastasis is to the vertebral column. The two physiological systems most affected are the genitourinary and musculoskeletal. An annual rectal examination is recommended for all men age 40 and older. It is the most inexpensive, quick, and easy method for early detection of prostatic cancer. To defer this examination is an unethical act from a humanitarian viewpoint. A six-month rectal examination should be performed on any male client with continuing urinary symptoms and with a family history of a blood relative who had prostate cancer. During the physical examination note any signs of vertebral compression, paresthesias, and pain. Carefully palpate the posterior lateral surfaces of the lobes of the prostate gland during the digital rectal examination. A mass may be detected or the midline furrow of the prostate gland may be obscured.

Testicular Carcinoma

Testicular carcinoma is the most common cancer of young men. An early childhood incidence peak is seen with a far greater peak occurring around the 16- to 35-year age group. It seldom occurs after the age of 40. It is frequently detected in screenings of aggregates of young men such as in the military, athletic teams, and in preschool and pre-employment physicals in university cities where there is an increased population of young men.

Reason for Seeking Health Evaluation

Detection of testicular masses usually occurs during a routine physical examination. The most common symptom of testicular carcinoma is an asymptomatic nodule or swelling, or a feeling of heaviness in the involved testicular area. These symptoms may not be enough to prompt a client to seek health evaluation. The knowledge of cancer of the testicles and of the process of performing self-testicular examination are educational goals to encourage men to seek medical attention in the presence of an enlargement or heavy feeling in the testes. Testicular carcinoma is not always painless, but less than 50% of the cases experience testicular pain. Symptoms due to metastasis can range from weight loss to dyspnea, anorexia, nausea, vomiting, abdominal pain, back pain, and urinary obstruction. Early detection is essential to survival, and all testicular lesions should be considered malignant until proven otherwise.

Sociocultural Aspects, Lifestyle and Habits

Another deterrent in seeking nursing and medical advice stems from cultural teaching that it is taboo to talk about one's genitals. Feelings of embarrassment and guilt often accompany afflictions of the genitalia. Teenagers and young adults especially are facing strong physiological sexual feelings and social mores that are causing conflict and confusion. As a result, it is quite difficult for the young man to reveal or want to discover abnormalities within his genitals, and this difficulty could prove to be deadly since testicular cancer is a disease of young men.

When investigating health habits it is very important to check whether the young to middle-age male client knows about testicular cancer and performs a self-testicular examination monthly. Risk factors for testicular carcinoma to be included in history-taking is to ascertain if the client has a past medical history of cryptorchid (undescended testicles), an inguinal hernia in childhood, mumps, and orchitis; the latter may have been associated with strenuous exercise or a sexually transmitted disease.

Physical Assessment

Massive pulmonary metastasis in testicular cancer may manifest in dyspnea and supraclavicular adenopathy, along with excessive use of the respiratory accessory muscles of the neck and chest. Cyanosis may be evident. Other symptoms may include abnormal fremitus findings, dull percussion notes within the lung fields, respiratory asymmetry, or adventitious lung sounds. Unequal diaphragmatic excursions may exist. Examination of the breasts may reveal gynecomastia. Vague abdominal pain may be found. Abdominal or back pain may result from metastasis with retroperitoneal adenopathy. Palpation of the testes of all young and middle-age men is a "must" in every physical examination. Clients should be instructed to seek immediate health evaluation for any change in previously normal testes. Swelling in the testicular area may be secondary to a mass or a hydrocele. Any swelling should be subject to the technique of transillumination. A hydrocele (collection of edema) will transilluminate whereas a testicular lesion will not transilluminate. Examination of the urinary system includes attention to any signs of urinary obstruction such as urinary retention with overflow, dysuria, frequency, and change in the size or force of stream.

Sexual Dysfunction

Common types of sexual dysfunction may encompass penile erection difficulties, loss of libido, ejaculatory problems, and inability to achieve orgasm. The occurrence of one or more symptoms within these patterns that denote sexual dysfunction is commonly referred to as "impotence." This term conveys the image of weakness, powerlessness, and worthlessness. Use of the term may prove to be detrimental to the client and may only reinforce or lead to poor self-esteem. This can only add to the psychological stress that often accompanies any sexual problem. Even as a health professional, there is most likely the unrecognized but biased impression of the client who is impotent as being a poor, weak, dejected, "less than a man" individual. Society has fostered the concept that "power" lies in the genitals and male sexual prowess (Farrell 1986). It is suggested for this reason that the use of the term "impotence" best be avoided in the nurse-client interactions and those of health care providers themselves.

Most clients do not readily talk about sexual problems and concerns unless questioned or unless discussion is initiated by the nurse. Sexual shortcomings are generally devastating to a client's self-esteem and confidence. If sexual difficulties are anticipated because of specific therapies and certain medical conditions, you have a professional obligation to discuss this with the client. Even if the client displays signs of embarrassment, a matter-of-fact and caring approach will help ease the discomfort and will be truly appreciated by the client. Furthermore, the client will perceive you as a knowledgeable and competent nurse.

The following are mythical sexual beliefs commonly held by American men and identified by Zilbergeld (Roberts 1990, p. 259):

1. Men should not have, or at least not express, certain feelings.
2. In sex, as elsewhere, it's performance that counts.
3. The man must take charge of and orchestrate sex.
4. A man always wants and is always ready to have sex.
5. All physical contact must lead to sex.
6. Sex equals intercourse.
7. Sex requires an erection.
8. Good sex is a linear progression of increasing excitement terminated only by orgasm.
9. Sex should be natural and spontaneous.
10. In this enlightened age, the preceding myths no longer have any influence on us.

Etiologies of Sexual Dysfunction

There are many possible causes of sexual difficulties, and often a single factor cannot be identified; the most common etiology is an anxiety or depressive state. Other than psychic causes, sexual dysfunction can result from organic causes and from the effects of certain drugs. The primary diagnostic goal is to determine whether the etiology is psychologically induced or is secondary to organic factors.

The inability to achieve orgasm is generally a result of psychogenic causes. Surrounding circumstances may be marital problems, disinterest in sexual partner, and stresses of work, play, family, and finances. Fear of rejection or sexual inadequacy, along with concern of pleasing a partner, contribute to the added pressure to perform. Other cognitive interferences may take the form of intense emotions (e.g., anger, chronic worry, anxiety, uncertainty of masculinity, self-consciousness, achievement-consciousness). A decrease in libido may result from stress as well. Other interacting factors that constitute psychological cause of sexual difficulties include religious orthodoxy and homosexuality. Surprisingly, nocturnal erections occur more frequently and are of a longer duration in males who have psychogenic sexual dysfunctions compared to sexually healthy males. Erections that occur during REM sleep begin in early childhood and continue through the eighth decade. If the neurological and cardiovascular systems that mediate erection are intact, nocturnal penile tumescence (NPT) will be experienced, and the etiology is probably psychogenic in nature.

Penile erection difficulties and ejaculatory problems, particularly premature ejaculation, may be related to psychosocial factors as well as to organic causes. Fatigue also may impact on sexual performance. Because organic causes of sexual dysfunction can arise from a large number of diseases and types of trauma, only the more common ones will be mentioned.

Hypogonadism (chromosomal, pituitary, or testicular) displays itself as the non-development or the regression of secondary sexual characteristics, decreased libido, the inability to obtain or maintain an erection, and absence of emission. The latter sign can be due also to retrograde ejaculation. Sexual dysfunction commonly occurs in such endocrine disorders as Klinefelter Syndrome, hemochromatosis (an inherited disease characterized by iron deposits in the pituitary gland), pituitary gigantism, acromegaly, hypothyroidism, Addison's Disease, Cushing's Syndrome, and diabetes mellitus. Within the first six years of the onset of diabetes mellitus, 50% of the male clients will develop sexual difficulties. The manifestation of *unexplained* erectile difficulties should prompt testing for *latent diabetes mellitus*. Signs of sexual dysfunction may be the first clinical signs of diabetic neuropathy.

The inability to obtain or maintain the erect state also might be secondary to insufficient blood flow to the penis, which could be caused by a penile thrombus. Severe arteriosclerosis also could be an etiology, and in addition, arteriosclerosis may hamper cognitive functioning and decrease sensation which could interfere with libido or thought process in planning and executing the sexual act. Mental retardation may influence the degree of understanding of sexual behavior and activities. Some clients with an abdominal aortic aneurysm may experience erectile difficulties as well. Other cardiovascular problems that may interfere with erection are sickle cell, Leriche Syndrome, and leukemia.

Peyronie's Disease, in which hard nodules develop beneath the skin on the dorsum and occasionally on the sides of the penis, causes a painful, arching distortion of the penile shaft; the deformity makes it virtually impossible to perform coitus. Another penile disease that interferes with sexual functioning is priapism (a painful, persistent erection that may often be unrelated to sexual activity). Additionally, penile trauma may result in sexual problems. Trauma from accidents and surgery can impact on sexual functioning.

With head injury there is the possibility of the client developing sexual dysfunction as long as several years following the accident. The incidence most often follows blows to the back of the head like those that are frequently experienced in boxing matches. Erectile problems and loss of sexual sensation may occur with spinal cord injuries and tumors with sacral and cauda equina destruction. In cord injuries of a higher level, some degree of reflex erections can occur. A transection above the sacral level results in the loss of sexual sensation; however, in some cases tactile stimulation of the penis, cremasteric region, perineum, and anus can produce a reflexogenic erection. Problems with sexual functioning also can occur with injuries such as herniated disks and "crushed" pelvic fractures.

Yeager (1980) stated that 15% of men under age 50 and 100% of men older than 70 experienced sexual dysfunction symptoms following abdominoperineal resection and proctocolectomy. Lower gastrointestinal tract surgery and prostate surgery carry the risk of sexual dysfunction secondary to nerve damage and disrupted blood flow. With such surgeries as colostomy, ileostomy, and suprapubic prostatectomy, the potential neurological and cardiovascular damage is commonly combined with psychic trauma; this makes it difficult to separate the cause and effect on sexual dysfunction as being solely due to the surgical trauma or resulting from the psychological responses to the illness (depression, anxiety) and associated poor self-image.

Krane (1988) pointed out that sexual dysfunction can occur from testicular atrophy if the testicular arteries are ligated during the surgical repair of a hernia. He also noted that radiation and chemotherapy could cause sexual dysfunction if destruction of the testes, hypothalamus, and pituitary gland occurred. In addition, he cited that a lumbar sympathectomy performed on older men yielded a 50% incidence of erectile problems. Ejaculatory capacity also may be disrupted following a sympathectomy and rhizotomies. A sympathectomy is sometimes performed to treat hypertension. Krane also stated that a 50% incidence of sexual dysfunction occurred in clients that had a pudendal neurectomy for neurogenic bladder.

Sociocultural Aspects, Lifestyle and Habits

Sexuality is a cultural phenomenon. Our beliefs and attitudes are socially learned and impact on our sexual behaviors. How a client views sexuality, sexual roles and sexual practices has roots in his culture and his life experiences. Assessment of cultural variables may provide a crucial piece in diagnosing sexual dysfunction. Other areas that require exploration are occupational, exercise, and leisure activities, drug use (including alcohol), diet, family history, and past medical history.

Carefully listen to the client's conversation; the content and specific words used will be clues to his attitudes and beliefs. Discussion of masculine and feminine roles and current events related to sexuality issues will aid in assessment of individual, culturally-influenced beliefs regarding sexual expectations and behavior. What does "being a man" mean to a client? How were incidents and discussions regarding sexual matters handled by his parents? What type of early sexual experiences did the client have? What style of parenting did the client grow up under?

More explicit to sexual functioning would be to ascertain if the client is sexually active. At this point you need to be aware of slang terms that the client may use in his conversation with you (see Table 24-1). If you are unsure of a term used by the client, ask him to explain what he means. Is he able to have sex? Is sex an important part of his life? Do any physical defects or illnesses interfere with his sexual experiences? Does he have any difficulty having or maintaining an erection (hard-on)? Is there any problem with ejaculation (coming)? Has drugs or drunkeness ever seemed to have interfered with his sexual performance? What role/actions does he

Table 24-1. Slang Expressions for Sexual Terms

Formal term	Slang expression
Breasts	Tits, sacks, front, headlights, knockers, boobs, bosom, bonkers, bust, jugs, buds
Climax	Come, go off, shoot, cream, blast off; the clouds and the rain (Oriental)
Clitoris	Bad fellow, little gem, badge of shame, gaiety, madness, narrow strip
Cunnilingus	Eating it, going down, eating pussy
Erection	Hard on, stiff, done, boner, hot rocks, lover's nuts
Fellatio	Going down, sucking, blowing, getting a blow job, giving head, cocksucking
Homosexual	Fairy, fag, faggot, gay, queen, nellie, homo, swish, pervert, pansy, back door artist, lez, sister, lesbo, dyke, bull dyke
Hymen	Cherry, membrane, maidenhead
Impotence	Couldn't get it up, couldn't get a hard on
Intercourse } Coitus	Make love, screw, fuck, get down, ball, make it, get laid, mess around, score, bang, jive, grig, get a piece, sleep with, get some tail; schtup (Yiddish)
Masturbation	Jack off, jerk off, pocket pool, hand fuck, circle jerk, beat the meat, hand job
Mutual oral-genital stimulation	Sixty-nine, give head, go down on
Orgasm	Come, climax, bust a nut, get a nut
Penis	Joystick, worm, dick, prick, stick, peter, rod, john, third leg, middle leg, joint, glans, cock, organ, thing; schmuck, putz (Yiddish); yang, steaming stalk (Oriental)
Pubic hair	Beaver, bush, pubes
Semen	Come, juice, egg white, gizzum, cum
Sexual choice	Straight (heterosexual), gay (homosexual), AC-DC (bisexual)
Sexual desire	Horny, cold fish (decreased libido), nympho (increased female libido)
Testes	Balls, nuts, cojones
Vagina	Pussy, hole, cunt, cat, pocketbook, treasure, twat, furburger, box, beaver, snatch, tunnel; yin, jade gate, golden gulley (Oriental)

Adapted from *Human Sexuality: A Nursing Perspective*, by R. Hogan (Ed.). Copyright © 1980 by Appleton-Century-Crofts. Reprinted by permission.

believe a man (and a woman) should assume in the sex act?

Since extreme fatigue may impinge upon sexual functioning, it is important to assess extent and stress of occupational activity and responsibility, amount and regularity of exercise regimens, and leisure activities. Regular sleep pattern and whether there has been changes in sleep pattern are investigated. Does the client use any medications or practices to induce sleep?

The number of drugs that interfere with male sexual functioning keeps growing. Smoking habits need to be assessed, as nicotine has been associated with erectile failure. Long term use of marijuana is thought to have an impact on erectile function, secondary to its effect on diminishing serum testosterone levels. Medications commonly associated with male sexual dysfunction are listed in Table 24-2 (Compiled from Braunwald et al 1987; Krane 1988).

Sexual dysfunction may be caused by anxiety, or it could be the side effect of a psychotropic medication that has been prescribed to treat anxiety. The antihypertensives Regitine and Dibenzyline are known to have specifically caused inhibitory ejaculation. The drug Reglan can cause hyperprolactinemia, which frequently is associated with hypogonadism and decreased serum testosterone levels. The result is the absence of emission.

Chronic use of drugs of habituation tend to be associated with erectile failure (e.g., cocaine, heroin, methadone, codeine, merperidine, marijuana, nicotine, and alcohol). Acute alcoholic episodes also may affect erectile function. Alcoholism effects diet, and the secondary malnutritional vitamin deficiency of poor diet in alcoholism (thiamine, niacin, vitamin B12) can compound sexual dysfunction via pelvic neuropathy.

Lastly, data on family history (diabetes mellitus, peripheral vascular disease, hypertension) and the client's past medical history (endocrine problems, genital disease, trauma and surgery, neurological damage, lower gastrointestinal surgery, cardiovascular system problems, severe depression, anxiety, nervous breakdown) need to be collected and analyzed.

Clients with multiple sclerosis may experience absence of emission, a "dry" orgasm, due to retrograde ejaculation (secretions flow backward into the bladder). Retrograde ejaculation may be an early sign of diabetes mellitus—as much as a year prior to diagnosis. It also may occur following surgery on the neck of the bladder. Surgery involving the penis, prostate gland, rectum, or testicles could result in neurologic damage and sexual functioning problems. Genital trauma from accidents or cystoscopy and vasectomy procedures could give rise to sexual functioning problems as well. Furthermore, temporal lobe lesions and temporal lobe epi-

Table 24-2. Drugs Associated With Male Sexual Dysfunction

- Antabuse
- Anticholinergics (Norpace, Probanthine, Tagamet, Xantac)
- Antihistamines
- Amphetamines
- Antihypertensives
  - Sympatholytics (Aldomet, Calapres, Serpasil, Sandril, Ismelin)
  - Alpha-Adrenergic Blocking Agents (Minipress, Dibenzylene, Regitine)
  - Beta-Adrenergic Blocking Agents (Inderal, Propranolol, Visken, Tenormen, Lopressor, Trandate, Normodyne)
  - Vasodilators (Apresoline, Loniten)
  - Diuretics (Diuril, Hydrodiuril, Hygroton, Aldactone)
- Chemotherapy Drugs
- Corticosteroids
- Digoxin
- Estrogen
- Lioresol (Rx of MS)
- Psychotropic Agents
  - Minor Tranquilizers (Valium, Librium, Milltown, Sexax, Tranxene, Tybatron)
  - Major Tranquilizers (Mellaril, Serentil, Thorazine)
  - Antidepressants (Tofranil, Elavil, Asenden, Desyrel, Norpramine, Vivactile, Eskalith, MAO inhibitors)
  - Psychedelics

lepsy have been associated with erectile problems and inability to achieve orgasm. Injury with neurogenic bladder dysfunction or that associated with diabetes mellitus could contribute to sexual functioning problems. Whether vascular problems such as priapism and intermittent claudication exist needs to be identified, as these may suggest an insufficient penile blood flow which will impede attainment and maintenance of the erect state of the penis. Krane (1988) stated that 60% of men on chronic hemodialysis experience erectile problems. This is thought to be due to azotemic effects on the neurological system, and from hyperprolactinemia and decreased serum testosterone due to endocrine alterations. Additionally, the psychological response to the chronicity of the illness adds to the stress.

Mental Status Assessment

Since many sexual difficulties are caused by psychological factors it is necessary to assess mental status. For instance, premature ejaculation is primarily related to a psychological state; it could be due to unreasonable performance expectations, to an emotional disorder, or to extreme anxiety or excitation in the sexual situation.

The client's self-concept is assessed. What is his perception of his sexual abilities? Has he had successful and unsuccessful sexual experiences? What are his usual sexual practices? Investigate his values of "right and wrong" surrounding sexual issues and activities in his cultural and societal realms and for himself. Does he have anxieties regarding sexual activity or ability? Does he practice safe sex? Explore relationships with his partner(s). How does he describe his ideal sexual partner? How does this ideal compare with his actual sexual partner(s)? Is there any evidence of marital discord? What turns him on? What turns him off? Is he under extreme pressure to sexually perform? Does he express any signs of feeling rejected or inadequate? How would he describe himself as a sexual partner? Does he express fear of sexual encounters and incompetence? Does he display any signs of chronic anxiety, guilt, or depression?

Physical Assessment

Examination of the skin may reveal abnormal body hair distribution and sparseness of hair, which may be a sign of hypogonadism. With vascular etiology, the examination of the eyegrounds may reveal changes consistent with vascular insufficiency and diabetes mellitus (e.g., narrowed arteries, hemorrhages, and exudates). If gynecomastia is observed, ask if the client is on digoxin. Digoxin's chemical structure is similar to the sex steroids, and some clients have exhibited increased estrogen and decreased testosterone levels as side effects to digoxin. When assessing the cardiovascular system, note weakness and absence of pulses. To check the penile pulse, palpate the penile body between your thumb and forefinger on either side of the midline. A doppler check may be warranted. On examination of the genitourinary system note any signs of dribbling, weakness of urinary stream, urgency, or frequency. Question the client about the existence of a "dry" orgasm and milky postcoital urine that would indicate retrograde ejaculation. When sexual dysfunction is associated with neurological deficits, you may detect poor anal sphincter tone, loss of perineal sensation, and weakness or absence of the bulbocavernosus reflex; this reflex, when present, is the anal sphincter constriction that is elicited by squeezing the glans penis (tip). Also with neurologic alterations you may find distal muscle weakness, absent deep tendon reflexes in the lower extremities (particularly the achilles deep tendon reflex), diminished or absent vibratory and position sense, and decreased or absent tactile and pain sensation.

Summary

This chapter explored cultural impact on male identity and associated interactional practices. The traditional perception of masculinity in Western society was discussed in light of its impact on men interacting with health professionals, and on men in health professional roles. The issues of masculinity and gender surrounding morbidity and mortality rates included the lack of preventive health practices, longevity less than that of women, and specific health problems and types of accidents that have a greater incidence in men. The selected health problems of men presented were cardiovascular disease, lung cancer, benign prostatic hyperplasia and prostatic carcinoma, testicular cancer, and sexual dysfunction. The associated symptomatology of these selected health problems that is inherent in sociocultural aspects, lifestyle and habits, mental status, and physical assessment was identified. Special health needs of men were highlighted, and a holistic view of the male client was emphasized.

Discussion Questions/Activities

1. Identify sexual values and beliefs learned from your cultural background.
2. Share your impression of society's prevailing views of masculinity.
3. Discuss the issues of masculinity associated with male morbidity and mortality rates.
4. Identify nursing prescriptions (approaches, interventions) to improve men's health.
5. Discuss (or role play) the data collection phase with a client experiencing sexual dysfunction.
6. List the variables pertinent to data collection in each of the following selected health problems of men: cardiovascular disease, lung cancer, benign prostatic hyperplasia and prostatic carcinoma, testicular cancer.

CHAPTER 25

Family Health Assessment

LEARNING OBJECTIVES

1. Discuss family structure, family function and family roles.
2. Why is it important to understand the concepts of family roles when carrying out a family health assessment?
3. Describe the communication patterns exhibited by healthy families.
4. What are the hallmarks of good family communication?
5. Describe dysfunctional communication.
6. Describe how a family's values affect the health of that family.
7. Discuss at least two types of family social support.
8. What is meant by family form?
9. Discuss the stages of family development.
10. List the basic components of the family health assessment.

Structure and Function of the Family

Health is greatly influenced by societal factors (see Chapters 1 and 2). The family unit and dynamics are closely related to the health of the family as a whole and the health of each individual within the family. The family is the basic unit of society. As such, it is imperative that the health of this unit be maintained and the level of wellness promoted to the optimal level. To aid in the assessment of the family unit, it is important to understand the following concepts that affect family functioning:

Family Structure

The family can be considered as one or more individuals, related by marriage, blood, or friendship. This could include cohabitating adults of either sex, blended families, single parents and children as well as the most well-known—the nuclear family. The unit needs to be broadly defined and not limited to household or age cohort. The family should not be defined or restricted by legal or residential boundaries (Mallinger 1989). The latter is especially important in the area of health care because it is within the family that health and illness behaviors are learned and supported. Family members are usually involved in all stages of illness and in all areas of health promotion. As a nurse, you must be aware that there is no right or wrong family unit and that the family must be provided health care as it is constituted.

Family Function

The family functions largely in relation to its cultural background. In Chapter 2 a discussion of cultural considerations states that an individual's response to health and illness must be viewed in the context of culture. Several areas in relation to culture and ethnicity that you must be aware of in carrying out health assessment are discussed. Additional concepts influenced by culture and related to family functions are family roles, communication patterns, family values and family social support systems.

Family Roles

To promote and encourage family health you must understand the family and its roles. These roles are often complex and multiple. There is much written on role theory, and there will be no attempt in this text to review these. The works of Sarbin (1954), Hardy and Conway (1978) and Biddle and Thomas (1966) have defined and described role theories. Role is defined as a pattern of wants, goals, beliefs, feelings, attitudes, values, and actions which members of a community expect as characteristic of the typical occupant of a position. The behaviors of a role are learned intentionally by instruction and incidentally by observation. Family role behavior is developed over time and is part of interaction within the social environment.

Role socialization is the process by which an individual acquires skills, knowledge, attitudes, values, and motives necessary for the performance of social roles (Brim 1968). Roles change as individuals grow, but are first learned within the family as the individual experiences such roles as that of being a boy, girl, good or bad, and observes the roles of the father, mother, and friend (Bomar 1989). There are a number of problems that effect the way role is carried out by different members of a family. These are role stress and role conflict. Role stress occurs when individuals experience difficulty in meeting role expectations and obligations. It can be described in terms of the individual feeling worried, anxious, or guilty (Nye 1976). Role conflict, another type of role stress, occurs when the individual experiences multiple roles with intense demands, and these roles are viewed as competitive with the individual's expectation as to what the role should be. The conflict stems from external issues as does role stress. Roles within the family are assessed to ascertain how the family is functioning. Family roles may expand or change when illness occurs in the family. Support and information needed to promote holistic family functioning can be identified from analysis of this data. The role assessment data is shared with the family to assist family members in identifying and ultimately reducing role stress and conflict when it occurs.

Communication Patterns

Communication within the family is a very important aspect of family functioning and cohesiveness. Communication refers to the process of exchanging feelings, desires, needs, information, and opinions (McCubbin 1985). Each family has a unique communication style or pattern through which societal needs and the needs of the family are met. Through this vehicle, family members develop healthy self-esteem.

Poor communications are believed to be a major contributor to poor family functioning (Holman 1983) (see Table 25-1 for a brief synopsis of dysfunctional family communications). A survey of family therapists showed that 85% of couples seeking family therapy cited poor family communications as the primary problem causing them to seek therapy (Beck and Jones 1983, as cited in Goldenberg and Goldenberg 1985). Healthy families are defined as untroubled and nurturing; they exhibit the following communication patterns: self-worth is high; communication is direct, clear, specific, and honest; rules are flexible, appropriate, and subject to change; and the linking to society is open and hopeful (Satir 1972). Curran (1983) proposed three hallmarks for good family communications. One of these hallmarks was that parents share the family power equally, and the second was the ability to listen. Of equal importance was the ability to recognize non-verbal messages. Healthy families use signs, symbols, body language, smiles, and other physical gestures to express feelings of caring and love. Families with dysfunctional communication are seriously troubled.

Dysfunctional communication is defined as unclearly transmitted or received messages and/or messages with incongruent content and command aspects (Friedman 1986). The dysfunc-

Table 25-1. Dysfunctional Family Communication

Unrealistic expectations

Parent requires more self-control from child than age, development or circumstances make reasonable.

Parent expects immediate obedience.

Parent enforces too many rules at once or provides no rules. (Children need rules for behavior and will seek them elsewhere, often in gangs.)

Parents request social skills of the child that they do not model owing to lack of knowledge or experiences.

Inconsistency

Family disharmony.

Parents lack a united front in goals, values, parenting philosophy, or moral stance about right and wrong.

Parents model behaviors and values incongruent with what they teach verbally and in rules established.

Enforcement is not consistently carried out.

Distortions in communication—too vague, too long, contradictory or void.

Extremes in style, methods

No limits established or no guidance and reinforcements to help child comply with limits; overpermissive.

Lack of firmness; parent not respected as authority.

Limits too rigid; power replaces authority and fear or anger replaces respect.

Reinforcements (positive or negative) do not match deed; too excessive, too long, teach wrong lesson.

Primary disciplinary methods employed are bribes, promises, threats, sarcasm.

Disturbed relationships

Parent is too close to child to permit growth—intrusive control, dominance—exemplified by parent who always (1) wants to change child, (2) demands to know child's activities and conversation, (3) interferes in child's problem-solving or decision making, (4) reminds child of his misdeeds.

Basically unfriendly or ambivalent interaction.

Interaction inappropriate for child's age, stage or temperament.

Parent is too distant for child to develop respect (1) parent preoccupied with self and own activities or wishes, (2) child feels isolated or unwanted.

From Tackett, J. J. "Parenting for the Socialization of Children." *In:* Tackett, J. J.; and Hunsberger, M. (Eds.). *Family-Centered Care of Children and Adolescents.* Philadelphia: W. B. Saunders, 1981, p. 57. Copyright © 1981 by Appleton-Century-Crofts. Reprinted with permission.

tional family often avoids communication. A low self-esteem in the family, and in individual family members, is a factor that creates dysfunctional communications. Friedman (1986) described self-centeredness, lack of empathy, and need for total agreement as a family as some issues that perpetuate low self-esteem in family members. Assessment of family communications can assist in the planning of therapeutic interventions (see also Chapter 3: Communication in Health Assessment).

Family Values

Values held by family members influence family function and are standards that people use to assess behavior. The family's culture is the prime source of a family's value system and norms. Comprehensive assessment of the family requires attention to values, because values guide the family's development of norms or rules. Values are inferred from behavior—what a person attaches value to, what a person believes, and the choices that are made under varying conditions. Values serve to clarify the purpose and meaning of life, and they set a standard of culturally acceptable behavior (Friedman 1986). Values are not static; they change over time. Changes occur as the family is exposed to different subcultures, as societal values undergo change, and as the family developmentally evolves over time. A family will shift priorities in response to new situations (Pender 1982).

It is important to consider the family members' value of health. The value placed on health is personal and appears to affect the frequency and intensity with which health protecting and health promoting behaviors are practiced. A variety of interacting variables influence daily behaviors to promote or thwart the achievement of high level wellness. Variables related to active participation in health care include the importance of the value of health, upper socioeconomic status, being married, and being employed. An important stressor in the relationship of nurse and family is a disparity in basic beliefs and values. Therefore it is important for you to recognize your own values, beliefs, and attitudes, and how these may affect family-centered assessment and care.

Family Social Support Systems

Every family and individual needs social support linkages to assist in the development of self-image, a sense of belonging, and a feeling of group satisfaction (MacElveen 1978). Social support can have many components; each serves a number of supportive functions. Emotional support includes intimacy, the ability to confide in one another, and a sense of attachment, contributing to a feeling that one is cared about or that one is a member of the group. Tangible support involves direct aid or services such as providing money or goods, providing a caretaking function, and performing a service. Informational support includes providing advice or information to assist in problem-solving, and giving feedback concerning an individual's progress (Shafer et al. 1981).

Support systems consist of kin, friends, neighbors, employers, fellow employees, classmates, teachers, groups, organizations, and communities of identity. Communities of identity are community groups in which a family shares common interests, goals, lifestyles, or social identity (Friedman 1986). In times of illness or trouble, the family support system becomes crucial in assisting families to cope successfully. Knowing a client's support system can help you plan interventions to further develop, strengthen, and facilitate the process of the family network.

Family Health Assessment

A family health assessment begins with the collection of a family health history. This data is then analyzed, and nursing diagnoses and subsequent plans for family assistance and care are developed. For a more detailed discussion of the health history see Chapter 4. A family health history consists of bibliographic data, developmental information, environmental data, and social role information.

Bibliographical Data

This should include the family name, address, first names, ages, sex, and birthdates of all members. Information about adult family members should come first, followed by oldest child and by each succeeding child in order of birth. The relationship of each family member to the other, as well as birthplace, occupation, and education should be listed. It should also contain information about marital status, current occupation, religion, race, and ethnic origins of all members. In describing ethnic background, the degree of acculturation should be assessed through such things as the language spoken at home, country of origin, as well as length of time in the country in which they now preside. Additional exploratory questions might include asking them to describe their social network, neighborhood, and especially the family's use of folk practitioners. It also helps to know how actively the family is involved in their particular religious organization, and in what religious practices the family engages. Information about neighborhood, education, occupation, and financial status can give a clue to the social class status of the family. Inquire as to who is (are) the breadwinner(s) in the family and if the family considers their income to be adequate.

Family Form

Describe the composition of the family unit. Is it a nuclear family, that is, one marriage with parenthood as an expectation, composed of a husband, wife and their immediate children (natural, adopted, or both)? Or is the family an extended family, in which the nuclear family and other kin share household arrangements and responsibilities? If it is a nuclear family, do strong bonds exist with kin even if they do not live in the same geographic area? Is the family form one that is variant? The variant family includes all variations from the traditional nuclear family and the extended family (e.g., single parent, homosexual partners, non-married heterosexual couple, commune family). Types of family forms are listed in Table 25-2.

Health Background

The health background of the family would include the past medical history of injuries, hospitalizations, and surgeries of each family member. It would also establish blood relationships and family history of individuals. Lifestyle and personal habits of each member of the family would be investigated (see Chapter 4). Lifestyle of a family may include examining the forms of decision-making used, and under what circumstances particular forms are employed. Do family decisions arrive through consensus, mandate, compromise, bargaining, negotiation, and/or coercion? Who is involved in decision-making? Is (are) some individual(s) the ultimate decision-maker(s) for the family?

Table 25-2. Family Forms

Traditional nuclear:
Consists of mother, father, and children, living in a common household established through the legal and social sanction of marriage. One or both partners employed outside the home.

Reconstituted nuclear:
Remarried man and woman living in a common household with children from one or both previous marriages, and children from current marriage. One or both partners employed outside the home.

Middle-aged or aging couple:
Husband as provider, wife at home, or both may be employed outside the home. Children have been "launched" into college, career, or marriage.

Dyadic nuclear:
Childless husband and wife. One or both partners employed outside the home.

Single parent:
One parent, as a consequence of separation, divorce, death, or abandonment, usually including children. Parent may or may not be employed outside the home. Support may come from government funds, extended family, or life insurance, savings, or financial settlement.

Dual career:
Husband and wife both have careers, may or may not have children; generally share household responsibilities.

Dual career (commuter marriage):
Husband and wife both have careers that take one or both of them some distance from home. Couple may see each other only at designated intervals; e.g., weekends, holidays. May or may not have children.

Single adult:
Lives alone; usually has a career; may or may not desire to marry.

Three-generation:
Three generations or more living in a common household.

Institutional:
Children or adults in orphanages, residential facilities, or correctional institutions.

Communal:
Household consisting of two or more monogamous couples with children, sharing common facilities, resources and appliances; socialization of children is shared by all adults.

Group marriage:
Household of adults and offspring known as one family, where all individuals are "married" to one another and all are parents to the children.

Unmarried parent and child:
Usually mother and child where marriage is not desired or possible; child may be natural or adopted.

Unmarried couple and child:
Usually a common-law marriage with natural or informally adopted children.

Homosexual couple:
Homosexual couple (male or female) living together with or without children. Children may be informally or legally adopted, or may be natural children of one of the partners.

Cohabitating retired couple:
Unmarried retired couple living together, usually because financial hardships would result if they married (retirement benefits would decrease).

Extended:
The nuclear family and other related (by blood) persons who are most commonly members of the family of orientation of one of the nuclear family mates. These are "kin"; e.g., grandparents, aunts, uncles, and cousins.

Developmental History

Havinghurst (1952) first used the term "developmental task." He identified a task as something that takes place at or about a certain period in the life of the individual. He theorized that successful achievement of a task leads to happiness and success in later tasks, whereas failure leads to unhappiness in the individual, disapproval by the society, and difficulty with later tasks. Families also have developmental tasks, delineated as responsibilities for growth that must be achieved by a family during each stage of its development in order to meet biological requirements, cultural demands, and its own aspirations and values. Duvall (1977) developed an eight-stage paradigm to describe family developmental tasks (see Table 25-3).

Beginning families (Stage I) have the developmental tasks of developing trust and understanding as mates. Roles and responsibilities are tested and determined, and the family focuses on deciding whether children will become a part of the family unit. In the early childbearing families (Stage II) the roles and responsibilities of parenting are developed. Providing for work satisfaction, child care, adequate living quarters, and an environment in which to rear a child are primary tasks. The family with preschool children (Stage III) has the tasks of feeling close to relatives in the larger family and helping the

Table 25-3. Family Developmental Tasks

Stage of the family life cycle	Positions in the family	Stage-critical family developmental tasks
1. Married couple	Wife Husband	Establishing a mutually satisfying marriage Adjusting to pregnancy and the promise of parenthood Fitting into the kin network
2. Childbearing	Wife-mother Husband-father Infant daughter or son or both	Having, adjusting to, and encouraging the development of infants Establishing a satisfying home for both parents and infant(s)
3. Preschool-age	Wife-mother Husband-father Daughter-sister Son-brother	Adapting to the critical needs and interests of preschool children in stimulating, growth-promoting ways Coping with energy depletion and lack of privacy as parents
4. School-age	Wife-mother Husband-father Daughter-sister Son-brother	Fitting into the community of school-age families in constructive ways Encouraging children's educational achievement
5. Teenage	Wife-mother Husband-father Daughter-sister Son-brother	Balancing freedom with responsibility as teenagers mature and emancipate themselves Establishing postparental interests and careers as growing parents
6. Launching center	Wife-mother-grandmother Husband-father-grandfather Daughter-sister-aunt Son-brother-uncle	Releasing young adults into work, military service, college, marriage, etc., with appropriate rituals and assistance Maintaining a supportive home base
7. Middle-aged parents	Wife-mother-grandmother Husband-father-grandfather	Rebuilding the marriage relationship Maintaining kin ties with older and younger generations
8. Aging family members	Widow/widower Wife-mother-grandmother Husband-father-grandfather	Coping with bereavement and living alone Closing the family home or adapting it to aging Adjusting to retirement

From Duvall, E. M., *Marriage and Family Development*, 5th ed. Philadelphia: J. B. Lippincott, 1977, p. 179. Reprinted with permission.

child develop knowledge and relationships with kin (e.g., grandparents, uncles, aunts, cousins). They also must plan for the beginning of formal education for the children. Families with school children (Stage IV) have the developmental tasks of providing for children's activity and parents' privacy, and cooperating to get things done. The parents need to continue to satisfy each other as marriage partners. Members of families with teenagers (Stage V) have widely different needs that include working out tasks, responsibilities of family living, and money matters with spouse and teenagers. Teenagers are establishing themselves with peer groups and, in regard to the family, have the task of maintaining communication systems and family contact among all family members. All are growing into the world as family and as individuals. The launching stage (Stage VI) tasks are to get the young adult(s) launched successfully into the world, while simultaneously maintaining a home base for the younger children in the home. Responsibilities are reallocated among grown and growing children. Widening the family circle is done by releasing young adult children who, in turn, acquire mates that are brought as new members of the family by marriage. The empty nest family (Stage VII) has the developmental tasks of drawing closer as a couple and keeping in touch with grown children's families and with siblings and aging parents. During this stage, security for later years needs to be assured in addition to maintaining a comfortable and pleasant home. The task of reaffirming the values of life that have real meaning is addressed. The final stage of family development is the family in retirement and old age (Stage VIII). The tasks briefly include nurturing each other as husband and wife, establishing comfortable household routines, caring for elderly relatives, adjusting to retirement time and income, maintaining contact with children and grandchildren, keeping an interest in people outside the family, finding meaning in life, and facing bereavement and the loss of a spouse. The areas included in a developmental assessment of the family are as follows:

1. The family's present developmental stage. This can be accomplished by using Duvall's eight stages.
2. The extent to which the family is fulfilling the development tasks appropriate for the present developmental stage.
3. The families of origin. Both mates' histories should be described from inception through present day, including developmental history, specific health problems, and health-related events such as deaths, divorces, and losses that happened in the families. This also would include what life with the family of origin was like, and the present and past relationships with parents.
4. The couple's relationship before marriage and the reason(s) for the couple's decision to get married. It is important to know if there were any obstacles to the couple's marriage and the families' responses to the union. This is an area where religion and culture may have a significant impact.
5. How marriage was before children and how the couple established their roles and tasks.
6. A list of any other persons who live or have lived with the family. Describe the relationships with these people and their role in the family. It is common in several ethnic groups for extended family to live together and frequently they have an important role in child raising.
7. The relationships between each mate and his/her parents and siblings. What was each mate's original position in the family? There is evidence to suggest that there are differences in the first born as opposed to the middle or youngest child.
8. The plans made for, and the arrival of, each new child. Determine if the children were planned and what impact the new child's arrival had on all family members.
9. The amount of time the family spends together. Include information about the family's daily routine and how family members think of and feel about each other.

Environment

An environmental perspective in family nursing is crucial. Individuals and families contribute to the environment and are influenced by it. Killien (1985) explained the benefits of this perspective in these words:

> The practice of nursing from an environmental perspective broadens the assessments, diagnoses, interventions, and evaluations made by the nurse to include not only the client but also the environmental systems surrounding the client. As a result, there is increased understanding of client's health behavior, additional intervention strategies become available and interventions may be more successful when the focus of practice is exclusively client focused.

The following information should be included in the family environmental assessment:

1. The neighborhood and community in which the family lives. Include the following types of information:
   a. The type and condition of the dwellings in the area.
   b. The safety of the area. What is the incidence of crime in the area?
   c. The demographic characteristics of the area. For example, is there a mixture of ethnic groups or does one or two ethnic groups dominate the area? What are the predominant occupations of the residents? How heavily or sparsely is the neighborhood populated? Is it an urban or rural area? What kind of industry is located there? Is there a high level of unemployment?
   d. Kinds of health and other basic services located in the area. Is there a hospital or clinic that serves the neighborhood? Are there shopping facilities within easy reach? Is there an accessible transportation system?
   e. Length of time the family has lived in the area. Have they moved frequently? If they have moved a lot, why?
2. Description of the family home. What type—single or multiple dwelling, high rise, flat? What condition is the dwelling in? Is the

dwelling large enough to accommodate all the members? Describe the water supply, sanitation, and adequacy of refrigeration. Are there refrigeration and cooking facilities? Are there adequate bathing and toilet facilities, and are they used just by the family or shared? What are the sleeping arrangements? Are there problems with vermin or rodents? Describe the safety of the dwelling by looking at the condition and placement of furniture, rugs, stairways, handrails, lights, appliances, and painted surfaces. Describe the conditions of fire and drugs and poison safety [e.g., matches, medicines, cleaning solutions, poison storage (are they out of children's reach), safety tops, smoke detectors, fire extinguishers].

Family Support Systems

The family social network consists of all the family members, friends, all helping persons or organizations who stand by to help the family, and all the linkages among these people. Healthy families have meaningful ties with friends, relatives, and social support groups. Relevant information to the assessment of support systems includes the following:

1. The ties the family has with friends, relatives, and social support groups. Does the family perceive that the people and groups identified provide assistance, support and guidance when needed? Is this family unable to identify family or friends who can assist them when needed? The following format has been suggested to elicit information about social supports:

> Who helps you with . . . ? If you had any problems about . . . who would you talk to to get help? Asking first general and then more specific questions is helpful. For example, who helped you through retiring from your job? Who or what kind of help have you had with financial concerns? Another useful question is, who has helped you through a tough situation in the past? (Hogue 1977)

2. The types of health-related resources used in the past and present, and the family's knowledge of available resources. Figure 25-1 and Table 25-4 are examples of tools developed for assessing family function.

Table 25-4. Guidelines for Assessment of Family Structure and Function

Structural element	Assessment data
Subsystems	Identify the executive subsystem. Identify the sibling subsystem.
Roles and power	How are the following roles provided in the family and by whom: provider, protector, disciplinarian, nurturer, dependent, main spokesperson, main decision maker, learner, others? Are members of the executive subsystem dependent? Are members of the sibling subsystem given executive powers?
Interactions	Describe the interactional patterns of the family. Include verbal and nonverbal behavior. Is the atmosphere of interaction mostly relaxed or tense? Give examples. Who answers most questions? Are all members of the family allowed to speak for themselves? Do family members speak to one another? Do they maintain eye contact with one another?
Values	Describe the major values of the family in the areas of work, recreation, health, religion, education. What other values does the family hold?
Environmental influences	Describe how the following outside influences affect the family: extended family, school, church, community organizations, other resources.

Client Family ______________________

Date of Assessment ______________________

Family functions	Observed behavior	Assessed need level	Suggested nursing responses
I. Management Function A. Use of power for all family members			
B. Rule making clear, accepted			
C. Fiscal support adequate			
D. Successful negotiations with extrafamilial systems			
E. Future planning present			
II. Boundary Function A. Clear individual boundaries			
B. Clear generational boundaries			
C. Clear family boundaries			
III. Communication Function A. Straight messages			
B. No manipulation			
C. Expression of positive and negative feelings safely			
IV. Emotional–Supportive Function A. Mutual positive regard			
B. Deals with conflict			
C. Uses resources for all family members			
D. Allows growth for all family members			
V. Socialization Function A. Children growing and developing in a healthy pattern			
B. Mutual negotiation of roles by age and ability			
C. Parents feel good about parenting			
D. Spouses happy with each other's role behavior			

Need levels

Level I: Current needs being met; no behaviors likely to lead to future problems.

Level II: Behaviors likely to lead to future problems; some needs recognized by nurse but not by client.

Level III: Current needs not being met.

Level IV: Unmet needs threaten survival.

Figure 25-1 Family Function Checklist. (F. B. Roberts, © 1982, reprinted with permission.)

Summary

This chapter has focused on factors that are important for the nurse to consider in the assessment of the family. In all areas of care, nurses should be aware of the importance of the family. The major thrust of family nursing is health promotion and maintenance. There is a great deal of current nursing literature related to family health. This chapter only attempts to provide the basic information that is gathered to assist the nurse in developing a nursing diagnosis and subsequent plan of care to support the family in developing or maintaining wellness.

Example of Family Health Assessment

The Milligan family was referred to Community Health Clinic by a community health nurse when she discovered that the two youngest children had not been immunized. Mr. Milligan had been out of work for two years and no longer had health insurance. He had been feeling very "tired and down" for the past few months. Mrs. Milligan believed she might be pregnant (about three months), but had not made an appointment with an appropriate health care provider.

Bibliographic Data

Family Name: Alison and Brian Milligan and 4 children

Address: 12½ High Street

Ages: Brian Milligan 41 years
Alison Iannopollo Milligan 36 years
Joseph Milligan 11 years
Jennifer Milligan 9 years
Ned Milligan 4 years
Margaret Milligan 18 months

Education: Mr. Milligan completed 12th grade
Mrs. Milligan completed 10th grade

The Milligans have been married for 16 years. The oldest two children attend a neighborhood Catholic school. It is the same grammar school that Mr. Milligan attended. Ned Milligan will be eligible to attend a Head Start Program this year.

Occupation: Mr. Milligan was a sheet metal worker for 20 years but was laid off two years ago when the company relocated. The Milligans were offered the opportunity to move but did not want to leave the area. Mr. Milligan was also offered job retraining and attended the local community college for about 6 months with the idea of becoming a computer programmer. He told me he left because he had a hard time concentrating and studying.

Mrs. Milligan is a housewife. She expressed the desire to complete the high school equivalency exam because she always wanted to be a teacher. She says her grades through school were always very high and that she dropped out because she was bored.

Religion: The family are practicing Catholics and at times have been active in parish activities. They plan on sending all the children to the parish school but worry about how they will pay for this.

Race and Ethnic Origins: The family is caucasian. Mrs. Milligan comes from a large, first generation Italian family. She has seven brothers and sisters and parents who live nearby. She was never encouraged to complete school but recalls that it was important that her brothers finished high school. She feels very close to her family and gets a lot of support from them. They have been critical about her husband's inability to find a job. They feel he "should dig ditches if necessary." Mr. Milligan's family are of Irish extraction. They are not Catholic and were unhappy when Mr. Milligan joined the Catholic Church. He has several sisters and describes himself as being close to all family members, especially his father. His father is a college graduate and was always disappointed that his son did not go on with his schooling. He encourages him to return to school and cannot understand why the son is so "lackadaisical" about the whole issue. Mrs. Milligan's family speaks a combination of Italian and English in the home, and the Milligans speak only English.

Social Class Status and Income: The family can be classified as lower middle class. The Milligan in-laws can be considered as upper middle class which appears to cause some conflict. Both parents describe their current income as being unsatisfactory. Mr. Milligan receives $250 each week for unemployment. Mrs. Milligan receives $5.35 per hour and usually works about 20 hours per week at McDonalds. They receive food stamps, and the elder Milligans help out with school tuition and clothes for their grandchildren. Income and employment is a major concern of the family.

Family: This is a nuclear family with strong kinship bonds.

Family Health Background

Father—Childhood illness: mumps age 8, chickenpox the same year, measles (not sure of year); immunizations DPT.
Allergies: none.
Past illness: appendectomy age 11; automobile accident age 17 (fractured left femur, concussion). Treated for depression in late 20's and 30's.

Mother—Childhood illness: measles age 7; does not remember any others; thinks she received immunizations.

Joseph—Childhood illness: immunized for DPT, polio, and mumps.
Past illness, surgery: T/A age 3 due to enlargement with recurrent ear infections. Miringotomy age 4, redone age 5. Tubes out at age 5½. Has had two right ear infections since at age 7 and 7½; treated with antibiotics. Joseph is in 5th grade; he talked about his friends and seems to be a healthy, well-developed boy; normal for his age and developmental stage.

Jennifer—No Childhood illness: immunized for DPT, polio, and mumps. Gets a cold about 1–2 times per year, treated with rest and liquids. Has had no surgery. Jennifer is in 3rd grade and according to her has almost all A's and plans to be a nurse when she grows up. Appears normal for her age and developmental stage.

Ned—Has had no communicable disease in spite of not having been immunized. Has an occasional cold which is treated with fluids and rest. Will begin Head Start soon. Appears well developed both physically and emotionally.

Margaret—Has not been immunized. Appears to be in good health. Began walking at one year. Very alert and active.

Developmental History

The Milligan family is in Duval's Stage IV. They appear to be fulfilling the developmental tasks of that stage. The parents are promoting school achievement in the three oldest children. They appear to have a satisfying marital relationship although there is the strain of unemployment and a possible unplanned pregnancy. This will have to be investigated more closely as nursing intervention is planned with the family.

Both parents describe very happy childhoods and good relationships with siblings and parents. They describe the usual disagreements with parents as teenagers but in retrospect believe their parents, although strict, were correct.

The couple met at a softball game 14 years ago. They dated for two years and then were married. Both sets of parents were upset about the religious differences but were supportive when the couple decided to marry. Mr. Milligan had since become a Catholic, and his family did object, but relationships remain friendly.

Mr. and Mrs. Milligan planned the first four of their children and state they always wanted at least four children. If Mrs. Milligan is pregnant it is unplanned, and there is concern because of Mr. Milligan's unemployment. However, terminating the pregnancy would be out of the question due to religious and personal beliefs. The family spends time together at meals and on weekends. In the summer the family camps at places not too far from home where there is swimming and other sports. During the school year, Sunday dinner is at the home of one of their parents.

Environmental Assessment

The Milligans describe their neighborhood and community as old but comfortable with most homes in good condition. Most of the homes are single or double and are owned by the people who live in them. Their house is a double, and they live on the first floor and rent the upstairs to a family with three children about the same ages as their own children. Their flat has four bedrooms, 1½ baths, kitchen, dining and living rooms, and an extra room used as a combination den and TV room. They own the house and have been able to keep up the payments with occasional help from their parents. They also receive $500 monthly rent from the tenants, which the Milligans say "helps." The neighborhood is urban with a mix of ethnic groups, mostly Italian and Irish. There is only some light industry in the area. They feel the crime rate is low but do keep doors locked and would not want their children out alone at night. Mrs. Milligan feels that the services they need (a hospital, clinic and grocery stores) are close. They live on a major bus route so she can get around when Mr. Milligan is using the car. The Milligans seem very proud of their home.

Assessment of Social Support

Throughout our discussions the Milligans referred to their close-knit family. Sisters, brothers, and parents are supportive, and most of the recreation of the family involves these people. Both sets of parents have been of great help during this period of unemployment. Mr. Milligan bowls once a week with friends and enjoys going to Buffalo Bills' football games. Mrs. Milligan plays cards with women in the neighborhood and often has coffee and talks with the woman upstairs and her next door neighbor.

Summary

This is a relatively brief assessment of a fictional family, but it is enough information to develop nursing diagnoses and to begin planning to meet some of the family's health needs. You may talk to families in a clinical setting and may feel it important to meet the families in their home settings at a later time. Observing a family functioning in the home environment may provide additional, pertinent data regarding family health.

APPENDIX A

Abbreviations Commonly Used in Assessment Documentation

AAL anterior axillary line
AC>BC air conduction greater than bone conduction
ad lib freely
A&P anterior and posterior
AP anterior-posterior
ARF acute rheumatic fever
ASA aspirin
ASHD arteriosclerotic heart disease
A/V artery/vein ratio
A/W alive and well
BMR basal metabolic rate
BP blood pressure
BRP bathroom privileges
BS bowel sounds
BSP bromsulphalein
BUN blood urea nitrogen
c̄ with
CBC complete blood count
CC chief complaint
CCU coronary care unit
CHF congestive heart failure
CNS central nervous system
CN cranial nerves
C/O complains of
COLD chronic obstructive lung disease
CPR cardio-pulmonary resuscitation
C&S culture and sensitivity
CSF cerebral spinal fluid
CVA costal vertebral angle (may also refer to cerebral vascular accident)
CVP central venous pressure
D/C discontinued
DD disc diameter (optic)
DJD degenerative joint disease
DM diabetes mellitus
DTR deep tendon reflex
DUB dysfunctional uterine bleeding
Dx diagnosis
ECG or **EKG** electrocardiogram
EEG electroencephalogram
EOMs extra ocular movements (muscles)
ER emergency room
ETOH alcohol
EUA examination under anesthesia
F.H.R. fetal heart rate
fx fracture
GU genito-urinary
GYN gynecology
HBP high blood pressure
Hct hematocrit
HCVD hypertensive cardiovascular disease
HEENT head, eyes, ears, nose, throat
Hgb hemoglobin
HJR hepato jugular reflux
HPI history of present illness
Hrt heart
ht. height
Hx history
IBW ideal body weight
ICS intercostal space
ICU intensive care unit
I&D incision and drainage
I&O intake and output
IPPB intermittent positive pressure breathing
IUD intra-uterine device
IV intravenously
IVP intravenous pyelogram
JVD jugular venous distention
JVP jugular venous pressure (pulse)
KUB kidney, ureters, bladder
LCBD left cardiac border dullness
LLQ left lower quadrant
LMP last menstrual period
LOC level of consciousness
LP lumbar puncture
LUQ left upper quadrant
ⓜ murmur
MAL mid axillary line
MCL mid clavicular line
MI myocardial infarction
MOM milk of magnesia
M&R measure and record
MSL mid sternal line
ⓝ normal
NAD no acute distress
NC/AT normcephalic, atraumatic
N/G naso-gastric
NPN non-protein nitrogen
NSR normal sinus rhythm
Ø or **ō** none or no
OB obstetrics
OBS organic brain syndrome
OD right eye
OOB out of bed
OPD out-patient department
OR operating room
OS left eye
OU both eyes
PAL posterior axillary line
P&A percussion and auscultation
PARR post anesthesia recovery room
PAT paroxysmal atrial tachycardia
PE physical exam
PERRLA pupils equal, round, react to light and accommodation
PMI point of maximum impulse or intensity
PND paroxysmal nocturnal dyspnea
PP patient profile
PPD packs per day (may also refer to TB skin test)
prn as needed
PVCs premature ventricular contractions
qod every other day
qs quantity sufficient
R right
RBC red blood count
RCM right costal margin
RHD rheumatic heart disease
RLL right lower lobe
R/O rule out
ROM range of motion (movement)
ROS review of systems
RUL right upper lobe
s̄ without
SEM systolic ejection murmur
SLE systemic lupus erythematosus
Stat immediately
T&A tonsils and adenoids
TB or **TBC** tuberculosis
TLC total lung capacity (may also refer to tender, loving care)
TM tympanic membrane
TPR temperature, pulse, respirations
URI upper respiratory infection
UTI urinary tract infection
VF ventricular fibrillation
V.S. vital signs
WBC white blood count
WD/WN well developed, well nourished
WNL within normal limits
wt. weight
< less than
Δ change
~ apparently

APPENDIX B

Developmental Aspects

B-1. Weight According to Frame, Women of Ages 25 and Over
B-2. Weight According to Frame, Men of Ages 25 and Over
B-3. Developmental Tasks in Ten Categories of Behavior from Birth to Death
B-4. Freud's Psychosexual Stages
B-5. Two Major Stage Theories of Development
B-6. Erikson's Eight Stages of Development
B-7. Maslow's Characteristics of a Self-Actualized Person
B-8. Characteristics of Infants' Thinking: Sensorimotor Stage
B-9. Characteristics of Toddlers' and Preschoolers' Thinking: Preoperational Stage
B-10. Characteristics of School-Age Children's Thinking: Concrete Operational Stage
B-11. Characteristics of Adolescents' Thinking: Formal or Abstract Operational Stage

Table B-1. Weight According to Frame (Indoor Clothing), Women of Ages 25 and Over*

Height†			Small frame		Medium frame		Large frame	
Feet	Inches	cm	Pounds	Kilograms	Pounds	Kilograms	Pounds	Kilograms
4	10	147.3	92–98	41.7–44.5	96–107	43.5–48.5	104–119	47.2–54.0
4	11	149.9	94–101	42.6–45.8	98–110	44.5–49.9	106–122	48.1–55.3
5	0	152.4	96–104	43.5–47.2	101–113	45.8–51.3	109–125	49.4–56.7
5	1	154.9	99–107	44.9–48.5	104–116	47.2–52.6	112–128	50.8–58.1
5	2	157.5	102–110	46.3–50.0	107–119	48.5–54.0	115–131	52.2–59.4
5	3	160.0	105–113	47.6–51.3	110–122	49.9–55.3	118–134	53.5–60.8
5	4	162.6	108–116	49.0–52.6	113–126	51.3–57.2	121–138	54.9–62.6
5	5	165.1	111–119	50.3–54.0	116–130	52.6–59.0	125–142	56.7–64.4
5	6	167.6	114–123	51.7–55.8	120–135	54.4–61.2	129–146	58.5–66.2
5	7	170.2	118–127	53.5–57.6	124–139	56.2–63.0	133–150	60.3–68.0
5	8	172.7	122–131	55.3–59.4	128–143	58.1–64.9	137–154	62.1–69.9
5	9	175.3	126–135	57.2–61.2	132–147	59.9–66.7	141–158	64.0–71.7
5	10	177.8	130–140	69.0–63.5	136–151	61.7–68.5	145–163	65.8–73.9
5	11	180.3	134–144	60.8–65.3	140–155	63.5–70.3	149–168	67.6–76.2
6	0	182.9	138–148	62.6–67.1	144–159	65.3–72.1	153–173	69.4–78.5

*For women between 18 and 25, subtract 0.5 kg (1 pound) for each year under 25.

†With shoes on—5.1 cm (2-inch) heels

Courtesy of the Metropolitan Life Insurance Company.

Table B-2. Weight According to Frame (Indoor Clothing), Men of Ages 25 and Over

Height*			Small frame		Medium frame		Large frame	
Feet	Inches	cm	Pounds	Kilograms	Pounds	Kilograms	Pounds	Kilograms
5	2	157.5	112–120	50.8–54.4	118–129	53.5–58.5	126–141	57.2–64.0
5	3	160.0	115–123	52.2–55.8	121–133	54.9–60.3	129–144	58.5–65.3
5	4	162.6	118–126	53.5–57.2	124–136	56.2–61.7	132–148	59.9–67.1
5	5	165.1	121–129	54.9–58.5	127–139	57.6–63.0	135–152	61.2–68.9
5	6	167.6	124–133	56.2–60.3	130–143	59.0–64.9	138–156	62.6–70.8
5	7	170.2	128–137	58.1–62.1	134–147	60.8–66.7	142–161	64.4–73.0
5	8	172.7	132–141	59.9–64.0	138–152	62.6–68.9	147–166	66.7–75.3
5	9	175.3	136–145	61.7–65.8	142–156	64.4–70.8	151–170	68.5–77.1
5	10	177.8	140–150	63.5–68.0	146–160	66.2–72.6	155–174	70.3–78.9
5	11	180.3	144–154	65.3–69.9	150–165	68.0–74.8	159–179	72.1–81.2
6	0	182.9	148–158	67.1–71.7	154–170	69.9–77.1	164–184	74.4–83.4
6	1	185.4	152–162	68.9–73.5	158–175	71.7–79.4	168–189	76.2–85.7
6	2	188.0	156–167	70.8–75.8	162–180	73.5–81.6	173–194	78.5–88.0
6	3	190.5	160–171	72.6–77.6	167–185	75.8–83.9	178–199	80.7–90.3
6	4	193.0	164–175	74.4–79.4	172–190	78.0–86.2	182–204	82.6–92.5

*With shoes on—2.5 cm (1-inch) heels.

Courtesy of Metropolitan Life Insurance Company.

Table B-3. Developmental Tasks in Ten Categories of Behavior from Birth to Death

	Infancy (birth to 1 or 2)	**Early childhood (2–3 to 5–6–7)**	**Late childhood (5–6–7 to pubescence)**
I. Achieving an appropriate dependence-independence pattern	1. Establishing oneself as a very dependent being 2. Beginning establishment of self-awareness	1. Adjusting to less private attention; becoming independent physically (while remaining strongly dependent emotionally)	1. Freeing oneself from primary identification with adults
II. Achieving an appropriate giving-receiving pattern of affection	1. Developing a feeling for affection	1. Developing ability to give affection 2. Learning to share affection	1. Learning to give as much love as one receives; forming friendships with peers
III. Relating to changing social groups	1. Becoming aware of alive as against inanimate, and familiar as against unfamiliar 2. Developing rudimentary social interaction	1. Beginning to develop ability to interact with age-mates 2. Adjusting in family to expectations it has for the child as a member of social unit	1. Clarifying adult world as over against child's world 2. Establishing peer groupness and learning to belong

From Lida F. Thompson, Michael H. Miller, and Helen F. Bigler, *Sociology—Nurses and Their Patients in a Modern Society*, 9th ed. (St. Louis: C. V. Mosby, 1975).

Early adolescence (pubescence to puberty)	Late adolescence (puberty to early maturity)	Maturity (early to late active adulthood)	Aging (beyond full powers of adulthood through senility)
1. Establishing one's independence from adults in all areas of behavior	1. Establishing oneself as an independent individual in an adult manner	1. Learning to be interdependent, now leaning and now succoring others, as needs arise 2. Assisting one's children to become gradually independent and autonomous beings	1. Accepting graciously and comfortably help needed from others as powers fail and dependence becomes necessary
1. Accepting oneself as a worthwhile person really worthy of love	1. Building a strong mutual affectional bond with a (possible) marriage partner	1. Building and maintaining a strong and mutually satisfying marriage relationship 2. Establishing wholesome affectional bonds with one's children and grandchildren 3. Meeting wisely the new needs for affection of one's own aging parents 4. Cultivating meaningfully warm friendships with members of one's own generation	1. Facing loss of one's spouse, and finding some satisfactory sources of affection previously received from mate 2. Learning new affectional roles with own children, now mature adults 3. Establishing ongoing, satisfying affectional patterns with grandchildren and other members of extended family 4. Finding and preserving mutually satisfying friendships outside family circle
1. Behaving according to a shifting peer code	1. Adopting an adult-patterned set of social values by learning a new peer code	1. Keeping within reasonable balance activities in various social, service, political, and community groups and causes that make demands on mature adults 2. Establishing and maintaining mutually satisfactory relationships with in-law families of spouse and married children	1. Choosing and maintaining ongoing social activities and functions appropriate to health, energy, and interests

(continued on page 606)

Table B-3. *Continued*

	Infancy (birth to 1 or 2)	Early childhood (2–3 to 5–6–7)	Late childhood (5–6–7 to pubescence)
IV. Developing a conscience	1. Beginning to adjust to expectations of others	1. Developing ability to take directions and to be obedient in presence of authority 2. Developing ability to be obedient in absence of authority where conscience substitutes for authority	1. Learning more rules and developing true morality
V. Learning one's psychosociobio-logical sex role		1. Learning to identify with male adult and female adult roles	1. Beginning to identify with one's social contemporaries of same sex
VI. Accepting and adjusting to a changing body	1. Adjusting to adult feeding demands 2. Adjusting to adult cleanliness demands 3. Adjusting to adult attitudes toward genital manipulation	1. Adjusting to expectations resulting from one's improving muscular abilities. 2. Developing sex modesty	
VII. Managing a changing body and learning new motor patterns	1. Developing physiological equilibrium 2. Developing eye-hand coordination 3. Establishing satisfactory rhythms of rest and activity	1. Developing large muscle control 2. Learning to coordinate large muscles and small muscles	1. Refining and elaborating skill in use of small muscles

Early adolescence (pubescence to puberty)	Late adolescence (puberty to early maturity)	Maturity (early to late active adulthood)	Aging (beyond full powers of adulthood through senility)
	1. Learning to verbalize contradictions in moral codes, as well as discrepancies between principle and practice, and resolving these problems in a responsible manner	1. Coming to terms with violations of moral codes in the larger, as well as in the more intimate social scene, and developing some constructive philosophy and method of operation 2. Helping children adjust to expectations of others and to conform to moral demands of culture	1. Maintaining a sense of moral integrity in face of disappointments and disillusionments in life's hopes and dreams
1. Strong identification with one's own sex mates 2. Learning one's role in heterosexual relationships	1. Exploring possibilities for a future mate and acquiring "desirability" 2. Choosing an occupation 3. Preparing to accept one's future role in manhood or womanhood as a responsible citizen of larger community	1. Learning to be a competent husband or wife and building a good marriage 2. Carrying a socially adequate role as citizen and worker in community 3. Becoming a good parent and grandparent as children arrive and develop	1. Learning to live on a retirement income 2. Being a good companion to an aging spouse 3. Meeting bereavement of spouse adequately
1. Reorganizing one's thoughts and feelings about oneself in face of significant bodily changes and their concomitants 2. Accepting reality of one's appearance	1. Learning appropriate outlets for sexual drives	1. Making a good sex adjustment within marriage 2. Establishing healthful routines of eating, resting, working, and playing within pressures of adult world	1. Making a good adjustment to failing powers as aging diminishes strengths and abilities
1. Controlling and using a "new" body		1. Learning new motor skills involved in housekeeping, gardening, sports, and other activities expected of adults in community	1. Adapting interests and activities to reserves of vitality and energy of aging body

(continued on page 608)

Table B-3. *Continued*

	Infancy (birth to 1 or 2)	Early childhood (2–3 to 5–6–7)	Late childhood (5–6–7 to pubescence)
VIII. Learning to understand and control the physical world	1. Exploring physical world	1. Meeting adult expectations for restrictive exploration and manipulation of an expanding environment	1. Learning more realistic ways of studying and controlling physical world
IX. Developing an appropriate symbol system and conceptual abilities.	1. Developing preverbal communication 2. Developing verbal communication 3. Rudimentary concept formation	1. Improving one's use of symbol system 2. Enormous elaboration of concept pattern	1. Learning to use language actually to exchange ideas or to influence one's hearers 2. Beginning understanding of real causal relations 3. Making finer conceptual distinctions and thinking reflectively
X. Relating oneself to the cosmos		1. Developing a genuine, though uncritical, notion about one's place in the cosmos	1. Developing a scientific approach

Early adolescence (pubescence to puberty)	Late adolescence (puberty to early maturity)	Maturity (early to late active adulthood)	Aging (beyond full powers of adulthood through senility)
		1. Gaining intelligent understanding of new horizons of medicine and science sufficient for personal well-being and social competence	1. Mastering new awareness and methods of dealing with physical surroundings as an individual with occasional or permanent disabilities
1. Using language to express and to clarify more complex concepts 2. Moving from the concrete to the abstract and applying general principles to the particular	1. Achieving level of reasoning of which one is capable	1. Mastering technical symbol systems involved in income tax, social security, complex financial dealings, and other contexts familiar to Western man	1. Keeping mentally alert and effective as long as is possible through later years
	1. Formulating a workable belief and value system	1. Formulating and implementing a rational philosophy of life on basis of adult experience 2. Cultivating a satisfactory religious climate in home as spiritual soil for development of family members	1. Preparing for eventual and inevitable cessation of life by building a set of beliefs that one can live and die with in peace

Table B-4. Freud's Psychosexual Stages

Age	Stage	Aspects of development
Birth to about one year	Oral stage	Pleasure centers around the mouth—eating, sucking, spitting, biting, chewing. Adults who fixate at this level may displace their oral impulses by being gullible, possessive, sarcastic, or argumentative, for example.
One year to three years	Anal stage	Pleasure centers around the retention and expulsion of feces; type of toilet training can affect the child's personality—depending on whether the training is too strict or too permissive, the child may become (as an adult) obstinate and stingy, or destructive and messy, or creative and productive, for example.
Three years to six years	Phallic stage	The child discovers and derives pleasure from his genitals; the Oedipal conflict and castration anxiety occur.
Six years to about eleven years	Latency period	To relieve the anxiety stemming from the Oedipal conflict, the child represses his desire for his opposite-sexed parent and identifies with his like-sexed parent, repressing all erotic impulses toward the opposite sex.
Adolescence	Genital stage	Egocentric and incestuous love is replaced by heterosexual love and sexuality; the adolescent prepares for adulthood by channeling his drives into group activities and preparation for work and marriage.

Table B-5. Two Major Stage Theories of Development

Theorist	Infant	Toddler	Preschool	School-age	Adolescent	Young adult
Piaget (Cognitive)	"Sensorimotor" (birth to 2 years) Uses senses, motor skills, reflexes to explore Object permanence, trial and error, and "insight" problem solving Syncretic reasoning	"Preoperational" (2 to 7 years) Self-centered; other centeredness begins Perception from own point of view: centering, artificialism, animism, irreversibility, number is name, literal interpretation of works and actions Judges things for outcome, consequence to self Transductive reasoning		"Concrete Operations" (7 to 11 years) Interpersonal collaboration and competition Social reciprocity and sense of fairness Uses elementary logic by manipulating actual objects and experiences Inductive-deductive reasoning	"Formal Operations" (12 years +) Sees world from many and different perspectives Thought is independent of concrete reality, is flexible, and manipulates abstract concepts and ideas Uses formal logic, manipulates symbols; forms hypotheses, theories Hypotheticodeductive/experimental reasoning Morally reasons on basis of what is right for best of world or for the majority of people and situations Abstract Reasoning	
Kohlberg (Moral Reasoning)	"Premoral" (birth—approximately 4 years) No idea of right or wrong regarding rules or authority Good = what is pleasant or exciting Bad = what is painful or fearful Impulses rule behavior		"Stage 1" (4 years + requires beginning concrete operational thinking) Punishment and Obedience Defer to power and authority Life valued for number and power of possessions	"Stage 2" (up to approximately 10 years, requires advanced concrete operational thinking) Bargaining Right fair deal Life valued for how one can satisfy other's needs "Stage 3" (10–13 years, requires transition into beginning formal operational thinking) Good Boy or Nice Girl Act to please; helps others Life valued for how good one's relations with others are	"Stage 4" (13 years + requires that most skills of formal operations have been attained) Law and Order Right to do duty, show respect for authority Follow fixed rules; life valued in terms of social or religious laws	"Stage 5" (after formal operations attained) Social Contract/ Individual Rights Emphasis on legal view but will change laws to uphold life, liberty, and emerging cultural values Must uphold social contracts Moral and legal views conflict

Source: This table was developed by Sherry Pontious, R.N., Ph.D.

Table B-6. Erikson's Eight Stages of Development

Age	Stage	Result of success	Result of failure
Early infancy (birth to about one year) (corollary to Freudian oral stage)	Basic trust vs. mistrust	Trust results from affection and gratification of needs, mutual recognition.	Mistrust results from consistent abuse, neglect, deprivation of love, too early or harsh weaning, autistic isolation.
Later infancy (one to three years) (corollary to Freudian muscular anal stage)	Autonomy vs. shame and doubt	Child views self as person in his own right apart from parents but still dependent.	Child feels inadequate, doubts self, curtails learning basic skills like walking, talking, wants to "hide" inadequacies.
Early childhood (about ages four to five years) (corollary to Freudian phallic locomotor stage)	Initiative vs. guilt	Child has lively imagination, vigorously tests reality, imitates adults, anticipates roles.	Child lacks spontaneity, has infantile jealousy "castration complex," is suspicious, evasive, suffers from role inhibition.
Middle childhood (about ages six to eleven years) (corollary to Freudian latency stage)	Industry vs. inferiority	Child has sense of duty and accomplishment, develops scholastic and social competencies, undertakes real tasks, puts fantasy and play in better perspective, learns world of tools, task identification.	Child has poor work habits, avoids strong competition, feels doomed to mediocrity; is in lull before the storms of puberty, may conform as slavish behavior, has sense of futility.
Puberty and adolescence (about ages twelve to twenty years)	Ego identity vs. role confusion	Adolescent has temporal perspective, is self-certain, is a role experimenter, goes through apprenticeship, experiences sexual polarization and leader-followership, develops an ideological commitment.	Adolescent experiences time confusion, is self-conscious, has a role fixation, and experiences work paralysis, bisexual confusion, authority confusion, and value confusion.
Early adulthood	Intimacy vs. isolation	Person has capacity to commit self to others, "true genitability" is now possible, *Lieben und Arbeiten*—"to love and to work"; "mutuality of genital orgasm."	Person avoids intimacy, has "character problems," behaves promiscuously, and repudiates, isolates, destroys seemingly dangerous forces.
Middle adulthood	Generativity vs. stagnation	Person is productive and creative for self and others, has parental pride and pleasure, is mature, enriches his life, establishes and guides next generation.	Person is egocentric, nonproductive, experiences early invalidism, excessive self-love, personal impoverishment, and self-indulgence.
Late adulthood	Integrity vs. despair	Person appreciates continuity of past, present, and future, accepts life cycle and life style, has learned to cooperate with inevitabilities of life, "death loses its sting."	Person feels time is too short; finds no meaning in human existence, has lost faith in self and others, wants second chance at life cycle with more advantages, has no feeling of world order or spiritual sense, fears death.

Table B-7. Maslow's Characteristics of a Self-Actualized Person

Characteristic	Explanation
1. More efficient perception of reality and more comfortable relations with it	The self-actualized person judges others accurately, detects falseness in others, and is capable of tolerating uncertainty and ambiguity.
2. Acceptance of self and others	He accepts himself as he is and is not defensive. He has little guilt, shame, or anxiety.
3. Spontaneity	Self-actualizers are spontaneous in both thoughts and behavior.
4. Problem centering	The problems with which the self-actualized person concerns himself are not of a personal nature, but instead are outside of himself.
5. Detachment; the need for privacy	Although he enjoys others, he does not mind solitude and sometimes seeks it.
6. Autonomy: independence of culture and environment	He is relatively uninfluenced by local customs.
7. Continued freshness of appreciation	He derives ecstasy, inspiration, and strength from the basic experiences of life. Acts that serve biological functions, such as eating and sexual behavior, are relatively unimportant in the total scheme of things but when enjoyed are done so wholeheartedly. There is no accompanying anxiety to detract from the intense pleasure.
8. Mystical experience	The self-actualizer, much more commonly than others, has experiences during which he feels simultaneously more power and more helpless than ever before.
9. Social interest	There is a feeling of identification, sympathy, and affection for others.
10. Interpersonal relations	Relationships with others are few, but they are deep and meaningful. The self-actualizer does on occasion get angry, but he does not bear long-lasting grudges.
11. Democratic character structure	He respects people irrespective of birth, race, blood, and family.
12. Discrimination between means and ends	Most people work only in order to receive the paycheck at the end of the week. The self-actualizer enjoys his work.
13. Sense of humor	He has a sense of humor that is both philosophical and nonhostile.
14. Creativeness	Maslow felt that everybody is potentially creative. He was not referring to great works of art or science, but rather to expressiveness, spontaneity, and perceptiveness in everyday life.
15. Nonconformity	Self-actualized people swim against the mainstream. They are open to new experiences.

Table B-8. Characteristics of Infants' Thinking: Sensorimotor Stage

Major task

Conquest of object.

Throughout this stage, infants are unable to think. Intelligence proceeds from directly acting, as a whole, on the environment to more goal-directed attending to and action on particular objects to make specific events occur. All the senses and motor skills are actively used to define and interpret objects and events.

Perception

Birth to 3 months: View of world and self undifferentiated; unconscious of self.

4 to 6 months: View of world centered around body; self-centered.

After 6 months: View of world as centered around objects.

6 to 12 months: Self seen as separated from objects.

12 to 18 months: Objects seen to have constancy and permanence.

18 to 24 months: Represents spatial relationships between objects and between objects and self (e.g., knows smaller things fit inside larger things).

Thought

Birth to 3 months: Not present. Uses inborn reflexes and senses.

4 to 6 months: Questions presence of thought. Uses combination of reflexes and senses purposively. Develops habits.

6 to 12 months: Knows objects by how he or she uses them. Knows objects have constant size before knows objects have same form; serially acts out two previously separate behaviors in goal-directed sequences.

12 to 24 months: Object permanence stimulates purposive, intentional use of behaviors to find hidden objects and to cause event via trial and error—problem solve via "insight"; can now see effect when given the cause (e.g., knows where train will come out when goes into tunnel). Symbolism and memory begin—uses deferred imitation to discover new ways of acting (e.g., when "pretends" sleep means "know" symbolic sleeping).

Reasoning

Birth to 6 months: Not present.

6 to 24 months: Syncretism: (1) perceives "whole"—impression without analysis of parts or synthesis of relations, (2) lacks systematic exploratory behavior until end of stage, (3) begins to connect series of ideas together into a confused whole.

Language

Birth to 3 months: Undifferentiated cry. Use of different intensities, patterns, and pitches of cry for different feelings (e.g., pain, hunger, fatigue).

6 to 8 weeks: Cooing: contented and happy sounds.

3 to 6 months: Babbling: repeated various sounds for sensation of pleasure. *Laughing:* when happy or excited.

6 to 12 months: Spontaneous vocalization: imperfect imitation. *Echolalia:* conscious imitation of sounds.

12 to 18 months: Expressive jargon: use of information, rhythms, and pauses to imitate sentence sounds. *Holophrases:* use of one word to convey meaning. *Gestures* substitute for or add meaning to speech.

18 to 24 months: Telegraphic speech: use of noun and verb to convey many meanings.

Play

Birth to 6 months: Exercise play: repetition of actions and sounds for pleasure (e.g., rolling over, babbling).

6 to 12 months: Exploratory play: pleasure from causing effect and reconfirming skill (e.g., "peek-a-boo," "drop and retrieve," "pat-a-cake").

12 to 24 months: Deferred imitation: imitates previously observed actions (not reasons for or purposes of actions) from memory (e.g., pretends to be "Daddy" and goes through getting dressed, shaving, then walks outside, and gets in the "car").

From Servonsky/Opas: *Nursing Management of Children*, © 1987 Boston: Jones and Bartlett Publishers.

Table B-9. Characteristics of Toddlers' and Preschoolers' Thinking: Preoperational Stage

Major task

Conquest of symbol

Thought is influenced almost completely by the child's own perceptions, personal actions, and experiences. Thinking moves from perceptual illusion and egocentricity (from the child's own viewpoint and in the child's own way) toward the beginning of sociocentricity (socially validated ideas from others' perspectives) and manipulating symbols.

Perception

2 to 5 years

Views world in terms of own perspective and as it appears. Self is focus and purpose of things in world. Refuses others' viewpoints because unaware other person can have viewpoint different from own.

5 to 8 years

Less egocentric, begins to appreciate other person's point of view and feelings although does not comprehend other's viewpoints when there is conflict with own perspective.

Thought

2 to 5 years

Perceptually bound (has perceptual illusions), distorts information to make it fit own viewpoint, centers on one status characteristic of objects and events, thinks in present tense.

Centering: attends to only one aspect of object or event.

Artificialism: believes natural events are created by human beings.

Animism: believes all things have consciousness and other human qualities.

Absolutism: believes things are right or wrong, black or white, work or don't work, hurt or don't hurt.

Irreversibility: believes actions and thoughts can't be reversed or compensated for.

Words and numbers: knows and uses only one name or label per object or event.

5 to 8 years

Views world in terms of a combination of own and beginning awareness of others' perspectives. World exists independent of self, but all events still have a purpose.

Decentering begins: can focus on two or more aspects of an event at the same time; begins to seriate and classify by dominant feature.

Animism: believes only things that move have consciousness.

Words and numbers: Begins understanding concepts of number and spatial relations.

Reasoning

2 to 5 years

Syncretism: connects ideas and events into confused whole.

Transductive: looks at parts, not whole; parts connected with "and" or "because."

Judgmental: makes judgments on basis of outcomes or consequences to self or on outward appearance.

5 to 8 years

Systematic trial-and-error problem solving and reasoning begins.

Judgments still made based on outcomes for self but now verbalizes intent behind actions.

Language

2 to 5 years

Words: represent labels (name of, one aspect of, or use of objects); imitates words others use without understanding concept or meaning; no understanding of relativity (e.g., more, less).

Self-conversations: talk without trying to convey ideas.

Questions: asked to satisfy curiosity, gain attention, or help to "label" or learn "purpose" of things.

5 to 8 years

Words: represent one or more common names or uses of things; still understands words more generally and less completely than adults; has learned the power of words (words more effective in creating reactions than actions are).

Questions: asked now to learn about the "how" of things and to express frustration.

Play

2 to 5 years

Deferred imitation: pretending based on what has been perceived (e.g., playing "house" or "school").

Parallel: reconfirms skill or releases tensions via exploratory play in presence of others without interacting with them (e.g., sand or water play, riding tricycles).

Social: plays simple games where rules are sacred, has fun only when wins (e.g., Candyland or hide and seek).

5 to 8 years

Symbolic: satisfies self needs and means of coping with conscious or unconscious conflicts by transforming what is real into what is wished was real (e.g., via painting, drawing, puppets, plays).

Social: plays games where rules are collectively made up so everyone wins and has fun (e.g., hopscotch, jumprope, tag).

From Servonsky/Opas: *Nursing Management of Children*, © 1987 Boston: Jones and Bartlett Publishers.

Table B-10. Characteristics of School-Age Children's Thinking: Concrete Operational Stage

Major task

Mastery of classes, quantities, and relations.

Thought processes are not internalized so that overt actions on objects or experiences are not essential; thought is limited by dependence on reality and past experiences, therefore it is of limited complexity; observation is now accurate (not perceptually bound) and objective.

Perception

View of world is concrete but objective and can encompass a variety of perspectives of others.

Thought

Animism is now confirmed to natural phenomena, but loss of animism causes need to cope with concept of death.

The following concepts are mastered.

Reversibility: can perform opposite or compensating act to undo first one

Measurement: and use of various measuring devices

Association, combination, negation

Causality: as different from association or combination

Classification and seriation

Conservation: mass of an object remains the same even if the form and shape change

The following concepts are attained at the approximate ages indicated.

6–7 years
length, number, amount, distance

7–8 years
substance, area, space, mass

9–10 years
weight, time

11 + years
volume, speed (time plus distance), velocity, density

Reasoning

1. Is concrete: mental experiments are done on things that were actually sensed previously or currently by directly organizing immediately given or remembered data
2. Lacks ability to transfer learnings immediately because the learning is still tied to particular objects and situations
3. Progresses from inductive reasoning (8–11 years) to deductive reasoning (11 and over) and uses elementary logic
4. Judges actions by logical effect; separates cause and intent from outcome

Language

Symbols now truly represent real objects and events as well as those concepts attained so far; structure of language now more important; progresses toward increasingly more sociocentric verbal exchanges, sharing ideas among people.

Play

Symbolic play continues

Collaborative play in groups (detailed rules to maintain equality and mutual respect) progresses toward competition (object is to win after "fair" play)

From Servonsky/Opas: *Nursing Management of Children*, © 1987 Boston: Jones and Bartlett Publishers.

Table B-11. Characteristics of Adolescents' Thinking: Formal or Abstract Operational Stage

Major task

Conquest of abstract thought.

Thinks beyond the present, beyond own realistic world and beliefs; has abilities to think about symbols, possible permutations, and combinations.

Perception

Views world beyond the concrete present to include future possibilities, abstractions, and contrary-to-fact propositions.

Thought

Thinking is flexible, powerful, effective, and independent of concrete reality; forms complex concepts that may violate reality; is future-oriented; uses formal logic to operate abstractly and with symbols, therefore comprehends metaphors, irony, satire, proverbs, and parables.

Reasoning

Uses true experimental method and hypothetical deductive and propositional reasoning to act on problems in the following manner:

1. Analyzes the problem, identifies all possibilities, develops hypotheses about what *might* happen
2. Designs experiment to test hypotheses systematically
3. Isolates and controls variables accurately and objectively; observes results
4. Draws appropriate conclusions and can prove assertions
5. Draws appropriate implications of possible statements, and forms unique synthesis

Judges right by what is best for the majority of group.

Language

1. Uses precise and flexible manipulation of language
2. Sees abstract relationships (not just relationships among things); develops concepts of concepts
3. Makes verbal use of symbols of thinking (philosophy, logic, algebra)
4. Deals with form of argument, not just content; may ignore content.

Play

Competitive, complex, and detailed games; thought puzzles or twisters; video or computer games, especially if they require strategy development.

From Servonsky/Opas: *Nursing Management of Children*, © 1987 Boston: Jones and Bartlett Publishers.

APPENDIX C

Childhood Infectious Diseases

Table C-1. Childhood Infectious Diseases

Disease	Incubation period	Transmission	Communi-cability period	Behavioral assessment	Nursing management and medical therapy	Immuniza-tion	Complications
Bacterial infections							
Diphtheria (*Coryne-bacterium diphtheriae*)	2–6 days	Direct contact with infected person or carriers; indirect contact with contaminated articles	Less than 2 weeks, (2 days in treated cases)	Sore throat and membranous covering of tonsils, pharynx, and larynx; malaise; fever; hoarse, brassy cough with stridor.	Maintain strict isolation during period of communicability. Administer antibiotics (penicillin or erythromycin) for bacterial infection. Maintain fluid and electrolyte balance. Encourage bedrest; ensure adequate tissue oxygenation (by suctioning, positioning, humidity). Offer soft foods. Provide quiet, diversionary activities.	DTP; active immunization; one episode usually gives immunity	Produces toxin that has affinity for renal, nerve, and cardiac tissue. Most serious complications are myocarditis and neuritis. May also cause paralysis of the soft palate, larynx, and pharynx; respiratory paralysis; and delirium.
Pertussis (whooping cough) (*Bordetella pertussis*)	5–21 days; usually 7–10 days	Direct contact with respiratory droplet secretions; indirect contact with articles contaminated with respiratory secretions	4 weeks, highest from 1–14 days (during catarrhal stage)	Catarrhal stage with nonspecific respiratory behaviors for 10–14 days progressing to paroxysmal cough, inspiratory whoop, and vomiting; cough worse at night.	Maintain strict isolation, especially of respiratory secretions. Administer antibiotics (erythromycin or ampicillin) for bacterial infection and sedatives (barbiturates) for relief of paroxysms. Minimize coughing episodes. Keep quiet. Promote rest. Provide adequate fluid intake and diet for age.	DTP; active immunization; one episode usually gives immunity	Bronchopneumonia most serious. Also may cause otitis media, atelectasis, bronchietasis, hemorrhage from paroxysms of coughing, encephalitis and permanent brain damage.

Tetanus (lockjaw) (*Clostridium tetani*)	2 days to 3 weeks; usually 7–10 days	Wound contamination by soil containing *C. tetani* bacteria	None; not transmitted from person to person	Tonic spasms of skeletal muscles followed by paroxysmal contractions; muscle stiffness, involving the jaw (lockjaw), neck (sardonic grin), opisthonotos and general body stiffness. Any excitant may precipitate painful paroxysmal spasms lasting from a few seconds to several minutes. Sensorium is clear. Tachycardia, profuse sweating, and low-grade fever may also be present.	Minimize environmental stimuli by keeping room quiet, dark. Prevent overstimulation of child by visitors. Arrange nursing care when child is sedated. Maintain patent airway and adequate ventilation. Provide adequate fluid intake and diet. Give fluids IV, if necessary. Administer antitoxins to neutralize toxin, antibiotics for wound infection, and sedatives or muscle relaxants to reduce muscle contractions and convulsions. Cleanse and debride wound.	DTP; active immunization; no natural immunity; Td booster every 10 years	Produces toxin that has affinity for nervous system. Complications result from interference with pulmonary ventilation by laryngospasm, respiratory muscle spasm, or increased accumulation of pulmonary secretions causing pneumonia, atelectasis, respiratory arrest, and death. May also cause pulmonary emboli, acute gastric ulcers, flexion contractures, and cardiac arrhythmias.
Scarlet fever (group A beta hemolytic streptococci)	2–5 days	Direct contact with infected person or carrier, by droplet spread	10–20 days	Fever, headache, sore throat, exudative tonsillitis, difficulty in swallowing, tender and swollen cervical lymph nodes, erythematous macular rash over body (except face); abdominal pain, anorexia, vomiting	Maintain isolation during period of communicability. Administer antibiotics (penicillin or erythromycin) for infection and analgesics (acetaminophen) for fever and discomfort. Encourage fluids and soft foods that are nonirritating to child's sore throat. Keep in bed while febrile.	None; one episode usually gives immunity	Pneumonia, glomerulonephritis, and rheumatic fever.

(continued on page 622)

Table C-1. *Continued*

Disease	Incubation period	Transmission	Communicability period	Behavioral assessment	Nursing management and medical therapy	Immunization	Complications
Meningococcemia (meningitides)	2–10 days	Direct contact with oral-nasal secretions of infected persons or carriers	While organisms are present in nose and throat	Sepsis with fever, headache, vomiting, malaise, irritability, petechial purpuric rash of skin and mucous membranes; occasionally joint pain.	Maintain isolation during period of communicability, especially of respiratory secretions. Administer antibiotics (penicillin, chloramphenicol, or sulfadiazine) for infection, and analgesics (acetaminophen) for fever and discomfort. Maintain adequate nutrition, hydration, and electrolyte balance.	Vaccines against some bacterial groups exist but are only given in epidemics; one episode provides immunity of unknown duration to bacterial group causing disease	Meningitis, septic arthritis, pneumonia, otitis media, pericarditis, interstitial myocarditis, disseminated intravascular coagulation (DIC), and death.
Cellulitis (*Staphylococcus aureus*; group A beta hemolytic streptococci—most commonly, *Haemophilus influenza* as seen in periorbital cellulitis)	Variable; depends on causative organism	Organism gains entrance through break or trauma to skin	Noninfectious after 24 hr of treatment	Purplish-red coloring, warmth, swelling, pain, tenderness, and limitation of motion at site of involvement. Fever, periorbital swelling, if cellulitis of the eye orbit.	Maintain wound isolation during period of communicability. Keep affected area immobilized. Minimize pain to area with warm compresses and analgesics (acetaminophen). Provide quiet, diversionary activities. Prepare child for incision and drainage procedure, if necessary. Administer antibiotics (penicillin, ampicillin) for infection. Maintain IV for drug administration. Provide adequate fluids and nutrients.	None	Osteomyelitis, septic arthritis.

Botulism (*Clostridium botulinum*)	12–36 hours	Ingestion of improperly canned food containing toxin produced by *C. botulinum* in children and adolescents Germination of spores or vegetative cells of *C. botulinum* in intestine without ingestion of apparent drug or contaminated food source in infants; however, organism has been detected in honey ingested by some affected infants	None; not transmitted from person to person	Weakness, dryness of mouth, motor nerve paralysis, nausea, vomiting, diarrhea, abdominal pain in children. Constipation, lethargy, difficulty feeding and swallowing, poor muscle tone and head control, inability to handle oral secretions in infants.	Support respiratory system (resuscitation, oxygen, maintenance on respirator). Suction oropharyngeal secretions. Administer antitoxin and antibiotics (sodium penicillin G) to children. Most infants respond to antibiotics without antitoxin. Assist in gastric lavage and catharsis. Provide parenteral fluids and nutritional support. Avoid ingestion of honey in infants.	None	Produces toxin that causes a curarelike action on motor endplate resulting in respiratory paralysis, arrest, and death in 1–8 days.
Anthrax (*Bacillus anthracis*)	Less than 7 days	Direct contact with animal products or soil, or eating contaminated meat Enters via broken skin, mucous membrane, or inhalation	While lesions are active	Painless, erythematous papule on skin changing to a vesicle and forming a black eschar; enlarged lymph nodes; abdominal pain; fever; rales in lungs; headache; malaise.	Maintain strict isolation. Administer antibiotics (penicillin, erythromycin, tetracycline, chloramphenicol) for infection. Provide good skin care. Maintain adequate fluids and nutrition.	Vaccine available for children at risk to exposure from infected animals or animal products	Pneumonitis, septicemia.

(*continued on page 624*)

Table C-1. *Continued*

Disease	Incubation period	Transmission	Communicability period	Behavioral assessment	Nursing management and medical therapy	Immunization	Complications
Sepsis or septicemia (*E. coli*, group B beta hemolytic streptococci most common)	Variable; depends on causative organism	Direct contact with infected organisms from maternal genitourinary tract at birth Indirect contact with organisms in environment	Noninfectious after 24 hr of treatment	Poor feeding, failure to thrive, irritability, jaundice, fever, vomiting, diarrhea, dyspnea, cyanosis.	Provide periods of uninterrupted rest. Ensure adequate nutrition and hydration. Maintain IV fluids. Administer antibiotics as appropriate (penicillin, ampicillin for group B streptococci: gentamicin, kanamycin for *E. Coli*). Prevent spread of infection with good handwashing technique. Keep clean and dry. Change position frequently for maximum lung expansion.	None	Meningitis, pneumonia.
Viral infections							
Rubeola (measles)	7–14 days, usually 10–12 days	Direct contact with airborne droplet spread of oropharyngeal secretions	From 4 days before to 4 days after rash	Fever, coryza with a brassy cough, conjunctivitis, enlarged lymph nodes, photophobia and Koplik's spots (small red spots with bluish white centers on buccal mucosa) 2–5 days before rash. Koplik's spots usually disappear 2 days after rash, which is a generalized maculopapular eruption (small reddish brown or pink macules changing to papules) that fade on pressure.	Maintain respiratory isolation during communicability period. Prevent respiratory infection by minimizing exposure to organisms and persons harboring them. Provide adequate nutrition. Liquefy secretions by providing fluids and humidity. Minimize discomfort with analgesics (acetaminophen). Comfort eyes by dimming lights. Maintain rest during febrile stage.	MMR; active immunization, one episode usually gives immunity	Otitis media, deafness, pneumonia, tracheobronchitis, encephalitis, brain damage.

				Rash begins behind ears or on forehead or cheeks, progresses to extremities, and lasts about 4 days.			
Rubella (German measles)	2–3 weeks; average 16 days	Direct or indirect contact with droplets, secretions, blood, urine, or stools of infected persons	From 1 week before to 1 week after rash	Slight fever, mild coryza, diffuse macular rash lasting 3 days; postauricular and occipital lymph node enlargement; occasionally, headaches and conjunctivitis; arthralgias.	Maintain isolation during communicability period. Caution against exposure to pregnant women. Minimize discomfort with analgesics (acetaminophen). Provide adequate hydration and nutrition.	MMR, active immunization, one episode usually gives immunity	Complications are rare (encephalitis may occur). Rubella is a mild disease in childhood; greatest danger is birth defects to fetus when contracted during pregnancy.
Varicella (chickenpox)	2–3 weeks; average 13–17 days	Direct contact with droplets. Indirect contact with skin lesion, discharges, or nasal pharyngeal secretions	From 5 days before rash until all lesions have crusted	Fever, fatigue, malaise, headache; pruritic rash starting as erythematous, progressing to macular, papular, vesicular, and scabs with eventual crusting (usually in less than a week); rash begins on the head and progresses to rest of body.	Maintain isolation while communicable. Assure adequate hydration by encouraging fluids. Provide adequate nutrition. Prevent secondary skin infection by keeping area clean and dry and minimizing itching. Relieve itching with calamine lotion, tepid sponge baths, and oral antipruritic or antihistamine medications. Keep fingernails trimmed and clean. Apply mittens or gloves, if necessary. Keep pajamas and linens clean and smooth. Provide diversionary activities.	None, one episode usually gives immunity	Bacterial skin infection, Reye's syndrome, pneumonia, and encephalitis. Children at risk for severe, and often fatal, varicella are those receiving corticosteroids or antimetabolites.

(continued on page 626)

Table C-1. *Continued*

Disease	Incubation period	Transmission	Communi-cability period	Behavioral assessment	Nursing management and medical therapy	Immuniza-tion	Complications
Parotitis (Mumps)	12–26 days; usually 18 days	Direct contact, droplet spread Indirect contact, secretions of oral cavity or respiratory tract	From 1 week prior to swelling until swelling subsides	Low-grade fever and malaise followed by swelling and pain in one or more (often bilateral) salivary glands (usually parotid); difficulty in swallowing; earache; pain and swelling of glands usually lasts 6–10 days.	Maintain strict isolation during period of communicability. Provide adequate rest until swelling subsides. Minimize discomfort with analgesics (acetaminophen) and cool or warm compresses. Provide fluids and soft, bland diet (foods that do not need much chewing and are not sour or spicy). Give mouth care frequently.	MMR; active immunization; one episode usually gives immunity	Encephalitis, orchitis, pancreatitis, oophoritis, deafness, and (rarely) arthritis, myocarditis. When contracted by adolescent and adult males, it can cause sterility.
Poliomyelitis	3–35 days; usually 10–12 days	Direct contact—fecal-oral and pharyngeal-oropharyngeal routes	Up to 6 weeks or longer	Initially, headache, fever, nausea, vomiting, diarrhea (flulike behaviors); then, intense headache, stiff neck, meningeal irritation, and muscular pain and tenderness progressing to paralysis, if severe.	Maintain isolation with enteric precautions. Keep on strict bedrest during acute stage. Support respirations with assisted ventilation if necessary. Position in correct body alignment to prevent contractures. Turn frequently to prevent decubitus ulcers. Perform range of motion exercises to extremities. Encourage flexion and contraction of muscles and movement.	TOPV; active immunization	Paralysis, usually asymmetrical and flaccid. Death from pulmonary paralysis.

					Maintain adequate nutrition and hydration.		
Rabies	10 days to 8 weeks; occasionally up to 1 year	Saliva of rabid animal entering a break in the skin	Depends on amount, virulence, and site of inoculation	Initially, pain, numbness, or tingling around wound; headache; fever; vomiting; sore throat; drowsiness; restlessness; irritability. Then photophobia, paralysis, muscle spasms of pharyngeal and laryngeal muscles causing inability to swallow and excessive salivation; extreme excitation; hydrophobia.	Maintain strict isolation. Prevent unnecessary stimulation. Maintain hydration via IV fluids. Ensure adequate oxygenation. Suction excess salivary secretions. Turn frequently to prevent pooling of secretions. Protect from injury. Support family. Medical prophylaxis therapy after exposure includes: prompt and thorough cleansing of the wound; quarantine the offending animal; inoculation for passive antibody with human rabies immune globulin (preferred treatment) or equine antiserum (anaphylaxis occurs in 25 percent of recipients sensitive to equine antiserum, which is derived from horse serum); and active immunization with human diploid cell vaccine (HDCV).	Preexposure prophylaxis with human diploid cell vaccine (HDCV) for child at risk to rabid animal exposure.	Once behaviors of the disease develop, outcome is usually fatal. Laryngospasm, respiratory paralysis, and death within 1 week.

(*continued on page 628*)

Table C-1. *Continued*

Disease	Incubation period	Transmission	Communicability period	Behavioral assessment	Nursing management and medical therapy	Immunization	Complications
					Children should be told to avoid all stray or wild animals, such as dogs, squirrels, and raccoons, even though they may appear to be tame.		
Influenza	1–4 days	Direct contact, airborne droplet spread	1 day prior to 1 week after onset of behaviors	Fever, chills, rhinorrhea, sneezing, cough, coryza, sore throat, nausea, vomiting	Provide adequate rest while behaviors are present. Increase oral fluid intake. Administer analgesics (acetaminophen) for pain and discomfort, nasal decongestants, cough suppressants, expectorants, and/or antihistamines as necessary. Remove nasal drainage (with bulb syringe in infants). Maintain adequate nutrition.	Influenza virus vaccine; active immunization for high-risk individuals	Otitis media, pneumonia, sinusitis, pulmonary edema, Reye's syndrome, cardiac failure.
Mononucleosis	7–50 days; 2–6 weeks	Direct contact with oral secretions	During acute illness; up to 6 months after	Fever, fatigue, enlarged lymph nodes (especially cervical lymph nodes), sore throat, malaise, enlarged liver and spleen, periorbital edema, maculopapular rash.	Maintain adequate rest. Prevent fatigue. Avoid activity causing blunt trauma to the abdomen. Administer analgesics (acetaminophen) for discomfort and corticosteroids, if indicated, during acute presenting behaviors of the disease. Provide adequate nutrition.	None; one episode usually gives immunity	Hepatitis, myocarditis, meningoencephalitis.

Cytomegalovirus infection (CMV)	Unknown	Transplacental at birth Postnatal (exact route unknown through contact with infectious secretions (e.g., urine, semen, saliva, tears, breast milk)	Unknown, may be several years	Usually without presenting behaviors, unless congenital; then failure to thrive, jaundice, petechial rash, deafness, enlarged liver and spleen, respiratory distress.	Maintain strict isolation of infants. Provide adequate fluids and nutrition. Administer blood transfusions, if necessary. Administer medications (adenine arabinoside), if indicated. Provide adequate rest and sensory stimulation.	None	Encephalitis, mental retardation, blindness, deafness, microcephaly in congenital CMV. Bone marrow depression, pneumonia, encephalitis, and hepatitis in acquired CMV.
Exanthem subitum (roseola)	7–17 days; usually 10 days	Unknown	Unknown	High fever (above 40.6°C) for several days before appearance of diffuse maculopapular rash largely confined to the trunk; fever breaks before appearance of rash.	Prevent convulsions due to high fever. Lower temperature with tepid sponge baths, antipyretics (acetaminophen). Provide adequate fluid and nutritional intake. Prevent injury during convulsions (should they occur when febrile).	None	Febrile seizure disorder.
Fungal infections							
Histoplasmosis (*Histoplasma capsulatum*)	5–18 days	Inhalation of airborne spores	Not usually transmitted from person to person	Initially, without presenting behaviors, then malaise, slight fever, cough, headache, irritability (mild, self-limited respiratory disease)—can progress to fever, prostration, dyspnea, chest pain, erythema nodosum, enlarged liver and lymph nodes, mouth and gastrointestinal ulcerations (disseminated disease).	Ensure maximum aeration of lungs. Provide adequate hydration (either by mouth or parenterally). Turn, cough, and deep breathe frequently. Administer analgesics (acetaminophen) for discomfort. Administer antibiotic (amphotericin B) for infection if indicated.	None	Pneumonia, chronic pulmonary disease, hepatitis, meningitis, endocarditis, death.

(continued on page 630)

Table C-1. *Continued*

Disease	Incubation period	Transmission	Communicability period	Behavioral assessment	Nursing management and medical therapy	Immunization	Complications
Coccidioidomycosis (valley fever) (*Coccidioides immitis*)	1–3 weeks; average 10–16 days	Inhalation of spores in dust or rarely, entry through injured skin	Not usually transmitted from person to person	Without presenting behaviors, or slight fever, cough, headache that may progress to erythema nodosum with granulomatous formations of the skin, lungs, and other organs.	Maintain bedrest. Ensure adequate aeration of lungs. Provide adequate hydration. Turn, cough, and deep breathe frequently. Minimize discomfort. Administer antibiotic (amphotericin B) for infection if indicated.	None	Lung lesions and abscesses throughout the body.
Candidiasis, moniliasis (thrush) (*Candida albicans*)	Variable; usually within 1 week	Direct contact—person to person (infants contract it during passage through vagina at birth) or by self-inoculation Indirect contact with contaminated articles	While lesions present	Oral thrush—white placques on erythematous macular lesions on buccal membrane and tongue surface. Cutaneous—erythematous macular, sharply circumscribed, raw, angry-looking lesions of skin (especially diaper area in infants). Vagina—thick, white discharge.	Maintain isolation during period of communicability. Administer antifungal medication to area of involvement (nystatin solution orally, nystatin ointment topically, nystatin suppositories vaginally). Maintain adequate nutrition. Clean mouth frequently. Expose skin lesions to air and heat. Keep skin lesions clean and dry.	None	Pneumonia, endocarditis.

Rickettsial infections							
Rocky Mountain spotted fever (*Rickettsia rickettsii*)	2–12 days, usually 4–8 days	By vector—wood and dog ticks	Not transmitted from person to person	History of tick bite, fever, chills, anorexia, headache 3–4 days prior to appearance of rash. Rash—peripheral, maculopapular, purpuric, and petechial, involving ankles, wrists, and lower legs and spreading centrally. Periorbital edema progressing to generalized edema of extremities.	Complete removal of the entire tick from child's skin. Minimize discomfort with positioning and analgesics (acetaminophen). Maintain adequate hydration. Ensure adequate output. Protect edematous skin from trauma. Keep skin dry and clean. Maintain adequate circulation. Administer antibiotics to control infection (tetracycline, chloramphenicol), and antipyretics for fever (acetaminophen). Maintain adequate nutrition.	Vaccine available for high-risk individuals but is of dubious efficacy.	Involvement of liver, kidneys, brain, and heart resulting in residual damage, possibly death.

From Servonsky/Opas: *Nursing Management of Children*, © 1987 Boston: Jones and Bartlett Publishers.

APPENDIX D

Mental Health Assessment Tools

D-1. Semantic Differential Scale for Assessing Patients' Feelings

Table D-1. Semantic Differential Scale for Assessing Patients' Feelings

DIRECTIONS: To help give you better care, we'd like to know how you feel about yourself at this time. One way to do this is to measure what certain words mean to you.

On this questionnaire, 12 pairs of adjectives are separated by lines composed of 7 boxes. On each line, place a check in the box that most closely describes your feelings about yourself. For example, which box below best describes you at this time?

Short 1	2	3	4	5	6	Tall 7

Score values:		
	1 Very short	5 Slightly tall
	2 Short	6 Tall
	3 Slightly short	7 Very Tall
	4 Neutral	

If you think you are very tall, place a check in box #7. If you are just tall, place a check in box #6.

The answers you give should apply only to how you feel right now. You may feel differently tomorrow. There are no wrong answers.

	1	2	3	4	5	6	7	
Changeable	☐	☐	☐	☐	☐	☐	☐	Stable
Uncertain	☐	☐	☐	☐	☐	☐	☐	Confident
Dejected	☐	☐	☐	☐	☐	☐	☐	Happy
Detached	☐	☐	☐	☐	☐	☐	☐	Involved
Confused	☐	☐	☐	☐	☐	☐	☐	Organized
Inattentive	☐	☐	☐	☐	☐	☐	☐	Concerned
Indifferent	☐	☐	☐	☐	☐	☐	☐	Enthusiastic
Passive	☐	☐	☐	☐	☐	☐	☐	Active
Uninterested	☐	☐	☐	☐	☐	☐	☐	Interested
Lonely	☐	☐	☐	☐	☐	☐	☐	Friendly
Uncomfortable	☐	☐	☐	☐	☐	☐	☐	Comfortable
Nervous	☐	☐	☐	☐	☐	☐	☐	Calm

L. J. Avillo, "Semantic Differential Scale for Assessing Patients' Feelings," *Instruments for Measuring Nursing Practice and Other Health Care Variables.* Vol. 1, 1978, 209–211, Health Manpower References, U.S. DHEW Publication No. HRA 78–53. Reprinted with permission.

APPENDIX E

Skin Alterations, Assessment, and Nursing Management

Table E-1. Viral, Bacterial, and Fungal Skin Alterations

Alteration	Epidemiology and etiology	Pathophysiology	Behavioral assessment
Aphthous stomatitis (canker sores)	May be an autoimmune disorder Occurs in all ages, less in children May be precipitated by emotional stress, trauma, hormonal changes (e.g., menstruation)	Exact source of aphthous stomatitis is unknown, but *Streptococcus sanguis* has been found in some lesions. Erosions and ulcerations invade the oral mucous membrane.	Prior to appearance of lesions, child may feel tingling or stinging sensation. Local erythema develops 24–48 hr later, followed by tiny superficial grayish white erosions. Area increases in size, evolving into shallow ulcers covered by gray membrane, surrounded by sharp borders and bright red areola. Lesions measure 3–6 mm in diameter and heal spontaneously in 8–12 days.
Cellulitis	Usually the result of *Hemophilus influenzae*, a bacterium endemic in some communities Usually occurs in children ages 1 month to 4 years Often associated with septicemia; often follows wound or trauma	Bacteria usually reside in nasopharynx, then spread locally or via bloodstream, causing acute inflammation of skin, especially deeper subcutaneous tissues.	Erythema, swelling, and tenderness of the area are seen. Child may be extremely ill and toxic, with an upper respiratory infection and septicemia. In 50% of *H. influenzae* cases, lesion is dusky red, bluish, or purplish red; common sites are the face or cheek, neck, periorbital area, possibly the extremities.
Furuncles/ carbuncles (boils)	Occur usually in children, adolescents, and young adults; usually males Occur in chronic staphylococcal "carriers," in people who wear tight collars or belts, and in people who suffer from obesity, diabetes, scabies, pediculosis, and abrasions	A furuncle is an acute, deep-seated, inflammatory nodule that develops in and around a hair follicle. A carbuncle is a necrotizing infection of the skin and subcutaneous tissue, composed of a cluster of furuncles, with multiple drainage sinuses.	Child has throbbing pain, extreme tenderness, low-grade fever, malaise. Lesion is red, firm, nodular, then fluctuant; then ruptures into ulcer with red halo. Usually round, scattered, isolated or few multiple lesions; occur only at hair follicles or in areas subject to friction and sweating; nose, neck, face, axillae, buttocks, paronychia (area around the nail). A carbuncle is a larger, draining version of a furuncle.
Tinea capitis (ringworm of the scalp)	Occurs primarily in children, rarely in adults Spreads from child to child, and via barber, hats, theater seats, pets	*Microsporum* and *Trichophyton* fungi invade hair shaft, causing inflammation, scaling, and broken shafts.	Alopecia with "black dot" appearance may be seen where hair shaft broke off. Lesions may be round or oval, sometimes irregular, 1–6 cm diameter. More severe types appear as boggy, elevated, purulent, inflamed nodule. Favus types may cause cutaneous atrophy, scarring, baldness, crusts.

Diagnostic criteria	Medical therapy	Complications and prognosis	Nursing management
Diagnosis by inspection; cannot detect any virus or bacteria on culture	Treatment is usually palliative. Most effective appears to be tetracycline suspension four times a day for 5 to 7 days. May also use lidocaine viscous. Silver nitrate may also be used, as well as topical corticosteroids.	No complications; lesions heal spontaneously in 10 to 14 days even if not treated.	Discuss with child possible causes of lesions, to help avoid recurrence.
Diagnosis by needle aspiration for gram stain and bacterial culture	Treated with antibiotics, usually ampicillin; if staphylococci detected, penicillinase-resistant penicillins are used; if organism cannot be identified, both antibiotics are used.	May develop septicemia; otherwise, prognosis is good.	Observe for behaviors of septicemia, as well as behaviors of drug toxicity or resistance.
Pustules may be aspirated for gram stain, culture, and antibiotic sensitivity studies; blood cultures may be done if septicemia suspected	*Simple:* Local warm, moist compresses often help. Severe or persistent infections may require systemic antibiotics, then incision and drainage. *Carbuncles:* Treated with systemic antibiotics and incision and drainage. *Recurrent:* Patient may be harboring staphylococci in nares, perineum or body folds. Controlled with frequent showers with iodine soap (no baths) and daily antibacterial ointment in nares.	May develop septicemia or tendency for recurrence; if treated properly, prognosis is good.	Teach child and family how to apply compresses of local heat; avoid burning. Observe for behaviors of septicemia. Discuss methods of preventing reinfection.
Some organisms that cause tinea capitis flouresce under Wood's lamp; may also see fungus in potassium hydroxide wet-mount and fungal cultures	Systemic griseofulvin, which attaches to newly formed keratin in hair and becomes fungistatic, is given for 6–8 weeks or more. Topical antifungal agents are ineffective.	Griseofulvin may cause several side effects (e.g., hypersensitivity, aplastic anemia, gastrointestinal disturbances, headaches, dizziness).	Since griseofulvin absorbs better after a fatty meal, give with milk or ice cream. Advise child and family to continue full course of medication, even if behaviors of the alteration disappear, it prevents recurrences. Discuss methods to prevent spread of infection.

Table E-1. *Continued*

Alteration	Epidemiology and etiology	Pathophysiology	Behavioral assessment
Tinea corporis (ringworm of the body)	Occurs in all ages, especially those who work with animals Occurs more often in warm, humid climates, or in people with leukemia, diabetes	Same organisms as in tinea capitis invade the superficial layers of the skin.	Small to large scaling may occur, with sharply marginated plaques with or without pustules or vesicles. Lesions are annular, with peripheral enlargement and central clearing. Single and occasionally multiple scattered lesions appear on the exposed areas of the body.
Tinea pedis (athlete's foot)	Unusual in young children; most common ringworm infection in adolescents and adults Most often caused by *Trichophyton* fungus	Fungus causes inflammation, primarily in intertriginous areas.	Erythemia, scaling, and vesiculopustular eruption occur, with maceration and peeling of skin. Lesions usually localized to interdigital webs and sides of toes; dorsum of foot usually remains clear.

From Servonsky/Opas: *Nursing Management of Children*, © 1987 Boston: Jones and Bartlett Publishers.

Diagnostic criteria	Medical therapy	Complications and prognosis	Nursing management
Diagnosis is based on classic circular shape, but may be masked by steroids and confused with several other disorders Also same techniques as used for tinea capitis	Antifungals such as clourimazole, haloprogin, micronazole, or tolnaftate are rubbed in twice a day. Application is continued for 2–3 weeks, even if lesions clear, if resistant, may need griseofulvin.	No complications; prognosis is very good with treatment.	Advise child and family to continue full course of medication, even if lesions disappear. Discuss methods to avoid recurrences (e.g., avoid pets until they have been checked and treated for ringworm).
Diagnosis by inspection; confirmed by potassium hydroxide mount and fungal cultures	Undecylenic acid (Desenex) or tolnaftate (Tinactin) foot powder is used, and feet are kept dry. If severe, systemic griseofulvin is used. May also use wet compresses of Burow's solution (aluminum acetate).	No complications, unless lack of treatment leads to more widespread infection; prognosis is excellent if treated.	Discuss with child and family methods to keep feet dry; thorough drying after bathing, avoiding occlusive footwear, exposing to air frequently, avoiding nylon socks, changing cotton socks twice a day. Suggest wearing rubber thongs in shower to avoid spreading fungus.

Table E-2. Summary Nursing Care Plan for a Child with Impetigo

Assessment	Nursing diagnosis	Patient goal	Nursing management
Vesicles, pustules, and bullae form on skin; yellow crusts are present	Impairment of skin integrity	The child's lesions will heal and disappear.	Teach and assist child and family in cleansing skin and removing crusts, and applying ordered topical ointment. If oral antibiotics are ordered, instruct child and family that child must take entire prescription; i.e., to continue medication even when lesions disappear (to avoid resistant strain of bacteria).
Areas of eczema and scabies Environmental history of crowded living conditions, poor hygiene, neglected minor trauma	Potential for injury related to infection	Child's lesions will be contained within originally infected area. Child's lesions will not become worse through rubbing or scratching. Child's lesions will not be spread to other people.	Discuss with child and family methods to prevent spread of infection; e.g., do not touch lesions, wash hands if lesions are accidentally touched, use separate washcloths, and so on. Encourage child not to rub or scratch lesions: this causes spread of lesions and secondary changes (e.g., excoriations). Recommend that young child wear mittens, especially while sleeping. Examine close contacts for lesions; refer to physician for treatment.
Child states that "these sores look bad"	Disturbance in self-concept	Child will develop or maintain a healthy self-concept	Involve child in care of lesions as much as possible, to give some sense of control Explain that lesions are only temporary if treated properly Praise positive accomplishments of child Provide nursing management to the child in a nonjudgmental manner to enhance the child's dignity. Encourage child to groom self and wear clothing that enhances physical appearance and emotional self-esteem.

From Servonsky/Opas: *Nursing Management of Children*, © 1987 Boston: Jones and Bartlett Publishers.

Table E-3. Insect Infestations

Alteration/parasite	Epidemiology and etiology	Pathophysiology	Behavioral assessment
Harvest mite (red bug, chigger); similar appearance to scabies	Most common in southern United States Live in grain stems, grasses, bushes Attach selves to skin near belts, bras, boots or shoe tops	Only larvae cause behaviors of infestation; attach to skin, inject secretion that causes itching	Intense itching a few hours after exposure, reaching peak on second day, decreasing next 5–6 days Bright red papules, 1–2 mm in diameter; also scratch marks, urticaria, diffuse erythema May last for months
Papular urticaria (lichen urticatus)	Common disease of childhood, caused by sensitivity reaction to bites of fleas, mosquitoes, bedbugs, other insects May be seen as young as age 2 weeks, but usually at 2–7 years, especially if history of allergies Usually occurs in late spring and summer	Sensitivity reaction to bites causes intercellular and intracellular edema and infiltration of lymphocytes	Lesions group in clusters on exposed areas of body; lesions are 3–10 mm firm papules with wheals Persist 2–10 days, or 3–4 years if exposure to insects continues Secondary changes include excoriation, lichenification, infected crusts, and ulcerations from rubbing or scratching
Pediculosis (lice); six-legged, wingless insects with translucent, gray, or grayish white 1–4 mm bodies Body lice are large, pubic lice are crablike; ova or nits are oval, grayish or yellowish white in color, 0.3–0.8 mm	Lice are an ancient plague, occurring in times of stress or overcrowding, and spreading by human contact and infested objects (e.g., clothes, furniture)	Louse pierces skin and secretes a poisonous salivary secretion; combination of puncture and saliva causes pruritic dermatitis May also transmit diseases such as typhus and trench fever	Moderate to severe pruritus; possible secondary pyoderma from scratching; possible wheals, excoriations, lymphadenopathy Blue spots (maculae caeruleae) may appear on pubic area, abdomen, or thighs, possibly from altered blood pigments or saliva from the louse Nits may attach to hair shafts on head or pubic area: these differ from dandruff in not being easily moved along shaft with comb or fingernail

Diagnostic criteria	Medical therapy	Complications and prognosis	Nursing management
Diagnosis by inspection and histologic examination	Treatment primarily symptomatic, with antihistamines, cool baths or compresses, topical steroids; clear nail polish may provide immediate relief by asphyxiating the mite If secondary infection, antibiotics used Insect repellants or toxicants (benzyl benzoate) used to prevent bites	Pruritus may persist for months Secondary infection may occur	Discuss with child and family methods for avoiding bites (not walking in grassy or bushy areas without proper clothing and repellant). Reinforce physician's instructions for symptomatic relief.
Diagnosis based on history of bites and microscopic examination	Antipruritics, topical calamine lotion, or corticosteroids used for symptomatic relief Prevention involves spraying household, especially baseboards, basements, bedframes, and upholstery, and spraying affected pets	May develop secondary infection from scratching; otherwise prognosis is very good	Discuss with family the need for spraying house and pets. Advise avoiding unsprayed animals, especially if a child is susceptible to alteration.
Diagnosis based on inspection of lice and nits in hair and clothing, as well as microscopic examination; Wood's lamp may be used (lice appear fluorescent)	Most popular and effective treatment is 1.0% gamma benzene hexachloride (Kwell) lotion or shampoo Proper hygiene and laundering are promoted, as lice live mainly in clothing	Possible drug toxicity; prognosis is very good if treated	Assess children for presence of lice and nits. Observe for behaviors of toxicity. Advise family to wash clothing and bedding. Advise against child sharing hats or combs with friends. Advise family to remove all dead nits after Kwell; some larvae may lie dormant. Allow family to air concerns about social embarrassment; state that lice have no respect for social class or income level.

(continued on page 644)

Table E-3. *Continued*

Alteration/parasite	Epidemiology and etiology	Pathophysiology	Behavioral assessment
Scabies (itch mite); pinpoint, oval, eight-legged, translucent, pearly gray, 0.5-mm-long parasite	Found most often in children under 5 or young adults (often through sexual contact) Spreads by skin-to-skin contact Epidemics occur in cycles every 30 years (latest began in 1971, began subsiding in 1982) Incubation period 1 month	Female mite burrows into stratum corneum and lays eggs in burrows, causing sensitization of host	*Primary lesions:* "Burrows" with gray or skin-colored ridges 0.5–1.0 cm long, linear or wavy with minute vesicle or papule at end of burrow; after months, possible brownish-red indurated nodules (1–2 cm); child may have severe pruritus *Secondary lesions:* Excoriations, crusts of bacterial infection, urticarial papules, eczematous plaques *Sites:* Burrows on palms (90%), wrists, penis, nipples, axillae, natal cleft (between buttocks, above anus); vesicles on sides of fingers; nodules on scrotum, penis, buttocks, groin, axillary folds, upper back, abdomen, thighs
Ticks (hard and soft); large, globular arachnids with short legs and hard leathery skin	Live in grass, shrubs, vines, bushes, animals Female tick attaches self to skin and sucks blood from superficial blood vessels	Toxin secreted by tick may cause pyrexia Neurotoxin injected during several days of tick engorging itself on blood may cause paralysis; may cause Rocky Mountain spotted fever	Initial bite usually painless but develops into infiltrated lesion with surrounding erythematous halo; persists 1–2 weeks Tick mouth parts in the wound cause small, pruritic nodules *Pyrexia:* Fever, chills, headache, vomiting, abdominal pain. Improvement 12–36 hr after tick removed *Paralysis:* Flaccid, ascending motor paralysis; death may result from respiratory paralysis

Diagnostic criteria	Medical therapy	Complications and prognosis	Nursing management
Diagnosis based on history of itching, distribution of lesions, microscopic examination; burrows are very diagnostic	Topical application of 1.0% gamma benzene hexachloride (Kwell) used most often; 10% Crotamiton, sulfur in petrolatum, 12.5–25% benzyl benzoate also used Ointment is applied for 12 hr, then washed off to avoid toxic level of absorption; may be repeated 1 week later if more larvae are detected Antipruritics and antibiotics used as needed	Possible drug toxicity Secondary infection from streptococci may lead to nephritis	Instruct child and family on proper use of medications. Observe for behaviors of toxicity (eczema, urticaria, aplastic anemia, alopecia, irritability, nausea, vomiting, amblyopia, headache, dizziness, convulsions; these usually occur if medication ingested or overused. Discuss with family the need to launder clothing, bedding, curtains. Overbathing may cause skin irritation. Pets may carry scabies; advise family to consult veterinarian.
Diagnosis based on history of tick bite or observation of tick on skin	Tick removed by heat, nail polish, mineral oil, petrolatum, ether, chloroform, or liquid nitrogen; removal of mouth parts must be ensured (may need punch biopsy) Paralysis disappears spontaneously 24 hr after tick removed Prevent with repellants	Respiratory paralysis may cause death if tick not removed; Rocky Mountain spotted fever can be a serious complication; otherwise, prognosis is good	Advise child and family to avoid tick-infested areas, or to use effective repellants. If child has progressive paralysis of unknown origin, examine entire body for hidden tick.

From Servonsky/Opas: *Nursing Management of Children*, © 1987 Boston: Jones and Bartlett Publishers.

Table E-4. Animal and Insect Inflicted Injuries

Injury	Behavioral assessment	Complications	Nursing management
Human bite	Localized redness and edema, teeth marks, potential break of the skin and bleeding	Secondary infection from streptococci or staphylococci	Culture wound, cleanse wound with high-pressure flow of normal saline, administer ordered antibiotics, culture the mouth and throat of the identified assailant, teach wound care and behaviors of secondary infection.
Dog bite	Localized redness and edema, teeth marks, potential break or tearing of the skin and bleeding, absence of tissue	Secondary infection from *Pasturella multocida*	Remove clothing and cleanse wound with high-pressure flow of normal saline; administer ordered analgesics, antibiotics, and tetanus vaccine; teach wound care and behaviors of secondary infection; teach children to stay away from dogs who are unknown, eating, or irritable.
Wild animal bite	Same as for dog bites	Rabies (rare), secondary infection from *Streptobacillus moniliformis* or *Spirillum minus*	Cleanse wound with high-pressure flow of normal saline; administer ordered analgesics, antibiotics, and antitoxins; teach wound care and behaviors of secondary infection; teach children to keep a distance between themselves and all wild animals.
Cat scratch	Localized redness and edema, claw marks, potential break of the skin and bleeding	Secondary infection from *Pasturella multocida, Staphylococcus epidermidis, Streptococcus viridans* and diptheroides	Cleanse wound with normal saline or soap and water, teach wound care and behaviors of secondary infection.
Venomous snake bite	Localized edema, presence of fang marks, progressive edema, paresthesia, and paralysis	Paralysis, respiratory insufficiency, disseminated intravascular coagulation, cardiac arrest	Know the endemic venomous snakes for the area, observe the site for fang marks, observe every 15 minutes for progression of neurologic behaviors, administer ordered antivenin, keep area immobilized and child quiet, release tourniquet every 15 minutes, check nailbeds for capillary refill, do not apply ice, have resuscitation equipment available, teach children precautions for hiking in deserts.
Venomous spider bite	Localized redness, nausea, sweating and fever, headache, muscle cramps, apprehension, paresthesias or hyperestheias	Ulceration and necrosis of the bite area, coma	Observe the site for an inoculation (puncture), assess every 15 minutes for progression of neurologic behaviors and induration, administer ordered antivenin (if available), teach care of ulceration, administration of ordered antibiotics for prophylaxis of secondary infection, and precautions for children's play areas.
Nonvenomous spider bite	Localized redness and itching	Localized infection from skin abrasion	Observe site for an inoculation, observe for unexpected systemic behaviors, teach children precautions for play in basements, sheds, and wood piles.

Table E-4. *Continued*

Injury	Behavioral assessment	Complications	Nursing management
Jellyfish sting	Painful stinging sensation, localized redness and itching, chills and fever, nausea and vomiting, weakness	Respiratory failure and death	Cleanse area with water; to cause diffusion of the venom through the skin, apply seaweed, wet teabags, or lime juice; teach children to observe for sealife when walking on beaches and in the ocean.
Bee sting	Localized itching, appearance of a stinger, histamine response	Anaphylaxis, respiratory failure and death	Remove stinger, apply a paste of baking soda to draw out the stinger, administer ordered antihistamines, observe for behaviors of anaphylaxis, apply topical antihistamines (such as calamine lotion) for localized itching and irritation.
Mosquito bite	Localized itching, histamine response	Localized infection from skin abrasion	Teach prophylactic use of mosquito repellants, apply topical antihistamines for localized itching and irritation.
Flea bite	Localized itching, histamine response	Localized infection from skin abrasion	Teach family to keep home and pets free of fleas and to change clothes and bedding when fleas are uncontrolled, apply topical antihistamines for localized itching and irritation, cut fingernails to prevent secondary infections from skin abrasion, teach children good health habits.

From Servonsky/Opas: *Nursing Management of Children*, © 1987 Boston: Jones and Bartlett Publishers.

APPENDIX F

Common Laboratory Values

Table F-1. Blood Gas Studies

Substance determined	Normal values	Clinical implications: Increase	Clinical implications: Decrease
Alveolar to oxygen gradient (A-a DO_2 ratio)	9 torr or less in a patient breathing room air	Mucus plugs Bronchospasm Airway collapse in: Asthma Bronchitis Emphysema Hypoxemia caused by: Pneumothorax Atelectasis Emboli Edema	
Base excess/ Deficit	(Plus or minus 3 mEq./l.)	Nonvolatile acid deficit	Nonrespiratory or metabolic disturbance nonvolatile acid accumulation due to a dietary intake, lactic acid, ketoacidosis
Blood pH	Arterial blood—7.35–7.45 Venous blood—7.34–7.41	Alkalemia Loss of gastric juice Vomiting Potassium or chloride depletion Excessive bicarbonate or lactate administration Hyperventilation Hysteria Lack of oxygen Toxic stimulation of the respiratory centers: High fever Cerebral hemorrhage Excessive artificial respiration Salicylates	Acidemia Renal failure Diabetic ketoacidosis Lactic acidosis Anaerobic metabolism Hypoxia Diarrhea Depression of respiratory centers: Drug overdose Barbiturate toxicity Anesthetics Interference with mechanized function of thoracic cage Deformity of thoracic cage Kyphoscoliosis Airway obstruction: Extra thoracic tumors Asthma Bronchitis Emphysema Circulatory disorders; Congestive heart failure Shock
Carbon dioxide (CO_2) Total carbon dioxide (CO_2)	24–30 mEq./l.	Severe vomiting Emphysema Aldosteronism Mercurial diuretics	Severe diarrhea Starvation Acute renal failure Salicylate toxicity Diabetic acidosis Chlorothiazide Diuretics
Oxygen (O_2) content	Arterial blood—15–22 Vol % Venous blood—11–16 Vol %		Chronic obstructive lung disease Respiratory complications postoperatively Flail chest Kyphoscoliosis Neuromuscular impairment Obesity hypoventilation

Source: From Fishbach, F. *Manual of Laboratory Diagnostic Tests for Nurses.* Philadelphia: Lippincott, 1980. Used with permission.

Table F-1. *Continued*

Substance determined	Normal values	Clinical implications: Increase	Clinical implications: Decrease
Oxygen saturation (SO_2)	(SaO_2) 95% or higher (S_vO_2) = 75%		
Partial pressure of carbon dioxide (PCO_2)	$PaCO_2$ 35–45 torr P_vCO_2 41–51 torr	Hypoventilation Obstructive lung disease Chronic bronchitis Emphysema Reduced function of respiratory center Over reaction Head trauma Anesthesia Pickwickian syndrome	Hyperventilation Hypoxia Nervousness Anxiety Pulmonary emboli Pregnancy
Partial pressure of oxygen (PO_2)	PaO_2 80 torr or greater P_vO_2 30–40 torr	Polycythemia Hyperventilation Increased frequency of breathing	Anemias Cardiac decompensation Insufficient atmospheric oxygen Intercardiac shunts Chronic obstructive or restrictive pulmonary disease Hypoventilation due to neuromuscular disease Decreased arterial PO_2 With normal or decreased arterial blood PCO_2 Tension in: Diffuse interstitial Pulmonary infiltration Pulmonary edema Pulmonary embolism Postoperative extracorporeal circulation

Table F-2. Average Range of Normal Blood Values Measured at Different Ages

Component	Premature	Full-term	2 days	7 days	14 days	2 months
Hemoglobin, gm/100 ml	13–18	13.7–20	18–21.2	196	13–20	
RBC/cu mm, in millions	5–6	5–6	5.3–5.6	5.3	5–5.1	
Nucleated RBC, %	5–15	1–5	1–2	0*		
Hematocrit, gm/100 ml	45–55	43–65	56.1	52.7	30–66	
WBC/cu mm, in thousands	15	9–38	21–22	5–21	5–21	5–21
Neutrophils, %	40–80	40–80	55	40	36–40	36–40
Eosinophils, %	2–3	2–3	5	5	2–3†	
Lymphocytes, %	30–31	30–31	20	20	48–53	48–53
Monocytes	6–12	6–12	15	15	8–9	8–9
Immature WBC, %	Over 10	3–10	5	0*		
Platelets/cu mm, in thousands	50–300	100–350	400	400	300–400	300–400
Reticulocytes, %	Up to 10	4–6	3	3	0.5–1.6†	

*Not normally found in the circulating blood after this age.

†Remains approximately the same for succeeding age levels.

From G.M. Scipien et al. *Comprehensive Pediatric Nursing* (New York: McGraw-Hill, 1975).

Table F-3. Miscellaneous Blood Measurements

RBC measurements	
Diameter	5.5–8.8 microns (newborn: 8.6)
Mean corpuscular volume	82–92 cu. microns (newborn: 106)
Mean corpuscular hemoglobin	27–31 micro-micrograms (newborn: 38)
Mean corpuscular hemoglobin concentration	32–36%
Color, saturation, and volume indices, each	1
Miscellaneous	
Bleeding time	1–4 min. (Duke) 1–9 min. (Ivy)
Circulation time, arm to lung (ether)	4–8 sec.
Circulation time, arm to tongue (sodium dehydrocholate)	9–16 sec.
Clot retraction time	2–4 hrs.
Coagulation time (venous)	6–10 min. (Lee & White) 10–30 min. (Howell)
Fragility, erythrocyte (hemolysis)	0.44–0.35% NaCl
Partial thromboplastin time	68–82 sec. (standard) 32–46 sec. (activated)
Sedimentation rate	
Men	0–9 mm. per hr. (Wintrobe)
Women	0–20 mm. per hr. (Wintrobe)

From *S K & F Pocket Book of Medical Tables*, 25th ed., © 1979 by SmithKline Corporation.

6 months	1 year	2 years	4 years	8–12 years	Adult Male	Adult Female
10.5–14	11–12.2	11.6–13	12.6–13	11–19	14–18	12–16
4.6	4.6–4.7	4.7–4.8	4.7–4.8	4.8–5.1	5.4	4.8
33–42	32–40	34–40	36–44	39–47	42–52	37–47
1–15	4.5–13.5	9–12	8–10	8	5–10	5–10
30–45	40–50	40–50	50–55	55–60	35–70	35–70
					2–3	2–3
48–60	48–53	48–50	40–48	30–38	30–35	30–35
5	5	5–8	5–8	5–8	5–8	5–8
					250–350	250–350
250–350†					0.5–1.6	0.5–1.6

Table F-4. Blood Chemistry

Constituent	Material	mg./dl. (mg. %)–or as noted
Aldolase	S	0.8–3 I.mU./ml
Ammonia	P	20–150 mcg/dl
Amylase	S	60–160 units (Somogyi)
		0.06–0.34 I.mU./ml
α-1-Antitrypsin	S	210–500
Ascorbic acid	B	0.4–1.5
Bilirubin		
Direct	S	up to 0.4
Indirect	S	0.4–0.8
Total	S	up to 1.2
Bromide	S	Toxic level about 15 mEq./L.
Bromosulphalein (5 mg./Kg.)	S	5% dye or less at 45 minutes
Calcium (ionized)	S	4.5–5.5 mEq./L. 2.4–2.9 mEq./L.@ pH 7.4
Carbon dioxide content	S	24–30 mM./L.
Carotene	S	50–300 mcg./dl.
Ceruloplasmin	S	23–50
Chloride	S	98–109 mEq./L.
Cholesterol, total	S	150–250
Cholesterol esters	S	60–75% of total
Cholinesterase	S	0.5 pH unit/hour or more
		2–5.3 I.U./ml
Creatine		
Males	S	0.2–0.6
Females	S	0.6–1.0
Creatine phosphokinase (CPK)		
Males	S	5–50 I.mU./ml
Females	S	5–30 I.mU./ml
Creatinine	S	0.8–1.2

Constituent	Material	mg./dl. (mg. %)–or as noted
Ferritin		
Males	S	27–329 ng/ml
Females	S	9–125 ng/ml
Fibrinogen	P	160–415
Folate	S	5–21 ng/ml
Gastrin	S	0–20 pg/ml
Glucose	S	60–100 (Nelson-Semogyi)
Glucose-6-phosphate dehydrogenase (G6PD)	red cells	5–10 I.U./g.Hb./30°C
γ-Glutamyl transpeptidase		
Males	S	<28 I.mU./ml
Females	S	<18 I.mU./ml
α-Hydroxybutyric dehydrogenase	S	0–180 I.mU/ml
17-Hydroxycorticosteroids		
Males	P	7–19 mcg/dl
Females	P	9–21 mcg/dl
After 25 units ACTH, i.m.		35–55 mcg/dl
Immunoglobulins	S	800–1500
IgG	S	50–200
IgA	S	40–120
IgM		
Iodine, protein-	S	4–8 mcg/dl
bound	S	50–150 mcg/dl
Iron	S	250–410 mcg/dl
Iron-binding capacity		
Isocitric dehydrogenase	S	50–260 units

(continued on page 652)

B = whole blood; P = plasma; S = serum; I.U. = international units; I.mU. = international milliunits.

From *S K & F Pocket Book of Medical Tables*, 25th ed., © 1979 by SmithKline Corporation.

Table F-4. *Continued*

Constituent	Material	mg./dl. (mg. %)– or as noted
Isozymes		

American	European	Myocardium	Liver	Muscle	RBC
5	1	4+	±	±	3+
4	2	4+	±	±	3+
3	3	±	+	+	+
2	4	±	2+	2+	±
1	5	±	4+	4+	±

Constituent	Material	mg./dl. (mg. %)– or as noted
17–Ketosteroids		
Males	P	40–150 mcg/dl
Females	P	38–130 mcg/dl
Lactic acid	B	6–20
Lactic dehydrogenase (LDH)	S	0–300 I.mU./ml
Lipase	S	0.2–1.5 units/ml (N/20 NaOH)
Lipids, total	S	400–800
Cholesterol		
Total	S	115–340
Esterified	S	70%
Free fatty acids	S	0.3–0.8 mEq./L.
Phospholipids	S	130–380
Triglycerides (neutral fat)	S	10–190
Lithium (therapeutic level)	S	0.5–1.0 mEq./L.
Magnesium	S	1.5–2.4 mEq./L.
Nonprotein nitrogen	S	25–40
Osmolality	S	280–290 mOsm/Kg plasma water
pH	P	7.35–7.45 glass electrode method
Phenylalaline	S	0–2
Phosphatase, acid	S	0.1–1.0 units (Bodansky) 0–11 I.mU./ml

Constituent	Material	mg./dl. (mg. %)– or as noted
Phosphatase, alkaline		
Children	S	5–14 units (Bodansky) 15–20 units (King-Armstrong)
Adults	S	1.4–4.1 units (Bodansky) 4–13 units (King-Armstrong) 20–48 I.mU./ml
Phosphorus		
Children	S	2.3–3.8 mEq./L.
Adults	S	1.45–2.76 mEq./L.
Potassium	S	3.6–5.5 mEq./L.
Proteins (electrophoresis)		
Albumin	S	3.2–5.6 g/dl
α_1 Globulin	S	0.1–0.4 g/dl
α_2 Globulin	S	0.4–1.2 g/dl
β Globulin	S	0.5–1.1 g/dl
γ Globulin	S	0.5–1.6 g/dl
Renin activity by RIA	P (EDTA)	0.4–4.5 ng/ml/hr.
Salicylates (therapeutic level)	S	20–25 (toxic >30)
Sodium	S	135–145 mEq./L.
Transaminase		
Glutamic oxalecetic (SGOT)	S	6–40 units (Karmen) 0–15 I.mU./ml
Glutamic pyruvic (SGPT)	S	6–36 units (Karmen) 0–15 I.mU./ml
Urea	S	17–42
Urea nitrogen	S	8–20
Uric acid		
Males	S	2.1–7.8
Females	S	2.0–6.4
Vitamin A	S	65–275 I.U./dl
Vitamin B_{12}	S	330–1025 pg/ml

Table F-5. Color Variations in Urine

Color	Cause
Straw-colored (dilute urine)	Nervous conditions, diabetes insipidus, granular kidney, large fluid intake
Dark yellow or amber (concentrated urine)	Acute febrile diseases, small fluid intake, vomiting, diarrhea
Turbid or smoky	Blood, chyle, spermatozoa, prostatic fluid, fat droplets
Red or red-brown	Porphyrin, hemoglobin, myoglobin, erythrocytes, transfusion reaction, hemorrhage, bleeding in urogenital tract, pyrvinium pamoate (Povan)
Orange-red or orange-brown	Drugs such as phenozyopyridine (Pyridium), urobilin
Yellow-brown or green-brown	Jaundice, obstruction of bile duct, phenol poisoning
Dark brown or black	Methylene blue medication, chorea, typhus
Cloudy	Pus, blood, epithelial cells, fat, phosphate bacteria, colloidal particles, urates, all-vegetable diet

Table F-6. Normal Urine Values*

Constituent	24-hour excretion or as noted
Aldosterone	2–10 mcg
Ammonia nitrogen	20–70 mEq
Amylase	35–260 Somogyi units/L.
Calcium	
200 mg diet	<7.5 mEq
Catecholamines	
Free, epinephrine and norepinephrine	<100 mcg
Metanephrine	<1.3 mg
VMA	<8 mg
Chloride	110–250 mEq
Coproporphyrin	100–300 mcg
Cortisol	2–10 mg
Free cortisol	7–25 mg male 4–15 mg female
Creatine	
Adult male	<50 mg
Adult female	<100 mg
Higher in children and pregnancy	
Creatinine	1–1.6 Gm (15–25 mg Kg)

Constituent	24-hour excretion or as noted
5-HIAA	2–9 mg
Lead	<120 mcg
Phosphorus	0.9–1.3 Gm
Porphobilinogen	<2 mg
Potassium	25–100 mEq
Protein	<50 mg
Sodium	100–260 mEq
Urea nitrogen	6–15 Gm
Uric acid	0.2–0.6 Gm
Urobilinogen	1–3.5 mg

	Estrone	Estradiol in mcg.	Estriol
Estrogens			
Female postpubertal	5–20	2–10	5–30
Female postmenopausal	0.3–2.4	0–14	2.2–7.5
Male / Female prepubertal	0–15	0–5	0–10

*Specific gravity: 1.015–1.025; pH: 4.8–8.5; volume: 600–2500 ml/24 hr.

Adapted from: *Harrison's Textbook of Medicine*, 8th edition, McGraw-Hill, 1977; *Textbook of Medicine*, Besson P., McDermott, W., 14th edition. W. B. Saunders Company, 1975.

Table F-7. Kidney Function Tests

Constituent or factor	Normal values	Remarks
Endogenous creatinine clearance (glomerular filtration primarily)	With normal physical activity: 90–130 ml/min. per 1.73 sq. meters body surface	Calculated from concentration of substance in urine and plasma, and the volume of urine excreted per min. in ml
Insulin clearance (glomerular filtration exclusively)	Male: 130 ± 20 Female: 120 ± 15 ml/min. per 1.73 sq. meters body surface	Short duration test; administered intravenously
Urea clearance (glomerular filtration and partial tubular reabsorption)	Maximum: 60–90 ml. per minute Standard: 40–65 ml/min.	Calculated number of ml blood completely cleared of urea as blood passes through kidneys during 1 min.; diuresis over 2 ml/min.
Phenolsulfonphthalein (chiefly tubular secretion, partially glomerular filtration)	25% or more in 15 min. 40–60% in 1 hr. 60–85% in 2 hr.	Administered intravenously; since tubular transport mechanism is not saturated by dose used, the test is mainly a reflection of renal blood flow
Concentration and dilution	Sp. gr. 1.025–1.032 (concentration) Sp. gr. 1.001–1.003 (dilution)	After fluids withheld for 10 hr. or more, administer 1500 ml of water; it is totally excreted in 2–4 hr., most during first hr.
Diodrast clearance (effective renal plasma flow and tubular function)	Male: 600–800 Female: 500–700 ml/min. per 1.73 sq. meters body surface 20–30% excretion in 15 min.	Rapidly and actively secreted by renal tubules
p-Aminohippurate clearance (effective renal plasma flow and tubular function)	Male: 600–800 Female: 500–700 ml/min. per 1.73 sq. meters body surface	Rapidly and actively secreted by renal tubules

From *SK & F Pocket Book of Medical Tables*, 25th ed., © 1979 by SmithKline Corporation.

Table F-8. Pulmonary Function Tests

Substance determined	Normal values	Clinical implications: Increase	Clinical implications: Decrease
Body plethysmography	Men: 0.081 (H)–2.94 Women: 0.135 (H)–0.008 (W)–4.74 TGV = approx. 2400 ml (thoracic gas volume) C = 0.2 L/cm H_2O RAW = 0.6 to 2.4 cm/H_2O/l/sec.	C—obstructive diseases TGV—obstructive pulmonary disease RAW—asthma, emphysema, bronchitis and other forms of obstruction	C—Fibrotic diseases, restrictive diseases, pneumonia, congestion, atelectasis
Carbon dioxide response	3-fold increase		Unresponsiveness suggests disturbance in normal physiological pathway of ventilatory changes and hypercapnia
Carbon monoxide diffusing capacity of the lung (DLCO)	Approximately 25 ml/min./torr		Multiple pulmonary emboli Emphysema Anemia Lung restriction Pulmonary fibroses Sarcoidosis Scleroderma Systemic lupus erythematosus Asbestosis
Closing volume (CV)	About 10% of vital capacity	In diseases in which the airway is decreased, in pulmonary edema, in chronic smokers, and in old patients	
Expiratory reserve volume (ERV)	Approximately 1200–1500 ml		Chest wall restriction due to nonpulmonary causes Elevated diaphragms as seen in massive obesity, ascites, or pregnancy Massive enlargement of the heart, pleural effusion, kyphoscoliosis, and thoracoplasty
Flow volume loops	Normal loops are characteristic of absence of lung disease		Abnormal flow volume loops are indicative of: obstructive lung disease; small airway obstructive disease as in emphysema and asthma; large airway obstructive disease such as tumors of trachea and bronchioles; restrictive diseases when the disease is far advanced.
Forced vital capacity (FVC) or forced expiratory volume (FEV)	Approximately 4800 ml	Restrictive lung disease can be normal or elevated	Obstructive lung disease such as emphysema, pulmonary fibrosis, and asthma

(continued on page 658)

From Fishbach, F. *Manual of Laboratory Diagnostic Tests for Nurses*. Philadelphia: Lippincott, 1980. Used with permission.

Table F-8. *Continued*

Substance determined	Normal values	Clinical implications: Increase	Clinical implications: Decrease
Functional residual capacity (FRC)	Approximately 2400–3000 ml	Obstructive airway disease represents hyperinflation from emphysematous changes, asthmatic or fibrotic obstruction of the bronchioles, compensation for surgical removal of lung tissue, or a thoracic deformity	Restrictive disease
Inspiratory capacity (IC)	Approximately 2500–3600 ml.	Changes usually parallel increases or decreases in the vital capacity	
Maximum voluntary ventilation (MVV)	Approximately 170 l./min.		Obstructive defects, chronic pulmonary disease (COPD), abnormal neuromuscular control, and poor patient effort
Methacholine challenge	Negative response	Asthma	
Peak expiratory flow rate (PEFR)	An average 300 l./min.		Obstructive disease such as emphysema; usually normal in restrictive lung disease, except in severe restriction, when it is reduced
Peak inspiratory flow rate (PIFR)	An average of at least 300 l./min.		Neuromuscular disorders, weakness, poor effort, and extrathoracic airway obstruction; substernal thyroid, tracheal stenosis and laryngeal paralysis
Residual volume (RV)	1200–1500 ml	Young asthmatics Emphysema Chronic air trapping Chronic bronchial obstruction	Sometimes in diseases that occlude many alveoli
Total lung capacity (TLC)	Approximately 5500 ml	Obstructive defect Normal or increased in broncheolar obstruction with hyperinflation and in emphysema	Edema Atelectasis Neoplasms Pulmonary congestion Pneumothorax or thoracic restriction
Vital capacity (VC)	4000–4800 ml		Depression of the respiratory center in the brain, neuromuscular diseases, pleural effusion, ascites, pneumothorax, pregnancy, limitations of thoracic movement due to pain
Volume of isoflow (V_{Iso})	Values cover a wide range based on age and sex	Mild airway obstruction Small airways disease	

Table F-9. Liver Function Tests

Test	Normal	Clinical functions
I. *Pigment studies*		
A. Serum bilirubin, direct B. Serum bilirubin, total C. Urine bilirubin D. Urine urobilinogen. E. Fecal urobilinogen (infrequently used)	0.–0.3 mg/ml 0.–0.9 mg/ml 0 0–1.16 mg/24 hrs. 40–280 mg/24 hrs.	These are measures of ability of liver to conjugate and excrete bilirubin. They are abnormal in liver and biliary tract disease, causing jaundice clinically.
II. *Dye clearances*		
A. Bromosulphalein excretion (BSP test)	<5% retention 45 minutes after dye injection of 5 mg/kg body weight	BSP binds to albumin in blood. Liver cells unbind BSP, conjugate it and excrete it in bile. Normal clearance depends on hepatic blood flow, functioning liver cell mass and lack of obstruction. Retention is increased in liver cell damage or decreased liver blood flow.
B. Indocyanine green	500–800 ml/sq. m. body surface/min.	Extracted from blood and excreted by liver. Depends on hepatic blood flow, functioning liver cells, and lack of obstruction.
III. *Protein studies*		
A. Total serum protein B. Serum albumin C. Serum globulin D. Serum protein electrophoresis	7.0–7.5 gm % 3.5–5.5 gm % 1.5–3.0 gm % Albumin 63–69% of total Alpha 1 Glob. 3.9–7.3% Alpha 2 Glob. 3.9–7.3% Alpha 2 Glob. 6.9–11.8% Beta Glob. 6.9–11.8% Gamma Glob. 9.8–20%	Proteins are manufactured by the liver. Their levels may be affected in a variety of liver impairments. Albumin: Cirrhosis, Chronic hepatitis, Edema, ascites Globulin: Cirrhosis, Liver disease, Chronic obstructive jaundice, Viral hepatitis
IV. *Prothrombin time*		
Response of prothrombin time to vitamin K	100% return to normal	Prothrombin time may be prolonged in liver disease. It will not return to normal with vitamin K in severe liver cell damage.
V. *Serum alkaline phosphatase*	Varies with method. 2–5 Bodansky units	Manufactured in bones, liver, kidneys, intestine. Excreted through biliary tract. In absence of bone disease, it is a sensitive measure of biliary tract obstruction.
VI. *Serum transaminase studies*		
A. SGOT B. SGPT C. LDH	10–40 units 5–35 units 165–400 units	Based on release of enzymes from damaged liver cells. These enzymes are elevated in liver cell damage.
VII. *Blood ammonia* (arterial)	20–50 mg/100 ml.	Liver converts ammonia to urea. Ammonia level rises in liver failure.

(continued on page 660)

From L. S. Bruner and D. S. Suddarth. *Textbook of Medical-Surgical Nursing*. 3rd ed. Philadelphia: Lippincott, 1975, p. 597. Used with permission.

Table F-9. *Continued*

Test	Normal	Clinical functions
VIII. *Flocculation tests*		
A. Cephalin flocculation	0–1 +	Depend on ability of serum proteins to stabilize colloidal suspension. Abnormal in liver and other diseases. Positive thymol turbidity also produced by elevated gamma globulin levels.
B. Thymol turbidity (these protein reactions are too nonspecific to be of great value)	0–5 units	
IX. *Cholesterol*	150–250 mg/ml	Elevated in biliary obstruction (each of excretion). Decreased in parenchymal liver disease.
Ester	60% of total	
X. *Radiologic studies*		
A. Barium study of esophagus		For varices. Varices in esophagus indicate increased portal pressure.
B. Plain film of abdomen		To determine gross liver size.
C. Liver scan with radio-tagged iodinated rose bengal, gold or technetium		To show size, shape of liver. To show replacement of liver tissue with scars, cysts, or tumor.
D. Cholecystogram and cholangiogram		For gallbladder and bile duct visualization.
E. Celiac axis arteriography		For liver and pancreas visualization.
F. Splenoporetogram (Splenic portal venography)		To determine adequacy of portal blood flow.
XI. *Peritoneoscopy*		Direct visualization anterior surface of liver, gallbladder and mesentery.
XII. *Liver biopsy*		To determine anatomic changes in liver tissue.
XIII. *Measurement of portal pressure*		Elevated in cirrhosis of the liver.
XIV. *Esophagoscopy*		To search for esophageal varices.
XV. *Electroencephalogram*		Abnormal in hepatic coma and impending hepatic coma.

Table F-10. Normal Values for Gastric Analysis

	Conventional units	Factor	S.I. units
Basal gastric secretion (1 hour)			
Concentration	(Mean ± 1 S.D.)		(Mean ± 1 S.D.)
Males	25.8 ± 1.8 mEq./liter	1.0	25.8 ± 1.8 mmol/l
Females	20.3 ± 3.0 mEq./liter		20.3 ± 3.0 mmol/l
Output	(Mean ± 1 S.D.)		(Mean ± 1 S.D.)
Males	2.57 ± 0.16 mEq./hr.	1.0	2.57 ± 0.16 mmol/h
Females	1.61 ± 0.18 mEq./hr.		1.61 ± 0.18 mmol/h
After histamine stimulation			
Normal	Mean output 11.8 mEq./hr.	1.0	Mean output 11.8 mmol/h
Duodenal ulcer	Mean output 15.2 mEq./hr.		Mean output 15.2 mmol/h
After maximal histamine stimulation			
Normal	Mean output 22.6 mEq./hr.	1.0	Mean output 22.6 mmol/h
Duodenal ulcer	Mean output 44.6 mEq./hr.		Mean output 44.6 mmol/h
Diagnex blue (Squibb):		1.0	0–0.3 mg in 2 h
Anacidity	0–0.3 mg in 2 hrs.		0.3–0.6 mg in 2 h
Doubtful	0.3–0.6 mg in 2 hrs.		Greater than 0.6 mg in 2 h
Normal	Greater than 0.6 mg in 2 hrs.		
Volume, fasting stomach content	50–100 ml	—	0.05–0.1 liter
Emptying time	3–6 hrs.	—	3–6 h
Color	Opalescent or colorless	—	Opalescent or colorless
Specific gravity	1.006–1.009	—	1.006–1.009
pH (adults)	0.9–1.5	—	0.9–1.5

From Conn, R. B., Jr.: Laboratory reference values of clinical importance. In Conn, H. F.: *Current Therapy 1981.* Philadelphia, W. B. Sanders, 1981.

Table F-11. Normal Values for Stools

Constituent	24-hour excretion or as noted
Fat	
Total	10–25% of dry matter and <5 g/24 hr.
Neutral	1–5% of dry matter
Free fatty acids	5–13% of dry matter
Combined fatty acids	5–15% of dry matter
Urobilinogen	40–200 mg/24 hr.

From *S K & F Pocket Book of Medical Tables*, 25th ed., © 1979 by SmithKline Corporation.

Table F-12. Gastrointestinal Absorption Tests

Test	Conventional units	Factor	S.I. units
d-Xylose absorption test	After an 8-hour fast, 10 ml/kg body weight of a 0.05 solution of d-xylose is given by mouth. Nothing further by mouth is given until the test has been completed. All urine voided during the following 5 hours is pooled, and blood samples are taken at 0, 60, and 120 minutes. Normally 0.26 (range 0.16–0.33) of ingested xylose is excreted within 5 hours, and the serum xylose reaches a level between 25 and 40 mg/100 ml after 1 hour and is maintained at this level for another 60 minutes.		No change
Vitamin A absorption	A fasting blood specimen is obtained and 200,000 units of vitamin A in oil is given by mouth. Serum vitamin A level should rise to twice fasting level in 3 to 5 hours.		No change

From Conn, R. B., Jr.: Laboratory reference values of clinical importance. In Conn, H. F.: *Current Therapy 1981.* Philadelphia, W. B. Saunders, 1981.

Table F-13. Cerebrospinal Fluid Tests

Substance determined	Normal values	Clinical implications: Increase	Clinical implications: Decrease
A/G ratio (albumin to globulin)	8:1		
Bilirubin	Negative		
Calcium	2.1–2.7 mEq./l.	Tuberculous meningitis	
Chloride	118–132 mEq./l.		Tuberculous meningitis Bacterial meningitis
Cholesterol	0.2–0.6 mg/dl		
Color	Crystal clear, colorless	Abnormal in: Subarachnoid Cerebral hemorrhage Bilirubinemia Subarachnoid block Acute meningitis Cloudiness Cryptococcal infection	
Creatinine	0.5–1.2 mg/dl		
Glucose	45–85 mg/dl (20 mg/dl less than blood level)	Mump encephalitis Cerebral trauma Brain tumors accompanied by increased intracranial pressure Hypothalamic lesions	Pyrogenic, tuberculous, and fungal meningitis Toxoplasmosis Sarcoidosis Subarachnoid hemorrhage Primary brain tumors Lymphomas Leukemia Melanoma Viral meningoencephalitis

(continued on page 664)

Table F-13. *Continued*

Substance determined	Normal values	Clinical implications: Increase	Clinical implications: Decrease
Pressure	75–150 mm H_2O	Intracranial tumors Purulent or tuberculous meningitis Low-grade inflammatory processes Encephalitis Neurosyphilis	Hydrocephalus when there is a small pressure drop that is indicative of a large CSF pool
Protein	15–45 mg/dl (lumbar) 15–25 mg/dl (cisternal) 5–15 mg/dl (ventricular)	Purulent meningitis Guillain-Barre syndrome Froin's syndrome Tuberculous meningitis Aseptic meningitis Syphilis Brain tumors and abscesses Subarachnoid hemorrhage Congenital toxoplasmosis	
Total cell count and differential cell count of CSF	0–8 mm^3	Purulent infection Viral infections Syphilis of CNS Tuberculous meningitis Multiple sclerosis Tumor or abscess Subarachnoid hemorrahge	Abnormal cells in: Brain tumors Inflammatory processes Multiple sclerosis Leukoencephalitis Delayed hypersensitivity responses Subacute viral encephalitis Meningitis (tuberculous or fugae) Cranial infarcts Surgical procedures or trauma to the central nervous system
Urea	7–15 mg/dl	Uremia	
Urea nitrogen	6–16 mg/dl		
Uric acid	0.5–4.5 mg/dl		

APPENDIX G

Nutritional Aspects

Table G-1. Nutrients for Health

Nutrient	Important sources of nutrient	Some major physiological functions		
		Provide energy	**Build and maintain body cells**	**Regulate body processes**
Protein	Meat, poultry, fish Dried beans and peas Egg Cheese Milk	Supplies 4 calories per gram	Constitutes part of the structure of every cell, such as muscle, blood, and bone; supports growth and maintains healthy body cells.	Constitutes part of enzymes, some hormones and body fluids, and antibodies that increase resistance to infection.
Carbohydrate	Cereal Potatoes Dried beans Corn Bread Sugar	Supplies 4 calories per gram Major source of energy for central nervous system	Supplies energy so protein can be used for growth and maintenance of body cells.	Unrefined products supply fiber—complex carbohydrates in fruits, vegetables, and whole grains—for regular elimination. Assists in fat utilization.
Fat	Shortening, Oil Butter, margarine Salad dressing Sausages	Supplies 9 calories per gram	Constitutes part of the structure of every cell. Supplies essential fatty acids.	Provides and carries fat-soluble vitamins (A, D, E, and K).
Vitamin A (Retinol)	Liver Carrots Sweet potatoes Greens Butter, margarine		Assists formation and maintenance of skin and mucus membranes that line body cavities and tracts, such as nasal passages and intestinal tract, thus increasing resistance to infection.	Functions in visual processes and forms visual purple, thus promoting healthy eye tissues and eye adaptation in dim light.
Vitamin C (Ascorbic Acid)	Broccoli Orange Grapefruit Papaya Mango Strawberries		Forms cementing substances, such as collagen, that hold body cells together, thus strengthening blood vessels, hastening healing of wounds and bones, and increasing resistance to infection.	Aids utilization of iron.
Thiamin (B_1)	Lean pork Nuts Fortified cereal products	Aids in utilization of energy		Functions as part of a coenzyme to promote the utilization of carbohydrate. Promotes normal appetite. Contributes to normal functioning of nervous system.

Courtesy of National Dairy Council

Table G-1. *Continued*

Nutrient	Important sources of nutrient	Some major physiological functions		
		Provide energy	Build and maintain body cells	Regulate body processes
Riboflavin (B_2)	Liver Milk Yogurt Cottage cheese	Aids in utilization of energy		Functions as part of a coenzyme in the production of energy within body cells. Promotes healthy skin, eyes, and clear vision.
Niacin	Liver Meat, poultry, fish Peanuts Fortified cereal products	Aids in utilization of energy		Functions as part of a coenzyme in fat synthesis, tissue respiration, and utilization of carbohydrate. Promotes healthy skin, nerves, and digestive tract. Aids digestion and fosters normal appetite.
Calcium	Milk, yogurt Cheese Sardines and salmon with bones Collard, kale, mustard, and turnip greens		Combines with other minerals within a protein framework to give structure and strength to bones and teeth.	Assists in blood clotting. Functions in normal muscle contraction and relaxation, and normal nerve transmission.
Iron	Enriched farina Prune juice Liver Dried beans and peas Red meat	Aids in utilization of energy	Combines with protein to form hemoglobin, the red substance in blood that carries oxygen to and carbon dioxide from the cells. Prevents nutritional anemia and its accompanying fatigue. Increases resistance to infection.	Functions as part of enzymes involved in tissue respiration.

Table G-2. Basic Four Food Groups Throughout the Growing Years

Food group	Servings per day	Average-size servings for age			
		Toddler	Preschool	School	Adolescent
Milk or equivalent	4	½–¾ cup	¾ cup	¾–1 cup	1 cup
1 cup milk equals:					
2 tbsp powdered milk					
1 oz cheese					
¼ cup evaporated milk					
½ cup cottage cheese					
1 serving custard (4 servings from 1 pt milk)					
½ cup milk pudding					
½ cup yogurt					
Meat, fish, poultry, or equivalent	2 or more	3 tbsp	4 tbsp	3–4 oz (6–8 tbsp)	4 oz or more
3 oz meat equals:					
1 egg, 1 frankfurter					
1 oz cheese,* 1 cold cut					
2 tbsp peanut butter, cut meat					
¼ cup tuna fish or cottage cheese*					
½ cup dried peas or beans					
Vegetables and fruits to include citrus fruit or	4 or more				
equivalent	1 or more	4 oz	4 oz	4–6 oz	4–6 oz
1 citrus fruit serving equals:					
½ cup orange or grapefruit juice					
½ grapefruit or cantaloupe					
¼ cup strawberries					
1 medium orange					
½ citrus fruit serving equals:					
½ cup tomato juice or tomatoes, broccoli, chard, collards, greens, spinach, raw cabbage, brussels sprouts					
1 medium tomato, 1 wedge honeydew					
Yellow or green vegetable or equivalent	1 or more	4 tbsp	4 tbsp	⅓ cup	½ cup
1 serving equals:					
½ cup broccoli, greens, spinach, carrots, squash, pumpkin					
5 apricot halves					
½ medium cantaloupe					
Other fruits and vegetables	2 or more				
Other vegetables, including potatoes		2–3 tbsp	4 tbsp	⅓–½ cup	¾ cup
Other fruits including apples, banana, pears, peaches		½ med apple	½-1 med apple	1 med apple	1 med apple
Breads and cereals or whole grain or enriched equivalent	4 or more				
1 slice bread equals		½ slice	1 slice	1–2 slices	2 slices
¼ cup dry cereal		½ cup	¾ cup	1 oz	1 oz
½ cup cooked cereal, rice, spaghetti, or macaroni		2 tbsp	¼–½ cup	½–1 cup	1 cup or more
1 roll, muffin, or biscuit					

* If cottage or cheddar cheese is used as a milk equivalent, it should not also be counted as a meat equivalent.

From *Infant Feeding Guide*, for use by professional staffs, Washington State Department of Social and Health Services, Health Services Division, Local Health Services, Nutrition Unit, 1972.

Table G-3. Fat-Soluble and Water-Soluble Vitamins

Vitamin	Deficiency	Behavioral assessment	Medical therapy and nursing management
Fat soluble			
A	Nyctalopia	Night and low-light blindness	Vitamin A supplementation in conjunction with a high-protein diet
	Xerophthalmia	Abnormal dryness and thickening of the surface of the conjunctiva and cornea leading to blindness Stages of progression are: dryness of conjunctiva (xerosis); foamy gray, triangular spots of keratinized epithelium on the conjunctiva (Bitot's spots); dryness of the cornea (xerosis); softening and necrosis of the cornea (keratomalacia); inflammation, ulceration, and perforation of the cornea	Diet instruction: encourage intake of foods high in vitamin A, such as liver, carrots, sweet potatoes, spinach, squash, broccoli, apricots, and cantaloupe
D	Rickets	Bowed legs in toddlers Widening of wrists, knees, and ankles Craniotabes (softening of the cranial bones, prominence of frontal bones) Harrison's groove (depression on lower edge of thorax) Lethargy, hypotonicity, joint hyperextensibility, motor retardation Convulsions and tetany Steatorrhea	Vitamin D supplementation Encourage daily exposure to sunlight Diet instruction: small amounts of vitamin D are contained in butter, cream, egg yolk, and liver Encourage use of vitamin D fortified dairy products
E	Hemolytic anemia	Excessive hemolysis of red blood cells, especially in premature infants	Vitamin E supplementation of formulas with a vegetable oil fat source
K	Hemorrhagic disease of the newborn	Hemorrhage Increased bleeding tendency	Vitamin K prophylactically at birth
Water soluble			
Thiamine (B_1)	Beriberi	Restlessness and crying (infants) Emesis of breast milk Abdominal distention, flatulence, constipation, insomnia Peripheral neuritis with tingling and burning Paresthesias of toes and feet Leg muscle tenderness and cramping	Thiamine administration If breast-fed, treat both mother and infant with thiamine Administration of other B vitamins Diet instruction: increase intake of pork, wheat germ, organ meats, poultry, and legumes

(continued on page 670)

Table G-3. *Continued*

Vitamin	Deficiency	Behavioral assessment	Medical therapy and nursing management
Riboflavin (B_2)	Ariboflavinosis	Angular stomatitis (cracks at the corner of the mouth) Cheilosis (painful cracks on the lips) Glossitis (smooth tongue) Conjunctivitis Photophobia Seborrheic dermatitis	Administration of riboflavin Diet instruction: increase intake of milk, cheese, green, leafy vegetables, and organ meats
Niacin	Pellagra	Early: anorexia, lassitude, weakness, numbness, burning sensations, dizziness Later: dermatitis, dementia, diarrhea Symmetrical erythema of exposed skin with sharp demarcation from healthy skin Red and painful mouth and tongue Gastrointestinal inflammation: dysphagia, nausea, vomiting, diarrhea	Niacin supplementation Diet instruction: increase intake of protein-rich foods (poultry, meats, and fish) Instruction on necessity of avoiding exposure to sun while skin lesions are active Skin care, especially with soothing lotions
Pyridoxine (B_6)	Seizure condition	Seizures are myoclonic Gastrointestinal distress Irritability Aggravated startle response	Pyridoxine administration Diet instruction: increase intake of meats, poultry, fish, and whole grains
Folic Acid (B_9)	Megaloblastic anemia	Weakness Pallor Anorexia and failure to gain weight Diarrhea Irritability Concomitant behaviors of scurvy may be present	Administration of folic acid and ascorbic acid Diet instruction: increase intake of wheat germ, bran, liver, and egg yolk
Cobalamin (B_{12})	Pernicious anemia	Severe anemia Irritability Anorexia Listlessness Smooth, red, painful tongue Ataxia, paresthesias, hyporeflexia, positive Babinski response, clonus, coma	Administration of vitamin B_{12} parenterally Vitamin B_{12} maintenance Therapy throughout life by IM injection
Ascorbic acid (C)	Scurvy	Irritability, tachypnea, anorexia, gastrointestinal disturbance General tenderness, especially in the legs Gums bluish purple, with spongy swelling of the mucous membranes Sternal depression Petechiae, hematuria, melena, orbital or subdural hemorrhage Delayed wound healing	Administration of ascorbic acid Diet instruction: increase intake of fresh fruits and vegetables

Source: Developed by Gayle Giboney Page, R.N., M.N., Children's Hospital of Los Angeles.

Table G-4. Minerals*

Mineral	Primary function in man	Food source	Daily requirement
Calcium (Ca)	Building material of bones and teeth; regulation of body functions; heart muscle contraction, blood clotting	Dairy products, leafy vegetables, apricots	Men: .8 grams Women: .8 grams
Phosphorus (P)	Combines with calcium to give rigidity to bones and teeth; essential in cell metabolism; serves as a buffer to maintain proper acid-base balance of blood	Peas, beans, milk, liver, meat, cottage cheese, broccoli, whole grains	Men: .8 grams Women: .8 grams
Iron (Fe)	Component of the red blood cell's oxygen and carbon dioxide transport system; enzyme constituent necessary for cellular respiration	Liver, meat, shellfish, lentils, peanuts, parsley, dried fruits, eggs	Men: 10 mg. Women: 18 mg.
Iodine (I)	Essential component of the thyroid hormone, thyroxin, which controls the rate of cell oxidation	Iodized salt, seafood	Men: 140 mcg. Women: 100 mcg.
Sodium (Na)	Regulates the fluid and acid-base balance in the body	Table salt, dried apricots, beans, beets, brown sugar, raisins, spinach, yeast	Men: 500–1000 mg. Women: 500–1000 mg.
Chloride (Cl)	Associated with sodium and its functions; a component of the gastric juice hydrochloric acid; the chloride ion also functions in the starch splitting system of saliva	Same as sodium	Men: 500–1000 mg. Women: 500–1000 mg.
Potassium (K)	Component of the system that controls the acid-base and liquid balances; is probably an important enzyme-activator in the use of amino acids	Readily available in most foods	
Magnesium (Mg)	Enzyme-activator related to carbohydrate metabolism	Readily available in most foods	Men: 400 mg. Women: 350 mg.
Sulfur (S)	Component of the hormone insulin and the sulfur amino acids; builds hair, nails, skin	Nuts, dried fruits, barley and oatmeal, beans, cheese, eggs, lentils, brown sugar	?
Manganese (Mn)	Enzyme-activator for systems related to carbohydrate, protein, and fat metabolism	Wheat germ, nuts, bran, green leafy vegetables, cereal grains, meat	?
Copper (Cu)	The function of copper has not been fully resolved although it is known to function in the synthesis of the red blood cell and the oxidation system of the body	Kidney, liver, beans, Brazil nuts, wholemeal flour, lentils, parsley	?
Zinc (Zn)	The function is unknown although it is a component of many enzyme systems and is an essential component of the pancreatic hormone insulin	Shellfish, meat, milk, eggs	?
Cobalt (Co)	A component of the vitamin B_{12} molecule	Vitamin B_{12}	?
Fluorine (F)	Essential to normal tooth and bone development and maintenance; excesses are undesirable	Drinking water in some areas	1 part per million in drinking water

*Several trace minerals—chromium, silenium, nickel, molybdenum, vanodium, and tin—are now known to be required in very small amounts by experimental animals (studies have not been done on man). Their distribution in food varies considerably, depending in part on the composition of the soil in which plants are raised.

Values are taken from *Recommended Dietary Allowances*. 7th ed. Washington, D.C.: National Academy of Sciences Publication 1694, 1968.

Table G-5. Recommended Daily Dietary Allowances (RDAs) for the United States

Age (years)	Weight (kg)	Weight (lb)	Height (cm)	Height (in)	Protein (g)	Fat-soluble vitamins: Vitamin A (μg RE)*	Vitamin D (μg)†	Vitamin E (mg α-TE)‡
Infants								
0.0–0.5	6	13	60	24	kg × 2.2	420	10	3
0.5–1.0	9	20	71	28	kg × 2.0	400	10	4
Children								
1–3	13	29	90	35	23	400	10	5
4–6	20	44	112	44	30	500	10	6
7–10	28	62	132	52	34	700	10	7
Males								
11–14	45	99	157	62	45	1,000	10	8
15–18	66	145	176	69	56	1,000	10	10
19–22	70	154	177	70	56	1,000	7.5	10
23–50	70	154	178	70	56	1,000	5	10
>51	70	154	178	70	56	1,000	5	10
Females								
11–14	46	101	157	62	46	800	10	8
15–18	55	120	163	64	46	800	10	8
19–22	55	120	163	64	44	800	7.5	8
23–50	55	120	163	64	44	800	5	8
>51	55	120	163	64	44	800	5	8
Pregnant					+30	+200	+5	+2
Lactating					+20	+400	+5	+3

From *Recommended Dietary Allowances*, 9th ed. (Washington, D.C.: National Academy of Sciences, 1980).

Note: The allowances are intended to provide for individual variations among most normal persons as they live in the United States under usual environmental stresses. Diets should be based on a variety of common foods in order to provide other nutrients for which human requirements have been less well defined. See text for detailed discussion of allowances and of nutrients not tabulated.

*Retinol equivalents. 1 retinol equivalent = 1 μg of retinol or 6 μg of β-carotene.

†As cholecalciferol. 10 μg of cholecalciferol = 400 IU of vitamin D.

‡α-tocopherol equivalents. 1 mg of *d*-α-tocopherol = 1 α-TE

§1 NE (niacin equivalent) is equal to 1 mg of niacin or 60 mg of dietary tryptophan.

Table G-6. Estimated Safe and Adequate Daily Dietary Intakes of Additional Selected Vitamins and Minerals for the United States, 1980

	Age (years)	Vitamins: Vitamin K (μg)	Biotin (μg)	Pantothenic acid (mg)	Trace elements: Copper (mg)	Manganese (mg)	Fluoride (mg)
Infants	0–0.5	12	35	2	0.5–0.7	0.5–0.7	0.1–0.5
	0.5–1	10–20	50	3	0.7–1.0	0.7–1.0	0.2–1.0
Children and adolescents	1–3	15–30	65	3	1.0–1.5	1.0–1.5	0.5–1.5
	4–6	20–40	85	3–4	1.5–2.0	1.5–2.0	1.0–2.5
	7–10	30–60	120	4–5	2.0–2.5	2.0–3.0	1.5–2.5
	>11	50–100	100–200	4–7	2.0–3.0	2.5–5.0	1.5–2.5
Adults		70–140	100–200	4–7	2.0–3.0	2.5–5.0	1.5–4.0

From *Recommended Dietary Allowances*, 9th ed. (Washington, D.C.: National Academy of Sciences, 1980).

Note: Because there is less information on which to base allowances, these figures are not given in the main table of the RDAs and are provided here in the form of ranges of recommended intakes.

*Since the toxic levels for many trace elements may be only several times usual intakes, the upper levels for the trace elements given in this table should not be habitually exceeded.

Water-soluble vitamins							Minerals					
Vitamin C (mg)	Thiamin (mg)	Riboflavin (mg)	Niacin (mg NE)[§]	Vitamin B_6 (mg)	Folacin[‖] (μg)	Vitamin B_{12} (μg)	Calcium (mg)	Phosphorus (mg)	Magnesium (mg)	Iron (mg)	Zinc (mg)	Iodine (μg)
35	0.3	0.4	6	0.3	30	0.5[¶]	360	240	50	10	3	40
35	0.5	0.6	8	0.6	45	1.5	540	360	70	15	5	50
45	0.7	0.8	9	0.9	100	2.0	800	800	150	15	10	70
45	0.9	1.0	11	1.3	200	2.5	800	800	200	10	10	90
45	1.2	1.4	16	1.6	300	3.0	800	800	250	10	10	120
50	1.4	1.6	18	1.8	400	3.0	1,200	1,200	350	18	15	150
60	1.4	1.7	18	2.0	400	3.0	1,200	1,200	400	18	15	150
60	1.5	1.7	19	2.2	400	3.0	800	800	350	10	15	150
60	1.4	1.6	18	2.2	400	3.0	800	800	350	10	15	150
60	1.2	1.4	16	2.2	400	3.0	800	800	350	10	15	150
50	1.1	1.3	15	1.8	400	3.0	1,200	1,200	300	18	15	150
60	1.1	1.3	14	2.0	400	3.0	1,200	1,200	300	18	15	150
60	1.1	1.3	14	2.0	400	3.0	800	800	300	18	15	150
60	1.0	1.2	13	2.0	400	3.0	800	800	300	18	15	150
60	1.0	1.2	13	2.0	400	3.0	800	800	300	10	15	150
+20	+0.4	+0.3	+2	+0.6	+400	+1.0	+400	+400	+150	#	+5	+25
+40	+0.5	+0.5	+5	+0.5	+100	+1.0	+400	+400	+150	#	+10	+50

[‖]The folacin allowances refer to dietary sources as determined by *Lactobacillus casei* assay after treatment with enzymes (conjugases) to make polyglutamyl forms of the vitamin available to the test organism.

[¶]The recommended dietary allowance for vitamin B_{12} in infants is based on average concentration of the vitamin in human milk. The allowances after weaning are based on energy intake (as recommended by the American Academy of Pediatrics) and consideration of other factors, such as intestinal absorption.

[#]The increased requirement during pregnancy cannot be met by the iron content of habitual American diets nor by the existing iron stores of many women; therefore the use of 30 to 60 mg of supplemental iron is recommended. Iron needs during lactation are not substantially different from those of nonpregnant women, but continued supplementation of the mother for 2 to 3 months after parturition is advisable in order to replenish stores depleted by pregnancy.

Trace elements*			Electrolytes		
Chromium (mg)	Selenium (mg)	Molybdenum (mg)	Sodium (mg)	Potassium (mg)	Chloride (mg)
0.01–0.04	0.01–0.04	0.03–0.06	115–350	350–925	275–700
0.02–0.06	0.02–0.06	0.04–0.08	250–750	425–1,275	400–1,200
0.02–0.08	0.02–0.08	0.05–0.1	325–975	550–1,650	500–1,500
0.03–0.12	0.03–0.12	0.06–0.15	450–1,350	775–2,325	700–2,100
0.05–0.2	0.05–0.2	0.1–0.3	600–1,800	1,000–3,000	925–2,775
0.05–0.2	0.05–0.2	0.15–0.5	900–2,700	1,525–4,575	1,400–4,200
0.05–0.2	0.05–0.2	0.15–0.5	1,100–3,300	1,875–5,625	1,700–5,100

Table G-7. Mean Heights and Weights and Recommended Energy Intakes for the United States, 1980

Category	Age (years)	Weight (kg)	Weight (lb)	Height (cm)	Height (in.)	Energy needs (with range) (kcal)	Energy needs (with range) (MJ)
Infants	0.0–0.5	6	13	60	24	kg × 115 (95–145)	kg × .48
	0.5–1.0	9	20	71	28	kg × 105 (80–135)	kg × .44
Children	1–3	13	29	90	35	1,300 (900–1,800)	5.5
	4–6	20	44	112	44	1,700 (1,300–2,300)	7.1
	7–10	28	62	132	52	2,400 (1,650–3,300)	10.1
Males	11–14	45	99	157	62	2,700 (2,000–3,700)	11.3
	15–18	66	145	176	69	2,800 (2,100–3,900)	11.8
	19–22	70	154	177	70	2,900 (2,500–3,300)	12.2
	23–50	70	154	178	70	2,700 (2,300–3,100)	11.3
	51–75	70	154	178	70	2,400 (2,000–2,800)	10.1
	>76	70	154	178	70	2,050 (1,650–2,450)	8.6
Females	11–14	46	101	157	62	2,200 (1,500–3,000)	9.2
	15–18	55	120	163	64	2,100 (1,200–3,000)	8.8
	19–22	55	120	163	64	2,100 (1,700–2,500)	8.8
	23–50	55	120	163	64	2,000 (1,600–2,400)	8.4
	51–75	55	120	163	64	1,800 (1,400–2,200)	7.6
	>76	55	120	163	64	1,600 (1,200–2,000)	6.7
Pregnancy						+300	
Lactation						+500	

From *Recommended Dietary Allowances*, 9th ed. (Washington, D.C.: National Academy of Sciences, 1980).

Notes: The data in this table have been assembled from the observed median heights and weights of children together with desirable weights for adults for the mean heights of men (70 in.) and women (64 in.) between the ages of 18 and 34 years as surveyed in the U.S. population (Health, Education and Welfare/National Center for Health Statistics data).

The energy allowances for the young adults are for men and women doing light work. The allowances for the two older age groups represent mean energy needs over these age spans, allowing for a 2% decrease in basal (resting) metabolic rate per decade and a reduction in activity of 200 kcal/d for men and women between 51 and 75 years, 500 kcal for men over 75 years, and 400 kcal for women over 75. The customary range of daily energy output is shown for adults in parentheses, and is based on a variation in energy needs of ± 400 kcal at any one age emphasizing the wide range of energy intakes appropriate for any group of people.

Energy allowances for children through age 18 are based on median energy intakes of children these ages followed in longitudinal growth studies. The values in parentheses are 10th and 90th percentiles of energy intake, to indicate the range of energy consumption among children of these ages.

Table G-8. U.S. Recommended Daily Allowances (U.S. RDAs)

Nutrient	Adults and children (4 years or older)	Infants (birth to 1 year)	Children (under 4 years)	Pregnant or lactating women
Required				
Protein (g)	45 or 65*	18 or 25*	20 or 28*	45 or 65*
Vitamin A (IU)	5,000	1,500	2,500	8,000
Vitamin C (mg)	60	35	40	60
Thiamin (mg)	1.5	0.5	0.7	1.7
Riboflavin (mg)	1.7	0.6	0.8	2.0
Niacin (mg)	20	8	9	20
Calcium (mg)	1,000	600	800	1,300
Iron (mg)	18	15	10	18
Optional				
Vitamin D (IU)	400	400	400	400
Vitamin E (IU)	30	5	10	30
Vitamin B_6 (mg)	2.0	0.4	0.7	2.5
Folic acid (mg)	0.4	0.1	0.2	0.8
Vitamin B_{12} (μg)	6	2	3	8
Phosphorus (mg)	1,000	500	800	1,300
Iodine (μg)	150	45	70	150
Magnesium (mg)	400	70	200	450
Zinc (mg)	15	5	8	15
Copper (mg)	2	0.6	1	2
Biotin (mg)	0.3	0.05	0.15	0.3
Pantothenic acid (mg)	10	3	5	10

From Food and Drug Administration, Washington, D.C.

*Lower value if protein efficiency ratio is equal to or greater than that of casein; higher value if protein efficiency ratio is less than that of casein, but greater than 20%.

Table G-9. High-Sodium Foods

Breads	
Biscuits	Pancakes
Bread sticks	Salted crackers
Cornbread	Stuffing mix
Flour, self-rising	Waffles
Cereals	
Instant hot cereal	
Quick cooking cereal	
Convenience foods	
Canned foods (any)	Instant breakfast drinks
Canned soup (any)	Macaroni and cheese
Dried soup	Pizza
Frozen foods (including TV dinners)	Shake and bake mixes
	Spaghetti
Condiments and seasonings	
Salts	Gravy (either packaged or canned)
M.S.G. (meat tenderizer)	Mustard
Barbeque sauce	Party dip
Catsup	Sauces (most)
Chili sauce	
Dairy products	
Cheese	
Meats and meat substitutes	
Anchovies	Liverwurst
Bacon	Lunch meats
Beef jerky	Meat spreads
Bologna	Pastrami
Canadian bacon	Peanut butter
Caviar	Salami
Chipped beef	Salt pork
Corned beef	Sausage
Dried fish	Scallops
Ham	Smoked fish and meat
Hot dogs	
Vegetables	
Canned (most)	Pickles
Frozen (most)	Sauerkraut
Instant mashed potatoes	Vegetable juices
Olives	

Table G-10. Potassium-Containing Foods

High-potassium foods

Fruits	*Vegetables*		*Others*
Apricots	Artichokes	Parsnip	Chocolate
Bananas	Avocado	Potatoes	Cocoa
Casaba melons	Beans (most)	Pumpkin	Nuts
Dates	Brussels sprouts	Spinach	Salt substitute
Honeydew melons	Chard	Squash	Tomato paste
Nectarines	Greens (fresh)	(winter varieties)	Tomato sauce
Oranges		Tomatoes	Milk
Prunes			Yogurt
Raisins			Cottage cheese
Rhubarb			

Medium-potassium foods

Fruits		*Vegetables*	
Apples	Grapes	Asparagus	Greens (frozen)
Blackberries	Papayas	Broccoli	Mushrooms
Cantaloupes	Peaches	Beets	Okra
Cherries	Plums	Cauliflower	Radish
Figs	Pineapples	Celery	Squash
Fruit cocktail	Strawberries (frozen)	Corn	(summer varieties)
		Eggplant	Turnip

From Servonsky/Opas: *Nursing Management of Children*, © 1987 Boston: Jones and Bartlett Publishers.

Glossary

abscess a collection of purulent exudate, commonly with local symptoms of inflammation.

acromegaly disease of adults from hyperfunction of the anterior pituitary, causing an increase in growth hormone; Marie's disease.

Addison's disease destruction of adrenal cortex tissue, resulting in decreased resistance to infections, fatigue, anorexia, hypotension, hyponatremia, and hypoglycemia.

agraphesthesia not possessing the sense of graphesthesia.

alopecia absence or loss of hair. Common causes are heredity, aging, radiation, chemotherapy, acute nervous disorders, debilitating disease, and endocrine disorders.

Alzheimer's disease presenile dementia with decreased frontal and occipital lobe functioning, resulting in memory loss, disorientation, decreased intellectual functioning, and apathy.

amenorrhea absence of menstrual bleeding.

amyotrophic lateral sclerosis (ALS) a generally fatal motor neuron disease involving degeneration of the pyramidal tract, brain stem, and spinal cord; manifested by muscular atrophy, weakness, and spasticity.

anemia decrease in red blood cells, hemoglobin, and hematocrit levels in the blood; can be due to many causes, including hemorrhage, iron deficiency, hemolytic disease, and loss of bone marrow. *See also* pernicious anemia.

aneurysm weakened wall of a blood vessel or heart chamber, resulting in localized outpouching or dilation; may result from congenital defect, infection, or trauma.

angina pain; e.g., angina pectoris is chest pain.

anisocoria unequal pupils, resulting from a congenital defect, localized lesions, or trauma to the nervous system.

ankylosing stiffening and fusing of a joint.

anomaly an abnormality; anything contrary to general rule.

anorexia loss of appetite.

anorexia nervosa extreme weight loss, fear of becoming obese, and extreme dieting, commonly seen in young females; thought to be of psychological origin.

anosmia loss of smell.

anoxia absence or complete lack of oxygen.

aphasia inability to communicate; receptive aphasia is the inability to understand communication; expressive aphasia is the inability to express oneself in any form of communication.

arrhythmia an irregular heartbeat, usually due to problems with the cardiac conduction system. *See also* sinus arrhythmia, tachyarrythmia.

arteriosclerosis thickening of the arterial walls, resulting in ischemia of tissues and organs; arteries become stenotic and lose their elasticity.

arthritis inflammation of a joint, generally accompanied by pain and swelling; may be seen with rheumatic fever, ulcerative colitis, gout, osteoarthritis, fibromyositis, or infection.

ascites fluid within the peritoneal cavity.

asthma bronchial spasm accompanied by wheezing, dyspnea, and bronchial secretions; attacks may be initiated by allergens, strenuous exercise, infection, irritants, and emotional stress.

asymmetrical not balanced; uneven.

atelectasis a collapsed lung.

atherosclerosis laying down of lipid and cholesterol deposits within the inner layers of the blood vessels. Pathogenesis is unclear. Atherosclerosis is commonly seen with aging, hypertension, obesity, and diabetes mellitus and may lead to angina pectoris, coronary artery disease, peripheral vascular disease, and myocardial infarction.

atrial septal defect an opening between the two atria; a congenital anomaly characterized by harsh systolic murmur and right atrial and ventricular hypertrophy; diagnosis is made by cardiac catheterization.

atrophy a wasting away and decrease in size.

azotemia increased nitrogenous bodies, especially urea, in the blood.

bacterial endocarditis *see* endocarditis.

Bell's palsy affliction of the facial nerve by such things as infection, neoplasm, or trauma; manifested by facial paralysis that may be unilateral or bilateral, temporary or permanent.

benign not malignant.

bimanually using two hands.

bradycardia slow heart action relative to age; a heart rate of below 60 in an adult or below 70 in a child.

brain stem all of the brain except the cerebrum and cerebellum.

bronchiectasis chronic bronchial dilation, characterized by coughing of copious amounts of offensive purulent sputum, dyspnea, and coarse rales; treated with antibiotics and postural drainage.

bronchitis inflammation of the bronchi, manifested by initial dry cough progressing to productive mucopurulent cough, fever, and back pain. Chronic bronchitis is characterized by productive cough for 3 or more consecutive months in at least 2 successive years.

brucellosis undulant fever; generally acquired from contaminated milk or milk products or through a break in the skin; common symptoms are fever, chills, diaphoresis, anorexia, weakness, headache, and joint pain.

bruit a venous or arterial sound; auscultated as a humming, crackling, rasping, blowing, or rubbing sound over blood vessels, organs, or glands.

Buerger's disease thromboangiitis obliterans; inflammatory vascular disease resulting in occulsion and related signs such as burning, numbness, tingling, loss of peripheral pulses.

bulimia a voracious craving for food; eating binges followed by purging, depression, and self-deprivation.

cachexia emaciation generally associated with malnutrition, a severe debilitating disease, or malignancy.

café au lait spots pale tan macular skin lesions that may be of no significance or may be associated with neurofibromatosis.

carbuncle inflammation in the skin manifested as a deep circumscribed pocket of purulent material that will suppurate; common sites are neck, upper back, and buttocks; occurs more frequently in men and diabetics.

carcinoma cancer; a growth within the epithelial tissue that tends to invade the adjacent areas and metastasize (spread) to other body parts via the lymph or blood system.

cardiomegaly enlargement of the heart.

cardiomyopathy disease of heart muscle generally due to an obscure etiology.

cerebral palsy upper motor neuron dysfunction developing from birth trauma or developmental defects; victim may exhibit dysphagia, difficulty sucking, athetosis or ataxia, spastic plegia, and impaired speech/vision/hearing. Mental ability is from normal to varying degrees of mental retardation.

cerebrovascular accident (CVA) ischemia of brain tissue caused by circulatory thrombosis, embolus, or hemorrhage (apoplexy); sequelae are focal. Severe symptoms diminish within a few days as brain tissue edema subsides.

cheilosis cracking and scaling of mouth and lips caused by deficient riboflavin intake.

chilblain red, edematous skin resulting from extreme cold exposure; skin area may burn and itch and could blister, crust, and ulcerate.

cholecystitis inflammation of the gallbladder, manifested by nausea, vomiting, food intolerance, right upper quadrant abdominal pain that may radiate to area between the scapulae, eructation, and flatulence; diagnosed by oral cholecystogram (x-ray).

cholera an acute bacterial infection involving the small intestines, resulting in severe fluid and electrolyte loss, vomiting, diarrhea (rice-water appearance), cyanosis, circulatory collapse, oliguria, and metabolic acidosis.

cholesteremia high level of cholesterol in the blood; also called cholesterolemia.

chronic obstructive pulmonary disease (COPD) a progressive irreversible disease of the lungs characterized by persistent dyspnea on exertion with or without cough and maximum breathing capacity cut in half; aggravated by tobacco, air pollutants; occurs secondary to bronchitis, chronic emphysema, and asthma. *See also* emphysema.

Chvotek's sign local muscular spasm in response to a tap on the side of the face over the area of the facial nerve (temporal-facial area); indicative of tetany.

circumoral around the lips.

cirrhosis chronic degeneration of the liver, manifested by anorexia, flatulence, ascites, light-colored stool, spider angiomas, abdominal pain, weight loss, weakness, portal hypertension, and esophageal varices; commonly caused by alcohol abuse, malnutrition, hepatitis, carbon tetrachloride and phosphorus poisoning, tumors/obstruction, animal parasites (especially schistosoma), tertiary syphilis, and congestion secondary to congestive heart failure (CHF).

cleft palate a fissure or elongated opening that divides the palate in half.

clonus alternating contraction and relaxation of muscles.

coarctation a stricture or narrowing of the lumen of a blood vessel, most commonly the aorta.

cognition act of abstracting and assimilating properties from the environment to acquire general and specific knowledge; the active process of perception, reasoning, and memory.

coitus sexual intercourse between a male and female involving penis insertion into the vagina.

congenital pertaining to a condition that one is born with, such as a birth anomaly.

conjunctiva mucous membrane that lines the inside of the eyelids and reflects onto the eyeball as a transparent covering over the sclerae of the eyes.

conjunctivitis inflammation of the conjunctivae; blood-shot eyes; results from bacterial infection, eyestrain, exposure to ultraviolet rays, irritation from heat, cold, or chemicals, presence of a foreign body, or trauma.

consolidation hardening; solidification.

contralateral on the opposite side.

cor pulmonale right-sided cardiac failure, manifested chiefly by edema, liver congestion, hepatomegaly, ascites, and high venous pressure.

coryza "cold" symptoms.

crepitation/crepitus a crackling sound heard in tissue palpation when air has entered, as around a tracheotomy; a grating sound with movement of the ends of a broken bone.

cretinism congenital thyroid hormone deficiency manifested by myxedema and arrested physical and mental development, resulting in dwarfism and mental retardation; treated with thyroid preparation.

cryptorchidism undescended testicle.

culture the symbols, rituals, ideas, values, traditions, and institutions of a specific population group.

Cushing's syndrome hypersecretion of adrenocortical hormones; the most common cause is pituitary tumor (Cushing's disease); manifested by "moonface," "buffalo hump," osteoporosis, amenorrhea, capillary fragility, edema, hirsutism, hypokalemia, muscle atrophy and weakness, purplish striae, and emotional changes.

cutaneous pertaining to the skin.

cyanosis bluish, gray-slate color to the skin and mucous membranes due to decreased blood hemoglobin, excessive deoxygenated hemoglobin, structural defects in the hemoglobin molecule (methemoglobin), or a congenital defect within the circulatory system (tetralogy of Fallot); especially apparent in nailbeds, on earlobes, at tip of nose, on buccal mucosa, and in conjunctivae.

cystic fibrosis hereditary disorder of the exocrine glands, affecting the sweat glands, respiratory system, and pancreas; manifested by viscous, foul-smelling stools, pancreatic insufficiency, and respiratory infections with thick mucous secretions.

decussation a crossing of fibers from one side to another, as with the optic chiasm and pyramidal tract fibers crossing over in the brain.

delusion a false belief; for example, a person may believe he is Napoleon or may not eat because he believes that he does not have a stomach.

dermatitis inflammation of the skin evidenced by pruritus, erythema, and various skin lesions.

dermatofibroma a nonmalignant skin nodule appearing as a gray or red, round, firm painless lesion, commonly on the extremities; sometimes seen in lupus erythematosus.

desquamation a flaking or sloughing off of epidermal cells of the skin.

diabetes mellitus a disorder of carbohydrate metabolism, manifested by polyuria, polyphagia, polydipsia, hyperglycemia, and glycosuria; results from inadequate production or use of insulin.

diaphoresis excessive sweating; copious perspiration.

diphtheria an acute infectious bacterial disease characterized by a false yellowish-white or gray membrane lining on any mucous surface (usually the throat), lymphadenopathy, fever, myocarditis, and late neuritis; is often fatal.

diplopia double vision.

distal toward the extremities of the body.

diverticulosis presence of sacs or pouches within the walls of a canal or organ, particularly the colon; may become inflamed (diverticulitis).

Down's syndrome congenital condition characterized by mental deficiency, small head and slanting eyes, and a fissured tongue that is usually large and protruding; caused by chromosomal abnormality.

dynamic active; changing, moving rapidly.

dyschezia painful defecation.

dyscrasia a synonym for disease.

dysmenorrhea painful menstruation.

dyspareunia painful coitus.

dyspepsia indigestion.

dysphagia difficulty swallowing.

dyspnea difficulty breathing; labored respirations.

dystonia impaired muscle tone.

ecchymosis bruised skin; bleeding into tissue from trauma, a bleeding disorder, or condition with bleeding tendency.

eczema an acute or chronic dermatitis with erythema, papules, pustules, vesicles, crusts, or scales alone or in combination; more a symptom than a disease.

edema an excessive amount of fluid within the interstitial compartment of the body; may be localized or generalized.

edentulous having no teeth.

effusion escape of fluid into a part, such as a cavity or tissue.

ejaculation emission of seminal fluid from the male urethra.

embolus a moving mass in a blood or lymphatic vessel; may consist of air bubbles or of solids such as tumor cells, blood plaques, tissue, or clumps of bacteria.

emphysema a condition in which the aveoli of the lungs are distended, the lungs lose their elasticity, and expiration becomes difficult.

empyema pus in a body cavity, especially the pleural cavity.

encephalitis inflammation of the brain; may be a specific disease caused by an arbor virus or may follow measles, influenza, chickenpox, smallpox, or other diseases; may also result from metal poisoning, such as lead poisoning.

encephalopathy any dysfunction of the brain.

endocarditis inflammation of the membrane lining the heart (endocardium) as a result of bacterial invasion.

endorphins polypeptides synthesized in the brain that act as opiates, producing analgesia and raising the threshold for pain.

enuresis bedwetting.

epididymitis inflammation of the epididymis, characterized by local edema, fever, chills, and inguinal pain; may be associated with prolonged use of an indwelling catheter or may be a complication of mumps, gonorrhea, syphilis, urethritis, prostatitis, or trauma.

epigastric pertaining to the area at the costal angle—the abdominal area inferior to the xiphoid process of the sternum.

epilepsy cerebral disorder characterized by seizures ranging from a fluttering of the eyes (petit mal seizure) to unconsciousness and sometimes incontinence. *See also* grand mal seizure.

epistaxis nosebleed; nasal hemorrhage.

Erb's point site at the left third or fourth intercostal space near the sternum.

erythema redness of the skin due to such things as wind, heat, inflammation, infection, or vasodilation.

erythema multiforme dark red papules appearing in successive eruptions of short duration, usually on the extremities; not accompanied by pruritus, burning, or joint pains.

erythroblastosis fetalis a hemolytic disease of the newborn marked by increased erythroblasts in the blood and characterized by anemia, jaundice, hepatomegaly, and splenomegaly; caused by Rh-negative antibodies developed in the mother against an Rh-positive fetus.

excoriation epidermal abrasion caused by heat, moisture, chemicals, trauma, or similar causes.

exfoliative dermatitis chronic inflammation of the skin accompanied by redness and the excessive scaling off of dead tissue; commonly involves the entire body surface; etiology is unknown.

exophthalmos abnormal protrusion of the eyeballs, seen in thyrotoxicosis, ocular orbital tumor, trauma, aneurysm or other intracranial lesions, Cushing's disease, acromegaly, leukemia, and other conditions.

extravasation escape of fluid—usually blood, serum, or lymph—into surrounding tissues.

exudate a fluid containing cells, protein, and solid material that accumulates in a cavity or oozes through the tissues, usually as the result of an inflammatory condition.

facies the expression or appearance of the face, such as the masklike expression in Parkinsonism, the pinched-drawn appearance in scleroderma, or the dull-coarse lethargic look in myxedema.

fasciculations involuntary twitching of small muscle fiber bundles, commonly seen with eyelid twitching due to eyestrain but clinically reflective of lower motor neuron damage.

feces stools; body waste discharged from the bowels.

fibrillation quivering or spontaneous contraction of muscle fibers, especially atrial or ventricular; contractions are rapid, tremulous, and ineffectual for adequate functioning.

fibroma a fibrous connective tissue tumor that is irregular in shape, of a firm consistency, and slow growing; pain occurs only with pressure or cystic degeneration.

fibrosis abnormal formation of fiber-containing tissue; can be seen to occur in the uterus, in muscles (dystrophies), and following pulmonary disease.

fissure crack in the skin or mucosal tissue.

fistula a tubelike passage from one cavity to another or to a free surface.

flaccid relaxed, flabby; having little or no muscle tone.

flatulence accumulation of intestinal gas, occasionally causing abdominal distention.

fluorescein a red crystalline powder used to detect foreign bodies in the eye or corneal lesions.

focal pertaining to a focus—a specific point or location.

foramen ovale an opening between the two atria of the heart that normally closes shortly before or after birth.

fremitus palpable vibration of air passing through the lung tissue with vocalization.

frenulum a fold of mucous membrane connecting two parts; for example, the frenulum of the tongue attaches the lower surface of the tongue to the gum.

furuncle a boil; an acute staphylococcal infection of a gland or hair follicle characterized by pain, erythema, and edema, usually suppurating with necrotic tissue present.

gait manner of walking.

gas gangrene a necrosis or tissue death in a wound infected by a gas bacillus.

gastric pertaining to the stomach.

gastroenteritis inflammation of the gastrointestinal tract (stomach and intestines).

Gaucher's disease a rare chronic familial disorder of fat metabolism associated with hepatomegaly, splenomegaly, skin hyperpigmentation, and bone lesions.

gene a basic unit of heredity occupying a certain place on a chromosome; sex-linked genes are contained within the X chromosome.

glabella frontal bone; forehead.

glaucoma a disease of the eye resulting in increased intraocular pressure; untreated, it will lead to optic disk atrophy and blindness. The classic early symptom of glaucoma is seeing halos around lights.

glossectomy removal of the tongue.

glycosuria sugar (glucose) in the urine.

goiter enlargement of the thyroid gland; may be due to dietary iodine deficiency, inflammation, tumors, or hyperfunction or hypofunction of the thyroid.

gonadotropins gonad-stimulating hormones such as follicle-stimulating hormone (FSH), luteinizing hormone (LH), and interstitial cell–stimulating hormone (ICSH); they stimulate ovarian and testicular functioning.

gout hereditary metabolic disease involving uric acid crystal deposits in the skin and joints; manifested by attacks of painful gouty arthritis.

grand mal seizure a seizure characterized by unconsciousness, tonic spasm followed by clonic movements, frothing at the mouth, and facial cyanosis.

graphesthesia the ability to perceive outlines, numbers, words, or symbols traced or written on the skin.

Graves' disease hyperthyroidism due to pituitary dysfunction; exophthalmos is the primary clinical sign.

gravida a pregnant state; usually seen in documentation to record a woman's number of pregnancies, whether or not they were carried to delivery of a child. *See also* para.

Guillain-Barré syndrome an idiopathic polyneuritis usually occurring after a viral infection or immunization for flu; characterized by muscular weakness that may lead to paralysis; resolution of affliction is seen in a few weeks to a few months.

gustatory pertaining to the sense of taste.

gynecomastia breast enlargement in the male.

hallucination a false perception, lacking any exterior stimuli; may be visual, auditory, olfactory, kinetic, microptic, somatic, or teleologic.

heart block blockage of nerve impulses from the atrium to the ventricles; characterized by arrhythmias.

heart murmur *see* murmur.

heave upward lift or rising of the chest, particularly of the precordial area, due to cardiac problems.

hematemesis vomiting of blood.

hematuria blood in the urine.

hemianopsia blindness of half the field of vision in one or both eyes.

hemiparesis slight paralysis of one side of the body.

hemiplegia paralysis of one side of the body.

hemochromatosis a rare disease characterized by excess iron deposits throughout the body, a bronze hue to the skin, hepatomegaly, diabetes mellitus, and frequently cardiac failure; occurs more commonly in males.

hemodialysis by-passing the kidneys using a machine containing semipermeable membranes to remove drugs or toxic chemicals from the blood.

hemolytic referring to the breaking down of red blood cells.

hemophilia a sex-linked condition characterized by a markedly prolonged blood coagulation time; occurs almost exclusively in males.

hemoptysis expectorating or coughing blood.

hepatic pertaining to the liver.

hepatitis inflammation of the liver caused by a virus or toxin; characterized by jaundice and by hepatomegaly, fever, chills, pruritus, nausea, vomiting, liver tenderness, headache, or general weakness.

hepatomegaly enlargement of the liver.

heredity transmission of genetic characteristics.

hernia protrusion or projection of an organ or part of an organ through the wall of the cavity that normally contains it. Weakness of the wall may be caused by debilitating disease, injury, increased pressure resulting from heavy lifting or from coughing, old age, or prolonged distention, as from tumors, ascites, or pregnancy.

herniated intervertebral disk a prolapsed nucleus pulposus (the cushion portion of an intervertebral disk), which allows the spinal nerves to be compressed and perhaps damaged; also called ruptured or slipped disk.

herpes simplex a cold sore or fever blister; vesicles caused by herpes simplex virus.

herpes zoster a painful vesicular eruption along the course of a nerve; caused by the varicella-zoster virus (the same virus that causes chickenpox); is almost always unilateral.

hiatal hernia protrusion of the stomach upward through the hiatus (opening) of the diaphragm; characterized by burning, dyspeptic symptoms.

hirsutism excessive growth of hair; can be hereditary or due to hormonal dysfunction or medication (especially testosterone); seen in porphyria.

Hodgkin's disease a disease of unknown cause producing lymphadenopathy, beginning in the cervical region, then proceeding to the axillary, inguinal, mediastinal, and mesenteric regions. Associated manifestations include hepatomegaly, splenomegaly, and anemia.

Homan's sign pain in the calf of the leg upon dorsiflexion of the foot; an early sign of deep venous thrombosis.

Horner's syndrome pupillary constriction, partial ptosis of the eyelid, enophthalmos, and sometimes loss of sweating over the involved side of the face; caused by paralysis of the cervical sympathetic nerve.

Huntington's chorea a hereditary disease with onset in the third to fifth decades of life; characterized by progressive chorea and dementia.

hydatidiform mole multiple cystic involvement of the chorionic villi of the uterus; can occur during pregnancy; characterized by uterine bleeding, nausea, edema, hypertension, hyperthyroidism, and anemia.

hydrocephalus increased accumulation of fluid within the ventricles of the brain or within the subdural spaces; may result from developmental anomalies, infection, injury, or brain tumors.

hydronephrosis collection of urine in the renal pelvis due to lower urinary tract obstruction, causing nephron destruction and impaired renal function.

hypercapnia high levels of carbon dioxide in the blood.

hypercholesteremia high blood levels of cholesterol.

hyperesthesia increased sensitivity to touch stimuli.

hyperglycemia increased level of glucose in the blood; high blood sugar.

hyperkeratosis overgrowth of the horny epidermal layer of the skin; overgrowth of the cornea of the eye.

hypernephroma a renal tumor that to the naked eye resembles adrenal tissue.

hyperplasia enlargement of a part as a result of an increase in the number of cells.

hyperprolactinemia increased secretion of prolactin believed to be a result of hypothalamic-pituitary dysfunction.

hyperthermia unusually high fever (hyperpyrexia); treatment of disease by raising bodily temperature.

hypertrophy enlargement of a part as the result of an increase in the size of the individual cells.

hypoglycemia decrease in the glucose level in the blood; low blood sugar.

hypogonadism decreased functioning of the sex organs (i.e. testes, ovaries).

hypokalemia decrease of potassium level of the blood resulting in weakness and cardiac rest in diastole.

hypovolemia oligemia; decreased volume of blood in the body.

hypoxia decreased oxygen content or tension.

ideation formation of ideas; the process of thinking.

idiopathic a disease or condition without a recognized cause; no clear pathogenesis known.

imperforate without an opening; for example, with an imperforate anus there is no lower opening from the intestinal tract.

impetigo a skin disease characterized by pustules that become crusted and rupture, usually around the mouth and nostrils; commonly caused by staphylococci or streptococci or a combination of both.

incontinence inability to retain urine, feces, or semen as a result of loss of sphincter control or of cerebral or spinal lesions.

induration an area of hardened tissue.

infarction an area of necrosis within the body.

infectious mononucleosis an infectious viral disease characterized by enlarged, often tender lymph nodes, splenomegaly, increased mononuclear leukocytes in the blood, fever, sore throat, and heterophile antibodies in the blood.

inguinal pertaining to the region of the groin.

insufficient inadequate for its purpose.

integument the skin, hair, and nails.

intention tremors tremors that are initiated upon movement.

intermittent claudication calf muscle pain occurring with walking and subsiding with rest; due to inadequate blood supply or venous return.

intertrigo a superficial dermatitis in the folds of the skin.

intraductal within a duct.

ipsilateral of the same side; affecting the same side of the body.

iritis inflammation of the iris, characterized by pain, photophobia, decreased vision, lacrimation, and an irregularly shaped and sluggish pupil.

ischemia local and temporary lack of blood to a body part caused by obstruction of circulation to the part.

jaundice *see* obstructive jaundice.

keratitis inflammation of the cornea.

keratosis overgrowth of cornified epithelium, characterized by horny growths on the skin, buccal mucosa, hair follicles, and sweat pores (especially on the palms and soles); also dry, gray, layered lesions of the aged, warts.

ketoacidosis accumulation of ketone bodies resulting from incomplete metabolism of fatty acids, generally from carbohydrate deficiency or inadequate utilization. Commonly observed in diabetes mellitus, starvation, high-fat diets, and pregnancy and following ether anesthesia.

17-ketosteroids steroids, produced by the adrenal cortex and gonads, that appear normally in the urine. A hyperexcretion or hypoexcretion level in the urine is indicative of endocrine disorder.

kinesthesia the ability to discriminate the extent, direction, or weight of one's movement.

Klinefelter syndrome a chromosomal abnormality estimated to occur in 1 out of 700 live male births. Testicular failure manifests in atrophied testes, gynecomastia, abnormally long legs, and subnormal intelligence.

Korsakoff's syndrome syndrome characterized by psychoses, amnesia, memory defects, insomnia, hallucinations, bilateral foot drop, and painful extremities; may occur as sequel to alcoholism. Also called polyneuritic psychosis. Associated with vitamin B complex deficiency, especially deficiencies of thiamine and B_{12}.

Kussmaul breathing an extreme rate and depth of respirations; commonly observed in ketoacidosis.

lacrimation the production of tears; usually refers to excessive tearing.

lactation the production and secretion of breast milk in the period of suckling.

lamina cribrosa the flat plate (cribriform plate) of the ethmoid bone.

Leriche syndrome absent or weak femoral pulses, sexual dysfunction, and ischemic pain in the buttocks and legs due to a thrombus at the aortic-femoral artery bifurcation.

lethargic drowsy, sluggish, stuporous.

leukemia a blood cancer of unknown cause characterized by an elevated leukocyte (WBC) count and the presence of immature leukocytes; occurs in both acute and chronic forms.

leukopenia a decrease in white blood cells; results in increased vulnerability to infection.

leukoplakia a white circumscribed plaque formation that is precancerous; may occur on the lips, buccal mucosa, tongue, vulva, or penis; needs referral for biopsy.

libido sexual urge, drive, or desire.

lift *see* heave.

lipoma a fatty tumor; frequently multiple but not metastatic.

lupus erythematosus a chronic and usually fatal systemic disease of unknown etiology characterized by a butterfly-pattern skin rash across the nasal bridge and cheeks, fever, arthritis, and usually varying degrees of renal, lung, and heart involvement; occurs primarily in females.

lymphadenopathy disease involvement of the lymph nodes.

lymphangitis inflammation of the lymph system, frequently due to streptococci, marked by fever, chills, moderate swelling, and pain; may be manifested by deep general flush of the affected area if the infection is in the deep layers of the skin.

lymphocytes lymph cells that can occur as B cells or T cells and are active in immune reactions.

lymphosarcoma a malignant disease of lymphatic tissue; may clinically appear similar to Hodgkin's disease.

maceration softening process caused by a seeping in of fluid.

malaria an infectious protozoan disease manifested by chills, pyrexia, diaphoresis, anemia, and splenomegaly; can be transmitted via infected blood transfusion or hypodermic needle.

malnutrition nutritional disorder caused by lack of adequate nutrient intake, malabsorption, or deficient body utilization of food.

mastitis inflammation of the breast.

mastoiditis inflammation of the air cells of the mastoid process; manifested by fever, chills, tenderness, leukocytosis, and sepsis.

melena dark tarry stool resulting from upper gastrointestinal bleeding.

menarche onset of menstruation; age when first menstrual period occurred.

meningioma a slow-growing tumor arising from arachnoidal tissue; may occur following head injury; results in brain tissue compression.

meningitis inflammation of the membranes of the spinal cord or brain due to bacteria, viruses, or other organisms; may be manifested by anorexia, irregular fever, intense headache, pupillary contraction, light and sound intolerance, opisthotonos, delirium, convulsions, and coma.

menorrhagia abnormally excessive amount of menstrual flow.

metastasis spread of bacteria or body cells (especially cancer cells) from one part of the body to another; usually applied to a secondary malignant growth in a new body location.

methemoglobinemia the presence in the blood of methemoglobin, a compound related to oxyhemoglobin that is useless as an oxygen carrier; follows poisoning by certain substances.

metrorrhagia bleeding between menstrual periods.

moniliasis a fungal infection of the skin, mucous membranes (mouth, vagina, bronchi, lungs), or nails; may also invade the bloodstream. Moniliasis is caused by yeastlike fungi of the *Candida* species, chiefly *Candida albicans*.

monocyte a large leukocyte (white blood cell).

monogamy marriage to only one person at any one time.

mononucleosis *see* infectious mononucleosis.

morbidity pertaining to illness; disease rates or occurrences.

mortality pertaining to death; death rates related to cause, age, sex, and other similar variables.

mucopurulent pertaining to drainage consisting of mucus and pus.

multiple myeloma malignant bone marrow growth characterized by progressive bone destruction, resulting in anemia, bone fractures, weight loss, proteinuria, and kidney failure; generally fatal.

multiple sclerosis a disease characterized by muscular weakness, lack of coordination, paresthesias, speech disturbances, and visual problems; caused by demyelination of portions of the white matter in the central nervous system.

murmur a soft blowing or rasping sound heard on auscultation; it is caused by vibrations produced by movement of blood within the heart and adjacent large blood vessels. The presence of a murmur does not necessarily indicate organic pathology.

muscular dystrophy genetically transmitted disease characterized by wasting away and atrophy of the muscles, weakness, and deformities.

myasthenia gravis a disease that results from a lack of acetylcholine or an excess of cholinesterase at the myoneural junction; characterized by extreme muscular weakness (without atrophy) and progressive fatigability. Ptosis of the eyelids is usually present. Symptoms are worse in the evening. Occurs most frequently in women and between the ages of 20 to 50.

myelin a fatlike substance composed of cholesterol, cerebrosides, phospholipids, and fatty acids; it is the principal component of the myelin sheath of nerve fibers.

myocardial pertaining to the heart muscle.

myositis ossificans an inherited disease in which bone tissue replaces muscle tissue, resulting in neck and spine stiffness that progresses to extremities.

myotonia tonic muscular spasms; spastic, stiff muscles that do not relax readily following contraction.

myxedema hypofunction of the thyroid occurring secondary to anterior pituitary hypofunction, dietary iodine deficiency, atrophy of the thyroid gland, surgical excision of the thyroid gland, or excessive use of antithyroid drugs. It is manifested by lethargy, mental apathy, large tongue, slow speech, coarse edematous skin, puffy hands and face, alopecia, coarse dry hair, and increased sensitivity to cold.

natal pertaining to the labor and delivery phase of pregnancy.

necrosis death of tissue or bone cells surrounded by healthy parts; a dead mass.

neoplasm a new growth; a mass.

nephritis inflammation of the kidney cells.

neurectomy partial or total resection of a nerve.

neuritis inflammation of a nerve.

neuroasthenia nervousness, irritability, anxiety, depression, chronic fatigue; nervous exhaustion; anxiety neurosis.

neurodermatitis pruritic skin disorder usually with lichenification and excoriations; common with family history of allergies.

neurogenic has origin in nerves; resulting from nerve impulses.

neuropathies diseases affecting the nerves; inflammation and degeneration of the peripheral nerves due to such causes as impaired circulation, trauma, toxic and chemical irritation, and infection.

neurosis maladaptation and coping in regard to anxiety.

neurosyphilis syphilis affecting the nervous structures, such as dementia paralytica and tabes dorsalis.

nevus a vascular skin tumor, usually congenital, caused by hyperplasia of the blood vessels; congenital pigmentation of a circumscribed area of the skin, such as a birthmark or mole.

niacin water-soluble vitamin of the B complex group that is not stored in the body. Good sources are poultry, fish, liver, kidney, eggs, nuts, and wheat germ.

Niemann-Pick disease a hereditary disease involving a disturbance in lipid metabolism; characterized by hepatomegaly, splenomegaly, anemia, lymphadenopathy, and progressive mental and physical deterioration; death usually occurs before age three.

nocturia the need to urinate during the night.

noncompliance lack of participation or cooperation.

nonpathologic not constituting a diseased state.

normal range within the parameters of normalcy.

nulliparous referring to a woman who has never had a viable offspring; para 0.

nystagmus constant involuntary oscillatory movement of the eyeball, which may be in any direction; appearance of the eyes rapidly darting back and forth in a vertical or horizontal plane.

obesity two times the IBW (ideal body weight).

obstructive jaundice yellow coloration of the hard palate, sclerae, and skin as a result of mechanical block of the flow of bile from the liver to the duodenum.

occlusion relation of the teeth when the jaws are closed; may also pertain to obstruction or closure of a passage, such as coronary occlusion—blockage of a coronary artery.

oculist a physician who specializes in diagnosing and treating diseases of the eye.

oliguria decreased amount of urine formation.

ophthalmologist a medical doctor who specializes in diseases of the eye.

ophthalmos protrusion of the eyeballs, sometimes to the extent that the eyelids will not close, creating danger of corneal drying and ulceration.

opisthotonos a body position characterized by an arched back with feet and head on the floor; seen in severe meningitis and tetanus.

organomegaly enlargement of a body organ.

orthopnea the inability to breathe while lying in a flat position.

Osler-Weber-Rendu disease an autosomal dominant inherited disease involving hemorrhagic telangiectasia; bleeding may be spontaneous or from minor trauma.

osmosis the transport of water from an area of greater concentration to one of lesser concentration.

osteodystrophy defective bone development.

osteogenesis imperfecta an autosomal dominant inherited disease involving disturbance in connective tissue; characterized by brittle bones, multiple fractures, blue sclerae, deafness, hypoplasia of the teeth, epistaxis, and diaphoresis.

osteomalacia softening of the bones so that they become flexible and brittle, resulting in deformities; caused by vitamin D deficiency or by deficiency or loss of calcium salts. It occurs in adults and mainly in women.

osteomyelitis infection of bone and bone marrow, characterized by pain, fever, diaphoresis, leukocytosis, and possibly suppuration.

osteoporosis increased porosity of the bone, predisposing to fractures and deformities; often occurs with immobilization and in postmenopausal women.

otitis externa inflammation of the pinna (auricle) of the ear.

otitis media inflammation of the middle ear.

otosclerosis ankylosis (fusing or growing together) of the stapes and oval window in the middle ear; characterized by chronic progressive deafness, especially for low tones; more common in females.

palpebral conjunctiva *see* conjunctiva.

palsy temporary or permanent loss of the ability to move or to control movement.

pancreatitis inflammation of the pancreas.

papilledema edema and inflammation of the optic nerve head due to increased intracranial pressure.

papilloma a benign epithelial tumor of the skin or of a mucous membrane; includes polyps, warts, condylomas.

para term used to document that a viable baby has been produced. *See also* parous.

paradoxical conflicting with expectation; seemingly contradictory.

paralysis loss of voluntary motor function.

paralytic ileus paralysis of the intestines, with resulting distention and symptoms of acute obstruction; the absence of peristalsis may be a postoperative complication, particularly of abdominal surgery.

paranoia the possession of persecutory delusions, usually centered on a major theme, such as an unfaithful spouse, a job situation, or finances; behaviors observed include aloofness, seclusion, resentment, aggressiveness, and hostility.

paraplegia paralysis of the lower portion of the body and both legs.

parasomnia a sleep disorder, mostly affecting children, consisting of night terrors, sleepwalking, and bedwetting that occur either individually or in combinations.

paresis partial or incomplete paralysis.

paresthesia abnormal sensation without objective cause, such as numbness, tingling, "crawling," or prickling sensations; heightened sensitivity.

Parinaud's syndrome palsy in which the individual is unable to look up or down; also conjunctivitis of bacterial cause accompanied by preauricular lymph node enlargement and tenderness.

Parkinson's disease a chronic nervous disease characterized by masklike facies, resting tremors, slow measured speech, muscular weakness and rigidity, forward inclination of the body with fast-shuffling gait, and a pill-rolling motion of the fingers.

parous having given birth.

paroxsymal nocturnal dyspnea (PND) awakening suddenly in the middle of the night unable to "get one's breath"; sudden dyspneic attack that wakes one up in the middle of sleep.

parturition childbirth.

patency the state of being open; not obstructed.

patent ductus arteriosus persistence of the foramen ovale after birth.

pathognomic see pathologic.

pathologic constituting a disease or disease process.

pavor nocturnus night terrors.

pemphigus an acute or chronic disease of adults manifested by successive eruptions of bullae, which appear suddenly and disappear leaving pigmented spots; may be accompanied by pruritus and burning; the etiology is unknown.

peptic ulcer a breakdown and ulceration of the gastric mucosa; manifested by burning epigastric pain that can usually be relieved by food or antacids.

pericarditis inflammation of the pericardium (the sac enclosing the heart), characterized by moderate fever, precordial pain, dry cough, dyspnea, palpitations, and a pulse that is initially rapid and forceful, then weak and irregular.

periodontitis inflammation or degeneration or both of dental periosteum, alveolar bone, cementum, and adjacent gingivae, wherein teeth become loose and gingivae recess; suppuration is common. It usually follows chronic gingivitis, Vincent's infection, or poor dental hygiene. May be predisposed by systemic factors.

peripheral vascular disease pathologic involvement of the blood vessels in the periphery of the body; when severe can lead to ischemia of tissue, ulceration, and necrosis of local areas.

peristalsis an involuntary progressive wavelike movement that occurs in the hollow tubes of the body, especially the alimentary canal.

peritonitis inflammation of the peritoneum (the lining of the abdominal cavity).

pernicious anemia macrocytic anemia due to achlorhydria (decreased secretion of intrinsic factor by the stomach for intestinal absorption of Vitamin B_{12}).

Perthes' disease a degenerative disease of the head of the femur, characterized by pain and a limp; occurs primarily in male adolescents.

petechiae small purplish, hemorrhagic spots on the skin that do not blanch with applied pressure.

Peyronie's Disease distortion or flexion of the penis due to the hardening of the corpora cavernosa; sexual intercourse is impossible or limited without augmented devices and medical, surgical, and/or radiologic therapy.

phenylketonuria (PKU) a recessive genetic condition in which the body is unable to oxidize the amino acid phenylalanine to tyrosine; it is characterized by tremor, convulsions, mental deficiency, hyperactivity, eczema, and offensive odor of urine and sweat.

pheochromocytoma an adrenal medullary tumor that produces catecholamines (norepinephrine and epinephrine), which in turn cause hypertension, pounding headaches, sweating, palpitation, flushing of the face, nausea and vomiting, and tingling of the extremities.

phlebitis inflammation of a vein, manifested by pain, erythema, skin hot to touch, and tenderness along the course of the vein; inflammatory swelling and acute edema occur below the inflammatory obstruction. Homan's sign (pain upon dorsiflexion of the foot) is present.

phonation the process of uttering vocal sounds.

photophobia the inability to tolerate light; commonly observed in measles, rubella, meningitis, and inflammation of the eyes.

Pick's disease see Alzheimer's disease.

pityriasis rosea macular yellow-salmon or red lesions, somewhat scaly, erupting on the trunk obliquely to the ribs, or reddish ring-shaped patches symmetrically distributed over the extremities.

placenta previa condition in which the placenta is attached at the lower uterine segment covering the cervical os; it is the most common cause of painless bleeding in the third trimester of pregnancy.

plantar wart viral-caused wart on the sole of the foot, appearing as a hyperkeratotic ring with soft central core.

pleural pertaining to the thoracic cavity; within the chest cavity.

pleural effusion *see* effusion.

pleurisy inflammation of the pleura (the membrane lining the lungs).

pleximeter the finger that is tapped with the plexor in the indirect method of percussion.

plexor a finger that applies the blow or tap in the indirect method of percussion.

pneumonectomy removal of a lung.

pneumonia bacterial or viral infection of the lungs characterized by chills, fever, chest pain, and productive mucopurulent cough, occasionally with headache, cyanosis, gastrointestinal disorders, or herpes simplex.

pneumothorax a collection of air or gas in the pleural cavity, causing a severe stabbing pain in the side, marked dyspnea, absence of breath sounds, and unilateral distention of the chest.

poliomyelitis a viral infection of the motor horns of the spinal cord, characterized by severe upper respiratory symptoms or by gastrointestinal disturbances that may come on gradually and by a slight fever, frequently lasting not more than three days. Paralysis may or may not occur at the end of this period. Extent of paralysis depends on the degree of nerve involvement. Small groups of muscles of one or all extremities or respiratory muscles may be involved.

polycystic having many cysts.

polycythemia an excess of red blood cells, characterized by weakness, fatigue, vertigo, tinnitus, flushing of the face, ecchymosis, redness and pain of the extremities, and splenomegaly; etiology is unknown.

polydipsia excessive thirst.

polyp a tumor on a stem that bleeds easily and may become malignant.

polyuria excessive amount of urine excreted.

postnatal occurring after birth; postpartal.

preeclampsia a toxemia of pregnancy characterized by hypertension, edema, headaches, proteinuria, irritability, and hyperreflexia; occurs in 5–7% of pregnancies.

prenatal prior to birth; antepartal; antenatal.

priapism painful constant erection of the penis because of disease, usually without sexual desire; may be due to organic irritation of nerve tracts or nerve centers and cord lesions above the lumbar region; sometimes observed with acute leukemia.

proctocolectomy removal of the rectum and colon.

prognosis estimation of course and end of disease; prediction of chance for recovery.

prostaglandins fatty acid derivatives that have a potent action on target organs, including the uterus, prostate, brain, lung, kidney, and pancreas.

prostatitis inflammation of the prostate gland; acute prostatitis is characterized initially by frequent urination, later by urine retention and by discomfort and pain in the perineal area.

proximal nearest to the center of the body; opposite of distal.

pruritus itching.

psoriasis a genetically determined dermatitis appearing as flat-topped papules covered by thin, grayish-white scaling; under the dry scales are red bleeding points.

psychosis any mental disorder manifesting personality disintegration and loss of contact with reality; usually characterized by delusions and hallucinations.

psychosomatic pertaining to bodily symptoms thought to be etiologically related to emotional factors.

ptosis dropping or drooping of an organ or part; usually applied to drooping of the eyelids because of paralysis or muscle weakness.

pulmonary pertaining to the respiratory system.

pulmonary embolus *see* embolus.

purpura ecchymotic areas characterized by hemorrhages into the skin; hemorrhages may also be in the mucous membranes, internal organs, and other tissues.

purulent pertaining to yellow, thick, puslike fluid.

pyloric pertaining to the opening between the stomach and the duodenum.

pyramidal tract tract arising from the giant pyramid-shaped cells of Betz present in the motor area of the cerebrum and descending the spinal cord.

pyrexia fever.

pyrosis heartburn; burning sensation in the epigastric and esophageal region.

pyuria pus present in the urine.

quadriplegia paralysis affecting all four limbs.

rationale explanation; reason; theory base.

Raynaud's disease a condition, common in young females, in which cold temperatures or emotional stress cause an abnormal degree of vasospasm in the extremities. Symptoms are relieved by heat.

regurgitation return of blood backward through a defective heart valve. Also, return of solids or fluids to the mouth or nose from the stomach.

rehabilitation the process of restoring a person who has been ill or handicapped to useful life or restoring a dysfunctional part to usefulness.

renal rickets a disturbance in epiphyseal growth during childhood caused by severe chronic renal insufficiency, resulting in persistent acidosis, dwarfism, and failure of gonadal development.

retrograde moving backward.

rheumatic fever a systemic febrile disease preceded by a group A beta hemolytic streptococcal infection. It is frequently followed by serious heart or kidney disease. The client is especially susceptible to subsequent attacks. The most common onset is sudden occurrence of fever and joint pain.

rhizotomy cutting of a spinal nerve.

riboflavin a water-soluble B vitamin found in milk and milk products, organ meats, fish, eggs, green leafy vegetables, whole grains, and legumes; deficiency is characterized by cheilosis, glossitis, face and scalp seborrheic dermatitis, photophobia, corneal opacities, edema, trembling, sluggishness, vertigo, vaginal pruritus, and urinary hesitancy.

rickets a disease characterized by abnormal shape and structure of bones, due chiefly to vitamin D deficiency, which affects calcium and phosphorus absorption from the intestine and phosphorus reabsorption by the renal tubules; may also result from inadequate calcium intake or excessive calcium loss.

rubella German measles (three-day measles); characterized by a short course, slight fever, and freedom from sequelae.

rugae folds in mucous membranes.

salpingitis inflammation of a fallopian tube.

scabies a highly communicable skin disease caused by an arachnid (*Sarcoptes scabiei*); most commonly affects the hands, the area between the fingers, the wrists, the axillae, the genitals, the area beneath the breasts, and the inner aspects of the thighs; characterized by papules, vesicles, pustules, burrows, and intense pruritis resulting in eczema.

scaphoid concave shape; sunken.

schistosomiasis a parasitic infection contracted by contact with fresh water contaminated with human feces; symptoms are focal to the body part infected—gastrointestinal, urinary, or respiratory tract.

schizophrenia a psychosis manifesting as gross distortion of reality, withdrawal, delusions, hallucinations, emotional lability, and other bizarre behaviors.

scleroderma a progressive skin disease affecting the collagen tissue, resulting in atrophied, smooth, waxy, stretched, edematous skin, which becomes indurated, yellowish, and adherent to underlying tissue, causing masklike facies or clawlike appearance of hands (sclerodactylia); may eventually show respiratory, cardiac, and renal involvement. The etiology is unknown; disease progression is usually slow.

scoliosis lateral curvature of the spine; an S curve as viewed from the back of the client.

sebaceous glands oil-secreting glands of the skin, often associated with hair follicles.

seborrhea a disease of the sebaceous glands marked by increased sebaceous secretion, leading to dandruff or greasy crusts and scales.

seizure a convulsion; a sudden attack of certain symptoms. *See also* grand mal seizure.

sensorium level of consciousness.

septicemia blood poisoning; absorption of septic products or pathogenic bacteria into the blood and tissues; characterized by fever, chills, petechiae, purpuric pustules, and abscesses.

sequelae conditions following and resulting from a disease.

shock a clinical syndrome (pallor, cyanosis, weak and rapid pulse, increased and shallow respirations, decreased or unobtainable blood pressure, oliguria, and dilated pupils) of varying degrees of diminished oxygen supply to the tissues and venous return to the heart; can be caused by many conditions, including hemorrhage, heart damage, injury, infection, drug reaction, poisoning, dehydration, and insect bites.

sickle-cell anemia a hereditary chronic hemolytic anemia occurring mostly in Blacks and persons of Mediterranean descent. Characterized by severe dyspnea and muscular pains.

sinus arrhythmia an irregular heart rhythm in which the heart rate increases with inspiration and decreases with expiration; common in children and young adults; nonpathological except in older adults.

somnambulism sleepwalking.

spastic pertaining to stiffness and muscular rigidity resembling spasms.

splenomegaly enlargement of the spleen.

spondylosis stiffening and fusing of the segments of the vertebral column.

squamous cell carcinoma malignant growth of the flat, scaly epithelial cells.

Starling's law law stating that the length of the heart fibers determines the force of the heartbeat/contraction.

stasis stagnation or pooling of the flow of fluids, such as venous blood, urine, or intestinal contents.

Stein-Leventhal syndrome an anovulatory ovarian follicle disorder manifested by menstrual abnormality, infertility, and hirsutism in about 50% of clients; of unknown etiology, but excess circulating androgen, such as testosterone, appears to be a factor.

stenosis constriction or narrowing of a passage or orifice; stricture.

stereognosis the ability to discriminate between shape, size, and relative weight of objects.

stomatitis inflammation of the buccal mucosa.

stools feces; waste matter discharged from the bowels.

strabismus squint; the inability to direct both eyes to the same object simultaneously because of the lack of muscular coordination. The prime factors leading to squint are hypermetropia and myopia.

stasis dermatitis hyperpigmentation and dry flakes of skin generally observed on the lower legs due to poor blood supply or venous return.

strial atrophia pinkish-white or gray lines of thin skin seen in parts of the body where the skin has been stretched, as with pregnancy, obesity, a tumor, or edema.

subacute less than acute but having some acute features.

subarachnoid pertaining to beneath the arachnoid meninge. Subarachnoid hemorrhage is bleeding into the subarachnoid space.

sublingual beneath the tongue; the sublingual glands, the smallest of the salivary glands, are located on either side of the frenulum between the tongue and the mandible.

suppuration the liquidification and accumulation of dead cells (forming pus) and discharge of the pus; accompanied by localized redness, swelling, heat, and pain.

suprapubic superior to the pubic symphesis.

syncope fainting; temporary, short loss of consciousness.

syndrome a cluster or group of signs and symptoms.

symmetrical even; balanced.

syphilis an infectious chronic sexually transmitted disease. The primary stage has skin lesions with lymphadenopathy about 2 weeks later; the secondary stage is characterized by headache, fever, anorexia, alopecia, bone or joint pain, and condylomata papules that appear 2 months after the primary lesions; the tertiary stage involves damage to various tissues such as the myocardium, heart valves, nerves, and brain.

systemic pertaining to the whole body or a whole system, as in systemic circulation.

tabes dorsalis locomotor ataxia; a form of neurosyphilis involving progressive degeneration of sensory neuron fibers of the posterior columns of the spinal cord and usually the dorsal roots and ganglia of spinal nerves.

tachyarrhythmia an irregular heartbeat that is of a rapid rate.

tachycardia abnormally rapid heart rate relative to age.

tamponade pathologic compression of an organ, especially the heart, by an external agent.

Tay Sachs disease an autosomal recessive inherited disease characterized by neurological deterioration and by blindness, convulsions, cherry red spots on maculae, spasticity, dementia, paralysis, and death usually before age 4.

telangiectasia dilation of small blood vessels that are more prone to trauma; also, a hereditary thinning of blood vessel walls of the nose, skin, and gastrointestinal tract, with a tendency to hemorrhage.

teratogenic harmful to the embryo or fetus.

tetanus an acute infectious disease caused by the toxins of *Clostridium tetani*, an anaerobic bacterium, at the site of an injury; manifested by stiffness of jaw, neck, and esophageal muscles, leading to a persistent painful state of muscle contraction (lockjaw, opisthotonos) and high fever. Usually but not always fatal.

tetany intermittent tonic muscular spasms induced by changes in the pH and extracellular calcium, as occurs with alkalosis, parathyroid deficiency or inadvertent removal of the parathyroids during thyroidectomy (removal of the thyroid), and vitamin D deficiency. Characterized by numbness, tingling of the extremities, muscle cramp (especially of the hands), nervousness, irritability, and apprehension. Diagnostic signs are Chvostek's sign, Trousseau's sign, and the peroneal sign.

Tetralogy of Fallot a congenital heart anomaly consisting of four defects: (1) pulmonic stenosis, (2) ventricular septal defect, (3) overriding of the aorta, and (4) right ventricular hypertrophy.

thrill a palpable murmur; the murmur is grade IV or louder and is of such intensity that palpable vibrations of the sound can be detected.

thrombocytopenic purpura a hemorrhagic disorder in which there is a lessening of the number of platelets in the blood; manifested by bleeding and ecchymosis upon slight injury; also called purpura hemorrhagica or Werlhof's disease.

thrombus a clot that is attached to the wall of a blood vessel, sometimes large enough to result in stenosis; may become dislodged and travel, at which time it is called an embolus.

thrust *see* heave.

thyroidmegaly enlargement of the thyroid gland.

thyrotoxicosis a toxic condition caused by the hyperfunction of the thyroid gland; manifested by tachycardia, tremors, increased basal metabolic rate, enlarged thyroid gland, exophthalmos, nervous symptoms, and loss of weight.

tic an involuntary spasmodic muscular twitch or contraction, commonly involving the face, head, neck, or shoulder muscles.

tic douloureaux dysfunction of the trigeminal nerve, with stabbing pains of the face; also called trigeminal neuralgia.

timbre quality of a sound other than pitch or intensity; vibratory quality.

tinea corporis ringworm; fungal skin inflammation in which central portions are clear, while new patches, in the form of red papules and vesicles, spring up in the periphery; often causes intense pruritus.

tinnitus a subjective ringing in the ears that may be due to a variety of causes, including impacted cerumen, myringitis, otitis media, labyrinthitis, Meniere's disease, otosclerosis, hysteria, and drug use (quinine, streptomycin).

tonometry measurement of the tension of a part, such as intraocular tension, using a special instrument called a tonometer.

tophi urate crystal deposits in the skin, often seen with gout; commonly detected on the helix of the ear and on the elbows and knees.

torticollis wryneck; congenital or acquired stiff neck, drawing the head to one side with the chin pointing to the other side; twisted neck.

tracheotomy surgical opening into the trachea, usually for insertion of a tube to overcome tracheal obstruction; tracheostomy.

trachoma a chronic contagious form of conjunctivitis caused by a virus transmitted directly by contact with secretions or indirectly by contaminated articles (towels, handkerchiefs, and so forth); occurs mostly in Asia and Africa but is also seen in the southwestern United States; a major cause of blindness.

trauma an injury (physical or emotional) or wound.

tremor quivering; shaking; trembling; may be fine or coarse, rapid or slow, aggravated or initiated with movement or upon resting of the body part.

trichinosis a disease contracted by eating raw or insufficiently cooked pork containing *Trichinella spiralis;* manifested by pain, nausea, vomiting, and serious diarrhea; in one to two weeks swollen, painful muscles develop, along with dyspnea, high fever, diaphoresis, and eosinophilia.

Trousseau's sign muscular spasm produced when pressure is applied to the nerves and vessels of the upper arm; indicative of late tetany; also occurs in osteomalacia.

tuberculosis an infectious disease caused by the tubercle bacillus; characterized by inflammation, tubercle formation, caseation, necrosis, abscesses, fibrosis, and calcification. It most commonly affects the respiratory system but may also infect the gastrointestinal tract, genitourinary tract, bones, joints, nervous system, lymph nodes, and skin.

ulcer an open sore or lesion of the skin or of a mucous membrane.

ulcerative colitis a chronic intestinal inflammatory disease marked by exacerbations and remissions. Acute symptoms are profuse watery diarrhea containing blood, mucus, and pus, accompanied by tenesmus, severe abdominal cramps, anemia, and weight loss.

umbilicus the "belly button"; the depressed point in the mid-abdomen that marks former attachment of the umbilical cord to the fetus.

uremia retention of nitrogenous substances normally excreted by the kidneys, producing a toxic state manifested by nausea, vomiting, headache, urinous odor to perspiration, lethargy, coma or convulsions, and azotemia; caused by renal disease or disturbances in circulation, fluid balance, or metabolism.

urticaria hives.

vascular pertaining to or composed of blood vessels.

vasectomy excision bilaterally of part or all of the vas deferens.

ventricular pertaining to a ventricle, especially either of the two lower chambers of the heart.

vertigo dizziness; a whirling feeling in the head; stationary vertigo refers to the sensation of the room or environment whirling about the person.

vertex the top of the head; vertex presentation is delivery of a fetus with the head presenting or born first.

viscus (plural: viscera) any internal organ enclosed within a cavity such as the abdomen or thorax.

vitiligo milk-white areas of the skin found in dark-skinned people. The cause is unknown.

wen a cyst, varying in size from that of a pea to a large walnut, that is painless, is rather soft, and contains a yellowish-white caseous mass; caused by retention of secretions in a sebaceous gland; slowly appears on scalp, face, or back.

Werlhof's disease *see* thrombocytopenic purpura.

Wilms' tumor a childhood malignant tumor of the kidney.

Wilson's disease a rare disease thought to be the result of abnormal copper metabolism; characterized by degeneration of the corpus striatum and cirrhosis of the liver; manifested by tremors and muscle distortion increased by activity.

xanthoma patches of yellow-appearing lipid deposits in tissues, usually accompanied by hyperlipidemia/hypercholesteremia; commonly observed with uncontrolled diabetes mellitus. It is called Hand-Schüller-Christian disease when present throughout the body, especially on the face, in tendon sheaths, and in mucous membranes.

Bibliography

Allen, D. G. and Whatley, M. 1986. Nursing and men's health—some critical considerations. *The nursing clinics of North America* 21(1):3–13.

Allend, A. 1970. *Adaptation in cultural evolution: an approach to medical anthropology.* New York: Columbia University Press.

Allison, S. D., and Wong, K. L. 1968. Skin cancer: some ethnic differences. In *Environments of man,* ed. J. B. Bresler. Reading, Mass.: Addison-Wesley.

Allport, G. W., and Vernon, P. E. 1960. *Study of Values.* 3rd ed. Boston: Houghton Mifflin.

American Medical Association Conference on Mental Retardation. Jan. 18, 1965. *Composite developmental inventory for infants and young children: a conference report. J.A.M.A.* 191: 153–154.

Apgar, V. 1985, 1958. *J.A.M.A.* 168.

Armstrong, B.; Van Merwyk, A. J.; and Coates, H. 1977. Blood pressure in Seventh Day Adventist vegetarians. *Am. J. Epidemiol.* 105 (5):444–449.

Audy, J. R., and Dunn, F. L. 1974. Health and disease. In *Human ecology,* ed. F. Sargent. New York: American Elsevier.

Beck, D. F., and Jones, M. A. 1985. *Family therapy, in overview.* 2nd ed. Eds. Goldenberg, I., and Goldenberg, H. Monterey, CA: Brooks/Cole.

Beckman, M.; Zentner, R.; and Proctor, J. 1979. *Nursing concepts for health promotion.* 2nd ed. Englewood Cliffs, N.J.: Prentice-Hall.

Bellack, J. P., and Bamford, P. A. 1984. *Nursing assessment: a multidimensional approach.* Boston: Jones and Bartlett.

Bello, T. A. Feb. 1976. The third dimension: cultural sensitivity in nursing practice. *Imprint* 23:36–38, 45.

Ben Leslies, S., and Short, M. 1983. The effects of physical exercise on self-attitudes. *Occupational Therapy in Mental Health* 3:11–28.

Bernard, J., and Thompson, L. F. 1970. *Sociology: Nurses and their patients in a modern society.* St. Louis: C. V. Mosby.

Biddle, B. J. and Thomas, E. S. 1966. *Role theory: concepts and research.* New York: Wiley.

Blattner, B. 1981. *Holistic nursing.* Englewood Cliffs, N.J.: Prentice-Hall.

Blood, R. A., and Wolfe, D. M. 1960. *Husbands and wives.* New York: Free Press.

Bomar, P. J. 1989. *Nurses and family health—concepts, assessment, and intervention.* Baltimore: Williams and Wilkins.

Bozett, F. W. and Forrester, D. A. 1989. A proposal for a men's health nurse practitioner. *IMAGE: Journal of Nursing Scholarship* 21(3):158–16?.

Braunwald, E.; Isselbacher, K.; Petersdorf, R.; Wilson, J.; Martin, J.; and Fauci, A. 1987. *Harrison's principles of internal medicine.* 11th ed. New York: McGraw-Hill Book Company.

Brill, E. L., and Kilts, D. F. 1986. *Foundations for nursing.* 2nd ed. Norwalk, Conn.: Appleton-Century-Crofts.

Brim, O. G. 1968. Adult socialization. In *Socialization and society,* ed. J. A. Clausen. Boston: Little Brown.

Brosnan, J. 1976. A proposed diabetic program for Puerto Ricans in New York City. In *Transcultural nursing: a book of readings,* ed. P. J. Brink. Englewood Cliffs, N. J.: Prentice-Hall. 263–275.

Brown, M. S. 1976. A cross-cultural look at pregnancy, labor, and delivery. *O.G.N.* 5.

Burch, T. A.; Comess, L. J.; and Bennett, P. H. 1968. The problem of gallbladder disease among Pima Indians. In *Biomedical challenges presented by the American Indian,* Pan American Health Organization scientific publication no. 165. Washington, D.C.: World Health Organization.

Burnside, I. 1980. *Psychosocial nursing care of the aged.* 2nd ed. New York: McGraw-Hill.

Burnside, I. 1984. *Working with the elderly—group process and techniques.* 2nd ed. Boston: Jones and Bartlett.

Byrne, M., and Thompson, L. 1978. *Key concepts for the study and practice of nursing.* 2nd ed. St. Louis: C. V. Mosby.

Cadoret, R. J., and King, L. J. 1974. *Psychiatry in primary care.* St. Louis: C. V. Mosby.

Caldwell, W. E., and Malloy, H. C. 1933. Anatomic variations in the female pelvis and their effect in labor, with a suggested classification. *Am. J. Obstetrics and Gynecology.* 26:479.

Caplan, D. 1974. *Support systems and community mental health.* New York: Behavioral Publications.

Carolenuto, R., and Bullock, J. 1980. *Physical assessment of the gerontologic client.* Philadelphia: F. A. Davis.

Carpenito, L. J. 1983. *Nursing diagnosis application to clinical practice.* Philadelphia: J. B. Lippincott.

Cassem, N. H., and Hackett, T. P. 1971. Psychiatric consultation in a coronary care unit. *Ann. Internal Med.* 75:9–14.

Center for Disease Control. 1972. *Ten state nutrition survey. 1968–1970. I. Historical development. II. Demographic data.* U. S. Department of Health, Education and Welfare. Publication No. (HSM) 72-8130. Atlanta: Center for Disease Control.

Chesler, P. 1972. *Women and madness.* New York: Doubleday.

Chinn, P. and Jacobs, M. 1987. *Theory and nursing—a systematic approach.* St. Louis: C. V. Mosby Company.

Clark, M. 1970. *Health in the Mexican-American culture.* Berkeley: University of California Press.

Clark, M.; Gosnell, M.; Hager, M.; and Shapiro, D. July 13, 1981. The mystery of sleep. *Newsweek.* 98:48–51.

Cohen, Y. 1968. *Man in adaptation: the biosocial background.* Chicago: Aldine.

Combs, A. W.; Avila, D. L.; and Purkey, W. W. 1971. *The helping relationship sourcebook.* Boston: Allyn & Bacon.

Cormier, W. H., and Cormier, L. 1979. *Interviewing strategies for helpers: a guide to assessment, treatment, and evaluation.* Monterey, Calif.: Brooks/Cole.

Curran, G. 1983. *Traits of a healthy family.* New York: Ballantine Books.

Damon, A. 1977. *Human biology and ecology.* New York: W. W. Norton.

Dean, Kathryn 1989. Self-care components of lifestyles: the importance of gender, attitudes, and the social situation. *Social Science Medicine* 29(2): 137–152.

DeAngelis, C. 1984. *Pediatric primary care.* 3rd ed. Boston, Toronto: Little, Brown.

Dingle, J. H.; Badger, G. F.; and Jordan, W. S. 1964. *Illnesses in the home: a study of 25,000 illnesses in a group of Cleveland families.* Cleveland: Case Western Reserve University.

Doll, R., and Peto, R. 1981. The causes of cancer: quantitative estimates of avoidable risks of cancer in the United States today. *Journal of the National Cancer Institute* 66:1193–1308.

Dougherty, M. C. 1976. Health agents in a rural black community. *J. Afro-Amer. Issues* 4(1):44.

Dubos, R. 1965. *Man adapting.* New Haven: Yale University Press.

Dunn, H. L. High-level wellness for man and society. *J.N.M.A.* 49:225–235.

Duvall, E. 1971. *Family development.* Philadelphia: J. B. Lippincott.

Duvall, E. M. 1977. *Marriage and family development.* 5th ed. Philadelphia: Lippincott.

Earnest, D. L., and Fletcher, G. P. 1969. Danger of rectal examination in patients with acute myocardial infarction: fact or fiction? *New Eng. J. Med.* 281: 238–241.

Ebersole, P., and Hess, P. 1981. *Toward healthy aging.* St. Louis: C. V. Mosby.

Edelman, G. N. November 1983. When kids won't sleep. *Parents.* 58:74–76.

Ekman, P.; Sorenson, E. R.; and Friesen, W. V. April 1969. Pan cultural elements in facial displays of emotion. *Science* 164:3875.

Erikson, E. H. 1950. *Childhood and society.* New York: W. W. Norton.

Erikson, E. H. 1968. *Identity, youth, and crisis.* New York: W. W. Norton.

Falls, H. B.; Baylor. A.; and Dishman, R. 1980. *Essentials of Fitness.* Philadelphia: Saunders College/ Holt, Rinehart and Winston.

Farrell, W. 1986. *Why men are the way they are.* New York: McGraw Hill.

Fast, J. 1971. *Body language.* New York: Pocket Books.

Fink, D. July 1976. Holistic health: Implications for health planning. *A.J.H.P.* 1:23–31.

Fink, R.; Shapiro, S.; and Soldensohn, S. S. 1969. The filter-down process to psychotherapy in a group practice medical care program. *Am. J. Pub. Health* 59:245–260.

Fire, M., and Baker, C. 1976. A smile and eye contact may insult someone. *J. Nurs. Ed.* 15:15.

Flynn, P. A. R. 1975. *Holistic health: the art and science of care.* Bowie, Md.: Robert J. Brady Company.

Fogel, C. I., and Woods, N. F. 1981. *Health care of women.* St. Louis: C. V. Mosby.

Foreman, M. D. 1986. Cardiovascular disease: a men's health hazard. *The nursing clinics of North America* 21(1):65–73.

Forrester, D. A. 1986. Myths of masculinity: impact upon men's health. *The nursing clinics of North America* 21(1):15–23.

Fredrich, J. A. 1977. Tension control techniques. In *Guide to fitness after fifty,* eds. R. Harris and L. W. Frankel. New York: Plenum Press. 337–338.

Freeman, H. E.; Levine, S.; and Reeder, L. G. 1972. *Handbook of medical sociology.* Englewood Cliffs, N.J.: Prentice-Hall.

Freiberg, K. 1983. *Human development: a life-span approach.* 2nd ed. Boston: Jones and Bartlett.

Fried, M. 1969. Social differences in mental health. In *Poverty and health,* ed. J. Kosa, A. Antonovsky, and I. K. Zola. Cambridge, Mass.: Harvard University Press.

Friedl, J., and Chrisman, N. J. 1975. *City ways: a selective reader in urban anthropology.* New York: Thomas Y. Crowell.

Friedman, M. M. 1986. *Family nursing: theory and assessment.* 2nd ed. Norwalk, CT: Appleton-Century-Crofts.

Friedman, M. M. 1981. *Family nursing: theory and assessment.* New York: Appleton-Century-Crofts.

Getchell, B. 1979. *Physical fitness: a way of life.* 2nd ed. New York: Wiley.

Getchell, B., and Anderson, W. 1982. *Being fit: a personal guide.* New York: Wiley.

Gibbs, C. E.; Martin, H. W.; and Gutierrez, M. J. 1974. Patterns of reproductive health care among the poor of San Antonio, Texas. *Am. J. Pub. Health* 64.

Goldston, I. ed. 1963. *The family: a focal point in health education.* New York: International Universities Press.

Goldston, I. ed. 1963. *Man's image in medicine and anthropology.* New York: International Universities Press.

Gordon, M. 1982. *Nursing diagnosis, process and application.* New York: McGraw-Hill.

Green, T. H. 1977. *Gynecology: essentials of clinical practice.* 3rd ed. Boston: Little, Brown.

Gribbin, K.; Schaie, K. W.; and Parham, I. A. 1980. Complexity of life style and maintenance of intellectual abilities. *J. Social Issues* 36:47–61.

Griffith, J., and Christensen, P. 1982. *Nursing process, application of theories, framework and models.* St. Louis: C. V. Mosby.

Griggs, W. 1978. Sex and the elderly. *Am. J. Nurs.* 77:1352–1354.

Groen, J. J. 1973. Gaucher's disease: hereditary transmission and racial distribution. In *Ethnic groups of America—their morbidity, mortality and behavior disorders*, ed. A. Shiloh and I. C. Selevan. Springfield, Ill.: Charles C Thomas.

Hales, D. 1981. *The complete book of sleep.* Reading, Mass.: Addison-Wesley.

Hall, E. T. 1960. Language of space. *Landscape* 10:41–42.

Hall, E. T. 1969. *The hidden dimension.* New York: Anchor Press.

Hall, E. T. 1973. *The silent language.* New York: Anchor Press.

Hall, E. T. 1976. *Beyond culture.* New York: Anchor Press.

Hammond, P. B. 1969. *Cultural and social anthropology.* London: Macmillan.

Harburg, E., et al. 1973. Sociocultural stressor areas and black-white blood pressure in Detroit. *J. Chron. Dis.* 26:595–611.

Hardy, M. and Conway, M. 1978. *Role theory perspective for health professionals.* Norwalk, CT: Appleton-Century-Crofts.

Havighurst, R. J. 1952. *Developmental tasks and education.* New York: David McKay.

Hertzog, C.; Schaie, K. W.; and Gribbin, K. 1978. Cardiovascular disease and changes in intellectual functioning from middle to old age. *J. Gerontology* 33:872–883.

Herzlich, C. 1973. *Health and illness: a social psychological analysis.* New York: Academic Press.

Hill, R. 1968. Social stress on the family. In *Sourcebook in marriage and the family,* ed. M. B. Sussman. New York: Houghton Mifflin.

Hogue, C. C. 1977. Support systems for health promotion. In *Distributive nursing practice: a systems approach to community health.* 2nd ed. Eds. J. Hall and B. Weaver. Philadelphia: Lippincott.

Hollingshead, A. B., and Redlich, F. C. 1958. *Social class and mental illness: a community study.* New York: Wiley.

Holman, A. M. 1983. *Family health assessment for understanding and intervention.* Beverly Hills, CA: Sage Publications.

Holmes, T. H., and Rahe, R. H. 1967. The Social Readjustment Rating Scale. *J. Psychosom. Res.* 11:213.

Horton, P. B. 1965. *Sociology and the health sciences.* New York: McGraw-Hill.

Howard, J., and Holman, B. L. 1970. The effects of race and occupation on hypertension mortality. *Millbank Memorial Fund Quarterly* 48:263–296.

Howe, J. 1980. *Nursing care of adolescents.* New York: McGraw-Hill.

Hui, Y. H. 1983. *Human nutrition and diet therapy.* Boston: Jones and Bartlett.

Iliff, A., and Lee, V. A. 1952. Pulse rate, respiratory rate, and body temperature of children between 2 months and 18 years. *Child Development.* 23:237.

Insel, P. M., and Moos, R. H. 1974. *Health and social environment.* Lexington, Mass.: Lexington Books, D. C. Heath.

Iyer, P. W.; Taptich, B. J.; and Bernocchi-Losey, D. 1986. *Nursing process and nursing diagnosis.* Philadelphia: W. B. Saunders.

Janosik, E. H. 1984. *Crisis counseling, a contemporary approach.* Boston: Jones and Bartlett.

Jenkins, C. D. 1971. Psychologic and social precursors of coronary disease. *New Eng. J. Med.* 284(5): 244–255.

Jourard, S. 1971. *The transparent self.* New York: Jossey Bass.

Kalisch, B. J., and Kalisch, P. A. 1981. *Politics of nursing.* Philadelphia: F. A. Davis.

Kark, S. L. 1974. *Epidemiology and community medicine.* New York: Appleton-Century-Crofts.

Katz, S. H., and Schall, J. 1979. Fava bean consumption and biocultural evolution. *Medical Anthropology* 3:459–477.

Kavanagh, H. B. May 1980. Some appraised instruments of values for counselors. *Personnel and Guidance Journal.* 613–617.

Keesing, R., and Keesing, F. 1971. *New perspectives in cultural anthropology.* New York: Holt, Rinehart and Winston.

Kellerman, H. 1981. *Sleep disorders: insomnia and narcolepsy.* New York: Brunner/Mazel.

Kelley, E. C. 1977. The fully functioning self. In *Human dynamics in psychology and education,* ed. D. E. Hamacheck. Boston: Allyn & Bacon.

Kephart, W. M. 1961. *Family, society and the individual.* Boston: Houghton Mifflin.

Killien, M. G. 1985. An environmental approach to nursing practice. In *Distributive nursing practice: a systems approach to community health.* 2nd ed. Ed. J. E. Hall. Philadelphia: Lippincott.

Kilwein, J. H. Jan. 1975. Social class differences in family attitudes: are they diminishing among young people? *J. School Health* 45:27–29.

Kim, M., and Moritz, D. A. 1982. *Classification of nursing diagnoses, proceedings of the third and fourth national conferences.* New York: McGraw-Hill.

Kinney, J., and Leaton, G. 1982. *Understanding alcohol.* New York: C. V. Mosby.

Koos, E. L. 1954. *The health of Regionville.* New York: Columbia University Press.

Koshi, P. T. 1976. Cultural diversity in the nursing curricula. *J. Nursing Ed.* 15(2):14–21.

Krane, R. J. 1988. Impotence. *The urologic clinics of North America* 15(1). Philadelphia: W. B. Saunders Company.

Kreigh, H. Z., and Perko, J. E. 1979. *Psychiatric and mental health nursing: commitment to care and concern.* Reston, Va.: Reston Publishing.

Kübler-Ross, E. 1975. *Death: the final stage of growth.* Englewood Cliffs, N.J.: Prentice-Hall.

Lebowitz, M. D. 1975. Social environment and health. *Pub. Health Rev.* 4:327–351.

Leighton, D. C., et al. 1963. *The character of danger.* New York: Basic Books.

Leininger, M. 1963. *Transcultural nursing: concepts, theories and practices.* Chicago: W. and J. Stone Foundation.

Leininger, M. 1970. *Nursing and anthropology: two worlds to blend.* New York: Wiley.

Levin, A. 1979. City diseases that can kill you. In *Culture, Cures, and Contagion,* ed. N. Klein. Novato, Calif.: Chandler and Sharp.

Levin, R. 1975. *Clinical pharmacy and therapeutics,* eds. E. T. Herfindal and J. Hirschman. Baltimore: Williams & Wilkins.

Lewis, C. M. 1984. *Basic and family nutrition: a self-instructional approach.* Philadelphia: F. A. Davis.

Lienhardt, G. 1966. *Social anthropology.* 2nd ed. New York: Oxford University Press.

Louie, T. T. T. 1976. Exploratory thinking in Chinese Americans. In *Transcultural nursing: a book of readings,* ed. P. J. Brink. Englewood Cliffs, N. J.: Prentice-Hall. 240–246.

McArdle, W. D.; Katch, F. I.; and Katch, V. L. 1981. *Exercise physiology.* Lea and Febiger.

McCubbin, H. and Dahl, B. 1985. *Marriage and family: individuals and life cycles.* New York: John Wiley.

McElroy, A., and Townsend, P. K. 1979. *Medical anthropology in perspective.* Boston: Duxbury Press.

MacElveen, P. M. 1978. Social networks. In *Clinical practice in psychosocial nursing: assessment and intervention,* eds. D. C. Longo and R. A. Williams. New York: Appleton-Century-Crofts.

MacGregor, F. C. 1960. *Social science in nursing.* New York: Russell Sage Foundation.

Mallinger, K. M. 1989. The American family: history and development. In *Nurses and family health promotion,* ed. P. J. Bomar. Baltimore: Williams and Wilkins.

Martin, H., and Prange, A. 1962. The stages of illness: psychosocial approach. *Nursing Outlook* 10(3).

Maslow, A. H. 1954. *Motivation and personality.* New York: Harper & Row.

Mausner, J. S., and Bahn, A. K. 1974. *Epidemiology: an introductory text.* Philadelphia: W. B. Saunders.

Mead, M. 1956. Understanding cultural patterns. *Nursing Outlook* 4(5):260–262.

Mead, M. 1964. *Anthropology: a human science.* Princeton, N. J.: D. Van Nostrand.

Mechanic, D. 1968. *Medical sociology: a selective view.* New York: Free Press.

Mizner, W. 1955. In *Speaker's handbook of epigrams and witticisms,* ed. H. V. Prochnow. New York: Harper.

Morgan, W. L., and Engel, G. I. 1969. *The clinical approach to the patient.* Philadelphia: W. B. Saunders.

Morris, M. G. 1968. Maternal claiming-identification processes: Their meaning for mother-infant mental health. In *Parent-child relationships: the role of the nurse.* Presented at Continuing Education Program for Nurses Workshop, eds. A. Clark, et al. New Brunswick, N.J.: Rutgers University, The State University of New Jersey. 34–35.

Myrianthopoulos, J. C., and Aronson, S. M. 1973. Population dynamics of Tay-Sachs disease—I. Reproductive fitness and selection. In *Ethnic groups of America—their morbidity, mortality, and behavior disorders,* ed. A. Shiloh and I. C. Selevan. Springfield, Ill.: Charles C Thomas.

Neel, J. V. 1967. Current concepts of the genetic basis of diabetes mellitus and the biological significance of the diabetic predisposition. *Excerpta Medica Internat. Congr.* Series no. 1725.

Niswander, J. D. 1968. In *Biomedical challenges presented by the American Indian,* Pan American Health Organization scientific publication no. 165. Washington, D. C.: World Health Organization.

Nye, F. I. 1976. *Role structure and analysis of the family.* Beverly Hills, CA: Sage Publications.

Oliver, John. 1974. *Clinical sexuality.* 3rd ed. Philadelphia: J. B. Lippincott.

Orque, M. 1981. Cultural components. In *Maternity care: the nurse and the family,* eds. M. Jensen, S. R. Bensom, and I. Bobak. St. Louis: C. V. Mosby.

Ostfeld, A. M., and Shekelle, R. B. 1967. Psychological variables and blood pressure. In *The epidemiology of hypertension,* ed. J. Stamler, R. Stamler, and T. Pullman. New York: Grune & Stratton.

Oswald, I. 1972. *Sleep.* Baltimore: Penguin Books.

Parad, H., and Caplam, G. 1965. A framework for studying families in crisis. In *Crisis intervention,* ed. H. Parad. New York: Family Service Association of America.

Peacock, J. L., and Kirsch, T. A. 1973. *The human direction.* New York: Appleton-Century-Crofts.

Pender, N. J. 1982. *Health promotion in nursing practice.* Norwalk, Conn.: Appleton-Century-Crofts.

Pettigrew, A. H., and Pettigrew, T. F. 1974. Race, disease and desegregation: a new look. In *Ethnic groups of America: their morbidity, mortality and behavior disorders,* vol. II., ed. A. Shiloh and I. C. Selevan. Springfield, Ill.: Charles C Thomas.

Phillips, D. C. 1976. *Holistic thought in social science.* Stanford: Stanford University Press.

Pilette, W. L. Aug. 1983. Caffeine: psychiatric grounds for concern. *P.N.M.H.S.* 21(8):19–24.

Preston, D., and Grimes, J. 1987. Study in differences in social support. *Journal of Gerontological Nursing* 13(2):36–40.

Raths, L. E.; Harmin, M.; and Simon, S. B. 1978. *Values and teaching.* 2nd ed. Columbus, Ohio: Merrill Publishing.

Ravin, A. 1967. *Auscultation of the heart.* 2nd ed. Chicago: Yearbook Medical Publishers.

Reitz, R. 1977. *Menopause: a positive approach.* New York: Penguin Books.

Roberts, A. 1990. *Crisis intervention handbook: assessment, treatment, and research.* Belmont, CA: Wadsworth Publishing Company.

Rokeach, M. M. 1973. *The nature of human values.* New York: Free Press.

Rosenberg, F. 1977. Lactose intolerance. *Am. J. Nurs.* 77.

Rosenthal, D., and Frank, J. D. 1958. The fate of psychiatric clinic outpatients assigned to psychotherapy. *J. Nerv. Ment. Dis.* 127:330–343.

Rousseau, J. J. 1913. *The social contract and discourses.* London: J. M. Dent and Sons.

Samouar, L., and Porter, R. 1976. *Intercultural communication: a reader.* 2nd ed. Belmont, Calif.: Wadsworth.

Sarbin, T. R. 1954. Role theory. In *Handbook of social psychology,* ed. G. Lindzey. Cambridge: Addison-Wesley.

Satir, V. 1972. *Peoplemaking.* Palo Alto, CA: Science and Behavior Books.

Saunders, L. 1954. *Cultural differences and medical care.* New York: Russell Sage Foundation.

Schaefer, C.; Cogne, J. C.; and LaZuras, R. S. 1981. The health related functions of social support. *Journal of Behavioral Medicine* 4:381–405.

Schaie, K. W. 1984. Midlife influences upon intellectual functioning in old age. *Intl. J. Beh. Dev.* 7:463–478.

Schaie, K. W. 1985. *Adult intellectual development in a life-span context.* 2nd Annual Research Lecture. College of Human Development. The Pennsylvania State University.

Scipien, G.; Barnard, M. U.; Chard, M.; Howe, J.; and Phillips, P. J. 1975. *Comprehensive pediatric nursing.* New York: McGraw-Hill.

Seaman, B., and Seaman, G. 1977. *Women and the crisis in sex hormones.* New York: Rawson Associates.

Seeman, M., and Evans, J. 1963. Alienation and learning in a hospital setting. *Am. Soc. Rev.* 27(6).

Sellew, G. 1962. *Sociology and its use in nursing service.* Philadelphia: W. B. Saunders.

Seltzer, C. C., and Mayer, J. A. 1965. Simple criterion of obesity. *Post Graduate Medicine.*

Selye, H. 1956. *The stress of life.* New York: McGraw-Hill.

Selye, H. 1965. The stress syndrome. *Am. J. Nurs.* 65:98.

Servonsky and Opas. 1988. *Nursing management of children.* Boston: Jones and Bartlett Publishers.

Shostrum, E. L. 1963. *The personal orientation inventory.* San Diego: Educational and Industrial Testing Service.

Simmons, O. G. 1979. Implications of social class for public health. In *Culture, curers, and contagion,* ed. N. Klein. Novato, Calif.: Chandler and Sharp.

Smith, M. B., and Hobbs, N. 1966. The community and the community mental health center. *Am. Psychologist* 21:499–509.

Smitherman, C. 1981. *Nursing actions for health promotion.* Philadelphia: F. A. Davis.

Smuts, J. C. 1926. *Holism and evolution.* New York: Macmillan.

Snow, L. L. June 1976. "High blood" is not high blood pressure. *Urban Health* 5:54–56.

Snow, L. L. 1974. Folk medical beliefs and their implications for care of patients: a review based on studies among Black Americans. *Ann. Intern. Med.* 81:82–96.

Spratlen, L. P. 1976. Introducing ethnic-cultural factors in models of nursing: some mental health care applications. *J. Nurs. Ed.* 15(2):23–29.

Syme, S. L.; Borhani, N. O.; and Baechley, R. W. 1965. Cultural mobility and coronary heart disease in an urban area. *Am. J. Epidemiol.* 82:334–346.

Syme, S. L.; Hyman, M. M.; and Enterline, P. E. 1964. Some social and cultural factors associated with the occurrence of coronary heart disease. *J. Chronic Dis.* 17:277–289.

Syme, S. L.; Hyman, M. M.; and Enterline, P. E. 1965. Cultural mobility and the occurrence of coronary heart disease. *Health Human Behavior* 6:178–189.

Tanner, J. M. 1962. *Growth in adolescence.* 2nd ed. Oxford: Blackwell.

Thomas, C. L. 1981. *Taber's cyclopedic medical dictionary.* 14th ed. Philadelphia: F. A. Davis.

Thomas, W. L. 1963. *The differential value profile.* Chicago: W. and J. Stone Foundation.

Thompson, L. F.; Miller, M. H.; and Bigler, H. F. 1975. *Sociology—nurses and their patients in a modern society.* 9th ed. St. Louis: C. V. Mosby.

Tyroler, H. A.; Heyden, S.; and Hames, C. G. 1975. Weight and hypertension—Evans County studies of blacks and whites. In *Epidemiology and the control of hypertension,* ed. P. Oglesby. New York: Stratton International.

U. S. Congress American Indian Policy Review Commission. 1976. *Task force six: Indian health.* Washington, D. C.: U. S. Government Printing Office.

U. S. Senate Select Committee on Nutrition and Human Needs. Dec. 1977. *Dietary goals for the United States.* Washington, D.C.: Government Printing Office.

Vaillot, M. C. 1966. Existentialism: a philosophy of commitment. *Am. J. Nurs.* 66:500–505.

Vaughan, C., and McKay, R. J. 1975. *Nelson textbook of pediatrics.* 10th ed. Philadelphia: W. B. Saunders.

Waldron, I. 1982. An analysis of causes of sex differences in mortality and morbidity. In *The fundamental connection between nature and nurture,* ed. W. Gove and G. R. Carpenter, p. 69. Lexington, MA: Lexington Books.

Wallace, H. M. 1973. The health of American Indian children: a survey of current problems and needs. *Clin. Ped.* 12:83–87.

Webb, W. B. 1975. Sleep: the gentle tyrant. Englewood Cliffs, N. J.: Prentice-Hall.

Weinberg, J. S. 1982. *Sexuality: human needs and practice.* Philadelphia: W. B. Saunders.

West, K. M. 1974. Diabetes in American Indians and other native populations in the new world. *Diabetes* 23:841–855.

Whillam, V. Nov. 1970. The autistic child. *Canadian Nurse* 66:44–47.

Williams, R. A. 1975. *Textbook of black-related diseases.* New York: McGraw-Hill.

Wolfe, D. M. 1959. Power and authority in the family. In *Studies in social power,* ed. D. Cartwright. Ann Arbor: Institute for Social Research, University of Michigan.

Yamamoto, J., and Goin, M. K. 1966. Social class factors relevant for psychiatric treatment. *J. Nerv. Ment. Dis.* 142:332–339.

Yeager, E. B., and Van Heerden, J. A. 1980. Sexual dysfunction following proctocolectomy and abdominoperineal resection. *Annuals of Surgery* 191:169.

Zborowski, M. 1952. Cultural components in responses to pain. *J. Social Issues* 8 (14):16–30.

Index

COLOR PLATES 16 THROUGH 22

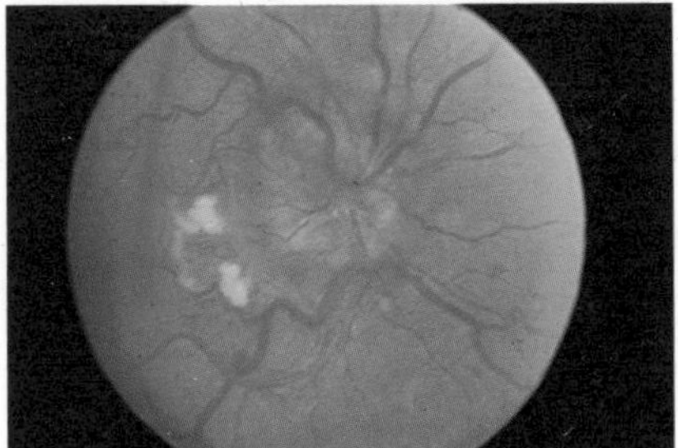

Plate 16. Papilledema with hard exudates.

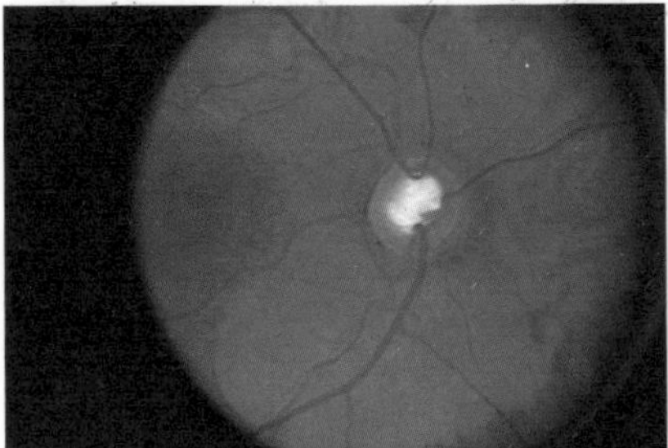

Plate 17. Glaucomatous cup.

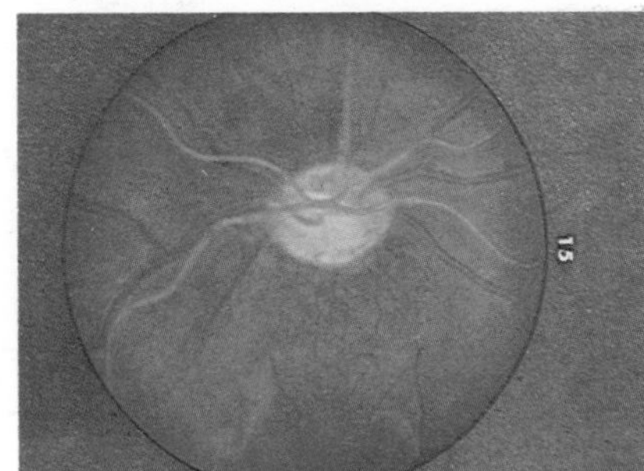

Plate 18. Copper-wire arteries.

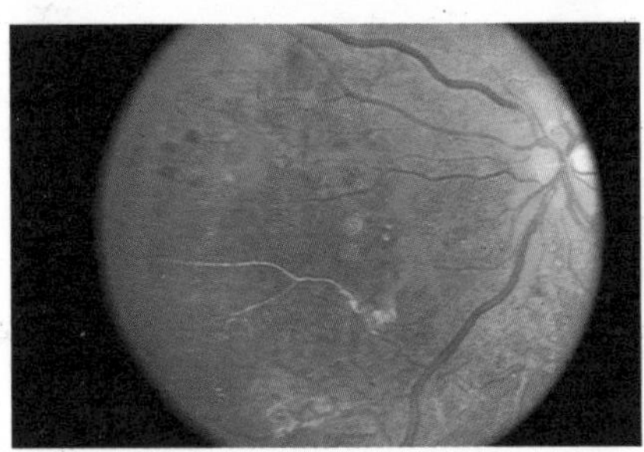

Plate 19. Silver-wire arteries and microaneurysms.

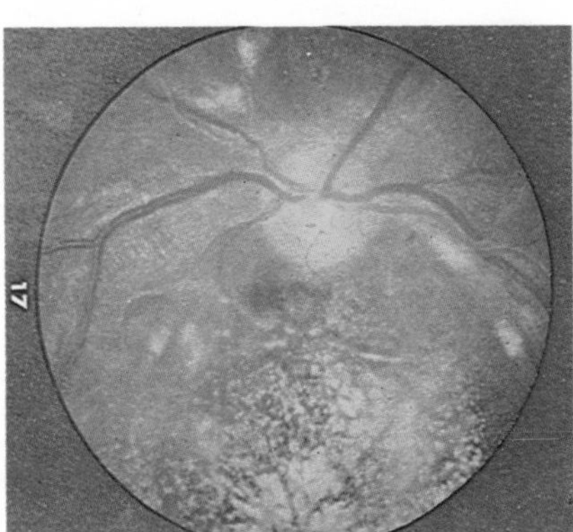

Plate 20. AV nicking.

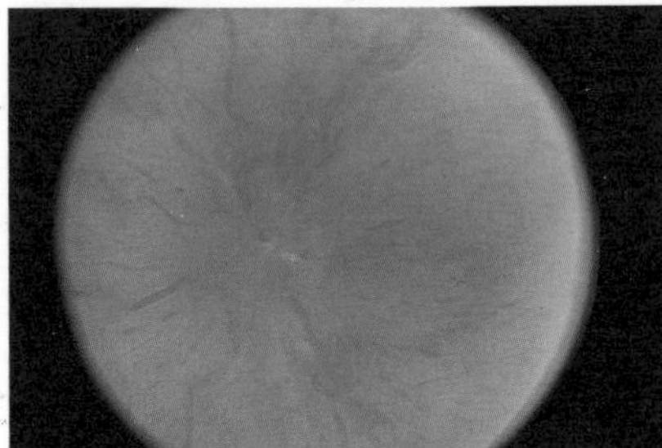

Plate 21. Tortuous venous distention.

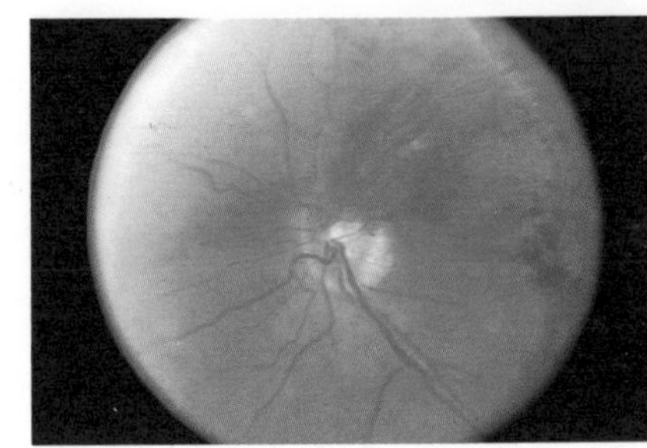

Plate 22. Blotchy hemorrhage.